W9-BTR-841

THIRD EDITION

LANGUAGE
INTERVENTION
STRATEGIES
IN
ADULT
APHASIA

THIRD EDITION

LANGUAGE INTERVENTION STRATEGIES IN ADULT APHASIA

Editor

Roberta Chapey, Ed. D.

Professor, Department of Speech
Brooklyn College
The City University of New York
Brooklyn, New York

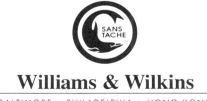

Williams & Wilkins

BALTIMORE • PHILADELPHIA • HONG KONG
LONDON • MUNICH • SYDNEY • TOKYO

A WAVERLY COMPANY

Editor: John P. Butler
Managing Editor: Linda S. Napora
Copying Editor: Melissa Andrews
Designer: Norman W. Och
Illustration Planner: Lorraine Wrzosek
Production Coordinator: Charles E. Zeller

Accurate indications, adverse reactions, and dosage schedules for drugs are provided in this book, but it is possible that they may change. The reader is urged to review the package information data of the manufacturers of the medications mentioned.

Printed in the United States of America

First Edition 1981
Second Edition 1986

Library of Congress Cataloging-in-Publication Data

[N2 Dept.—insert catalog card when received from the Library of Congress]
Language intervention strategies in adult aphasia / editor, Roberta Chapey.—3rd ed.
p.   cm.
Includes bibliographical references and indexes.
ISBN 0-683-01513-3
1. Aphasic persons—Rehabilitation. 2. Language disorders. I. Chapey, Roberta.
[DNLM: 1. Aphasia—Therapy. 2. Language Therapy—methods. WL 340.5 L287]
RC425.L37   1994
616.85'5206—dc20
DNLM/DLC
for Library of Congress

92-48908
CIP

97 98
4   5   6   7   8   9   10

This book is dedicated to the memory of my dad, Robert (Bob) Chapey, for his boundless generosity, kindness, love, understanding, tolerance, support, humanness, and humor—and for his truly brilliant strategies for living, He was a super parent.

R.C.

Preface

The first edition of this book was published in 1981 and the second edition was published in 1986. Both editions grew out of the realization that the discussion of aphasia therapy had become a major theme in clinical aphasiology literature but that the specification of numerous types or strategies of intervention was of fairly recent origin. All three texts grew out of the belief that there continues to be a substantial number of approaches applicable to the remediation of the language-disordered adult that must be brought together and shared. They are also grounded in the realization that a variety of different therapeutic principles and approaches need to be articulated, assembled, applied, and critiqued in order to strengthen the quality of future work in our field. The major purpose of the present book is to bring together significant thoughts on intervention and to stimulate further developments in the remediation of adult aphasic patients. It should be noted, however, that some of the models presented in this book still need to be supported by controlled studies and long-term clinical application.

The present text contains 33 chapters. Section I covers basic considerations such as the incidence of stroke and aphasia, definitions of aphasia, the role of the aphasiologist, quality assurance in aphasia, medical aspects of stroke rehabilitation, brain imaging and its application to rehabilitation, and the assessment and differential diagnosis of aphasia.

Section II is the largest section of the text and presents 15 chapters on language and communication intervention approaches to rehabilitation with adult aphasic individuals. A number of these chapters are classified as stimulation approaches since they emphasize the reorganization of language through stimulation or increased cortical activity through problem solving rather than the teaching of specific responses to particular stimuli. Some of the chapters in this section do teach specific responses to stimuli. Language and communication strategies for specific impairments such as fluent aphasia, Broca's aphasia, reading and writing disorders, and apraxia of speech are discussed in Section III of the text.

Section IV contains suggestions for the remediation of disorders that frequently accompany aphasia or are related to or confused with aphasia; namely, dysphagia, right hemisphere damage, dementia, and closed head injury. Section V contains a discussion of professional considerations that are important to the treatment of adult aphasic individuals. Chapters cover the application of research to intervention, interdisciplinary team intervention, and contemporary and future professional issues in clinical aphasiology.

Language Intervention Strategies in Adult Aphasia, third edition, can be used in classes for advanced undergraduate and graduate students in speech language pathology. Clinical aphasiologists who are no longer formal students, but who desire to keep abreast of new ideas in their field will also find the material of interest. Further, the material will be valuable to students and professionals in nursing, medicine, and other health-related disciplines.

ROBERTA CHAPEY, ED.D.

Acknowledgments

To those who have contributed to my personal life and professional career, past and present, I express my deep appreciation. I am also grateful to the authors and publishers who granted me permission to quote from their works.

Many concerned and dedicated people have helped bring this book to fruition. Sincere appreciation is extended to each of them. First and foremost, to my husband and best friend, Kris Thiruvillakkat: I thank him for being so extremely supportive and loving toward me, and for being so very easy on the eye, particularly warming to the heart, and especially nurturing to the soul. Thanks for being my hero, my Knight in Shining Armor. And to my three stepsons, Kris, Michael and David, for their support and friendship and for making life fun, I extend special thanks.

To the faculty and staff of Marymount Manhattan College for giving me an absolutely outstanding undergraduate education, I extend special thanks. Thanks, too, to my parents, who were generous and paid for my education.

With the passing of Dr. Edward Mysak, former Chairman of the Department of Speech Pathology and Audiology at Columbia University, the field has lost an outstanding leader. I have lost a friend who was extremely supportive of my doctoral studies and my academic career. I am, indeed, saddened by his passing.

Drs. Eleanor Morrison and Seymour Rigrodsky, professors at Columbia, are owed special thanks for their inspiring contribution to my academic development and growth.

My appreciation goes to Laura Brodsky, Jerry Crump, Joseph Chapey, Sr. William Daley, R.S.H.M., Sandra Dupuy, Sandy Milton, and Milton and Arlene Salzberg for deep emotional support.

Contributors

Judith B. Amster, Ph.D.
Associate Professor, School of Education
Director, Learning Disabilities Program
New York Institute of Technology
Old Westbury, New York

Walter W. Amster, Ph.D.
Professor, Department of Speech
Brooklyn College
City University of New York
Brooklyn, New York
Program in Speech and Hearing Sciences
Graduate Center
The City University of New York
New York, New York

James L. Aten, Ph.D.
Retired Chief, Audiology and Speech Pathology
Long Beach Veterans Administration Medical Center
Assistant Clinical Professor
University of California, Irvine
Long Beach, California

Donna L. Bandur, M. Cl. Sc.
Manager
Department of Speech-Language Pathology
University of Western Ontario
London, Ontario, Canada

Kathryn A. Bayles, Ph.D.
Associate Professor
Department of Speech and Hearing Sciences
The University of Arizona
Assistant Director
National Center for Neurogenic Communication Disorders
Tucson, Arizona

David R. Beukelman, Ph.D.
Professor, Department of Special Education and Communication Disorders

University of Nebraska-Lincoln
Lincoln, Nebraska

Roberta Chapey, Ed.D.
Professor, Department of Speech
Brooklyn College
City University of New York
Brooklyn, New York

Sandra B. Chapman, Ph.D.
Research Scientist
Callier Center
University of Texas at Dallas
Adjunct Instructor in Neurology
University of Texas Southwestern Medical Center, Dallas
Dallas, Texas

Chris Code, Ph.D.
School of Communication Disorders
The University of Sydney
Faculty of Health Sciences
Lidcombe, New South Wales, Australia

John W. Deck, Ph.D.
Speech Pathology Service
Veterans Affairs Medical Center
Indianapolis, Indiana

Joseph R. Duffy, Ph.D.
Consultant, Speech Pathology
Division of Neurology
Mayo Clinic
Professor, Mayo Graduate School of Medicine
Rochester, Minnesota

Neva L. Frumkin, Ph.D.
Research Speech-Language Pathologist
Veterans Administration Medical Center
Instructor
Department of Neurology
Boston University School of Medicine
Boston, Massachusetts

Kathryn L. Garrett, Ph.D.
Department of Special Education and Communication Disorders
University of Nebraska-Lincoln
Lincoln, Nebraska

Argye Elizabeth Hillis, M.A.
Research Associate
Department of Cognitive Science
The Johns Hopkins University School of Medicine
Baltimore, Maryland

Jennifer Horner, Ph.D.
Associate Professor and Director
Speech and Language Pathology Program
Department of Surgery
Duke University Medical Center
Durham, North Carolina

Monica Strauss Hough, Ph.D.
Assistant Professor
Department of Speech-Language and Auditory Pathology
East Carolina University
Greenville, North Carolina

Karen Hux, Ph.D.
Department of Special Education and Communication Disorders
University of Nebraska-Lincoln
Lincoln, Nebraska

Richard C. Katz, Ph.D.
Chief, Audiology and Speech Pathology Service
Carl T. Hayden Veterans Administration Medical Center
Phoenix, Arizona

Kevin P. Kearns, Ph.D.
Chairman
Department of Speech and Language
North Eastern University
Boston, Massachusetts

Michael L. Kimbarrow, Ph.D.
Director, Speech-Language Pathology
Rehabilitation Institute of Michigan
Associate Professor
Department of Physical Medicine and Rehabilitation
Wayne State University School of Medicine
Detroit, Michigan

Jeri A. Logemann, Ph.D.
Professor
Departments of Otolaryngology and Neurology
Professor and Chairman
Department of Communicative Disorders
Northwestern University
Evanston, Illinois

Russell J. Love, Ph.D.
Professor
Division of Hearing and Speech Sciences
Vanderbilt University School of Medicine
The Bill Wilkerson Center
Nashville, Tennessee

Felice L. Loverso, Ph.D.
Executive Vice President, Clinical Affairs
Braintree Hospital Rehabilitation Network
Braintree, Massachusetts

Associate Research Professor, Neurology
Boston University
Assistant Professor
Speech/Language Pathology
Northeastern University
Boston, Massachusetts

Rosemary Lubinski, Ed.D.
Associate Professor
Department of Communication Disorders and Sciences
University of Buffalo
Amherst, New York

Robert C. Marshall, Ph.D.
Chief, Audiology and Speech Pathology Service
Veterans Affairs Medical Center
Associate Professor
Department of Neurology
Oregon Health Sciences University
Portland, Oregon

Ruth E. Martin, Ph.D.
Research Scientist
Toronto Hospital–Western Division
Assistant Professor
Post-doctoral Fellow Oro-facial Motor Control Laboratories
Faculty of Dentistry
University of Toronto
Toronto, Ontario, Canada

E. Jeffrey Metter, M.D.
Medical Officer
Baltimore Longitudinal Study of Aging
Gerontology Research Center
National Institute on Aging
Baltimore, Maryland

Anthony G. Mlcoch, Ph.D.
Audiology and Speech Pathology
Hines Veterans Affairs Medical Center
Hines, Illinois

Penelope S. Myers, Ph.D.
Section of Speech Pathology
Division of Neurology
Mayo Clinic
Rochester, Minnesota

Margaret A. Naeser, Ph.D.
Associate Research Professor of Neurology
Boston University School of Medicine
Aphasia Research Center
Boston Veterans Administration Medical Center
Boston, Massachusetts

Carole L. Palumbo, B.A.
Research Associate
Aphasia Research Center
Department of Neurology
Boston University School of Medicine
Boston, Massachusetts

Richard K. Peach, Ph.D.
Associate Professor
Departments of Otolaryngology & Bronchoesophagology and Neurological Sciences
Rush Medical College
Department of Communication Disorders and Sciences
College of Health Sciences
Rush University
Rush-Presbyterian-St. Luke's Medical Center
Chicago, Illinois

Robert S. Pierce, Ph.D.
Professor
School of Speech Pathology and Audiology
Kent State University
Kent, Ohio

Bruce E. Porch, Ph.D.
Associate Professor
Department of Communicative Disorders
Speech and Hearing Center
University of New Mexico
Albuquerque, New Mexico

Paul R. Rao, Ph.D.
Director, Speech-Language Pathology Service
Co-Director, Stroke Recovery Program
National Rehabilitation Hospital
Adjunct Professor, Department of Audiology and Speech
Pathology
Gallaudet University
Washington, DC
Adjunct Professor, Department of Speech Pathology
Loyola College
Baltimore, Maryland
Adjunct Professor
Department of Hearing and Speech Science
University of Maryland, College Park
College Park, Maryland

Leslie Gonzalez Rothi, Ph.D.
Staff Speech Pathologist
Veterans Affairs Medical Center, Gainesville
Adjunct Associate Professor
Departments of Neurology, Clinical and Health Psychology,
and Communicative Processes and Disorders
University of Florida
Gainesville, Florida

Scott S. Rubin, Ph.D.
Assistant Professor
Department of Communication Sciences and Disorders
The University of Georgia
Athens, Georgia

Cynthia M. Shewan, Ph.D.
Senior Vice President
Research, Analysis and Development Division
American Physical Therapy Association
Alexandria, Virginia

Robert W. Sparks, M.Sc.
Chief, Speech Pathology/Audiology (Retired)
Veterans Affairs Medical Center
Boston, Massachusetts

Paula A. Square, Ph.D.
Chair
Graduate Department of Speech Pathology
Faculty of Medicine
University of Toronto
Toronto, Ontario, Canada

Shirley F. Szekeres, Ph.D.
Associate Professor
Nazareth College of Rochester
Rochester, New York

Cynthia K. Thompson, Ph.D.
Associate Professor
Communication Sciences and Disorders
Northwestern University
Evanston, Illinois

Connie A. Tompkins, Ph.D.
Associate Professor
Dept. of Communication
University of Pittsburgh
Pittsburgh, Pennsylvania

Professor Hanna K. Ulatowska, Ph.D.
Callier Center
University of Texas at Dallas
Dallas, Texas

Wanda G. Webb, Ph.D.
Assistant Professor
Division of Hearing and Speech Sciences
Vanderbilt University
Director of Speech Pathology
Vanderbilt University Medical Center
Nashville, Tennessee

Mark Ylvisaker, Ph.D.
Assistant Professor
Department of Communication Disorders
College of St. Rose
Albany, New York

Contents

SECTION TWO
LANGUAGE AND COMMUNICATION INTERVENTION APPROACHES IN ADULT APHASIA

SECTION ONE
BASIC CONSIDERATIONS

CHAPTER 1
Introduction to Language Intervention Strategies in Adult Aphasia

ROBERTA CHAPEY

According to the National Institutes of Health (NIH), stroke is the third leading cause of death in the United States and the most common cause of adult disability (Zivin and Choi, 1991). Zivin and Choi (1991, p. 56) note that "Of the approximately 500,000 new victims each year, roughly 30 percent die, and 20 to 30 percent become severely and permanently disabled." Thus, for at least 40% of those who survive, stroke is a seriously crippling disease—physically and often communicatively. It is marked by the obvious signs of a sagging face, a dangling arm, and a tortured gait and frequently by aphasia, the impairment or loss in ability to use language to communicate or comprehend and exchange thoughts and feelings. Aphasic individuals may also have difficulty reading, writing, using numbers, or making appropriate gestures (Brody, 1992). Each year 80,000 Americans develop aphasia, leaving more than a million Americans with this seriously handicapping condition (Brody, 1992).

Within a matter of minutes, the lives of stroke/aphasia victims change completely. They become prisoners in their own bodies, prisoners in their own minds. They want to move and walk but can't; they want to think and talk and communicate but are significantly limited in their ability to do so.

The prevalent negative attitude toward the communicatively and physically handicapped in the United States and around the world results in additudinal barriers, marginal social status, suspicion, rejection, distrust, stigmatization and loss of esteem. Stroke victims are often condemned to live as pariahs, are met with outright public rejections, and are shunned, ostracized and isolated by all but those most devoted to them (Brody, 1992; Love, 1981; Post and Leith, 1983; Sahs and Hartman, 1976).

Stroke and aphasia victims may "be unable to do the jobs they were trained for and be forced to retire, a further assault on their egos that typically adds to feelings of isolation, frustration and worthlessness" (Brody, 1992, p. C13). Many people with aphasia are lonely, desperate, and even suicidal (Brody, 1992).

Advancing age is the factor most consistently associated with stroke (Sahs and Hartman, 1976). This is particularly alarming in light of the demographic statistics released by the U.S. Census Bureau that strongly predict the aging of the American population (Herbers, 1981). Indeed, by 2025, the medial age in the United States is expected to be 42, and 22% of the U.S. population is expected to be in the 65 plus age group

(Fein, 1983). The aging of the U.S. population brings with it increased risks for catastrophic disease, illness, and disability (Marge, 1991), including adult aphasia. To offset this trend, we need to encourage the development and specification of new methods to prevent stroke, to rehabilitate stroke and aphasia victims, and to increase the effectiveness of our intervention efforts.

The present text represents the editor's desire to assemble a reasonably accurate and coherent picture of language intervention as it currently exists and to make it available in useful form. Uppermost is the desire to bring significant thoughts on language intervention together and to stimulate further study concerning the effectiveness of the approaches that are presented.

However, before proceeding with the discussion of specific intervention strategies, it may be useful to consider several general issues that are relevant to clinical aphasiology. Specifically, the following topics will be considered: definitions of adult aphasia, a rationale for providing language therapy to persons with aphasia, specification of the settings in which language intervention is performed, the role of the clinical aphasiologist, the characteristics of an effective aphasiologist, and major issues affecting the delivery of aphasia therapy.

DEFINITIONS OF ADULT APHASIA

A number of definitions of adult aphasia appear in our literature. Several of these definitions will be presented below.

Propositional Definition

Jackson's concept of aphasia is intrinsically linked to his notion of propositional language (Head, 1915). This is an intellectual, volitional, rational language that involves the use of linguistic symbols for the communication of highly specific and highly appropriate ideas and relationships. In a proposition, both the words and the manner in which they are related and refer to one another are important. Jackson contrasts propositional language with subpropositional language, which he characterized as inferior, automatic, highly learned responses (Head, 1915).

According to Jackson, aphasia is an impairment in one's ability to make propositions. The aphasic individual's chief difficulty is the inability to communicate specific meaning and to integrate

Table 1.1.
The Abstract-Concrete Model of Aphasia[a]

Abstract	Concrete
• Adaptive behavior	• Adaptive behavior
• Propositional	• Nonpropositional (automatic, serial content, social gesture)
• Assumes a mental set voluntarily and volitionally, and a conceptual framework	• Unable to assume a mental set . . . interruption disrupts behavior
• Takes initiative (begins performance)	• Unreflexive, passive
• Actions determined by the way the individual thinks about them	• Actions determined by objects
• Shifts voluntarily from one aspect of a situation to another, making a choice	• Reactive, unable to shift to a new situation, perseverates (no rule to change)
• Keeps various aspects of a situation in mind simultaneously	• Impressed by one property exclusively—experiences only this one and reacts to it
• Reacts to two stimuli that do not belong intrinsically together	• Cannot react to two stimuli that do not belong intrinsically together
• Conscious, aware, volitional, rational, reasoning	
• Grasps essential of given whole	• Cannot grasp essential of given whole
• Permits use of past experience to form rules and to continue	• Reacts to "here and now" only
• Breaks whole into parts, isolating them voluntarily and combining them to wholes	• Cannot grasp essentials of a given whole
• Abstracts common properties, transcends the immediate	• Deals with "here and now"; deals with the specific or immediate sense impressions
• Plans ahead ideationally	• Deals with the "here and now"; no rule to change
• Assumes an attitude toward the merely possible	• Thinking and acting are determined by the immediate claims made by the particular aspect of an object or situation
• Able to account to oneself, to verbally account for what one does	
• Thinks and performs symbolically	
• Detaches ego from the outer world and inner experience	• Cannot detach ego from inner experience; reacts to "here and now"—immediate sense impressions
• Permits inhibition	• Reacts to "here and now"

[a] From Goldstein, K. (1948). *Language and language disturbances*. New York: Grune & Stratton.

words into particular contexts in order to express specific relationships. Some patients may know words, but they habitually use them incorrectly and are unable to embed these words in a variety of sentences. Jackson noted that, even when propositional language is impaired, many patients will retain subpropositional, automatic language. The individual will be able to name the days of the week, to complete sentences such as "The grass is ____," or to produce highly learned responses such as "Hi. How are you?"

The individual who is impaired in propositional language is unable to use spontaneous language in order to communicate specific meaning. The more specific the communication requirements, the more the patient will be impaired.

Within the context of this definition, assessment involves an analysis of the patient's ability to use spontaneous speech in order to propositionalize or communicate specific ideas. Intervention focuses on stimulation of the patient's ability to communicate such ideas, or to use propositional language.

Concrete-Abstract Definition

Goldstein (1948) observed that use of an abstract attitude implies an ability to react to things in conceptual manner. This attitude is necessary to isolate properties that are common to several objects and for the formulation of concepts as opposed to sensory impressions of individual objects. It is also used to comprehend relationships between objects and events in the world. An abstract attitude gives the individual the power to inhibit action or reactions and to use past experiences. These experiences help the individual to organize perceptual rules and therefore to create and continue interactions or ways of relating to people.

Language that reflects an abstract attitude is propositional language. In contrast, in the concrete attitude, the individual passively responds to reality and is bound to the immediate experience of objects and situations. Concrete language consists of speech automations, emotional utterances, sounds, words, and series of words (Goldstein, 1948) (see Table 1.1).

In general, impairment in abstract attitude is reflected in propositional language. If one cannot abstract, one cannot symbolize or embed symbols in a number of specific relationships. The individual will be unable to produce a variety of concepts, to consider things that are only possibilities rather than actualities, to keep in mind simultaneously various aspects of a situation, to react to two stimuli that do not belong intrinsically together, to inhibit reactions, and to ideationally isolate parts of a whole.

Goldstein and Scheerer (1941) and their associates developed a number of "tests of ability to assume the abstract attitude." Specifically, they discuss the following tests in their monograph: the Goldstein-Scheerer Cube Test, the Gelb-

Goldstein Color Sorting Test, the Gelb-Goldstein-Weigl-Scheerer Object Sorting Test, the Weigl-Goldstein-Scheerer Color Form Test, and the Goldstein-Scheerer Stick Test. For example, subsequent to the administration of the Object Sorting Test, one may analyze responses to determine if the individual sorted according to color, form, use (function), texture, and so on. Then one may ask, Is the sort concrete (perceptual) or abstract (conceptual)? Can the individual verbally account for his or her sort (abstract)? Can he or she verbally account for a sort presented by the examiner (abstract)?

The intervention implications of this definition would be to stimulate the patient to comprehend and produce language that is increasingly more abstract and propositional. The individual would be stimulated to produce a larger number and variety of categories, to consider things that are only possibilities rather than actualities, to keep in mind simultaneously various aspects of a situation, and so forth.

Unidimensional Definition

Definitions of aphasia that relate language behaviors to a single common denominator and that view the language mechanism as a unitary process support the solidarity of the expressive and receptive, as well as the semantic and syntactic, components of language. Such definitions suggest that damage to such a mechanism results in general language impairment in which there is equivalent or symmetrical damage in all aspects of language. Such definitions, then, are the antitheses of definitions that conceptualize a Broca's-Wernicke's, sensory-motor, receptive-expressive, input-output dichotomy in the language process and in aphasia.

One of the most popular and in-depth unidimensional definitions—that proposed by Schuell and her colleagues (1964)—defined aphasia as a general language impairment that crosses all language modalities: speaking, listening, reading, and writing. These authors noted that the behaviors that are impaired in aphasia involved kinds of integrations that cannot be attributed merely to organization of motor responses or to events in outgoing pathways; rather, they involved use of an ability that was dependent on higher-level integrations.

According to this definition, aphasia is not modality specific. Rather, it is the inability to retrieve words and rules of an acquired language for communication (Schuell et al., 1964). The aphasic person has lost functional, spontaneous language, or the ability to use connected language units to communicate according to the established conventions of the language.

Schuell's concept of the cause of this general language breakdown—an impairment of ability to reauditorize or analyze and integrate language sequences (Schuell et al., 1955)—similarly reflects a broad and dynamic view of the language process. It also appears to encompass far more than a language mechanism that can generate only highly learned input-output responses.

The assessment implications of this definition involve an analysis of patient ability to comprehend and produce language within all four modalities—an analysis of the ability to retrieve words and rules of the acquired language and to use functional, spontaneous, connected language units in order to communicate. Schuell's test, the Minnesota Test for Differential Diagnosis of Aphasia (MTDDA) (Schuell, 1973) is based on this model (see Chapters 4, 5, and 7).

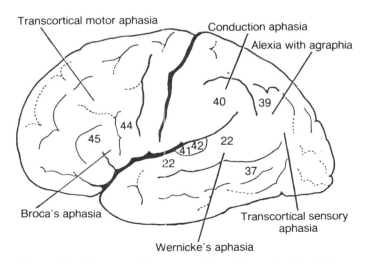

Figure 1.1   Diagrammatic representation of the major loci of lesions in the principal types of aphasia. Brodmann's areas 44 and 45 correspond to the classic Broca's area, area 22 to Wernick's area. Areas 41 and 42 correspond to the primary auditory cortex; these extend into the depth of the sylvian fissure. Area 40 = supramarginal gyrus. Area 39 = angular gyrus. Area 37, principally located in the posterior sector of the second temporal gyrus, does not have correspondence in gyral nomenclature.

The intervention implications are similarly unidimensional and multimodality and focus on the use of strong, controlled, and intensive auditory stimulation of the impaired symbol system in order to maximize patient reorganization of language. The clinician manipulates and controls specific dimensions of stimuli in order to make complex events happen in the brain and thus aid the patient in making maximal responses.

A majority of the approaches to therapy in the clinical aphasiology literature and of those that are presented in this text are stimulation approaches.

Multidimensional Definitions

Some individuals in the area of adult aphasia have conceptualized aphasia as a dichotomy, such as a Broca's-Wernicke's, fluent-nonfluent, or semantic-syntactic dichotomy. Frequently, these definitions are associated with the cerebral localization of aphasia (Fig. 1.1). However, before these definitions are discussed, the term "paraphasia" will be defined.

According to A. Damasio (1981), **paraphasia** is a central symptom of aphasia: "It consists of an incorrect and unintended word or sound for a correct one" (p. 55). This author refers to several different types of paraphasia. **Global** or **verbal** paraphasia occurs when the entire word is substituted. In this instance, the paraphasia may or may not be related to the target word. If the word belongs to the same semantic field, it is **semantic** paraphasia; if not, it is **random** paraphasia. When paraphasias involve the substitution of an entirely novel word, it is called **neologistic** paraphasia. **Phonemic** or **literal** paraphasia occurs when a phoneme is added or substituted for the correct phoneme. When too many global paraphasias appear in the individual's speech, it is **jargon**.

Fluent Aphasias

There are three basic types of fluent aphasia: conduction aphasia, Wernicke's aphasia, and transcortical sensory aphasia (TSA) (see Fig. 1.1).

Conduction Aphasia. The speech of conduction aphasics is fluent, although less abundant than that of Wernicke's aphasia (Damasio A., 1981). However, fluency may be restricted to brief runs of speech (Goodglass and Kaplan, 1983). Repetition of words and sentences is "disproportionately severely impaired in relation to the level of fluency in spontaneous speech and the near normal level of auditory comprehension" (Goodglass and Kaplan, 1983, p. 86). Most patients "repeat words with phonemic paraphasias, but often they will omit or substitute words, and they may fail to repeat anything at all if function words rather than nouns are requested" (Damasio, A., 1981. p. 61). Thus, their major impairment is the proper choice and sequencing of phonemes (Goodglass and Kaplan, 1983). Their literal paraphasia repeatedly interferes with speech.

Wernicke's Aphasia. The critical features of Wernicke's aphasia are impaired auditory comprehension and fluently articulated but paraphasic speech (Goodglass and Kaplan, 1983) in which syntactic structure is preserved. The uncorrected paraphasias are in the form of sound transpositions and word substitutions (Goodglass et al., 1964). Patients also experience naming difficulty that is disproportionately severe in relation to their fluent small talk (Goodglass et al., 1964). These individuals also have difficulty in repeating words and in both reading and writing (Damasio, A., 1981).

Transcortical Sensory Aphasia (TSA). Aphasic individuals with TSA have "fluent and paraphasic speech (global paraphasias predominate over phonemic ones) and a severe impairment in . . . (auditory) comprehension" (Damasio, A., 1981, p. 61). Speech is well articulated, but irrelevant paraphasias, including neologisms, occur (Goodglass and Kaplan, 1983). Confrontation naming is quite impaired, and the patient may offer an irrelevant response or echo the words of the examiner (Goodglass and Kaplan, 1983). Thus, repetition is intact.

Nonfluent Aphasias

There are three basic types of nonfluent aphasia: Broca's aphasia, transcortical motor aphasia (TMA), and global aphasia.

Broca's Aphasia. The essential characteristics of Broca's aphasia are "awkward articulation, restricted vocabulary, restriction of grammar to the simplest, most overlearned forms, and relative preservation of auditory comprehension" (Goodglass and Kaplan, 1983, p. 75). Writing is usually at least as severely impaired as speech. However, reading is only mildly affected.

Transcortical Motor Aphasia (TMA). The term "transcortical" implies that "repetition" is particularly intact in a setting of otherwise limited speech" (Goodglass and Kaplan, 1983, p. 94). This type of patient exhibits phonemic and global paraphasias, perseveration (Damasio, A., 1981), and difficulty imitating and organizing responses in conversation (Goodglass and Kaplan, 1983). Confrontation naming is usually preserved, but auditory comprehension is impaired.

Global Aphasia. Global aphasia is a disorder of language in which the patient does not respond verbally to stimuli or responds with an automatized word, phrase, or phoneme sequence. Patients have little or no understanding along any modality and little or no ability to communicate (Wepman and Jones, 1961).

Another multidimensional definition of aphasia was formulated by Wepman and Jones (1961). These authors identified five types of aphasia: pragmatic, semantic, syntactic, jargon, and global.

Pragmatic Aphasia. Pragmatic aphasia is a disruption in recognizing and comprehending incoming signals by failing to associate incoming signals with appropriate concepts. Patients with this type of aphasia convey little meaning in their speech; are constricted in their vocabularies, using fewer low-frequency words than would be expected; show an excess of neologisms; have inadequate feedback along all modalities; and rarely recognize their errors. However, they maintain a flow of language and retain the melody and pitch changes of normal speech. There is little, if any, agrammatism (Wepman and Jones, 1961).

Semantic Aphasia. Semantic aphasia is a disorder of symbol formulation in which the patient has difficulty in attaching a meaningful verbal sign to a previously acquired concept and in recalling and using previously acquired forms applicable to such a concept. Such patients have great difficulty remembering and using substantive words (nouns, verbs, adjectives), and they often use pauses, repetitions, or circumlocutions when trying to recall the appropriate word. However, they retain function words (articles, demonstratives, pronouns, prepositions, and so on) and highly frequent substantive words, as well as normal speech melody and pitch (Wepman and Jones, 1961).

Syntactic Aphasia. Syntactic aphasia is a disorder of symbol formulation in which patients are unable to use their previously acquired grammatical structure. These patients misuse or omit the function words (articles, demonstratives, pronouns, prepositions, auxiliary verbs) and grammatical inflections (markers of tense, plurality, and so on). They cannot form sentences or smaller syntactic constructions such as prepositional phrases, noun phrases, or verb phrases but speak telegraphically using single substantive words. They retain little speech melody; however, they retain many substantive words (nouns, verbs, adjectives) (Wepman and Jones. 1961).

Jargon Aphasia. Jargon aphasia is a disorder of symbol formulation and expression in which previously acquired sequences of phonemes making up intelligible units of speech are no longer available, and unintelligible ones (i.e., jargon) are used in their place. Patients use sequences of phonemes that are unlike any specific words of their previously acquired language but that generally follow the overall phonemic patterns of that language (i.e., its consonants, vowels, and their permitted combinations) as well as its accentual and pitch patterns (Wepman and Jones, 1961).

Global Aphasia. (see above)

For individuals who hold a multidimensional view of aphasia, assessment involves determining what symptomatology is present and subsequently classifying a patient in one category or another. The Boston Diagnostic Aphasic Examination (BDAE) (Goodglass and Kaplan, 1983), the Western Aphasia Battery (Kertesz, 1982; Kertesz and Poole, 1974), and the Language Modalities Test for Aphasia (Wepman and Jones, 1961) reflect such classification systems. Intervention would be oriented toward the deficit. That is, the clinician would attempt to rehabilitate the specific language modality (such as speaking) or behavior (such as confrontation naming or phonemic production) that was found to be impaired (for example, see Cubelli et al., 1988).

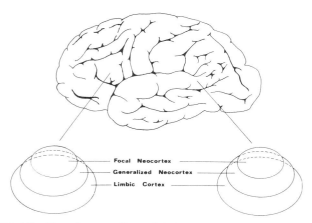

Figure 1.2 The microgenetic model of language organization. The Broca and Wernick zones (focal neocortex) are specified out of surrounding regions of generalized neocortex, which in turn evolve from limbic neocortex. Evolutionary and maturation growth trends construct a hierarchical system in the anterior and posterior hemisphere that elaborates stages in language processing.

Microgenetic Definition*

Wernicke (1874) portrayed the surface of the brain as "a mosaic of [elementary psychic functions] which are characterized by their anatomical connections with the periphery of the body" (Brown and Perecman, 1986). Brown (1972, 1977, 1979) and Brown and Perecman (l986) challenged this classical model, rejecting the notion that language production can be explained by postulating a "mosaic" of cortical speech centers and connecting pathways that convey "cognitive packets," that is, memory images, from one processing center to another. These authors proposed an alternative conceptual framework in which language processing is conceived as an event that emerges over evolutionarily sequential brain levels rather than across cortical areas. Specifically, the limbic mechanisms mediate early stages in psychological and linguistic representation, and the left lateralized focal neocortex (including Broca's area and Wernicke's areas), the more recently evolved areas of the brain, mediate the final stages in cognition and linguistic processing (see Figure 1.2). Second, language is processed simultaneously by complementary systems in the anterior and posterior divisions of the brain rather than by means of rostral conveyance of nerve impulses. These anterior and posterior language zones both develop out of a common limbic core, establishing a fundamental unity of the two systems. The emergence of language in these systems is characterized by a progressive specification of linguistic information. Therefore, lesions of brain structures that mediate evolutionary stages in the emergence of language give rise to a progression of aphasias corresponding to the succeeding stages in the differentiation of language in each of these systems. Third, pathways serve to "maintain in phase" different regions of the brain rather than to convey information. These neutral pathways between homologous levels in the anterior and posterior systems of the same hemisphere, as well as commissural connections to the corresponding anterior or posterior level of the opposite hemisphere,

serve to link up temporally, that is, maintain in phase, homologous levels of different brain regions. Language processes occur simultaneously in the anterior and posterior sectors. The corticocortical fibers relate to timing or phase relations in separate, conically organized systems and do not serve as conduits for the transfer of linguistic information.

According to Brown and Perecman (1986), a lesion in one of the language areas of the brain alters the flow of activity from one stage in the processing continuum of language to another; the effect of a lesion is to give rise to a relative prominence of a preliminary stage of language processing. The aphasic symptom is thus a magnification of the processing events that, in normal language, are mediated by the lesioned area.

Two basic claims about the organization of language in the brain are implicit in this approach: (*a*) that both speech and speech perception differentiate out of the same deep organization, no matter how highly distinct their end products, and (*b*) that bilateral lesions are essential for aphasic symptom formation at early structural and functional brain levels. As brain organization becomes more differentiated functionally, and as language becomes more lateralized, symptoms occur with unilateral focal lesions. According to Brown and Perecman (1986), treatment focuses on a facilitation of the transition from one stage to the next in the microgenetic sequence.

Thought Process Definition

Wepman (1972a) noted that the aphasic patient frequently substitutes a word that is associated with a word he or she is attempting to produce, and that the remainder of the individual's communicative effort often relates to the approximated rather than to the intended word. In addition, the aphasic person's inaccurate verbal formulation may feed back an altered message to the thought process and change the thought process so that it is in consonance with the utterance. For example, if the patient is trying to say "circle" and instead utters "square," his concept of circle may change so that it agrees with his utterance, and he will begin to think of a circle as a square. Wepman (1972a) suggested that aphasia may be a thought process disorder in which impairment of semantic expression is the result of an impairment of thought processes that "serve as the catalyst for verbal expression" (p. 207).

Individuals who cannot retrieve the most appropriate lexical symbol for a context are impaired in their ability to communicate a number and variety of specific propositional ideas. When the remainder of the communication relates to the approximated rather than the intended word, spontaneous language will be even more impaired, since, in this instance, aphasic patients become incapable of using the learned code to communicate their true feelings and thoughts.

Within a thought process definition, assessment involves determining if individuals can follow a train of thought in their communication or spontaneous language and/or expand on topics and ideas. For Wepman (1972b, 1976), the first stage of therapy is thought-centered or content-centered discussion therapy in which patients are stimulated to attend to their thoughts and remain on a topic. During the second stage of therapy, patients are encouraged to elaborate on various topics.

(*This section is taken from Brown and Perecman, 1986)

A Psycholinguistic Definition

Language has three highly interrelated and integrated components: cognitive, linguistic, and communicative (Muma, 1978).

1. *Cognitive* refers to the manner in which individuals acquire a knowledge of the world and in which they continue to process this knowledge. The two most important cognitive processes involved in adult language are thinking and memory. Thinking is the act or process of reasoning or of conceiving ideas; memory is the power, act, or process of remembering.
2. *Linguistic* refers to language form and content. A form is a system of rules for communicating meaning. Three rule systems of language are phonology, morphology, and syntax. Language content is the meaning, topic, or subject matter involved in an utterance.
3. *Communicative* is the use, purpose, or function that a particular utterance serves at any one time. For example, the same content and form "How are you?" can be used to question a statement, request information, greet a friend, and so on.

According to Chapey (1986), aphasia may be defined as an acquired impairment in language and the cognitive processes that underlie language. Aphasia is caused by organic damage to the brain and is characterized by a reduction in and dysfunction of language *content* or meaning, language *form* or structure, and language *use* or function and the cognitive processes that underlie language, such as recognition, understanding, memory, and thinking. This impairment is manifested in listening, speaking, reading, and writing—although not necessarily to the same degree in each.

Chapey (1986) believes that assessment would involve an analysis of the cognitive, linguistic, and communicative abilities and impairments of a patient. Intervention is the stimulation of these abilities, but especially the stimulation of the cognitive processes underlying language comprehension and production. Emphasis is on the communication of meaning, since meaning is the essence of language (see Chapter 11).

RATIONALE FOR LANGUAGE INTERVENTION

A rationale for language intervention with persons who have aphasia is based on the belief that language constitutes what is considered the human essence and that therapy can, in most cases, effect a change in a patient's language performance.

Language: The Human Essence

The need for socialization is the core of human existence, and the desire to communicate with others is the essence of that socialization. Language is the basic form of this communication and is what Chomsky (1972) calls the human essence. Language is *the* distinctive quality of the mind that is unique to humans and that which makes humans unique. Indeed, "the possession of language, more than any other attribute, distinguishes man from other animals" (Fromkin and Rodman, 1974, p. 1). Language is the source of human life and power. It is the most basic characteristic of the intellect and the very means through which the mind matures and develops. Language enables individuals to describe and clarify their thoughts for themselves and others (Fromkin and Rodman, 1974).

Human experience and interaction are welded to language. According to Goodman (1971), the ability to share experience through language is a means of homeostasis that enables human beings to maintain and/or restore an equilibrium in which they can survive. Goodman (1971) also observes that language is the basis of personality and that personality consists largely of one's language habits. Language, he observes, reveals our inner being and our psychic ties with the world.

Language is also the essence of maturity, which is defined as an ability to relate warmly to and intimately with others—with their goals, aspirations, and hopes. It involves a "fitting in" and carrying one's share of personal and social responsibility. The mature individual is self-reliant, self-actualized, and task- and other-oriented rather than self-oriented. Thus, definitions of maturity involve and indeed revolve around the ability to use language effectively.

Aphasia is an impairment in language. Insofar as persons with aphasia are impaired in their ability to use language, they are impaired in their human essence—their ability to be human. The very core of human existence—a need for socialization and communication with others—is lessened. Part of the personality is lost and the ability to maintain interpersonal relationships, to convey wants and needs, and to be a mature, self-reliant, self-actualized person is impaired. When individuals lose language, they are reduced as fully functioning, mature adults. Equilibrium is devastated.

Aphasia cannot be cured, but intervention enables many individuals to be able to comprehend and produce language and to communicate more effectively. Intervention is an attempt to heighten each person's potential to function maximally within the environment in order to facilitate feelings of self-esteem and to restore dignity.

In addition, the goal is to help patients find a purpose in life, despite their specific impairments. This is done, in part, by giving them the opportunity to be goal-oriented and responsible. The aphasiologist, therefore, establishes goals for and with patients and expects them to take an active part in reaching those goals. Responsibility and subsequent success act in a circular feedback relationship to increase a patient's self-esteem. Clinicians very frequently find that even a small amount of amelioration in the language impairment does a great deal in allowing persons to regain some part of their personality, their maturity, and their dignity. Conversely, failure to provide intervention often results in the rejection of the patient by those in the environment or in the patient becoming infantilized and irritable (Wepman, 1972a).

It is unfortunate that many potentially rehabilitative post-trauma and poststroke patients are left untreated. Many of these individuals have the capacity to communicate more effectively and yet are never encouraged to do so. The field of rehabilitative medicine must recognize that quality health care means going beyond the provision of basic physical maintenance care and giving quality and dignity to human life. Rehabilitation should, whenever possible, be continued until the patient's maximum language and communicative functions have been achieved. Individuals should be granted the right to be treated by the best techniques within the society—to the fullest extent of which they are capable (Keith, 1975). We must give living dignity by giving greater independence through quality rehabilitation. For, not to allow persons to communicate to the best of their ability is to deprive them of living as human beings. However, individuals who do not wish to be treated should have their wishes respected. Each individual has the right to make this decision for himself or herself.

LANGUAGE INTERVENTION SETTINGS

Speech-language pathologists rehabilitate adult aphasic patients in a variety of settings such as hospitals, rehabilitation centers, skilled nursing facilities, nursing homes, clinics, their own private offices, and the patient's own home.

Hospitals

Most major community hospitals have a comprehensive program for stroke rehabilitation including a basic rehabilitation team that includes a physician, a rehabilitation nurse, a social worker, a physical therapist, an occupational therapist, and a speech-language pathologist. Optimally, a physiatrist, a psychologist, and a rehabilitation counselor should also be part of this team. The acute, immediately poststroke patient is frequently placed in an acute medical area and may receive speech-language evaluation, intervention, and counseling at the bedside. In most instances, convalescent stroke patients are separated from acute medical and surgical patients so that they may receive appropriate attention, so that their beds can be placed close to rehabilitation services, and so that the area can have appropriate handrails and specially designed toilets and bathtubs. Typically, hospitals have a specific area which that properly equipped for rehabilitation. Within this area, "special attention is given to the facilities and personnel required for the speech-language rehabilitation because of the complex problems involved." (Sahs and Hartman, 1976, p. 210). Adequate space and equipment are usually provided to ensure high-quality evaluation, treatment, and counseling services, which are rendered for both inpatients and outpatients.

The advantage of providing speech-language services in this setting is that a hospital provides an integrated, coordinated, comprehensive team management for stroke and aphasia. The same may be said for rehabilitation centers.

Rehabilitation Center

Rehabilitation centers can be a component of a hospital or can exist as a separate, independent facility that has a close working relationship with one or more hospitals. In either case, there are usually both inpatient and outpatient services that provide comprehensive team rehabilitation (Sahs and Hartman, 1976). For patients who have recovered from the acute state poststroke, the decision as to whether they should receive rehabilitation in a rehabilitation service as an outpatient or inpatient or be transferred to another facility depends on several variables, such as the extent of disability (e.g., speech-language impairment) and therefore the need for integrated comprehensive therapy, the economic situation, the degree of family involvement, and the nature of available resources (Sahs and Hartman, 1976).

Skilled Nursing Facility

Skilled nursing facilities provide less intensive services than those available in a hospital or rehabilitation center but more than exist in a nursing home. This type of setting is best for individuals who still require certain limited therapeutic services but whose level of need does not justify hospitalization or when outpatient care is not feasible (Sahs and Hartman, 1976). These facilities typically provide occupational therapy, physical therapy, and speech-language therapy and attempt to meet the social and emotional needs of the patient.

Nursing Home

The level of care provided by nursing homes is variable. Some offer only custodial care, whereas others with a "rehabilitation orientation have the services and capabilities for providing long-term management programs to maintain or improve the functional level of stroke patients" (Sahs and Hartman, 1976, p. 211). In most instances, these homes provide social and environmental stimulation and attempt to meet the patient's social and emotional needs.

Independent Speech and Hearing Centers: The Speech-Language Pathologist's Office

Independent speech and hearing clinics are often located within university settings. Independent speech-language pathologists who are in private practice will have a private office. In both instances, services are provided for a variety of communicative disorders. Typically, both settings have suitable rooms and proper equipment in order to provide appropriate assessment, intervention, and counseling services to patients.

In most instances, there is no formal structure of a rehabilitation team. However, individual speech-language clinicians often refer patients to other appropriate and necessary rehabilitation professionals and establish close communication with other professionals who are working with the patient. In addition, many private practices are established with other rehabilitation personnel or are located in a building that houses other rehabilitation personnel.

The Patient's Home

Many stroke and aphasia patients return to their home after the acute medical emergency has subsided or after a period of therapy at a rehabilitation center. When this happens, community-based home health care agencies provide a variety of services to the patient through a well-structured, closely coordinated program. Indeed, home care services to the elderly are growing rapidly because of the pressure on hospitals to reduce costs (ASHA, 1986; Hamilton, 1991) Insurers like such services because they are cost-effective, and most elderly consumers prefer it because they like to receive such services in their own home (ASHA, 1986). According to Kerr (1992), community-based programs provide reasonable prices and high-quality care and have better long-term results than residential facilities, since skills do not have to be transferred back to the home environment because they are taught where they will be used. In addition, independence and self-reliance are fostered. The range of services may include visiting physician care; visiting nurse service; physical therapy; occupational therapy; speech-language evaluation and therapy; psychiatric, psychological, and social work evaluation and therapy; special assistive devices; financial help for medical/rehabilitation and maintenance requirements; dietary counseling; and homemaker or household assistance.

ROLE OF THE SERVICE PROVIDER

Regardless of the professional setting in which the clinician is employed—a hospital, nursing home, college or community clinic, or home health care—the clinical aphasiologist performs many of the same functions. The most common functions of this clinician are (*a*) identification and selection of clients, (*b*) assessment, (*c*) intervention, (*d*) administration, (*e*) consultation, (*f*) counseling, (*g*) education, and (*h*) research.

Identification and Selection of Clients

The method employed to locate individuals who have aphasia varies from setting to setting. In most instances, however, persons with aphasia are identified when another member of the rehabilitation team refers the patient to the aphasiologist. While the team referral technique enjoys the widest popularity in some settings (Chapey et al., 1979), this method is dependent on the team member's ability to recognize the language impairment and his or her interest in reporting the problem to the speech pathologist. Therefore, dependency on this approach is sometimes ineffective in locating the target population.

In some residential settings, the clinician may screen each individual who enters the facility (Chapey et al., 1979). The purpose of the screening is to identify those who have language problems. Once persons with aphasia have been identified, a more detailed assessment is performed. Case selection is dependent on the attitude of the patient, the family, and others concerning the need for intervention, the client/clinician ratio, economic factors, and prognostic factors.

Assessment

Assessment and intervention are the most important functions of the aphasiologist. The purpose of assessment is to provide an in-depth description of each client's cognitive, linguistic, and communicative behaviors in order to identify existing problems, determine the goals of intervention, and define the factors that should be taken into account in order to stimulate the patient's use of language (see Chapters 4 and 5).

Intervention

Stroke rehabilitation in general is

a complex, dynamic process of comprehensive patient care beginning at the time of the acute stroke and continuing until the maximum physical, psychological, social (language), and vocational functions for each individual have been achieved. The rehabilitation of the stroke patient is based upon the concept that every disabled individual has the right to be treated by the best techniques available so that he may again participate within his society to the fullest extent of which he is capable (Sahs and Hartman, 1976, p. 205).

Language intervention is also a complex, flexible, organized, goal-directed, dynamic process that is aimed at restoring or reestablishing the individual's previously learned language through treatment and/or training. It is a process that is designed to change language behavior—not only within the domain of the clinical cubicle but also in life. It involves the stimulation of the brain through the presentation of stimuli in a hierarchy of difficulty at the point where performance just begins to break down and immediately involves transfer of performance to real-life situations. Recovery, then, is not stimulus-response behavior nor the muttering of a new word or two as a light flashes, but the spontaneous, intentful use of verbal expressions

(Wepman, 1972b). The goal is to empower the aphasic patient with language.

Intervention is also not confined to language and communication alone. Specifically, the clinician should help patients to gain a positive attitude, to increase their morale, to maintain their social contacts, to gain insight into their impairment and to develop a feeling of acceptance, optimism, and emotional stability (Darley, 1982). Therefore, the entire "program must be individually patterned, uniquely presented, and continuously tailored to signs of progress and signs of failure" (Darley, 1982, p. 238).

Intervention is an innovative process that responds to the neurological, linguistic, and social needs of each client (Wepman, 1972b). It involves comprehensive patient care that begins at the time of the trauma or stroke and continues until maximum physical, psychological, social, vocational, and communicative functions have been achieved (Keith, 1975). The focus is on function. Intervention is also called language rehabilitation or language therapy.

Administration

Program administration or management usually encompasses record keeping and report writing, scheduling and grouping clients, and ordering supplies.

Records and **reports** play a significant role in an aphasiology program. The primary purpose for keeping records is to generate an account of the clinical services provided and to support the planning of future assessment and intervention goals. The system of record keeping that is chosen should be one that can easily be interpreted by other professionals. Some of the specific types of records and reports that may be used are assessment records, session plans (including goals, methods, type of therapy, and an evaluation of the client's responses), conference records, release of information forms, referral forms, master schedules, statistical summaries of cases, progress reports, and quarterly disposition reports. The primary purpose of preparing reports is to disseminate information. Accurate, clear, and timely records and reports are essential to providing a continuity of service and a cumulative account of each individual's assets, limitations, and progress in therapy. In addition, paperwork is often the only basis on which other professionals evaluate a clinician's effectiveness and is also essential to program development and justification. It also serves to facilitate performance assessment to evaluate customer satisfaction (see Appendix 1.1) and the quality, cost-effectiveness, efficiency, productivity, and competitiveness of the clinician and facility.

Thorough documentation is also the vehicle that determines Medicare, Medicaid, and other insurance reimbursement. Toward that end, a speech-language assessment must contain a complete history; a clear statement of the problem; a plan of action to address the problem, including long-term and short-term goals that are describable and documentable; and tasks, modalities, and expected results of intervention—preferably in terms of skills and abilities that facilitate independent functional behavior, reduce depression, and increase confidence (Slominski, 1985a). Functional recovery in ADLs (activities of daily living), facilitation of independent behavior, and reduction of depression are highly regarded (Slominski, 1985a). The potential for progress is essential for reimbursement. Indeed, one common reason for denying service delivery is that the condition is too chronic or is degenerative. In addition, speech-language pathologists need to know each insurer's goals for consumers so that they can relate their documentation to these goals (Slominski, 1985a).

As treatment continues, progress should be recorded in detail. For example, a visual aid to describe change can add clarity to the report (Slominski, 1985a). The report should also contain a description of how the individual has improved intellectually, emotionally, and socially (Slominski, 1985a). Has motivation changed? Have there been changes in preexisting conditions?

Documentation should be logical and sequential. Each report should be strongly tied to the preceding and subsequent ones. Whenever possible, statements from patients and their families or significant others (SOs) should be a component of progress notes or revisions of goals and procedures (Slominski, 1985a). Reimbursement documentation must be excellent, since we are often our patients' only advocate for continued funding of rehabilitation (Slominski, 1985a). However, while documentation can continue reimbursement, professionals must not permit funding agencies to dictate what treatment goals they select or what treatment procedures they use.

Scheduling involves preparing a timed plan for the year and each week. Scheduling for the year involves determining the dates of legal holidays and professional conventions and conferences, providing time for inservice training sessions, vacation time for each member of the staff, and so forth. In planning a weekly schedule, time must be reserved for traveling, holding conferences, writing reports, preparing sessions, coordinating activities, performing inservice education, and reading current professional literature. The largest amount of time should be invested in patient assessment and intervention. Scheduling of individual patients is dependent on such things as the severity of the disorder, geographic availability, client/clinician ratio, and financial considerations.

Relevant equipment, materials, and supplies are also ordered by the clinician, depending on their perceived usefulness and the availability of funds for such purchases. Items that are frequently obtained include standard tests, textbooks, workbooks, prepared therapy materials, tape recorders, audiotapes, videotape recorders, videotapes, computers, paper, and so forth.

Consultation/Collaborative Care

The clinical aphasiologist also functions as a member of a rehabilitative assessment-intervention team in order to share knowledge and information with other professionals such as the occupational therapist, physical therapist, nurse, and family. This necessitates team development and real partnerships involved in decision making and collaboration. Topics might relate to case management of specific clients, coordination or execution of clinical services, aphasia in general, nutrition assessment and intervention, equipment selection, common problems with the elderly such as medication, management of behavior disorders such as alcoholism, making sense of the human experience, and so on.

This interactive process is carried out so that the clinician may help each patient to be rehabilitated to his or her fullest possible potential. Interdisciplinary consultation, including inservice training programs and speaking before professional groups, generates better case management through knowledge, understanding, and cooperation.

Counseling/Education

The role of **counselor** or adviser involves exchanging ideas or opinions or conducting discussions with the patient, members of the family, other professionals, or the community. The specific content of individual or group counseling depends on the appropriateness to the individuals receiving the counseling. Topics such as the causes of strokes, types of medical/surgical/language rehabilitation services available, psychological and emotional impact of a stroke, and death and dying may be discussed.

In the role of **educator**, the aphasiologist supervises student clinicians and paraprofessionals and gives inservice training to administrators, home health aides, other health care staff, and family members. Patient education can involve empowering individuals by informing them about the array of medical, communicative, environmental, and social choices available to them (Winslow, 1992). The more individuals are involved in making decisions about their own care, the less they complain about it and the more they participate in it (Winslow, 1992). In addition, informing them about patient rights and discussing issues such as hope and its role in recovery (Goleman, 1991), stress management, self-esteem, and meaning in the lives of the elderly may be beneficial to treatment.

The clinical aphasiologist also educates the public and fosters self-protective, self-regulation of habitual actions that put the individual at greater risk for stroke. "Every year millions of people suffer and die of illnesses that could be cured or eliminated by altering patterns of personal behavior" (Ewart, 1991, p. 931). Therefore, the speech-language pathologist (SLP) seeks to empower individuals for self-change by stimulating a "sense of self control, mastery, and power to effect change" (Ewart, 1991, p. 940). Through education, they also encourage collective empowerment within the community for appropriate decision making concerning community resources and development of strategies to achieve better health patterns (Ewart, 1991).

Self-education is carried out in order to achieve advanced professional competence. Usually, enrichment programs are accomplished by reading professional journals and attending conferences, workshops, and courses. Topics might include the following: international perspectives on aphasia; current advances in assessment and intervention of perceptual motor, cognitive, linguistic, and emotional deficits; advances in medical management; community and vocational reentry systems; current issues in ethics and aphasia recovery; how to gain cooperation through effective communication; how to deal with conflict; how to motivate other people; substance abuse training; private-practice strategies (such as marketing, business law, contract negotiation, bookkeeping and accounting, personnel management); stress management; how to build self-esteem; legal aspects of aphasia; innovations in plan management; and promotion of quality self-audit by health care professionals.

Research

Clinicians need the knowledge and techniques that only research can produce. Indeed, Minifie (1983) believes that the destiny of our field is imminently tied to practitioners assuming a greater role in developing the clinical science and that mediocrity comes from a division between clinical and research programs. Research is inseparable from clinical service (Goldstein,

1984). Therefore, each aphasiologist has a responsibility to document his or her clinical successes and failures. To do this, clinicians need to be familiar with techniques of scientific research design, measurement, and analysis.

Treatment research needs to have greater design sophistication and be more directly and clearly related to specific behavioral, cognitive, communicative, and/or linguistic models of intervention (Kearns and Thompson, 1991). Too many of our present studies suffer from *"technical drift"*—that is, they are becoming more and more technical and less conceptual (Kearns and Thompson, 1991). According to Kearns and Thompson (1991), recovery is too documentation-oriented and therefore emphasizes unimportant but highly measurable issues rather than pragmatics and meaning. We urgently need to develop more efficient, powerful, meaningful, and functional quality assurance assessment techniques.

Intervention strategies need to be effective and cost-efficient in terms of time, personnel and other required resources and must result in the acquiring of a generalized communicative repertoire (Warren and Rogers-Warren, 1985). Traditional models that train specific lexical and syntactic items separately from their communicative functions do not usually facilitate generalization of this knowledge to new contexts. Therefore, we need to collect social validation data, or data that demonstrate that aphasic patients communicate better following treatment across behaviors, time, and contexts (Thompson and Kearns, 1991). It is essential to establish "how much and what kind of treatment is best and what changes constitute important treatment outcomes" (Thompson and Kearns, 1991, p. 52).

While the kind and quality of research that is undertaken is dependent on the availability of facilities and subjects and on the cooperative atmosphere provided by the administration and staff, it is also largely dependent on the commitment of the individual clinician to analyze the effectiveness of his or her work. An essential component of quality research is the creation of an environment that is conducive to risk taking. Thus, the quality, motivation, and personal relationships of the research staff and the style of management that is either supportive of creativity or critical of new ideas will influence the quality of research that is conducted (Ringel, 1982).

CHARACTERISTICS OF AN EFFECTIVE APHASIOLOGIST

The effective aphasiologist is a responsible, sensible, competent individual whose major goal is high-quality, first-rate patient care through the use of high-caliber assessment and intervention techniques. Therefore, this individual possesses a Certificate of Clinical Competence (C.C.C.) from the American Speech-Language-Hearing Association (ASHA) and, where appropriate, a state license as a speech pathologist. This clinician is intellectually competent and is therefore able to analyze and synthesize data accurately, to formulate problems, and to use logic, repetition, and drill to develop and test hypotheses. He or she is able to find and use knowledge effectively, to think and learn independently, to see clusters or relationships, and to think through a variety of alternatives. The effective clinician has the ability to develop relevant knowledge, approaches, insights, and models in order to plan and manage simple and complex cases (Falck, 1972).

A competent clinician demonstrates highly consistent yet flexible clinical behavior. Remedial procedures are carried out

effectively, and the clinician is able to accurately define why they were productive or, if they failed, why they were ineffective. Session goals and procedures reflect a thorough understanding of assessment results and current literature. Therapy is realistically planned in terms of time limitations, client characteristics, and availability of materials and equipment. In addition, therapy is paced realistically so that the client has an adequate opportunity to respond.

Effective clinicians have a rationale for everything they do and communicate that rationale, whenever possible, to the client. They foster responsible participation in the selection of goals, in ways of reaching those goals, and in the development of appropriate attitudes and skills such as personal responsibility for learning.

It is essential that the competent clinician have genuine motivation to help others (Minifie, 1983), be capable of intimacy and of genuine caring, and have a patient attitude, enthusiasm, a strong sense of humor, and an ability to make therapy interesting and fun (Post and Leith, 1983).

Competent aphasiologists are sensitive to each client's responses, reactions, and needs and react to them appropriately while leading the client to achievement of goals. Effective clinicians recognize that their primary responsibility is to the client and make every effort to foster maximum self-determination on the part of the client (Cormier and Cormier, 1991). They provide the environment and the freedom to learn and maintain an emotional climate that contributes positively to the therapeutic relationship (Rogers, 1969). They facilitate growth of attitudes and behaviors and provide inspiration, motivation, encouragement, and leadership to clients.

Efficient clinicians can renew and reform present systems creatively. Rogers (1969) identifies effective clinicians as persons who have learned how to learn and how to adapt and change. These individuals realize that no knowledge is secure, that only the process of seeking knowledge gives a basis for security. They rely on the process rather than on static knowledge (Rogers, 1969). They belong to a community of learners who attempt to free curiosity (their own and their clients), to unleash a sense of inquiry, to open everything to questioning and exploration (Rogers, 1969).

Productive language pathologists also have the capacity for self-renewal and self-supervision and realize that one must always continue to establish professional and personal goals and define ways of reaching those goals. Effective clinicians have successfully integrated the personal and scientific parts of themselves and achieved a balance of interpersonal and technical competence (Cormier and Cormier, 1991). Their intrapersonal/interpersonal knowledge encompasses *competence* of relevant subject areas and appropriate use of *power* and *intimacy* (Cormier and Cormier, 1991). Efficient clinicians are aware of their own assets and limitations because they supervise, critique, assess, monitor, and edit their own behavior. They realize that becoming an effective aphasiologist is a sequential learning experience that is never terminated. They seek to broaden and deepen their clinical training and/or ability to plan, implement, and evaluate their clinical behavior. They do this through (a) self-evaluation; (b) the establishment of clearly defined professional goals; (c) use of assessment, intervention, and supervisory models; (d) continuing education such as attending professional conferences and reading scholarly journals; (*e*) observation of peer clinicians; and (*f*) in-depth interdisciplinary team communication.

Efficient clinicians are able to interact effectively with the entire rehabilitation team. They treat colleagues with respect, courtesy, fairness, and good faith (Cormier and Cormier, 1991). They maintain records and reports accurately and completely and keep them up to date. In all instances, clinicians protect the client's privacy and confidentiality, initiate proper referrals and recommendations, and exhibit proper follow-through.

MAJOR ISSUES AFFECTING THE DELIVERY OF APHASIA THERAPY

Our health care system is in transition. The following issues are relevant to current and future service delivery in all settings.

Research on How the Brain Functions: How It Organizes Language

Recent research on the brain has been focusing on plotting a theory of brain function including its organization for language. One such theory, that of Gerald Edelman (cited in Hellerstein, 1988), proposes that the brain contains enormously variable nerve- cell connections that are "not inherently marked for prescribed function or meaning" (Hellerstein, 1988, p. 61, col. 3). Cell groups can perform a variety of functions, depending on their input. They can also reorganize rapidly. Input or experience strengthens certain combinations of connections between cells in specific groups. However, over time, the strength of the synaptic connections shifts and the movements are no longer random (Hellerstein, 1988). "After the connections are made, selection occurs to change the strengths—but not the patterns of the connections," Edelman says (cited in Hellerstein, l988, p. 61, cols. 1, 2). This process of selection continues throughout life such that every experience alters and shapes each individual's brain and the strengths of its connections. That is, each individual "learns to perceive."

Each person's brain pattern of organizing his or her language, then, is unique, since it is based on his or her experience and subsequent perception (Blakeslee, 1991). Although the left side of the brain is significantly predisposed to language, the brain does not have a single center for language. Rather, language processing is distributed widely across the brain (Blakeslee, 1991). These areas or patches for different aspects of language (such as regular and irregular verbs, proper nouns and common nouns, reading, identifying meaning of words, recalling words, processing the words and grammars of foreign languages) are connected to many other areas or patches located in distant parts of the brain. However, "These areas do not send their signals to a common destination for integration. Rather, language and perhaps all cognition is governed by some yet undiscovered mechanism that binds different brain areas together in time, not place" (Blakeslee, 1991, p. C1, col. 5).

According to Edelman, each brain contains functional "maps" or arrangements of cells (such as those for touch and vision) in various regions of the brain. The maps are connected to one another through a vast network of fibers such that these maps communicate or talk with one another—a process called reentry (Hellerstein, 1988). It is the communication by reentry, between maps of different qualities such as yellowness or roundness, that enables us to develop concepts. "The part of the human brain that sees red must communicate with the part

of the brain that sees edges and roundness before it can even begin to conclude that what it is seeing is an apple" (Hellerstein, 1988, p. 61, col. 2). Edelman's idea allows for coordination of perception and action—a kind of parallel processing of senses "without the necessity of a central area of the brain that puts everything together" (Hellerstein, 1988, p. 61, col. 2).

Blakeslee (1991) reports that some researchers such as Drs. Antonio and Hannah Damasio view the essential language areas as "convergence zones" where the key to the combination of components of words and objects is stored. This knowledge of words and concepts is "distributed widely throughout the brain but needs a third-party mediator—the convergence zone—to bring the knowledge together, during reactivation" (Blakeslee, 1991, p. C10, col. 5). For example, if you are asked to think of a tennis ball, you compose an internal image of a tennis ball drawn from its features (it is yellow, round, it bounces, it can be manipulated or thrown) (Blakeslee, 1991). When you reactivate a concept or name, you draw on distant clusters of neurons that separately store knowledge of each of its features. "Those clusters are activated simultaneously by feedback firing from a convergence zone" (Blakeslee, 1991, p. C10, col. 5).

This literature seems to reinforce our belief that frequency of use affects the individual's ability to retrieve and use language and reinforces Brown and Perecman's microgenetic theory, which suggests that areas of the brain are bound together in time, not place. The literature does not appear to support strict localization of language theories that hold that language occurs in a specific place. This information also suggests that, as clinicians, we need to give greater consideration to stimulating attributes or features of objects, events, and relationships (such as "Can you think of all of the objects that are soft and movable?"—a divergent thinking task), since it appears that features are so important in concept formation, identification, and use. As aphasia clinicians, we need to continue to learn about how the brain organizes language and to reflect on how this kind of knowledge can affect the growth and development of new approaches to therapy.

Gerontology: The Study of Normal Aging

The past two decades have brought an increasing interest in age-related changes in adults. Toward this end, numerous professionals have measured cognition, perception, sensation, mobility, communication, and other neurological and psychological systems in an attempt to identify key variables that may or may not change with age.

Some of this research has focused on positive changes with age and functioning in the elderly. Indeed, in an article titled "The Aging Brain: The Mind Is Resilient, It's The Body That Fails," Kolata (1991) reports that there is "no reason to believe that aging per se leads to decline and loss of cognitive and intellectual activities" (Kolata, 1991, p. C1). "The myth is that to be old is to be sick, sexless and senile" (Frady et al., 1985). The reality is that this is not true for most people. There has been a revolution in the health of the elderly. Indeed, the majority of those who are over 85 are continuing to care for themselves (Frady et al., 1985). Today, more elderly are more vigorous and more independent than ever before (Frady et al., 1985). The elderly who do not do as well on mental ability tests usually have something specifically wrong with them such as depression, amnesia, Alzheimer's disease, vitamin deficiencies, or alcoholism, or they may be hindered by medications including sedatives and/or nonsteroidal antiinflamatory drugs or by environmental insults such as pollution and stress (Allison, 1991; Kolata, 1991).

Evidence of positive changes that may come with age can be derived from animal research, which suggests that old rat brains are as capable of growing new connections between brain cells as younger rat brains. Researchers hypothesize that this is also true in humans (Kolata, 1991). Other experiments indicate that exposing young rats to mild but chronic stress accelerates brain changes and disrupts communication among neurons in the hippocampus (necessary for learning and memory), but does not cause cells to die (Allison, 1991). However, in old rats, the signaling ability of these neurons is not impaired by chronic stress. However, some neurons die (Allison, 1991). This suggests that "the brain adapts as it ages" (Allison, 1991, p. 7). Indeed, one type of neuron in the brain that is loaded with the enzyme acetylcholinesterase (which helps to burn the fuel necessary for communication among cells) "actually becomes more abundant during adulthood, and is preserved in healthy older people" (Allison, 1991, p. 7). Because higher thought processes take place in this region of the brain, Dr. Mesulam (cited in Allison, 1991) believes that such age-related changes may underlie "wisdom." This researcher suggests that "programmed neuronal death and the growth of new connections could be the brain's way of sculpting new and better pathways" (Allison, 1991, p. 8). Indeed, according to Mesulam (cited in Allison, 1991), dendrites (or branches of neurons) grow significantly in healthy older people.

Some studies do, however, indicate that older people have less intercommunication in their brain. For example, areas of the neocortex "that control judgment, language and orientation in time and place become less well connected" (Kolata, 1991, p. C10). However, Kolata (1991) suggests that one possible explanation for this might be that older individuals are better able to focus the brain's attention. Some people believe in the "use-it-or-lose-it hypothesis," she says—that using the mind can preserve it (Kolata, 1991). However, Kolata (1991) and Frady et al. (1985) state that, in general, the elderly do well and negative changes are simply not the norm.

It is hoped that animal and human brain research will facilitate the development of "strategies for halting disease processes or boosting the power of healthy brains" (Allison, 1991, p. 8). For example, experimental drugs such as cognitive enhancers—which usually "target the cholinergic system, a chemical communication channel connecting neurons" (Allison, 1991, p. 8)—might someday become effective. Today, however, they have only limited effects. Researchers hope that other drugs that might increase the brain's ability to use its own existing glucose (which is needed for cognitive activities such as memory) may also be developed and perfected (Allison, 1991). Although the secret of mental longevity lies largely in our genes, it is hoped that research not only can reverse brain damage but also can preserve and amplify the strengths of the older brain (Mesulam, cited in Allison, 1991).

Some gerontological research has been focusing on how individuals can age in a healthy manner. For example, the University of Connecticut Health Center in Farmington received a $1 million grant from Travelers Company Foundation to explore a proactive focus on life-style behaviors (including nutrition and finding meaning in the lives of the well elderly) and medical standards that support healthy aging.

Most of the research in health aging shows that controlling diet, exercise, and stress leads to the fountain of youth. By controlling these life-style choices, life can often be prolonged (Dunbar and Most, 1991; Robins, 1987, 1991). Indeed, according to Krinsky (1991), handling stress well may hold the key to "successful" aging. In addition, older people who remain active find a continuing sense of purpose and therefore age well (Krinsky, 1991). People need ongoing involvement with family, friends, and others to keep mentally alert. Conversely, "Isolation, boredom and lack of intellectual stimulation are often the forerunners to mental deterioration" (Krinsky, 1991, p. 12).

Therefore, a special branch of psychiatry, geropsychiatry was developed to help older persons cope with common psychological and personal changes associated with age such as reduction in independence, dignity, self-worth/self-esteem, motivation, intimacy and sexuality, and interest in social and work activities (Fox, 1991). Geropsychiatry attempts to alleviate depression, somatic complaints, and feelings of hopelessness, emptiness, and rejection (Fox, 1991). Assessment targets biological, spiritual, social, and psychological issues, which are an individual's emotional daily living skills (Fox, 1991). The goal is to use problem-solving and decision-making skills to help individuals realize that older people can be vital, productive members of society; that "life can begin at 80" (Fox, 1991); and that a significant part of the quality of life lies in the mind and heart of the individual.

But aging inevitably brings some decline in function. Therefore, parts of the gerontological literature have focused on the clinical aspects of aging and profiles diseases and other problems of the elderly. For example, the *Merck Manual of Geriatrics* (Abrams and Berko, 1990) discusses the following: (*a*) the aging process and its effect on the cardiovascular, pulmonary, gastrointestinal, genitourinary, hematological, musculoskeletal, metabolic and endocrine systems (*b*) infectious disease; (*c*) neurological disorders; (*d*) skin, eye, and ear, nose, and throat disorders; (*e*) fall and gait disorders; (*f*) problems of electrolyte imbalance; (*g*) fractures; (*h*) urinary incontinence; (*i*) pain; (*j*) sleep disorders; (*k*) pressure sores; (*l*) social issues: use of services, continua of care, financing health care; (*m*) mistreatment and malnourishment; (*n*) legal issues: do-not-resuscitate order, family issues, long-term care; (*o*) ethical issues; (*p*) allocation of resources; and (*q*) assessment instruments.

As providers of health care to the language-impaired elderly, we need to facilitate patterns of healthy aging in our patients and in the community and identify clinical aspects of aging in order to better understand our patients and to initiate referrals when necessary.

Prevention

Recent data from the 42-year-long Framingham Study conducted by the National Institutes of Health (They're Not Kidding, 1992) suggest that strokes are twice as likely to occur between 6 A.M. and noon than at any other time of the day and that more than half (especially hemorrhagic strokes) occur on Mondays. This knowledge should encourage employers to perform task analyses to determine their stress level and schedule stressful tasks in the afternoon and perhaps consider starting the workday (especially Mondays) later in the day. It should also encourage those over 50 to reduce their own stress levels as much as is possible, especially on Sunday night and Monday mornings. The data may also stimulate neurologists to develop a better understanding of "the risk factors and behaviors that precede and contribute to the often fatal attacks" (They're Not Kidding, 1992, p. 113).

Gerontology: Impact of Demographic and Social Trends

Although America is an aging society, current policies for retirement, health care, and long-term care are not equipped for our rapidly expanding older population (Frady et al., 1985).

Retirement

The early retirement revolution has been fueled by corporate and government needs to reduce costs. Older workers, who often make higher salaries, are targeted with early retirement incentives or are fired. This forces many into dependency and nonproductivity. Many of these individuals live for 20 to 30 years after they leave work. They may find themselves financially impoverished with many empty hours they had not expected (Frady et al., 1985). In addition, recruitment, hiring, and promotion policies are oriented toward youth—such that, for those over 45, the average length of unemployment is 35% longer than for younger workers (Frady et al., 1985). This age discrimination leaves many elderly shut out of the workplace. Many have no pension, leaving an estimated one-third of those over 65 living at or just above the poverty line (Frady et al., 1985).

One way to ease the poverty of the elderly might be to change the outdated policy of mandatory retirement (usually at 70). Reintegrating older Americans back into society would also ease their need for companionship and social interaction and give them a sense of being wanted, active, and productive. Retirement in the future should mean life flexibility, life transition, the opportunity to have both leisure and work; it should be a time to contribute, and not a time to sit back and be excluded from society (Frady et al., 1985).

Health Care

Medical health care insurance plans for retirees are not prevalent. Many middle-class and poor individuals cannot afford the continuing payments that Medicare health insurance requires. In addition, spiraling health care costs mean that Medicare and Medicaid are no longer able to pay for quality care and are beginning to ration the care they provide (Frady et al., 1985). Concomitantly, the medical system has become careless toward the elderly. Many are neglected, improperly diagnosed, overmedicated, or undermedicated; receive poor or dangerously deficient care; and/or are lost in the health care system (Frady et al., 1985). Many in the medical community are "untrained and uninterested in treating" (Frady et al., 1985, p. 13) the elderly because treatment of these patients "takes time and often can't be billed at the far higher prices for other procedures" (Frady et al., 1985, p. 13). The major incentives of the industry are financial. Therefore, health care for the elderly is in need of significant rethinking and nationwide planning.

Health Care Reimbursement

There are several reimbursement issues that affect services delivery in health care in general and speech-language services in particular.

1. *DRGs*: The federal government has instituted a cost-cutting measure, the DRG (Diagnostically Related Group) system of reimbursement, which pays hospitals a fixed fee for a specific diagnostic group for Medicare recipients. The DRG system has given hospitals a powerful incentive to save money, which has caused a general decline in the quality of medical care. For example, many elderly patients are released from hospitals earlier when they are still sick, since hospitals can no longer bill Medicare for each day the patient stays (Gilbert, 1990). Some patients are denied admission to the hospital (e.g., if they are too sick or have complications that would cost hospitals too much because they would stay in the hospital longer, or if their symptoms do not fit "squarely" into a DRG), while others are being denied specific kinds of treatment (e.g., when the reimbursement for a specific procedure or service such as cognitive/communicative training, sign/gestural communication, or group speech and language intervention [ASHA, 1990] is so low that the hospital would lose money). Several states have also adopted DRGs for administering Medicaid, the joint federal and state health care system for the poor (Gilbert, 1990).
2. *Insurance reimbursement*: Some private health insurance companies such as the Travelers and Aetna Life and Casualty are now using a payment system similar to the government's DRG system (Gilbert, 1990). Thus, many services such as speech and language services are excluded or restricted in many outpatient coverage policies (ASHA, 1990).
3. *HMOs and PPOs*: Health Maintenance Organizations (HMOs) and Preferred Provider Organizations (PPOs) specify coverage exclusions or arbitrary limitations that affect many services such as speech and language services for aphasic clients (ASHA, 1990).
4. *Writing for reimbursement*: Existing bill-coding systems do not adequately represent the scope of practice in many areas such as speech-language assessment and intervention procedures (ASHA, 1990). In addition, many professionals such as speech and language pathologists often do not have sufficient information on the type of documentation required by claims reviewers that make coverage decisions (ASHA, 1990). This may mean that some specific services will not be covered.

This current system of reimbursement is flawed in many ways. For example:

1. The system cares more for numbers than for patients (Frady et al., 1985).
2. The system cares more about "accountability" and paperwork than about efficacy of treatment. Accountability has come to mean cost containment and cost accounting rather than appropriate intervention.
3. The health care that is provided is often substandard.
4. The system will not pay for rehabilitation of complications; it will pay only for primary illness. It will not pay for what it considers nonessential services; however, improvement of complications and "nonessentials" are necessary to improved functioning for many individuals.
5. There is a disincentive for hospitals and nursing homes to care for seriously ill patients because they will exceed the Medicare timetable or are more costly to care for because they need more services such as physical therapy, occupational therapy, and speech therapy.

Clearly, the system needs to be revamped so that patients can receive the first-rate care they deserve and clinicians and physicians receive the professional respect and decision-making discretion they should. Difficult decisions lie ahead.

Moral Decisions in Health Care: Final Choices

During the 21st century, health care workers will increasingly be interacting with patients, family, and other health care workers and making decisions about the right to life, euthanasia, do-not-resuscitate (DNR) orders, the quality of life, and the right to unlimited health care. "The ultimate dilemma [is] who shall live, who shall die, who shall receive our limited health care funds" (Frady et al., 1985, p. 18). Some of the agonizing questions we will have to face are, Who has the right to decide how long a patient lives? How much of our very limited financial resources should be used to delay death? How much should be allocated to individuals with a better prognosis (Frady et al., 1985; PBS, 1991a)?

Long-Term Care

Some older Americans need help with routine custodial management such as food shopping, cooking, cleaning, and other activities of daily living. The percentage of those over the age of 65 is small, and by the age of 85, slightly less than half will need long-term care (Frady et al., 1985). The majority (70%) will find such care among their families. Others will receive care in day-care centers, in continuing-care retirement communities, or in nursing homes (Frady et al., 1985).

Currently, for seniors, it is increasingly difficult to be admitted into a nursing home because the homes with the best reputations for high-quality care have a vacancy rate of only 5% (Frady et al., 1985). These homes can choose who they want: the healthiest, most affable, affluent patients and/or those with long-term care insurance. The frailest, most vulnerable, heavy care, poor patients and those who have behavior problems are often at risk to go to homes that have reputations for abuse and neglect (Frady et al., 1985). According to Frady et al. (1985), family and community monitoring is essential to lower the problems in these substandard homes.

Institutionalization is both emotionally and financially devastating for individuals and their family. The cost of caring is high (PBS, 1991a). Currently, Medicare does not pay for long-term care (Frady et al., 1985). To qualify for Medicaid within the current guidelines, there are limits on income and assets. Therefore, most individuals need to "spend down" or give away their assets before they go into nursing homes, or they use most of their savings to pay for care (Freudenheim, 1992). Therefore, of those who are institutionalized, two-thirds will die as paupers (Frady et al., 1985).

Routine help in the home and adult day-care centers can forestall or eliminate such institutionalization for many elderly. For the elderly who do receive care from a family member, approximately half is provided by a spouse and half from adult children such as a daughter or daughter-in-law (Frady et al., 1985). However, by the year 2000, there will be as many adults over 80 as there are under 60, which will limit the number of adult children available to provide such care (Frady et al., 1985).

Clearly, there are a growing number of middle-aged employees who are providing long-term care for elderly parents or relatives, and the numbers are increasing. Indeed, according to Miller (1991), 40% to 50% of all employees in the United States expect to care for an elderly relative sometime in the next 5 years.

Women continue to shoulder most of the responsibilities involved in caregiving for both children and older parents (ASHA, 1990). Indeed, the average American woman now spends 17 years raising children and another 18 years caring for aged parents (Miller, 1991; Weinstein, 1989). Juggling caregiving, work, and social schedules often results in stress-related illness from fatigue, depression, and emotional strain, and also results in absenteeism, lateness, and loss of job productivity (Miller, 1991).

Therefore, in response to the child-care and elder-care crises, a growing number of companies are now providing flexible schedules, better leave policies, dependent-care spending accounts (FSAs = Flexible Spending Accounts), resource and referral services, counseling and long-term care insurance for staff and family members (Miller, 1991). Some employers have even created an "Office of Dependent Care" (Miller, 1991). Companies who provide such family-friendly benefits reap their own benefits from increased productivity; less absenteeism, lateness, and turnover; reduced health care costs; more positive employee attitudes toward their jobs and employer; and high morale.

Unfortunately, the U.S. government does not have a comprehensive policy to support elder care. Such a policy, Miller (1991) reports, would result in monetary savings of a larger tax base, fewer welfare and unemployment payments, and possibly reduced costs of the criminal justice system. The benefits of such a program would be especially good for women who lose pay as well as valuable pension, social security, and insurance benefits because they take less responsible jobs in order to provide caregiving (Miller, 1991). This may mean that the government will have to support most of them when they become elderly (Miller, 1991).

Today, as never before, there is a need to foster comprehensive, coherent, and realistic policies on retirement income, health care, and long-term care within our communities, within our companies and within our government so that clients will receive the high-quality, first-rate care they deserve and so that they can live with dignity and respect. We also need such policies because "The old are us. It's our future selves, you and me" (Dr. Butler, in Frady et al., 1985, p. 31).

Underserved Populations

Three groups of clients whose needs are just now beginning to become clearer in our literature are acquired immunodeficiency syndrome (AIDS) dementia clients, bilingual and bicultural aphasic individuals, and deaf and hard-of-hearing aphasic patients.

Clients with AIDS Dementia

An increasing number of our patients will have AIDS dementia, since more than 60% of people with AIDS eventually develop some impairment in thinking or remembering (Kolata, 1990). Severity can range from mild to severe (Kolata, 1990). This impairment is complicated by the fact that some patients may also have "a brain tumor, a brain abscess, a parasitic infection and infections with other viruses" (Kolata, 1990). We need to continue to develop and provide relevant intervention procedures to this expanding population (ASHA, 1989a; Flower and Sooy, 1987).

Hepatitis, HIV and AIDS. The rapid and ever-increasing spread of hepatitis, human immunodeficiency virus (HIV), and AIDS throughout the country and the world means that many of our clients are infected. According to the CDC (Center for Disease Control), the risk of the spread of HIV to health care workers in the workplace is negligible (Frattali, 1991), since it is usually transmitted by blood and semen. However, because these diseases are deadly, it is imperative that clinicians become familiar with the universal infection control precautions or guidelines from the CDC in order to protect their clients and themselves from contracting any infectious disease. All bodily fluids should be treated as vehicles of the virus and recommended precautions should be used with *all* patients.

There are also two legal/ethical issues related to these diseases: one is *confidentiality*; the other is *refusal to treat*. Specifically, clinicians cannot disclose the diagnosis of the infected individual to others unless it is professionally necessary and in the patient's best interest, and clinicians cannot refuse to treat an infected individual.

Bicultural/Bilingual Populations

According to Webster (1977), culture is the "integrated pattern of human behavior that includes thought, speech, action and artifacts" (Webster, 1977, p. 277). It is the "customary beliefs, social forms and material traits of a racial, religious or social group" (Webster, 1977, p. 277). Culture is one of the major determinants of people's life-styles, as well as their ideas about illness, disability, medical intervention, and death. Today, the American family is becoming increasingly more culturally, linguistically, and racially diverse. Clinical aphasiologists are serving these diverse populations, including ethnic minorities such as blacks, Hispanics, Asians and Native Americans.

Sensitivity to Differences. Clinicians need to familiarize themselves with the individual and cultural similarities and differences, to the extent that these variables affect service use and delivery. Workshops and courses in cross-cultural psychology or the study of the similarities and differences in individual psychology and social functioning in various cultures and ethnic groups (Castro, 1992) can help the clinician respond more appropriately to clients (ASHA, 1988, 1992b).

Biases. Clinicians should be alert and sensitive to the presence of biases—their own and those of others—and should examine the basis for any unreasoned distortion of judgment. Prejudice can sometimes be resolved through education, exposure, and sensitivity training.

Bilingual Clinicians. Many aphasic clients are also bilingual and need the services of a speech-language pathologist who is able to speak (or sign) their primary language with native or near-native proficiency (ASHA, 1989b) and who can provide assessment and treatment in their native language. (ASHA, 1992b; Grosjean, 1989; Lebrun, 1988; Mumby, 1988; Paradis, 1983, 1987). Currently, only 3.7% of ASHA members and certificate holders have identified themselves as minorities (ASHA, 1992b). This relative lack of persons from culturally diverse populations in our field is a major concern (ASHA, 1992b; Terrell et al., 1991). There is a strong need for "innovative and aggressive efforts to recruit, train, support and retain" multicultural clinicians (Wallace and Freeman, 1991, p. 60) in order to serve clients from these groups with maximum appropriateness (Wallace and Freeman, 1991).

Epidemiology. According to Kutzke (1985), there are a number of variables that suggest that these multicultural populations will have a high rate of neurological impairments. However, a very small number of neurologically impaired adults currently receiving speech-language services are from multicultural populations (Wallace and Freeman, 1991). Marketing of services targeted to these individuals may resolve this problem. The availability of bilingual/bicultural clinicians may also resolve this dilemma.

The Deaf and Hard of Hearing

There is also a strong need to develop appropriate assessment and therapy methods for *sign language aphasics* to stimulate the cognitive, communicative components of their language (Coelho, 1989; Handelman, 1990). We also need to recruit potential clinicians who know sign language and strongly encourage current practitioners to learn it and to become more familiar with appropriate methods of intervention with such clients.

Professional Status

It is increasingly difficult to recruit qualified individuals into the field of speech-language pathology (ASHA, 1990; Kovach and Moore, 1992). This is because the current

> state of our profession is not good. Our services are not valued. Our visibility within society is limited. Our economic and social status within our society is not commensurate with our training, and our professional prerogatives are violated too frequently by the medical . . . profession. . . . [We] are undervalued, underpaid and overregulated" (Cooper, 1982, p. 931).

Therefore, we need to attract new professionals—individuals who are energetic and resourceful (Carey, 1992a) and who are visionary, creative thinkers (Kovach and Moore, 1992). According to Ringel (1982, p. 401), "gifted scientists are individualistic, open-minded, freedom-loving, highly motivated, fiercely independent, imaginative, nonconformist and usually critical of the status quo." We need to identify and recruit individuals with these personality characteristics and we need to develop effective mentoring programs to develop increased leadership within our profession (Kovach and Moore, 1992).

Salaries

Wage rates are influenced primarily by the sex composition of specific occupations (Butler et al., n.d.). Indeed, Signer (1988) observes that low salary and low status are linked to the preponderance of women in a profession. Gender-based allocation of fiscal resources has been traditional in the United States, where women's work is less valued and they typically don't control scarce resources (Butler et al., n.d.).

Women make up 75% of the health care work force (Butler et al., n.d.). Therefore, throughout the health care professions, salaries are low. Some clinicians and clinics continue to provide services at a minimum fee. Not surprisingly, there is also a strong relationship between gender and status (Butler et al., n.d.). The health labor force is notorious for its hierarchical status and power structure, which features wide disparities of wealth and power between high-ranking and low-ranking workers (Butler et al., n.d.; Signer, 1988). For example, in ASHA,

88.8% of the members are women. However, 17% of male members are directors and heads of programs, whereas only 6.2.% of female members are administrators (Signer, 1988). Because women sometimes contribute only secondarily to income, they may not assert their right to a salary commensurate with their training and professional status. The lower salaries in our profession are also tied to inadequate marketing of our scope of practice and the value of our services (Holley, 1988).

Sex

There is a strong need to eliminate the sexist attitude that exists in our profession and in society and possibly a need to increase the ratio of males in our profession. As a largely female organization, we should take a leadership role in women's issues such as the role and status of women in the workplace and in religious and political organizations; adequate monetary compensation for women; the need for elder care and child care (two-thirds of ASHA members have dependents, either adults or children (Shewan and Blake, 1991), and ASHA members spend an average of more than 20 hours per week caring for their dependents) and the empowering of women to assume leadership roles in society.

Private Practice

In 1992, 53.1% of ASHA members were employed in educational facilities; 38.8% were employed in health care facilities (a total of 91.9%); and 73.6% were employed as clinical service providers (ASHA, 1992c). Therefore, there does not appear to be a strong private-practice base in our field. However, private practice is the backbone of all independent health-related professions. Economic survival underlies professional survival, which underlies public service. There is therefore a need to provide information related to methods of initiating and developing a private practice and a need to become direct Medicare providers. We also need stronger marketing.

Marketing

Marketing is the process of defining what a potential customer wants or needs, producing that service, and then letting others know the service is for sale (Mathews, 1988). The focus is on the detailed analysis of the customers' perceptions, wants, and needs (what is important to them, what they really want), the competition, and other external variables that will affect service delivery (Mathews, 1988). For example, one way to analyze customer perception is to administer a patient satisfaction questionnaire such as the one in Appendix 1.1. Customers can be either users of the service or referral sources for other people who influence decisions for users such as third-party payers (Mathews, 1988).

Promotion involves letting your target market know that you are special and that you have what they want (Mathews, 1988). It includes *personal selling*, or telling people about your service and convincing them to choose you; *public relations*, or tools to enhance and maintain your image (such as brochures, newsletters, educational pamphlets, and slide shows) and *advertising* or placing an ad in a newspaper, journal, or yellow pages or on the radio or television (Mathews, 1988).

Product/service development, price, and distribution are important components of marketing. Effective marketing strategies build a profession and a business. They result in increased volume, increased referral sources, and higher customer satisfaction (Mathews, 1988).

Hard work is not enough. We must advertise our availability, avoid complacency, and maintain our visibility. We need to make a personal commitment to develop widespread public information campaigns to educate the public, other professionals and third-party payers about the scope of practice within our profession, about the value of our service, and about the etiology, symptomatology, and significance of stroke and aphasia (ASHA, 1990; Cooper, 1982).

The overall goal is to develop efficient and effective marketing techniques in order to disseminate information about and to change attitudes and behavior toward stroke prevention and care, toward the patients themselves, and toward our profession as a whole.

Burnout

Burnout is a "reaction to chronic, job related stress characterized by physical, emotional and mental exhaustion" (Bucci, 1991, p. 18). It is an "imbalance between the individual's psychological resources and the demands of the job" (Bucci, 1991, p. 18). Burnout is characterized by anxiety, fatigue, tension, and exhaustion (Bucci, 1991, p. 18). Other factors include the stress of dealing with patients' families, inadequate staffing and work overload, an awareness of tremendous responsibility for others and concomitant feelings of incompetence and/or insecurity, and interpersonal conflicts with other health care workers and administrators (Bucci, 1991).

The first phase is detachment or depersonalization as opposed to respect for each human being (Tilke, 1990). The second phase is a reduced sense of accomplishment, and the third phase is emotional exhaustion (Tilke, 1990).

Diversification of job and role responsibilities is thought to be one of the most effective ways to ensure that burnout does not occur. Therefore, we need to create job diversification and greater role responsibility, to develop methods to increase our effectiveness as well as to decrease paperwork in order to prevent burnout. Burnout can also be lessened by self-renewal, such as spiritual growth, relaxation, vacations, self-nurturance, the development of hope or a positive mental attitude (Goleman, 1991), forgiving others, laughter, personal growth, development of skills in human relationships (Carnegie, 1952), social and professional friendships and support systems, continuing education, self-evaluation, yoga, and exercise.

Some helpful references are Farber (1983), Goldman et al. (1992), and *Catch the Creative Spirit Video Series* (1992). Slominski's (1985b) tape is particularly relevant, since it addresses finding lasting peace of mind, emotions at risk, and the need for creativity in the workplace. The book and video *Catch the Creative Spirit* also provide an excellent resource relevant to this topic. Reducing stress and avoiding burnout are ongoing processes that require regular assessment of what the "drainers and fillers" in each individual's life are (Tilke, 1990). "If you want to make your life better start now" (Slominski, 1985b).

Quality Assurance

Deep budget cuts and increased competitiveness from other businesses and professionals are forcing both private and public sectors of society to "suddenly have an incentive to embrace quality'' (Even Uncle Sam, 1991, p. 137). Quality has become the mantra for the decade (Even Uncle Sam, 1991). All sectors of society are attempting to deliver better, more competitive products and services more effectively or at least with a smile (Even Uncle Sam, 1991). Quality is seen as the competitive advantage.

The push for total quality management (TQM) involves paying attention to every one of the processes involved in delivering a service or making a product, involving employees in every one of these processes, and paying attention to the customer (Even Uncle Sam, 1991). The emphasis is on productivity, flexibility, efficiency, effective communication and consumer-driven services.

The word "total" in TQM emphasizes the enormous change that must take place if a service or product wants to remain competitive (Underhill, 1991). TQM is different because it seeks to build quality into the essence of an organization, not just inspect for it (Labovitz, 1991). It affects the total organization—the whole process and all its components or departments. It involves "active participation by every person in an enterprise" (Underhill, 1991). TQM enterprises have well-defined objectives and guidelines for every participant and are led by informed and active people. These institutions believe that it is people that make the difference.

The author of a recent article on TQM entitled "Big Q at Big Blue" (Bemowski, 1991) suggests that the key to the success of IBM (including its recent receipt of the Congressional Baldridge Award) was its founder's business philosophy rather than its innovations, marketing skills, or financial resources. Tom Watson, Sr.'s operating principles are:

1. People are the greatest asset of any organization. Therefore, individuals must be respected and helped to respect themselves. Institutions must "let employees know they make a difference, reward superior performance, promote from within and create a democratic environment (no titles on doors, executive washrooms, etc.)" (Bemowski, 1991, p. 19). They must empower people by education and by example and make heroes of people who take initiative (Bemowski, 1991).
2. "The customer must be given the best possible service" (Bemowski, 1991, p. 19). Organizations must let customers know how important they are and satisfy each customer's requirements. To accomplish this, "every employee's job description must be related to this goal and every employee must receive appropriate training and education in how to reach it" (p. 19).
3. "Excellence and superior performance must be pursued" (Bemowski, 1991, p. 19). The goal is perfection. To ensure such excellent performance, institutions must recruit educated, motivated individuals and then provide the necessary training and environment conducive to excellence (Bemowski, 1991).
4. Strong investments in research and development are essential to quality, as is a high readiness/receptiveness to change.

In all organizations, communication lines must be open before TQM concepts are introduced (McLaurin and Bell, 1991). Good communication is vital to the success of the total quality process (Varian, 1991). Indeed, the quality of communication among all members often determines the ultimate success of the total quality process (Varian, 1991). A supportive communicative environment facilitates TQM; a defensive one retards it (Varian, 1991) (see Table 1.2). Varian (1991) notes that celebration is a powerful TQM communication tool, since it informs members of progress toward a vision and goal.

According to Bemowski (1991), the United States "is not going to be a world leader if there isn't perfection in its businesses, its government, and its education system. There is no secret to being a world leader, and there is no shortcut" (Bemowski, 1991, p. 21). She states that "it takes an educated, dedicated work force; a commitment to excellence; a commitment to quality and perfection; and an execution that is really first rate in every regard" (p. 21).

Within government, for example, some cities such as Fairfield, California, conduct an annual "satisfaction" survey of its citizens to determine if various city departments meet customer needs (Even Uncle Sam, 1991).

Within education, TQM is giving teachers, parents, and principals a say over many more educational decisions and providing a greater variety of educational choices (Readin', Writin', and Reform, 1991). The assembly line education of the 1900s is not just being improved—it is being rebuilt to reflect the need for problem solving and innovation within society (Readin', Writin', and Reform, 1991). Therefore, multiple-choice tests are being replaced because they do not show whether an individual can apply and use learning (Readin', Writin', and Reform, 1991). Society needs individuals with such skills.

In colleges, students are the customers and education is the product. Therefore, colleges are showing interest in quality practices and are asking students how they can make the schedule better, use their facilities better, and use their human resources better (A New Lesson Plan, 1991). TQM colleges are gearing up to become the preferred suppliers for education in specific areas. Within these institutions, weekly critiques of professors give them prompt feedback on whether lectures are on target and meet students' needs (A New Lesson Plan, 1991). Further, TQM faculty research is more productive and responsive to consumer needs and concerns and targets improvement in the quality of the services delivered within specific fields.

Health care and other institutions where speech-language pathologists function need to demonstrate that professionals such as speech-language pathologists (SLPs), occupational therapists (OTs) and physical therapists (PTs) are the greatest asset of their respective facilities. This means showing respect for the professional prerogatives of these individuals. These professionals need to be able to exercise a greater degree of professional discretion in the decisions that they make in regard to patients, methodologies, and facilities and not have these issues dictated by the state, the institution, or the insurance company. Excellence also involves encouraging SLPs, OTs, and PTs to

Table 1.2.
Supportive and Defensive Communication

Supportive Communication Behavior	Defensive Communication Behavior
1. *Descriptive.* Objective perception	1. *Judgment.* Critical behavior
2. *Problem oriented.* Cooperative, oriented toward finding a solution	2. *Control-oriented.* Commanding, dictating
3. *Spontaneous.* Honest	3. *Strategic.* Manipulative
4. *Empathy.* Caring	4. *Neutrality.* Not involved
5. *Equality.* Respects others as equals	5. *Superiority.* Needs to be more powerful, intelligent
6. *Flexibility*	6. *Rigidity*

Table 1.3.
Survey of Facility and Organizational TQM

How do you define the service that you provide?
What is the vision of your organization? Was it arrived at collaboratively? Does everyone share that constancy of purpose?
Can everyone in your organization identify and specify the road maps and road blocks to quality and productivity for your service?
Is this facility/organization built on quality, excellence, and service?
Is the culture of the organization a heritage of ethical behavior, of expectations of excellence, of respect for "fellow employees"?
Do you have specific goals for quality, as you do for other key areas, such as fiscal containment?
Are you continuously striving for quality improvement and perfection?
What rewards do you provide for quality improvement by employees?
Is the employment environment conducive to excellence?
Is this facility a really enjoyable place to work?
Are people having fun working at this facility and working toward quality? Is it a fear-free environment?
Does the organization provide necessary continuing education and training?
How many layers of management are there?
Are upper-level managers readily accessible to the employees?
Has the company created a democratic environment (no titles on doors, no executive washrooms)?
Does the organization empower people?
Do the people closest to the customer make the decisions?
Do subordinates always have to check with supervisors before doing things?
Is there a "we" orientation or mindset of collaboration and not competition?
Is there true collegiality among the employees? Is there mutual trust?
Does your company delegate responsibility as aggressively as possible?
When problems arise, does the institution organize itself and dedicate resources to solving the problem?
Has your organization lost its direction and momentum?
Is it clear that people are the organization's greatest asset?
How does this facility communicate to its employees that they are respected? That they are the top priority? That they make a difference?
How does the organization promote growth of employees from within?
Does this facility recruit the most motivated, highly educated, competent professionals?
Do employees use their creative energies to satisfy and delight customers?
Do all employees think about conducting their business in a perfect way?
Are there vehicles within the organization that continually strive for work simplification, work elimination, and business process improvement?
Do people across this organization feel that everyone else is working as hard as they are?
Does the credit for the prosperity of the facility/organization go to the people?
What vehicles do you use to get people to take pride in their work?
Are all members of the organization involved in the quality effort?
How is superior performance rewarded?
Do individuals accomplish their tasks in a timely, effective, and high-quality manner?
Have you created a customer-centered culture?
Is every employee committed to try to delight each customer?
How often do you administer a consumer satisfaction survey? What were the results of this customer satisfaction study? What areas are you targeting for improvement as a result of this investigation? How have you translated customer needs into redesigning your service?
Is your purchaser confident in your (the supplier's) quality systems?
Is there a customer/supplier partnership?
Are service delivery, marketing, billing, and customer service processes reviewed and analyzed regularly to determine if they can be improved?
Do you search for changes in services to create a competitive advantage?
Have you determined your customer's prioritized expectations related to service (such as ease of use, timeliness, certainty, and outcome specifics) (Lawton, 1991)?

think independently and creatively. Productivity through people (Peters and Waterman, 1982) or creating in all SLPs, OTs, and PTs the awareness that they really do make a difference, that their best efforts are essential, and that they will share in the success of the facility and the field is essential to TQM.

A critical part of health care TQM is solving problems by communicating with, involving, and giving decision-making power to the people who actually deal with the process (Labo-

vitz, 1991). Involving people in the process makes solutions last longer, and the solutions tend to be more effective (Labovitz, 1991). According to Labovitz (1991), this type of TQM process is more like preventive medicine than rehabilitation. Intercommunication with all workers is essential. It is important to inform all workers of as many aspects of the functioning of an institution as possible. Intercommunication can transform employees "from hired hands to hired heads" (Labovitz, 1991,

p. 47). "Human resources are and will be the competitive edge, the key to any organization's growth" (Labovitz, 1991, p. 47).

Within health care in general and speech-language pathology in particular, there is a need to define what makes a TQM program (see Table 1.3). We need to define our customers in very specific terms. Who are we serving: insurance companies, facilities, the state, the patient? Specifically, what are their needs? How can we become more responsive to these needs? What constitutes success in a TQM facility? What is our vision? What are our goals?

To be excellent, we must stay close to our customers, learn their preferences, and cater to them (Peters and Waterman, 1982). We need to assess consumer satisfaction (see Appendix 1.1) (Chapey, 1977) and ask how we can make their schedule better, use our facilities better for their benefit, and use our human resources better in order to be the preferred provider of cognitive, linguistic, and communicative services to our patients. The customer must be given the best service possible. Excellence and superior performance must be pursued. Such service becomes a way to keep existing customers and to attract new ones (If the Service, 1992). Indeed, to compete effectively in today's marketplace, you need "to create an environment where you encourage customers to complain" (If the Service, 1992, p. 9). Resolving such complaints fosters good will with customers (If the Service, 1992). Service is becoming the buzzword of the 1990s as businesses rediscover that the customer is always right (If the Service, 1992).

As a field, we also need a strong investment in research and development to create quality assurance measures that assess the vast complexity of patient language and cognition and subsequently our efficacy or success with these patients. We need to move away from assembly line, operationally written goals and paperwork toward professional decision making and innovation because this will serve our customers more effectively.

In addition, we need to mandate that *all* SLPs, regardless of setting, have adequate professional training or an M.A., a C.C.C., and a state license. We need to be cohesive as a group and not be duped into thinking that these credentials are not important if one is working with "just children" or "just adults." We should insist that those without these credentials be called "speech aides" and not speech-language pathologists. Continuing education and development of each professional must be stressed. Our clients have complex, multifaceted impairments and deserve to interact with qualified professionals. That's the hallmark of TQM.

TQM also demands that we heighten ASHA's responsibility to us, its membership and customers, more than to its organizational hierarchy. ASHA needs to focus on issues that are important to its members/customers (such as working more aggressively and effectively against use of New York State Certification as a Teacher of Speech and Hearing Handicapped—a B.A. level credential—as the professional credential of choice in 90% of New York State facilities). ASHA presently considers state issues such as this issue outside the realm of its operating policy. We need to communicate our satisfaction with such a stand. The essential question is, Are our customers getting top-priority service when they receive speech-language service from a B.A.-level individual? Does that show respect for our customer? Does that reflect the pursuit of excellence and superior performance? Write to ASHA and inform them about your satisfaction and/or dissatisfaction with their performance. You are their customer. Remember, "The squeaky wheel does get the grease" (If the Service, 1992, p. 9).

In TQM organizations, involvement is empowerment. If you don't get involved in your facility, state, and professional organization, no one is going to do it for you. You have the power to influence the decision-making process in these institutions. Your inertia is a signal that you don't care about yourself or your clients and that you don't really want quality. Your involvement is your empowerment. You are ASHA. You are the state. You are your facility. Vote for quality with your hands, head, and feet. People do make the difference.

Health care and containment of health care costs will be the political issue of the 21st century. The winners in this competition "will not necessarily be the cheapest health care facilities, but those that meet customer needs by delivering quality care" (Labovitz, 1991, p. 46). We need to integrate TQM into our decision of the kind of changes that we believe are essential to the highest quality service (see Table 1.3).

LANGUAGE INTERVENTION STRATEGIES IN ADULT APHASIA

The major purpose of the present text is the specification of various models of intervention for adult aphasia patients and for patients with related disorders. Such models can provide a framework to focus therapy, to generate intervention tasks, and to analyze empirically the efficiency of rehabilitation efforts.

Some of these therapeutic strategies have appeared in part or in whole in previous literature; others have not. It should be recognized, however, that it is not the purpose of this text to assess any of the models or to resolve the inconsistencies in these approaches. These functions are better performed in appropriate professional journals or through further experiments. It is hoped that this text will provoke theoretical speculation and that those chapters that are rich conceptually will prompt the collection of further data and generate the production of new approaches. The readings are organized into sections to give the reader perspective on the field. However, the sections of the book—and indeed the chapters—can be used in any order.

References

Abrams, W. and Berko, R. (1990). *The Merck manual of geriatrics.* Rahway, NJ: Merck, Sharpe & Dhomme Research Laboratories.

Allison, M. (1991, October). Stopping the brain drain. *Harvard Health Letter,* *16*(12), 6–8.

American Speech-Language-Hearing Association. (1986). The delivery of speech-language and audiology services in home care. *ASHA, 28*(5), 49–52.

American Speech-Language-Hearing Association. (1988). Definition: Bilingual speech language pathologists and audiologists. *ASHA, 30*(5), 53.

American Speech-Language-Hearing Association. (1989a). AIDS/HIV: Implications for speech-language pathologists and audiologists. *ASHA, 31*(6-7), 33–37.

American Speech-Language-Hearing Association. (1989b). Committee on the status of racial minorities. Definition: bilingual speech language pathologists and audiologists. *ASHA, 31*(3), 93.

American Speech-Language-Hearing Association. (1990). Women, stress, karoski. *ASHA, 2,* 11–12.

American Speech-Language-Hearing Association. (1991). Omnibus survey results. Rockville, MD: American Speech-Language-Hearing Association.

American Speech-Language-Hearing Association. (1992a). ASHAs proposed long-range strategic plan. *ASHA, 34*(5), 32–36.

American Speech-Language-Hearing Association. (1992b). Our multicultural agenda. *ASHA, 34*(5), 37–53.

American Speech-Language-Hearing Association. (1992c). ASHA facts. *ASHA 34*.(3), 20.

Bemowski, K. (1991, May). Big Q at big blue. *Quality Progress, 24*, 17–21.

Blakeslee, S. (1991, September 10). Brain yields new clues on its organization for language. *New York Times*, p. C1, cols. 1–5, p. C10, cols. 3–5.

Brody, J. (1992, June 10). When brain damage disrupts speech. *New York Times*, p. C13.

Brown, J. W. (1972). *Aphasia, apraxia and agnosia: Clinical and theoretical aspects*. Springfield, IL: Charles C. Thomas.

Brown, J. W. (1977). *Mind, brain and consciousness*. New York: Academic Press.

Brown, J. W. (1979). Language representation in the brain. In H. Steklis and M. Raleigh (Eds.), *Neurobiology of social communication in primates*. New York: Academic Press.

Brown, J. W. and Perecman, E. (1986). Neurological basis of language processing. In R. Chapey (Ed.), *Language intervention strategies in adult aphasia*. Baltimore MD: Williams & Wilkins.

Bucci, E. (1991, May 13). Stress of health care employees gains increased attention. *Advance for Physical Therapists*, pp. 18–19.

Butler, I., Carpenter, E., Kay, B., and Simmons, R. (n.d.). *Sex and status in the workforce*. Washington, DC: American Public Health Association. Carey, A. (1992a). Leadership. *ASHA, 34*(1), 32. Carnegie, D. (1952). *How to win friends and influence people*. New York: Simon & Schuster.

Castro, N. (1992). Cultural issues in the treatment of head injury. *NHIF Newsletter for the New York City Region, 1*(1), 3.

Catch the creative spirit video series: Inside creativity, creative beginning, creative work, creative community. (1992). Alexandria, VA: PBS Video (1-800-343-4727).

Chapey, R. (1977). Consumer satisfaction in speech-language pathology. *ASHA, 19*, 829–832.

Chapey, R. (1986). An introduction to language intervention strategies in adult aphasia. In R. Chapey (Ed.), *Language intervention strategies in adult aphasia*. Baltimore, MD: Williams & Wilkins.

Chapey, R., Lubinski, R., Salzberg, A., and Chapey, G. (1979). Survey of speech, language and hearing services in nursing home settings. *Long-Term Care Health Services Administration Quarterly, 3*, 307–316.

Chomsky, N. (1972). *Language and mind*. New York: Harcourt, Brace & World.

Coelho, C. A. (1989). Communication skills in an aphasic deaf adult. *Archives of Physical Medicine and Rehabilitation, 70*, (2), 159–161.

Cooper, E. (1982). The state of the profession and what to do about it. *ASHA, 24*, 931–936.

Cormier, W. H. and Cormier, L. S. (1991). *Interviewing strategies for helpers* (3rd ed) Pacific Grove, CA: Brooks/Cole.

Cubelli, R., Foresti, A., and Consolini, T. (1988). Reeducation strategies in conduction aphasia. *Journal of Communication Disorders, 21*, 239–249.

Damasio, A. (1981). The nature of aphasia signs and syndromes. In M. T. Sarno (Ed.), *Acquired aphasia*. New York: Academic Press.

Damasio, H. (1981). Cerebral localization of the aphasias. In M. T. Sarno (Ed.), *Acquired aphasia*. New York: Academic Press.

Darley, F. L. (1982). *Aphasia*. Philadelphia: W. B. Saunders.

Dunbar, L., and Most, S. (1991). *Healthy aging*. Lifeguides Video. Los Angeles, CA: KCET.

Even Uncle Sam is starting to see the light. (1991). *Business Week*, pp. 133–137.

Ewart, C. (1991). Social action theory for a public health psychology. *American Psychologist, 46*(9), 931–942.

Falck, V. (1972). The role and function of university training programs. *ASHA, 14*, 307–310.

Farber, B. (Ed.). (1983). *Stress and burnout in the human service professions*. Palo Alto, CA: Consulting Psychologists Press.

Fein, D. (1983). Population data from the U.S. Census Bureau. *ASHA, 25*, 47.

Flower, W., and Sooy, C. (1987). AIDS: An introduction for speech language pathologists and audiologists. *ASHA, 29*(11), 25–30.

Fox, S. (1991, March 25). Gero-psychiatry. Life can begin at 80. *Advance for Occupational Therapists*, p. 15.

Frady, M., Gerdau, R., Lennon, T., Sherman, W. and Singer, S. (1985, December 28). *Growing old in America*. ABC News Close-Up.

Frattali, C. (1991). Professional practices perspectives on infection control. *ASHA, 33*(5), 10.

Freudenheim, M. (1992, May 3). Medicaid plan promotes nursing-home insurance. *New York Times*. p. 1, cols. 1–2; p. 45, col. 1.

Fromkin, V., and Rodman, R. (1974). *An introduction to language*. New York: Holt, Rinehart & Winston.

Gilbert, S. (1990, April 29). ''Is America abandoning sick patients?'' *New York Times, Good Health Magazine*, pp. 22, 30.

Goldman, D. Kaufman, P., and Ray, M. (1992). *Catch the creative spirit*. Dalton, Penguin.

Goldstein, K. (1948). *Language and language disturbances*. New York: Grune & Stratton.

Goldstein K., and Scheerer, M. (1941). Abstract and concrete behavior in experimental study with special tests. *Psychological Monograph, 53*, 2.

Goldstein, R. (1984). To be or not to be? Kansas City, Missouri, Luncheon Address, Silver Anniversary Convention, Missouri Speech, Language, Hearing Association.

Goleman, D. (1991). Hope emerges as key to success in life. *New York Times*, p. C1, cols. 3–5; p. C7, cols. 1–5.

Goodglass, H., and Kaplan, E. (1983). *The assessment of aphasia and related disorders*, (2nd ed). Philadelphia: Lea & Febiger.

Goodglass, H., Quadfasel, F., and Timberlake, W. (1964). Phrase length and type and severity of aphasia. *Cortex, 1*, 133–153.

Goodman, P. (1971). *Speaking and language: Defense of poetry*. New York: Random House.

Grosjean, F. (1989). Neurolinguistics beware! The bilingual is not two monolinguals in one person. *Brain and Language, 36*(1), 3–15.

Hamilton, M. (1991, May 6). Cost containment program in U.S. health care system under fire. *Advance for Physical Therapists*, p. 22.

Handelman, D. (1990). *Sign language aphasia*. Brooklyn, NY: Brooklyn College student term paper.

Head, H. (1915). Hughlings Jackson on aphasia and kindred affections on speech. *Brain, 38*, 1–27.

Hellerstein, D. (1988, May 22). Plotting a theory of the brain. *New York Times Magazine*, pp. 16–20, 27, 28, 55, 61, 64.

Herbers, H. (1981, May 24). Rise of elderly population in 70's portends vast changes in nation. *New York Times*, p. 1, cols. 5–6; p. 44. cols. 3–6.

Holley, S. (1988). Marketing your services. President's page. *ASHA, 30*(9), 37–38.

If the service is poor, don't get mad, get even. (1992, September 5). *New York Times*, p. 9.

Kearns, K. and Thompson, C. (1991). Technical drift and conceptual myopia. In T. Prescott (Ed.), *Clinical Aphasiology Conference Proceedings*, 19. Austin, TX: Pro-Ed.

Keith, R. (1975). The effectiveness of treatment in aphasia. Discussion. In R. Brookshire (Ed.), *Clinical Aphasiology Conference Proceedings*. Minneapolis, MN: BRK.

Kerr, P. (1992, April 3). Cutting costs of brain injuries. *New York Times*, p. D1, col. 3; p. D2, cols. 1–4.

Kertesz, A. (1982). *Western Aphasia Battery*. New York: Grune & Stratton.

Kertesz, A., and Poole, E. (1974). The aphasia quotient: The taxonomic approach to the measurement of aphasic disability. *Canadian Journal of Neurological Science, 1*, 7–16.

Kolata, G. (1990, December 14). AIDS researchers find clues to how virus attacks brain. *New York Times*, p. A34, cols, 1, 2.

Kolata, G. (1991, April 16). The aging brain: The mind is resilient, it's the body that fails. *New York Times*, p. C1, col. 1; p. C10, cols. 2–6.

Kovach, T., and Moore, S. (1992). Leaders are born through the mentoring process. *ASHA, 34*(1), 33–34.

Krinsky, R. (1991, June 10). Getting old—is it all in your mind? *Advance for Occupational Therapists*. p. 12.

Kutzke, J. (1985). Epidemiology of cerebrovascular disease. In F. McDowell and L. Caplan (Eds.), *Cerebrovascular survey report*. pp. 1–34. Bethesda, MD: National Institute of Neurological and Communicative Disorders and Stroke.

Labovitz, G. (1991). The total quality health care revolution. *Quality Process, 24*(9), 45–50.

Lawton, R. (1991). Creating a customer-centered culture in service industries. *Quality Process, 24*(9), 69–74.

Lebrun, Y. (1988). Multilingualism and aphasia. *Review of Laryngology, Otology and Rhinology*(Bard), *109*(4), 299–306.

Love, R. J. (1981). The forgotten minority: The communicatively disabled. *ASHA, 23*, 485–490.

Mathews, C. (1988). Marketing your services: Strategies that work. *ASHA, 30*, 22–25.

McLaurin, D., and Bell, S. (1991). Open communication lines before attempting total quality. *Quality Process, 24*(6), 25–28

Miller, C. (1991). Dependent care in the 1990's: Business and government share the working family's burden. Part 1. Defining the need. *Current Contents*, pp. 5–10.

Minifie, F. (1983). ASHA from adolescence onward. *ASHA, 25,* 17–24.

Muma, J. (1978). *Language handbook: Concepts, assessment and intervention.* Englewood Cliff, NJ: Prentice-Hall.

Mumby, K. (1988, December 23). An adaptation of aphasia screening test for use with Panjabi speakers. *British Journal of Disorders of Communication, 3,* 267–292.

A New Lesson Plan for College (1991). *Business Week,* 144-145.

Paradis, M. (Ed.). (1983). Readings on aphasia. In *Bilinguals and Polyglots.* Quebec: Didier.

Paradis, M. (1987). *The assessment of bilingual aphasia.* Hillsdale, NJ: Lawrence Erlbaum.

PBS. (1991a). *The cost of caring.* Lifeguides Video. Los Angeles, CA: KCET.

PBS. (1991b). *Final choices.* Lifeguides Video. Los Angeles, CA: KCET.

Peters, T., and Waterman, R. (1982). *In search of excellence.* New York: Warner Books.

Post, J., and Leith, W. (1983). I'd rather tell a story than be one. *ASHA 25,* 23–26.

Readin', Writin', and Reform. (1991). *Business Week,* pp. 140–141.

Ringel, R. (1982). Some issues facing graduate education. *ASHA, 24,* 399–404.

Robins, J. (1987). *Diet for a new America: Your health, Your planet.* Walpole, NH: Stillpoint Publishers.

Robins, J. (1991). *Diet for a new America: Your health, Your planet.* Lifeguides Video. Los Angeles, CA: KCET.

Rogers, C. (1969). *Freedom to learn.* Columbus, OH: Charles E. Merrill.

Sahs, A. L., and Hartman, E. C. (Eds.). (1976). *Fundamentals of stroke care.* Washington, DC: U.S. Department of Health, Education and Welfare.

Schuell, H. (revised by J. Sefer) (1973). *Differential diagnosis of aphasia with the Minnesota test.* Minneapolis, MN: University of Minnesota Press.

Schuell, H., Carroll, V., and Street, B. (1955). Clinical treatment of aphasia. *Journal of Speech and Hearing Disorders, 20,* 43–53.

Schuell, H., Jenkins, J. J., and Jiminez-Pabon, E. (1964). *Aphasia in adults.* New York: Harper Medical Division.

Shewan, C., and Blake, A. (1991). Caregiving: A common role for ASHA members. *ASHA, 33*(2), 35.

Signer, M. (1988). The value of women's work. *ASHA, 30,* 24–25.

Slominski, T. (1985a). *Medicare and speech pathology: Reimbursement strategies* (an audiocassette tape). Gaylord, MI: Northern Speech Services.

Slominski, T. (1985b). *The speech and language pathologist: Emotions at risk.* (an audiocasette tape). Gaylord, MI: Northern Speech Services.

Snyder, M., and Ware, J. (n.d.). *A study of twenty-two hypothesized dimensions of patient attitudes regarding medical care.* Pub. No. PB 239-518/AS. Springfield, VA: National Technical Information Service.

Terrell, S., Mueller, P., and Conley, L. (1991). Sister programs: Historically black and majority white universities. *ASHA, 33*(9), 45–48.

They're not kidding when they say "Blue Monday". (1992, May 18). *Business Week,* p. 113.

Thompson, C., and Kearns, K. (1991). Analytical and technical directions in applied aphasia analysis: The Midas touch. In T. Prescott (Ed.), *Clinical aphasiology,* (Vol. 19, pp. 41--54). Austin, TX: Pro-Ed.

Tilke, B. (1990, April 23). Administrators, OTs can reduce stress, potential burnout factors. *Advance for Occupational Therapists,* p. 17.

Underhill, B. (1991). "Total" remains bread and butter of total quality management. Letter to editor. *Quality Process, 24,* 8.

Varian, T. (1991). Communicating total quality inside the organization. *Quality Progress, 6,* 30–31.

Wallace, G., and Freeman, S. (1991). Adults with neurological improvement from multicultural populations. *ASHA, 33*(6–7), 58–60.

Ware, J., and Snyder, M. (1975). Dimensions of patient attitudes regarding doctors and medical care services. *Medical Care, 13,* 669–682.

Ware, J., Snyder, M., McClure, E., and Jarrett, I. (n.d.). *The measurement of health concepts.* Pub. No. PB 239-508/AS. Springfield, VA: National Technical Information Service.

Ware, J., Snyder, M., and Wright, W. (1973). *Patient perceptions of health care services. Implications for the academic medical community.* Technical Report No. MHC 73-2. Carbondale, IL: Southern Illinois University School of Medicine.

Warren, S., and Rogers-Warren, A. (1985). *Teaching functional language: Generalization and maintenance of language skills.* Austin, TX: Pro-Ed.

Webster. (1977). *Webster's New Collegiate Dictionary.* Springfield, MA: G. & C. Mirriam Co.

Weinstein, G. W. (1989, October). Help wanted—the crises of elder cares. *Ms.* 18(4), 72–79.

Wepman, J. (1972a). Aphasia therapy: A new look. *Journal of Speech and Hearing Disorders, 37,* 203–214.

Wepman, J. (1972b). Aphasia therapy: Some "relative" comments and some purely personal prejudices. In M. Sarno (Ed.), *Aphasia—selected readings.* New York: Appleton-Century-Crofts.

Wepman, J. (1976). Aphasia: Language without thought or thought without language. *ASHA, 18,* 131–136.

Wepman, J. and Jones, L. (1961). *Studies in aphasia: An approach to testing: The Language Modalities Test for aphasia.* Chicago: Education-Industry Service.

Wernicke, C. (1874). Der aphasische Symptomenkomplex. Cohen and Weigart, Breslau. Also as the Symptom Complex of Aphasia. (1969). In R. Cohen and M. Wartofsky (Eds.), *Studies in the philosophy of science.* (Vol. IV). Durdrecht, Reidel.

Winslow, R. (1992, February 25). Videos, questionnaires aim to expand role of patient in treatment decisions. *Wall Street Journal,* p. B1, cols. 3–5.

Zivin, J., and Choi, D. (1991, July). Stroke therapy. *Scientific American, 265*(1), 56–63.

APPENDIX 1.1[a]

Consumer Satisfaction in Speech-Language Pathology

by ROBERTA CHAPEY

QUESTIONNAIRE

The questionnaire presented in the following list is an adaptation of the Patient-Satisfaction Questionnaire (PSQ) developed by Ware and his colleagues (Snyder and Ware, n.d.; Ware and Snyder, 1975; Ware, Snyder, and McClure, and Jarrett, n.d.; Ware, Snyder, and Wright, 1973).

1. Speech-language pathologists consider the patient's feelings.

2. I can reach a speech-language pathologist to ask questions.

3. Speech-language pathologists are careful to explain the probable outcome of the treatment they prescribe for a particular patient.

4. The care I have received from the speech-language pathologist includes everything it should.

5. Speech-language pathologists are sensitive to client responses, reactions, and needs.

6. When a speech-language pathologist does not know the answer to a question he will help you find the answer.

[a]Reprinted by permission from Chapey, R. (1977). *ASHA, 19,* 826–832.

7. Speech-language pathologists are thorough in giving a complete diagnostic examination.
8. There are enough speech-language pathologists in our vicinity.
9. Speech-language pathologists check up on the problems I have had before.
10. Speech-language pathology sessions are carefully planned and have a specific goal.
11. The cost of the speech service is reasonable.
12. Speech-language pathologists meet with family members to help them understand the nature of the client's disorder.
13. Speech-language pathologists keep records of the treatment you have received.
14. Speech-language pathologists recommend a client to a specialist (for example, a doctor, a dentist) when it is necessary.
15. Speech-language pathologists respect privileged communication (reports, interviews with clients, test scores).
16. Speech-language pathologists have their speech diplomas posted in their office or clinic.
17. Speech-language pathologists seem concerned about the whole person, not just a person's speech or language.
18. Speech-language pathologists explain why they recommend or refer a client to a specialist.
19. People who work in speech-language pathologists' offices are courteous and friendly.
20. I am satisfied with the speech care I receive.
21. You can get a medical insurance plan that pays for all of the speech-language pathology expenses a person might have.
22. Speech-language pathologists examine their clients carefully before deciding what is wrong.
23. My speech-language pathologist's office is complete with all the necessary facilities.
24. People are usually kept waiting a long time when they are at the speech-language pathologist's office.
25. Speech-language pathologists are real and genuine people who like and understand their clients.
26. Speech-language pathologists conduct research to help them learn more about different speech and language disorders.
27. Speech-language pathologists have their offices in very convenient locations.
28. Speech-language pathologists usually explain a client's speech problem to him.
29. Speech-language pathologists give clear instructions about how and when to do assignments.
30. Speech-language pathologists know of the broad range of health services available in the area and refer clients to them.
31. Speech-language pathologists are warm, friendly, and easy to talk to.
32. Speech-language pathologists do their best to keep you from worrying.
33. Speech-language pathologists are as thorough as they should be.
34. Speech-language pathologists meet with family members to help them understand the type of therapy that a client receives.
35. When a speech-language pathologist does not know the answer to a question, he will admit that he does not know.
36. Speech-language pathologists treat their clients with respect.
37. Speech-language pathologists tell a client the purpose of every lesson and assignment.
38. Speech-language pathologists have a sensitive awareness of the way the process of speech-language pathology seems to the client.
39. When speech-language pathologists are unsure of what's wrong with you, they refer you to a specialist.
40. You can get an appointment to see your speech-language pathologist right away.
41. Speech-language pathologists always avoid unnecessary expenses for the client.
42. Speech-language pathologists provide information about normal speech and language development to people in our community.
43. I see the same speech-language pathologist every time I go to the clinic.
44. Speech-language pathologists try to explain the procedures used in therapy so the client won't worry.
45. Speech-language pathologists keep up on all of the latest discoveries in their field.
46. Speech-language pathologists let their clients tell them everything that is important.
47. You get what you pay for with medical insurance.
48. Speech-language pathologists tell clients what to expect during treatment.
49. Clinic hours when you can get speech-language services are good for most people.
50. Speech-language pathologists meet with family members to help them learn about the client's progress.

ITEM GROUPING FOR THE CLIENT QUESTIONNAIRE

Grouping	Item	Content
Access and convenience		
Access	2	Is available to answer questions
	40	Has frequent open appointments
Convenience	27	Is in a convenient location
	49	Has convenient office hours
	24	Keeps people waiting
Availability of resources	8	Are enough clinicians available?
	43	Is the same clinician each session

Grouping	Item	Content
Finances		
Cost of care	11	Cost of care is reasonable
	41	Avoids unnecessary expenses
Insurance	21	Insurance coverage is adequate
	47	Services are adequate when paid by insurance
Speech-language pathologist's conduct		
Client centeredness and humanness		
Respect	15	Respects privileged information
	36	Treats client with respect
Sensitivity to client	5	Is sensitive to client responses/reactions/needs
	38	Is sensitive re: how therapy affects client
Real person	25	Is real/genuine—likes/understands client
	31	Is warm/friendly/easy to talk to
Considers more than disorder	1	Considers patient's feelings
	17	Is concerned about whole person
	32	Tries to avoid patient anxiety
	46	Listens to client concerns
Quality/Competence		
Thorough diagnosis and therapy	7	Gives thorough diagnosis
	9	Checks previous history
	10	Plans therapy/goal oriented
	13	Keeps records
	22	Gives thorough diagnostic
	29	Gives clear instructions re: assignment
	37	Explains rationale: therapy
	44	Explains procedures: therapy
Referrals	24	Recommends specialist when necessary
	30	Knows health services available
	39	Makes appropriate referrals
Information to client	3	Explains outcome of treatment
	6	Helps client find information
	16	Posts diploma
	18	Explains reason for referral
	28	Explains disorder to patient
	35	Admits lack of knowledge
	48	Explains process of therapy
Information to family/community	12	Gives family counseling: nature of disorder
	34	Gives family counseling: type of therapy
	42	Educates community
	50	Gives family counseling: progress in therapy
Professional activities	26	Conducts research
	45	Keeps up on latest discoveries
Speech facilities		
Adequacy	19	Staff courteous/friendly
	23	Office complete
General satisfaction		
Adequacy	4	Care includes what it should
	20	Satisfied with care
	33	Generally thorough

SCORING

Each item can be scored by a client as follows: strongly agree 5; agree, 4; uncertain (or do not know), 3; disagree, 2; or strongly disagree, 1. Scores can be computed from the simple algebraic sum of scores for items (contained in each scale) as shown below. For example, the speech-language pathologist's facilities scale (SPFS) can be constructed from the 50-item form as follows: SPFS = Item 19 + Item 23. Thus, SPFS is the simple algebraic sum of scores for Items 19 and 23.

16 Scales and Five Global Scales Constructed from the 50-Item Questionnaire

Scale Name	Scale Label	Formula for Scale
Accessibility	Var 1	Item 2 + Item 40
Convenience	Var 2	Item 27 + Item 49 + Item 24
Availability of resources	Var 3	Item 8 + Item 43
Total access and convenience	Var 17	Var 1 + Var 2 + Var 3
Cost of care	Var 4	Item 11 + Item 41
Insurance	Var 5	Item 21 + Item 47
Total finances	Var 18	Var 4 + Var 5
Clinician's respect	Var 6	Item 15 + Item 36
Clinician's sensitivity	Var 7	Item 5 + Item 38
Clinician as a person	Var 8	Item 25 + Item 31
Notices whole person	Var 9	Item 1 + Item 17 + Item 32 + Item 46
Total client centeredness/humanness	Var 19	Var 6 + Var 7 + Var 8 + Var 9
Quality diagnosis/therapy	Var 10	Item 7 + Item 9 + Item 10 + Item 13 + Item 22 + Item 29 + Item 37 + Item 44
Quality referrals	Var 11	Item 14 + Item 30 + Item 39
Information to client	Var 12	Item 3 + Item 6 + Item 16 + Item 18 + Item 28 + Item 35 + Item 48
Information to family/community	Var 13	Item 12 + Item 34 + Item 42 + Item 50
Professional activities	Var 14	Item 16 + Item 45
Total quality	Var 20	Var 10 + Var 11 + Var 12 + Var 13 + Var 14
Speech facilities	Var 15	Item 19 + Item 23
General satisfaction	Var 16	Item 4 + Item 20 + Item 33
Total satisfaction	Var 21	Var 15 + Var 16 + Var 17 + Var 18 + Var 19 + Var 20

CHAPTER 2
Medical Aspects of Stroke Rehabilitation

ANTHONY G. MLCOCH AND E. JEFFREY METTER

Stroke is the most common cause of aphasia. "Stroke" is not a technical medical term but rather is a general one that refers to a number of related disorders. It is "a sudden action or event" (*Webster's New World Dictionary*, 1973). According to *Dorland's Illustrated Medical Dictionary* (1965), it is "a sudden and severe attack, as of apoplexy or paralysis." The term refers to the suddenness of onset of a prominent and frequently persistent neurological deficit. Specifically, it refers to illnesses resulting from damage to the circulation to the brain. Another commonly used term is "cerebrovascular accident" (CVA), which implies a vascular etiology and differentiates it from other brain disorders that are not related to circulation but have a strokelike onset.

Because all strokes are not a result of vascular disease, it is important for health professionals other than the physician to have a basic understanding of differences between disorders and their patterns of presentation. These professionals might be the first to recognize that a given case may be unusual, that is, not typical for a CVA.

Appropriate aphasia treatment requires close communication between the physician and other members of the rehabilitation team in order to allow for prompt, integrative, and cost-efficient patient care that will optimize the rate and extent of possible recovery. Such communication can also be a vehicle to alert the physician if unusual changes occur or new problems develop that can affect the patient's well-being. Thus all members of the rehabilitation team need a thorough understanding of the basic aspects of the pathophysiology, diagnosis, and treatment of stroke.

The physician should be the head of the rehabilitation team because stroke victims frequently have complex medical problems that restrict the extent and nature of therapies that can be applied at a given time. In some circumstances, particularly following the acute aspects of the illness, the physician may assume a less centralized and active role.

The primary role of the speech-language pathologist following stroke is the treatment of a resulting aphasia and/or dysarthria. This entails not only helping patients recover their speech and language skills as quickly as possible but also educating and counseling the family, physician, nurses, and other health professionals as to the nature and extent of the disorder as well as what they can do to enable patients to communicate more efficiently. This is especially important during the acute phase of stroke, since patients, at this time, are often confused and disoriented and, when aphasic, are faced with a disability that interferes with their ability to indicate their wants and needs. The physician and nursing staff on an acute neurological or medical ward are frequently too busy either to counsel the family or to reorient patients to their environment and circumstances. This responsibility falls on the speech-language pathologist, who must help patients cope with their disorder. The speech pathologist also advises the family as to what to expect now and over time and tells them how they can best assist patients in their recovery. In addition, speech pathologists must advise and educate the staff as to how they can best work with the patient.

In addition to the patient's rehabilitation, the speech-language pathologist is also responsible for the initial diagnosis of the patient's communication disorder. In the case of aphasia, this entails a careful examination of the patient's receptive and expressive language skills, making certain the symptom complex demonstrated is consistent with a diagnosis of aphasia and not another type of neurogenic disorder that may mimic aphasia (i.e., acute confusional state, dementia, locked in syndrome, akinetic mutism, etc.). This information, in turn, can assist the physician in determining the extent of the cerebral damage (i.e., focal or diffuse) and provide clues as to the neuroanatomical site of the insult. A detailed evaluation can also help determine the stroke patient's overall prognosis. A poor prognosis may be in store for the aphasic who is experiencing severe to profound receptive and expressive language deficits, while the individual who demonstrates a specific type of aphasia may have a better prognosis. In any case, a thorough speech and language evaluation is needed to establish a baseline that can be used to gauge the patient's progress.

In order for speech-language pathologists to provide diagnostic, therapeutic, and counseling services to the patient, the patient's family, and other health professionals, they must be knowledgeable about the medical management of stroke. Speech pathologists must be aware of how strokes are manifested, their etiology, and the treatment approaches and tools that the physician uses to diagnose and treat stroke. The remainder of this chapter will provide this information.

EPIDEMIOLOGY

Stroke ranks third behind heart disease and cancer as an underlying cause of death in the United States. The current death rate from stroke is approximately 1 person per 1000 population per year and accounts for 10% to 12% of all deaths (Bonita, 1992). The annual incidence is between 1 and 2 per 1000, while the prevalence rates are between 4 and 6 per 1000 (Kurtzke, 1980). These numbers imply that for a population of 230 million people, approximately 1 million individuals at a given time will be living after suffering from a stroke, while 250,000 to 500,000 will suffer from a stroke annually, and half this number will die related to the stroke. The total cost of stroke, as estimated by a President's Commission (1964), was greater than $1 billion. In today's dollars and with advancing technology, the current annual loss to society is more likely at least $5 billion to $10 billion.

The incidence of stroke increases geometrically with age and is primarily a disorder of aging. Thus, for individuals under age 50, the incidence is less than 1 per 1000 annually, while by age 70 it approaches 10 per 1000 and by age 80 is about 20 per 1000 (Kurtzke, 1980). About 1 in 4 men and 1 in 5 women aged 45 will have a stroke if they live to an age of 85 (Bonita, 1992).

Recent epidemiological studies (see Whisnant, 1983) demontrated that the annual incidence of strokes has been declining over the past 50 years. From 1980, though, the rates have been increasing. For example, in Rochester, Minnesota, the incidence of stroke increased from 1980 to 1984 (Broderick et al., 1989). The authors attributed the increase to improved diagnostic methods caused by the introduction of computed tomography (CT) scanning. In some populations, the increases are attributed to a rising incidence of hemorrhagic strokes (Mayo, et al., 1991).

Preventive measures may contribute to lowering the incidence of major disability. Life-style changes, proper counseling, and earlier recognition of changes in patient health status have contributed to the trend. There is some evidence that the rate of hemorrhagic strokes has been increasing over the past few years (Mayo et al., 1991). One major factor for the long downtrend has been increased public awareness of hypertension and its association with the development of stroke. The improved treatment of hypertension by lowering blood pressure has been shown to decrease the incidence of stroke and myocardial infarctions (Veterans Administration Cooperative Study Group on Antihypertensive Agents, 1967, 1970). Other risk factors include heart disease (Kannel, 1971), arrhythmias (Wolf et al., 1978), diabetes mellitus (Lavy et al., 1973), cigarette usage, obesity, and dietary patterns. The recognition of transient ischemic attacks (described below) can also forewarn of impending disaster, and appropriate referral becomes critical. Improved recognition and treatment of such factors have helped to reduce the incidence of stroke.

Stroke-related mortality most frequently results from other vascular disease, particularly coronary artery disease and associated heart attacks. Mortality is typically considered as being early within the initial hospitalization, or from 3 to 4 weeks postonset, or late. Early mortality varies between 17 and 34% during the first month poststroke (Bonita, 1992). The most significant factors associated with early mortality have been alteration in consciousness, which implies a greater and more extensive stroke and increasing age (Truscott, et al., 1974). Myocardial infarction, congestive heart failure, and hypertension have been correlated with early mortality in some studies (Ford and Katz, 1966). Late mortality occurs after the initial hospitalization and is much higher than for the general age-adjusted population. Terent (1989) noted a 1-year fatality rate of 33% during the years 1983 to 1987, and a 3-year rate of 34%. This was an improvement from the rates in 1975 to 1979, where the 1-year fatality rate was 41%. Marquardsen (1969) reported a 3-year mortality of 46% in those who survived beyond 3 weeks. The average annual mortality remained constant for at least 10 years after the stroke, with an average annual rate of 17%. This number approaches that of the general population after about 10 years (Eisenberg et al., 1964; Pincock, 1957).

The scope of the problem becomes clearer when examining what becomes of stroke survivors. Marquardsen (1969), in an extensive review of the literature noted that of unselected stroke survivors, 1% to 25% were able to return to work, 50% to 75% were able to walk unaided and were discharged home, and 20% to 30% required continued institutionalization. In his study, of 407 immediate survivors, 52% were restored to independence in self-care, 15% were able to walk unaided but required some help with personal needs, and 33% were dependent for walking and self-care. Of the patients employed prior to the stroke, about one-third returned to work. Seventy-five percent of the patients were able to return home. Thorngren and Westling (1990) found a similar rate of survivors living at home 1 year postonset of stroke in 1986. Held (1975) notes, ''The percentage of patients who can resume their capability to earn wages is lower than in virtually all other handicaps, physical or intellectual.'' From these observations, it is apparent that stroke will have a devastating effect on the patient and the entire family.

STROKE ETIOLOGY

The most common cause of strokelike illnesses is related to vascular disease. Each minute, approximately 800 mL of blood circulates to the brain, which represents 15% to 20% of the total body blood supply for an organ, which represents 1% to 2% of the body's weight. Loss of circulation results in rapid disruption of the ability of brain neurons to function properly and, if severe and persistent, in the death of neuronal tissue. Resulting symptoms depend on the area of the brain damaged and the effect that the damaged region has on the remainder of the brain.

The circulation to the brain arises from two pairs of arteries: the internal carotids and the vertebrals. The carotid arteries course in the anterior aspects of the neck. At the level of the superior border of the thyroid cartilage, both arteries divide into an external and internal branch. The internal carotid artery enters the cranium and supplies much of the forebrain. The carotid artery bifurcates into the anterior and middle cerebral arteries, which supply the cerebral hemispheres over the anterior and much of the lateral surfaces (Gray, 1967; Truax and Carpenter, 1969).

The vertebral artery is the first branch of the subclavian artery. It enters the vertebral foramen of the sixth cervical vertebra then proceeds upward through the corresponding vertebral foramina and enters the posterior fossa of the cranium through the foramen magnum. The two vertebral arteries unite at the pontomedullary border to form the basilar artery. The basilar artery continues along the midline of the pons. At the upward end of the pons, the artery divides into two posterior cerebral arteries, which proceed posteriorly to the inferior medial surfaces of the hemispheres to the occipital lobes. The artery supplies blood to those regions where it passes, including the brain stem, the inferior and medial aspects of the hemispheres, and the occipital area.

At the base of the brain, interconnections occur between the carotid and vertebral arteries, forming a circular passage that allows for mixing of blood from the anterior and posterior circulations. This interconnection is called the circle of Willis and forms a major source of collateral circulation for the brain.

Collateral circulation refers to the ability of blood from separate brain arteries to redistribute to other brain areas. The brain has extensive collaterals, which include the circle of Willis, connections between the external and internal carotids, connections between the left and right anterior cerebral arteries via the anterior communicating artery, and connections between the three cerebral artery systems. This is particularly important when the principal artery to a region becomes compromised. If collateral circulation is adequate, no brain damage may occur. It is clear that in some individuals the internal carotid can be occluded without significant functional deficit. This is accounted for by the ability of collateral arteries to take over and supply adequate blood to the affected internal carotid (Gillilan, 1980). Strokes are typically divided into two types: ischemic and hemorrhagic. Ischemic cerebrovascular accidents result from the sudden loss of cerebral blood flow with an interruption to the blood supply to the brain. Hemorrhagic strokes result from bleeding from an artery within the intracranial space.

Ischemic Strokes

Ischemic strokes occur with the complete or partial occlusion of arteries. When blood flow to a region falls below a critical level needed to maintain cellular function and to remove accumulating toxic waste (e.g., lactic acid), cells begin to die and an infarct develops with necrosis and loss of tissue bulk (Plum and Posner, 1980; Raichle, 1983). When circulation returns to the region, body mechanisms will remove the dead tissue, leaving a residual cystic cavity. Occlusion of the internal carotid artery typically leads to greater damage than occlusion to a distal blood vessel in the middle cerebral artery distribution. The amount of collateral circulation available to the ischemic region if adequate can prevent infarction from occurring. Typically, in ischemic regions, there will be an inner zone of infarction with a surrounding zone of ischemia. Most research on treatment attempts to protect the ischemic zone to prevent the extension of the inner zone of infarction and thus limit functional disability.

The most common cause of ischemic strokes are thrombotic and/or embolic occlusion of the artery related to atherosclerosis. Atherosclerosis is a proliferation of the smooth muscle cells in the intima of the arterial wall with an expansion and deposition of lipid within the associated connective tissue (Ross, 1980; Ross and Glomset, 1973). Atheroma deposition within the arterial wall results in narrowing or stenosis of the artery. If the stenosis

reaches a critical level, usually considered greater than about 70%, changes occur in distal blood flow. As stenosis increases and flow becomes stagnant, the likelihood of thrombosis within the artery increases. A second change results from injury to the friable and easily damaged atherosclerotic lesion with the development of an ulcer. The blood system responds to the ulcer as it would to any other injury within the arterial wall, with the laying down of fibrin material, platelet adhesion, and trapping of blood cells. This deposition is called a thrombus. It can either occlude the blood vessel called a thrombosis or break apart and be released into the bloodstream as an embolus, which can occlude a distal artery. Embolism can result from thrombus formed for any reason and not just from an ulcerated arterial lesion. Another site of embolic material is the left ventricle of the heart when the chamber has been significantly damaged by a myocardial infarction. These two mechanisms—thrombosis and embolus—are the principal causes of ischemic strokes.

The clinical picture with ischemic stroke as with any neurological disorder, depends on the regions of the brain damaged and the involved artery. Internal carotid artery occlusion typically results in infarction within the middle or anterior cerebral artery cortical regions. With middle cerebral artery distribution infarctions, patients will show some or all of the following, including contralateral hemiparesis or plegia, hemisensory loss, homonymous hemianopsia, aphasia, and perceptual dysfunction.

Anterior cerebral artery occlusion results in infarction of the anterior and mesial portions of the frontal lobes. With this stroke, the patient may show hemiparesis but with greater weakness of the leg than of the upper extremity. This pattern is the opposite to what is observed with middle cerebral artery occlusion. In addition, the patients are frequently mute and are indifferent to their environment, with little spontaneous activity.

Brain stem and cerebellar infarctions result from occlusion of the vertebral, the basilar, or a branch artery. A variety of clinical symptoms can occur in many combinations. These include weakness and/or sensory loss involving any combination of extremities, vertigo, abnormalities in vision, changes in breathing pattern, dysphagia, dysarthria, ataxia, coma, and abnormalities in eye movements. What is most characteristic is involvement of cranial nerve functions as these nerves arise within the brain stem.

Hemorrhagic Stroke

Hemorrhagic strokes result from the rupture of a blood vessel within the intracranium. The hemorrhage can occur within three different spaces: the parenchyma of the brain, the subarachnoid space or the subdural space. The most frequent type of hemorrhage that would result in consultation with a speech-language pathologist would be an intraparenchymal hemorrhage. Such hemorrhages occur secondary to rupturing of a small artery within the brain, or occasionally by bleeding from a complex of abnormally formed blood vessels called an arteriovenous malformation. Intraparenchymal hemorrhages most frequently occur within the putamen (60%), thalamus (10%), pons (10%), and cerebellum (10%). Intracerebral hemorrhage causes symptomatology by mass displacement of brain tissue, increased pressure in adjacent and distal brain regions, and tissue destruction at the site of bleeding. In the past, the prognosis of surviving from an intracerebral hemorrhage was thought to be quite low, with an overall mortality of 80 to 90% (Gilroy and Meyer,

1975). This observation was based on difficulty in identifying small hemorrhages. Those hemorrhages that were diagnosed were large, massive bleeds associated with poor prognosis. With the advent of x-ray computed tomography (CT), small hemorrhages are now being identified that have a good prognosis.

Clinical features are relatively distinct, depending on type and location of the hemorrhage. The onset frequently occurs during activity or exertion. The patient has the sudden onset of a severe headache, with rapid development of alteration of consciousness. Putaminal hemorrhages result in contralateral hemiplegia, hemisensory loss, and homonymous hemianopsia. Typically, with recovery there is sparing of cortical functions, including language, spatial perception, and cognition. Studies have shown occasional language abnormalities associated with deep lesions involving the basal ganglia and thalamus (Alexander and LoVerme, 1980; Damasio et al., 1982; Naeser et al., 1982). Thalamic hemorrhages result in paresis of vertical eye gaze, small pupils, severe primary sensory loss, and hemiparesis. Pontine hemorrhages present with rapid development of coma, quadriparesis, and loss of or severely aberrant eye movements. Cerebellar hemorrhage consists of the abrupt onset of dizziness, nausea, vomiting, and incoordination of the extremities. There is gradual loss of consciousness over several hours. The recognition of this latter syndrome is important because early drainage of the cerebellar hematoma can result in good recovery (Ott et al., 1974).

Transient Ischemic Attacks

Transient ischemic attacks (TIAs) are particularly important for the speech-language pathologist to understand because an individual who has such an attack is at a high risk of having a stroke. In fact, there is a 10% to 20% chance of having a stroke within 1 year and a 30% to 60% chance of having one in 5 years. A number of investigators (see Brust, 1977) have found great variability in the incidence of stroke in TIA patients. Part of the difference is related to the definitions used for accepting a patient as having a TIA. For such reasons, when reading papers on TIAs, it is extremely important to read clinical criteria carefully and to understand the group of patients actually being studied. A TIA is a brief focal cerebral event in which the symptoms develop rapidly. The duration of an attack ranges from 2 to 30 minutes, to as long as 24 hours, while most are less than 2 to 3 hours in duration. The patient may have two or more such attacks over a variable period of time (Joint Committee for Stroke Facilities, 1974). During a TIA, part of the brain has temporarily become ischemic, resulting in the clinical symptoms. With resolution of the ischemia, the symptoms disappear.

Carotid territory TIAs show one or more of the following (Joint Committee, 1974): (a) hemiparesis—muscular weakness or clumsiness of an arm and/or leg on one side of the body; (b) hemisensory changes; (c) transient aphasia; (d) amaurosis fugax—transient loss of vision in one eye; and/or (e) homonymous hemianopsia—transient loss of vision with an inability to see one side of the visual field.

Vertebral-basilar TIAs show a different combination of symptoms determined by the structures that receive their blood flow from this arterial complex. Symptoms include one or more of the following: (a) motor dysfunction involving one or more extremities; (b) sensory changes involving one or more extremities, usually including the face; (c) visual loss, both total or partial loss of vision; (d) gait or posture instability with ataxia, imbalance, or unsteadiness but not vertigo; and/or (e) double vision (diplopia), swallowing problems (dysphagia), dysarthria, or vertigo occurring in combination with the above.

The following are not considered as TIAs since each of the symptoms commonly occurs and is not associated with stroke: (a) altered consciousness or faints; (b) dizziness; (c) amnesia alone; (d) confusion alone; (e) seizure activity; (f) march (progression) of motor or sensory symptoms; (g) vertigo alone; (h) diplopia alone; (i) dysphagia alone; (j) dysarthria alone; or (k) symptoms associated with migraine, such as scintillating scotomata (Joint Committee, 1974).

Treatment for a TIA is successful at decreasing the risk of impending strokes. It attempts to prevent the formation of thrombus and the release of emboli. Two major approaches are being used. The surgical approach is to remove the atheromatous material from within the carotid artery; this is called endarterectomy. Recent cooperative studies have shown that carotid endarterectomies are beneficial to patients with recent hemispheric or retinal transient ischemic attacks (Barnett et al., 1991; European Carotid Trialists' Collaborative Group, 1991; Mayberg et al., 1991). Patients with stenosis >70% of the vessel lumen to their symptomatic carotid artery were less likely to incur a stroke after undergoing an endarterectomy than if they had received only antiplatelet treatment (e.g., aspirin). However, there is a risk from the arteriogram required to define the anatomy of the blood vessels and from the surgical procedure itself (Whisnant et al., 1983). Endarterectomy seems warranted only when overall morbidity and mortality from the angiogram and surgical procedure are less than 5% (Sundt et al., 1975). Low morbidity and mortality are dependent primarily on the skills and experience of the angiographer and the surgeon. Rates have been reported as high as 20% (Easton and Sherman, 1977).

The second treatment approach is medical and consists of preventing thrombus formation. Immediately following a first TIA, a patient is treated with heparin and then placed on an anticoagulant for a variable period of time (Sandok et al., 1978). Anticoagulants prevent the formation of the thrombus, thus preventing the release of emboli. The risk of anticoagulants is bleeding, and this can be a high risk. In using these medications, bleeding parameters of the blood, primarily the prothrombin time, need to be carefully followed and adjusted. In general, the physician attempts to keep the value at 1.5 to 2.0 times normal, which minimizes the bleeding risk. Because of the high risk of bleeding, anticoagulants are typically used for periods of 3 to 6 months. The second medical treatment has been use of antiplatelet agents such as aspirin. Aspirin decreases the stickiness of platelets so that they will not adhere to the atheromatous lesions. Several studies have shown that the use of aspirin lowers the risk of subsequent TIAs, strokes, and death, particularly in males (Canadian Cooperative Study Group, 1978; Fields et al., 1977). At present, one aspirin or less a day seems to be an appropriate dose. The low risk of complications (other than gastrointestinal complications) makes this an appealing treatment.

Other Causes

A large number of other disorders can result in strokelike syndromes (Levine and Swanson, 1969). Such illnesses include brain tumors, chronic subdural hematoma (Moster et al., 1983), infections of the brain, multiple sclerosis, and residual of head trauma. At times there are clinical clues that what appears to be a stroke may be something else. The key is that over time the patient is not showing normal recovery but rather is becoming worse. Clinical symptoms include slowly increasing weakness, seizures, increasing confusion, aphasia, or the development of new signs or symptoms that were not noted previously.

DIAGNOSIS

Diagnosis refers to "the art of distinguishing one disease from another" or "the determination of the nature of a case of disease" (*Dorland's Illustrated Medical Dictionary*, 1965). A key point here is that it is an "art" and requires a degree of skill and an ability to obtain information from a patient. At times, patients have difficulty in expressing their problem, making diagnosis difficult. A diagnosis is made based on a history, physical examination, and diagnostic studies. The history is the most important part of the evaluation. Without adequate information, the physician typically does not know what to look for.

In making a neurological diagnosis, answers are needed to several key questions. The first question is whether the problem is based on a nervous system dysfunction. For example, a patient being seen because of a sudden episode of loss of consciousness lasting 2 to 3 minutes could have had a seizure that is of neurological origin, or a syncopal episode (faint), which is usually not neurological but is more likely of cardiovascular origin. The second question asks where in the nervous system the dysfunction occurs. Can the clinical picture be explained by a single lesion or multiple lesions? The third question is what the etiology of the lesion is. The answers to these three questions dictate the nature and extent of intervention.

History

The history is the most important part of the neurological evaluation. It alerts the physician as to the problem and gives direction for evaluation and treatment. After taking the history, the physician can usually make an accurate diagnosis. The remainder of the evaluation is meant to prove or disprove and at times to modify the initial impression (DeJong, 1980).

Initially, the history consists of obtaining the reason the patient has come to the physician, followed by a thorough history of the problem. Much of the questioning needs to be open ended to allow patients to state the problems in their own words. Skill is needed to keep the patient on important information, but in general, specific questions are not asked until the full picture has been described, and then the questions are used to understand the details. Next, questions are asked about specific neurological and other body systems to look for other problems that may be directly or indirectly related to the patient's complaint. A review of medication, job history, and social and medical history is also taken to understand the patient.

At times the patient either cannot give or does not know the history. Under such circumstances, the physician has to obtain information from family members or from individuals who have observed the event. As an example, an elderly male complained of loss of vision with graying that lasted seconds to a minute. He had been diagnosed as having TIA and had a

carotid endarterectomy. Following the surgery, his symptoms persisted. On talking to the patient, it sounded like he was having TIAs, but when the story was checked with the patient's wife, it was discovered that during the visual gray-outs, he was unresponsive to other stimuli. The diagnosis became obvious, and the patient was evaluated and treated for a seizure disorder.

Physical Examination

The purpose of the physical examination is to confirm the history. The exam includes a full survey of the neurological systems, a general medical, and a mental status evaluation. The neurological examination includes the cranial nerves, the motor system, the sensory system, the cerebellar system, and the reflexes. The general medical evaluation includes heart, lung, abdomen, rectum, vascular systems, and the extremities. The mental status evaluation includes state of awareness, orientation, speech, language, memory, cognition, and perception.

Diagnostic Studies

The role of diagnostic studies in stroke patients is to help identify the location, etiology, and pathophysiology of the problem. Stroke is associated with disease in a number of other body organs and is caused by other medical conditions. As an example, prior to the advent of antibiotics a frequent cause of strokelike illnesses was syphilis (Holmes et al., 1984). At present, syphilis is an unusual cause of stroke, but it needs to be examined for in all stroke patients.

Laboratory Evaluation

A variety of nonatherosclerotic causes of stroke syndromes can occur (Levine and Swanson, 1969). Routine tests are usually done to define hematologic, connective tissue, and inflammatory disorders. Typically, blood studies include counts of the red and white blood cells. A screening panel is done that examines blood electrolytes (sodium, potassium, chloride, bicarbonate, calcium), glucose, and liver and kidney function. Other blood tests include syphilis serology, as well as screening tests for connective tissue diseases. Routine studies also include an electrocardiogram and chest x-ray to evaluate the heart. These tests are done because of their low cost, safety, and high return of information that may not be available from other sources.

Noninvasive Carotid Studies

Since carotid endarterectomy has become an appropriate therapy for nonhemorrhagic strokes related to atherosclerotic disease, techniques are needed to evaluate the extent of disease at the carotid bifurcation. The ideal would be to have a procedure that would be 100% accurate in detecting the extent of disease and would carry no risk. The accepted procedure to evaluate this area is cerebral angiography, but this carries a definite risk. A battery of tests have been developed that can evaluate the carotid bifurcation with 80% to 90% accuracy and far less risk, with 3% to 5% false positives in experienced laboratories. Noninvasive studies are most appropriately used during the evaluation of patients when there is some question as to whether carotid angiography (see below) should be performed to define the detail of vascular structure.

Two major noninvasive approaches are used to study the carotid bifurcation. The first uses Doppler imaging devises and is based on the Doppler effect; that is, a sound source that moves toward you has a higher pitch than if it is standing still, and it has a lower pitch if it is moving away from you (Borowitz and Beiser, 1966). Doppler imaging registers echoes of ultrasound waves in relation to the velocity of blood flow. It presents an image of the vessel lumen and in particular the blood column. The second approach uses B-scan mode ultrasonography, which registers echoes related to variations in the ''acoustical impedance of tissues'' (Ackerman, 1980). It images the vessel wall instantaneously as a real-time image. Current equipment allows for the simultaneous evaluation of blood flow velocity by Doppler and arterial anatomy by ultrasound. Batteries of noninvasive testing offer a reasonable means to evaluate the carotid arteries in selected patients to make the decision whether angiography is indicated.

Recently, Doppler techniques have been applied to the study of intracranial arteries. The procedures allow for the estimation of whether intracranial arterial stenosis, aneurysm, or arteriovenous malformations are present. The procedure is valuable in assisting the physician in understanding the blood flow dynamics in patients with complex cerebrovascular problems (Asslid, 1992).

Cerebral Angiography

Cerebral angiography at present represents the ''gold standard'' for determining the nature and extent of the vascular abnormality in cerebral blood vessels. Angiography is particularly necessary when considerations are being made to do a surgical procedure, or where clinical diagnosis is uncertain. Typically, the procedure is carried out by placing a small-bore tubing into the femoral artery in the groin and passing it up the artery to the aortic arch and into the appropriate arteries, including both carotid arteries and a vertebral artery. When in place, contrast medium is forced through the tubing and into the arterial circulation, while x-ray pictures are taken in rapid sequence over a 10- to 20-second period. Pictures are taken in several planes, resulting in three-dimensional reconstruction of the arteries (Peterson and Kieffer, 1976). In the hands of a good angiographer, the risk is typically less than 1% morbidity and mortality, the major risk being the development of a stroke during or shortly after the procedure.

Digital subtraction angiography offers an alternate method to examine the arterial circulation by allowing the use of computers to improve resolution and quality of pictures. This approach has been available for almost 10 years and as yet has not replaced standard angiographic methods, even though it has the advantage of not requiring the catheterization of specific arteries (e.g., carotid or vertebral artery), thus decreasing the risk of stroke or death associated with the procedure. Following the intravenous injection of contrast material, serial x-ray pictures are taken and digitalized into a computer. The quality of the pictures obtained varies but frequently allows for adequate visualization of extracranial circulation. Intracranial circulation can be studied but less reliably. The major problems with the procedure rest with the amount of contrast media that has to be given during intravenous injections. The media is eliminated from the body through the kidneys and has some renal toxicity. Most reports note that if the technique is done in patients who are well hydrated, renal complications have been at a minimum (DeFilipp et al., 1983; Kempczinski et al., 1983; Little et al., 1982).

Recently, magnetic resonance angiography has been developed that takes advantage of the power of magnetic resonance imaging (see below and Chapter 3). This technique offers the advantage of imaging carotid and intracerebral circulation without the use of injected contrast media. At present, its role in clinical practice has not been established (Ruggieri et al., 1991).

Brain Imaging

The techniques examined so far have studied what occurs within the blood vessel. An important issue for the physician is the kind and nature of the damage to the brain. Over the past 10 years, improved methods have been developed to examine structural and physiological changes in the brain. Using these technologies, two types of neuroimaging methods have emerged that enable the physician to obtain three-dimensional images of the central nervous system: those that measure the transmission of energy through tissue such as computed transmission tomography and those producing images from natural or introduced energy sources, including magnetic resonance imaging, positron emission tomography, and single photon emission computed tomography (Fig. 2.1).

Transmission tomography examines differential tissue absorption of externally administered energy and includes standard radiography and CT. In standard radiography, the brain is irradiated by x-ray. The x-rays that are unabsorbed or transmitted through the brain are recorded by sensitive film or a video image device (fluoroscopy). This provides a planar or two-dimensional image that has excellent spatial but poor contrast resolution (i.e., the ability to distinguish white matter from gray matter). CT is the only transmission technique employed by the physician to obtain three-dimensional images of the brain. This is done by measuring the amount of transmitted radiation using multiple detectors that rotate around the brain. The amount of transmitted radiation at each integral point (pixel) is then calculated using a dedicated computer. A three-dimensional image of the brain is constructed using this information.

CT studies brain structure, pathology, and anatomy. Contrast between structures depends on the amount x-ray absorbed and on the thickness, density, and atomic number of the structures. For example, bone that contains a high concentration of calcium absorbs x-ray much more readily than other tissues and is clearly delineated by both conventional radiography and CT. Distinctive structures within the brain are more difficult to see because specific gravity differences between adjacent structures are small. CT is capable of differentiating tissues with small absorption differences. With standard x-ray, resolution is basically continuous, while with CT it is dependent on pixel size, since each pixel represents an average value of transmitted radiation within its borders. Current scanners have a resolution on the order of 1 mm (Oldendorf, 1981; Peterson and Kieffer, 1976).

Emission tomography produces images using data from internal energy sources. Such sources include magnetic radionuclides injected intravenously, intraarterially, or by inhalation, and the electrophysiological characteristics of the brain. Emission techniques include magnetic resonance imaging (MRI), positron emission tomography (PET), single photon emission computed tomography (SPECT), and brain electrical activity mapping (BEAM).

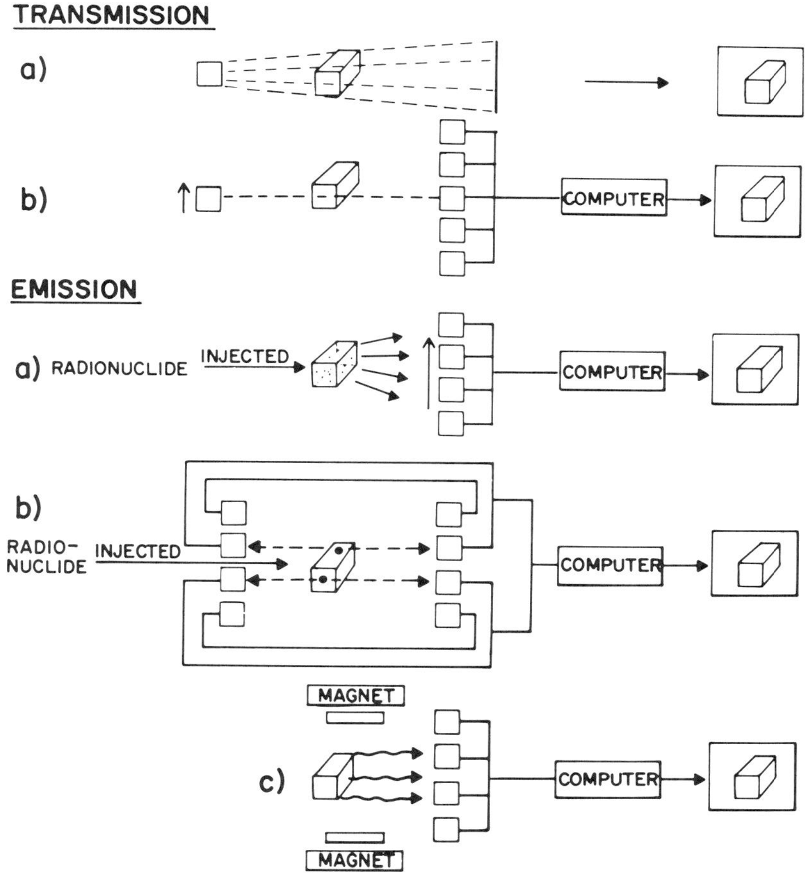

TRANSMISSION

EMISSION

Figure 2.1. Transmission and emission methods of neuroimaging. Transmission: (**a**) standard planar radiography; (**b**) computed transaxial tomography. Emission: (**a**) Single photon emission computed tomography; (**b**) positron emission tomography; and (**c**) magnetic resonance imaging.

MRI is the most recent development in brain imaging. It does not use radioactive substances but examines the response of selected elements in response to a large magnetic field. Current techniques are concerned primarily with the study of proton distribution, that is, water. The resolution of MRI is on the order of CT but has better contrast in distinguishing gray matter from white matter. The technique is particularly useful in studying the posterior fossa, where CT has difficulty.

MRI uses a very different set of physical properties, taking advantage of the behavior of nuclei as small dipoles or very weak magnets. Under normal circumstances, the axes of the nuclei point in random directions. In a strong magnetic field, the nuclei line up so that their dipoles are either parallel or antiparallel with the field. The nuclei can flip back and forth between the parallel and antiparallel positions, which requires energy absorption and the emission of a radiowave. MRI uses this property, by applying a radiofrequency wave, to the fixed magnetic field, encouraging nuclei to flip back and forth (resonate) between parallel and antiparallel positions and measuring the radiowaves emitted in the process (Bradley, 1982; Crooks et al., 1981).

Each element in a magnetic field resonates at specific frequencies, making the physical properties of the fields specific to a given element. Hydrogen is most commonly scanned because of its excellent resonating ability and abundance in tissue as a component of water and all organic molecules.

Two measures usually studied are magnetic relaxation times "T1" and "T2," which are dependent on nuclear density and

environment. T1 is the "thermal relation" or "spin-lattice" reaction time and represents the time for the nuclei to become aligned and magnetized when placed in a magnetic field. T1 depends on the physical properties of the sample; for example, liquids are held together by looser forces than are solids, and will become magnetized more quickly than solids, and will have a shorter T1.

T2 is the "spin-spin" or "transverse" relaxation time. Nuclei tend to spin much as does a top. As a top spins, it points perpendicular to the ground when under stable conditions. If a second energy source is applied (as by touching it with a finger), it begins to wobble. The wobble represents a torque, which describes a second axis of rotation for the top. Nuclei in a strong magnetic field, when pulsed by a radiofrequency wave, behave in a similar manner. T2 is a measure of how well and how long this wobble is maintained following the radiofrequency pulse. For solids, T2 is very short because of the fixed rigid structure of the molecules, whereas it is long for liquids (Bradley, 1982).

Contrast has been striking with MRI. Principal advantages include improved contrast between gray and white matter and the ability to examine the posterior fossa. The contrast is 10 times better than that found with CT (Crooks et al., 1981). In stroke, MRI demonstrates infarction and edema as early as 90 minutes after occlusion (Spetzler et al., 1983). An extensive review of the method and literature pertaining to MRI and CT will be made in Chapter 3.

PET and SPECT are two tomographic techniques based on the technology of detecting gamma ray emissions from intravenous injected radioisotopes. Unlike CT and MRI, which are essentially limited to identifying structural changes to the brain, PET and SPECT are designed to measure functional changes such as regional cerebral blood flow (rCBF) and metabolism. These methods are distinguished by the type of radiopharmaceuticals and equipment each employs. PET is unique, since the isotopes it uses can provide quantitative measures of a substantial number of different neurophysiological and biochemical processes. The half-lives of these isotopes are usually short, necessitating the availability of a cyclotron, which adds considerable expense to the procedure. These isotopes are also unique, since the annihilation of their electrons produces two gamma photons that discharge at 180 degrees from each other. Detection of both photons is made by a gamma camera with a series of parallel gamma ray detectors. Using a dedicated computer, the sites at which the dual photons were emitted are located with excellent accuracy. Current PET equipment has a spacial resolution of 3 to 4 mm.

SPECT also employs isotopes that are injected intravenously. At present, there are only two SPECT radioisotopes approved by the Federal Drug Administration for clinical use: N-isopropyl-p-iodoamphetamine (IMP) and 99mTc hexamethylpropylene amine oxide (HMPAO). These radiotracers have relatively long half-lives and do not require an on-site cyclotron. They either are made from kits or are shipped directly from the manufacturer. They also differ from those isotopes used by PET in that they emit one gamma photon after binding to a specific receptor site or are entrapped within a neuron. The site at which the photon was emitted is located by using a collimator, which is a lead shield with a series of holes cut into it. The collimator is mounted on the head of the gamma camera and acts as a filter, allowing only those photons that directly pass through unimpeded to be detected. Spatial resolution depends on the number of gamma counts generated and the diameter and length of the holes in the collimator. At present, using a single-head rotating gamma camera with a high-resolution collimator, SPECT has a resolution of 1.5 cm. A resolution of 7 to 9 mm has been obtained with the newer rotating three-headed gamma cameras.

Electroencephalolography (EEG) has been long used to diagnose various structural and functional brain lesions. The effectiveness of this technique to detect underlying brain dysfunction has been questionable, since the amount of electrical brain activity measured is too much to be easily assimilated by visual inspection alone. BEAM is a direct outgrowth from EEG (Duffy et al., 1979). In this technique, EEG and evoked potential data (i.e., brain electrical activity evoked from sensory or cognitive stimulation) recorded from a standard array of scalp electrodes are statistically interpolated. This information is then graphically displayed as a transaxial section of the brain on a color video screen in real time. The image is color coded depending on whether the brain area was deactivated (i.e., cerebral infarct), compromised (i.e., ischemia or deafferentation), or activated (i.e., seizure or sensory stimulation). At present, BEAM has not been used extensively by the physician to diagnose stroke. Instead it has been employed in the investigation of those neurological disorders that have no evidence of structural brain lesions, such as seizure disorders (Gregory and Wong, 1984), dyslexia (Duffy and McNulty, 1990), spasmodic dysphonia (Finitzo and Freeman, 1989), Alzheimer's disease (Duffy et al., 1984), and schizophrenia (Pool et al., 1988).

X-Ray Computed Tomography. CT has been a powerful tool in correlating brain structural abnormalities with speech and language pathology. CT has the capability of detecting even relatively small and long-standing cerebrovascular lesions. The size and location of intracerebral hemorrhages have been identified by CT with a precision heretofore unattainable (Walshe et al., 1977). Prior to the development of CT, only large and usually lethal hemorrhages were easily identified clinically. Now, strokes that which previously would have been called infarcts are being identified as hemorrhages by CT.

Studies have described the relationship between lesion site, as revealed by CT, and type of aphasia (Hayward et al., 1977; Kertesz et al., 1979; Mazzocchi and Vignolo, 1979; Naeser and Hayward, 1978; Noel et al., 1980). Specific lesions have resulted in specific aphasia syndromes in a manner consistent with classical descriptions. The prerolandic/postrolandic separation of nonfluent and fluent aphasias seems well supported by CT (Kertesz et al., 1979; Naeser and Hayward, 1978). A number of cases do not fit within the model (Mazzocchi and Vignolo, 1979; Metter et al., 1981). It has been demonstrated that the location of brain lesions can be predicted from aphasia type with reasonable accuracy; however, the reverse does not appear to be true (Noel et al., 1980). In general, larger lesions result in poorer outcome and more severe aphasia than do small, single lesions (Kertesz et al., 1979; Yarnell et al., 1976). Lesion localization independent of size may also be critical for recovery, as noted by the poor prognosis of lesions involving the posterior superior temporal and infrasylvian supramarginal regions, which are associated with poor comprehension (Selnes et al., 1983). Some large lesions are less devastating than very critically placed smaller lesions. The value of knowing the site of brain lesions in predicting the recovery potential of aphasia patients has been demonstrated (Selnes et al., 1983). Such information may be of value in planning language therapy for aphasic patients. Patients without lesions in specific areas may benefit from early intensive therapy to facilitate recovery. This concept will be fully reviewed in Chapter 3.

Serial studies have shown little change in the size of an infarct once it appears on CT (Kertesz et al., 1979). Frequently, within the first few hours postonset, no lesions are seen by CT. This has been a limitation in the use of CT in acute stroke. From 24 to 48 hours, edema may occur, which obscures the true boundaries of the lesion. Mazzocchi and Vignolo (1979) have indicated that aphasia mirrors the effect of the lesion most faithfully in the period between the 21st and 60th day postonset. It is about this time that the lesion becomes well demarcated and easier to localize.

CT has been particularly valuable in the identification of subcortical lesions and their correlation to language disturbance. Subcortical infarctions of the dominant hemisphere with basal ganglia involvement have resulted in aphasia that is characterized by word-finding difficulties, phonemic paraphasia, intact repetition and rapid recovery (Brunner et al., 1982). More severe and long-lasting aphasic symptoms were observed when subcortical lesions appeared in combination with cortical lesions. Nonhemorrhagic infarctions of the anterior limb of the internal capsule and of the striatum in the dominant hemisphere have produced aphasia syndromes that do not correspond to the classical descriptions of cortical aphasia (Damasio et al.,

1982). Recovery of aphasic symptoms tended to occur rapidly with these lesions. A specific type of ''thalamic speech'' has also been recognized, with paucity of spontaneous speech, hypophonia, anomia, perseveration, and neologisms with intact comprehension and word repetition characterizing the aphasia associated with thalamic CT lesions (Alexander and LoVerme, 1980). Further support for a role of subcortical structures in aphasia was found by Naeser et al. (1982). They report that patients with capsular/putaminal lesion sites with anterior-superior white-matter lesion extension had good comprehension; slow, dysarthric speech; and lasting right hemiplegia. On the other hand, patients with capsular/putaminal lesion sites with posterior white-matter lesion extension had poor comprehension and fluent Wernicke-type speech. It is the hope of investigators that identification of specific syndromes may lead to specific and improved treatments.

Positron Emission Computed Tomography. PET is the most advanced of the radionuclide scanning techniques. At present, PET is an experimental tool. The limitation for its widespread use is the short half-life of the radionuclide, which requires the presence of a cyclotron for isotope production. Models are available for studying several parameters (e.g., rCBF, local cerebral metabolic rates for oxygen [LCMRO2], or local cerebral metabolic rates for glucose [LCMRGlc]) (see Phelps et al., 1982b).

The spatial resolution of PET does not approach that of CT or MRI and in the future may be on the order of 1 to 2 mm (Phelps et al., 1982a). Most deep structures are not well resolved (Hoffman et al, 1979; Mazziotta et al., 1981b). The ability to see a structure depends on the object size, shape, and influence of neighboring structures. These factors must be considered in trying to understand reported data. Partial volume effects (i.e., the possibility of a structure occupying only part of a pixel) remain a problem for quantitative determination of tracer concentration. To circumvent such difficulties as much as possible, corresponding regions in both hemispheres are compared. This assumes that the partial volume effects are relatively similar for structures in each hemisphere in relationship to their imaging. The limitations are not so great as to negate the usefulness of the approach, but they must be considered in any interpretation.

PET has been used to study speech and language performance in normal subjects while subjects are resting or doing specific tasks. Resting studies also have been done in patients with neurological disorders. LCMRGlc can be measured by the fluorodeoxyglucose (FDG) method, where subjects are injected with the radionuclide, and then after 40 minutes scanning begins. During the 40 minutes while the FDG is taken up by the brain, the subject can either be resting or be doing a specific task. The long period of uptake restricts the value of FDG for studying how the brain responds to specific behavioral tasks. For this reason, shorter scans obtained using (O15)-water as a measure of cerebral blood flow may prove more ideal when brain activation is to be studied. In normal subjects, changes in cerebral blood flow are tightly coupled to changes in cerebral metabolic rates and neuronal activity (DesRosiers et al., 1974; Freygang and Sokoloff, 1958; Roy and Sherrington, 1990; Salford et al., 1973).

Under resting conditions without sensory deprivation, cerebral glucose metabolism is symmetric in the left and right hemispheres, while there is a slight decline in glucose use with

increasing age (Kuhl et al., 1982). Sensory deprivation studies (Mazziotta et al., 1982a) have shown that plugging both ears and covering both eyes resulted in significant right hemisphere hypometabolism that was not apparent when only eyes or ears were occluded. These findings demonstrated the importance of knowing how any physiological study is performed and that all resting states are not equivalent. The degree of visual input also has been found to be important, as seen by varying the degree of complexity of visual inputs (Phelps et al., 1981a; Phelps et al., 1981b).

Auditory stimulation has shown differences in glucose use based on the nature of the stimulus (Mazziotta et al., 1982b) and in some cases the strategy employed in carrying out the task. Listening to a story produced diffuse left-sided and bilateral transverse and posterior temporal increases in metabolism, as well as increases in the left frontal regions and thalamus. Nonverbal stimuli with chords produced diffuse right-sided as well as bilateral inferior parietal activation. Tone sequences produced variable responses that seemed dependent on the subject's strategy in analyzing the data. Individuals using highly analytical strategies showed greater left posterior temporal activations, while a nonanalytical strategy had right-sided activations. These studies demonstrated that FDG can be used to create differential maps of metabolism that depend on task and strategy.

Most functional activation studies are using cerebral blood flow rather than metabolism. The advantage is that these scans take only a few minutes to complete. What is sacrificed by the short scans is spatial resolution. Improvements in PET equipment, better computer algorithms, and better techniques are enhancing the quality of the images. Techniques to subtract one set of images from a second set allow for the direct comparison of two brain states, such as the difference in brain function in seeing a word and in naming a word. The assumption is that a linear increase in blood flow occurs as a brain region increasingly processes information. The major question in interpreting such studies is understanding the characteristics and implication of a change in blood flow for a specific brain region and task. The assumption of linearity may not be correct for all brain regions. Several reports have shown that visual and auditory word recognition do not specifically activate the parietal lobe according to the assumption of linearity, arguing against a role for the angular and supramarginal gyri in the processing of words (Peterson et al., 1988; Zatorre et al., 1992). Such observations are at odds with aphasia research, where focal parietal lesions are typically associated with such tasks.

FDG PET studies have demonstrated that cerebral glucose metabolism in stroke patients extends beyond the zone of infarction as determined by CT (Kuhl et al., 1980; Metter et al., 1981). Figure 2.2 shows an example of the distant effects that may be seen with cerebral infarction (Metter et al., 1985). In this case, the CT study, 1 month postevent and 1 week before the patient's death shows several lacunar infarcts in the left and right internal capsule/basal ganglia regions. The same lesions can be seen on the gross section of the brain. The FDG scan shows similar but subtler changes in the regions. In addition, there is prominent metabolic depression in the left frontal region, where there is no evidence of structural changes on CT or the gross brain specimen. The case seems to demonstrate a disconnection syndrome in which the left frontal region has been disconnected from its input and output that runs through

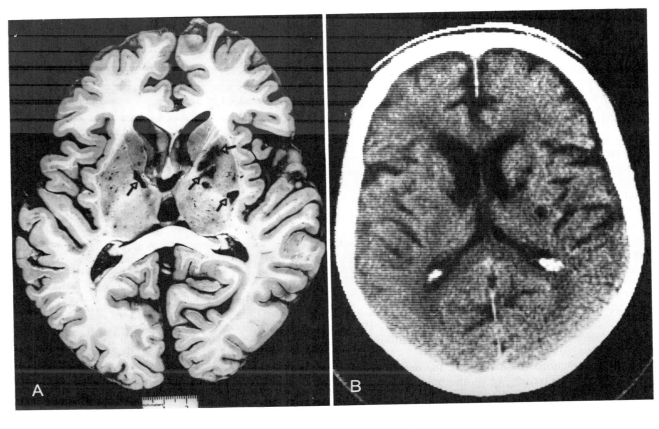

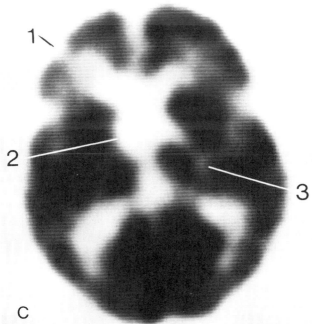

Figure 2.2. Comparison of imaging techniques in a patient with multiple brain infarctions. The three sections are taken from the same level of the brain. **A,** Gross brain section. Arrows have been added to point out four regions of lacunar infarction. Note that the overlying cortex in this brain section appears to be normal. **B,** CT scan of the same section. Note that each area of lacunar infarction found on the brain section can be seen in this scan. The scan and brain agree closely in anatomy. **C,** FDG PET scan of the same section. *Arrows 2* and *3* point out the areas of lacunar infarction noted in **A** and **B**. In addition an abnormality can be seen in the left frontal region (*arrow 1*). This metabolic abnormality does not correspond to any structural abnormality demonstrated in the gross brain section **A** or CT scan **B**. The metabolic at *1* represents the effect of disconnecting the left frontal region from its input and output caused by the lesion in the left internal capsule (the arrow on the left in **A**). The PET scan gives physiologic information that allows for the understanding of the effects of structural lesions that can be demonstrated using CT.

the internal capsule. The left internal capsule has been destroyed by the lacunar infarct in the internal capsule. Similar remote changes have been found in all stroke cases studied. Remote effects have been reported, including decreased activity in the ipsilateral thalamus in both acute and chronic stages following stroke, ipsilateral cortex adjacent and at a distance from the lesion, cerebellar hemisphere contralateral to the cortical lesion, and hemisphere contralateral to supratentorial infarctions (Baron et al., 1981; Kuhl et al., 1980; Lenzi et al., 1981; Martin and Raichle, 1983; Metter et al., 1981; Metter et al., 1987). The presence of distant regions with hypometabolism suggests that function in undamaged tissue may be aberrant and might account for some aspects of the aphasic language disturbance.

Models of the pathoanatomy of aphasia have been based on comparing the nature of language disruption following a stroke with the areas of the brain that has been damaged by infarction or hemorrhage. Studies that examine brain blood flow and metabolism demonstrate that focal brain regions have clear effects on other parts of the brain. Such observations appear to allow for more unifying concepts regarding the development of aphasia following stroke. For example, it has been found that essentially all aphasic patients studied by FDG PET demonstrated metabolic abnormalities in the left temporoparietal regions independent of where the structural lesion causing the aphasia is located (Metter et al., 1990). Furthermore, Wernicke's, Broca's, and conduction aphasias were found to differ on the extent of metabolic abnormalities in the prefrontal cortex, a part of the brain not thought to be directly responsible for most aphasias (Metter et al., 1989). The data also suggested that language function may not be attributable only to the structural lesion but rather to what occurs in other brain areas when the perisylvian region (which functions as a unit involved with language function) is structurally damaged. Adjacent language areas may have assumed increasing importance in the remaining language function in these aphasic patients (Metter, 1987).

Studying brain metabolism has also demonstrated aspects of the role of subcortical brain structures in aphasia (Metter, 1992). Differences in the location of subcortical structural damage are associated with differences in the location changes in overlying cortex. As shown in Figure 2.2, lesions of the anterior internal capsule result in frontal lobe hypometabolism. For most middle cerebral artery distribution strokes, the presence of subcortical extension of the infarct will be associated with frontal lobe hypometabolism. These metabolic changes and the associated subcortical structural changes are associated with the expressive aspects of the aphasia (Metter et al., 1988). Metabolic changes in the left caudate in aphasic patients were found to correlate with Porch Index of Communicative Ability (PICA) language measures, which suggested a caudate language role related to phonetic recognition for simple, over-learned materials, including simple syntax, low levels of abstraction, and identification or sequencing of phonetic and semantic material. The role appeared related but independent of Broca's area and inferior frontal lobe function. An alternative explanation was that caudate function may involve cortical organization of planned movement (Metter et al., 1988). The studies demonstrated that the head of the caudate may be of particular importance in the ability of Broca's and inferior frontal areas to work together with other brain regions, which may reflect on its role in speech and language. This relationship

is consistent with known anatomical connections of the caudate head (Yeterian and Van Hoesen, 1978).

Single Photon Emission Computed Tomography. SPECT has been employed primarily to measure rCBF. Historically, the first measurement of cerebral blood flow was made by Kety and Schmidt (1948) in 1948. After a subject inhaled nitrous oxide, its concentration in the jugular veins was measured. Unfortunately, because the blood sampled was from cerebral as well as extracerebral tissue, the values from each vein were different. In 1961, Ingvar and Lassen (1961), using the gamma emitter Krypton'79, were able to observe the blood flow differences between gray and white cerebral matter. Localization was poor, however, since a single gamma ray detector was used.

In 1975, two-dimensional sagittal views of the cerebral cortex were made (Obrist et al., 1975) using a multidetector camera system and Xenon (Xe) gas, which could be either inhaled or intravenously injected. Through this technique, different speech and language tasks such as reading, word perception, and speaking were found to activate different patterns of rCBF on both the left and right cerebral cortex (Larsen et al., 1978). One striking finding has been the presence of superior frontal and right hemisphere activation that could not be predicted from previous anatomical studies, indicating limitations in the anatomical model of brain organization of language. Auditory-processing tasks in normal subjects produced significant increases over the left posterior sylvian region, with a trend for the verbal task to evoke a wider area of activation than the nonverbal task (Knopman et al., 1980).

The multidetector/Xenon method has also been applied to the study of patients with aphasia secondary to stroke (Maly et al., 1977; Soh et al., 1978). These studies revealed that while the areas of diminished rCBF were more widely distributed than would have been predicted, these patterns tended to be in regions in agreement with classical aphasia theory (Soh et al., 1978). Mean left hemispheric blood flow was also found to differ based on the type of aphasia, with global aphasic patients having the lowest flow and anomic aphasic patients having the highest. Wernicke's aphasia patients generally have higher focal and hemisphere flow measures than patients with Broca's aphasia (Maly et al., 1977).

Prognosis for recovery from aphasia has shown a strong relationship to measurements of rCBF during psychophysiological activation tests (Yamaguchi et al., 1980). Yamaguchi et al. (1980) indicated that poor prognosis for recovery was associated with failure of an increase in bilateral frontotemporal regions during behavioral activation by motor speech (counting), conversation, and listening to music. Better prognosis for aphasia recovery was associated with rCBF increases from the resting state in the area homologous to Broca's area in the nondominant hemisphere, suggesting the possibility of some transfer of speech functions to the nondominant hemisphere in patients with good recovery of speech. Knopman et al. (1983) have found that aphasic patients with poor recovery develop an increase of rCBF in the right inferior frontal region in response to a listening condition over a 3- to 9-month period; this increase was not found in aphasic patients with good recovery.

Although the multidetector/Xenon method has yielded important information pertaining to the neuroanatomical substrates of speech and language processing in general and specifically to aphasia, the technique has limited clinical use, since it can only provide two-dimensional views of the lateral cerebral cortex of one hemisphere. Cerebral blood flow information from within deep cortical and subcortical regions known to be important to speech and language functioning cannot be observed.

In 1975, SPECT was developed. Using a camera capable of detecting gamma emissions from intravenous infected technetium 99m isotope while rotating 360 degrees around the head, Kuhl et al. (1975) were able to obtain three-dimensional tomographic images of the brain, including views of subcortical regions. Since this development, SPECT neuroimaging has provided important information about strokes that could not be obtained through CT, MRI, or the Xenon method. In the case of acute infarction, SPECT scans show areas of reduced rCBF earlier and usually larger than those seen on CT (Hayman et al., 1989; Hill et al., 1984). Like PET, areas of hypoperfusion remote from the lesions identified on CT are often observed. These include subcortical infarcts resulting in cortical hypoperfusion as well as cortical frontoparietal lesions resulting in contralateral cerebellar diaschisis (Bogousslavsky et al., 1988; Vallar et al., 1988). In chronic cerebral infarctions, two zones of abnormalities can be identified on SPECT scans: a central zone with markedly reduced rCBF, which is the infarcted area seen on CT, and an area of hypoperfusion immediately surrounding the central zone called the ischemic penumbra. The ischemic penumbra is not seen on CT and is probably a result of deafferentation (Raynaud et al., 1987). Occasionally, an area of hyperemia (increased blood flow) is observed in an area surrounding the cerebral infarction (Bushnell et al., 1987).

The utility of SPECT scans to predict recovery after cerebral infarction has also been studied (Bushnell et al., 1989; Defer et al., 1987; Giubilei et al., 1990; Gupta et al., 1991; Lee et al., 1984; Limburg et al., 1991; Mountz et al., 1990). For the most part, these investigations have shown that the size of the rCBF defect is inversely correlated with stroke recovery. That is, the larger the defect, the less likely the patient will exhibit good recovery. Equivocal conclusions have been reached as to whether other SPECT parameters, such as the number of gamma counts within the hypoperfused area, the redistribution parameters, or the difference in the defect size seen on SPECT and CT, are useful in the prediction of stroke recovery.

SPECT has not been used extensively to investigate cerebral processing of speech and language information in normal individuals. One interesting study was conducted by Goldenberg et al. (1987). While undergoing a SPECT procedure with IMP, they found that the pattern of rCBF activity exhibited by the patient in response to a word memory task was dependent on the type of memory strategy employed. When the patient used a visual imagery strategy to remember words presented auditorily, the left superior temporal region as well as the superior frontal regions bilaterally tended to activate. A no-imagery strategy, on the other hand, was associated with right hemisphere activation. A correlation analysis showed that the performance of all word memory tasks was strongly associated with the activity of the hippocampal and inferior temporal regions of both hemispheres as well. These results indicate that while the memorization of words in general is a bilateral cerebral process, the left hemisphere is most likely responsible for the imagery of words. Lang et al. (1987) also used SPECT and IMP to study the rCBF patterns associated with word memorization in normal subjects. They used several paradigms including one requiring the subject to use mental imagery. In response to the imagery task, a significant increase of rCBF was found in both superior frontal lobe regions.

Aphasia has also been investigated using SPECT. Tikofsky et al. (1985) studied the resting patterns of five aphasic patients who demonstrated either improved language function or no improvement 1 year after stroke onset. Two patients who showed little change in their aphasia quotients (AQ) on the Western Aphasia Battery demonstrated large rCBF defects associated with infarcted tissue with little or no surrounding ischemia. The three remaining patients with improved AQs showed reduced but not absent cerebral blood flow in the cortical language regions of the left hemisphere. Tikofsky et al. also noted that in some of the improved patients, evidence of slightly increased rCBF in regions of the right cerebral hemisphere was present. In a subsequent investigation, these researchers attempted to determine whether the rCBF response to cognitive stimulation might distinguish chronic aphasic patients who continue to show language improvement from those who do not (Tikofsky, 1988). Using the Boston Naming Test, they found no discernible visual evidence of change between the rCBF patterns obtained during the naming of objects and the patterns obtained during rest. However, improving patients showed greater rCBF activity in response to the naming task compared with normals, while the activity of the unimproved aphasic patients was lower than the normals.

In a series of investigations, Walker-Batson and her colleagues (1987, 1988, 1989) studied the utility of SPECT and Xenon in research on aphasia. In one study, the rCBF patterns of normal and aphasic subjects were examined during rest, during a passive listening task where the subject listened to a series of consonant-vowel syllables, and during a phoneme detection task that required the subject to identify a particular phoneme when it was heard. A hemispheric difference was not found for either group. However, the majority of the normal subjects demonstrated bilateral mesial frontal activation in response to the phoneme detection task, while the aphasic patients showed no distinct cortical or subcortical activation pattern. One interesting finding was that activation did occur in either the ipsilateral region or the contralateral cerebellar region in response to the detection task for the aphasic patients. Walker-Batson suggests that this might indicate that the frontal-motor system or the corticocerebellar loop was activated during the phoneme detection task. In another investigation, Walker-Batson et al. (1988) studied the rCBF patterns of a man with crossed aphasia (i.e., aphasia in a right-handed patient resulting from a right hemisphere lesion) who showed significant improvement over a 10-year period. The investigators studied rCBF responses to a resting state, (silent answers to questions from the Wechsler Adult Intelligence Scale (WAIS) information subscale), to a mental arithmetic task, and to a phoneme detection task. Cerebral activation occurred primarily in the right hemisphere, indicating that the patient was processing language information in this side of his brain. For the math task, rCBF increases to the right parietal and temporal lobes were found. Activation of the central and right temporal lobes was obtained for the WAIS task, while increases to both frontal lobes were observed for the phoneme detection task.

At present, there are only two studies that have looked at whether SPECT can be used to either explain or predict recovery from the acute onset of aphasia. Vallar et al. (1988) studied the recovery of aphasia secondary to subcortical lesions. Six aphasic patients with either an ischemic or hemorrhagic lesion confined to the subcortical regions were given neurological and SPECT assessments within the first 33 days and again at 3 months postonset. All patients showed marked language improvement. Cortical hypoperfusion was seen for all patients in their initial SPECT images. The 3-month scans showed significant increases of blood flow in the anterior and middle cortical region indicating that recovery from subcortical aphasia is most likely due to the reduction of cortical hypoperfusion. Bushnell et al. (1989) administered the PICA to 10 aphasic patients within 30 days and again at 3 months poststroke. SPECT scans were obtained at the time of initial clinical testing to determine whether these images could predict aphasia recovery. Of all the parameters measured, including the volume, count density, and redistribution characteristics of the IMP defect, only the volume of the defect was found to be predictive of recovery. Those patients (n = 5) who demonstrated at least a 50% improvement of their overall PICA percentile scores had small IMP defects of 10% or less, while the poor-recovery patients had relatively large areas of reduced rCBF (25% or more of the damaged cerebral hemisphere). A significant negative correlation (r = -.81) was obtained, indicating that the larger the rCBF defect the less likely the aphasic patient will exhibit good language recovery at 3 months poststroke.

The studies reviewed suggest that language requires the interaction of a number of highly integrated systems of the brain. This interaction involves both hemispheres as well as cortical and subcortical structures. Subcortical areas associated with arousal, attention, and sequenced planning of response seem particularly important in language and speech. Future studies with SPECT as well as PET and other imaging procedures should allow for an improved understanding of brain function in normal and diseased states.

Brain Electrical Activity Mapping. Since its inception nearly 13 years ago (Duffy et al, 1979), BEAM has been used primarily to investigate those seemingly neurological and neuropsychiatric disorders whose etiology has not been readily explained by CT or MRI. These include developmental dyslexia (Duffy and McNulty, 1990; Duffy et al., 1980), Alzheimer's disease (Duffy et al., 1984), schizophrenia (Pool et al., 1988), seizure disorders (Gregory and Wong, 1984), and spasmodic dysphonia (Finitzo and Freeman, 1989). Stroke has not been extensively studied using BEAM. In the few studies that have studied this, it has been shown that BEAM often detects focal brain abnormalities that are undetected by other neuroimaging methods (Jonkman et al., 1985; Nagata et al., 1986; Nuwer et al., 1987). For instance, Nagata et al. (1986) have shown that while the electrophysiological measures from BEAM are significantly correlated with rCBF measures from PET, BEAM often uncovers brain abnormalities not seen on PET images. In two patients, one with global aphasia and the other with Broca's aphasia, PET neuroimages showed a marked reduction of rCBF in the whole left cerebral hemisphere and the left frontal lobe, respectively. Electrophysiological defects, on the other hand, were seen in the frontal lobes bilaterally for both patients. In a third case, which involved a sensory aphasia, BEAM showed diffuse abnormalities, whereas PET localized the rCBF defect to the left temporal lobe. The authors believe that these undetected defects may be indicative of deafferentation or the isolation of the cerebral cortex from afferent influences.

Only two studies to date have used BEAM to study aphasia. Employing 100 stroke patients, Chapman et al. (1989) found that the electrophysiological information obtained from BEAM images could be used to differentially diagnose aphasia, which generally agreed with established anatomoclinical principles. Aphasic patients could be distinguished from nonaphasic stroke patients based on the presence of an electrophysiological deficit to their left perisylvian region, while the presence of a left temporoparietal deficit differentiated global from nonglobal aphasic patients. Severely nonfluent aphasic patients showed defects to their left inferior frontal/anterior temporal regions, while patients with severely impaired auditory comprehension or expression had abnormalities to their left posterior temporoparietal cortex. Using the same population, Finitzo et al., (1991) found that the information obtained from BEAM images could also be used to predict aphasic behavior. The presence of aphasia could be predicted in 96% of all cases when electrophysiological abnormalities occurred in the left parietal region with normal activity in the right temporal areas. Likewise, the classification of a comprehension deficit was associated with aberrant activity in the left parietal region. Eighty-six percent of all patients with a severe comprehension loss were correctly classified using this criteria. In contrast, if the patient demonstrated an electrophysiological defect to the left inferior frontal/anterior temporal lobes, the patient was then classified as severely nonfluent. This criteria correctly classified 89% of all cases.

TREATMENT

The treatment of a patient who has developed a stroke can be divided into two parts. The initial, or acute, therapy is directed to preserving life and to preventing expansion of the disability associated with stroke. The second part of therapy is directed toward rehabilitation, with the reestablishment of as normal a life-style as possible. Once a stroke has occurred, both acute and chronic therapy are relatively limited. The treatment of intracerebral hemorrhage parallels that of ischemic disease and will not be discussed separately. The best treatment for stroke is prevention. Aspects of prevention have already been discussed in relation to TIA.

ACUTE THERAPY

Medical treatment is limited and for the most part is involved with the preservation of life (Byer and Easton, 1980). Appropriate treatment is dependent on the establishment of the etiology and associated disorders including myocardial infarction, congestive heart failure, arrhythmias, and so on (Moss, 1984; Sherman et al., 1984). The proper identification and treatment of underlying problems will decrease mortality. Many stroke patients die of factors not directly related to brain damage; these factors are most frequently of cardiac origin. Thus, evaluation of cardiac status is important (Brott and Reed, 1989). Currently, patients with stroke secondary to cardiac emboli are anticoagulated to prevent further embolization. Evidence suggests that such treatment reduces overall morbidity and mortality (Easton and Sherman, 1980).

During the acute phase, careful reevaluation of the patient is important, as some will show progression of deficit. This situation is called "stroke in evolution" or "progressing stroke." Evidence exists that the use of anticoagulants, in particular heparin, can prevent further progression of disability (Millikan, 1980). Under any circumstance where the physician plans to use an anticoagulant, intracerebral hemorrhage has to first be ruled out by CT and, depending on circumstances, with a lumbar puncture. The presence of hemorrhage is an absolute contraindication for the use of an anticoagulant, which increases the risk of further bleeding.

With ischemic strokes, there is a region of infarction surrounded by an ischemic zone whose tissue can either recover or progress to infarction. Extensive effort has been made to protect the ischemic region and to improve its blood flow. Vasodilators are drugs that cause the blood vessels to enlarge and increase blood flow. They have been tried with no major effect. The idea is that a dilator will cause the blood vessels to the ischemic region to enlarge and blood flow will return. In reality, the blood vessels to ischemic tissue lose their normal reactivity and do not respond to such drugs, while other blood vessels do. This results in a "steal" phenomenon, where the blood is taken from rather than supplied to the desired region. An alternate approach has been to increase perfusion pressure by increasing mean arterial pressure in an attempt to force blood into the ischemic area. Extensive studies have not examined this form of therapy. Calcium channel blockers have likewise not been found to be particularly useful. Another approach has been volume expansion, which has not proved beneficial.

A problem that develops in many stroke patients 1 to 3 days postictus is the development of swelling within the brain secondary to water accumulation. The cause of the edema is related primarily to the beginning of necrosis within the infarcted tissue. The accumulation of water can act as a large mass within the brain and result in symptom progression and alteration of consciousness (Anderson and Cranford, 1979). If edema is severe, death can follow from brain herniation. Corticosteroids are known to be very effective for removing edema associated with brain tumors. This form of edema is secondary to changes in the blood vessels with increased permeability. Unfortunately, the edema associated with infarction is not caused by these vasogenic changes but rather by cytotoxic factors (i.e., the breakdown of cells). Infarction edema does not respond well to corticosteroids, but interestingly, these agents are used extensively in stroke therapy. Agents that have greater effect on infarction edema are hyperosmolar agents, including urea and mannitol as well as hyperventilation. They decrease the swelling in the brain on a transient basis. The difficulty is that a rebound phenomenon with increasing edema can occur, causing physicians to shy away from the treatment.

Surgical approaches to the treatment of acute stroke are relatively limited. In recent years, there has been renewed interest in doing acute surgery in selected subjects. If a patient can be seen within 1 to 2 hours following an internal carotid artery occlusion, an emergency endarterectomy to remove the new thrombus seems to improve overall recovery (Goldstone and Moore, 1976). In patients with intracranial hemorrhage, if the individual is deteriorating and the hemorrhage is relatively superficial, then removal of the clot may save the patient's life.

Chronic Therapy

Chronic therapy begins during and after the acute therapy phase. As soon as a patient has had a stroke, a rehabilitation program should begin. Initially, the goal is to prevent contractions and decubiti in those patients who are seriously disabled.

Passive ranging of the hemiplegic arm and leg should be done several times a day. It is important that this be gentle to prevent soft-tissue damage to the shoulder and hip. Such activity is typically done by the physical therapist or nurse. The patient should also be routinely rotated in bed so that excessive irritation does not occur on bony prominences and pressure points, which will quickly result in decubiti.

As soon as the patient is medically stable, it is important to start getting him or her out of bed into a lounging or wheelchair. Initially, this may be for only a few minutes at a time, but gradually, the time is increased.

When the patient is medically stable and out of the acute phase of the illness, a formal rehabilitation program can be started. Such a program includes interactions between physicians, nurses, physical therapists, occupational therapists, social service workers, psychologists, speech-language pathologists and vocational therapists. The rehabilitation program will be discussed elsewhere in the text. At this point, we will focus on those factors within the patient that may affect outcome and recovery.

One of the key problems for the rehabilitation team, particularly in the current emphasis on cost efficiency, is to identify factors that are prognostic for recovery. Two questions seem to be most relevant. First, what predictive factors are most important in evaluating a patient for possible rehabilitation potential? The better that the extent of possible improvement can be predicted, the more realistic the establishment of appropriate individual programs can be. Second, what types of programs should be used in the treatment and rehabilitation to allow for the greatest degree of improvement with the least expense? A number of studies have evaluated one or more factors associated with recovery. These have included motor return, cooperation, age, complicating illnesses, perceptual or cognitive dysfunction, homonymous hemianopsia, and persistent incontinence (Adler and Tal, 1965; Feigenson et al., 1977; Gersten et al., 1970; Gordon et al., 1978; Held, 1975; Lehmann et al., 1975).

The most significant factor in overall outcome for recovery is the extent of motor strength that returns, in relationship to the degree of spasticity (Gersten et al., 1970; Lorenze et al., 1958). Hemiparesis is extremely frequent in stroke. In general, the upper extremity shows the greater involvement but recovers the least (Held, 1975). A possible explanation for the high percentage of arm weakness and disability is that in the cerebral cortex, the arm is located in the middle region of the middle cerebral artery circulation, while the leg receives its greatest circulation from the anterior cerebral artery. A second factor is that the arm requires fine-motor movements in order to be functional, while the leg requires only gross movements for ambulation.

Twitchell (1951) studied the recovery from hemiplegia and noted that immediately after the onset of weakness, there was a loss of voluntary movement associated with a decrease or absence of reflexes and loss of tone. Within 48 hours, there was a gradual increase in reflexes, and shortly thereafter a gradual increase in the resistance, initially involving palmar and plantar flexures followed by the adductors and flexures of the upper extremity and the adductors and extensors of the lower extremity. Voluntary movement begins to appear within 6 to 30 days, with slight flexion in the shoulder and hip and then a gradual proximal-to-distal progression of improvement.

With improved strength, there develops a total flexor pattern of movement at all joints, called a "flexor synergy," which is followed by an extensor synergy. Gradually, a decrease in spasticity occurs and also a breakdown in the flexor and extensor synergies, allowing for movement at a single joint. Twitchell believed that the recovery of movement could be divided into three stages: (*a*) proprioceptive reactions, followed by (*b*) contractual reactions, followed by (*c*) independent movement. In studying recovery, the most reliable prognostic sign was the occurrence of proprioceptive facilitation and a proximal traction response. Proprioceptive facilitation consists of attempted willed movement during a proprioceptive reaction such as a finger jerk. Attempted willed movement can bring out a reflex that normally would not be present. A proximal traction response consists of increased flexion in fingers, wrist, elbow, and shoulder to a stretch applied to the flexures of each joint one at a time. It becomes apparent from Twitchell's study that recovery from hemiplegia follows a uniform pattern that may break down or cease to advance further in a given patient.

Recovery from hemiparesis seems to be dependent on a number of factors. Patients with hemiparesis show greater improvement in less time than patients do with hemiplegia (Gray et al., 1990; Stern et al., 1971). Essentially, all neurological improvement occurs within 14 weeks after the onset, but overall recovery may continue for years (Dombovy and Bach-y-Rita, 1988). Recovery begins as early as the first week but not later than the seventh. The average interval to 80% recovery was 6 weeks. Similar findings have been found in regard to the upper extremity.

Sensory losses are common to some degree in most subjects. Patients with sensory loss tend to be hospitalized longer and to have a worse prognosis for recovery. The effect of sensory loss seems closely tied to the degree of perceptual problems.

Pharmacological Treatment

One area that has not been adequately investigated is the treatment of aphasia pharmaceutically. In ancient times, neurological disorders were been treated by many different remedies, including wine, berries, roots, and herbs (LaPointe, 1983). In the modern era, researchers have looked for pharmaceutical agents that might influence language recovery in aphasia. These agents include sodium amytal (Bergman and Green, 1951; Billow, 1949; Linn, 1947; Linn and Stein, 1946), stimulants such as meprobamate (West and Stockel, 1965) and Ritalin, and the depressant Librium (Darley et al., 1977). These drugs either have yielded equivocal findings or have shown no beneficial effect. However, within the past 5 years, two drugs, d-amphetamine and bromocriptine, have shown some promise for the treatment of aphasia.

D-amphetamine is an agonist to the central nervous system neurotransmitter norepinephrine. Significant improvements in motor function have been reported in animals who have received d-amphetamine early after experimental lesions were induced (Boyeson and Feeney, 1984; Feeney et al., 1982; Feeney and Hovda, 1983; Hovda and Feeney, 1984). Interestingly, this improvement occurred only when the administration of amphetamine was given simultaneously with motor training. D-amphetamine treatment alone did not improve motor function. Similar findings have been observed in humans. Crisostomo et al., (1988) showed that stroke patients who received d-amphetamine with physical therapy demonstrated a rate of improvement 40% greater than the patients who received physical therapy and a placebo.

Walker-Batson and her colleagues (1991, 1992) have studied the effects of amphetamine on aphasia recovery in a small group of stroke patients. The investigators used an experimental paradigm similar to the one employed in the animal and human studies. Six patients, within 30 days of their strokes, were given 10 to 15 mg of d-amphetamine followed by a 1-hour session of intensive speech and language therapy every fourth day for 10 sessions. The PICA was administered 3 days prior to initiation of treatment, 1 week after the treatment was terminated, then again at 3-months poststroke. Comparisons of their 3-month PICA overall scores and their 6-month predicted overall PICA scores were made. Of the six patients, four had achieved over 94% of their projected 6-month score at the end of their 10 weeks of d-amphetamine and language therapy sessions. At 3 months postonset, five of the six aphasic patients demonstrated over 100% of their 6-month predicted score. Although these results are preliminary at best, they indicate that d-amphetamine might increase the rate of language recovery in aphasia. Whether this agent enhances the overall extent of aphasia recovery is not known.

Bromocriptine, on the other hand, is a pharmaceutical agent that has been used for many years to improve the initiation and ease of movement in patients with Parkinson's disease. It acts to excite dopaminergic receptor sites, which are located primarily in the mesial frontal cortex, which is part of the limbic system. The role that the limbic system plays in the recovery of language is not well understood. However, some indirect evidence shows that the limbic system may drive the production of speech. Robinson (1976), for example, reported on a man with a nonfluent aphasia who also had a history of manic-depressive illness. During the manic stage, the patient's speech became fluent. In contrast, when under medication that improved his manic symptoms, the patient's nonfluent speech returned.

Lesions resulting in aphasia are usually limited to perirolandic and perisylvian regions and do not involve the mesial frontal cortex. Investigators believe that bromocriptine excites the receptor sites within the mesial frontal cortex, enhancing the limbic system's ability to drive the production of speech and language in aphasic patients. Albert et al. (1988) reported the effects of bromocriptine on a man who had incurred a transcortical motor aphasia 3.5 years prior to treatment. Using a single-subject, open-labeled, test-retest design, these investigators reported that after 43 days and a maximum 30-mg daily dose, the patient demonstrated improvement in speech fluency, including a decrease in response latency and the number of pauses produced between and within utterances. The number of content words and grammatical morphemes also was reported to increase to normal during drug treatment. However, 28 days after bromocriptine treatment was discontinued, the patient's language skills returned to pretreatment levels. Bachman and Morgan (1988) investigated the effects of bromocriptine on two additional patients, one with a mixed anterior aphasia and the other with a Broca-type aphasia. While the patients did not show any obvious changes in their performance on the Boston Diagnostic Aphasia Examination (BDAE), both patients displayed a reduction in the number of pauses between and within utterances in connected discourse. In addition, the patients and their wives reported the use of novel words and the ability to initiate conversations more readily. While these results are promising, Bachman and Morgan warn that these changes might reflect improvement in areas other than language processing, such as cognitive functioning or mood.

Bromocriptine therapy for aphasia was investigated by Gupta and Mlcoch (1992) also using a clinical open-labeled, unblinded design. In their study, two patients, one with Broca's aphasia for 18 months and the other with a transcortical motor aphasia for 10 years, were given progressively larger dosages of bromocriptine over a 3-month period. Speech and language evaluations were done before bromocriptine therapy and thereafter at 4-week intervals. Each evaluation consisted of samples of each patient's conversational and descriptive speech and the administration of the BDAE and the Boston Naming Test. The Broca's aphasic patient demonstrated steady improvement in his fluency over the course of the study. At pretreatment, he was able to speak, without pausing, with an average of 3.19 words per utterance. While on 30 mg of bromocriptine, his mean length utterance (MLU) climbed to 4.25 words. In addition his repetition of sentences and his ability to list animals had markedly improved. The transcortical motor aphasic patient also showed observable improvement. Interestingly, these changes appeared to be due to the level of dosage. At 10 mg, the patient's MLU had increased 1.95 words from 2.82 words at pretreatment to 4.77 words per utterance. At 30 mg, the patient's speech had deteriorated to 3.08 words per utterance. However, when his bromocriptine dosage was reduced to 10 mg, his overall speech fluency had again markedly improved to 4.44 words per utterance. While these results were impressive, the authors concluded that a double-blind study using a statistically significant number of patients must be performed before the efficacy of bromocriptine treatment of aphasia can be proved.

The only single-blind investigation of bromocriptine therapy was conducted by MacLennan et al. (1991). In this study, a 63-year-old man with a 4-year history of a transcortical motor aphasia secondary to a left cerebral infarct was given a 4-week period of placebo followed by 7 weeks of drug treatment during which he received a maximum 15-mg dose of bromocriptine. This was followed by a 4-week withdrawal phase. A test battery consisting of tests of the patient's visual reaction time, auditory comprehension, naming, word fluency, and connected speech was given at 2-week intervals during each phase of the investigation. During the drug phase, the patient's performance on the visual reaction time test, the Token Test, the Boston Naming Test, and the Word Fluency Measure was not substantially different from his performance during the placebo phase. The total number of words and the number of words the patient produced that were accurate, relevant, and informative to the listener were observably different during the drug phase. The patient produced more words and content words while taking bromocriptine than during the baseline or placebo phase. However, MacLennan et al. thought that because these changes began during the placebo phase and the rate of increase was unchanged during the drug phase, bromocriptine might not have been responsible. Although they did speculate as to why these findings occurred they suggest that to advocate the use of bromocriptine to treat aphasia is premature at this time.

Obviously, none of the studies reviewed provides conclusive proof that either d-amphetamine or bromocriptine is an effective treatment of aphasia. Most of the studies employ a single-subject test-retest design without adequate experimental controls such as including a placebo condition or blinding both the patient and the examiner as to what the patient is taking. At best, these single-subject investigations are based on seemingly strong neurophysiological and theoretical underpinnings. However, until a group study using either a control and a experimental group or a repeated design where each patient acts as his or her own control is undertaken, the efficacy of these agents for the treatment of aphasia can not be ascertained. It is hoped that within the near future, a double-blind group study addressing this clinically important question will be conducted.

FUTURE TRENDS

The trends in stroke research will be a continued effort to reduce the incidence, morbidity, and mortality. Preventive measures will be directed to improving life-style and identifying factors that are most associated with high risk of strokes. Improved understanding of the pathophysiology of atherosclerosis will result in improved prophylaxis for patients who demonstrate evidence for this disease. Daily treatment with aspirin or other platelet-inhibiting agents, improved dietary habits, regular exercise, and a decline in tobacco usage are important preventive measures.

Much effort is being directed to reduce the extent of functional damage associated with a stroke. At present, such therapeutic approaches have been of limited value. Further studies to understand the pathophysiology of the ischemic process should improve this effort. As part of the acute treatment, imaging techniques that study brain physiology may identify subgroups of stroke patients who might benefit from a given treatment approach. Until such subgroups are identified, it is difficult to develop therapeutic strategies that are directed enough to show benefits.

Rehabilitation techniques are not likely to improve significantly until a better understanding is obtained of what happens to the brain when it is damaged and how it changes during recovery. Studies using PET, SPECT, BEAM, and other imaging techniques would allow a better understanding of functional recovery and the correlation to structural damage. Improving resolution and techniques to evaluate other aspects of brain biochemistry including receptor and drug distribution, can allow for a more complex understanding of the effect of a stroke. Recognizing patterns of distributional changes of structure and biochemical markers may help identify patients who will most likely respond to specific forms of rehabilitation.

References

Ackerman, R. H. (1980). *Non-invasive diagnosis of carotid disease*. In Cerebrovascular Survey Report for Joint Council Subcommittee on Cerebrovascular Disease. National Institute of Neurological and Communicative Disorders and Stroke, and National Heart and Lung Institute.

Adler, E., and Tal, E. (1965). Relationship between physical disability and functional capacity in hemiplegic patients. *Archives of Physical Medicine and Rehabilitation, 46*, 745–752.

Albert, M. L., Bachman, D. L., Morgan, A., and Helm-Estabrook, N. (1988). Pharmacotherapy for aphasia. *Neurology, 38*, 877–879.

Alexander, M., and LoVerme, S. R. (1980) Aphasia after left hemispheric intracerebral hemorrhage. *Neurology, 30*, 1193–1202.

Anderson, D. C., and Cranford, R. E. (1979). Corticosteroids in ischemic stroke. *Stroke, 10*, 68–71.

Asslid, R. (1992). *Transcranial Doppler sonography*. New York: Springer-Verlag.

Bachman, D. L., and Morgan, A. (1988). The role of pharmacotherapy in the treatment of aphasia: preliminary results. *Aphasiology, 2*, 225–228.

Barnett, H. J. M., Taylor, D. W., Haynes, R. B., Sackett, D. L., Peerless, S. J., and Ferguson, G. G. (1991). Beneficial effect of carotid endarterectomy in symptomatic patients with high-grade carotid stenosis. *New England Journal of Medicine, 325*, 445–453.

Baron, J. C., Bousser, M. G., Comar, D., Duquesnoy, N., Sastre, J., and Castaigne, P. (1981). Crossed cerebellar diaschisis: A remote functional depression secondary to supratentorial infarction in man. *Journal Cerebral Blood Flow Metabolism, 1* (Suppl. 1), S500–S501.

Bergman, P. S., and Green, M. (1951). Aphasia: Effects of intravenous sodium amytal. *Neurology, 1*, 471–475.

Billow, B. W. (1949). Observation of the use of sodium amytal in the treatment of aphasia. *Medical Records, 162*, 12–13.

Bogousslavsky, J., Miklossy, J., and Regli, F. (1988). Subcortical neglect: Neuropsychological correlations with anterior choroidal artery territory infarction. *Annals of Neurology, 23*, 448–452.

Bonita, R. (1992). Epidemiology of stroke. *Lancet, 339*, 342–344.

Borowitz, S., and Beiser, A. (1966). *Essentials of physics: A text for students of science and engineering*. Reading, MA: Addison-Wesley.

Boyeson, M. G. and Feeney, D. (1984). The role of norepinephrine in recovery from brain injury. *Society of Neuroscience Abstracts, 10*, 638.

Bradley, W. G. (1982). *NMR tomography*. Diasonic Interactive Education Program. Militas, CA: Diasonics Inc.

Broderick, J. P., Phillips, S. J., Whisnant, J. P., O'Fallon, W. M., and Bergstralh, E. J. (1989). Incidence rates of stroke in the eighties: The end of the decline in stroke. *Stroke, 20*, 577–582.

Brott, T., and Reed, R. L. (1989). Intensive care for acute stroke in the community hospital setting. *Stroke, 20*, 694–697.

Brunner, R. J., Kornhuber, H. H., Seemuller, E., Suger, G., and Wallesch, C. W. (1982). Basal ganglia participation in language pathology. *Brain and Language, 16*, 281–299.

Brust, J. C. M. (1977). Transient ischemic attacks: Natural history and anticoagulation. *Neurology, 27*, 701–707.

Bushnell, D. L., Gupta, S., Mlcoch, A. G., and Barnes, E. (1989). Prediction of language and neurologic recovery after cerebral infarction with SPECT imaging using N-isopropyl-p-(I123) iodoamphetamine. *Archives of Neurology., 46*, 665–669.

Bushnell, D. L., Gupta, S., Mlcoch, A. G., Romyn, A., Barnes, E., and Kaplan, E. (1987). Demonstration of focal hyperemia in acute cerebral infarction with iodine-123 iodoamphetamine. *Journal of Nuclear Medicine, 28*, 1920–1923.

Byer, J. A., and Easton, J. D. (1980). Therapy of ischemic cerebrovascular disease. *Annals of Internal Medicine, 93*, 742–756.

Canadian Cooperative Study Group. (1978). A randomized trial of asp sulfinpyrazone in threatened stroke. *New England Journal of Medicine, 299*, 53–59.

Chapman, S. B., Pool, K. D., Finitzo, T., and Hong, T. (1989). Comparison of language profiles and electrocortical dysfunction in aphasia. In T. E. Prescott (Ed.), *Clinical aphasiology* (Vol. 18). Boston: College Hill.

Crisostomo, E. A., Duncan, P. W., Propst, M. A., Dawson, D. V., and Davis, J. N. (1988). Evidence that amphetamine with physical therapy promotes recovery of motor function in stroke patients. *Annals of Neurology, 23*, 94–97.

Crooks, L., Herfkens, R., and Kaufman, L. (1981). Nuclear magnetic resonance imaging. *Progressive Nuclear Medicine, 7*, 149–163.

Damasio, A. R., Damasio, H., Rizzo, M., Varney, N., and Gersch, F. (1982). Aphasia with nonhemorrhagic lesions in the basal ganglia and internal capsule. *Archives of Neurology, 39*, 15–20.

Darley F. L., Keith, R. L., and Sasanuma, S. (1977). The effect of alerting and tranquilizing drugs upon the performance of aphasic patients. In R. H. Brookshire (Ed.), *Clinical aphasiology: Conference proceedings 1977*. Minneapolis, MN: BRK.

Defer, G., Moretti, J. L., and Cesaro P. (1987). Early and delayed SPECT using N-isopropyl-p-iodoamphetamine iodine 123 in cerebral ischemia: A prognostic index for clinical recovery. *Archives of Neurology, 44*, 715–718.

DeFilipp, G. J., Pinto, R. S., Lin, J. P., and Kricheff, I. I. (1983). Intravenous digital subtraction angiography in the investigation of intracranial disease. *Radiology, 148*, 129–136.

DeJong, R. N. (1980). Case taking and the neurologic examination. In A. B. Baker and L. H. Baker (Eds.), *Clinical neurology*. Philadelphia: Harper & Row.

DesRosiers, M. H., Kennedy, C., and Potlak, C. S., (1974). Relationship between local cerebral blood flow and glucose utilization in the rat. *Neurology (Minn), 24*, 389.

Dombovy, M. L., and Bach-y-Rita, P. (1988). Clinical observations on recovery from stroke. *Advances in Neurology, 47*, 265–276.

Dorland's illustrated medical dictionary (24th Ed.) (1965). Philadelphia: Saunders.

Duffy, F. H., Albert, M. S., and McNulty, G. (1984). Brain electrical activity in patients with presenile and senile dementia of the Alzheimer type. *Annals of Neurology 16*, 439–448.

Duffy, F. H., Burchfiel, J. L., and Lombroso, C. T. (1979). Brain electrical activity mapping (BEAM): A method for extending the clinical utility of EGG and evoked potential data. *Annals of Neurology, 5*, 309–321.

Duffy, F. H., Denckla, M. B., Bartels, P. H., and Sandini, G. (1980). Dyslexia: Regional differences in brain electrical activity by topographic mapping. *Annals of Neurology, 7*, 412–420.

Duffy, F. H., and McNulty, G. (1990). Neurophysiological heterogeneity and the definition of dyslexia: Preliminary evidence for plasticity. *Neuropsychologia, 28*, 555–571.

Easton, J. D., and Sherman, D. G. (1977). Stroke and mortality rate in carotid endarterectomy: 228 consecutive operations. *Stroke, 8*, 565–568.

Easton, J. D., and Sherman, D. G. (1980). Management of cerebral embolism of ca origin. *Stroke, 11*, 433–442.

Eisenberg, H., Morrison, H. T., and Sullivan, P. (1964). Cerebrovascular accidents. Incidence and survival rates in a defined population, Middlesex County, Connecticut. *JAMA, 189*, 833–888.

European Carotid Trialists' Collaborative Group MRC/European Carotid Surgery Trial. (1991). Interim results for symptomatic patients with severe (70–99%) or with mild (0–29%) carotid stenosis. *Lancet, 1*, 1235–1245.

Feigenson, J. S., McCarthy, M. L., Meese, P. D., Feigenson, W. D., Greenberg, S. D., Rubin, E., and McDowell, F. H. (1977). Stroke rehabilitation. I. Factors predicting outcome and length of stay—an overview. *New York State Journal of Medicine, 77*, 1426–1434.

Feeney, D., Gonzales, J., and Law, W. (1982). Amphetamine, haloperidol and experience interact to affect rate of recovery after motor cortex injury. *Science, 217*, 855–857.

Feeney, D., and Hovda, D. A. (1983). Amphetamine and apomorphine restore tactile placing after motor cortex injury in the cat. *Psychopharmacology, 79*, 67–71.

Fields, W. S., Lemak, N. A., Frankoski, R. F., and Hardy, R. J. (1977). Controlled trial of aspirin in cerebral ischemia. *Stroke, 8*, 301–315.

Finitzo, T., and Freeman, F. J. (1989). Spasmodic dysphonia, whether and when: Results of seven years of research. *Journal of Speech and Hearing Research, 32*, 541–555.

Finitzo, T., Pool, K. D., and Chapman S. B. (1991). Quantitative electroencephalography and anatomoclinical principles of aphasia. In R. A. Zappulla, F. LeFever, J. Jaeger, and R. Bilder (Eds.), *Windows on the brain: Neuropsychology's technological frontiers*. New York: New York Academy of Sciences.

Ford, A. B., and Katz, S. (1966). Prognosis after strokes. *Medicine, 45*, 223–246.

Freygang, W. H., and Sokoloff, L. (1958). Quantitative measurement of regional circulation in the central nervous system by use of radioactive inert gas. *Advanced Biology, Medicine and Physiology, 6*, 263–279.

Gersten, J. W., Ager, C., Anderson, K., and Cenkovich, F. (1970). Relation of muscle strength and range of motion to activities of daily living. *Archives of Physical Medicine Rehabilitation, 51*, 137–142.

Gillilan, L. A. (1980). *Anatomy of the blood supply to the brain and spinal cord*. In Cerebrovascular Survey Report for Joint Council Subcommittee on Cerebrovascular Disease. National Institute of Neurological and Communicative Disorders and Stroke, and National Heart and Lung Institute.

Gilroy, J., and Meyer, J. S. (1975). *Medical neurology, (2nd ed.)*. New York: Macmillan.

Giubilei, F., Lenzi, G. L., and Dipiero, V. (1990). Predictive value of brain perfusion single photon emission computed tomography in acute ischemic stroke. *Stroke, 21*, 895–900.

Goldenberg, G., Podreka, I., Steiner, M., and Willmes, K. (1987). Patterns of regional cerebral blood flow related to memorizing of high and low imagery words—an emission computed tomography study. *Neuropsychologia, 25*, 473–485.

Goldstone, J., and Moore, W. S. (1976). Emergency carotid artery surgery in neurologically unstable patients. *Archives of Surgery, 111*, 1284–1291.

Gordon, E. G., Drenth, V., Jarvis, L., Johnson, J., and Wright, V. (1978). Neurophysiologic syndromes in stroke as predictors of outcome. *Archives of Physical Medicine Rehabilitation, 59,* 399–403.

Gray, C. S., French, J. M., Bates, D., Cartilidge, N. E., James, O. F., and Venables, G. (1990). Motor recovery following stroke. *Age and Ageing, 19,* 179–184.

Gray, H. (1967). *Anatomy of the human body, (28th ed.).* Philadelphia: Lea & Febiger.

Gregory, D. L., and Wong, P. K. (1984). Topographic analysis of the centrotemporal discharges in benign rolandic epilepsy. *Epilesia, 25,* 705–711.

Gupta, S., Bushnell, D., Mlcoch, A. G., Eastman, G., Barnes, W. E., and Fisher, S. G. (1991). Utility of late N-isopropyl-p-(I 123)-iodoamphetamine brain distribution in the predictive recovery/outcome following cerebral infarction. *Stroke, 22,* 1512–1518.

Gupta, S. R., and Mlcoch, A. G. (1992). Bromocriptine treatment of nonfluent aphasia. *Archives of Physical Medicine and Rehabilitation, 73,* 373–376.

Hayman, L. A., Taber, K. H., Jhingran, S. G., Killian, J. M, and Carroll, R. G. (1989). Cerebral infarction: Diagnosis and assessment of prognosis using 123 IMP-SPECT and CT. *American Journal of Nuclear Research, 10,* 557–562.

Hayward, R. W., Naeser, M. A., and Zatz, L. M. (1977). Cranial computed tomography in aphasia. *Radiology, 123,* 653–660.

Held, J. P. (1975). The natural history of stroke. In S. Licht (Ed.), *Stroke and its rehabilitation.* Baltimore, MD: 1975.

Hier, D. B., Mondlock, J., and Caplan, L. R. (1983). Behavioral abnormalities after right hemisphere. *Neurology, 33,* 337–344.

Hill, T. C., Magistretti, P. L., Holman, B. L., Lee R. G., O'Leary, D. H., and Uren, R. F. (1984). Assessment of regional cerebral blood flow (rCBF) in stroke using SPECT and N-isopropyl-(I-123)-p-iodoamphetamine (IMP). *Stroke, 15,* 40–45.

Hoffman, E. J., Huang, S. C., and Phelps, M. E. (1979). Quantitation in positron emission tomography. 1. Effect of object size. *J. Computer Assisted Tomography, 3,* 299–308.

Holmes, M. D., Brant-Zawadzki, C., and Simon, R. P. (1984). Clinical features of meningovascular syphilis. *Neurology, 34,* 553–556.

Hovda, D. A., and Feeney, D. (1984). Amphetamine and experience promotes recovery of locomotor function after unilateral frontal cortex injury in the cat. *Brain Research, 298,* 358–361.

Ingvar, D. H., and Lassen, N. A. (1961). Quantitative determination of regional cerebral blood flow in man. *Lancet, 2,* 806–807.

Joint Committee for Stroke Facilities. (1974). XI. Transient focal cerebral ischemia: Epidemiological and clinical aspects. *Stroke, 5,* 276–287.

Jonkman, E. J., Poorvliet, D. C., Veering, M. M., De Weerd, A. W., and John, E. R. (1985). The use of neurometrics in the study of patients with cerebral ischemia. *Electroencephalography Clinical Neurophysiology, 61,* 333–341.

Kannel, W. B. (1971). Current status of the epidemiology of brain infarction associated with occlusive arterial disease. *Stroke, 2,* 295–318.

Kempczinski, R. F., Wood, G. W., Berlatzky, Y., and Pearce, W. H. (1983). A comparison of digital subtraction angiography and noninvasive testing in the diagnosis of cerebrovascular disease. *American Journal of Surgery, 146,* 203–207.

Kertesz, A., Harlock, W., and Coates, R. (1979). Computer tomographic localization, lesion size and prognosis in aphasia and nonverbal impairment. *Brain and Language, 8,* 34–50.

Kety, S. S., and Schmidt, C. F. (1948). The nitrous oxide method for quantitative determination of cerebral blood flow in man: Theory, procedure and normal values. *Journal of Clinical Investigation, 27,* 476–483.

Knopman, D. S., Rubens, A. B., Klassen, A. C., Meyer, M. W., and Niccum, N. (1980). Regional cerebral blood flow patterns during verbal and nonverbal auditory activation. *Brain and Language, 9,* 93–112.

Knopman, D. S., Rubens, A. B., and Selnes, O. (1983). Right hemisphere participation in recovery from aphasia: Evidence from xenon-133 inhalation rCBF studies. *Cerebral Blood Flow Metabolism, 3,* (Suppl. 1), S250–S251.

Kuhl, D. E., Metter, E. J., Riege, W. H., and Phelps, M. E. (1982). Effects of human aging on patterns of local cerebral glucose utilization determined by the (18FDG) fluorodeoxyglucose method. *J. Cereb Blood Flow Metabolism, 2,* 163–171.

Kuhl, D. E., Phelps, M. E., Kowell, A. P., Metter, E. J., Selin, C., and Winter, J. (1980). Effect of stroke on local cerebral metabolism and perfusion: Mapping by emission computed tomography of 18FDG and 13NH3. *Annals of Neurology, 8,* 47–60.

Kuhl, D. E., Reivich, M., and Alavi, A. (1975). Local cerebral blood volume determined by three dimensional reconstruction of radio nuclide scan data. *Circulatory Research, 36,* 610–619.

Kurtzke, J. (1980). *Epidemiology of cerebrovascular disease.* In Cerebrovascular Survey Report for Joint Council Subcommittee on Cerebrovascular Disease. National Institute of Neurological and Communicative Disorders and Stroke, and National Heart and Lung Institute.

Lang, W., Lang, M., and Goldenberg, G. (1987). EEG and rCBF evidence for left frontocortical activation when memorizing verbal material. In R. Johnson, J. W. Rohrbaugh, and R. Parasuraman (Eds.), *Current trends in event related potential research* (pp. 328–334). New York: Elsevier.

LaPointe, L. L. (1983). Aphasia interventions with adults: Historical, present and future approaches. In J. Miller and D. Yoder (Eds.), *Contemporary issues in language intervention: ASHA reports 12.* Rockville, MD: American Speech-Language-Hearing Association.

Larsen, B., Skinhoj, E., and Lassen, N. A. (1978). Variations in regional cortical blood flow in the right and left hemispheres during automatic speech. *Brain, 101,* 193–209.

Lavy, S., Melamed, E., Cahane, E., and Carmon, A. (1973). Hypertension and diabetes as risk factors in stroke patients. *Stroke, 4,* 751–759.

Lee, R. G., Hill, T. C., and Holman, B. L. (1984). Predictive value of perfusion defect size using N-isopropyl-(I-123)-p-iodoamphetamine emission tomography in acute stroke. *Journal of Neurosurgery, 61,* 449–452.

Lehmann, J. F., DeLateur, B. J., Fowler, R. S., Warren, C. G., Arnhold, A., and Schertzer, G. (1975). Stroke rehabilitation: Outcome and prediction. *Archives of Physical Medicine and Rehabilitation, 56,* 383–389.

Lenzi, G. L., Frackowiak, R. S., and Jones, T. (1981). Regional cerebral blood flow (rCBF), oxygen utilization (CMRO2) and oxygen extraction ratio (OER) in acute hemispheric stroke. *Journal of Cerebral Blood Flow Metabolism, 1* (Suppl. 1), S504–S505.

Levine, J., and Swanson, P. D. (1969). Nonatherosclerotic causes of stroke. *Annals of Internal Medicine, 70,* 807–816.

Limburg, M., Royen, E. A., Hijdra, A., and Verbeeten, B. (1991). rCBF-SPECT in brain infarction: When does it predict outcome? *Journal of Nuclear Medicine, 32,* 382–387.

Linn, L. (1947). Sodium amytal in treatment of aphasia. *Archives of Neurology and Psychiatry, 58,* 357–358.

Linn, L., and Stein, M. (1946). The use of sodium amytal in the treatment of aphasia. *Bulletin of the U.S. Army Medical Department, 5,* 705–708.

Little, J. R., Furlan, A. J., Modic, M. T., and Weinstein, M. A. (1982). Digital subtraction angiography in cerebrovascular disease. *Stroke, 13,* 557–566.

Lorenze, E. J., DeRosa, A. J., and Keenan, E. L. (1958). Ambulation problems in hemiplegia. *Archives of Physical Medicine and Rehabilitation, 39,* 366–370.

MacLennan, D. L., Nicholas, L. E., Morley, G. K., and Brookshire, R. H. (1991). The effects of bromocriptine on speech and language function in a patient with transcortical motor aphasia. In T. E. Prescott (Ed.), *Clinical aphasiology* (Vol. 20, pp. 145–156). Boston: College Hill.

Maly, J., Turnheim, M., Heiss, W., and Gloning, K. (1977). Brain perfusion and neuropsychological test scores: A correlation study in aphasics. *Brain and Language, 4,* 78–94.

Marquardsen, J. (1969). The natural history of acute cerebrovascular disease. *Acta Neurologica Scandinavia, 45,* (Suppl. 38), 1–192.

Martin, W. R. W., and Raichle, M. E. (1983). Cerebellar blood flow and metabolism in cerebral hemisphere infarction. *Annals of Neurology, 14,* 168–176.

Mayberg, M. R., Wilson, S. E., Yatsu, F., Weiss, D. G., Messina, L., and Colling, C. (1991). Carotid endarterectomy and prevention of cerebral ischemia in symptomatic carotid stenosis. *JAMA, 266,* 3289–3294.

Mayo, N. E. Goldverg, M. S., Leve, A. R., Danys, I., and Korner-Bitensky, N. (1991). Changing rates of stroke in the province of Quebec, Canada. *Stroke, 22,* 590–595.

Mazziotta, J. C., Phelps, M. E., Carson, R. E., & Kuhl, D. E. (1982a). Tomographic mapping of human cerebral metabolism: Sensory deprivation. *Annals of Neurology, 12,* 435–444.

Mazziotta, J. C., Phelps, M. E., Carson, R. E., and Kuhl, D. E. (1982b). Tomographic mapping of human cerebral metabolism: Auditory stimulation. *Neurology, 32,* 921–937.

Mazziotta, J. C., Phelps, M. E., Miller, J., and Kuhl, D. E. (1981a). Tomographic mapping of human cerebral metabolism: Normal unstimulated state. *Neurology, 31,* 503–516.

Mazziotta, J. C., Phelps, M. E., Plummer, D., and Kuhl, D. E. (1981b). Quantitation in positron emission computed tomography. 5. Physical-anatomical effects. *Journal of Computer Assisted Tomography, 5,* 734–743.

Mazzocchi, F., and Vignolo, L. A. (1979). Localization of lesions in aphasia: Clinical–CT scan correlation in stroke patients. *Cortex, 15,* 627–653.

Metter, E. J. (1987). Neuroanatomy and physiology of aphasia: Evidence from positron emission tomography. *Aphasiology, 1,* 3–33.

Metter, E. J. (1992). Role of subcortical structures in aphasia: Evidence from resting cerebral glucose metabolism. In G. Vallar, S. F. Cappa, and C. W. Walesch (Eds.), *Neuropsychological disorders associated with subcortical lesions* (pp. 478–500). New York: Oxford University Press.

Metter, E. J., and Hanson, W. R. (1985). Brain imaging as related to speech and language. In J. Darby (Ed.), *Speech evaluation in neurology* (pp. 123–160). New York: Grune and Stratton.

Metter, E. J., Hanson, W. R., Jackson, C. A., Kempler, D., Van Lancker, D., and Mazziotta, J. C. (1990). Temporoparietal cortex in aphasia: evidence from positron emission tomography. *Archives of Neurology, 47,* 1235–1238.

Metter, E. J., Kempler, D., Jackson, C., Hanson, W. R., Mazziotta, J. C., and Phelps, M. E. (1989). Cerebral glucose metabolism in Wernicke's, Broca's, and conduction aphasias. *Archives of Neurology, 46,* 27–34.

Metter, E. J., Kempler, D., Jackson, C. A., Hanson, W. R., Riege, W. H., and Camras, L. R. (1987). Cerebral glucose metabolism in chronic aphasia. *Neurology, 37,* 1599–1606.

Metter, E. J., Mazziotta, J. C., Itabashi, H. H., Mankovich, N. J., Phelps, M. E., and Kuhl, D. E. (1985). Comparison of x-ray CT, Glucose metabolism and postmortem data in a patient with multiple infarctions. *Neurology, 35,* 1695–1701.

Metter, E. J., Riege, W. H., Hanson, W. R., Phelps, M. E., and Kuhl, D. E. (1988). Evidence for a caudate role in aphasia from FDG positron computed tomography. *Aphasiology, 2,* 33–43.

Metter, E. J., Wasterlain, C. G., Kuhl, D. E., Hanson, W. R., and Phelps, M. E. (1981). 18FDG positron emission computed tomography in a study of aphasia. *Annals of Neurology, 10,* 173–183.

Millikan, C. H. (1980). *Treatment of occlusive cerebrovascular disease.* Cerebrovascular Survey Report for Joint Council Subcommittee on Cerebrovascular Disease National Institute of Neurological and Communicative Disorders and Stroke, and National Heart and Lung Institute.

Moss, A. J. (1984). Atrial fibrillation and cerebral embolism. *Archives of Neurology, 41,* 707.

Moster, M. L., Johnston, D. E., and Reinmuth, O. M. (1983). Chronic subdural hematoma with transient neurological deficits: A review of 15 cases. *Annals of Neurology, 14,* 539–542.

Mountz, J. M., Modell, J. G., Foster, N. L., & Dupree, E. S. (1990). Prognostication of recovery following stroke using comparison of CT and technetium-99m HMPAO SPECT. *Journal of Nuclear Medicine, 31,* 61–66.

Naeser, M. A., Alexander, M. P., Helm-Estabrooks, N., Levine, H. L., Laughlin, S. A., & Geschwind, N. (1982). Aphasia with predominantly subcortical lesion sites. *Archives of Neurology, 39,* 2–14.

Naeser, M. A., and Hayward, R. W. (1978). Lesion localization in aphasia with cranial computed tomography and the Boston Diagnostic Aphasia Exam. *Neurology, 28,* 545–551.

Nagata, K., Tagawa, K., Shishido, F., and Uemura, K. (1986). Topographic EEG correlates of cerebral blood flow and oxygen consumption in patients with neuropsychological disorders. In F. H. Duffy (Ed.), *Topographic mapping of brain electrical activity.* Boston: Butterworth.

Noel, G., Bain, H., Collard, M., and Huvelle, R. (1980). Clinicopathological correlations in aphasiology by means of computerized axial tomography: Interest of using printout and prospective considerations. *Neuropsychobiology, 6,* 190–200.

Nuwer, M., Jordan, S., and Ahn, S. (1987). Evaluation of stroke using EEG frequency analysis and topographic mapping. *Neurology, 37,* 1153–1159.

Obrist, W. D., Thompson, H. K., and King, C. H. (1975). Determination of regional cerebral blood flow by inhalation of 133 XE. *Circulatory Research, 20,* 124–135.

Oldendorf, W. H. (1981). Nuclear medicine in clinical neurology: An update. *Annals of Neurology, 10,* 207–213.

Ott, K. H., Kase, C. S., Ojemann, R. G., and Mohr, J. P. (1974). Cerebellar hemorrhage: Diagnosis and treatment. *Archives of Neurology, 31,* 160–167.

Peterson, H. O., and Kieffer, S. A. (1976). Neuroradiology. In A. B. Baker and L. H. Baker (Eds.), *Clinical neurology.* Philadelphia: Harper & Row.

Peterson, S. E., Fox, P. T., Posner, M. I., Mintum, M., and Raichle, M. E. (1988). Positron emission tomographic studies of the cortical anatomy of single-word processing. *Nature, 331,* 585–589.

Phelps, M. E., Hoffman, E. J., Ricci, A., and Huang, S. C. (1982a). A new high resolution technology for positron CT: The signal amplification technique (SAT). *Journal of Cerebral Blood Flow Metabolism, 3* (Suppl. 1), S113–S114.

Phelps, M. E., Kuhl, D. E., and Mazziotta, J. C. (1981). Metabolic mapping of the brain's response to visual stimulation: Studies in humans. *Science, 211,* 1445–1448.

Phelps, M. E., Mazziotta, J. C., and Huang, S. C. (1982b). Study of cerebral function with positron computed tomography. *J Cerebral Blood Flow and Metabolism, 2,* 113–162.

Phelps, M. E., Mazziotta, J. C., Kuhl, D. E., Nuwer, M., Packwood, J., Metter, J., and Engel, J. (1981b). Tomographic mapping of human cerebral metabolism: Visual stimulation and deprivation. *Neurology, 31,* 517–529.

Pincock, J. G. (1957). The natural history of cerebral thrombosis. *Annals of Internal Medicine, 46,* 925–930.

Plum, F., and Posner, J. B. (1980). *The diagnosis of stupor and coma (3rd ed.).* Philadelphia: Davis.

Pool, K. D., Finitzo, T., Paulman, R. G., Judd, C., Gregory, R. R., and Raese, J. D. (1988). Brain electrical activity mapping in paranoid schizophrenia and related disorders. *Journal of Clinical and Experimental Neuropsychology, 10,* 332.

Presidents Commission on Heart Disease, Cancer and Stroke. (1964) Report to the President: A National Program to Conquer Heart Disease, Cancer and Stroke.

Raichle, M. E. (1983). The pathophysiology of brain ischemia. *Annals of Neurology, 13,* 2–10.

Raynaud, C., Rancurel, G., and Samson, Y. (1987). Pathophysiologic study of chronic infarcts with I-123 isopropyl iodoamphetamine (IMP): The importance of peri-infarct area. *Stroke, 18,* 21–29.

Robinson, R. G. (1976). Limbic influences on human speech. *Annals of the New York Academy of Science, 280,* 761–771.

Ross, R. (1980). *Atherosclerosis.* In Cerebrovascular Survey Report for Joint Council Subcommittee on Cerebrovascular Disease. National Institute of Neurological and Communicative Disorders and Stroke, and National Heart and Lung Institute.

Ross, R., and Glomset, J. A. (1973). Atherosclerosis and the arterial smooth muscle cell. *Science, 180,* 1332–1339.

Roy, C. S., and Sherrington, M. B. (1990). On the regulation of the blood supply of the brain. *Journal of Physiology, 11,* 85–108.

Ruggieri, P. M., Masayk, T., and Ross, J. S. (1991). Magnetic resonance angiography: Cerebrovascular applications. *Current Concepts of Cerebrovascular Disease and Stroke, 26,* 29–36.

Salford, L. G., Duffy, T. E., and Plum, F. (1973). Altered cerebral metabolism and blood flow in response to physiological stimulation. *Stroke, 4,* 351–362.

Sandok, B. A., Furlan, A. J., Whisnant, J. P., and Sundt, T. M. (1978). Guidelines for management of transient ischemic attacks. *Mayo Clinic Proceedings, 53,* 665–674.

Selnes, O. A., Knopman, D. S., Niccum, N., Rubens, A. B., and Larson, D. (1983). Computed tomographic scan correlates of auditory comprehension deficits in aphasia: A prospective recovery study. *Ann. Neurol., 5,* 558–566.

Sherman, D. G., Goldman, L., Whiting, R. B., Jurgensen, K., Kaste, M., and Easton, D. (1984). Thromboembolism in patients with atrial fibrillation. *Archives of Neurology., 41,* 708–710.

Soh, K., Larsen, B., Skinhoj, E., and Lassen, N. A. (1978). Regional cerebral blood flow in aphasia. *Archives of Neurology, 35,* 625–632.

Spetzler, R. F., Zabramski, J. M., Kaufman, B., and Yeung, H. (1983). NMR imaging: Preliminary laboratory and clinical evaluation of focal cerebral ischemia. *Journal of Cerebral Blood Flow Metabolism, 3,* (Suppl. 1), S87–S88.

Stern, P. H., McDowell, F., Miller, J. M., and Robinson, M. (1971). Factors influencing stoke rehabilitation *Stroke, 2,* 213–218.

Sundt, T. M., Sandok, B. A., and Whisnant, J. P. (1975). Carotid endarterectomy: Complications and preoperative assessment of risk. *Mayo Clinic Proceedings, 50,* 301–306.

Terent, A. (1989). Survival after stroke and transient ischemic attacks during the 1970s and 1980s. *Stroke, 20,* 1320–1326.

Thorngren, M., and Westling, B. (1990). Rehabilitation and achieved health quality after stroke. A population-based study of 258 hospitalized cases followed for one year. *Acta Neurological Scandinavia, 82,* 374–380.

Tikofsky, R. S. (1988). SPECT brain studies: Potential role of cognitive challenge in language and learning disorders. *Advances in Functional Neuroimaging, Spring,* 12–15.

Tikofsky, R. S., Collier, B. D., Hellman, R. S., Sapena, V. K., Zielonka, J. S., Krohn, L., and Gresch, A. (1985). Cerebral blood flow patterns determined by SPECT I-123 iodoamphetamine (IMP) imaging and WAB AQs in chronic aphasia: A preliminary report. Poster presented at the Academy of Aphasia, Nashville, TN.

Truax, R. C., and Carpenter, M. B. (1969). *Human neuroanatomy*, (6th ed.). Baltimore, MD: Williams & Williams.

Truscott, B. L., Kretschmann, C. M., Toole, J. F., and Pajak, T. F. (1974). Early rehabilitative care in community hospitals: Effect on quality of survivorship following a stroke. *Stroke, 5*, 623–629.

Twitchell, T. E. (1951). Restoration of motor function following hemiplegia in man. *Brain, 74*, 433–480.

Vallar, G., Perani, D., Cappa, S., and Messa, C., Lenzi, G. L., and Fazio, F. (1988). Recovery from aphasia and neglect after subcortical stroke: Neuropsychological and cerebral perfusion study. *Journal of Neurology, Neurosurgery, and Psychiatry, 51*, 1269–1276.

Veterans Administration Cooperative Study Group on Antihypertensive Agents. (1967). Effect of treatment on morbidity in hypertension. I. Results in patients with diastolic blood pressure averaging 115 through 129 mm Hg. *JAMA, 202*, 116–122.V

Veteran's Administration Cooperative Study Group on Antihypertensive Agents. (1970). Effect of treatment on morbidity in hypertension. II. Results in patients with diastolic blood pressure averaging 90 through 114 mm Hg. *JAMA, 213*, 1143–1152.

Walker-Batson, D., Devous, M. D., Bonte, F. J., and Oelschlaeger, M. (1987). Single-photon emission tomography (SPECT) in the study of aphasia: A preliminary report. In R. H. Brookshire (Ed.), *Clinical aphasiology: Conference proceedings* (pp. 313–318) Minneapolis, MN: BRK.

Walker-Batson, D., Devous, M. D., Curtis, S. S., Unwin, H., and Greenlee, R. G. (1991). Response to amphetamine to facilitate recovery from aphasia subsequent to stroke. In T. E. Prescott (Ed.), *Clinical aphasiology* (Vol. 20). Boston: College Hill.

Walker-Batson D., Devous M. D., Millay K. K., Reynolds S., Ajamani A. J., Grant D. E., and Bonte F. (1989). Tomographic regional cerebral blood flow activation during phoneme detection in normal and aphasic subjects. In T. E. Prescott (Ed.), *Clinical aphasiology* (Vol. 18, pp. 75–89). Boston: Little, Brown.

Walker-Batson, D., Unwin, H., Curtis, S., Allen, E., Wood, M., and Smith, P. (1992). Use of amphetamine in the treatment of aphasia. *Restorative Neurology and Neurosciences, 4*, 47–50.

Walker-Batson, D., Wendt, J. S., Devous, M. D., Barton, M. M., and Bonte, F. J. (1988). A long-term follow-up case study of crossed aphasia assessed by single photon emission tomography (SPECT), language, and neuropsychological testing. *Brain and Language, 33*, 311–322.

Walshe, T. M., Davis, K. R., and Fisher, C. M. (1977). Thalamic hemorrhage: A computed tomographic-clinical correlation. *Neurology, 27*, 217–222.

Webster's new world dictionary. New York: World Publishing Co. (1973).

West, R., and Stockel, S. (1965). The effect of meprobamate on recovery from aphasia. *Journal of Speech and Hearing Research., 8*, 56–62.

Whisnant, J. P. (1983). The role of the neurologist in the decline of stroke. *Annals of Neurology, 14*, 1–7.

Whisnant, J. P., Sandok, B. A., and Sundt, T. M. (1983). Carotid endarterectomy for unilateral carotid system transient cerebral ischemia. *Mayo Clinic Proceedings, 58*, 171–175.

Wolf, P. A., Dawber, T. R., Thomas, E. H., and Kannel, W. B. (1978). Epidemiologic assessment of chronic atrial fibrillation and risk of stroke: The Framingham Study. *Neurology, 28*, 973–977.

Yamaguchi, F., Meyer, J. S., Sakai, F., and Yamamoto, M., (1980). Case reports of three dysphasic patients to illustrate r-CBF responses during behavioral activation. *Brain and Language, 9*, 145–148.

Yarnell, P., Monroe, P., Sobel, L. (1976). Aphasic outcome in stroke: A clinical neuroradiological correlation. *Stroke, 7*.

Yeterian, E. H., and Van Hoesen, G. W. (1978). Cortico-striate projections in the rhesus monkey: The organization of certain cortico-caudate connections. *Brain Research, 139*, 43-e.

Zatorre, R. J., Evans, A. C., Meyer, E., and Gjedde, A. (1992). Lateralization of phonetic and pitch discrimination in speech processing. *Science, 256*, 846–849.

CHAPTER 3
Brain Imaging and Its Application to Aphasia Rehabilitation: CT and MRI

NEVA L. FRUMKIN, CAROLE L. PALUMBO, AND MARGARET A. NAESER

INTRODUCTION

Brief History of Brain Imaging

Prior to the late 1960s, the technique available for imaging the anatomy of the body and head was shadow radiography, also known as plain x-ray. A radiograph, or x-ray, depicted the amount of x-radiation that passed through the body. The amount of obstructed, or attenuated, x-ray was determined by the density of body structures through which the radiation passed. These differences in densities allowed visual differentiation of anatomical entities.

The value of plain radiographs as a diagnostic tool for disorders of the central nervous system has always been especially limited (Straub, 1984; Trapnell, 1967). The resolution of radiographs of the brain is limited to depicting differences in attenuation values that are more than 2% (Katz, 1984; Martin and Brust, 1985). Except for abnormally dense or abnormally thin areas within soft tissue, finer distinctions in densities are not visible on the plain-film radiographs (Trapnell, 1967). For example, the gray matter and white matter of the brain cannot be distinguished because of their similar absorption of x-rays. Cerebrospinal fluid and soft tissues, which constitute the bulk of the central nervous system, have similar radiographic densities; therefore, differentiation between these anatomical entities is also limited. Superimposition of structures was another major shortcoming of plain radiographs (Katz, 1984).

Within the last two decades, two imaging techniques became clinically available that revolutionized the field of neuroradiology. The imaging techniques of computed tomography (CT) and magnetic resonance imaging (MRI) substantially improved the ability to visualize structures of the body and, more specifically, the brain. This chapter reviews the neuroanatomical imaging technologies of CT and MRI, specifically as applied to the study of aphasia.

Computed Tomography

The first practical model of a computerized reconstructive scanner was developed by Godfrey Hounsfield and his colleagues in the late 1960s in Great Britain (Katz, 1984). Houns-field's interest in reconstruction techniques using the computer led to the development of the first clinically useful CT scanner (Seeram, 1982). This advancement in imaging was so significant that Hounsfield was awarded the Nobel Prize for physiology and medicine in 1979 (Martin and Brust, 1985). In 1973, approximately 5 years after its development, the first brain CT scanners were installed at the Mayo Clinic and the Massachusetts General Hospital (Seeram, 1982).

CT is a technique in which a computer reconstructs the internal structure of a selected body section (Weisberg et al., 1984). Many narrow beams of x-rays are directed into the selected body section from multiple directions. The amount of radiation that is absorbed by the different tissue densities is mathematically reconstructed to create a cross section of absorption values using a computer algorithm (Villafana, 1983). With the aid of a computer, the absorption information is collected as numerical values that are eventually converted into a gray-scale pictorial display (Oldendorf, 1985). Tomography, as in computed tomography, refers to the use of moving x-ray tubes, body parts, or x-ray image receptors to desuperimpose obstructing anatomy from the anatomy of interest (Carroll, 1985). This computerized display is quite different from the direct x-ray picture taken of a body section in plain radiograph films.

Attenuation in which the x-rays are reduced in intensity on passing through objects depends on structural densities (Carroll, 1985). The distribution of CT attenuation values has been established on a relative scale with the attenuation of water as a reference (De Groot, 1984). This scale is measured in Hounsfield units (HU), named for Hounsfield's contribution to the development of CT scanning technology. On the two extremes of the scale, bone and air have values of +1000 and −1000 Hounsfield units, respectively. Once the attenuation values are obtained, the numerical image can be converted to a gray-scale image. High-density bone is represented as white, since much of the CT x-ray beam is absorbed, and low-density air and cerebrospinal fluid are represented as black, since little of the x-ray beam is absorbed. All other values represent varying shades of gray (Seeram, 1982).

Attenuation coefficients are reconstructed for specific volume elements, or sections, of the object being scanned (Seeram, 1982). These volume elements are called voxels. A typical volume element in CT measures 10 mm in depth, 0.5 mm in width, and 0.5 mm in length. Thus, a voxel has three dimensions: depth, width, and length. Depth refers to slice thickness of the tissue that has been scanned. It is usually 10 mm in thickness but can be as thin as a few millimeters.

A pixel has only two dimensions: width and length. A pixel is a tiny picture element similar to the dots used to construct a photograph on newsprint. On the surface image of a CT scan, the image itself is reconstructed using pixels; the most common pixel used today is 0.5 mm (width) by 0.5 mm (length). CT scans produced in this manner are said to have a 512 by 512 matrix—for example, 512 pixels along the x-axis and 512 pixels along the y-axis. Each pixel is 0.5 mm in width and 0.5 mm in length. A CT scan that has been reconstructed on a 256 by 256 matrix has a pixel size that is 1.0 mm by 1.0 mm. The image reconstructed with a 512 by 512 matrix will be clearer than an image reconstructed with a 256 by 256 matrix because the pixel size on the 512 by 512 matrix is smaller (0.5 mm by 0.5 mm), thus allowing greater image resolution.

In addition to the intrinsic parameters specific to the CT technique, there are also extrinsic parameters specific to CT that are under operator control. The most important extrinsic parameters to CT studies of aphasia patients are image slice thickness and plane of image. The thickness of a slice of anatomical information chosen for a CT study is variable. The thicker the slice, the more information is mathematically averaged together within the section. Extremely thin slices, however, are generally not possible because of technical restrictions, nor are they advisable because of the dose of radiation (Alexander et al., 1986). Slice thickness in CT studies is generally 10 mm but can vary between 1 and 10 mm. CT slices are usually contiguous, with no space between slices. With regard to plane of image, the standard CT scan image is of the transverse axial plane. Although there is not universal agreement on a standard plane of section, the planes are often angled about 25° to the canthomeatal line (Hanaway et al., 1980).

CT scans can be obtained with or without contrast enhancement. Contrast enhancement refers to the method of improving visualization of certain structures and tissues by the use of iodinated contrast material (Seeram, 1982). In a contrast-enhanced study, radiopaque contrast material is injected intravenously prior to performing the CT scan (Martin and Brust, 1985). The injection of contrast material allows enhancement of regions of the brain that have either increased vasculature or an impaired blood-brain barrier. A contrast-enhanced area shows up as a lighter, white area on CT. Contrast enhancement is most effective in helping to visualize the presence of an area of cerebral infarction between approximately the fifth day after stroke onset and week 3 or 4 (Yock, 1985; Zulch, 1985).

Magnetic Resonance Imaging

The use of MRI in the medical field is relatively new; however, scientists have employed the technique of nuclear magnetic resonance in the laboratory for nearly 50 years (Gademann, 1984; Martin and Brust, 1985). The present surge of interest in medical applications for MRI stems from two studies done in the 1970s. Using rats, Damadian (1971) found that MRI could be used for discriminating between malignant tumors and normal tissue. Lauterbur (1973) found that an image of an object could be generated by coupling several projections of

magnetic fields and then selectively emphasizing certain of the fields. In the early 1980s, after years of intensive developmental work on the MRI systems, the focus of attention shifted from machine development to clinical application (Gademann, 1984). In 1984, the Food and Drug Administration (FDA) permitted two American companies to begin commercial sales of the devices to hospitals and physicians (Bydder and Steiner, 1982).

The concept of MRI is based on magnetic forces that inherently occur in the body (Gademann, 1984). Certain nuclei within the body (those with an odd number of protons) have their own individual magnetic properties. These nuclei spin on their own, creating randomly distributed small magnetic fields. The main component of the MRI system is a large superconducting magnet, which produces a strong external magnetic field. When a person is placed in the external magnetic field, the individual spinning nuclei become aligned with the main magnetic field. Once the nuclei are aligned, a specific radio frequency (RF) is applied to the field, and it tilts the resonant atoms at a specific angle. The nuclei now spin on a tilted axis to the main magnetic field. When the RF energy is switched off, the nuclei relax and emit their own specific RF signals. MR images are pictorial representations of the information emitted in these signals.

The appearance of structures in an MR image is based on four main intrinsic parameters that are specific to each tissue (Bradley, 1987; Breger and Kneeland, 1987). After the magnetic forces are applied to the body section of study, these four parameters determine to a large extent how the resulting images will appear. The four tissue characteristics are (a) the density of the spinning nuclei in the specific area of study (spin density); (b) the time it takes for the nuclei to relax back from their tilts to realign with the main magnetic field (T1); (c) the time it takes for the nuclei to dephase or lose their coherence with each other (T2); and (d) the flow characteristics of the substance (flow). These measurements vary according to the composition of the anatomical regions under study.

In addition to the inherent characteristics of body tissues, the appearance of images on MRI can be further adjusted or "weighted" by the operator's manipulation of the pattern and timing of the radio frequency pulses applied to an area of study (Crooks et al., 1982). The sequencing of radio frequency pulses can be adjusted to emphasize different degrees of spin density, T1 or T2 information in the resulting image. Specific adjustments can enhance various characteristics of tissues. For example, "T1-weighted images" provide excellent gray-matter/white-matter anatomical differentiation, while "T2-weighted images" are more sensitive to variations in fluids and pathology. Furthermore, adjustments can be made for various amounts of T1- or T2-weighting. For example, a lightly T2-weighted image versus a heavily T2-weighted image can demonstrate different characteristics of specific tissues.

Slice thickness available on commercial MRI scanners varies from 2 mm to 10 mm (Elster, 1986). As with CT, there is a trade-off between thickness of slice, signal intensity, and scanning time. Thinner slices, although they may demonstrate finer anatomical detail, require longer times to scan. The signal-to-noise ratio, or the proportion of noise to the signal, also becomes less desirable as the slices get thinner. The thicker the slice, however, the more anatomical information is averaged into an image. Typical options for slice thickness are 3, 5, 7, and 10 mm. Unlike standard CT, MRI image slices are usually not contiguous. Because there is some partial excitation of neighboring tissues outside of the area of study, it has been determined that inserting gaps between the slices is an effective correction for the overflow of magnetic force. Typically, an interslice space is 25% to 50% of the actual slice thickness, that is, a 2.5-mm gap for a study with 5-mm slice thickness (Field and Wehrli, 1990). Certain types of images can be obtained in MRI where interslice space is not necessary.

On all MRI scanners, an option exists for obtaining images in orthogonal (right angle) planes in the human head (Gademann, 1984). Axial, sagittal, and coronal images are directly obtainable from the digital data collected during the MRI study without the need to reposition the patient or perform computer reconstructions (Elster, 1986). Unlimited or oblique planes of study are also available, depending on the computer software capabilities of the respective system.

MR systems vary in the strength of their magnetic field. The strength of the magnet used has a direct influence on the quality of the images. This becomes important in the depiction of fine anatomical detail and the clarity of gray-matter/white-matter distinction (Jack et al., 1990). "Tesla" is a term that refers to the unit of magnetic field density used in MR imaging (Elster, 1986). One Tesla (T) is equal to 10,000 gauss or 10,000 times the approximate strength of the Earth's magnetic field on its surface. MRI systems using magnetic fields greater than 0.5 T are considered high field, and those with magnetic fields less than 0.5 T are considered low-field systems.

For a complete review of other operator-controlled MRI parameters, such as pulse sequences, pulse time intervals (time between the repetition of the radio frequency pulse [TR] and time to echo [TE]), matrix size, and number of signal averages (NEX), the reader is referred to Elster (1986) and to Field and Wehrli (1990).

Comparison of CT and MRI Technology

To review, CT is a technique in which a computer reconstructs the internal structure of a selected body section. The method used in CT is detection of radiation that passes through the body and is then mathematically reconstructed to create a cross section of absorption values by the use of a computer algorithm. Attenuation, in which the x-rays are reduced in intensity on passing through objects, depends solely on structural densities. MRI is a technique that uses the inherent property of spinning atomic nuclei in the body to obtain information. MR images are produced during relaxation of nuclei that are initially excited by various magnetic forces. The relaxing nuclei emit a signal, based on the density of the spinning nuclei, plus other magnetic properties of the tissues under study. Because of the intrinsic differences in the two imaging methods, there are certain contrasts that should be recognized when these techniques are used for the study of stroke.

Because CT is based on the use of x-radiation, the patient is exposed to a small amount of radiation during the study. In general, the radiation dose is related to the basic imaging parameters of the CT unit, which includes slice thickness of the images, collimation levels of the x-ray beams, and the x-ray detector efficiency. The maximum surface dose of radiation for a standard head CT scan is approximately 0.5 to 1.5 rads (Shapiro, 1990).

MR imaging does not employ the use of ionizing radiation; however, the entire process is based on the use of powerful magnets. Implanted ferromagnetic objects (those that contain iron), such as surgical clips, heart valves, orthopedic implants, or cochlear implants may be contraindicated for MR imaging. Most surgical clips, virtually all modern types of heart valves, and most orthopedic implants currently in use, however, are only weakly, if at all, ferromagnetic and pose no problems during MR examination (Pavlicek, 1988; Shellock and Schatz, 1991). Cardiac pacemakers have specifically been identified as a hazard for MR examination (Laakman et al., 1985; Pavlicek et al., 1983). The major concern with a pacemaker is possible damage to its electronic components as a result of the strong MR magnetization (Pavlicek, 1988).

MR images are not obscured by bone. There are no spinning nuclei in bone; therefore, bone is not affected by the magnetic forces applied to the brain and no signal can be emitted (Gademann, 1984). Because bone does not emit a signal and therefore does not obscure visualization of other anatomical areas of the brain, infarctions that are located on or near the cortex, in the cerebellum, or in the brain stem are well visualized on MRI (Kinkel et al., 1986). Since there is no signal emitted from bone, MR imaging likewise cannot demonstrate the extent and degree of calcifications in the brain, as can be demonstrated on CT.

Currently, it takes 20 to 30 minutes to complete a CT study of the brain. A routine MRI study of the brain takes approximately 1 hour, depending on the parameters of the study (slice thickness, number of planes of study, type of sequence of radio frequency pulses, etc.). For a patient who is unable to cooperate, is in an unstable condition, needs constant life support, or experiences claustrophobia, the time required to stay in the MR machine may be prohibitive. There are currently a variety of fast imaging techniques under investigation, however, that would decrease the time required to remain in the MRI machine (Cohen and Weisskoff, 1991).

As of April 1991, there were approximately 2000 MRI systems operating in the United States (Pollack, 1991). In contrast, many more hospitals own, or have access to, a CT scanner. MRI systems currently cost between $1 million and $2 million. The cost of an MRI study is also currently more than that of a CT study. These factors may currently make it more practical to obtain CT studies on stroke patients than MRI studies.

CHARACTERISTICS OF OCCLUSIVE INFARCT IN ADULT STROKE

Computed Tomography

A CT scan may appear almost or completely normal until 8 hours after stroke onset (Wang et al., 1988). At approximately 8 hours after stroke onset, depending on the size and location of the infarct, the first evidence of ischemia may appear. Between the 8 and 24 hours following stroke onset, a *noncontrast* CT may demonstrate a slight hypodense (dark) area with poor margins and a spotty appearance (Goldberg, 1983). Edema may cause effacement, or the smoothing-over appearance of cortical sulcal spaces (Weisberg et al., 1984). During this first 24 hours, there is little or no swelling or mass effect (Goldberg, 1983). Small lesions, without significant edema, may not become apparent until later in the chronic stage, when a cystic lesion forms (Goldberg, 1983).

After a few days, the hypodense area representing infarction becomes more distinct. It may take on a triangular, rectangular, trapezoid, round, or oval shape, depending on the occluded artery and the vascular territory involved (Bories et al., 1985). From the third to the fifth day after stroke onset, the low-density area becomes more homogeneous, with sharper edges, and the area of hypodensity increases (Goldberg, 1983). During this time, edema and tissue death are increasing and reaching their maximum. Swelling and mass effect depend on the size of the infarct. Some degree of mass effect is reported in 21% to 70% of infarcts and is most evident between the third and fifth days (Goldberg, 1983). Swelling, causing mass effect, and edema begin to decrease after the first week, and by the 12th to 21st day after stroke onset are usually completely resolved (Goldberg, 1983; Weisberg et al., 1984).

During the second and third weeks following stroke onset, curvilinear bands, which are either hyperdense (bright white) or isodense (same intensity as surrounding brain), often develop at the margins of or within the infarcted area (Goldberg, 1983). These bands are a result of new capillary ingrowth, improved circulation, or hemorrhage within the infarct. These bands cause the boundaries of the lesion to become less sharp than on earlier scans. Because of an increase in density of the lesion on CT during this time, the lesion may become isodense, making visualization of the lesion difficult. This phenomenon, which may occur during the second or third weeks after stroke onset, is called the "fogging effect" (Bories et al., 1985; Weisberg et al., 1984).

Starting at approximately 1 month after stroke onset, and continuing for 2 to 3 months, the resorption phase begins (Weisberg et al., 1984). The outline of the infarct becomes sharp, and the hypodense area begins to appear smaller because of absorption of the necrotic tissue and continued resolution of edema (Weisberg et al., 1984). Depending on the size and location of the infarct, atrophy from the necrotic brain tissue may cause the lateral ventricles to dilate and shift toward the infarcted area. There may also be a shift of the brain midline toward the side of the infarct. Atrophic change, demonstrated by a shrinking of the brain tissue and widening of the sulci, may be seen in the cortex overlying the infarct. Beginning in the fifth week poststroke, many necrotic infarcts become fluid-filled cysts that have a low attenuation value on CT similar to cerebrospinal fluid (Wang et al., 1988). By the end of the third month, chronic brain changes are usually complete (Goldberg, 1983; Weisberg et al., 1984). Figure 3.1 shows an example of the appearance of an infarct on a chronic (3.5 months postonset [MPO]) CT scan. (This same infarct, at 3.5 MPO on MRI, is explained and displayed in the next section.)

Magnetic Resonance Imaging

The strongest determinant of signal change on an MR image during the period of ischemia and subsequent infarction is the acute increase in the water content of tissue (Brant-Zawadzki, 1988). Water is composed chiefly of hydrogen elements (each water molecule has two hydrogen nuclei), and hydrogen is the nucleus most studied in magnetic resonance (Bradley, 1987). Water is the greatest contributor to the MR signal detected from a voxel of tissue (Bradley, 1987).

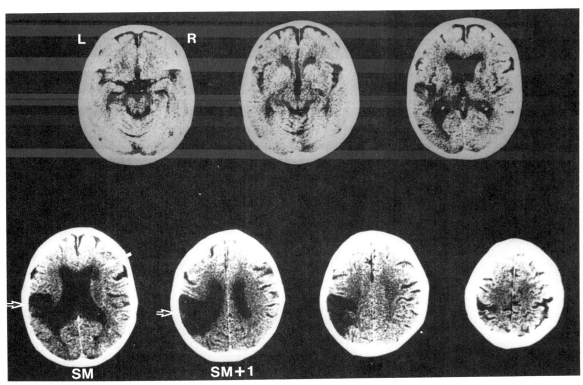

Figure 3.1.   CT scan performed at 3.5 months postonset (MPO) revealed bilateral lesions. The lesion in the left hemisphere was centered in the supramarginal and angular gyrus areas, the cortex, and subjacent white matter (slices SM and SM + 1, *black and white arrows*). There was a small right-hemisphere lesion in the anterior periventricular white matter deep to the lower motor cortex area for the mouth (slice SM, *white arrow*). The left hemisphere is shown on the left side of the figure (see *L* and *R* on the first slice). The language behavior for this 71-year-old female was consistent with conduction aphasia.

The concentration of brain water starts to change in the first hours after an ischemic event (Brant-Zawadzki, 1988). There is an accumulation of water within the cells of the affected area, which is referred to as cytotoxic edema (Brant-Zawadzki and Kucharczyk, 1987). Cytotoxic edema is a result of ischemia and is found in association with acute infarcts (Bradley, 1987). Within the first 30 minutes of ischemia, there is a 3% to 5% increase in the water content in the area (Brant-Zawadzki and Kucharczyk, 1987). These changes in water content allow MRI to detect pathology within the first hour or two following vascular occlusion (Brant-Zawadzki, 1988). By the sixth hour, the blood-brain barrier typically begins to break down, which allows additional leakage of water and protein from the vascular spaces (Brant-Zawadzki and Kucharczyk, 1987). This secondary process of edema is called vasogenic edema and continues to occur for the first few days after stroke onset, producing mass effect in and around the area of the infarct.

During the initial stage of ischemia, both the T1 relaxation rate (the time it takes for the nuclei to relax back from their tilts to realign with the main magnetic field) and the T2 relaxation rate (the time it takes for the nuclei to dephase or lose their coherence with each other) are prolonged on MRI, indicating water accumulation (Kinkel et al., 1986). Prolonged relaxation time on a T1-weighted image will cause the area of ischemia to look like a low-intensity (dark black) zone. On T2-weighted images, the area of ischemia will present as a high-intensity (bright white) zone. T2 images tend to be more sensitive to changes (cytotoxic edema) at the very earliest hours after stroke onset (Moseley, 1988; Sipponen et al., 1983). The ischemic evolution, including mass effects, progresses for the first 3 to 7 days and typically stabilizes in the second week (Kinkel et al., 1986; Sipponen et al., 1983).

Some ischemic infarcts may be complicated by hemorrhage. Up to 42% of patients who initially present with ischemic infarction develop secondary hemorrhage (Brant-Zawadzki, 1988). Within the evolution of infarction from mass effect to the resolution stage, usually in the second week following infarction, a small amount of leaking blood may escape from the site of damage. These hemorrhages are generally silent clinically. Acute hemorrhage within an area of infarction is demonstrated by an excessive shortening of T2 relaxation time, or a low-signal (dark black) area on T2-weighted images.

Whether combined with hemorrhage or not, after approximately the second week, infarcts evolve in a typical pattern (Brant-Zawadzki, 1988). By the third week, and into the chronic stage in the evolution of the infarct, mass effect and edema begin to resolve and subsequent atrophy develops (Brant-Zawadzki and Kucharczyk, 1987; Kinkel et al., 1986). Cells may die in the necrotic areas of the brain, and tissues may become soft because of greater water content. On T2-weighted images, encephalomalacia, or "soft brain," is demonstrated as high signal intensity (bright white), similar to the appearance of cerebrospinal fluid (CSF). This bright intensity area includes the central core of the chronic infarct combined with any additional surrounding edema. On T1-weighted images, the central core of the chronic infarct is demonstrated as low signal intensity (dark black), similar to the appearance of CSF, with less distinction of surrounding edema.

An example of the appearance of an infarct on a chronic (3.5 MPO) MRI scan is shown in Figure 3.2. T1- and T2-weighted images of this infarct are shown in Figure 3.2 (*top* and *bottom*, respectively).

LOCALIZATION OF LANGUAGE AREAS AND LESION SITE ANALYSIS

Computed Tomography

Most CT scans examined in our research are obtained at approximately 20° to the canthomeatal line, without contrast, with 10-mm slice thickness and 3-mm slice overlap through the ventricles beginning at the level of the suprasellar cistern. CT scan slices are contiguous and are obtained in the transverse axial plane. Figure 3.3 illustrates the location of cortical language areas in relationship to the ventricular system (in a lateral view diagram), with slices marked at 20° to the canthomeatal line, similar to CT scan slices. Numbers on this diagram refer to Brodmann's cortical areas as follows: 44 and 45, Broca's area; 22, Wernicke's area; 40, supramarginal gyrus area; 39, angular gyrus area. CT scan lesion site analysis currently includes cortical language areas as well as subcortical areas. These cortical and subcortical areas are diagrammed on the axial CT scan slices shown in Figure 3.4. These axial slices show the location of cortical and subcortical language areas in relationship to the shape of the ventricles on CT scan slices performed at 20° to the canthomeatal line. Most of these neuroanatomical areas are identified in various CT scan atlases (DeArmond et al., 1976; Hanaway et al., 1980; Matsui and Hirano, 1978).

The complete and final borders of an infarct are best visualized on chronic CT scans, that is, those scans performed after 2 or 3 months postonset. Acute CT scans that are performed earlier than 2 or 3 months postonset do not accurately reveal the final borders of an infarct and are not useful in making predictions for long-term recovery in speech and language functions after stroke. To use the information in this chapter, a CT scan should be obtained after 2 or 3 months after stroke onset, according to the protocol described above. CT scans performed in this manner will conform to the CT scan slice images shown in Figure 3.4.

The extent of lesion (amount of infarction) within each cortical and subcortical neuroanatomical area on the CT scan is visually assessed using a 0–5 point scale, where 0 = no lesion; 1 = equivocal lesion; 2 = small, patchy, or partial lesion; 2.5 = patchy, less than half of area has lesion; 3 = half of area has lesion; 3.5 = patchy, more than half of area has lesion; 4 = more than half of area has solid lesion; and 5 = total area has solid lesion. Lesion-extent values >3 (indicating lesion in greater than half of a specific area) are of special importance, since they have been observed to correlate with increased severity of language deficit (Naeser et al., 1987; Naeser et al., 1989; Naeser et al., 1990).

For a discussion of the localization of language areas and lesion site analysis on MRI scans, the reader is referred to the last section in this chapter, "Future Trends in Brain Imaging."

CLINICAL CT STUDIES AND RESULTS

This section focuses on the relationship between lesions in a select few of the cortical and subcortical areas on CT scan and two specific areas of language recovery in aphasia: (*a*) recovery of auditory language comprehension in Wernicke's

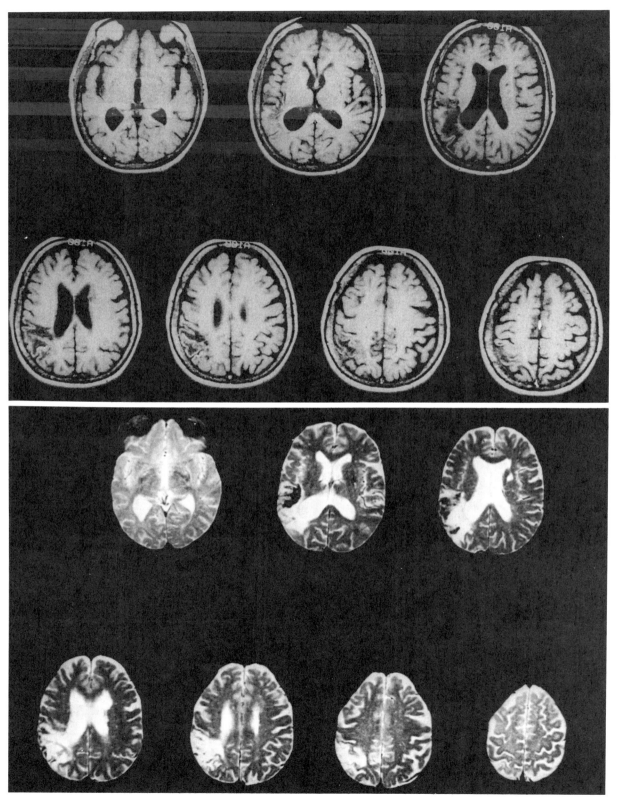

Figure 3.2.

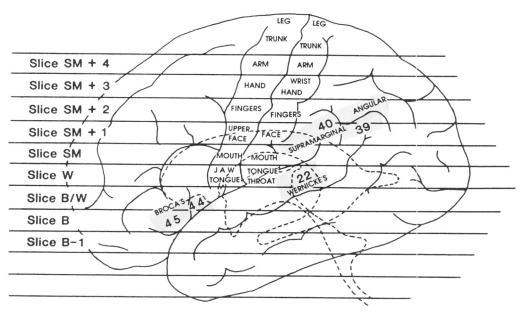

Figure 3.3. Lateral diagram of the location of cortical language areas in relationship to the ventricular system (*dotted lines*). The CT scan slices are marked at 20° to the canthomeatal line, similar to the angle at which they are performed. Numbers refer to Brodmann's areas as follows: 44 and 45, Broca's area; 22, Wernicke's area; 40, supramarginal gyrus area; 39, angular gyrus area. The different parts of the motor and sensory homunculi are labeled for each CT scan slice. *Note:* The motor cortex area for the mouth is located on CT scan slice SM.

aphasia patients and global aphasia patients, and (*b*) recovery of some functional spontaneous speech in patients with severe limitation in speech output. The emphasis in this section is not on aphasia syndromes per se but rather on recovery in the two aspects of language behavior mentioned above: auditory comprehension and spontaneous speech. The term "recovery" does not usually refer to "amount of change" or "rate of change" from early scores to late scores. The term "recovery" in this section usually refers to the actual language scores obtained by a patient after at least 6 MPO. Language behavior was measured with the Boston Diagnostic Aphasia Examination (BDAE) (Goodglass and Kaplan, 1983) and/or the Boston Assessment of Severe Aphasia (BASA) (Helm-Estabrooks et al., 1989b). The CT scans were performed at least 2 or 3 months after stroke onset.

Most material in this section is based on our CT scan research at the Boston University Aphasia Research Center, Boston VA Medical Center. The reader is referred to the original publica-

tions for complete speech and language data and complete CT scan data.

Recovery of Auditory Language Comprehension in Wernicke's Aphasia

In this retrospective study, CT scans and auditory comprehension scores were examined for 10 male Wernicke's aphasia patients classified after 6 MPO as mild, good recovery (GR) cases (*n* = 5), or moderate-severe, poor recovery (PR) cases (*n* = 5) (Naeser et al., 1987). Each patient was right-handed and had suffered single-episode left hemisphere occlusive-vascular stroke between the ages of 47 and 71 years (mean = 58.4, SD = 6.9), with no significant group differences. The CT scans used for lesion localization were performed between 3 and 36 MPO.

The auditory comprehension subtest scores and the Overall Auditory Comprehension Z-scores from the Boston Diagnostic Aphasia Exam (BDAE) (Goodglass and Kaplan, 1972) were examined from two time periods. Time 1 (T1) scores were

Figure 3.2. MRI scans of the same patient shown in Figure 3.1, performed 1 day after the CT scan (3.5 MPO). These MRI scans were performed using a 1.5 Tesla magnetic field. **Top,** The T1-weighted axial image (TR 500 msec, TE 20 msec) revealed bilateral lesions generally similar to those shown on the CT scan in Figure 3.1. The lesion appears black on a T1-weighted image. The lesion in the left hemisphere was centered in the supramarginal and angular gyrus areas. The lesion in the right hemisphere was located in the white matter deep to the lower motor cortex area for the mouth. These bilateral lesions appear to be smaller on the T1-weighted MRI images than on the CT scan images, because the T1-weighted MRI images primarily show only the cavity portion of the lesion. **Bottom,** The T2-weighted axial image (TR 2500 msec, TE 80 msec) revealed bilateral lesions generally similar to those shown on the CT scan in Figure 3.1 and on the T1-weighted MRI scan (at *top* of

this figure). The lesion appears white on a T2-weighted image. The lesion in the left hemisphere was centered in the supramarginal and angular gyrus areas. The lesion in the right hemisphere was located in the white matter deep to the lower motor cortex area for the mouth. These bilateral lesions appear to be larger on the T2-weighted MRI images than on the CT scan images, because the T2-weighted MRI images show the lesion plus surrounding gliosis, which may not be part of the actual lesion. Thus, these T2-weighted MRI images tend to exaggerate the borders of the lesion. *Note:* Hemosiderin (a breakdown product from blood) was present in the left hemisphere, anterior to the parietal lobe lesion, on this T2 MRI scan. Hemosiderin appears black on the MRI scan. The presence of hemosiderin in this case indicated that the patient experienced a partial hemorrhagic component to this stroke sometime during the first 3 months. (A CT scan performed at 3 days after stroke onset had not shown any bleeding.)

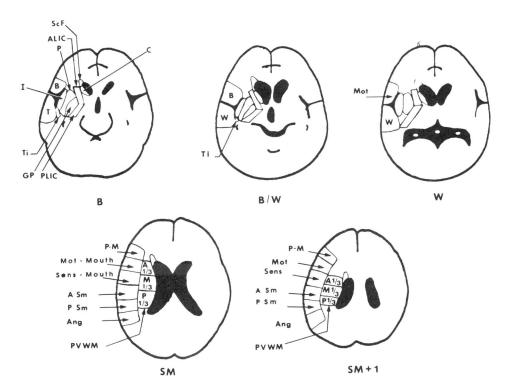

Figure 3.4. Location of specific neuroanatomical areas on CT scans that are analyzed for presence of lesion in the CT scan lesion site analysis. The CT scan slices B, B/W, W, SM, and SM + 1 are labeled according to the Naeser and Hayward (1978) slice labeling system. Each neuroanatomical area is examined for extent of lesion using a 0–5 point scale (0 = no lesion; 5 = entire area has solid lesion; see text). B = Broca's area (45 on slice B; 44 on slice B/W); T = temporal lobe anterior–inferior to Wernicke's area on slice B; Ti = temporal isthmus; I = insular structures including insula, extreme capsule, claustrum, external capsule; P = putamen; GP = globus pallidus; ALIC = anterior limb, internal capsule; PLIC = posterior limb, internal capsule; Sc F = medial subcallosal fasciculus; C = caudate; W = Wernicke's area (22); Mot = motor cortex; PM = premotor cortex; Sens = sensory cortex; A Sm = anterior supramarginal gyrus; P Sm = posterior supramarginal gyrus; Ang = angular gyrus; PVWM = periventricular white-matter area (A ⅓, anterior ⅓ PVWM; M ⅓, middle ⅓ PVWM; P ⅓, posterior ⅓ PVWM).

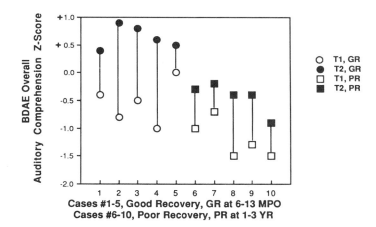

Figure 3.5. Time 1 (1–2 MPO) and Time 2 (6 MPO or 1–3 years). Overall Auditory Comprehension Z-scores for 10 Wernicke's aphasia patients. Graph shows that there was overlap in the T1 scores among some of the good recovery (GR) cases and poor recovery (PR) cases; thus the T1 test scores could not be used on a case-by-case basis to predict GR or PR after 6 MPO.

obtained at 1 to 2 MPO; Time 2 (T2) scores were obtained after 6 MPO.

Patients could not be differentiated on a case-by-case basis using only the early T1 test scores. The Time 2 testing was administered at 6 to 13 MPO for the mild group and at 12 to 38 MPO for the moderate-severe group. The T2 scores for the moderate-severe group were taken as long after onset as possible to extend the potential recovery period. Patients were differentiated on the basis of T2 scores as follows: (a) good recovery (GR) cases scored above 0 (above the 50th percentile) on the BDAE Overall Auditory Comprehension Z-score; (b) poor recovery (PR) cases scored below 0 (below the 50th percentile). (See Fig. 3.5.) The reader is referred to the original paper for exact T1 and T2 test scores for all 10 Wernicke's aphasia patients (Naeser et al., 1987).

The CT scans were analyzed with two methods: (a) the CT scan lesion site analysis described above, where the 0–5 extent-of-lesion scale was used to visually rate the degree of damage (amount of infarction) within each cortical and subcortical area, and (b) a computer-based lesion *size* analysis that quantified the total percent left-hemisphere temporoparietal lesion size (Jernigan et al., 1979; Naeser et al., 1981).

Since Wernicke's time, there have been multiple interpretations regarding the exact location and limits of the so-called "Wernicke's area" (Bogen and Bogen, 1976). For the purposes of this study, Wernicke's area was defined as the posterior two-thirds of the left superior temporal gyrus area. On CT scans, the anterior half of Wernicke's area (i.e., the middle third of the superior temporal gyrus area) was located lateral to the maximum width of the third ventricle on slice B/W (Fig. 3.4). In addition, the posterior half of Wernicke's area—that is, the posterior third of the superior temporal gyrus area—was located lateral to the roof of the third ventricle on slice W (Fig. 3.4). The supramarginal and angular gyrus areas in the parietal lobe were also analyzed on slices SM and SM + 1 (Fig. 3.4).

All GR Wernicke's patients with T2 Auditory Comprehension Z-scores above 0 had lesion in only half, or less than half, of Wernicke's area. All PR Wernicke's patients with T2 Auditory Comprehension Z-scores below 0 had lesion in more than half of Wernicke's area (see Fig. 3.6 [top]). The correlation between T2 BDAE Overall Auditory Comprehension Z-scores and extent of lesion within Wernicke's area was −.91 (p<.001).

The total percent left temporoparietal lesion size was not useful in distinguishing between cases with good recovery and those with poor recovery of auditory comprehension at T2 (see Fig. 3.6 [bottom]). The correlation between the T2 Auditory Comprehension Z-scores and total percent left temporoparietal lesion size was −.56, n.s. There was also no significant correlation between "amount of change" between T1 and T2 and extent of lesion within Wernicke's area (r = −0.494, n.s.), or total percent left-hemisphere temporoparietal lesion size (r = −0.013, n.s.). There was a significant correlation, however, between the total percent left temporoparietal lesion size and the T2 Visual Confrontation Naming scores from the BDAE (−.88, p<.001). This latter finding (naming) is in general agreement with Kertesz (1979), who found that the highest degree of correlation between total lesion size and severity of aphasia existed for anomic aphasia patients.

Case Examples

Figure 3.7 shows the CT scan of a Wernicke's aphasia patient with lesion in Wernicke's cortical area, *only* on slice W, and good recovery of auditory comprehension at 7 to 10 MPO (lesion in about half of Wernicke's total area). Figure 3.8 shows the CT scan of a Wernicke's aphasia patient with complete lesion in Wernicke's cortical area on both slice B/W and slice W, and poor recovery of auditory comprehension at 14 MPO (lesion in all of Wernicke's area).

Results from this study support the notion that careful examination of extent of lesion within Wernicke's area on a chronic CT scan (performed after 2 or 3 MPO) may be useful in predicting long-term recovery of auditory comprehension in Wernicke's aphasia patients. Those patients with lesion in only half, or less than half, of Wernicke's area have a better prognosis for recovery of auditory comprehension within the first year after stroke onset.

Recovery of Auditory Language Comprehension in Global Aphasia

In this retrospective study, CT scans and auditory comprehension scores were examined for 14 right-handed stroke patients with global aphasia (12 men and 2 women, ages 50 to 66 years) who had unilateral left-hemisphere ischemic infarcts (Naeser et al., 1990). All patients had been tested a minimum of twice with the BDAE (Goodglass and Kaplan, 1972). T1

testing ranged from 1 to 4 MPO. All patients had been classified as globally aphasic at T1 on the basis of the BDAE. All patients had BDAE Overall Auditory Comprehension Z-scores at T1 that were below −1.0; that is, they had severe auditory comprehension deficits. T2 testing was approximately 1 to 2 years after stroke onset.

All patients had CT scans that were obtained after 2 MPO (range, 2 to 110 MPO). CT scan lesion site analysis was performed. Most of the cortical and subcortical areas shown in Figure 3.4 were visually assessed for extent of lesion, including major frontal, parietal, and temporal lobe areas, as well as subcortical areas. Special emphasis was placed on analyzing lesion extent in Wernicke's cortical area (and immediate subjacent white matter) on CT scan slices B/W and W, as well as lesion extent in the subcortical temporal lobe structure, the temporal isthmus area, on CT scan slices B and B/W.

The subcortical temporal isthmus area contains auditory pathways from the medial geniculate body to Heschl's gyrus. Lesion in the temporal isthmus area has been associated with producing auditory language comprehension deficits since Nielsen (1946). Its location was defined as the white matter that is inferior to the sylvian fissure/insular area and superior to the temporal horn (Naeser et al., 1982; Nielsen, 1946). (See Fig. 3.9.)

Nielsen (1946, pp. 119–120) has described the following measurements of the small subcortical temporal isthmus area: "It measures from 10 to 15 mm across and is in height nearly equal to that of the thalamus. . . . The artery of supply of the isthmus is the anterior choroidal." In the present study, only the anterior half of the temporal isthmus was evaluated for extent of lesion in the auditory pathways; the posterior half of the temporal isthmus contains visual pathways.

On the basis of CT scan lesion site analysis, the subjects were classified into two groups. Group 1 global aphasia cases had cortical/subcortical lesion in the frontal, parietal, and temporal lobes, including Wernicke's cortical area. Each case in Group 1 (n = 9) had lesion in at least half of Wernicke's cortical area. Group 1 cases are labeled FPT cases to reflect cortical/subcortical lesion in the *f*rontal, *p*arietal and *t*emporal lobes.

Group 2 global aphasia cases (n = 5) also had cortical/subcortical lesion in the frontal and parietal lobes, but only subcortical lesion in the temporal lobe, including the subcortical temporal isthmus area (Ti). Group 2 cases are labeled FPTi cases to reflect cortical/subcortical lesion in the *f*rontal and *p*arietal lobes, but only subcortical temporal lobe lesion including the temporal isthmus (Ti). Both groups had similar mean lesion-extent values in frontal, parietal, and subcortical areas, including the subcortical Ti area. All cases in the FPT group had lesion in more than half of Wernicke's cortical area; none of the cases in the FPTi group had cortical lesion in Wernicke's area.

There was no significant difference in age at stroke onset between the two groups (FPT group: mean = 58.2 years, SD = 4.2; FPTi group: mean = 57.8 years, SD = 5.0). Each group had only one woman. There were no significant differences between the two groups in terms of MPO when T1 or T2 testing was performed.

The T2 Auditory Comprehension Z-scores were *above* −0.5 for four of the five FPTi cases and *below* −0.5 for eight of the nine FPT cases (Fig. 3.10). There was a significantly greater increase (p<.01) in the amount of recovery that had taken place

Figure 3.6. Top, Graph showing a highly significant correlation ($r = -91$, $p < .001$) between total extent of lesion within Wernicke's area on CT scan slices B/W and W, and T2 BDAE Overall Auditory Comprehension Z-scores for 10 Wernicke's aphasia patients. A total extent-of-lesion value of 10 reflects a rating of 5 (complete solid lesion) in Wernicke's area on both CT slices B/W and W. Patients with total extent-of-lesion values ≤6 have lesion in only half, or less than half, of Wernicke's area; these patients had good recovery after 6 MPO, and T2 BDAE Z-scores above 0 or above the 50th percentile. Patients with total extent-of-lesion values >6 have lesion in more than half of Wernicke's area; these patients still had poor recovery 1 to 3 years after stroke onset. **Bottom,** Graph showing no significant correlation ($r = -.56$, n.s.) between total percent left temporoparietal lesion size on CT scan slices B, B/W, W, SM, and SM + 1, and T2 BDAE Overall Auditory Comprehension Z-scores for 10 Wernicke's aphasia patients. There was overlap between the GR cases and the PR cases around the 10% lesion-size value. Total lesion size could not be used to separate all GR and PR cases at T2 testing. Only total extent of lesion within Wernicke's area could be used to separate all GR and PR cases at T2 testing (see Figure 3.6, *Top*).

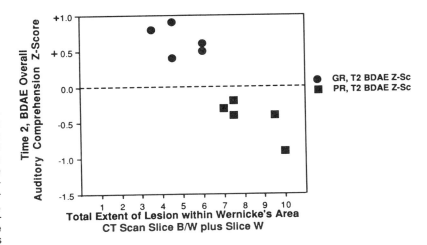

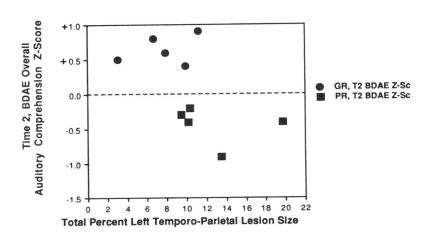

from T1 to T2 for the FPTi group versus the FPT group in the BDAE Overall Auditory Comprehension Z-score. The mean change from T1 to T2 for the FPTi group was +1.58. The mean change from T1 to T2 for the FPT group was only +0.65.

The FPTi cases had a significantly greater ($p<.01$) amount of recovery from T1 to T2 at the single-word level of comprehension (Word Discrimination and Body-Part Identification subtests) than did the FPT cases. Patients in the FPTi group actually had significantly higher ($p<.01$) Body-Part Identification absolute scores at T2 than did patients in the FPT group (T2 FPTi mean = 14.3, SD = 3.6; T2 FPT mean = 5.7, SD = 4.5).

Thus, most global aphasia cases with temporal lobe lesion that included at least half of Wernicke's cortical area had poor recovery of auditory comprehension at 1 to 2 years postonset, whereas most global aphasia cases with only subcortical temporal lobe lesion including the subcortical temporal isthmus had better recovery of auditory comprehension at 1 or 2 years poststroke.

There were no significant differences between the two groups in the amount of recovery that had taken place from T1 to T2 in the number of words per phrase length in spontaneous speech, single-word repetition, or naming. Most subjects in each group remained severely impaired in these three aspects of language behavior at T2. The reader is referred to the original paper for all exact T1 and T2 scores (Naeser et al., 1990).

Case Examples

Figure 3.11 shows the CT scan and BDAE Overall Auditory Comprehension Z-scores for an FPTi case, with relatively good recovery of auditory comprehension after 1 year postonset. Figure 3.12 shows the CT scan and BDAE Overall Auditory Comprehension Z-scores for an FPT case, with poor recovery of auditory comprehension even at 8 years after stroke onset.

Results from this study suggest that careful examination of cortical versus subcortical lesion in the temporal lobe on CT scan provides information regarding potential for recovery of some auditory language comprehension (especially single-word comprehension) after 1 year postonset in a subset of global aphasia patients. A majority of the patients (approximately 80%) with only subcortical temporal isthmus lesion in the temporal lobe (versus cortical lesion in Wernicke's area in the temporal lobe) had increased recovery of single-word comprehension after 1 year postonset.

The results from this study support the notion of Sarno and Levita (1979, 1981) that global aphasia patients are not a homogeneous group. These results suggest that careful examination of cortical versus subcortical lesion in the temporal lobe can result in information that may be useful in predicting a subset of global aphasia patients who have potential for in-

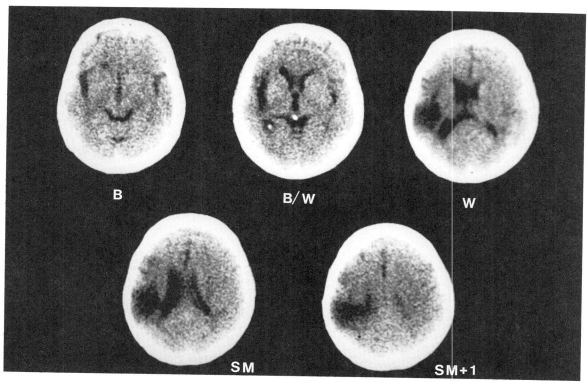

Figure 3.7. CT scan performed 24 MPO in a mild Wernicke's aphasia patient (Case 2) who had good recovery (+0.9 on BDAE Auditory Comprehension Z-score) at T2 testing (7 MPO). Lesion was present only in the posterior half of Wernicke's area on slice W (lesion-extent value, 4.5). There was additional parietal lobe lesion in the anterior and posterior supramarginal gyrus areas, surface and deep.

creased recovery of auditory comprehension 1 or 2 years after stroke onset.

Recovery of Spontaneous Speech

Our research and that of others has demonstrated that presence of lesion in certain subcortical white-matter areas on CT scan can have a profound effect on limiting spontaneous speech (Alexander et al., 1987; Hier et al., 1977; Naeser et al., 1982; Naeser et al., 1989). In our 1989 study, for example, we observed recovery of spontaneous speech to be related to amount of lesion in two specific white-matter areas *combined:* (*a*) the medial subcallosal fasciculus area, which is located deep to Broca's area on slices B and B/W; and (*b*) the middle one-third of the periventricular white-matter area, which is located deep to the motor/sensory cortex area for the mouth on slice SM. These two important areas are described in detail, later, within this section.

In this retrospective study, CT scans and number of words per phrase length in elicited spontaneous speech were examined for 27 right-handed aphasia patients (24 men and 3 women) with single-episode, left-hemisphere, occlusive-vascular strokes (thromboembolic infarcts) (Naeser et al., 1989). Their mean age at onset was 57.6 years (SD = 7.6; range, 35 to 69 years). Each patient had a CT scan performed between 2 months and 9 years following stroke onset.

The number of words per phrase length for spontaneous speech was determined from the elicited spontaneous speech sample for description of the Cookie Theft Picture from the

BDAE (Goodglass and Kaplan, 1972). These speech samples were obtained from the latest testing time available following stroke onset (6 MPO to 9 years), and they were used to assign patients to one of four groups, based on severity of impairment of spontaneous speech. The classification of patients according to severity of spontaneous speech was carried out independently from the CT scan analysis.

Group 1: No Speech or Only a Few Irrelevant Words. Group 1 consisted of seven patients (six men, one woman) who were able to provide either no speech or only a few irrelevant words in describing the Cookie Theft Picture. (See Table 3.1 for speech samples.) The speech samples for these patients were obtained at a variety of times postonset, ranging from 9 MPO to 8 years. For information on auditory comprehension, repetition, and naming for each patient, see Table 3.2. Not all cases were globally aphasic in all areas of language.

Group 2: Only Stereotypies. Group 2 consisted of 10 patients (all men) who were able to provide only stereotypies in describing the Cookie Theft Picture. (See Table 3.1 for speech samples.) The speech samples for these patients were obtained from 6 MPO to 9 years. This group, like Group 1, included cases who were not globally aphasic in all areas of language. For more information on each patient, see Table 3.2.

Group 3: A Few Words and/or Some Overlearned Phrases. Group 3 consisted of five patients (four men and one woman) who were able to provide a few words and/or some overlearned phrases in describing the Cookie Theft Picture. (See Table 3.1 for speech samples.) Their spontaneous speech was more difficult to classify and was considered "borderline" between the most severe cases in Groups 1 and 2 and the least severe cases in Group 4. The speech samples for these patients were obtained from 7 MPO to 4.5 years. This group was similar to

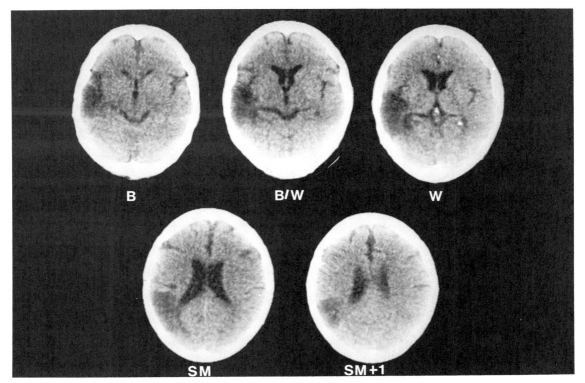

Figure 3.8. CT scan performed 7 MPO in a severe Wernicke's aphasia patient (Case 10) who had poor recovery (−0.9 on BDAE Auditory Comprehension Z-score) at Time 2 testing (14 MPO). Extensive lesion was present in Wernicke's area on both slices B/W and W (extent-of-lesion value, 5 on each slice = total extent-of-lesion value of 10). Large temporal lobe lesion was also present on slice B (extent-of-lesion value, 4.5), anterior and inferior to Wernicke's area. There was additional parietal lobe lesion in anterior and posterior supramarginal gyrus areas, surface and deep. There was also some lesion in the angular gyrus on slices SM and SM + 1.

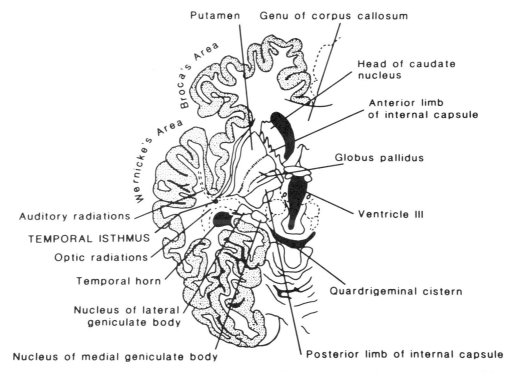

Figure 3.9. Schematic drawing of CT scan slice B/W (left hemisphere) showing location of the auditory radiations within the anterior half of the temporal isthmus (Ti). The Ti is located in the white matter inferior to the sylvian fissure and superior to the temporal horn.

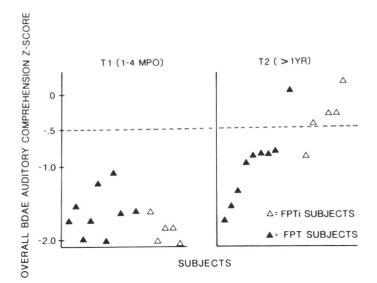

Figure 3.10. Graph of BDAE Overall Auditory Comprehension Z-scores for all cases at time 1 (T1) testing and time 2 (T2) testing. Note that at T1 testing, not one FPT case (cortical/subcortical lesion in the frontal lobe, parietal lobe, and temporal lobe, including Wernicke's cortical area) or FPTi case (cortical/subcortical lesion in the frontal and parietal lobes, but only subcortical temporal lobe lesion including the temporal isthmus) achieved a Z-score that was better than −1.0. At T2 testing, four of five FPTi cases achieved Z-scores better than −.05. At T2 testing, only one of nine FPT cases achieved a Z-score better than −0.5.

Groups 1 and 2 in that not all cases were globally aphasic in all areas of language. For more information on each patient, see Table 3.2.

Group 4: Nonfluent Broca's. Group 4 consisted of five patients (four men and one woman) who were able to provide verbal information relevant to the Cookie Theft Picture with reduced, hesitant, poorly articulated, agrammatical speech. (See Table 3.1 for speech samples.) The speech samples for these patients were obtained from 7 MPO to 6 years. This group was milder in all language modalities than the other three groups. For more information on each patient, see Table 3.2.

When t-tests were used to compare the BDAE scores between the groups, the patients in Group 4 had significantly higher ($p<.005$) Auditory Comprehension Z-scores and Visual Confrontation Naming scores than the patients in Groups 1, 2, or 3. In addition, the patients in Group 4 had significantly higher ($p< .005$) Word Repetition scores than the patients in Group 2. There were no other significant differences in auditory comprehension, word repetition, or naming among the groups.

CT scan lesion site analysis was performed. The cortical and subcortical areas on CT scan that were examined for extent of lesion for each patient are shown in Figure 3.4.

No significant differences (Mann-Whitney U-Tests, $p < .01$ and beyond) were observed in the extent-of-lesion data for specific lesion site areas, between the aphasia patients with no speech (Group 1) and those with stereotypies (Group 2). Therefore, the lesion site data from these two groups were combined, forming a no speech/stereotypies group ($n = 17$) for comparison with the nonfluent Broca's group ($n = 5$). (The lesion site data for patients who used only a few words and/or some overlearned phrases [Group 3] are discussed later.)

When the extent-of-lesion data for specific lesion site areas for each individual case were examined, there was no single

neuroanatomical area alone that could discriminate the 17 no speech/stereotypies cases from the 5 nonfluent Broca's cases. There were, however, two lesion site areas that, when *combined,* produced no overlap between the no speech/stereotypies cases and the nonfluent Broca's cases. These two lesion site areas were two subcortical white-matter areas, including (*a*) the medial subcallosal fasciculus area (M Sc F), mean lesion extent over slices B and B/W; and (*b*) the middle one-third periventricular white-matter area (M $\frac{1}{3}$ PVWM), slice SM. The locations of these two areas on CT scan are shown in the shaded areas in Figure 3.13 (*top*).

A graph showing the extent of lesion in these two white-matter areas, combined, for the no speech/stereotypies cases versus the nonfluent Broca's cases shows no overlap between these two groups (Fig. 3.13 [*bottom*]). All the no speech/stereotypies cases had summed lesion-extent scores above 7, and all the nonfluent Broca's cases had summed lesion-extent scores below 6. No other lesion site combination could be used to discriminate these 22 cases into the two groups.

The mean lesion-extent values in the M Sc F, alone, were not adequate to discriminate these two different groups of patients. The lesion-extent values in the M $\frac{1}{3}$ PVWM, alone, also were not adequate to discriminate these two different groups of patients. It was only when the lesion-extent values were combined for these two lesion site areas (M Sc F at slices B and B/W, plus the M $\frac{1}{3}$ PVWM at slice SM) that the two groups were successfully discriminated on the basis of CT scan lesion-extent values. The neuroanatomical connections contained within these two white-matter pathway areas are discussed briefly, below.

Medial Subcallosal Fasciculus Area

The M Sc F area is a narrow white-matter area surrounding the lateral angle of the frontal horn containing a pathway through which fibers pass from the supplementary motor area (SMA) and the cingulate gyrus area 24 to the caudate. The subcallosal fasciculus was first described by Muratoff (1893) in the dog brain as the ''fasciculus subcallosus.'' It is located under the corpus callosum. Dejerine (1895) has diagrammed it in the human brain and labeled the medial portion as substance *grise sous-ependymaire* (Sge). The medial portion of the M Sc F is very narrow, and in fact, it is only one-tenth the distance from the lateral border of the frontal horn to the cortical mantle. (This represents only approximately 1 millimeter on a CT scan.) Yakovlev and Locke (1961) have diagrammed these SMA and cingulate projections to the caudate in detail in the monkey brain. In their work, the most medial portion of the subcallosal fasciculus is labeled stratum subcallosum, St Sbc (Fig. 3.14).

Research by Benjamin and Van Hoesen (1982) using horseradish peroxidase injections in monkey brains has shown strong reciprocal connections between cingulate gyrus area 24 and the SMA. The importance of the SMA in ''the development of the intention to act'' has been reviewed by Goldberg (1985). Research by Barnes et al. (1980) using the autoradiography technique in monkey brains has shown that a major entry point for direct projections from the cingulate gyrus to the caudate (and indirect projections from the SMA to the caudate due to strong cingulate-SMA reciprocal connections) is in the most medial white matter surrounding the lateral angle of the frontal horn in its most rostral portion.

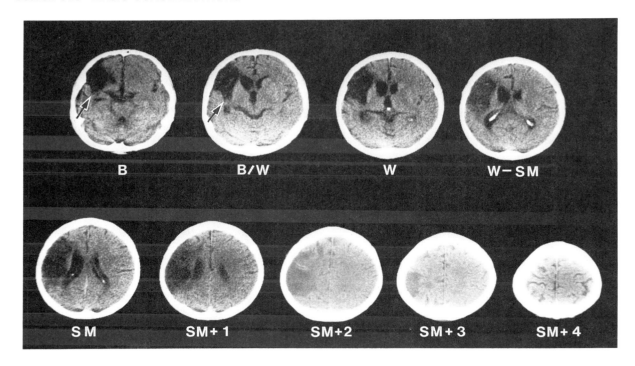

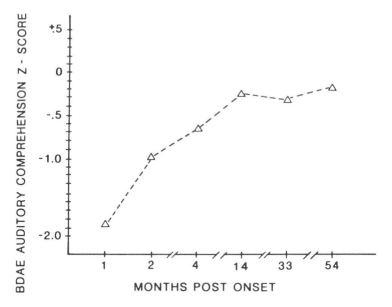

Figure 3.11.   Top, CT scan at 33 MPO of an FPTi case (age, 61 years) showing extensive cortical/subcortical lesion in the frontal and parietal lobes, but only subcortical temporal lobe lesion in the temporal isthmus at slices B and B/W (*arrows*). Note complete sparing of Wernicke's cortical area on slices B/W and W. **Bottom,** Graph showing this patient's BDAE Overall Auditory Comprehension Z-scores over a period of several months postonset. Note good recovery of auditory comprehension beginning at 2 to 4 MPO. His BDAE Auditory Comprehension Z-scores were −.24, −0.33, and −0.18 at 14, 33, and 54 MPO, respectively.

Jurgens (1984) has observed direct connections from the SMA to the caudate. These mesial frontal cortex projections then spread to the ventral and lateral portions of the caudate and to the lateral portion of the putamen. Thus, lesion located in the most medial white matter surrounding the lateral angle of the most rostral portion of the frontal horn (M Sc F) would be interrupting pathways from the cingulate gyrus area 24 and SMA, leading into the caudate and putamen. This would have an effect on the initiation, preparation for speech movements, and limbic aspects of spontaneous speech.

Middle One-Third Periventricular White-Matter Area

The M ⅓ PVWM area adjacent to the body of the lateral ventricle on CT scan slice SM is believed to contain, in part,

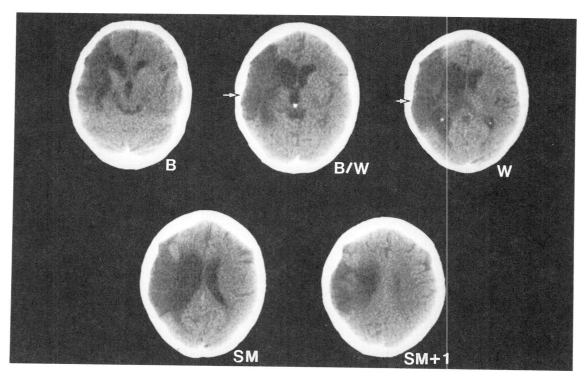

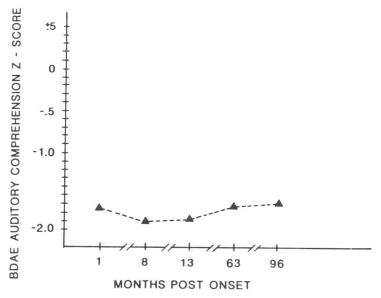

Figure 3.12. Top, CT scan at 8 MPO of an FPT case (age, 61 years), showing extensive cortical/subcortical lesion in the frontal, parietal, and temporal lobes, including Wernicke's cortical area, compatible with global aphasia. There was complete lesion in Wernicke's cortical area, including the immediately subjacent white matter on slices B/W and W (*arrows*). **Bottom,** Graph showing this patient's BDAE Overall Auditory Comprehension Z-scores over a period of several months postonset. A severe auditory comprehension deficit was still present at 12 years postonset (Z-score = −1.7).

the motor/sensory pathways for the mouth. These pathways are diagrammed coronally in Figure 3.15. The motor cortex projections for the mouth have recently been identified in an anterograde staining study with rhesus monkeys to project directly into the second quarter of the PVWM, adjacent to the body of the lateral ventricle (Schulz et al., in preparation). Thus the M ⅓ PVWM area probably contains the motor/sensory

projections for the mouth, immediately superior to their descent into the genu of the internal capsule.

In addition to containing the motor/sensory projections for the mouth, the M ⅓ PVWM area contains the body of the caudate nucleus and numerous other intra- and interhemispheric pathways. These pathways include, in part: (*a*) the descending pyramidal tract pathways for the leg and arm (Ross, 1980;

Table 3.1.
Spontaneous Speech Samples for Patients Studied Regarding Recovery of Spontaneous Speech

Case	Time Postonset	Spontaneous Speech Samples for Description of the Cookie Theft Picture
Group 1		
1	27 mo	"Yeah . . . yeah"
2	8 yr	No speech
3	9 mo	No speech
4	47 mo	"Juh . . . ah . . . jou . . . juhjuh . . . uhpai . . . uhnouer."
5	2.5 yr	No speech
6	15 mo	"No . . ." (and "grunts").
7	9 mo	No speech.
Group 2		
8	6 yr	"Boom . . . boom."
9	18 mo	"Ai . . . da tu . . . dididi."
10	13 mo	"Senny fenny."
11	9 yr	"I don't know . . . good good . . . yes, yes . . . tu, tu . . . no, no."
12	4 yr	"Wa, wa . . . for Christ sake."
13	15 mo	"Guhdi, guhdi . . . wazuh waz."
14	2 mo	"Bee bee . . . bye bye."
	(2 yr)	At this time there was almost no speech.
15	6 mo	"Yes, yes."
16	33 mo	"Morning, morning . . . boy, boy."
17	13 mo	"1, 2, 3, 4, 5 . . . boom, boom."
Group 3		
18	35 mo	Unintelligible vowel sound, "Siuhl . . . yeah down . . . un . . . cookies wash um um wahs eeah no water here, fuhee, no good over here."
19	7 mo	"Goddam . . . Chrissakes . . . I forgot it . . . well goddam."
20	15 mo	"There, too . . . there, too . . . um . . . I don't know . . . that's all I guess gee whiz. I don't know, that's all . . . well . . . that, too and there and there."
21	52 mo	"Well . . . uh . . . Duh um . . . glasses . . . run."
22[a]	8 mo	"Nothing. The kid break'in an . . . on an that one. He gonna get gett'in, gah. It's running. He given one to give one. She's dissing."
Group 4		
23	7 mo	"The wady is doing her dishes. Sink undis over uh . . . The window is open and the 'w' won . . . a very funny day outside . . . ook children . . . a boy and a girl."
24	7 mo	"A kids . . . a cookies . . . and uh, uh, fall down, . . . wash'in de dishes . . . un runn'in water . . . fish fash . . . uh foor . . . he was . . . girl a cookie."
25	24 mo	"The girl . . . uh, sh-sh sheez, the boy fall down . . . the ch-ch chair . . . the boy . . . is . . . cookies . . . the boy, the lady . . . is . . . raiping the dishes."
26	17 mo	"Well, wiss . . . watcheez, water, . . . uh, this kaitee jar . . . uh . . . do . . . eee . . . dee . . . deezeez . . . uh, ahniz . . . ahniz, uh, whoops . . . bay . . . birl . . . no . . . girl . . . boy . . . girl, I/ton/know."
27	6 yr	"Dis iz . . . bee out a lawn built up . . . This kid . . . fall down . . . This kid waking up here."

[a] At this time, the patient's speech output was almost compatible with nonfluent Broca's aphasia; however her comprehension was still too impaired for her to be considered a Broca's aphasic.

Schulz et al., in preparation); (*b*) the midcallosal pathways; (*c*) additional medial subcallosal fasciculus pathways with connections from the SMA and cingulate gyrus, to the body of the caudate (Dejerine, 1895; Muratoff, 1983; Yakovlev and Locke, 1961); (*d*) the occipitofrontal fasciculus (Dejerine, 1895); and (*e*) the superior lateral thalamic peduncle, which includes projections from the dorsomedial nucleus and the anterior nucleus to the cingulate (Mufson and Pandya, 1984) and projections from the ventrolateral nucleus to the motor cortex.

The lesion in the M ⅓ PVWM, deep to the lower motor/sensory cortex area for the mouth, may have interrupted the pathways necessary for motor execution as well as those pathways necessary for sensory feedback. Hence, we hypothesize that the lesion in the two deep subcortical white-matter pathway areas, the M Sc F and the M ⅓ PVWM, *combined*, effectively prevents any relevant spontaneous speech because there are no

available pathways for speech initiation, motor execution, or sensory feedback.

It is important to understand that the presence or absence of hemiplegia is not always a useful marker in predicting potential for long-term recovery of spontaneous speech (Case 16, Tables 3.1 and 3.2) (Naeser et al., 1989). For example, the descending pyramidal tract pathways for the leg are *most medial* within the *second and third quarters of the PVWM area* on CT scan and *immediately adjacent* to the body of the lateral ventricle (slices SM and SM + 1) (Naeser et al., in press; Schulz et al., in preparation). The descending pyramidal tract pathways for the arm are slightly more anterior and lateral within the PVWM. Thus, if the paralysis is due to lesion in the PVWM, it will be directly related to the *depth* of the PVWM lesion, *adjacent* to the body of the lateral ventricle, assuming absence of lesion in higher cortical motor pathways for the leg and arm,

Table 3.2.
Patient Data and Boston Diagnostic Aphasia Examination Test Scores for Patients Studied Regarding Recovery of Spontaneous Speech, Groups 1–4

Case	Sex	Age at Onset (yr)	Testing (time postonset)	BDAE Auditory Comprehension Z-Score	Auditory Comprehension Words (72)	Auditory Comprehension Commands (15)	Word Repetition (10)	Visual Confrontation Naming (105)
Group 1								
1 (SF)	F	66	27 mo	−1.60	28.5	2	5	0
2 (LP)	M	61	8 yr	−1.70	30.0	1	8	6
3 (HJ)	M	35	7 mo	−0.21	51.5	10	0	0
4 (TF)	M	65	4 yr (TF)	−1.19	15.5	9	5	0
5 (MW)	M	68	2.5 yr	−0.58	42.5	10	7	19
6 (LN)	M	52	15 mo	−1.0	22.5	6	0	0
7 (HL)	M	53	9 mo	−0.11	60.0	13	1	0
Group 2								
8 (WC)	M	53	3 mo	−1.90	11.0	4	0	0
9 (DA)	M	54	18 mo	−1.34	47.0	4	0	0
10 (DE)	M	56	13 mo	−0.60	53.0	7	1	0
11 (GP)	M	55	9 yr	+0.05	60.0	12	5	24
12 (HM)	M	58	8 yr	−0.90	35.0	9	5	4
13 (AG)	M	64	15 mo	−0.94	43.0	4	0	0
14 (JN)	M	53	2 yr	−0.21	50.0	9	0	0
15 (EH)	M	55	6 mo	−1.95	13.5	4	4	0
16 (KM)	M	59	33 mo	−0.33	60.0	8	0	0
17 (GJ)	M	59	13 mo	+0.09	57.0	10	7	0
Group 3								
18 (HD)	M	63	35 mo	+0.29	57.0	12	6	42
19 (CA)	M	69	7 mo	−2.10	10.5	2	0	0
20 (KW)	M	61	15 mo	−0.90	55.5	5	0	4
21 (AA)	M	58	52 mo	−0.70	41.0	8	9	13
22 (ZJ)	F	64	11 mo	−0.44	57.0	5	6	0
Group 4								
23 (WA)	M	50	7 mo	+0.75	66.5	14	9	83
24 (ME)	M	58	5 mo	+0.55	60.0	13	6	62
25 (ML)	F	56	24 mo	+0.93	71.0	15	9	85
26 (BJ)	M	67	17 mo	+0.84	70.0	15	DNT	101
27 (TH)	M	42	6 yr	+0.38	58.5	12	7	58

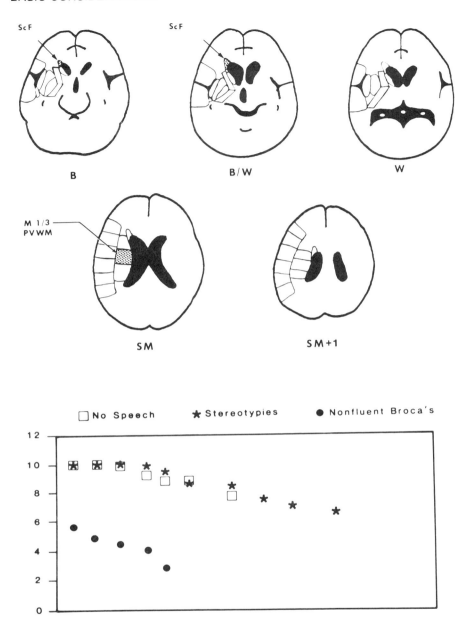

Figure 3.13.   Top, Location on CT scan slices of the two deep subcortical white-matter areas that, when examined for total extent of lesion *combined,* discriminated the cases with no speech or only stereotypies versus those with nonfluent Broca's aphasia. These two deep subcortical white-matter areas included (*a*) the medial subcallosal fasciculus, mean lesion extent at slices B and B/W plus (*b*) the white matter deep to the lower motor/sensory cortex area for the mouth, the middle ⅓ PVWM at slice SM. **Bottom,** Values for total lesion extent on the CT scan in the two deep subcortical white-matter areas *combined:* (*a*) the medial Sc F area (mean lesion extent at slices B and B/W) plus (*b*) the white-matter area deep to the lower motor/sensory cortex area for mouth, middle ⅓ PVWM at slice SM, for individual cases in three groups. Note that all cases with the most severe limitation in speech (Groups 1 and 2) had total lesion-extent values above 7; all cases with the least severe limitation in speech (Group 4, Broca's aphasia) had total lesion-extent values below 6: The summed maximum lesion-extent value on the graph represents maximum lesion-extent ratings of 5 (entire area has solid lesion) in each of the two deep subcortical white-matter areas combined. Open squares = no speech; stars = stereotypies; closed circles = nonfluent Broca's aphasia.

and absence of lesion in lower, subcortical motor pathways for the leg and arm (internal capsule and brain stem) (Naeser et al., in press).

A patient with no spontaneous speech may have lesion in the M Sc F and in more than half of the M ⅓ PVWM area,

yet the *deepest* portion of the M ⅓ PVWM area, *immediately adjacent* to the body of the lateral ventricle, may have no lesion and no paralysis. The CT scan of a patient without paralysis, but who also had no spontaneous speech, is shown in Figure 3.11 (*top*) in this chapter (Case 16, Naeser et al., 1989). Thus, both the severity of spontaneous speech and the severity of paralysis can be shown to have specific, separate lesion sites. Therefore, recovery from paralysis is often a separate issue from recovery of spontaneous speech.

In summary, the cases with the least recovery of spontaneous speech—that is, those with no speech or only stereotypies (Groups 1 and 2)—had combined lesion-extent values of above 7 for the M Sc F plus M $\frac{1}{3}$ PVWM. Those cases with better recovery of spontaneous speech—that is, those with nonfluent Broca's aphasia (Group 4), had combined lesion-extent values of below 6 for the M Sc F plus M $\frac{1}{3}$ PVWM. Those cases who fell in between these two groups in terms of severity of impairment of spontaneous speech—that is, those with a few words and/or some overlearned phrases—basically fell in between these two groups in terms of combined lesion-extent values (values around 6). There were exceptional cases at either extreme within Group 3. A few case examples and CT scans are presented below.

Case Example for Group 1: No Speech or Only a Few Irrelevant Words. Case 3, HJ, is a 35-year-old man who at 9 months following stroke onset still had no speech, although he could phonate and produce gruntlike sounds. He had a dense right hemiplegia with poor recovery (the second- and third-quarter PVWM lesion was *immediately adjacent* to the body of the lateral ventricle at slice SM). The CT scan in Figure 3.16 shows a primarily *subcortical* infarct that included extensive lesion in the M Sc F at slices B and B/W, and extensive lesion in the M $\frac{1}{3}$ PVWM at slice M. The total lesion extent in these two areas combined was 9.95 (see Fig. 16).

Case 3, HJ, is an aphasia case with primarily subcortical lesion sites. This patient had no spontaneous speech output, and a moderate comprehension deficit was present (−0.21 on the BDAE Auditory Comprehension Z-score at 7 MPO). (See Tables 3.1 and 3.2.) This moderate comprehension deficit is compatible with lesion in the anterior subcortical temporal isthmus area on slices B and B/W. (See the section on "Recovery of Auditory Language Comprehension in Global Aphasia," above.)

Case Example for Group 4: Nonfluent Broca's Aphasia. Case 23, WA, is a 50-year-old man who at 7 months following stroke onset produced nonfluent, agrammatical speech that was compatible with Broca's aphasia (see Tables 3.1 and 3.2). Mild hemiparesis was present initially, but there was good recovery of the paralysis (there was no lesion in the second and third quarters of the PVWM area immediately adjacent to the body of the lateral ventricle at slices SM or SM + 1). The CT scan in Figure 3.17 shows there was extensive lesion in the M Sc F at slices B and B/W, but only minimal lesion in the M $\frac{1}{3}$ PVWM at slice SM (small, patchy lesion). The total lesion extent in the two areas, combined, was 5.88 (Fig. 3.17).

This case had a typical lesion distribution associated with longer-lasting Broca's aphasia. (The Broca's aphasics who were included in this study were still nonfluent and agrammatical at 7 months to 6 years following stroke onset.) This lesion distribution usually includes infarction in parts of Broca's area that extends across to the border of the frontal horn (including M Sc F, slices B and/or B/W), plus superior lesion extension into the lower motor cortex area for the mouth (slices W and SM), which extends into the deep, anterior $\frac{1}{3}$ PVWM area and

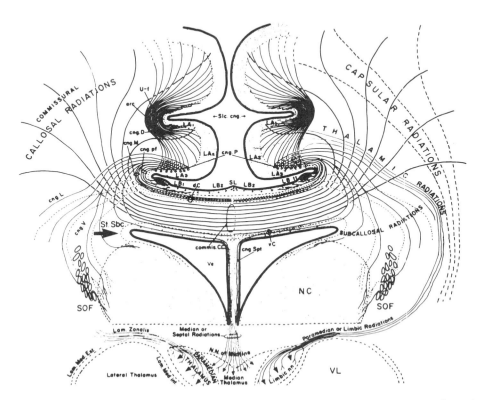

Figure 3.14. Drawing in coronal plane from Yakolev and Locke (1961, Fig. 6), showing location of the medial subcallosal fasciculus (stratum subcallosum, St Sbc) in the lateral angle of the frontal horn (*arrow*). Note that the connections from the cingulate gyrus and supplementary motor area to the head of the caudate are located within the St Sbc area immediately lateral to the frontal horn.

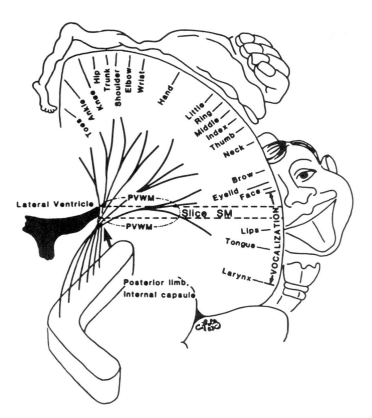

Figure 3.15. Coronal diagram showing location of descending pyramidal tract pathways in the deepest, subcortical periventricular white matter (PVWM) are immediately adjacent to the body of the lateral ventricle (*arrow*). On CT scan, these descending pyramidal tract pathways are located in the second and third quarters of the PVWM on slices SM and SM + 1. On the CT scan slices inferior to these, the pyramidal tract pathways are located in the posterior limb of the internal capsule (CT scan slices W, B/W, and B as labeled in Fig. 3.4).

sometimes part of the M ⅓ PVWM area (slice SM). In some cases, the lower motor cortex area lesion is absent (slices W and SM). The deep subcortical anterior ⅓ PVWM lesion, however, is usually always present. The cortical portions of this lesion are compatible with lesion sites in longer-lasting Broca's aphasia cases previously published by Mohr et al. (1978).

Comparison of the CT scan for Case 3 (Fig. 3.16), who had no speech at 9 MPO, with the CT scan for Case 23 (Fig. 3.17), who had functional, nonfluent spontaneous speech at 7 MPO, reveals that the less severe case (Case 23) actually had more *cortical* damage (including Broca's area on slices B and B/W, and the lower motor cortex area for mouth on slice SM) than did the more severe case (Case 3), who had no cortical lesion in either Broca's area or the lower motor cortex area for the mouth. Comparison of the CT scans for these two cases suggests that the lesion extent within the two subcortical white-matter areas (M Sc F and M ⅓ PVWM) is related to the severity of spontaneous speech output, not lesion extent within the cortex. Case 3, with no spontaneous speech, had complete lesion in the M Sc F at slices B and B/W, and complete lesion in the M ⅓ PVWM at slice SM. Case 23, with functional, nonfluent, spontaneous speech, had lesion in more than half of the M Sc F at slices B and B/W, but lesion in only a small part (less than half) of the M ⅓ PVWM at slice SM.

The 1989 study by Naeser et al. focused on spontaneous speech, and although all cases in Groups 1 and 2 had severe limitation in spontaneous speech, not all of these cases had complete cessation of speech (e.g., 10/17 cases in groups 1 and 2 could still repeat a few words, and 4/17 could correctly name some pictures to visual confrontation). Research has shown (Jurgens, 1984; Kirzinger and Jurgens, 1982; Smith et al., 1981) that lesion in the SMA has a direct effect on initiation of "spontaneous" motoric behavior patterns that are triggered internally, and not those triggered directly by external stimuli. Kirzinger and Jurgens (1982) observed, for example, that after the SMA was ablated in squirrel monkeys and these monkeys were placed in isolation, the number of vocal "isolation calls" emitted from the monkeys was reduced, although the acoustic structure remained intact. Thus, the absence of internally generated speech (spontaneous speech) in the presence of some externally generated speech (word repetition and naming) may be compatible, in part, with lesion directly affecting projections from the SMA. Further, variation in word repetition and naming ability observed across those subjects who otherwise had no meaningful spontaneous speech may have been due, in part, to variation in the extent of lesion in the projections from the SMA, as well as other areas. This would require further study.

Results from this study suggest that careful examination of lesion in the M Sc F area and the M ⅓ PVWM area is a basic starting point for assessing potential for long-term recovery of spontaneous speech in severely nonfluent stroke patients with infarction in the various branches of the left middle cerebral artery (LMCA). When working with patients who have lesion outside the distribution of the LMCA, especially in the left anterior cerebral artery (LACA), one must examine different structures. For example, in cases with LACA infarcts, it is possible that cortical lesion in the SMA and/or the cingulate gyrus area may combine with subcortical lesion in the M ⅓ PVWM to produce long-lasting impairment in speech, even when no lesion may be present in the M Sc F at slices B and B/W. Obviously, other cortical and/or subcortical lesion sites may also combine to produce severe limitation in spontaneous speech.

Implications for Treatment Decisions in Aphasia Therapy

We have recently completed two studies where results from the above-mentioned CT scan *recovery* studies were applied to *treatment* studies with aphasia patients who had severe limitation in spontaneous speech. The first study focused on CT scan lesion sites in patients with limited spontaneous speech who were treated with one specific verbal treatment program, melodic intonation therapy (MIT). The second study focused on CT scan lesion sites in patients with no functional spontaneous speech who were treated with one specific nonverbal treatment program, the computer-assisted visual communication program (C-ViC). Future research may indicate that the results from these CT scan studies with the MIT verbal treatment program and the C-ViC nonverbal treatment program may assist speech pathologists in future treatment planning decisions for their most severe aphasia patients.

Good Response Versus Poor Response to the Melodic Intonation Therapy Treatment Program

Melodic intonation therapy (MIT) is a treatment program for aphasia patients with limited spontaneous speech. In this retrospective study, CT scan lesion sites and good response versus poor response to MIT were examined for eight chronic stroke patients (Naeser et al., submitted 1992b).

The MIT program was designed to improve verbal expression in patients with severely limited, or nonfluent speech (Albert et al., 1973; Sparks and Holland, 1976). The program uses phrases and sentences that are slowly intoned, with continuous voicing, using simple high-note/low-note patterns based on normal speech prosody (Helm-Estabrooks et al., 1989a). Two studies have demonstrated that not all patients with limited verbal output respond positively to MIT (Helm, 1978; Sparks et al., 1974). Positive response to MIT is defined as improvement in number of words per phrase length as tested with the Cookie Theft Picture description from the BDAE (Goodglass and Kaplan, 1983).

Language data were collected from files on patients treated with MIT in the Audiology and Speech Pathology Service, Boston VA Medical Center. All patients were separated into two groups: good response (GR) to MIT and poor response (PR) to MIT. Good response to MIT was defined as an increase of *at least two words* per phrase length on the spontaneous speech characteristics rating scale as applied to the Cookie Theft Picture description, following a series of MIT treatments. Poor response to MIT was defined as *no increase* in the number of words per phrase length, following a series of MIT treatments.

Data were reviewed for eight male stroke cases who were treated only with MIT and who had chronic CT scans available for analysis. Each patient was right-handed and had suffered

single-episode left-hemisphere occlusive-vascular stroke between the ages of 24 and 65 years (mean = 49, SD = 14.2). One patient had an additional small lesion in the right parietal lobe that was not extensive enough to be considered the primary cause of the aphasia (Case WF). The CT scans used for CT scan lesion site analysis were performed between 3 and 36 MPO. All eight patients were treated with MIT during the chronic phase poststroke, beginning at 3 to 51 MPO.

Four patients had good response with MIT, and the other four patients had poor response with MIT. There were no significant differences between the GR cases and the PR cases in age at onset or MPO when the MIT treatments were begun. The mean age at onset for the GR cases was 49.5 years (SD = 12.3), and they began MIT treatments at a mean of 8.75 MPO (SD = 6.9). The mean age at onset for the PR cases was 48.75 (SD = 17.75), and they began MIT treatments at a mean of 16.25 MPO (SD = 23.17).

The language characteristics of aphasia patients who are good candidates for successful treatment with MIT have been under development since the first published papers (Albert et al., 1973; Sparks et al., 1974). These pre-MIT language characteristics were recently summarized by Helm-Estabrooks and Albert (1991), as follows:

1. Poorly articulated, nonfluent, or severely restricted verbal output that may be confined to a nonsense stereotypy (e.g., ''bika bika'')
2. At least moderately preserved auditory comprehension, exceeding the 45th percentile on the BDAE Rating Scale
3. Poor repetition, even for single words

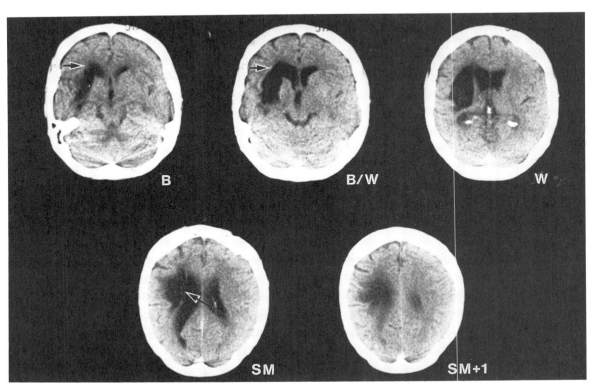

Figure 3.16. CT scan at 9 MPO for a 35-year-old man (Case 3) who had no speech at 7 MPO or even 2 years later (Group 1). A dense right hemiplegia was present. The left-hemisphere lesion is on the left side of the CT scan. Lesion extent in the medial SC F at slice B was rated 5, and at slice B/W, lesion extent was also 5 (*arrows*); mean was 5. Lesion extent in the middle ⅓ PVWM at slice SM was rated 4.95 (*arrow*); total lesion extent was rated 9.95. Note that the entire lesion is primarily subcortical.

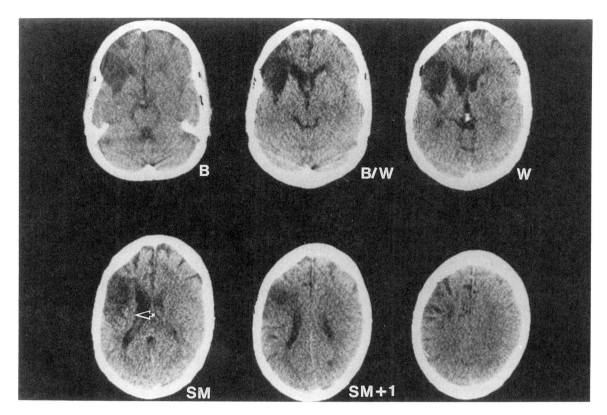

Figure 3.17. CT scan at 44 MPO for a 54-year-old man (Case 23) who had nonfluent agrammatical speech and Broca's aphasia at 7 MPO (Group 4). A mild hemiparesis was present, and there was good recovery. Lesion extent in the medial Sc F at slice B was rated 4; slice B/W was rated 3.75; and mean was 3.88. Lesion extent in the middle ⅓ PVWM at slice SM was rated only 2; total lesion extent was 5.88. The *arrow* at slice SM shows a minimal lesion in the middle ⅓ PVWM, which greatly reduced the combined total lesion extent to below 6, a value compatible with his mild limitation in speech. The mild hemiparesis with good recovery in this case was compatible with sparing of the deepest PVWM area immediately adjacent to the body of the lateral ventricle at slices SM and SM + 1. This deepest PVWM area contains, in part, the descending pyramidal tract pathways.

4. Poorly articulated speech, earning a rating of 3 or less for Articulatory Agility on the BDAE Profile of Speech Characteristics

These four language characteristics associated with good candidacy for successful treatment with MIT were refined over several years of experience with MIT at the Boston VA Medical Center, and several of the patients in the present study were treated with MIT prior to final development of these four characteristics. In the present study, all patients treated with MIT had met at least three out of four of these pre-MIT language characteristics. The decision to treat the patient with MIT was made by the speech pathologist treating the patient at that time; no CT scan lesion site information was used in the treatment decision.

The MIT treatment program is hierarchically structured and is divided into three levels. The decision to continue a patient in the MIT treatment program or to terminate the program was made by the speech pathologist based on the patient's scores at each level of the program (Helm-Estabrooks et al., 1989). A wide range for the total number of MIT treatments provided (6 to 115 treatments) was observed across the GR and PR groups. This wide range was due, in part, to the fact that if a patient could not complete Level I, treatment was terminated.

Pre-MIT. Mann-Whitney U-tests were performed on the pre-MIT spontaneous speech data for the GR group versus the PR group. The GR group had significantly better pre-MIT spontaneous speech scores for number of words per phrase length and grammatical form than the PR group (see *bottom* of Table 3.3). Although the GR group had significantly better pre-MIT spontaneous speech scores than the PR group, it should be remembered that each GR case and each PR case met at least three of the four pre-MIT language characteristics associated with good candidacy for successful treatment with MIT (Helm-Estabrooks and Albert, 1991).

Post-MIT. Mann-Whitney U-tests were also performed on the post-MIT spontaneous speech data for the two groups. As would be expected, the GR group had significantly better post-MIT spontaneous speech scores than the PR group (see *bottom* of Table 3.3). Paired *t*-tests were performed on the spontaneous speech data at T1 versus T2 for the GR cases. The GR group showed significant improvement post-MIT in number of words per phrase length ($p < .006$) and articulatory agility ($p < .03$). The PR group showed no significant improvement post-MIT on any of the spontaneous speech scores.

CT scan lesion site analysis was performed. The cortical and subcortical areas on CT scan that were examined for extent of lesion are shown in Figure 3.4.

Each of the four GR patients had a total extent-of-lesion value for the M Sc F area plus M ⅓ PVWM area that was ≤7

Table 3.3.
Spontaneous Speech Statistics for Good Response Group and Poor Response Group Treated with Melodic Intonation Therapy (MIT)

Mean and Standard Deviations for Pre-MIT and Post-MIT Spontaneous Speech Scores for the Good Response Group and the Poor Response Group						
	Pre-MIT		Post-MIT		Pre-Post Change	
	Mean	SD	Mean	SD	Mean	SD
Good Response Group						
No. words phrase length	3.0	2.3	5.8	1.9	+2.8	1.5
Articulatory agility	1.5	1.0	3.3	1.0	+1.8	1.9
Grammatical form	3.8	3.2	5.0	2.8	+1.3	1.9
Poor Response Group						
No. words phrase length	0.3	0.5	0.3	0.5	0	0
Articulatory agility	0.5	1.0	0.8	1.5	+0.3	0.5
Grammatical form	0.3	0.5	0.3	0.5	0	0

Mann-Whitney U-Test Comparisons for the Good Response Group versus the Poor Response Group				
	Pre-MIT		Post-MIT	
	Z Corrected for Ties	p-Level 1-Tail	Z Corrected for Ties	p-Level 1-Tail
No words phase length	2.14	.016	2.38	.008
Articulatory agility	1.52	.064	1.95	.025
Grammatical form	2.12	.017	2.25	.012

Table 3.4.
CT Scan Lesion Sites, and Extent-of-Lesion Data for Patients with Good Response, and Poor Response to Melodic Intonation Therapy (MIT)

Case	CT Scan (MPO)	Medial Subcallosal Fasciculus (mean B, B/W)	Mid. 1/3 PVWM (SM)	Total Extent of Lesion, M Sc F + M 1/3 PVWM (≤7 = GR)	Wernicke's Area (mean B/W, W)	Temporal Isthmus (mean B, B/W) (<3 = GR)	Occipital Length Asymmetry
Good Response							
ME	3.5	3.00	2.0	5.00	1	0.50	R
WA	44.0	3.25	2.5	5.75	0	0	L
TH	77.0	1.75	2.0	3.75	2	1.25	L
MJ	72.0	5.00	2.0	7.00	0	0	=
Poor Response							
GNJ	4.0	4.00	4.50	8.50	1.87	4.50	=
SF	3.5	5.00	4.90	9.90	2.87	4.00	L
RP	18.0	3.63	3.85	7.48	4.50	3.75	=
WF	100.0	4.90	4.80	9.70	5.00	5.00	R

(range 3.75 to 7). See Table 3.4 column, "Total Extent of Lesion M Sc F + M 1/3 PVWM." Each of the four PR patients had a total extent-of-lesion value that was >7 (range 7.48 to 9.9). It is of interest to note, in fact, that in this small study with eight patients, the GR patients could be separated from the PR patients on the basis of the M 1/3 PVWM extent of lesion rating *alone*, versus the lesion *combination* of M Sc F plus the M 1/3 PVWM. All four GR cases had M 1/3 PVWM extent-of-lesion ratings that were <3; all four PR cases had M 1/3 PVWM extent-of-lesion ratings that were <3.

The extent of lesion in Wernicke's area could not be used to discriminate between the GR cases and the PR cases, because although 4/4 GR cases had lesion in less than half of Wernicke's area, 2/4 PR cases also had lesion in less than half of Wernicke's area (see Table 3.4 column, "Wernicke's Area").

All four GR cases had extent-of-lesion ratings of <3 in the subcortical temporal isthmus area, whereas all four PR cases had extent-of-lesion ratings of >3 in the subcortical temporal isthmus area. The GR group had pre-MIT BDAE Auditory Comprehension Z-scores that were −0.46, +0.46, +0.75, and +1.0. The PR group had pre-MIT BDAE Auditory Comprehension Z-scores that were −2.33, −1.48, and −0.4 (one PR case was tested only with the BASA and therefore does not have a BDAE Auditory Comprehension Z-score available). There were too few subjects with complete data to permit statistical comparisons on auditory comprehension. However, prior to MIT treatment, 4/4 of the GR cases were *better* than −0.5 on the BDAE Auditory Comprehension Z-score, and only one of the PR cases was *better* than −0.5 on the BDAE Auditory Comprehension Z-score. The relatively greater deficit in auditory comprehension for most of the PR cases was probably related to lesion in the subcortical temporal isthmus area in 4/4 PR cases, and/ or to lesion in Wernicke's area in 2/4 of the PR cases.

There was no single *cortical* language area where the extent of lesion could be used to discriminate between all the GR cases versus all the PR cases, including extent of lesion in Broca's area, Wernicke's area, the supramarginal or angular gyrus areas, or the SMA.

Case Examples. The CT scan for one patient with good response to MIT is shown in Figure 3.18, and the CT scan for one patient with poor response to MIT is shown in Figure 3.19.

The results from this most recent study have expanded and revised the results from the Naeser and Helm-Estabrooks (1985) CT scan study with MIT. Results from the present study revealed that total extent of lesion in the M Sc F area plus the M ⅓ PVWM area discriminated 100% between patients with good response to MIT and patients with poor response to MIT. This included even those patients treated as late as 4 years after stroke onset. The importance of these two subcortical white-matter areas to the recovery (or nonrecovery) of spontaneous speech had not yet been recognized when our first CT scan study with MIT was published in 1985.

Results from our most recent CT scan study with MIT have revealed the following language behavior criteria and CT scan criteria regarding which nonfluent aphasia patients are likely

to be the best candidates for successful treatment with MIT: (*a*) *Language behavior criteria:* The patient will meet at least three of the four pre-MIT language characteristics listed earlier in this section (Helm-Estabrooks and Albert, 1991); (*b*) *CT scan criteria:* The patient will have a total extent-of-lesion value of <7 for the M Sc F area plus the M ⅓ PVWM area, and the patient will also have lesion in less than half of Wernicke's area and in less than half of the subcortical temporal isthmus area.

Good Response Versus Poor Response to the Nonverbal Computer-Assisted Visual Communication (C-ViC) Treatment Program

The nonverbal computer-assisted visual communication (C-ViC) treatment program enables patients with no spontaneous speech (or ability to read or write) to use pictures and icons on a computer screen to communicate needs and ideas. In a retrospective study, CT scan lesion sites and good response versus poor response to the C-ViC program were examined for seven severe aphasia patients with no ability to speak, read, or write (Naeser et al., submitted 1992a). These patients were treated with C-ViC beginning in the chronic phase poststroke.

Almost 20 years ago, the first systematic attempts to use a substituted language based on representational and arbitrary

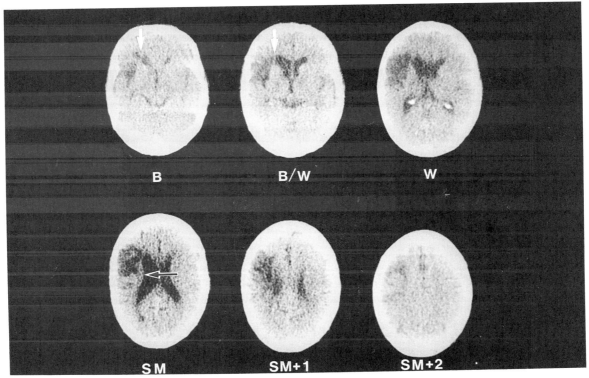

Figure 3.18. CT scan for a 58-year-old man (Case ME) who had good response to the melodic intonation therapy (MIT) treatment program beginning at 3 MPO. He improved from one to three words in phrase length after 3 months of MIT. The total extent-of-lesion value for the M Sc F *plus* the M ⅓ PVWM was 5. This total extent-of-lesion value was computed in the two areas as follows: (*a*) M Sc F at slice B = 2.5 (patchy lesion in less than half of the area, *white arrow*); M Sc F at slice B/W = 3.5 (patchy lesion in more than half of the area, *white arrow*); mean M Sc F at slices B and B/W = 3. (*b*) M ⅓ PVWM at slice SM = 2 (small, patchy, partial lesion, *black and white arrow*). Total extent-of-lesion value for M Sc F (3) + M ⅓ PVWM (2) = 5. CT scan is 3.5 MPO. *Note:* This patient had almost no lesion in Wernicke's area on slices B/W and W (mean lesion-extent value of 1) and almost no lesion in the subcortical temporal isthmus area on slices B and B/W (mean lesion-extent value of 0.5).

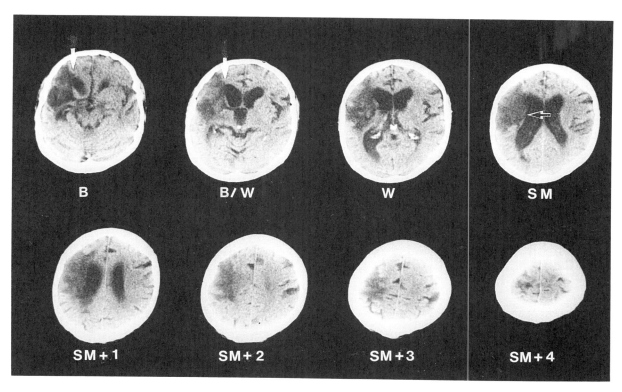

Figure 3.19. CT scan for a 65-year-old man (Case SF) who had poor response to the MIT treatment program beginning at 5 MPO. The total extent-of-lesion value for the M Sc F *plus* the M ⅓ PVWM was 9.9. This total extent-of-lesion value was computed in the two areas as follows: (*a*) M Sc F at slice B = 5 (entire area has solid lesion, *white arrow*); M Sc F at slice B/W = 5 (entire area has solid lesion, *white arrow*); mean M Sc F at slice B and B/W = 5. (*b*) M ⅓ PVWM at slice SM = 4.9 (almost the entire area has solid lesion, *black and white arrow*). Total extent-of-lesion value for M Sc F (5) + M ⅓ PVWM (4.9) = 9.9. CT scan is 3.5 MPO. *Note:* This patient had lesion in less than half of Wernicke's area on slices B/W and W; there was only small, partial lesion (mean lesion extent value of 2.87). Lesion was present in more than half the subcortical temporal isthmus area, however, on slices B and B/W (mean, 4).

icons were reported (Baker et al., 1975; Gardner et al., 1976). More recently, the iconic C-ViC "language" that can be carried in, and manipulated with, a minicomputer was developed (Steele et al., 1989; Weinrich et al., 1989a; Weinrich et al., 1989b). These investigators have demonstrated that severely aphasic patients can manipulate the computer "mouse" and button-click necessary for operation and can learn the rules of lexical organization. The patients learn to construct and comprehend complex "sentences" in the C-ViC pictorial "language." Not all severely aphasic patients, however, have been able to grasp the lexical and syntactic rules of the C-ViC communication system and use them to initiate communication independently.

In our study, CT scan lesion sites and GR versus PR to C-ViC were examined for seven severe stroke patients (Naeser et al., submitted 1992a). All seven patients had suffered a left-hemisphere cerebrovascular accident. The age at onset of stroke ranged from 43 to 65 years (mean = 56, SD = 7.5). One case was left-handed. All seven patients had severe right hemiplegia. One patient had a small right-hemisphere infarction in addition to the major left-hemisphere lesion.

The BASA (Helm-Estabrooks et al., 1989b) was performed immediately prior to C-ViC training and again at its termination. The BASA was designed for severely aphasic patients and probes for even very small improvement in auditory comprehension or language production. Most patients were also tested

with parts of the BDAE (Goodglass and Kaplan, 1983). Aphasia diagnosis prior to C-ViC treatment was severe aphasia with no spontaneous output—spoken or written—in conversation or picture description. Auditory comprehension was also substantially impaired. Table 3.5 summarizes language capacity.

All seven cases had been previously treated with one or more traditional treatment programs without success. These included verbal treatment programs such as melodic intonation therapy (Albert et al., 1973; Sparks and Holland, 1976); and/or nonverbal treatment programs such as bucco-facial, visual action therapy, which trains patients with severe oral apraxia to produce representational gestures using the oral musculature (Ramsberger and Helm-Estabrooks, 1988); and/or limb, visual action therapy, which trains patients with severe aphasia and limb apraxia to produce representational, purposeful gestures with the hand and arm (Helm-Estabrooks et al., 1982).

All patients were treated with C-ViC in the chronic phase poststroke, >3 MPO (range 4 MPO to 6 years). The patients were seen as outpatients for half-hour treatment sessions, usually twice per week. All patients were able to match objects to pictured icons on a computer screen (and vice versa), and all were able to use the computer "mouse" easily with the left hand.

The C-ViC training consisted of two phases (Baker and Nicholas, submitted). In Phase I, patients were trained to use the computer "mouse" to carry out commands presented in

Table 3.5.
Patient Data and Language Test Scores for Patients Treated with the Computer-Assisted Visual Communication (C-ViC) Treatment Program[a]

Case	Sex	Age at Onset (yr)	MPO When C-ViC Started	Months in Tx.		BDAE No. Wds. Phrase Length (7)	BDAE Aud. Comp. Z-Score	BASA Auditory Comprehension Raw Score (16)	BASA Total Raw Score (61)	BASA Oral-Gestural Expression Raw Score (21)	C-ViC Response Phase II Step 5 (PICA scale—16)[b]
Good Response											
BJ[c]	M	43	7	3	Pre	0	-0.8	13	49	14	15.0
					Post	1-2	+0.5	14	51	14	
DJ	M	54	6	6	Pre	0	-1.75	8	36	9	14.5
					Post	0	NA	7	39	14	
SH	F	65	4	18	Pre	0	NA	7	26	3	14.0
					Post	0	NA	10	37	5	
CA	M	49	72	9	Pre	0	-0.63	13	40	7	12.5
					Post	0	NA	13	40	8	
Poor Response											
RR	M	59	21	28	Pre	0	-0.61	6	25	3	9.0
					Post	0	NA	6	38	13	
FW	M	59	7	7	Pre	0	-1.60	9	31	6	8.5
					Post	0	-0.33	13	41	7	
SM	M	60	60	7	Pre	0	-1.74	4	24	7	8.0
					Post	0	-1.61	8	29	7	

[a] Patients are rank-ordered by response to Phase II, Step 5 of ViC program; see last column. Scores ≥13 reflect ability to initiate communication independently with the C-ViC program.
[b] The last step in Phase II, Step 5 of C-ViC requires the patients to initiate a question or command independently. Scores of 8 or 9 reflect inability to initiate a question or command independently.
[c] Left-handed but aphasic from left-hemisphere lesion.
NA Information is not available.

C-ViC (comprehension); to answer questions; and finally, to compose descriptions of simple acts (production). Phase II focused on real-life communicative acts, including expressing needs, making requests (giving commands), and asking questions. Variability in duration of C-ViC treatment in the present study reflected ongoing program development as well as patient availability.

The quality of the communications generated by patients using C-ViC in Phase I and Phase II was rated by the clinician, using the Porch Index of Communicative Ability (PICA) rating scale, which ranges from 1 to 16 (Porch, 1967). A PICA score of ≥13 represents *independently initiated* successful communication. Scores >13 were considered good C-ViC productions, whereas scores <13 were considered poor C-ViC productions.

To reach criterion at the end of Phase I and to be considered a GR case at the end of Phase II, the patient's communications generated with C-ViC must have reached scores of at least 13 on the PICA scale. A patient with a Phase II C-ViC score of <13 was considered to be a PR case. Three patients had GR, with Phase II scores ranging from 14 to 15; one patient had borderline GR, with a score of 12.5; and three patients had PR, with scores ranging from 8 to 9 (see Table 3.5, last column).

There was no significant correlation between the age at stroke onset and the Phase II C-ViC score ($r = -.482$), nor between the MPO when entering the C-ViC program and the Phase II C-ViC score ($r = -.352$). There was also no significant correlation between the number of months a patient received the C-ViC program and the Phase II C-ViC score ($r = -.275$).

One of the patients who had good response with C-ViC (Case SH) was able to remain at home with her spouse, rather than transferring to a nursing home, as a result of the new communication ability provided through C-ViC. Because of severe difficulties in communication and management, the necessity of a nursing home had been considered prior to C-ViC training. As a result of this patient's success with the C-ViC program, a Macintosh computer was placed in the home, and the patient was able to use the system to communicate her needs to her husband, including when she felt there was a need for her prescriptions to be refilled.

Even patients with poor response to C-ViC by PICA scoring were able to use C-ViC for some interactions not possible with speech or writing. Case RR was considered to have poor response to C-ViC because he was not able to initiate communications independently with C-ViC following Phase II training. He was, however, able to use C-ViC to answer specific questions posed by another person. For example, Case RR has the Macintosh computer in the home, and he can use it to respond to his wife's verbally presented question, "What do you want for breakfast?"

The BASA scores prior to C-ViC treatment had a general correspondence to level of response to C-ViC. The four GR cases had pre-C-ViC overall BASA scores of 26 to 49 out of 61 items, and auditory comprehension BASA scores of 7 to 13 out of 16 items. The three PR cases had pre-C-ViC overall BASA scores of 24, 25, and 32 out of 61 items, and auditory comprehension scores of 4, 6, and 9 out of 16 items. During post-C-ViC training, significant improvements on the BASA were observed among the patients as a group: overall BASA score ($p<.01$) auditory comprehension ($p<.05$), and oral-gestural expression ($p<.05$).

CT scan lesion site analysis was performed. The cortical and subcortical areas that were examined for extent of lesion are shown in Figure 3.4. The CT scans used for lesion site analysis were performed between 3 and 36 MPO.

There was no relationship between GR and PR to C-ViC and lesion extent in any single neuroanatomical area analyzed on CT scan. The 1989 study by Naeser et al. had observed that extensive lesion in the M Sc F area plus the M ⅓ PVWM area, *combined,* was compatible with no recovery of spontaneous speech. In fact, in this C-ViC study, all seven cases had no spontaneous speech, and all seven cases had total extent-of-lesion values that were >7 for the M Sc F and the M ⅓ PVWM combined (see column labeled, "Total Extent of Lesion M Sc F + M ⅓ PVWM" in Table 3.6). The GR and PR cases had complete overlap of total extent-of-lesion values in these two white-matter areas.

Only one combination of additional lesion extension in two extra areas completely discriminated between all GR cases and all PR cases treated with C-ViC. These two extra areas included the following: (*a*) extra area 1, the *supraventricular* area, including the SMA/cingulate gyrus area 24; and (*b*) extra area 2, the *temporal lobe* area, including Wernicke's area or the subcortical temporal isthmus. The PR patients had extensive lesion (extent-of-lesion value >3) in *each* of these two extra areas. The GR patients had extensive lesion (extent-of-lesion value >3) in *none,* or *only one* of these two extra areas (see Table 3.6).

Case Examples. The CT scan for one patient who had good response to C-ViC training is shown in Figure 3.20. The CT scan for one patient who had poor response to C-ViC training is shown in Figure 3.21.

The results from this study suggest that CT scan lesion site analysis may be useful in helping to identify severe nonverbal aphasia patients who probably will not recover spontaneous speech but who are likely to benefit from training with the nonverbal C-ViC treatment program or a similar nonverbal treatment program. Treatment with C-ViC seems to be appropriate for patients with total extent-of-lesion values >7 for the M Sc F area plus the M ⅓ PVWM area.

Furthermore, patients with extensive lesion in both of the two extra areas (extra area 1, the *supraventricular* area, including the SMA/cingulate gyrus area 24; and extra area 2, the *temporal lobe* area, including Wernicke's area or the subcortical temporal isthmus) appear to be unable to initiate communication independently with C-ViC. They require assistance, such as a repeated cue or repeated instructions.

Although some patients have poor response to C-ViC, this does not mean that these patients should not be trained to use C-ViC. The term "poor response" refers to communications that are rated below 13 on the PICA scale and to inability to initiate communications independently with C-ViC at the Phase II level. The expectations of outcome with the C-ViC program may be lowered to accommodate patients who cannot independently initiate C-ViC messages but who can use it with assistance to answer specific questions. Thus, practical use of C-ViC in the home, nursing home, or rehabilitation setting should be determined on an individual case-by-case basis.

Sarno and Levita (1981) have observed that the greatest recovery in severe aphasia patients occurs after 6 to 12 MPO. It is possible that with a severe, nonverbal aphasia patient, where treatment planning decisions may be difficult, obtaining a CT scan after 3 MPO could be helpful in better understanding

Table 3.6.
CT Scan Lesion Sites and Extent-of-Lesion Values for Patients Treated with the Computer-Assisted Visual Communication (C-ViC) Treatment Program

Case	CT Scan (months postonset)	Medial Subcallosal Fasc. (mean B, B/W)	Middle 1/3 PVWM (SM)	Total Extent of Lesion M ScF + M 1/3 PVWM (>7 = basic lesion, no recovery of spontaneous speech)	Two Extra Areas				Right Hemisphere Lesion	Occipital Length Asymmetry
					Extra Area 1 Supraventricular		Extra Area 2 Temporal Lobe			
					Supplem. Motor Area	Cingulate Gyrus Area 24	Wernicke's Area (mean B/W, W)	Temporal Isthmus (mean B, B/W)		
Good Response										
BJ[a]	12	5.0	4.90	9.90	0	0	0	0	No	=
DJ	13	5.0	4.25	9.25	Deep	Deep	1.00	0	Yes, high right frontal	=
SH	6	4.9	4.75	9.65	0	0	3.25	4.37	No	R
CA	72	3.5	5.00	8.50	0	0	4.55	4.50	[b]	R
Poor Response										
RR	49	4.75	4.90	9.65	Cortical and deep	Cortical and deep	2.50	4.50	No	L
FW	13	4.25	5.00	9.25	Cortical and deep	Cortical and deep	2.37	4.37	No	R
SM	60	2.37	4.75	7.12	Deep	Deep	4.90	5.00	No	L

[a] Left-handed but aphasic from left-hemisphere lesion.
[b] Shunt in right ventricle.

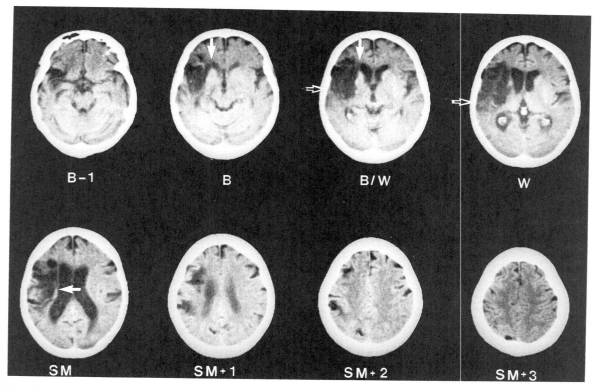

Figure 3.20 CT scan for patient SH, a 65-year-old woman who entered the C-ViC program at 4 MPO and had good response to the C-ViC treatment program. The basic lesion site pattern associated with no recovery of spontaneous speech was present in the M Sc F on slices B and B/W (*white arrows*), plus the M ⅓ PVWM at slice SM (*white arrow*). The total extent-of-lesion value for M Sc F plus M ⅓ PVWM was 9.65. In addition, extensive lesion was present in only one of the two extra areas. Lesion was present in extra area 2, the temporal lobe area, including Wernicke's area on slices B/W and W (*black and white arrows*) and the temporal isthmus on slices B-1 and B. No lesion was present in extra area 1, the supraventricular area, including the SMA/cingulate gyrus on slices SM + 2 or SM + 3. CT scan is 6 MPO.

the potential for long-term recovery of spontaneous speech and/or auditory comprehension. Therefore, the results from the CT scan could be used to help with treatment decisions for the 6 to 12 MPO treatment period, and beyond. Of course, other treatment approaches should be used earlier with severe aphasia patients, including helping the patient to use a basic communication board, drawing (Morgan and Helm-Estabrooks, 1987), or gesture (Rao, 1986; Skelly et al., 1974; Skelly et al., 1975).

FUTURE TRENDS IN BRAIN IMAGING AND ITS APPLICATION TO APHASIA RESEARCH

Since the advent of in vivo brain imaging with CT scans almost 20 years ago, the field of lesion localization and aphasia research has advanced markedly. Our current research has focused on the relationship between lesion location in certain cortical and subcortical areas on CT scan, and specific aspects of language recovery in aphasia, namely recovery of auditory language comprehension and recovery of spontaneous speech. Most recently, research from our laboratory has indicated that chronic CT scans performed after 2 or 3 MPO may be useful in identifying which aphasia patients may be appropriate for verbal versus nonverbal aphasia treatment programs. Thus, one exciting trend in applying the techniques of brain imaging to

aphasia research is to continue studying the anatomical correlates of prognosis for recovery from aphasia and prognosis for benefit from specific types of aphasia treatment programs.

Thus far, there have been only a few aphasia studies using MRI for lesion analysis (Caplan and DeWitt, 1988; DeWitt et al., 1985; Murdoch et al., 1991; Poncet et al., 1987; Tranel et al., 1987). Horizontal and coronal templates have been introduced that are marked with Brodmann's cortical areas and vascular territories, which may be useful for lesion site analysis on MRI scans (Damasio and Damasio, 1989; Frumkin et al., 1989a; Palumbo et al., 1990).

The proper timing of imaging studies for aphasia research is extremely important. CT scan lesion site information in stroke patients should be obtained after 2 to 3 MPO (Naeser, 1985; Poeck et al., 1984). It appears that the final borders of the area of infarction on MRI scan are also not complete until 3 MPO (Alexander et al., 1991). In this latter study, MRI scans were performed at 1 and 3 MPO for comparison with CT scans performed in the same stroke patients at 3 MPO (*n* = 15). The subacute MRI scans (≤1 MPO) showed the general location of the area of infarction, on both T1- and T2-weighted images. The T1-weighted MR images at ≤1 MPO, however, showed the lesion to be less extensive than it was on the 3 MPO CT scan; and the T2-weighted MR images ≤1 MPO showed the lesion to be more extensive than it was on the 3 MPO CT scan.

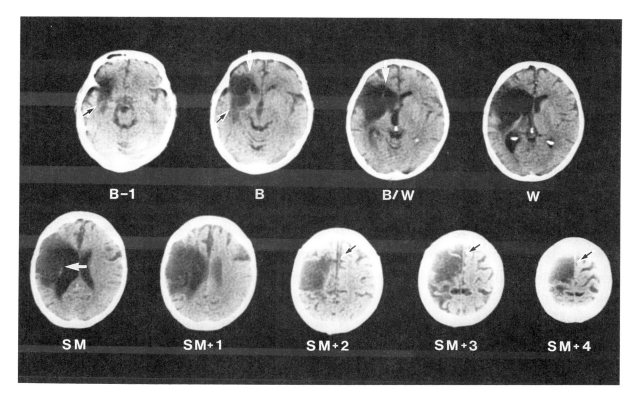

Figure 3.21. CT scan for patient RR, a 60-year-old man who entered the C-ViC program at 21 MPO and had poor response to the C-ViC treatment program. The basic lesion site pattern associated with no recovery of spontaneous speech was present in the M Sc F on slices B and B/W (*white arrows*), plus the M ⅓ PVWM at slice SM (*white arrow*). The total extent-of-lesion value for M Sc F plus M ⅓ PVWM was 9.65. In addition, extensive lesion was present in both of the two extra areas. Lesion was present in extra area 1, the supraventricular area, including the SMA/cingulate gyrus on slices SM + 2, SM + 3, SM + 4 (*black and white arrows*); and lesion was present in extra area 2, the temporal lobe area, including the temporal isthmus on slices B-1 and B (*black and white arrows*). CT scan is 4 years postonset.

The lesion location on the 3 MPO MRI scans was generally congruent with the lesion location on the 3 MPO CT scan. The 3 MPO T1-weighted MR images tended to show only the cavity of the lesion, however, and the 3 MPO T2-weighted MR images tended to exaggerate the borders of the lesion.

Based on results from the first 15 patients, the ≤1 MPO MRI scans were not clear enough to permit refined lesion site analysis that could be used to predict long-term potential for recovery in aphasia (Alexander et al., 1991). There is no question, however, that early MRI scans (≤1 MPO) will provide more information regarding general presence of an area of infarction than will an early CT scan (≤1 MPO) (Shuaib et al., 1992).

In summary, at this time, a 3 MPO CT scan is the neuroimaging procedure about which we know the most, regarding correlation with long-term potential for recovery in aphasia. Future studies with MRI, especially in the coronal plane, may help to further refine lesion site issues (Alexander et al., 1991; Frumkin, 1989; Frumkin et al., 1989b).

A future trend in lesion mapping and analysis is the combination of MRI technology with advancements in computers and brain imaging techniques (SiliconGraphics, 1991). One such combination is the development of three-dimensional MRI (Damasio and Frank, 1992). In this technique, raw data are collected after employing a special MRI protocol; then the brain is reconstructed and viewed as a three-dimensional whole, in hemispheres, or resliced into any two-dimensional plane. This reconstruction can be done for an anatomical structure or, more specifically, a lesion. Brain lesions can be analyzed for location and extent, both cortically and subcortically, in individual brains.

Another promising area of future MRI research is the application of MRI technology to regional cerebral blood volume (CBV) studies (Belliveau et al., 1991). These studies produce regional CBV maps of the brain during resting and activated states. This research demonstrates the potential of MRI for high-resolution mapping of brain areas involved in cognitive processing.

Significant advances in understanding neuroanatomical correlates of aphasia have occurred over the past 20 years, mainly because of the rapid evolution in the brain imaging techniques of CT and MRI. Future progress in lesion mapping and analysis should further promote our understanding of the correlation between language deficits and focal brain damage. By studying neuroimaging information in relation to clinical data, we may be able to improve language intervention strategies in the aphasia population while reducing the overall time and cost associated with long-term rehabilitation.

Acknowledgments

The authors would like to acknowledge the invaluable assistance of Sulochana Naidoo, M.S., for her assistance in data collection; and Claudia Cassano and Roger Ray, for assistance with manuscript preparation. We also thank the Radiology service of the Boston DVA Medical Center, including Drs. A. Robbins and R. N. Samaraweera; and the Medical Media Service, Boston DVA Medical Center for photography and illustrations (John Dyke and Mary Burke). This research was supported, in part, by the Medical Research Service of the Department of Veterans Affairs and by USPHS Grant DC00081.

References

Albert, M. L., Sparks, R., and Helm, N. (1973). Melodic intonation therapy for aphasia. *Archives of Neurology, 29,* 103–131.

Alexander, J., Kalender W., and Linke, G. (1986). *Computed tomography: Assessment criteria, CT system technology, clinical applications.* Berlin, Germany: Siemens Aktiengesellschaft.

Alexander, M. P., Naeser, M. A., and Palumbo, C. L. (1987). Correlations of subcortical CT lesion sites and aphasia profiles. *Brain, 110,* 961–991.

Alexander, M. P., Naeser, M., and Sweriduk, S. (1991, October). *Comparison of lesion profiles with CT and early and late MRI: Implications for aphasia research.* Paper presented at the 29th annual meeting of the Academy of Aphasia, Rome, Italy.

Baker, E., Berry, T., Gardner, H., Zurif, E., Davis, L., and Veroff, A. (1975). Can linguistic competence be dissociated from natural language functions? *Nature, 254,* 609–619.

Baker, E. H., and Nicholas, M. Computer-assisted visual communication (C-ViC) for severe nonverbal aphasia patients: A training manual. Submitted.

Barnes, C. L., Van Hoesen, G. W., and Yeterian, E. H. (1980). Widespread projections to the striatum from the limbic mesocortices in the monkey. *Society for Neuroscience Abstracts, 6,* 271.

Belliveau, J. W., Kennedy, D. N., McKinstry, R. C., Buchbinder, B. R., Weisskoff, R. M., Cohen, M. S., Vevea, J. M., Brady, T. J. and Rosen, B. R. (1991). Functional mapping of the human visual cortex by magnetic resonance imaging. *Science, 254,* 716–719.

Benjamin, D., and Van Hoesen, G. W. (1982). Some afferents of the supplementary motor area (SMA) in the monkey. *Anatomical Record, 202,* 15A.

Bogen, J. E., and Bogen, G. M. (1976). Wernicke's region: Where is it? *Annals of the New York Academy of Science, 280,* 834–843.

Bories, J., Derhy, S., and Chiras, J. (1985). CT in hemispheric ischaemic attacks. *Neuroradiology, 27,* 468–483.

Bradley, W. G. (1987). Pathophysiologic correlates of signal alterations. In M. Brant-Zawadzki and D. Norman (Eds.), *Magnetic resonance imaging of the central nervous system* (pp. 23–42). New York: Raven Press.

Brant-Zawadzki, M. (1988). MR imaging of the brain. *Radiology, 166,* 1–10.

Brant-Zawadzki, M., and Kucharczyk, W. (1987). Vascular disease: Ischemia. In M. Brant-Zawadzki and D. Norman (Eds.), *Magnetic resonance imaging of the central nervous system.* New York: Raven Press.

Breger, R., and Kneeland, J. B. (1987). Basic physics of magnetic resonance imaging. In D. L. Daniels, V. M. Haughton, and T. P. Naidich (Eds.), *Cranial and spinal magnetic resonance imaging. An atlas and guide.* New York: Raven Press.

Bydder, G. M. and Steiner, R. E. (1982). NMR imaging of the brain. *Neuroradiology, 23,* 231–240.

Caplan, L. R. and DeWitt, L. D. (1988). Determining the cause of aphasia. *MRI Decisions, 2,* 2–13.

Carroll, W. B. (1985). *Fuchs's principles of radiographic exposure, processing and quality control.* Springfield, IL: Charles C. Thomas.

Cohen, M. S., and Weisskoff, R. M. (1991). Ultra-fast imaging: A review. *Magnetic Resonance Imaging, 9,* 1–37.

Crooks, L. E., Mills, C. M., Davis, P. L., Brant-Zawadzki, M., Hoenninger, J., Arakawa, M., Watts, J., and Kaufman, L. (1982). Visualization of cerebral and vascular abnormalities by NMR imaging. The effects of imaging parameters on contrast. *Radiology, 144,* 843–852.

Damadian, R. (1971). Tumor detection by nuclear magnetic resonance. *Science, 171,* 1151–1153.

Damasio, H., and Damasio, A. R. (1989). *Lesion analysis in neuropsychology.* Oxford and New York: Oxford University Press.

Damasio, H., and Frank, R. (1992). Three-dimensional in vivo mapping of brain lesions in humans. *Archives of Neurology, 49,* 137–143.

DeArmond, S. J., Fusco, M. M., and Dewey, M. M. (1976). *Structure of the human brain: A photographic atlas* (2nd ed.). New York and London: Oxford University Press.

De Groot, J. (1984). *Correlative neuroanatomy of computed tomography and magnetic resonance imaging.* Philadelphia: Lea & Febiger.

Dejerine, J. (1895). *Anatomie des centres nerveux* (Vol. 1). Paris: Rueff.

DeWitt, L. D., Grek, A., Buonanno, F., Levine, D. N., and Kistler, J. P. (1985). MRI and the study of aphasia. *Neurology, 35,* 861–865.

Elster, A. D. (1986). *Magnetic resonance imaging: A reference guide and atlas.* Philadelphia: J. B. Lippincott.

Field, S. A., and Wehrli, F. W. (1990). *SIGNA applications guide.* Milwaukee: General Electric Co.

Frumkin, N. L. (1989). *MRI and CT analysis of occlusive infarct in adult stroke.* Unpublished doctoral dissertation, Michigan State University, East Lansing, Michigan.

Frumkin, N. L., Palumbo, C. L., Naeser, M. A., Stiassny-Eder, D., and Lydon, J. (1989a). *Location of cortical language areas on MRI scans versus CT scans.* Poster presented at the annual meeting of the Academy of Aphasia, Sante Fe, New Mexico.

Frumkin, N. L., Potchen, E. J., Aniskiewicz, A. S., Moore, J. B., and Cooke, P. A. (1989b). Potential impact of magnetic resonance imaging on the field of communication disorders. *ASHA, 31,* 95–99.

Gademann, G. (1984). *NMR-tomography of the normal brain.* Berlin: Springer-Verlag.

Gardner, H., Zurif, E. B., Berry, T., and Baker, E. H. (1976). Visual communication in aphasia. *Neuropsychologia, 14,* 275–292.

Goldberg, G. (1985). Supplementary motor area structure and function: Review and hypothesis. *Behavioral and Brain Sciences,* 567–615.

Goldberg, H. I. (1983). Stroke. In S. H. Lee and K. C. V. G. Rao (Eds.), *Cranial computed tomography* (pp. 583–658). New York: McGraw-Hill.

Goodglass, H., and Kaplan, E. (1972). *The assessment of aphasia and related disorders.* Philadelphia: Lea and Febiger.

Goodglass, H., and Kaplan, E. (1983). *The assessment of aphasia and related disorders* (2nd ed.). Philadelphia: Lea & Febiger.

Hanaway, J., Scott, W. R., and Strother, C. M. (1980). *Atlas of the human brain and the orbit for computed tomography.* St. Louis: Warren H. Green.

Helm, N. A. (1978). *Criteria for selecting aphasia patients for melodic intonation therapy.* Paper presented at the symposium, Language Rehabilitation in Aphasia, annual meeting of the American Association for the Advancement of Science, Washington, DC.

Helm-Estabrooks, N. A., and Albert, M. L. (1991). *A manual of aphasia therapy.* Austin, TX: Pro-Ed.

Helm-Estabrooks, N., Fitzpatrick, P., and Barresi, B. (1982). Visual action therapy for global aphasia. *Journal of Speech and Hearing Disorders, 47,* 385–389.

Helm-Estabrooks, N., Nicholas, M., and Morgan, A. (1989a). *Melodic intonation therapy program.* San Antonio, TX: Special Press.

Helm-Estabrooks, N., Ramsberger, G., Morgan, A., and Nicholas, M. (1989b). *Boston Assessment of Severe Aphasia.* San Antonio, TX: Special Press.

Hier, D. B., Davis, K. R., Richardson, E. P., and Mohr, J. P. (1977). Hypertensive putaminal hemorrhage. *Annals of Neurology, 11,* 152–159.

Jack, C. R., Berquist, T. H., Miller, G. M., Forbes, G. S., Gray, J. E., Morin, R. L., and Ilstrup, D. M. (1990) Field strength in neuro-MR imaging: A comparison of 0.5 T and 1.5 T. *Journal of Computer Assisted Tomography, 14,* 505–513.

Jernigan, T. L., Zatz, L. M., and Naeser, M. A. (1979). Semiautomated methods for quantitating CSF volume on cranial computed tomography. *Radiology, 132,* 463–466.

Jurgens, U. (1984). The efferent and afferent connections of the supplementary motor area. *Brain Research, Amsterdam, 300,* 63–81.

Katz, M. (1984). Principles and techniques of image reconstruction with CT. In L. Weisberg, C. Nice, and M. Katz (Eds.), *Cerebral computed tomography: A text atlas.* Philadelphia: W. B. Saunders.

Kertesz, A. (1979). *Aphasia and associated disorders: Taxonomy, localization and recovery.* New York and London: Grune & Stratton.

Kinkel, P. R., Kinkel, W. R., and Jacobs, L. (1986). Nuclear magnetic resonance imaging in patients with stroke. *Seminars in Neurology, 6,* 43–52.

Kirzinger, A., and Jurgens, U. (1982). Cortical lesion effects and vocalization in the squirrel monkey. *Brain Resarch, Amsterdam, 233,* 299–315.

Laakman, R. W., Kaufman, B., Han, J. S., Nelson, A. D., Clampitt, M., O'Block, A. M., Haaga, J. R., and Alfidi, R. J. (1985). MR imaging in patients with metallic implants. *Radiology, 157,* 711–714.

Lauterbur, P. C. (1973). Image formation by induced local interactions: Examples employing nuclear magnetic resonance. *Nature, 242,* 190–191.

Martin, J. H., and Brust, J. C. M. (1985). Imaging the living brain. In E. R. Kandel and J. H. Schwartz (Eds.), *Principles of neural science* (pp. 259–283). New York: Elsevier.

Matsui, T., and Hirano, A. (1978). *An atlas of the human brain for computerized tomography*. Tokyo: Igaku-Shoim.

Mohr, J. P., Pessin, M. S., Finkelstein, S., Funkenstein, H. H., Duncan, G. W., and Davis, K. R. (1978). Broca aphasia: Pathologic and clinical. *Neurology, 28*, 311–324.

Morgan, A., and Helm-Estabrooks, N. (1987). Back to the drawing board: A treatment program for nonverbal aphasia patients. In R. H. Brookshire (Ed.), *Clinical Aphasiology Conference proceedings.* (pp. 64–72). Minneapolis: BRK.

Moseley, I. (1988). Acute disturbances of cerebral function: Stroke and cerebro-vascular disease. In I. Moseley (Ed.), *Magnetic resonance imaging in diseases of the nervous system*. Oxford: Blackwell Scientific.

Mufson, E. J., and Pandya, D. N. (1984). Some observations on the course and composition of the cingulum bundle in the rhesus monkey. *Journal of Comprehensive Neurology, 225*, 31–43.

Muratoff, W. (1893). Secundare degeneration nach durchschneidung des balkens. *Neurologisches Centralblatt, 12*, 714–729.

Murdoch, B. E., Kennedy, M., McCallum, W., and Siddle, K. J. (1991). Persistent aphasia following a purely subcortical lesion: A magnetic resonance imaging study. *Aphasiology, 5*, 183–197.

Naeser, M. A. (1985). Quantitative approaches to computerized tomography in behavioral neurology. In M. M. Mesulam (Ed.), *Principles of behavioral neurology* (pp. 363–383). Philadelphia: F. A. Davis.

Naeser, M. A., Alexander, M. P., Helm-Estabrooks, N., Levine, H. L., Laughlin, S. A., and Geschwind, N. (1982). Aphasia with predominantly subcortical lesion sites—description of three capsular/putaminal aphasia syndromes. *Archives of Neurology, 39*, 2–14.

Naeser, M. A., Alexander, M. P., Stiassny-Eder, D., Galler, V., Hobbs, J., and Bachman, D. (in press). Real versus sham acupuncture in the treatment of paralysis in acute stroke patients—a CT scan lesion site study. *Journal of Neurologic Rehabilitation.*

Naeser, M. A., Frumkin, N. L., Baker, E. H., Nicholas, M., Palumbo, C. L., and Alexander, M. P. *CT scan lesion sites in severe nonverbal aphasia patients appropriate for treatment with a computer-assisted visual communication program (C-VIC).* Manuscript submitted for publication, 1992a.

Naeser, M. A., Frumkin, N. L., Fitzpatrick, P., and Palumbo, C. L. *CT scan lesion sites and good response versus poor response with melodic intonation therapy—a report of eight cases.* Manuscript submitted for publication, 1992b.

Naeser, M. A., Gaddie, A., Palumbo, C. L., and Stiassny-Eder, D. (1990). Late recovery of auditory comprehension in global aphasia: Improved recovery observed with subcortical temporal isthmus lesion versus Wernicke's cortical area lesion. *Archives of Neurology, 47*, 425–432.

Naeser, M. A., and Hayward, R. W. (1978). Lesion localization in aphasia with cranial computed tomography and the Boston Diagnostic Aphasia Exam. *Neurology, 28*, 545–551.

Naeser, M. A., Hayward, R. W., Laughlin, S. A., Becker, J. M. T., Jernigan, T. L., and Zatz, L. M. (1981). Quantitative CT scan studies in aphasia II: Comparison of the right and left hemispheres. *Brain and Language, 12*, 165–189.

Naeser, M. A., and Helm-Estabrooks, N. (1985). CT scan lesion localization and response to melodic intonation therapy with nonfluent aphasia cases. *Cortex, 21*, 203–223.

Naeser, M. A., Helm-Estabrooks, N., Haas, G., Auerbach, S., and Srinivasan, M. (1987). Relationship between lesion extent in "Wernicke's area" on CT scan and predicting recovery of comprehension in Wernicke's aphasia. *Archives of Neurology, 44*, 73–82.

Naeser, M. A., Palumbo, C. L., Helm-Estabrooks, N., Stiassny-Eder, D., and Albert, M. L. (1989). Severe non-fluency in aphasia: Role of the medial subcallosal fasciculus plus other white matter pathways in recovery of spontaneous speech. *Brain, 112*, 1–38.

Neilsen, J. M. (1946). *Agnosia, apraxia, aphasia: Their value in cerebral localization* (2nd ed., pp. 119–120). New York, NY: Hoeber.

Oldendorf, W. H. (1985). Principles of imaging structure by NMR. In L. Sokoloff (Ed.), *Brain imaging and brain function* (pp. 245–257). New York: Raven Press.

Palumbo, C. L., Naeser, M. A., and Verfaellie, M. (1990). *Location of memory areas and cortical language areas on MRI scans vs. CT scans.* Paper presented at the International Neuropsychological Society Meeting, Kissimmee, Florida.

Pavlicek, W. (1988). Safety considerations. In D. D. Stark and W. G. Bradley (Eds.), *Magnetic resonance imaging* (pp. 244–257). St Louis: C. V. Mosby.

Pavlicek, W., Geisinger, M., Castle, L., Borkowski, B. P., Meaney, T. F., Bream, B. L., and Gallagher, J. H. (1983). The effects of nuclear magnetic resonance on patients with cardiac pacemakers. *Radiology, 147*, 149–153.

Poeck, K., de Bleser, R., and von Keyserlingk, D. G. (1984). Computed tomography localization of standard aphasic syndromes. In F. C. Rose (Ed.), *Advances in neurology: Vol. 42. Progress in aphasiology* (pp. 71–89). New York: Raven Press.

Pollack, A. (1991, April 29). Medical technology "arms race" adds billions to the nation's bills: Concern over costs prompts limits on scanners. *New York Times*, pp. A1, B8.

Poncet, M., Habib, M., and Robillard, A. (1987). Deep left parietal lobe syndrome: Conduction aphasia and other neurobehavioral disorders due to a small subcortical lesion. *Journal of Neurology, Neurosurgery, and Psychiatry, 50*, 709–713.

Porch, B. E. (1967). *Porch Index of Communicative Ability.* Palo Alto: Consulting Psychologists Press.

Ramsberger, G., and Helm-Estabrooks, N. (1988). Visual action therapy for bucco-facial apraxia. *Clinical Aphasiology Conference proceedings.* San Diego: College Hill Press.

Rao, P. R. (1986). The use of Amer-Ind code with aphasic adults. In R. Chapey (Ed.), *Language intervention strategies in adult aphasia* (pp. 360–367). Baltimore: Williams & Wilkins.

Ross, E. D. (1980). Localization of the pyramidal tract in the internal capsule by whole brain dissection. *Neurology, 30*, 59–64.

Sarno, M. T., and Levita, E. (1979). Recovery in aphasia during the first year post stroke. *Stroke, 10*, 663–670.

Sarno, M. T., and Levita, E. (1981). Some observations on the nature of recovery in global aphasia after stroke. *Brain and Language, 31*, 1–12.

Schulz, M. L., Pandya, D., and Rosene, D. (in preparation). *The somatotopic arrangement of motor fibers in the periventricular white matter and internal capsule in the rhesus monkey.* Doctoral dissertation, Department of Behavioral Neuroscience, Boston University School of Medicine and Graduate School.

Seeram, E. (1982). *Computed tomography technology.* Philadelphia: W. B. Saunders.

Shapiro, J. (1990). *Radiation protection—a guide for scientists and physicians* (p. 88). Cambridge, MA: Harvard University Press.

Shellock, F. G., and Schatz, C. J. (1991). Metallic otologic implants: In vitro assessment of ferromagnetism at 1.5 T. *American Journal of Neuroradiology, 12*, 279–281.

Shuaib, A., Lee, D., Pelz, D., Fox, A., and Hachinski, V. C. (1992). The impact of magnetic resonance imaging on the management of acute ischemic stroke. *Neurology, 42*, 816–818.

SiliconGraphics: Computer Systems. (1991). A. M. Gambelin (Ed.), *Biomedical imaging: Brain surface mapping.* Mountain View, CA.

Sipponen, J. T., Kaste, M., Ketonen, L., Sepponen, R., Katevuo, K., and Sivula, A. (1983). Serial nuclear magnetic resonance (NMR) imaging in patients with cerebral infarction. *Journal of Computer Assisted Tomography, 7*, 585–589.

Skelly, M., Schinsky, L., Smith, R., Donaldson, R., and Griffin, J. (1975). American Indian Sign: Gestural communication for the speechless. *Archives of Physical Medicine and Rehabilitation, 56*, 156–160.

Skelly, M., Schinsky, L., Smith, R., Donaldson, R., and Griffin, J. (1974). American Indian Sign (Amerind) as a facilitator of verbalization for the oral-verbal apraxic. *Journal of Speech and Hearing Disorders, 39*, 445–456.

Smith, A. M., Bourbonnais, D., and Blanchette, G. (1981). Interaction between forced grasping and a learned precision grip after ablation of the supplementary motor area. *Brain Research, 222*, 395–400.

Sparks, R., Helm, N., and Albert, M. (1974). Aphasia rehabilitation resulting from melodic intonation therapy. *Cortex, 10*, 303–316.

Sparks, R., and Holland, A. L. (1976). Method: Melodic intonation therapy for aphasia. *Journal of Speech and Hearing Disorders, 41*, 287–297.

Steele, R. D., Weinrich, M., Wertz, R. T., Kleczewska, M. K., and Carlson, G. S. (1989). Computer-based visual communication in aphasia. *Neuropsychologia, 27*, 409–426.

Straub, W. H. (1984). Current diagnostic imaging methods: Relative strengths and limitations. In W. H. Straub (Ed.), *Manual of diagnostic imaging* (pp. 13–16). Boston: Little, Brown.

Tranel, D., Biller, J., Damasio, H., Adams, H. P., and Cornell, S. H. (1987). Global aphasia without hemiparesis. *Archives of Neurology, 44*, 304–308.

Trapnell, D. H. (1967). *Principles of x-ray diagnosis.* London: Butterworths.

Villafana, T. (1983). Physics and instrumentation. In S. H. Lee and K. C. V. G. Rao (Eds.), *Cranial computed tomography* (pp. 1–46). New York: McGraw-Hill.

Wang, A. M., Lin, J. C. T., and Rumbaugh, C. L. (1988). What is expected of CT in the evaluation of stroke? *Neuroradiology, 30,* 54–58.

Weinrich, M., Steele, R., Carlson, G. S., Kleczewska, M., Wertz, R. T., and Baker, E. H. (1989a). Processing of visual syntax in a globally aphasic patient. *Brain and Language, 36,* 391–405.

Weinrich, M., Steele, R., Kleczewska, M., Carlson, G. S., Baker, E. H., and Wertz, R. T. (1989b). Representation of ''verbs'' in a computerized visual communication system. *Aphasiology, 3,* 501–512.

Weisberg, L., Nice, C., and Katz, M. (1984). *Cerebral computed tomography: A text atlas.* Philadelphia: W. B. Saunders.

Yakovlev, P. I., and Locke, S. (1961). Limbic nuclei of thalamus and connections of limbic cortex. III. Corticocortical connections of the anterior cingulate gyrus, the cingulum, and the subcallosal bundle in monkey. *Archives of Neurology, 5,* 364–400.

Yock, D. H. (1985). *Computed tomography of CNS disease: A teaching file.* Chicago: Year Book Medical Publishers.

Zulch, K.-J. (1985). *The cerebral infarct: Pathology, pathogenesis, and computed tomography.* Berlin: Springer-Verlag.

CHAPTER 4
Assessment of Language Disorders in Adults

ROBERTA CHAPEY

Language has three highly interrelated and integrated components: cognitive, linguistic, and communicative (Muma, 1978) (see Fig. 4.1). **Cognitive** refers to the manner in which individuals acquire a knowledge of the world and in which they continue to process this knowledge. It refers to all of the processes by which sensory input is transformed, reduced, elaborated, stored, recovered, and used (Neisser, 1967). Through cognitive processes, we achieve knowledge and command of our world—we process information. According to Chapey (1983), these processes can be operationally defined as cognition or recognition/understanding, memory, convergent thinking, divergent thinking, and evaluative thinking.

Linguistic refers to language form and content. A form is a system of rules for communicating meaning. Three rule systems of language are phonology, morphology, and syntax. Language content is the meaning, topic, or subject matter involved in an utterance. **Communicative** refers to the use of language for the communication of meaning and involves a knowledge of how to converse with different partners and in different contexts (Craig, 1983); a knowledge of the rights, obligations, and expectations underlying the maintenance of discourse (Ochs and Schieffelin, 1979); and a knowledge of who can say what to whom in which way, where and when, and by what means (Prutting, 1979). It also refers to the use, purpose, or function that a particular utterance serves at any one time. For example, the same content and form "How are you?" can be used to question a statement, request information, greet a friend, and so on.

Within this context, **adult aphasia** is defined as an acquired impairment in language and the cognitive processes that underlie language caused by organic damage to the brain. It is characterized by a reduction in and dysfunction of language content or meaning, language form or structure, language use or function, and the cognitive processes that underlie language, such as recognition, comprehension, memory, and thinking. This impairment is manifested in listening, speaking, reading, and writing—although not necessarily to the same degree in each.

Aphasia does not include single-modality impairments (Darley, 1978), such as acquired isolated impairment in visual processing. The individual with a modality impairment or a disorder in which he or she performs better in one modality than

another—for example, visual versus auditory or gestural versus oral—has a transmissive type of problem called agnosia or apraxia (Darley, 1978; Wepman and Jones, 1961; Wepman and Van Pelt 1955). Aphasia, on the other hand, is an impairment in the individual's linguistic (content and form), communicative (use), and language-related cognitive systems (recognition, comprehension, thinking, and memory), regardless of which input or output modality is used (Fig. 4.1).

The transmissive impairment called **agnosia** is an inability to imitate, copy, or recognize the significance of incoming sensory information in the absence of perceptual deficits in the affected sensory modality (Darley, 1978; Wepman and Jones, 1961). That is, the individual might be unable to recognize a circle even though visual sensation is intact. In contrast, **apraxia** is an impairment in voluntary motor positioning and sequencing in the absence of an impairment in muscular control (Darley, 1978; Wepman and Jones, 1961). It is a motor speech disorder in which a disruption of central motor planning causes phonological errors that are variable and inconsistent. When a motor speech deficit is due to an impairment in muscular control, it is labeled **dysarthria**. In this instance, phonological errors are consistent.

Because aphasia, agnosia, apraxia, and dysarthria can occur in one individual, assessment involves determining which, if any, of these disorders exist and subsequently defining the nature and extent of the particular impairment.

ASSESSMENT

Assessment is defined as an organized, goal-directed evaluation of a variety of the three interrelated and integrated components of language cited above. Such an evaluation is carried out to determine the patient's abilities and impairments and the degree to which the impairments can be modified. It should explore "the nature of the language impairment and indicate what aspects of language performance are most appropriate for treatment" (Byng et al., 1990, p. 67).

According to Byng et al. (1990), Schuell (1970) described the roots of therapy in the following sources of knowledge: "(1) The clinician must know which cerebral processes are impaired and which are intact. (2) The clinician must know the

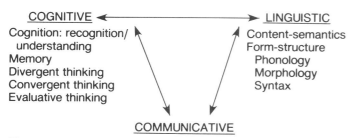

COGNITIVE ←————→ LINGUISTIC

Cognition: recognition/
understanding
Memory
Divergent thinking
Convergent thinking
Evaluative thinking

Content-semantics
Form-structure
Phonology
Morphology
Syntax

COMMUNICATIVE

Figure 4.1. Interrelated and integrated components of language.

level at which performance breaks down in each language modality. (3) The clinician must know the reason that performance breaks down when it does'' (p. 67).

A thorough, specific, and detailed assessment is essential if one is to see patterns of behavior, describe the complexity of the patient's language behavior, and develop a specific hierarchy of therapeutic goals that are appropriate to each patient. Specifically, there should be a strong connection between one's definition of language, one's description of the patient's language, and the goals that are established for therapy.

Therefore, the focus of this chapter is on the assessment of the language impairment in aphasia in relationship to the three interrelated and integrated components of language with particular reference to how findings may be used in organizing language therapy. Concerns are presented for accurate analysis of spontaneous language and knowledgeable presentation of tasks such as in standard tests of aphasia. The first section presents goals of assessment, a framework for classifying the data that are collected, and a list of what may be considered to be hallmarks of a quality assessment. These are followed by a discussion of components or procedures used in assessment. Last, the chapter is concerned with an analysis of each of the goals of assessment.

GOALS OF ASSESSMENT

The purposes of assessment are to describe language behaviors, to identify existing problems, to determine intervention goals, and to define factors that facilitate the retrieval of language. Specific goals are divided into etiologic goals, cognitive/linguistic/communicative goals, and intervention goals. In the present discussion, particular emphasis is placed on the evaluation of auditory comprehension and verbal language production, since these are the most essential components of language and, therefore, usually the focus of therapeutic activity.

Etiologic Goals

Etiologic goals are as follows:

1. Determination of the presence of aphasia
2. Identification and definition of factors that have precipitated or are maintaining the impairment to determine if they can be eliminated, reduced, or changed.

Cognitive/Linguistic/Communicative/Goals

In each of the following goals, behaviors are analyzed in order to specify the nature and extent of abilities and impairments in that particular behavior:

3. Analysis of ability to produce cognitive behaviors
4. Analysis of ability to comprehend the content of spoken language
5. Analysis of ability to comprehend the form of spoken language
6. Analysis of ability to produce the content of verbal language
7. Analysis of ability to produce the form of verbal language
8. Analysis of ability to communicate or use language for various functions

Intervention Goals

Intervention goals are as follows:

9. Determination of candidacy for therapy and prognosis in therapy
10. Specification and prioritization of a series of intervention goals

HALLMARKS OF A QUALITY ASSESSMENT

The nature of aphasic language deficit dictates the need to perform a high-quality, thorough assessment. Some of the characteristics that typify a quality evaluation are as follows: (*a*) It involves a current knowledge of significant characteristics and patterns of the language impairment in aphasia. This knowledge is based on firsthand experience with patients and a thorough knowledge of significant literature in aphasia and in language. (*b*) It is based on comprehensive and detailed language samples of patients performing tasks at various levels of difficulty. (*c*) It consists of repeated observation, abstraction of patterns of behavior, and formulation of theories to account for deficient performance. (*d*) It entails a quantitative and a qualitative or descriptive account of performance in order to generate information regarding the course, extent, and scope of therapy. (*e*) It involves respect for each individual patient, including that patient's past history and accomplishments.

INTERRELATED COMPONENTS OF THE ASSESSMENT PROCESS

Assessment in aphasia involves three interrelated processes: data collection, hypothesis formation, and hypothesis testing. Data collection is the process of obtaining information that is linked directly or indirectly to the language abilities and impairments of the individual. Hypothesis formation involves categorizing the data or forming taxonomies based on regularities or similarities observed in the information collected. It also entails interpreting the data and making decisions regarding the presence of aphasia, candidacy for therapy, prognosis, and goals of intervention. The third process consists of hypothesis testing or ongoing assessment and analysis of goals, methods, and progress in therapy.

Data Collection

The data that are collected are linked in some way to the language abilities and impairments of each patient. This information can be obtained through reported observations or direct observations.

Reported observations involve gathering data from other professional workers who have appraised a variety of aspects of the person's behavior or are familiar with the patient's history. In addition, persons who live with or who have frequent contact with the patient can provide valuable information concerning language. These individuals may be asked to keep a diary or complete checklists or rating scales that relate to their perception of the client's cognitive, linguistic, and/or communi-

Table 4.1.
Final 16 Items of the Communicative Effectiveness Index (CETI)[a]

Please Rate _____'s ability at . . .

1. Getting somebody's attention.
2. Getting involved in group conversations that are about him/her.
3. Giving yes and no answers appropriately.
4. Communicating his/her emotions.
5. Indicating that he/she understands what is being said to him/her.
6. Having coffee-time visits and conversations with friends and neighbors (around the bedside or at home).
7. Having a one-to-one conversation with you.
8. Saying the name of someone whose face is in front of him/her.
9. Communicating physical problems such as aches and pains.
10. Having a spontaneous conversation (i.e., starting the conversation and/or changing the subject).
11. Responding to or communicating anything (including yes or no) without words.
12. Starting a conversation with people who are not close family.
13. Understanding writing.
14. Being part of a conversation when it is fast and there are a number of people involved.
15. Participating in a conversation with strangers.
16. Describing or discussing something in depth.

[a] From Lomas, J., Pickard, L., Bester, S., Elbard, H., Finlayson, A., and Zoghaib, C. (1989). The Communicative Effectiveness Index: Development and psychometric evaluation of a functional communication measure for adult aphasia. *Journal of Speech and Hearing Disorders, 54,* 113–124. Reprinted by permission. © 1989, the American Speech-Language-Hearing Association.

Table 4.2.
Attitudes of Spouse Toward Persons with Aphasia: Rank Order of Items 1–10 and 61–70 Based on Spouses' Raw Score Data[a]

	Spouse Group		
Rank Order	Fluent Aphasia (N = 15)	Nonfluent Aphasia (N = 15)	Controls (N = 30)
1	Demanding	Demanding	Mature
2	Temperamental	Temperamental	Kind
3	Worrying	Immature	Sensitive
4	Nervous	Worrying	Good-natured
5	Emotional	Nervous	Friendly
6	Immature	Adaptable	Pleasant
7	Moody	Preoccupied	Warm
8	Impatient	Confused	Sexy
9	Confused	Intolerant	Thoughtful
10	Mannerly	Impatient	Intolerant
61	Optimistic	Self-controlled	Persistent
62	Aggressive	Optimistic	Worrying
63	Cold	Dependable	Nervous
64	Obnoxious	Affectionate	Gloomy
65	Self-confident	Thoughtful	Confused
66	Self-centered	Sexy	Cold
67	Intelligent	Intelligent	Slow
68	Mature	Mature	Obnoxious
69	Sexy	Capable	Demanding
70	Independent	Independent	Immature

[a] From Zraich, R. J., and Boone, D. R. (1991). Spouse attitude toward the person with aphasia. *Journal of Speech and Hearing Research, 34*(1), 123–128. Reprinted by permission. © 1991, The American Speech-Language-Hearing Association.

errors of aphasic patients vary independently across different communication contexts, contents, and tasks (Glosser, et al., 1988). Therefore, the examiner will want to elicit language in several contexts, such as unstructured, moderately structured, and highly structured contexts, and consider the effects of sampling methodology on the language elicited.

Unstructured Spontaneous Language Observation

In unstructured observation, the clinician describes the individual's cognitive, linguistic, and communicative behaviors in a natural setting when there is a minimum of control or interference. The setting should be familiar to the client and provide an opportunity for the individual to interact verbally with others.

Moderately Structured Spontaneous Language Observation

At times, the observer may take a moderately active role in structuring observations and use predetermined questions or tasks to elicit spontaneous language. For example, the client might be asked to retell a story, describe pictures, or answer direct questions or requests, such as "How do you make a cup of coffee?" "How do you make a phone call?" or "Describe the way you might get into your apartment if you have forgotten your key." The clinician and client may also role play specific situations, such as (*a*) ordering in a restaurant and paying the bill, (*b*) relating the date and time of a doctor's appointment,

cative behaviors. For example, the spouse might compile a diary of how her husband typically makes his needs and wants known during a certain period of time each day. Reported observations can take the form of an interview or written correspondence.

An excellent example of such a tool is the Communicative Effectiveness Index (CETI) (Lomas et al., 1989) (see Table 4.1), which allows significant others to rate their partner's performance in several functional communicative situations. It can be used at various time intervals and can therefore measure change in functional communication ability. Another measure that uses reported observations assesses spouse attitudes toward their aphasic partner with respect to **maturity** (Factor 1:48.9), **independence** (Factor 2:19.5), **desirability** (Factor 3:9.5), **compliance** (Factor 4:8.4), **egocentricity** (Factor 5:4.6), and **sociability** (Factor 6:3.7) (Zraich and Boone, 1991). Table 4.2 presents the rank order of the first and last 10 items of this measure for the three spouse groups studied by Zraich and Boone (1991).

During **direct observation**, the clinician observes the behavior of the client. Such assessment occurs during several sessions in order to maximize the patient's ability to respond and to minimize fatigue, stress, and failure. Obtaining several samples is also necessary, since the verbal complexity and language

or (c) answering the phone and relaying a message. Narrative, procedural, conversational, and expository types of discourse should be obtained, if possible, since Wambaugh et al. (1991) found that type of discourse significantly affected the aphasic individual's use of communicative functions.

The use of moderately structured observations permits the clinician to elicit and observe a larger language sample than might otherwise be possible and/or explore specific aspects of spontaneous language that had not emerged in a totally natural and unstructured context.

Highly Structured Spontaneous Language Observation

Direct observations that involve the use of highly stimulus–response tasks, such as "The sky is _____" or "Tell me the name of this object," are part of every assessment. In most instances, standard tests of aphasia form the major portion of highly structured observations.

The three most frequently used comprehensive tests of language ability are the Minnesota Test for Differential Diagnosis of Aphasia (MTDDA) (Schuell, 1965), the Boston Diagnostic Aphasia Examination (BDAE) (Goodglass and Kaplan, 1983), and the Porch Index of Communicative Ability (PICA) (Porch, 1967).

The MTDDA, developed by Hildred Schuell (1965), is the most comprehensive test for aphasia and focuses on the assessment of the patient's strengths and weaknesses in all language modalities (speaking, listening, reading, and writing) in order to facilitate the selection of intervention goals.

The test itself consists of 46 subtests that are divided into 5 sections: 9 subtests of visual and reading ability; 15 subtests of speech and language; 10 subtests of visuomotor and writing skills; and 4 subtests of numerical and arithmetic processes. Within each section, subtests range in length from 5 to 32 items, and items range from easy to difficult. A clinical rating scale from 0 to 6 can be used to quantify performance in the four modalities.

This test provides a classification system into one of five major and two minor groups. The categories are simple aphasia, aphasia with visual impairment, aphasia with persisting disfluency, aphasia with scattered findings, aphasia with sensorimotor involvement, aphasia with intermittent auditory imperception, and irreversible aphasia syndrome (see Chapter 7). This classification system is unique since it is not anatomically based but rather reflects Schuell's view that aphasia is a multimodality, unidimensional impairment. In addition, these classifications help identify the presence of additional problems that sometimes accompany aphasia, such as perceptual disorders, apraxia, or dysarthria. Results can also be interpreted in terms of prediction of recovery.

The BDAE was developed by Harold Goodglass and Edith Kaplan (1972, rev. 1983). This test provides a comprehensive exploration of a wide range of communicative abilities. It contains 27 subtests that are divided into sections: conversational and expository speech, auditory comprehension, oral expression, understanding written language, and writing. Supplementary tests are also provided.

Scoring of the conversational and expository speech section is accomplished with an aphasia severity rating scale from one (1) to seven (7), and a profile of speech characteristics: *melodic line* (intonational contour), *phrase length* (longest occasional uninterrupted word runs), *articulatory agility* (facility at phonetic and syllable level), *grammatical form* (variety of grammatical constructions, even if incomplete), *paraphasia* in running speech, *repetition* (score in high-probability subtest), *word finding* (information content in relation to fluency), and *auditory comprehension* (mean of percentiles on four auditory comprehension subtests).

Scoring of the auditory, oral, reading, and writing sections varies from plus-minus scores, 4-point scales, and counts of the number of paraphasias in the oral expression subtests. The total score varies on each subtest. Therefore, the scores are summarized on a subtest summary profile form. These scores are derived to allow for comparison of patient profiles with performances of a standard group. Results are also used to identify specific localization-based aphasic syndromes, namely Broca's, Wernicke's, anomic, or conduction aphasia (see Chapter 1).

This test does not interpret results in terms of prognosis. However, each of the above syndromes has been shown to have specific characteristics of recovery. Therefore, the individual clinician can use these classifications as a basis for predicting degrees and patterns of recovery (Davis, 1983).

The PICA was developed and standardized by Bruce Porch (1967). This test is not as comprehensive as the MTDDA or the BDAE and samples a limited number of language behaviors. However, it is a "sensitive and reliable measurement of degree of deficit and amount of recovery" (Davis, 1983, p. 160). The test contains 18 subtests: 4 verbal, 8 gestural, and 6 graphic. There are 10 common objects and therefore 10 tasks within each subtest. For each task, patient behavior is evaluated on a 16-point multidimensional scoring system that is intended to be sensitive to the completeness, accuracy, promptness, responsiveness, and efficacy of each response (see Table 4.3). The number assigned to each response in a subtest is averaged, yielding 18 subtest scores. These scores can be further averaged to provide a verbal, gestural, and graphic mean. Scores for the language functions of pantomime, reading, auditory, visual, writing, and copying can also be obtained. A total mean response level represents the patient's overall level of communicative ability. Percentile scores indicate how a patient compares with a larger standard sample of aphasic patients and can be interpreted in terms of prognosis.

Other comprehensive tests of language function include the Neurosensory Center Comprehensive Examination for Aphasia (Spreen and Benton, 1969, rev. 1977), the Language Modalities Test for Aphasia (Wepman and Jones, 1961), and the Western Aphasia Battery (Kertesz, 1982; Kertesz and Poole, 1974, rev. 1982). Two of the tests that measure language use are the Functional Communication Profile (Sarno, 1969) and Communicative Abilities in Daily Living (Holland, 1980).

A recent survey of aphasia clinicians (Jackson and Tompkins, 1991) found that the nine most frequently used supplemental aphasia tests in decreasing frequency of use are the Boston Naming Test (Goodglass and Kaplan, 1972, rev. 1983), the Reading Comprehension Battery for Aphasia (LaPointe and Horner, 1979), the Word Fluency Test (Borkowski et al., 1967), the Coloured Progressive Matrices (Raven, 1965), the Revised Token Test (McNeil and Prescott, 1978), the Peabody Picture Vocabulary Test—Revised (Dunn and Dunn, 1981), the Auditory Comprehension Test for Sentences (Shewan, 1979), the Nelson Reading Skills Test (Hanna et al., 1977), and the Reporter's Test (De Renzi and Ferrari, 1978). In another recent presen-

Table 4.3.
Multidimensional Scoring Categories[a]

Score	Level	Description
16	Complex	Accurate, responsive, complex, immediate, elaborative response to test item
15	Complete	Accurate, responsive, complete, immediate response to test item
14	Distorted	Accurate, responsive, complete, response to test item, but with reduced facility of production
13	Complete-Delayed	Accurate, responsive, complete response to the test item which is significantly slow or delayed
12	Incomplete	Accurate, responsive, response to test item which is lacking in completeness
11	Incomplete-Delayed	Accurate, responsive, incomplete response to test item which is significantly slowed or delayed
10	Corrected	Accurate response to test item self-correcting a previous error without request or after a prolonged delay
9	Repetition	Accurate response to test item after a repetition of the instructions by request or after a prolonged delay
8	Cured	Accurate response to test item stimulated by a cue, additional information, or another test item
7	Related	Inaccurate response to test item which is clearly related to or suggestive of an accurate response
6	Error	Inaccurate response to the test item
5	Intelligible	Intelligible response which is not associated with the test item, for example, perseverative or automatic responses or an expressed indication of inability to respond
4	Unintelligible	Unintelligible or incomprehensible response which can be differentiated from other responses
3	Minimal	Unintelligible response which cannot be differentiated from other responses
2	Attention	Patient attends to test item but gives no responses
1	No Response	Patient exhibits no awareness of test item

[a] From Porch, B. (1971). Multidimensional scoring in aphasia testing. *Journal of Speech and Hearing Research, 14,* 776–792. Reprinted by permission. © 1971, The American Speech-Language-Hearing Association.

tation (Helm-Estabrooks and Nicholas, 1991), it was reported that several new test protocols are being used with severe aphasic individuals. They are the Boston Assessment of Severe Aphasia (Helm-Estabrooks et al., 1989), the Aphasia Diagnostic Profiles (Helm-Estabrooks, 1991a), and the Test of Oral and Limb Apraxia (Helm-Estabrooks, 1991b).

When using any test of aphasia, the clinician should define the specific cognitive, linguistic, and communcative data that are obtainable from that measure. To facilitate this process, Appendix 4.1 presents an analysis of some of the above tests in terms of the cognitive, linguistic, and/or communicative behavior that may be ascertained from each.

Nonstandard observations are also used as data. These observations are highly structured observations that do not have published norms. They are typically cited as tasks in empirical research studies and doctoral dissertations and can easily be adopted for assessment purposes. Such measures can yield valuable insights into the individual's language and communication abilities and impairments.

For example, Shewan (1988a, 1988b) developed a comprehensive and in-depth method for analyzing spontaneous language samples in response to picture description tasks (see Table 4.4)—tasks that are part of the Western Aphasia Battery (WAB) (Shewan and Kertesz, 1980) and of the Minnesota Test for Differential Diagnosis of Aphasia (Schuell, 1965). Appendix 4.2 contains part of the scoring system for the language sample using the SSLA (Shewan Spontaneous Language Analysis) system.

Content Validity of Tests of Aphasia

Determining the content validity of a test involves deciding if the instrument is measuring what it should be measuring. The emphasis is on what is being evaluated (Kerlinger, 1964). Analysis is guided by the question, Is the content of the test representative of language as it is spoken and heard by adults who are actively engaged in communication? Does the test provide useful information about the nature of the underlying disorder (Byng et al., 1990; Kay et al., 1990)? Standard tests of aphasia have been questioned on this basis (Byng et al., 1990; David, 1990; Kay et al., 1990; Martin, 1977; Weniger, 1990) in part because there is no clear operational definition of what is being assessed and no specific model of language that is used as a basis of test construction. The conceptual schemata underlying tests have ignored the complexity factor in language (Byng et al., 1990; David, 1990; Kay et al., 1990; Martin, 1977; Weniger, 1990) and provide little opportunity for sentence creation (Taylor, 1965). Tests have not reflected the fact that the communication of meaning is the essence of language (Goodman, 1971), and results do not supply enough information about the content, context, intent, structure, relevance, and meaningfulness of utterances.

Indeed, Byng et al. (1990) suggest that standardized tests "neither clarify what is wrong with the patient, nor specify what treatment should be provided" (p. 67). Further, Byng et al. (1990) state that formal aphasia tests cannot meet Schuell's (1970) requirements cited above.

David (1990), Kay et al. (1990), and Weniger (1990) observe that standardized tests are clearly unsuitable measures of change (over time), "most having simply not enough items in the individual subtests to allow for sensitive and reliable measurement'' (David, 1990, p. 105). Indeed, real change made by the patient in specific areas of language functioning may not be represented in the overall test score, and the effectiveness of specific treatments may not therefore be adequately measured (Kay et al., 1990). David (1990) states that treatment of aphasic patients demands tools of the highest caliber because treatment based on findings obtained through inadequate assessment instruments or procedures ''will almost certainly lack focus or be misdirected'' (p. 106).

Nonetheless, valid tests that are properly constructed to take into account salient psycholinguistic variables should be a component of assessment (Kay et al., 1990). They are valuable because they enable the clinician to screen the aphasic individual's language ability and to obtain objectively specific information about selected types of language functioning in a relatively brief period of time. In addition, results allow the clinician to compare each patient to objective norms and to the behavior of other individuals who have aphasia.

However, before tests are selected for use with aphasic individuals, the goals and scope of particular tests must be reviewed:

Does the test allow for observation of patients when they are actively engaged in communication?

What model of language formed the basis of test construction (Byng et al., 1990)?

Does the test reveal the nature of the language impairment (Byng et al., 1990; Kay et al., 1990; Weniger, 1990)?

What is the rationale for each task in the test?

Does the test sample the complex and dynamic (or changing) components of language (Muma, 1983)?

Does the test assess the functioning of the components of the language processing system, that is, the modular independent subsystems and the connections between them (Byng et al., 1990; Kay et al., 1990)?

Does the test sample the crucial and representative aspects of language (Snyder, 1983)?

Which items in the test allow for evaluation of phonology, morphology, syntax, and semantics?

Do test results tell about context, content, relevance, form, meaningfulness, and use of the client's language?

Do results specify the conditions under which language comprehension and production are facilitated (e.g., the context in which it occurs, the partner with whom it occurs)?

Table 4.4.
Shewan Spontaneous Language Analysis (SSLA) System[a]

1. *Number of Utterances.* This is a measure of the total number of utterances spoken by a subject. An utterance represents a complete thought and frequently corresponds to a complete sentence. However, this correspondence is not one to one. The criteria used to segment the sample into utterances are detailed in Shewan (1988a)
2. *Time.* The total speaking time for the language sample is measured beginning with the first syllable and ending with the last syllable. Any spoken material such as interjections or prompts from the examiner are subtracted from the overall time so that only speaker time is included.
3. *Rate.* Rate of speech is defined as the total number of syllables spoken per minute by the subject.
4. *Length.* The length measure is calculated by dividing the number of utterances containing five or fewer words by the total number of utterances spoken and is expressed as a percentage.
5. *Melody.* The variables of melody, involving the rhythm of speech, the stress patterns employed, and the intonation contours expressed, deal in part with the suprasegmental aspects of phonology. However, the rating is independent of pauses, since they can be the result of a word-finding problem rather than a prosodic disturbance per se. The 7-point melody rating scale, similar to that on the BDAE, is used.
6. *Articulation.* Articulation is rated using a global judgment of articulatory accuracy. This includes imprecise speech and/or verbal dyspraxia. Determination of whether the errors represent articulatory or phonological disturbances or both is not made. The 7-point articulation rating scale, similar to that for articulatory agility on the BDAE, is used.
7. *Complex Sentences.* This syntactic variable measures the number of complex sentences relative to the total number of utterances in the sample. It is expressed as a percentage to account for the different number of utterances across subjects. A complex sentence is defined as one that contains at least one independent clause and at least one or more dependent clauses. Conjoined sentences and complementing and noncomplementing infinitive constructions are not considered complex sentences.
8. *Errors.* This variable measures syntactic and morphological errors. It reflects the number of errors produced relative to the number of utterances, expressed as a percentage. Therefore, if a subject makes more than one error per utterance, the percentage could exceed 100.
9. *Content Units.* This measure is very similar to that described by Yorkston and Beukelman (1977). A content unit is defined as a grouping of information expressed as a unit by normal speakers. The number of content units is a measure of the total amount of information conveyed by a speaker. Two major steps establish the content units (Appendix 4.1). Each major concept, which normal speakers expressed, was first listed. These included concepts such as *house, boy, girl, pond,* and so on. They might be likened to topics as described in the child language literature. Each additional grouping of information describing or modifying the major concepts was added as a content unit.
10. *Paraphasias.* The paraphasia measure is primarily a measure of substitution behavior to capture what an aphasic patient describes when he or she cannot produce the correct content. The percentage of paraphasias is a measure of the number of paraphasias relative to the total number of utterances. Similar to the Errors variable, the percentage can exceed 100 if a person makes more than one paraphasia per utterance. Paraphasias include several types: literal (phonemic), verbal (semantic), neologism, and jargon.
11. *Repetitions.* Repetitions are simply counted and a percentage is calculated.
12. *Communication Efficiency.* This variable, taken from Yorkston and Beukelman (1977), is a measure of the amount of information conveyed per unit of time or the rate of information transfer. It is computed by dividing the total number of content units by the time for the language sample (see Appendix 4.1).

[a] From Shewan, C. (1988). The Shewan Spontaneous Language Analysis (SSLA) system for aphasic adults: Description, reliability and validity. *Journal of Communication Disorders, 21,* 103–138.

Does the test assess the regularity or predictability of language, such as lexical status, word frequency, part of speech, imageability, and semantic relationships between items (Byng et al., 1990)? Are these controlled systematically?

Is the test ecologically valid (i.e., does it sample language in a natural environment) (Muma, 1983)?

Does the test assess ability to learn or to profit from language therapy? How therapeutically relevant is the content of the test (Byng et al., 1990)?

Hypothesis Formation

The information obtained during data collection needs to be organized, systematized, and condensed in a meaningful way. In this decision-making component of assessment, the diagnostician sifts through all of the information obtained, delicately balancing and blending the data to arrive at a penetrating understanding of a person's total behavior. Hypothesis formation, then, is a sophisticated clinical judgment applied to the information collected. It is an evaluation of the type, frequency, and pattern of behaviors produced by the individual and an exploration of the interrelatedness of various behaviors. Significant decisions must be made during this process. One decision involves a determination of the suitability of the patient for therapy. Further, a synthesis of the diagnostic findings will indicate priorities and specific plans for a program of intervention.

Characterization of Hypotheses

Many clinicians use one of the anatomically based classification systems available in the aphasia literature (such as fluent versus nonfluent, or Broca's, Wernicke's, or anomic aphasia) to categorize or label the results of their assessment. However, there is still no universally acceptable classification system (Holland et al. 1986; Kertesz, 1979). In addition, the validity of such classification systems has been called into question (Binder, 1984; Byng et al., 1990; Caramazza, 1984; David, 1990; Holland et al., 1986; Marshall, 1984; Metter et al., 1984; Schwartz; 1984, Swindell et al., 1984; Trupe, 1984; Weniger, 1990; Whitaker, 1984) for several reasons: (*a*) some patients cannot be fitted into one of the categories, (*b*) patients in these categories cannot be said to be homogeneously impaired, (*c*) a patient can evolve from one classification to another during the course of recovery, (*d*) discrepancies in interjudge reliability can possibly stem from lack of agreement as to how to assign and weight specific responses, (*e*) severity and/or education rather than site of lesion can possibly be responsible for the variability of patient behavior, (*f*) categories do not reveal the nature of the language impairment, and (*g*) syndrome classification in itself does not provide the basis for any comprehensive treatment program. In addition, according to Holland et al. (1986), agreement on the nature, type, and extent of secondary problems can confound the labeling of patients—even for "experts."

Some government agencies are encouraging clinicians to summarize patient data on rating scales such as the Functional Independence Measure (FIM) (Research Foundation, 1990) (see Table 4.5). The FIM, part of the Uniform Data Set for medical rehabilitation, was developed in part as a means to set reimbursement rates in response to cost-containment efforts by the government (Frattali, 1992). The brevity of description alone on this rudimentary, conceptually flawed measure makes it an

Table 4.5.
Functional Independence Measure (FIM)[a]

7	Complete Independence (Timely, Safely)	NO
6	Modified Independence (Device)	
L Modified Dependence		
E 5	Supervision	
V 4	Minimal Assist (Subject = 75%)	
E 3	Moderate Assist (Subject = 50%+)	HELPER
L Complete Dependence		
S 2	Maximal Assist (Subject = 25%+)	
1	Total Assist (Subject + 0%+)	

Self-Care	FOLLOW-UP
A. Eating	
B. Grooming	
C. Bathing	
D. Dressing—Upper Body	
E. Dressing—Lower Body	
F. Toileting	
Sphincter Control	
G. Bladder Management	
H. Bowel Management	
Mobility	
Transfer:	
I. Bed, Chair, Wheelchair	
J. Toilet	
K. Tub, Shower	
Locomotion	
L. *Walk/wheelchair*	w
	c
M. Stairs	
Communication	
N. Comprehension	a
	v
O. Expression	v
	n
Social Cognition	
P. Social Interaction	
Q. Problem Solving	
R. Memory	
	Total FIM: _____

NOTE: Leave no blanks; enter 1 if patient not testable due to risk.

[a]From Research Foundation. (1990). Guide for use of the Uniform Data Set for Medical Rehabilitation. Buffalo, NY: Research Foundation, State University of New York.

instrument of questionable reliability, validity, and sensitivity. Frattali (1992) believes that a more in-depth description of the individual's vocational and residential/environmental communication needs and his or her communication performance in a variety of contexts would yield a more valid functional independence measure. In addition, it is hoped that an instrument that contains a sufficient range of performance and is relevant to functioning outside the clinical setting would be more sensitive to change over time (Frattali, 1992).

Rather than summarize assessment results with two or three scores, Weniger (1990) observes that there is a growing tendency among clinicians to approach assessment from the perspective of information-processing models—to analyze what underlying impairment may be causing surface-level symptoms.

That is, clinicians increasingly seek to understand the nature of the deficit (Weniger, 1990)—to explore tasks so that they can consider language deficits in terms of the processing problems underlying them (Byng et al., 1990).

Specifically, to reach a hypothesis about the nature of the impairment, we need to assess performance on a variety of appropriate tasks; that is, we should assess the type(s) of errors made and the manner in which the patient goes about doing a task (Byng et al., 1990). We also need to break tasks (such as sentence comprehension, reading aloud single words, gesturing, hailing a bus, filling in a check, and turn taking) into their component processes and examine the functioning of each of those processes in detail (Byng et al., 1990) in order to derive hypotheses about the nature of the underlying processing problems of the language deficit. Such hypotheses can subsequently be tested in therapy.

In addition, since aphasia is a dynamic disorder and the symptomatology of a patient may change over time, many clinicians, such as David (1990), believe that it is essential to describe the way in which the pattern of the disorder may change during recovery. David (1990) suggests that this knowledge provides information that is essential in planning the direction of therapy.

Therefore, the present orientation emphasizes that it is more clinically relevant to describe and summarize the actual cognitive, linguistic (content and form), and communicative abilities and impairments of each individual (Table 4.6), since this type of information will clarify and facilitate the choice of intervention goals. Assessment should indicate the underlying processing needed to respond to tasks and the component processes that are impaired. Descriptive summaries should indicate the level at which (*a*) the individual is able to perform without error, (*b*) performance begins to break down, and (*c*) performance breaks down completely. For example, a patient might never produce the word "fork" in unstructured spontaneous language but might be able to say it inconsistently in an open-ended sentence such as "I eat with a knife and ____." The same individual might consistently recognize the word "fork." Thus, specific abilities and impairments are described and summarized, and the factors that facilitate and retard the retrieval of these behaviors are identified.

As noted above, results of testing are sometimes expressed as a quantitative score. However, this method of characterizing data has often been questioned (Frattali, 1992; Goldstein, 1948; Martin, 1977), since a numerical score gives little insight into what the patient still can and cannot do and is not the most meaningful information for establishing therapeutic goals.

A more appropriate description of data can be formulated by segmenting or dividing behaviors into various categories. For example, the clinician may have one category for all movable objects, one for all nonmovable objects, one for body parts, one for food, one for contingent utterances, one for discourse repairs/revisions, and so on. When findings are divided into such categories, they are called **taxonomies**. Frequency counts of each taxonomy are then tabulated to determine the number of times each category is produced.

Subsequently, the aphasiologist attempts to hypothesize about factors that appear to facilitate or retard the occurrence of particular behaviors within each taxonomy. For example, a patient may be able to use the words "is" and "are" in the greeting "How is everything?" and "How are you?" but not

Table 4.6.
Outline for Language Summaries

I. Cognitive Behavior

Thinking
a. Cognition (recognition/understanding), convergent thinking, divergent thinking, and evaluative thinking produced
b. Level at which performance begins to break down
c. Level at which performance breaks down completely
d. Factors that facilitate and retard performance

Memory
a. Memory skills demonstrated
b. Level at which performance begins to break down
c. Level at which performance breaks down completely
d. Factors that facilitate and retard performance

II. Linguistic Behavior

Auditory Comprehension
Content
a. Content comprehended
b. Level at which performance begins to break down
c. Level at which performance breaks down completely
d. Factors that facilitate and retard performance
Form
a. Form comprehended
b. Level at which performance begins to break down
c. Level at which performance breaks down completely
d. Factors that facilitate and retard performance

Language Production
Content
a. Content produced: lexical selection/use, topic selection/use, specificity/accuracy
b. Level at which performance begins to break down
c. Level at which performance breaks down completely
d. Factors that facilitate and retard performance
Form
a. Form produced
b. Level at which performance begins to break down
c. Level at which performance breaks down completely
d. Factors that facilitate and retard performance

III. Communicative Behavior

a. Speech acts produced
b. Topic selection, introduction, maintenance, and change
c. Turn-taking initiation, response, repair/revision, pause time, interruption/overlap, feedback to speakers, adjacent utterances, contingent utterances, quality/conciseness
d. Stylistic variations produced
e. Ability to relate to given and new information
f. Nonverbal communication produced
g. Level at which performance begins to break down
h. Level at which performance breaks down completely
i. Factors that facilitate and retard performance

IV. General Impression of the Effectiveness of Language
A summary of the client's interactions and behavior related to content/form/use and production/comprehension

to indicate possession in a sentence such as "This is mine." Another patient may be able to repeat a word if it is accompanied by a picture but be unable to repeat the same word in the absence of a visual cue.

Taxonomies are also described by comparing each individual's behavior with a predetermined standard of performance.

Such a standard may be operationally defined and criterion referenced. For example, descriptions might include the following: consistent use of the preposition ''on'' with common nouns; production of the name of a significant individual in the environment 50% of the time; and use of the verbs ''come'' and ''eat'' in their infinitive form in 25% of the patient's utterances, where appropriate. The objective of such description is to determine the degree to which a specific behavior is available. Therefore, these descriptions are helpful in determining the initial goal of therapy and in reassessing the patient to determine when goals have been reached (Bloom and Lahey, 1978; Lahey, 1988). Thus, when descriptive language summaries are accurately written, well organized, easy to understand, and free of professional jargon, slang, and vague terminology, they will clarify and facilitate the choice of therapeutic goals and strategies.

Hypothesis Testing

The results of hypothesis formation, and specifically the goals of intervention that are established, should be considered tentative and flexible enough to change as new evidence emerges. Hypothesis testing, then, enables the clinician to continue to secure additional data about the language abilities and impairments of each patient in order to determine the validity, accuracy, and appropriateness of hypotheses that were formulated. Separation of assessment and intervention allows for the presentation of information in an organized manner. However, in practice, assessment is an ongoing part of management and occurs at every phase of rehabilitation.

GOAL 1: DETERMINATION OF THE PRESENCE OF APHASIA

The presence or absence of aphasia frequently can be determined during an initial observation or interaction with the patient. When the language impairment is severe or moderate, the presence of aphasia is obvious and a diagnosis can be made within a brief period of time. The remainder of the assessment would then focus on specifying the nature and extent of the disorder. However, when symptoms are mild, it may be more difficult to confirm the presence of a language impairment. That is, language problems may not be apparent when conversation is limited and expected responses are convergent. In such cases, despite the presence of aphasia as identified by the family or the physician, persons with aphasia may be so mildly impaired that they achieve perfect or near-perfect scores on traditional or standard tests of aphasia. For these persons, a diagnosis of aphasia may be identified by describing the cognitive, linguistic, and communicative deficits that are exhibited. For example, an individual might experience difficulty in producing certain aspects of the content of spoken language such as infrequently used words like ''Tarrytown,'' the name of the city where he lives, and yet be able to produce frequently used words, such as ''knife,'' ''fork,'' and ''pen,'' without difficulty. At times, the final decision regarding the presence of aphasia in mildly impaired individuals is tentative and is based on carefully documented observation and clinical judgment.

In addition to determining the presence of aphasia, it is frequently the responsibility of the clinician to differentiate between the language impairment in aphasia and a language impairment that results from a different etiology. Careful analysis of the case history should be performed to confirm the fact that the language symptoms do not reflect right-hemisphere impairment, dementia, or closed head injury (see Chapters 5, 28, 29, and 30) or other neurological, pharmacological, or emotional disorders.

Right-Hemisphere Impairment (RH)

According to Myers (1984), RH patients are capable of functioning adequately on superficial communicative levels but experience difficulty in more complex and sophisticated communicative situations. Myers (1984) suggests that the patient is impaired in four areas: (a) lower-order perceptual problems, (b) problems with affect and prosody, (c) linguistic disorders, and (d) higher-order perceptual and cognitive deficits (see Chapter 28).

The lower-order perceptual deficits can include various visuospatial deficits (such as visual discrimination, visual memory, visual integration, visual imagery, facial recognition, topological, geographic and spatial orientation, left-side neglect, and visuoconstructive deficits) and difficulty in extracting meaning from sensory information because of inability to appreciate the external context in which the stimulus is embedded and inability to integrate it with internal associations (Myers, 1984). Patients may also have reading and writing deficits that can be perceptually based and/or linguistically based.

When affect is impaired, the individual may have difficulty in the discrimination and production of a normal range of facial expressions that express various emotions. Prosody impairments are also common, and the patient may be perceived as speaking in a monotone (Myers, 1984).

The linguistic deficits that are common in RH patients do not resemble those of the aphasic patient. Indeed, RH patients may have more difficulty on tasks that are easy for aphasics and less difficulty on tasks that are more difficult for aphasics (Myers, 1984). Myers (1984) suggests that impairments on aphasia tests may reflect visuospatial or neglect impairments, visual integration deficits, and problems in higher-order cognitive and perceptual processing rather than linguistic deficits per se. RH patients fall below the norm on various auditory comprehension and language production tasks and experience most difficulty when complexity (e.g., linguistic, extralinguistic, and cognitive complexity) increases.

Higher cognitive impairments are most apparent when the patient is engaged in open-ended, more sophisticated communication (Myers, 1984).

The less concrete and the more complex the task, the more likely the patient will manifest the following deficits: (a) difficulty in organizing information in an efficient, meaningful way; (b) a tendency to produce impulsive answers that are rife with tangential and related, but unnecessary, detail; (c) difficulty in distinguishing between what is important and what is not; (d) problems in assimilating and using contextual cues; (e) a tendency to overpersonalize eternal events; (f) a tendency to lend a literal interpretation to figurative language; and (g) a reduced sensitivity to the communicative situation and to the pragmatic or extralinguistic aspects of communication (Myers, 1984, p. 195).

RH patients have difficulty organizing, structuring, isolating, integrating, or interpreting relevant information. Because they

Table 4.7.
Types of Dementia (Foley's [1972] taxonomy with modifications noted by *)[a]

Remedial Nonvascular Causes
Intoxications
    Infections
    Metabolic disorders
    Nutritional defects (Korsakoff's syndrome)*
    Subdural hematoma
    Benign intracranial tumors
    Occult hydrocephalus (normal pressure hydrocephalus [NPH])
    Sensory deprivation
    Depression
Irreversible Nonvascular Dementia with Movement Disorder
    Parkinson's disease*
    Huntington's chorea
    Creutzfeldt-Jacob disease
    Progressive supranuclear palsy
    Progressive subcortical gliosis
Irreversible Nonvascular Dementia Without Movement Disorder
    Alzheimer's disease
    Pick's disease
    Senile brain atrophy
Vascular Dementia
    Multiple infarctions

---

[a] Modifications by Bayles, K. (1984). Language and dementia. In A. Holland (Ed.), *Language disorders in adults: Recent advances.* San Diego, CA: College Hill Press.

are unable to judge which details or parts matter, they catalog random, unimportant, or incidental facts (Myers, 1984; Wapner et al., 1981). They are unable to grasp the hierarchically appropriate key points or basic schema of a story and frequently retell stories verbatim rather than paraphrasing or recording them (Wapner et al., 1981).

RH patients also have difficulty in apprehending, relating to, or deriving meaning from contextual cues. For example, Rivers and Love (1980) found that, although RH patients are able to define and read words, they are impaired in their ability to use sentence clues to substitute a real for a nonsense word, and they are impaired in the ability to make up a story based on sequential pictures. RH patients also tend to be literal-minded, to miss nuances and subtlety, and to overlook intended and connotative meaning (Myers, 1984). They appear unresponsive to intended meaning and extralinguistic cues and seem unable to fully appreciate the speaker's intentions, the purpose of the exchange, or the listener's needs (Myers, 1984).

Dementia

Dementia, which is also called organic brain syndrome, is a condition of chronic progressive degeneration "of intellect, memory and communicative function resulting from organic brain disease" (Bayles, 1984, p. 209). Symptomatology varies from subtle changes during early dementia that may not be noticeable to profound changes during later states that may render the patient unable to function socially or occupationally (Bayles, 1984).

Foley (1972) classified dementia according to etiology (Table 4.7). All of these dementias are associated with neural

degeneration. The language profiles of each of these etiologically different dementia patients are discussed by Bayles (1984) (see also Chapter 29).

Albert (1978) discusses the language impairments of cortical and subcortical dementias. He indicates that, although they share certain deficits, such as lack of initiative to speak, perseveration, and naming impairment, each also has additional specific impairments. Specifically, **subcortical dementia** patients have a slow rate, low volume, decreased output on verbal fluency tests (divergent thinking), agraphia, impaired ability to make verbal abstractions, and disturbances in rhythm, pitch, and articulation.

In contrast, patients with **cortical dementia**, of which Alzheimer's disease is the primary type, have logorrhea, empty speech, verbal paraphasias, impaired naming, impaired comprehension, preserved repetition, and topic digression (Albert, 1978; Bayles, 1984). According to Obler and Albert (1981), cortical dementia patients have all the language problems of subcortical patients plus agnosias, apraxias, and aphasias and are likened to Wernicke's and anomic aphasias (Bayles, 1984).

Bayles (1984) describes the language disturbance during the progression of dementing disease. She indicates that, in the early stage, the patient is forgetful and disoriented for time but generally not for place or person, and that both long-term and short-term memory are affected. However, the language impairment is usually imperceptible in casual conversation. Specifically, Bayles (1984) observes that:

> Although the content of such discourse may be somewhat inappropriate due to word boundary erosion, dementia patients adhere to the rules of syntax and phonology. The combined effects of slight cognitive disorientation and semantic pragmatic impairment may result in an inability to detect humor and sarcasm. As the ability to produce and comprehend language deteriorates, there is greater reliance on cliches (Bayles, 1984, p. 227).

During the early stages, patients may also digress from the topic and ramble at length during conversation.

During the middle stages of dementia, the individual is "disoriented for time and place, but orientation to self is maintained" (Bayles, 1984, p. 228). Both long-term and short-term memory become impaired. The individual can no longer manage personal finances, employment, or medication (Bayles, 1984). Conversation becomes vague, empty, and often irrelevant, and syntactic forms affecting meaning are likely to be misused:

> Semantic paraphasias are more common than phonemic, and there is an obvious loss of the more specific and abstract semantic features of words. Individuals are no longer able to generate verbal sequences of meaningfully related ideas, and become increasingly apathetic towards other individuals and their environment. Language becomes egocentric, and there is less adherence to the conversational maxims that govern normal conversations. Affected individuals neither ask questions of their conversational partners nor comment on their utterances. Verbal perseverations are frequent, particularly ideational repetition, the repetition of an idea after another idea has been expressed (Bayles, 1984, pp. 228–229).

In the later stages of dementia, the patient is disoriented for time, place, and person:

> No longer can the person care for himself, and assistance with dressing, washing, feeding, and toileting is needed. Many severe

dementia patients wander aimlessly and require placement in a protective environment. Life may seem to become a continuously fading dream, as one is unable to form new, lasting memories. Persons may be mute, echolalic, palilalic, use only jargon, or produce bizarre nonsensical utterances. Symptom variations probably reflect differences in the distribution of neural lesions. Pragmatic competencies of language may be so devastated that eye contact must be established before these dementia patients recognize that they are being spoken to. Syntax and phonology are grossly disrupted, particularly among jargon and palilalic patients (Bayles, 1984, pp. 229–230).

Closed Head Injury (CHI)/Head Trauma

''CHI'' is a term used to indicate that the primary source of brain injury is one of blunt trauma to the skull. ''There may or may not be concurrent fracture of the skull and/or discontinuity of neural substance'' (Hagen, 1984, p. 250). The term excludes etiology of brain-penetrating wounds, cerebral vascular insult, and space-occupying lesions (Hagen, 1984).

It is estimated that 75% or more of CHI patients have a language disturbance (McKinley, 1981). However, language is not disturbed in typically aphasic ways. According to Darley (1982), this ''language of confusion'' has a pattern of ''a high degree of irrelevance of content coupled with paradoxically adequate syntax and fluency that differentiates the language performance of the confused patients from that of aphasic patients'' (p. 25). While both groups are impaired in speaking, listening, reading, and writing, Holland (1982) notes that aphasic patients have an impairment of form, whereas CHI patients have a disorder of language use or pragmatics. They have problems of ''digressiveness, difficulty in self-monitoring that includes impetuousness and disinhibition, difficulty in attending to topic, disorganization, difficulty in initiating speech and its converse problem—once initiated, speech is difficult to stop—and difficulty in changing topic'' (p. 347).

Conversational language is frequently fragmented and tangential and often drifts to irrelevant topics (Levin et al., 1979). Thought content is confused, seldom relevant to the discussion, and inappropriate in length. According to Hagen (1984), language disorganization is more frequently the cause of impaired ability to communicate than is the presence of a categorical linguistic deficit. However, the patient does have word-retrieval problems. These naming errors are qualitatively different than aphasic naming errors. In addition to the circumlocutions, paraphasias, and reduced word fluency that are typical of both groups, CHI patients make naming errors that are related to their personal situation or to the nature of the stimulus, or they make errors of confabulation (Holland, 1982).

Cognitive problems are central to the CHI patient's problems. These patients experience

> impairments in concentration, attention, memory, nonverbal problem solving, part/whole analysis and synthesis, conceptual organization, abstract thought and speed of processing. Because these cognitive abilities are inextricably involved in language formulation and processing it would seem reasonable to assume that post-CHI language dysfunction is heavily influenced, and in some instances created, by cognitive dysfunction (Hagen, 1984, p. 249).

Hagen (1984) suggests that the characteristics of this cognitive-language disorganization result in a disruption of the seven cognitive processes: attention, memory, discrimination and sequential organization of, categorization of, association/integra-

tion of, and analysis/synthesis of stimuli and throughts (see Chapter 30). The Rancho Los Amigos Scale (Hagen and Malkmus, 1979) classifies each patient in terms of severity in these areas:

Level I: No response
Level II: Generalized response
Level III: Localized response
Level IV: Confused and agitated response
Level V: Confused, inappropriate, and nonagitated response
Level VI: Confused and appropriate response
Level VII: Automatic and appropriate response
Level VIII: Purposeful and appropriate response

A more in-depth discussion of differential diagnosis of aphasia is contained in Chapter 5.

GOAL 2: IDENTIFICATION OF THE FACTORS THAT HAVE PRECIPITATED OR ARE MAINTAINING THE IMPAIRMENT TO DETERMINE IF THEY CAN BE ELIMINATED, REDUCED, OR CHANGED

The clinician aids in determining which factors precipitated and which are continuing to contribute to the language problem. The purpose of this assessment is to determine what variables can be reduced, eliminated, or changed in order to facilitate language retrieval.

To define the precipitating and maintaining factors affecting language, the clinician should assess areas such as educational history, medical history, family history, psychological history, perceptual-motor history, occupational history, and past and present communication environment. Numerous texts contains forms for obtaining this type of information.

The patient's medical chart and preinterview or referral forms such as those in Appendices 4.3 and 4.4 of this chapter can also be used to obtain information from other members of the intervention team such as the family, the physician, and sometimes the patients themselves (see Appendix 4.5). Use of such forms to exchange information can often save time and provide a focus and direction for subsequent interviews.

During subsequent interviews, specific areas that seem unclear or that need greater specificity may be explored. Interviews provide an opportunity to verify and clarify information obtained on the preinterview forms or to pursue data that may be pertinent to the nature of each client's communication problem but that is not included on the form. For example, the clinician may attempt to determine the degree to which the verbal and nonverbal behavior of individuals in the environment facilitates or impedes language recovery. Other areas that may be described are the relationship among the persons in the environment, the social role change of the client and family subsequent to aphasia, patient and family attitudes toward aphasia and rehabilitation, needs and expectations concerning intervention, and the realistic or unrealistic nature of these expectations.

In an attempt to define the factors that have precipitated or are maintaining the impairment, the clinician often works closely with members of the assessment–intervention team who have evaluated some aspect of the client's physical, psychological, or emotional functioning. Such a team may be composed of the attending physician and nurse(s), a neurologist, a physiatrist, an occupational therapist, a physical therapist, a psychologist, and family members. Their goal in working together is to determine the factors that can be eliminated, reduced, or changed and thus, to provide a high-quality assessment and intervention program for the patient.

The clinician should obtain much of the information regarding the individual's personal and medical history prior to the initial patient contact. This enables the aphasiologist to formulate an opinion concerning the possible areas that need greater specificity during testing.

Definition of Complicating Conditions

During testing of the aphasic patient, the evaluator should be alert for signs of dysfunction in areas that do not appear to be generally equivalent in severity with overall performance. This is done to determine if there are conditions that may interfere with recovery. More detailed assessment of these areas should subsequently be made in order to determine the presence of complicating areas of deficit. Testing included in this category would be behaviors frequently associated with right-hemisphere functions such as visual, spatial, and nonverbal. In addition, auditory sensitivity and ability to recognize auditory stimuli are assessed.

Right-Hemisphere Functions

It is important to determine that the individual's visual acuity and visual fields are intact enough that they will not pose significant problems for the rehabilitation program. When such a defect is suspected, the individual is referred to an ophthalmologist for testing.

Nonverbal impairments such as inability to recognize music rhythms or forms may also interfere with the therapeutic process. Other frequent problems that are noted are (*a*) **constructional apraxia**, or a deficit in the ability to draw or construct three-dimensional figures (Goodglass and Kaplan, 1972, rev. 1983); (*b*) **prosopagnosia** or a deficit in the ability to recognize faces (Brookshire, 1973); and (*c*) **autopagnosia**, or a difficulty in recognizing body parts (Brookshire, 1973).

Auditory Sensitivity

Assessment of auditory sensitivity includes several measures such as (*a*) threshold for the awareness of sound; (*b*) standard pure-tone threshold—both air and bone conduction; (*c*) speech reception thresholds; and (*d*) speech discrimination scores. Aphasia is not a problem in auditory sensitivity but rather an impairment in the comprehension of language. Peripheral hearing losses do not account for language impairments. However, the necessity of testing hearing sensitivity is made obvious by the fact that many individuals are older and therefore at high risk of peripheral hearing disorders (see ASHA, 1989; Bess et al, 1989; Cranford, et al., 1990; Helfer and Wilber, 1990; Orchik, 1981; Ventry and Weinstein, 1983). It should also be noted that testing the hearing acuity of some aphasic patients may be very difficult if they are severely language impaired and therefore unable to understand test instructions or to grasp the nature of the response requirements.

Auditory Agnosia

Occasionally, clients with aphasia are also impaired in their ability to recognize auditory stimuli, although they may recognize the same stimuli in other modalities. For example, a patient would recognize the printed word "hat" but not the spoken word "hat." This impairment occurs in the absence of perceptual deficits in hearing. In diagnosing agnosia, it is important to exclude (*a*) sensory deficits in the affected modality, (*b*) comprehension deficits, (*c*) expressive disturbances, and (*d*) unfamiliarity with test stimuli (Brookshire, 1973).

Poststroke Clinical Depression

Some patients suffer from poststroke clinical depression, which is a serious medical problem that can compromise the overall rehabilitative process, including speech-language therapy (Hammons and Swindell, 1987). Therefore, speech-language pathologists need to identify stroke patients who might possibly be clinically depressed and make appropriate referrals for psychological assessment and intervention.

GOAL 3: ANALYSIS OF COGNITIVE BEHAVIORS

"Cognition" is a generic term for any process whereby an organism becomes aware of or obtains knowledge of an object (English and English, 1958). It "refers to all the processes by which sensory input is transformed, reduced, elaborated, stored, recovered, and used" (Neisser, 1967, p. 4). It is a group of processes by which we achieve knowledge and command of our world, that is, a method of processing information. It is "the activity of knowing: the acquisition, organization, and use of knowledge" (Neisser, 1967, p. 1).

Chapey (1983) reinterpreted Guilford's (1967) structure-of-intellect (SOI) model and suggests that cognition can be operationally defined as the use of the five mental operations within this SOI model (see Chapter 11).

Mental Operations

The five mental operations are cognition, memory, convergent thinking, divergent thinking, and evaluative thinking or judgment.

Cognition

Cognition involves knowing, awareness, immediate discovery or rediscovery and recognition of information in various forms, and comprehension or understanding. Recognition involves acknowledgment that something has been seen or perceived previously (Guilford, 1967).

Memory

Memory is the power, act, or process of fixing newly gained information in storage. It involves the ability to insert new information into memory and to retain the new information (Guilford, 1967).

Convergent Thinking

Convergent thinking is the generation of logical conclusions from given information, where emphasis is on achieving the conventionally best outcomes. Usually, the information given fully determines the outcome (Guilford and Hoepfner, 1971). Convergent production is in the area of logical deductions or compelling inferences. It involves the generation of logical necessities.

Divergent Thinking

Divergent production involves the generation of logical alternatives from given information where emphasis is on variety, quantity, and relevance of output from the same source. It is concerned with the generation of logical possibilities, with the ready flow of ideas and with the readiness to change the direction of one's responses (Guilford, 1967). It involves providing ideas in situations where a proliferation of ideas on a specific topic is required. Such behavior necessitates the use of a broad search of memory storage, and the production of multiple possible solutions to a problem. It is the ability to extend previous experience and knowledge or to widen existing concepts (Cropley, 1967). Divergent behavior is directed toward new responses—new in the sense that the thinker was not aware of the response before beginning the particular line of thought (Gowan et al., 1967).

Divergent questions are open-ended and do not have a single correct answer. Responses are scored according to the number of ideas produced (fluency) and the variety of ideas suggested (flexibility). They can also be scored according to originality or the unusualness of the response and/or elaboration or the ability to specify numerous critical details in planning an event or making a decision (Guilford, 1967).

Evaluative Thinking or Judgment

According to Guilford (1967), judgment involves the ability of the individual to use knowledge to make appraisals or comparisons or to formulate evaluations in terms of known specifications or criteria, such as correctness, completeness, identity, relevance, adequacy, utility, safety, consistency, logical feasibility, practical feasibility, or social custom.

The Guilford SOI model also has contents and products (see Chapter 11).

Contents

There are four broad, substantive, basic kinds (or areas) of information, material, or content that the organism discriminates. They are figural, symbolic, semantic, and behavioral. The two that are relevant to assessment in aphasia are semantic and behavioral.

Semantic Content

Semantic content pertains ''to information in the form of conceptions or mental constructs to which words are often applied.'' Therefore, it involves thinking and verbal communication. However, it need not necessarily be dependent on words (Guilford and Hoepfner, 1971).

Behavioral Content

Behavioral content pertains to the psychological aspects—to information essentially nonfigural and nonverbal—involved in human interactions, where the attitudes, needs, desires, moods, intentions, perceptions, and thoughts of others and of ourselves are involved. Some of the cues that the human organism obtains about the attention, perception, thinking, feeling, emotions, and intentions of others come indirectly through nonverbal means.

Products

The six types of products are units, classes, relations, systems, transformations, and implications. These products are thought to replace the time-honored concept of association. That is, products represent the way in which things are associated (see Chapter 11). The present writer views the products as a possible continuum from simple to complex and/or from concrete to abstract.

Units: Units are relatively ''segregated or circumscribed items or 'chunks' of information having 'thing' character'' (Guilford and Hoepfner, 1971). Units are things to which nouns are often applied.

Classes: Classes are ''conceptions underlying sets of items of information grouped by virtue of their common properties'' (Guilford and Hoepfner, 1971). That is, they involve common properties within sets.

Relations: Relations are meaningful connections or ''connections between items of information based upon variables or points of contact that apply to them'' (Guilford and Hoepfner, 1971).

Systems: Systems are organized patterns or ''structured aggregates of items of information; complexes of interrelated or interacting parts'' (Guilford and Hoepfner, 1971).

Transformations: Transformations are changes of various kinds (such as redefinitions, shifts, transitions, or modifications) in existing information.

Implications: Implications are ''circumstantial connections between items of information, as by virtue of contiguity, or any condition that promotes 'belongingness' '' (Guilford and Hoepfner, 1971). Implications involve information expected, anticipated, suggested, or predicted by other information.

Assessment of Cognition

Since cognition is the way in which or the process by which language is learned and used, each of the cognitive processes should be assessed. Further, the aphasic patient's ability to produce semantic and behavioral units, classes (concepts), systems, relations, transformations, and implications should be explored in some depth. The tests developed by Guilford and his colleagues can be used for this purpose (see Chapter 11). In addition, other tests that tap these abilities can be used. For example, cognition (or recognition/understanding) and convergent thinking are assessed on many standard tests of aphasia. The Test of Problem Solving (Zachman et al., 1983), developed to measure reasoning abilities in children, can also be used to describe some aspects of cognitive-semantic behavior in adult aphasic patients, such as explaining inferences, determining causes, answering negative questions, determining solutions, and avoiding problems.

GOAL 4: ANALYSIS OF ABILITY TO COMPREHEND THE CONTENT OF SPOKEN LANGUAGE

Language content is the meaning, topic, or subject matter involved in conversation and the characterization or conceptualization of topics according to how they relate or are similar to one another in different messages. A topic is the particular idea expressed in a message—such as comments about a specific *object* (e.g., a pipe); a particular *action* (e.g., eating lunch); or a specific *relation* (such as between Harry and his pipe or a patient and his shoes) (Bloom and Lahey, 1978; Lahey, 1988).

Topics also include content categories such as *possession* or comments about having or owning an object, quality, or ability; *recurrence* or utterances about the reappearance of an object or event; and *rejection*, or comments that indicate opposition to an action or object (see Appendix 4.6).

The literature in clinical aphasiology indicates that the ability to comprehend the content of spoken language is always impaired in aphasia. Such deficiencies are impairments in assigning meaning to incoming auditory messages or to understanding words as they relate to objects, persons, ideas, and experiences. For many patients, this impairment is confounded by deficiencies in auditory memory or the ability to retain or remember stimuli as length increases. Assessment, therefore, centers on analyzing auditory memory and the comprehension of language content.

Auditory Retention Span

The assessment of auditory memory or retention includes the use of digit memory tasks (e.g., "Now repeat: 7, 2, 9, 5"), word memory tasks (e.g., "Point to the circle, square, and triangle"), and sentence recall tasks (e.g., "Now repeat: The cat jumped over the book"). In most instances, several variables are manipulated, such as the number and length of stimuli presented, the associative strength between stimuli, and the length of time allowed before a response is permitted. Ability is measured in terms of the number and length of items remembered and the length of time items can be retained (see Appendix 4.2 and Table 4.8). Responses are analyzed to identify patterns of impairment, such as remembering only the beginning or end of material or the production of random errors.

Auditory Comprehension of Content in Isolated Words

Receptive vocabulary is assessed by asking patients to point to real or pictured concrete and abstract objects, events, and relationships, and categories of objects, events, and relationships (e.g., "Point to car," "Show me fruit," or "Point to running"). Knowledge of language categories is also assessed by requiring the patient to point to words that belong to a specific class or group of words (e.g, "Which words belong together: apple, house, banana and pear?") and to identify rhyme words, synonyms, and antonyms (see Appendix 4.1 and Table 4.8). Word frequency, length, and picturability are varied to assess the influence of each of these variables on understanding.

Auditory Comprehension of Content in Sentences and Paragraphs

Comprehension of labels for objects, events, and relationships and of categories of objects, events, and relationships is also assessed in structures such as sentences and paragraphs (see Appendix 4.1 and Table 4.8). The aphasiologist evaluates the patient's ability to point to common objects by function (e.g., "Point to something we eat with") and/or to follow directions or commands (e.g., "Stop writing") (see Appendix 4.1 and Table 4.8). Testing also includes assessment of ability to understand concrete and abstract sentences. For example, in evaluating concrete sentences, the clinician might ask, "Is this a pencil?" Abstract sentence comprehension includes items such as "Will ice cubes melt in snow?" "Is it possible for a good swimmer to be drowned?" or "Is your mother's brother your aunt?" (see Appendix 4.1 and Table 4.8). Ability to understand sentences about content categories is evaluated by presenting items such as "Point to the woman's coat" to test comprehension of possession or "Point to the cup that is not yellow" to evaluate understanding of denial (see Table 4.8).

During highly structured assessment of both content and form response requirements are carefully controlled to be sure that success or failure are dependent on the stimulus characteristics and not on an inability to respond. The individual is therefore required to respond by pointing to a word or picture or by producing a one-word answer such as "yes/no" or "true/false." Abilities and impairments can then be ascribed to the specific input parameter that is being systematically controlled.

Comprehension of narrative stories can also be performed. For example, one might attempt to determine if the individual's comprehension is affected by story structure—that is, ability to retell a greater proportion of information units that are central to the story structure than information units that are peripheral to the story structure (Ernest-Baron et al, 1987).

Auditory Comprehension of Content During Spontaneous Language

Ability to understand meaning in unstructured, spontaneous language is determined by noting the content that appears to be understood, as demonstrated by appropriate responses to conversation. For example, if an individual hears the statements "No, this belongs to the nurse," "Is this hers?" and "This is mine. Please give it to me" and responds appropriately, the observer begins to hypothesize that the patient comprehends the relationship of possession. Taxonomies can be constructed for various types of content that the individual understands (see Table 4.9 and Appendix 4.6).

GOAL 5: ANALYSIS OF ABILITY TO COMPREHEND THE FORM OF SPOKEN LANGUAGE

Language form includes syntax or a system of rules used to relate words to one another in order to express ideas (Pei and Gaynor, 1954). In aphasia, impairments in ability to understand syntax are common. Deficiencies are observed in the ability to understand both form words and syntactic structures. Form words can be of two types: substantive words and relational words. Substantive words include verbs, nouns, pronouns, adjectives, adverbs, and so forth. Relational words are words such as prepositions, conjunctions, and articles. Use of syntactic structures involves ordering words within an utterance or the use of rules to construct sentences such as active, passive, negative, and negative passive sentences. Assessment involves an analysis of ability to understand both form words and syntactic structures.

Comprehension of Form Words

Ability to comprehend the meaning of both substantive and relational words is assessed through the use of picture verification tasks in which the individual sees a picture, hears a word or phrase, and points to the best picture for a word or phrase. For example, a picture verification task to evaluate comprehension of prepositions might include stimuli such as, Point to (*a*)

Table 4.8.
Auditory Retention and Comprehension Tasks

Task	Example	Input[a]	Output[a]
Auditory Retention Tasks			
Recognition or repetition of digits	Point to: 8, 4, 2	A	G
	Say after me: 9, 3, 7	A	V
Recognition or repetition of words	Touch the red square and blue circle	A	G
	Say after me: man, cup, hat, dog	A	V
Recognition or repetition of noun phrases	Point to: The man	A	G
	Say after me: The man	A	V
Recognition or repetition of verb phrases	Point to: Ate the lunch	A	G
	Say after me: Ate the lunch	A	V
Recognition or repetition of sentences	Point to: The man ate the sandwich	A	G
	Say after me: The man ate the sandwich	A	V
Auditory Comprehension Tasks			
Recognition of objects named	Point to the hat	A	G
Recognition of events named	Point to running	A	G
Recognition of relationships named	Point to family	A	G
Recognition of two or more objects, two or more events, or two or more relationships named	Point to the quarter and the comb	A	G
	Point to washing and to eating	A	G
	Point to family and to in front of	A	G
Recognition of categories named	Point to fruit	A	G
Recognition of two or more categories named	Point to clothing and to food	A	G
Recognition of objects when given the function of the object	Point to the one that is used for writing	A	G
Recognition of two objects when given the function of the objects	Point to the one that is used to buy things and the one that is used to comb hair	A	G
Recognition of an event described	Point to the one that shows what we do every night (sleep)	A	G
Recognition of two events described	Point to the one that shows food being prepared and the one that shows going to work	A	G
Recognition of semantically similar objects, events, relationships (2, 3, 4)	Point to the ones that go together: shopping, walking, cooking	A	G
Recognition of rhyme words	Point to a picture that rhymes with the word peas	A	G
Recognition of antonyms	Point to the opposite of up	A	G
Recognition of synonyms	Point to a word that means the same as sob	A	G
Following directions	Ring the bell	A	G
Understanding concrete sentences	Is this a cup?	A	G
Understanding abstract sentences	Will a stone sink in water?	A	G
Understanding complex or abstract relationships in sentences (adapted from Wiig and Semel (1976))			
a. Comparative relationship	Are towns larger than cities?	A	G/V
b. Possessive relationship	Does the hat belong to the girl?	A	G/V
c. Spatial relationship	Is the man walking in front of the cat?	A	G/V
d. Temporal relationship	Does lunch come before breakfast?	A	G/V
e. Inferential relationship	The man cut the steak. Did the man use a knife?	A	G/V
f. Familial relationship	Is your mother's brother your aunt?	A	G/V
g. Part-whole relationship	Does milk come from cows?	A	G/V
h. Object to action relationship	Can a car be driven?	A	G/V
i. Cause-effect relationship	Can smoke cause fire?	A	G/V
j. Sequential relationship	Were the Indians in this country before the white men came?	A	G/V
k. Degree relationships	Are inches larger than feet?	A	G/V
l. Antonym relationship	Is day the opposite of night?	A	G/V
m. Synonym relationship	Does sob mean the same as cry?	A	G/V
Comprehension of content categories			
a. Existence	Point to the hat	A	G/V
b. Nonexistence	Point to: "The pie is all gone"	A	G/V
c. Recurrence	Point to: "The man returns"	A	G/V
d. Rejection	Point to: "He doesn't want a bath"	A	G/V
e. Denial	Point to: "The cup is not yellow"	A	G/V
f. Possession	Point to the woman's coat	A	G/V
g. Attribution	Point to the large red circle	A	G/V
Understanding paragraphs	(Read paragraph) Questions: In this story, did Lucy find a bird?	A	G/V

[a] A = auditory; G = gestural; V = verbal.

Table 4.9.
Suggested Taxonomies of Objects, Events, and Relationships

Objects	Events	Relationships
Objects that move	Cooking	Interclass relations
Objects that do not move	Sports	Intraclass relations
Animate objects	Travel	Interevent relations
Inanimate objects	Work	Intraevent relationships
Body parts	News	Spatial relations
Furniture	Entertainment	Temporal relations
Food	Feelings	Sequential relations
Clothes	Activities of daily living	Familial relations
Colors		
Geometric forms		
Personal care objects		
Health		
Kitchen utensils		
People		
Places or locations		
Transportation		
Occupations		
Nature		

the cup is on the table; (b) the cup is under the table; or (c) the cup is near the table (see Table 4.10). In each instance, responses are analyzed to determine the type and frequency of words the individual is able to understand, the length of stimulus that can be understood, and the latency or length of time needed to comprehend the material.

Comprehension of Syntactic Structures

The patient's ability to comprehend basic sentence types is also determined. Assessment usually takes the form of a picture sentence verification task in which the individual decides if a phrase or sentence is true or false or if it answers the question yes or no. For example, the individual might be presented with a picture of a boy pushing a girl. He would be required to point to the printed word "true" or "false" after each of the following sentences: The boy is pushing the girl; the girl is pushing the boy; the boy is not pushing the girl; the girl is not pushing the boy; and so forth. In some instances, the individual is required to point to the words that best go together or to arrange two, three, or four movable cards into a grammatically correct phrase or sentence.

In determining the complexity of structures that the patient can comprehend, the five levels of syntactic complexity presented in Appendix 4.7 of this chapter may be helpful. Although these levels are based on normal developmental psycholinguistic research by Bloom (1970), Brown (1973), and others, and need further empirical investigation with aphasic individuals, they may serve as a possible framework to describe the structures that the patient can comprehend and to identify the approximate level at which the individual is functioning (see Appendix 4.7). Structures that are frequently assessed are comprehension of two words, morphological inflections, phrase structure rules, transformations, and complex sentences.

Conditions That Modify or Facilitate Auditory Comprehension

Comprehension of content and form are inversely proportional to the level of abstraction, intellectual complexity (Shewan and Canter, 1971; Siegel, 1959), length, frequency, semantic relatedness, imageability (Kay et al., 1990), salience and rate (Nicholas and Brookshire, 1986), and personal significance of the material. The context (Darley, 1977), topic of conversation, and grammatical class or part of speech also influence comprehension. Nicholas and Brookshire (1986) found that all subjects comprehend main ideas better than detail and stated detail better than implied detail. In addition, performance may increase when sentences are preceded by an introductory alerter such as "Tell me something" (Green and Boller, 1974) and by task instructions that are highly direct, specific, and clear. The influence of each of these variables and of rehearsal, repetition, and redundance is specified.

Ability to benefit from auditory analysis of errors is also evaluated. In addition, clinicians may ask themselves, How does comprehension change as a result of modeling, prompting, and/or expansion? For example, do prompts of a symbolic or realistic nature such as models, photographs, or demonstration of the use of an object facilitate comprehension?

The nonlinguistic behaviors that contribute to success and failure in comprehension are also defined. Specifically, the degree to which comprehension is facilitated or retarded by gesture, tone of voice, intensity, stress, speed, pauses at intervals, prolongation of words, and/or combined auditory and visual stimulation is determined.

GOAL 6: ANALYSIS OF ABILITY TO PRODUCE THE CONTENT OF VERBAL LANGUAGE

Impairments in ability to produce language content are always part of aphasia. Deficiencies are observed in the appropriate use of vocabulary words relating to objects, events, relationships, and content categories. The individual has difficulty in word finding, labeling, and categorizing and/or in the spontaneous selection or substitution of one appropriate word for another. It is not just a loss of nouns but a reduction in vocabulary that is inversely related to the frequency of word usage (Howes, 1964). Therefore, assessment involves an analysis of ability to label or name objects, events, and relationships in response to highly structured tasks and to produce the same content in spontaneous language.

Naming in Response to Highly Structured Tasks

An important component of content evaluation involves determining ability to name objects, events, and relationships at various levels of difficulty and across a continuum of word frequency. Several levels of naming difficulty are (a) defining referents, (b) confrontation naming, (c) automatic closure naming, (d) automatic serial naming, (e) recognition naming, and (f) repetition naming (see Appendix 4.1). For each level, the frequency, picturability, and abstractness of labels are varied to enable the aphasiologist to specify the nature and extent of the impairment.

Defining referents: Ability to define words is assessed by asking the client questions such as "What does 'robin' mean?" What does 'history' mean?" Responses are analyzed to determine the type of

Table 4.10.
Tasks Used to Assess Auditory Comprehension of Syntax

Task	Example	Input[a]	Output[a]
	Understanding Substantive Words		
Pronouns			
a. Personal	Point to: "She ate the cake"	A	G
b. Reflexive personal	Point to: "She kept it to herself"	A	G
c. Indefinite	Point to: "Is there any left?"	A	G
d. Demonstrative	Point to: "This is the cake"	A	G
e. Interrogative	Point to: "Which one won the race?"	A	G
f. Negative	Point to: "Nobody is interested"	A	G
Adjectives (attribution)			
a. Color	Point to the blue one	A	G
b. Size	Point to the large one	A	G
c. Shape	Point to the square one	A	G
d. Length	Point to the short one	A	G
e. Height	Point to the tall one	A	G
f. Width	Point to the narrow one	A	G
g. Age	Point to the new one	A	G
h. Taste	Point to the sour one	A	G
i. Speed	Point to the slow one	A	G
j. Temperature	Point to the cold one	A	G
k. Distance	Point to the one that is near	A	G
l. Comparatives	Point to the larger one	A	G
m. Superlatives	Point to the largest one	A	G
Adverbs			
ly adverbs	Point to the friendly one	A	G
	Understanding Relational Words		
Prepositions			
a. Locative	Put the hat in the box	A	G
b. Directional	Push the book under the table	A	G
c. Temporal	Do you go to church on Sunday?	A	G
Conjunctions	Point to ice cream and cake	A	G
Articles	Point to a cake	A	G
	(Picture of a boy hitting a girl)		
a. Active declarative	The boy has hit the girl	A	G/V
b. Yes/no question	Did the boy hit the girl?	A	G/V
c. Wh question	Whom has the boy hit?	A	G/V
d. Negative	The boy has not hit the girl	A	G/V
e. Negative question	Has the boy not hit the girl?	A	G/V
f. Passive	The girl has been hit by the boy	A	G/V
g. Passive question	Has the girl been hit by the boy?	A	G/V
h. Negative passive	The girl has not been hit by the boy	A	G/V
i. Negative passive question	Has the girl not been hit by the boy?	A	G/V
j. Complex sentences	Is this sentence complete or incomplete: "The nurse who comes in the morning"	A	G/V

[a] A = auditory; G = gestural; V = verbal.

explanation produced, such as definition by usage, by location, by classification, and so forth. Ability to name words that are defined can also be explored.

Confrontation naming: Naming in response to visual presentation is assessed by presenting objects, events, and relationships or pictures of these that vary in frequency and type of category. For example, naming of objects, geometric forms, letters, animals, colors, body parts, and actions is almost always evaluated.

Automatic closure naming: Capacity to complete an open-ended sentence such as "The sky is ____" is often a component of assessment.

Automatic serial naming: Ability to produce rote material is appraised. For example, the patient is asked to count to 20, name the days of the week, and/or recite well-known prayers or poems.

Recognition naming: When clients are unable to name an item, the correct word can be offered to them to determine if they are capable of recognizing words they cannot name. Evidence of ability to recognize names auditorially is almost always gathered (e.g., "Show me car" or "Point to car"). This involves comprehension of content.

Repetition naming: Repetition of words is assessed to determine if the individual can repeat words that he or she cannot name. For example, the examiner says "Now repeat: man."

Assessment of Content in Connected Language

Ability to retrieve precise words for objects, events, and relationships during unstructured, spontaneous language is important to the communication of meaning. Therefore, utterances are analyzed to determine the accuracy, responsiveness, completeness, promptness, and efficiency of such naming. Two excellent systems for quantifying the spontaneous language of aphasic patients were developed by Yorkston and Beukelman (1977) (see Table 4.11) and Shewan (1988a, 1988b) (see Table 4.4 and Appendix 4.2).

Assessment also involves forming taxonomies or categories to determine the frequency and complexity of utterances about various objects, events, and relationships. Examples of possible taxonomies are presented in Table 4.9 and Appendix 4.6. The frequency with which each of these categories is produced is determined by counting the number of comments about a specific topic. For example, an individual may produce eight utterances about food and two about cooking.

The phenomenon of content complexity is a more elusive and subjective concept that relates to the appropriateness and specificity of a word to a particular situation. For example, an individual who says ''the thing that you put the things on'' instead of the word ''shelf'' has not chosen the most appropriate specific vocabulary. Mathematical linguistic phenomena such as word frequency and length as well as abstractness are used to specify content complexity. Word frequency is the frequency of occurrence of a word in the English language estimated on the basis of the Carroll et al. (1971), the Kucera (1967), or the Thorndike-Lorge (1944) word counts. ''Man'' and ''hat'' are examples of frequently used words. Abstractness, on the other hand, is a concept that is difficult to define. Brown (1958) used the term to indicate a superordinate-subordinate relationship, such as *apple* vs. *fruit*. Spreen (1968) indicates that it may also relate to a lack of sense experience with the item, for example, *liberty* as abstract, *dime* as concrete.

Other objective descriptions may also be employed. For example, patient descriptions of objects, events, and/or relationships could be classified as:

1. *Enumerative* descriptions (naming people, objects, and physical surroundings)
2. *Literal* descriptions (simply a reproduction of visual stimuli without attempting to establish relationships or continuity)
3. *Imaginative* descriptions (introduction of unseen figures and objects that are incorporated into a story)
4. *Interpretative* descriptions (attempts to explain motives or action; introduces forms of analysis and synthesis) (adapted from Berry, 1969)

For each taxonomy, the stimulus relationship is determined. That is, ability to talk about objects, events, and relationships that are not perceptually present but are expected to be or have just been present (past or future) is determined. The clinician asks himself or herself, To what degree is language linked to ongoing activity? Does the individual talk about thoughts concerning objects rather than just the objects themselves (Goldstein, 1948)? How frequently does language relate to groups of objects, events, and relationships?

Categories

Ability to classify semantically related words and concepts (such as ''apple,'' ''banana,'' and ''strawberry'') is assessed in various word-frequency categories. Client ability to categorize in his or her own language is often described as **perceptual** (or relevant to the sensory quality of a stimulus, such as shape or color) or **conceptual** (or relating to a generalized idea of a class of objects such as fruit); **concrete** or **abstract** (e.g., ''hat'' versus ''peace'' or ''hope''); and **superordinate** or **subordinate** (e.g., ''furniture'' versus ''chair''). An example of an explanation that is perceptual rather than conceptual and that is concrete rather than abstract is as follows:

E: Do you have a different outfit for every three days?

Table 4.11.
Concepts Elicited from Normal Speakers Describing the "Cookie Theft" Picture[a]

Two	little	mother	in the kitchen (indoors)
children	girl	woman (lady)	general statement about disaster
little	sister	children behind her	lawn
boy	standing	standing by sink	sidewalk
brother	by boy	washing (doing)	house next door
standing	reaching up	dishes	open window
on stool	asking for	drying	curtains
wobbling (off balance)	cookie	faucet on	
3-legged	has finger to mouth	full blast	
falling over	saying "shhh" (keeping him quiet)	ignoring (daydreaming)	
on the floor		water	
hurt himself	trying to help (not trying to help)	overflowing	
reaching up	laughing	onto floor	
taking (stealing)		feet getting wet	
cookies		dirty dishes left	
for himself		puddle	
for his sister			
from the jar			
on the high shelf			
in the cupboard			
with the open door			
handing to sister			

[a] From Yorkston, K., and Beukelman, D. (1977). A system for quantifying verbal output of high-level aphasic patients. In R. Brookshire (Ed.), *Clinical Aphasiology Conference proceedings.* Minneapolis, MN: BRK. Reprinted by permission.

S: Tomorrow, . . . ah brown, all brown, and rust slacks. Ah brown, ah ah ah yellow ah ah orange . . . yea? Brown, yea.

A patient who produces subordinate rather than superordinate parts of a category might say something like "Then, Charlotte, ah Artie ah Susan, ah ah Spain, Israel, Caribbean, London, nice. . . ."

In an attempt to explore client ability to talk about categories, variations of the object-sorting task described by Goldstein (1948) are sometimes used. Clients sort objects into categories and are then asked to explain the rationale for their sort. At times, they may also be asked to explain a sort produced by the examiner. Explanations can be grouped according to object use (e.g., smoking utensils), situation (belonging together in a particular context such as eating), color (e.g., red), form (e.g., oblong), or the material the objects are made of (e.g., wool) (Goldstein, 1948).

Observation of categories also includes (a) finding the names of an object category (e.g., "What name would include all of these objects: apple, banana, grapes?"); (b) naming as many words as possible that belong to a category (e.g., "Can you think of all of the objects that could be used in cooking?"); and (c) producing word associations (e.g., "What is the first word that you think of when I say 'house'?") (Albert et al., 1973).

Analysis of Responses

The clinician compares availability of words at each level of difficulty and within various word-frequency groups (Kay et al., 1990). The presence of verbal paraphasias, or the substitution of inappropriate or incorrect words for a target word, and the pattern or type of error produced are analyzed. For example, when the individual is unable to retrieve a specified word, the clinician determines if it is (a) a **phonological** confusion—or a confusion of words that sound alike; (b) a **semantic** confusion—or the production of words that are associated in meaning or experience; or (c) an **unrelated** response that is not a direct associate of the target word. When semantic confusions occur, the error word is analyzed to determine if it is an **antonym** ("buy" for "sell"), a **synonym** ("pretty" for "beautiful"), or from the same category ("arm" for "leg") as the target word (Rinnert and Whitaker, 1973).

Whenever possible, errors are assigned to one of the following categories: **category/instance** ("holiday" for "Easter"); **object/description** ("wet" for "boy"); **part/whole** relations confusion ("door" for "room"); **action** and **outcome** confusion ("walk" for "arrival at a destination"); **spatial contiguity** confusion ("hair" for "head"); **instrument** and **function** confusion ("to light" for "match"); and **shape** and **size** analogy confusion ("shovel" for "spoon") (Rinnert and Whitaker, 1973).

Many clinicians also evaluate the word-retrieval or self-correction skills of the individuals. According to Marshall (1976), word-retrieval skills can be arranged in a hierarchical order of efficiency. The success with which skills facilitate production of an intended word appears to be strongly related to the severity of aphasia. In order of their efficiency, they are **delay**, or patient request for additional time to produce the word; **semantic association**, or patient production of one or more words that are semantically related to the desired word; **phonetic association**, or patient production of a word or words that are phonetically similar to the desired word; **description**, or subject attempts to produce the desired word by describing what he or she is talking about; and **generalizations**, or individual production of general words or empty words in place of the desired word. Self-correction strategies can be analyzed using the same hierarchy.

General Comments

In addition to taxonomies of the frequency and complexity of utterances about objects, events, relationships, and content categories, general comments about qualitative aspects of the content of language can be made. Some of these comments relate to language use or function. Observations may refer to questions such as:

To what degree does the patient
* have meaningful conversations and keep the meaning going in conversations?
* use spoken symbols to communicate specific ideas or elicit specific responses?
* express ideas clearly and with variety and order ideas sequentially toward a purpose?
* hold the thread of discussion in mind in order to identify main ideas and distinguish between the relevant and irrelevant information?
* verbalize a variety of possibilities and perspectives?
* take the role or see the viewpoint of another?

Cohesion Analysis

Various authors, including Lemme et al. (1984), suggest that we explore semantic cohesion in the spontaneous speech of aphasic adults. These authors define cohesion as semantic relations that "tie" linguistic items (such as one main clause and all subordinate clausal and nonclausal elements attached or embedded in it) together, thereby creating meaningful interdependencies among the words in a text (such as narrative). Cohesion can also relate to surface structures that contribute to coherence. These authors cite five types of cohesive ties:

1. *Reference*—reference items refer to something else for their interpretation
   a. Pronominals   I, me, we, us, you
   b. Definite articles   the
   c. Demonstratives   this, these, those
   d. Comparatives   same, more, better
2. *Lexical*—vocabulary selection
   a. Reiteration/repetition
   b. Synonyms
   c. Superordinates
   d. Collocatives
3. *Conjunction*
   a. Additive   and
   b. Temporal   then
   c. Causal   so
   d. Continuative   now, after all
4. *Substitutions*—replacement of one item with another
   a. Nominal   "This box is small." "I must get a larger *one*."
   b. Verbal   "Does John run in marathons?" "I think they all *do*."
   c. Causal   "Is there going to be rain?" "It says *so*."
5. *Ellipsis*—omission of an item that can be presupposed from the previous text
   a. Nominal
   b. Verbal
   c. Lexical

d. Operator

e. Clausal

To analyze the degree of clausal coherence in oral language, Gutierrez-Clellen and Iglesias (1992) recommended using coding conventions for narrative samples: A = action; PS = physical state; MS = mental state; M = motivation; R = resultant; I = imitation; G = goals; UR = unrelated statements; and E = enablement. These codes might prove helpful in analyzing aphasic language.

The amount of cohesion in an individual's language can be either appropriate or inappropriate (Piehler and Holland, 1984); therefore, there is a need to explore the relationship between the quality of intelligibility and clarity of a message and the amount of cohesion it contains.

Variables that Facilitate or Retard the Production of Linguistic Content

Variables that facilitate or impede the production of language content are determined. For example, topics that facilitate and those that retard the amount of meaningful speech, jargon, and/or neologisms are noted. The level of abstraction, intellectual complexity, length, and frequency of these topics are ascertained.

The aphasiologist also determines if the production of content is related to the requirements of the task. For example, is it easier to complete an open-ended sentence (e.g., "The sky is ____''), next easiest to name a picture, and most difficult to name an item subsequent to a description? Can the individual produce names when objects are more realistic or colorful? Do prompts of a symbolic or realistic nature (e.g., models, photographs, or demonstration of the use of the object) facilitate production of language content?

Evaluation also includes an analysis of the patient's ability to use clinician-produced and/or self-generated cues such as the first phoneme in a word or an associated error word (Berman and Peelle, 1967), to use an alternative modality such as visual rather than auditory, to respond to loud or intense rather than soft auditory stimulation, or to use combined auditory and visual stimuli to produce a correct target word.

GOAL 7. ANALYSIS OF ABILITY TO PRODUCE THE FORM OF VERBAL LANGUAGE

Linguistic form includes syntax and phonology.

Syntax

Syntactic impairments in verbal production are common in aphasic patients. Indeed, according to Schuell et al. (1969), aphasic subjects experience difficulty in combining words into both simple and complex constructions in order to express relationships. Patients demonstrate restricted use of sentence types and use few, if any, sentence transformations. Deficiencies are also noted in the use of relational words such as articles, prepositions, and conjunctions and in the production of personal pronouns. In addition, morphological inflections such as plural /-s/ and possessive /-s/ are frequently lost. This impairment occurs in the order of grammatical rather than phonological complexity (Goodglass and Berko, 1960) (see Appendix 4.7). Some patients will also substitute infinitive verb stems for inflected verb forms (Goodglass and Berko, 1960).

Assessment focuses on an analysis of language to determine the availability, complexity, frequency, and consistency of various syntactic structures.

Availability and Complexity

The clinician determines the specific syntactic structures that are available to each patient. This process of writing rules for the language produced by each patient is a complex task that is complicated by the fact that there are no simple procedures for doing so. Therefore, the aphasiologist needs a text that describes basic sentence types and modifications of these types. Three sources that offer assistance in this endeavor are *Government-Binding Theory and Some of its Applications* (Leonard and Loeb, 1988), *English Transformational Grammar* (Jacobs and Rosenbaum, 1969) and *Syntax, Speech and Hearing* (Streng, 1972). Structures that are frequently assessed are two-word constructions, morphological inflections, phrase structure rules, transformations, and complex sentences (see Appendix 4.7).

Some clinicians also assess syntax by identifying the specific forms that are used to express content or meaning. That is, they establish content taxonomies and subsequently write rules for language used to talk about different topics. This method of evaluation allows the aphasiologist to explore the interaction of content and form in order to determine if particular content classifications facilitate the production of specific forms.

The type of errors that are produced are specified as the aphasiologist determines if errors are a substitution or omission of target structures. Omission errors might, for example, involve production of verbs in their infinitive form—without agreement or tense—or the omission of a whole group of words such as relational words or substantive words. Substitution errors would be the interchangeability of constituents. For example, the individual might confuse nouns with adjectives or adverbs. Analysis involves a determination of whether sentences are understandable in spite of omissions and substitutions.

Frequency

The frequency of production of various syntactic structures is evaluated to determine which structures are frequently, infrequently, or never used. For example, during 3 hours of testing, P. used plural /-s/ 18 times and past /-ed/ twice. The morphemes /-er/ and /-est/ were never used.

Consistency

The consistency with which each construction is produced is defined. The aphasiologist may ask, When rules are not used consistently, do semantic complexity, frequency of word usage, and/or context affect production? For example, P. used a question intonation or a raising inflection rather than a question transformation or a *wh* question word to ask most questions. However, she produced the word "what" when she was unable to understand what the examiner was saying and doing.

Phonology

Phonology has two components: a segmental part that consists of phonemes and syllables and a suprasegmental part that includes intonation, stress, and pauses.

Table 4.12.
Items of Paired-Word Intelligibility Test Listed by Phonetic Contrast[a]

Category of Feature	Pair 1	Pair 2	Pair 3
Initial voicing	bee–pea	do–two	goo–coo
Final voicing	add–at	buzz–bus	need–neat
Vowel duration	eat–it	gas–guess	pop–pup
Stop vs. fricative	see–tea	sew–toe	do–zoo
Glottal vs. null	high–eye	hit–it	has–as
Fricative vs. affricate	shoe–chew	shop–chop	ship–chip
Stop vs. nasal	dough–no	bee–me	buy–my
Alveolar vs. palatal	see–she	sew–show	sip–ship
Tongue height	eat–at	soup–soap	eat–eight
Tongue advancement	hat–hot	tea–two	day–dough
Stop place	pan–can	dough–go	bow–go
Diphthong	buy–boy	high–how	aisle–oil
r/l	ray–lay	rip–lip	raw–law
w/r	way–ray	row–woe	won–run
Liquid vs. vowel	string–stirring	spring–spurring	bring–burring
Cluster with one intrusive vowel	blow–below	plight–polite	claps–collapse

[a] From Kent, R., Weismer, B., Kent, J., and Rosenbeck, J. (1989). Toward phonetic intelligibility testing in dysarthria. *Journal of Speech and Hearing Disorders, 54*(4), 493.

Segmental Phonology

Aphasia is frequently accompanied by a segmental phonological disorder or an impairment in ability to produce the distinctive sound elements of a word or syllable in the standard manner. Segmental phonological disorders are frequently diagnosed as dysarthria or apraxia. Both disorders are frequent accompaniments of aphasia. According to Darley (1978), **dysarthria** is

> ... a generic term which embraces a large family of expressive speech problems resulting from a lesion of some motor portion of the central or peripheral nervous system. Because of the lesion, muscles innervated by the affected nerves operate inefficiently, displaying a degree of weakness (a severe degree would be called paralysis), slowness of movement, lack of coordination, alteration of muscle tone, or some combinations of these changes. These alterations of function may be manifested in any or all of the basic processes involved in the execution of speech—respiration, phonation, resonance, articulation, and prosody. A severe degree of impairment of motor function which renders the patient essentially speechless is called anarthria (Darley, 1978, p. 493).

The hallmark of dysarthria is that there is some impairment in the innervation of specific muscle groups (Darley, 1978). Examination reveals slowness, weakness, incoordination, or changes in the tone of muscles involved in respiration, phonation, resonance, articulation, and/or prosody (Darley, 1978). Phonological errors are consistent and are usually simplifications of the act of articulation.

Kent et al. (1989) have developed a word intelligibility test proposed for use with dysarthric speakers. The test is "designed to examine 19 acoustic–phonetic contrasts that are likely to (a) be sensitive to dysarthric impairment and (b) contribute significantly to speech intelligibility" (p. 482) (see Table 4.12). The authors discuss the therapeutic implications of their test.

Apraxia of speech (AOS), on the other hand, is an articulatory impairment in the ability to program the positioning and sequencing of muscle movements for voluntary production of speech. This disorder need not be accompanied by significant weakness, slowness, or incoordination, although such difficulties may be present because of coexisting dysarthrias. The same muscles may be used without difficulty in reflex or automatic acts (Darley, 1964; Johns and Darley, 1970). AOS is a disorder of skilled movement despite the intactness of muscle strength (Darley, 1978). Errors are variable and inconsistent and often appear to be complications of the act of articulation rather than simplifications (Darley, 1978; Shankweiler and Harris, 1966).

Consonant distortions, primarily involving timing abnormalities, exceed all other error types including sound substitutions (Odell et al., 1990). Errors predominate in the medial position of words (Odell et al., 1990). More errors occur "that involve place of articulation than either manner or voice, the most vulnerable place features were dental and palatal, the place feature most likely to serve as a substitution was alveolar, and the majority of substitutions and distorted substitutions were close approximations to the target" (Odell et al., p. 356). Distortions are attributed to impairment of a peripheral stage of motor processing. Indeed, according to Odell et al. (1990), "Substitutions, with the possible exception of those sequencing errors of pre- and postpositioning and metathesis, are traditionally thought to reflect a linguistic disorder involving a planning stage of speech production" (p. 355).

Phonological variability in AOS is sometimes related to word length (Darley, 1978), word frequency (Goodglass and Kaplan, 1972, rev. 1983), word meaning (Martin and Rigrodsky, 1974), the context of the utterance, and the nature of the task being performed. Increased effort tends to aggravate the problem so that difficulty is encountered when the individual attempts to produce discrete responses on request.

When either apraxia or dysarthria is present, phonology is assessed in detail. The data collected include (a) phoneme errors produced during unstructured spontaneous language and the phonological context of those errors, (b) errors produced on a standard articulation test, (c) results of patient stimulability or ability to modify production of error phonemes following auditory and visual stimulation, and (d) results of an evaluation of the peripheral speech mechanism.

Suprasegmental Phonology

The suprasegmental components of phonology, intonation, stress, and pauses are also frequently impaired in aphasic patients.

Intonation is the modulation of the voice, pitch, or tone quality, or the musical flow of speech (Pei and Gaynor, 1954). Ability to produce normal melodic intonation or prosodic qualities is assessed to determine if the patient has lost speech melody as an indicator of grammatical segmentation (Goodglass, 1968), such as at the end of a phrase or at the end of a sentence.

Stress is the force or prominence of a particular sound (Pei and Gaynor, 1954). The aphasiologist determines if the individual uses normal stress patterns or if he or she manifests incorrect stress placement and subsequent reduction of vowels that would normally have been stressed. The evaluator may also ask, Can the person start an utterance with an unstressed word, or does he or she gravitate to the first stressed or salient word, such as a noun or principal verb (Goodglass, 1968)?

A **pause** is an interruption in the flow of language that usually occurs in those places where in writing one would use a comma (Osgood and Miron, 1963). The clinician analyzes the appropriateness of pauses and the continuity of word sequences. Specifically, the appropriateness of filled pauses (ahs, ums, and so forth), unfilled pauses, repeats, and false or corrected starts is determined. For example, P. used pauses inappropriately. That is, she often used filled and unfilled pauses in place of an action word or verb:

> **E**: How do you make a cup of coffee?
> **P**: Water and ah . . . cup . . . ah . . . Savarin and ah . . . 10 minutes . . . ah . . . then, a cup of coffee. Cream . . . and ah . . . two sugars.

The continuity of word sequences is evaluated by calculating the rate of speech or the number of words per minute.

The specific suprasegmental phonological variables that the client can produce or that he or she can be stimulated to produce are determined. Those that can be used to facilitate or increase the intelligibility of speech or the communicating of meaning are taken into account in formulating therapeutic goals.

GOAL 8. ABILITY TO COMMUNICATE OR USE LANGUAGE FOR VARIOUS FUNCTIONS

Communication is an assertive act of coping. It is a constant attempt to vary the content, form, and acceptability of a message; to switch or shift sets of reference as topics change (Muma, 1975); and to be sensitive to the influence of one's communicative partner and the physical context in which communication occurs (Prutting and Kirchner, 1983) in order to achieve a message of best fit and thus effective and efficient communication (Muma, 1975).

Communicative competence implies a knowledge of how to converse with different partners and in different contexts (Craig, 1983) and a knowledge of the rights, obligations, and expectations underlying the maintenance of discourse (Ochs and Schieffelin, 1979). It is a knowledge of who can say what to whom, in what way, where and when, and by what means (Prutting, 1979).

Pragmatics involves the acquisition and use of such conversational knowledge and of the semantic rules necessary to communicate an intent in order to affect the hearer's attitudes, beliefs, or behaviors (Lucas, 1980). This semantic knowledge develops and is used within the context of a **speech act**, a theoretical unit of communication between a speaker and a hearer (Lucas, 1980). According to Searle (1969), the speech act includes what the speaker means, what the sentence (or other linguistic elements) uttered means, what the speaker intends, what the hearer intends, what the hearer understands, and what the rules governing linguistic utterances are. Speech acts include making promises, statements, requests, assertions, and so forth. In Searle's (1969) theory, the **proposition** is the words or sentences produced, and the **illocutionary force** of this proposition is the speaker's intent in producing the utterance.

Thus, pragmatics involves the interactional aspects of communication, including a sensitivity to various aspects of social contexts (Prutting and Kirchner, 1983). It is an analysis of the use of language for communication. The emphasis is not on sentence structure but on how meaning is communicated—how units of language function in discourse (Prutting and Kirchner, 1983).

A number of cognitive/pragmatic products or discourse structures have been identified. They include physical context variables, communication partner variables, communication of intent, and turn-taking rules (including topic selection, maintenance and change, and code switching) (see Table 4.13).

Physical Context Variables/Partner Variables: Definition of the Communication Environment

Communication is a reciprocal act of sending and receiving information that is profoundly influenced by the environment in which it is used. That is, both communicative contexts and communicative partners are dynamic components of the communication itself.

Because communicative **contexts** are dynamic, language varies with each context. Indeed, the language produced by an individual at any point in time will be an interactive product of contextual variables and the individual's structural linguistic knowledge (Gallagher, 1983). Various conversational settings

Table 4.13.
Discourse Structures

1. Physical context variables
2. Communicative partner variables
3. Communication of intent

Label	Greeting	Attention
Response	Repeating	Protesting (Dore, 1974)
Request	Description	

Request	Order	Warn (Searle, 1969)
Assert	Argue	
Question	Advise	

3. Turn taking
   A. Initiation of speech act
   B. Maintenance of communication
      i. Role switching/turn taking
      ii. Sustaining a topic
         (a) Contingent utterances
         (b) Adjacent utterances
         (c) Feedback to speaker
         (d) Repair/revision
         (e) Code switching

may affect the length, complexity, redundancy, fluency, responsiveness (such as elaborations of comments), and semantic relatedness of comments.

Interestingly, Glosser et al. (1988) found that verbal complexity and language errors varied significantly with different contents and contexts of communication. For example, in conditions that restricted usual contact between speaker and listener, aphasic patients produced fewer communicative gestures and more complex verbalizations. Thus, "aphasic patients show appropriate and predictable linguistic changes in response to nonlinguistic social contextual variables" (p. 115).

Therefore, assessment involves an analysis of how the individual's linguistic behavior changes with various contexts and how specific contexts affect the number and variety of the individual's communicative behaviors. We ask, Which contexts facilitate communication? Which act as barriers to communication? What rules does the patient have for various contexts?

Specific communicative **partners** may also affect the length, complexity, redundancy, fluency and responsiveness of comments (such as elaborations of comments); the semantic relatedness of comments; and the amount of eye contact during an utterance (Gallagher, 1983). Partner characteristics such as age, sex, familiarity, and status will affect communication. Therefore, we need to determine whether a particular patient has anyone with whom to talk, and/or we need to identify who the frequent and infrequent communicative partners are and how they affect communicative behavior. We ask, How do content and form vary with different communicative partners?

Successful communication involves having the opportunity to communicate. It is not related to the length or complexity of the semantic-syntactic utterance. Rather, it "is the feeling of fulfillment gained when a message is sent and received" (Lubinski, 1981, p. 351). It is the opportunity to transmit highly personal feelings and the awareness that the message transmitted is valued. Successful communication gives the individual the feeling of social connectedness (Lubinski, 1981). Conversely, the communication-impaired environment is one in which there are few opportunities for successful, meaningful communication. It is one where there is a lack of sensitivity to the value of interpersonal communication, few reasons to talk, lack of privacy, no viable communication partner, and/or lack of stimulation in general (Lubinski, 1981). Therefore, we evaluate the communication opportunities afforded the individual and the barriers to such communication. The Profile of the Communication Environment of the Adult Aphasic, developed by Lubinski (see Chapter 13), provides a useful tool for assessing the communication environment—both opportunities and barriers.

Other tools for assessing the communicative environment or interaction are the Family Interaction Analysis by Florence (1981) (see Table 4.14) and the Process Evaluation Form by Loverso et al. (1982) (see Table 4.15). Use of such nonstandardized assessment techniques can help the aphasiologist to identify the physical or contextual and psychosocial factors that promote successful communication interaction and those that contribute to a communication-impaired environment. Subsequently, the aphasiologist can help the individual and his or her significant communication partners create a positive and rewarding communication environment that contains stimulating activities and a variety of interesting communication partners.

Table 4.14.
Family Interaction Analysis: Scoring Form[a,b]

Significant Other Behaviors	S	U	R
Nonfacilitative			
1. Inattentive posture.	___	___	___
2. Incongruent affect	___	___	___
3. Lengthy response	___	___	___
4. Self-focus	___	___	___
5. Inappropriate topic change	___	___	___
6. Advice giving	___	___	___
7. Judgmental response	___	___	___
8. Premature confrontation	___	___	___
9. Interrupting	___	___	___
10. Guessing	___	___	___
11. Repeating	___	___	___
12. Simple language	___	___	___
13. Loud voice	___	___	___
14. Abrupt topic change	___	___	___
15. Speaking for patient	___	___	___
Facilitative			
16. Closed question	___	___	___
17. Verbal following	___	___	___
18. Minimal encouragers	___	___	___
19. Open question	___	___	___
20. Paraphrasing content	___	___	___
21. Reflecting feeling	___	___	___
22. Summarizing content	___	___	___
23. Summarizing feeling	___	___	___
24. Sharing	___	___	___
25. Confrontation	___	___	___
26. Interpretation	___	___	___
27. Verbal cueing	___	___	___
28. Gesturing	___	___	___
29. Instruction	___	___	___
30. Labeling	___	___	___
31. Modeling	___	___	___
32. Physical cue	___	___	___
33. Request for attention	___	___	___

[a] From Florence, C. (1981). Methods of communication analysis used in family interaction therapy. In R. Brookshire (Ed.), *Clinical Aphasiology Conference proceedings.* Minneapolis, MN: BRK.
[b] S = successful; U = unsuccessful; R = rejection.

Communication of Intent

Language is a tool which is used to communicate a variety of intentions. Dore (1974) specified the following intents:

Label:	The intention to name an object or action, but the act is not addressed to listener
Response:	The intention to attend to another's utterance
Request:	The intention to address another for help
Greeting:	The intention to convey a conventional greeting
Protesting:	The intention to object to another person's behavior, or to reject or resist the action, statement, or command of another
Repeating:	The intention to imitate another person's speech or action
Description:	The intention to give a mental image of something seen or heard
Attention:	The intention to point something out to another person

Table 4.15.
Process Evaluation Form Based on Consolidation of Task, Maintenance, and Nonfunctional Role Descriptors[a]

Role	Descriptor	Individual No. 1	2	3	4	5	6	7	8
Task	Evaluating	___	___	___	___	___	___	___	___
	Initiating	___	___	___	___	___	___	___	___
	Elaborating	___	___	___	___	___	___	___	___
	Summarizing	___	___	___	___	___	___	___	___
	Information giving	___	___	___	___	___	___	___	___
	Information seeking	___	___	___	___	___	___	___	___
Maintenance	Encouraging	___	___	___	___	___	___	___	___
	Harmonizing	___	___	___	___	___	___	___	___
	Gatekeeping	___	___	___	___	___	___	___	___
	Standard setting	___	___	___	___	___	___	___	___
	Following	___	___	___	___	___	___	___	___
Nonfunctional	Blocking	___	___	___	___	___	___	___	___
	Self-directing	___	___	___	___	___	___	___	___
	Disrupting	___	___	___	___	___	___	___	___
	Disorting	___	___	___	___	___	___	___	___

Evaluating = determine group difficulties and/or evaluate group progress
Initiating = suggestion of ideas, new definitions of problem
Elaborating = clarifying, envisioning an idea if adopted
Summarizing = restating ideas after discussion
Information giving = offering facts or opinions, restating experiences
Information seeking = asking for ideas, wanting feedback
Encouraging = willing to hear others, supportive to group
Harmonizing = relieving dispute, compromising
Gatekeeping = making sure all members are heard
Standard setting = expressing standards for group after discussion
Following = going along with group norms and discussions
Blocking = arguing, rejecting ideas before they are heard
Self-directing = hidden agendas, self-aggrandizement
Disrupting = group clown, jokester
Distorting = distorting facts, ideas or decisions

Remarks:

[a] From Loverso, F., Young-Charles, H., Tonkovich, H. (1982). The application of a process evaluation form for aphasic individuals in small group setting. In R. Brookshire (Ed.), *Clinical Aphasiology Conference proceedings*. Minneapolis, MN: BRK.

The intents specified by Searle (1969) are as follows:

Request: The intention occurs when the speaker addresses another for help.

Assert: The intention occurs when the speaker points out to another that some statement or proposition is true; this intent includes a subset called *affirm*, which includes instances in which the speaker is agreeing with or confirming a proposition.

Question: The intention occurs when the speaker does not know if the proposition is true, or does not have the information needed, and thinks the listener may be able to provide the information. This intent also occurs when the speaker wants to know if the listener knows the answer.

Order: The intention occurs when the speaker believes that the listener is capable of performing the act and may not perform it in the normal course of events and the speaker perceives himself or herself to be in a position of authority over the listener.

Argue: The intention occurs when the speaker believes some proposition and wishes the proposition to be believed by the listener, who does not seem to know it is true.

Advise: The intention occurs when a speaker believes some act will benefit the listener and it is not obvious that the listener will perform the act in the normal course of events.

Warn: The intention occurs when the speaker believes that some event will occur that is not in the listener's interest and it is not obvious to the listener that the event will occur.

Many of these intents are used in one or more of the four communication categories proposed by Lomas et al. (1989) (see Table 4.1).

1. **Basic need**: Communication is required to meet basic needs (e.g., toileting, eating, grooming, positioning).
2. **Health threat:** Physical well-being or health is dependent on effective communication (e.g., calling for help after falling, giving or receiving information about one's medical condition).
3. **Life skill:** Giving or receiving information that is necessary to accomplish everyday living (e.g., shopping, home maintenance, use of telephone, understanding traffic symbols).
4. **Social need:** Communication that is primarily social in nature (i.e., communication with others as an end in and of itself such as engaging in dinner table conversation, playing cards, or writing a letter to a friend) (p. 123).

All language intents may be communicated and comprehended through semantic-syntactic utterances and/or by previous or subsequent utterances. In addition, intent may be expressed (and comprehended) through facial expression or accompanying actions, gestures, or tone of voice. What is not said may also communicate intent. We can also say one thing and mean another. Individuals frequently use their knowledge of the physical context variables and the communicative partner variables to help them decipher between what is said and what is meant.

Assessment involves analyzing the ability to communicate and comprehend various speech acts or intents. Does the individual communicate and comprehend a variety of intents? How? Can he or she distinguish between what is said and what is meant? Can he or she work out the implications of sentences and relate appropriately to new and old information? Can he or she use nonverbal means to communicate intents?

Turn Taking

The reciprocal nature of communication involves a number of aspects, including the initiation of the speech act and the maintenance of communication.

Initiation of the speech act (as speaker) includes topic selection and introduction and/or change of topic. The communicative act should contain new, relevant, and what is judged to be sincerely wanted information. The speaker must determine what, if any, information is shared by various listeners. Thus, topical or referential identification involves searching one's long-term memory for information that is judged to be relevant to the partner, wanted by the partner, and perhaps interesting.

Maintenance of communication involves role taking or the variation of roles as speaker-initiator and listener-respondent. The listener's role is to comprehend the speaker's message. It is indicated with a nonverbal response, such as nodding the head or leaning forward, or a short and usually affirmative verbal response such as "yes." It is characterized by visual orientation rather than gaze avoidance (Davis, 1981). Assisting the speaker in conveying a message involves the ability of the listener to monitor and evaluate the speaker's message and provide feedback to the speaker concerning his or her effectiveness and acceptability.

Nonverbal cues are usually used by partners to signal a wish to maintain or change roles (Harrison, 1974; Rosenfeld, 1978). The speaker usually retains his or her role by gaze avoidance and a hand gesture that is not maintained or not returned to a resting state through a phonetic clause juncture (Rosenfeld, 1978). When a speaker wants a listener's reaction, he or she signals "with a pause between clauses" or "with a rising or falling pitch at the end of a phonemic clause" (Davis, 1981,

p. 171). The listener maintains his or her role by visual orientation to the speaker.

Role switching may occur as a result of the speaker's desire to relinquish the role. Thus, the listener needs to formulate a judgment concerning the speaker's willingness to switch roles. When role switching occurs in the absence of the speaker's readiness to switch, it may be accompanied by overloudness and a shift of the head away from the speaker (Davis, 1981).

Repair and/or **revision** are also part of discourse maintenance and regulations. This involves the speaker's sensitivity to cues provided by the listener and the ability to respond to such cues by repeating and/or modifying the message when necessary. Moves by the speaker and the listener to repair sequences and respond to such regulatory devices as requests for clarification are essential to the maintenance of communication (Fey and Leonard, 1983). Repair variables may be classified and analyzed according to the following categories proposed by Purcell and Liles (1992): (*a*) type of repair: grammatical and text meaning, and (*b*) cohesion repairs: categories (personal, demonstrative, comparative, lexical, conjunction), frequency, success, and location.

Maintenance of communication may also involve a response that sustains a topic—one that involves a specific response to the speech act (as listener). For example, **contingent utterances** are utterances that share the same topic with the preceding utterance and that add information to the prior communication act. It is an elaboration of the speaker's topic. Sequential organization of topics is also a component of communication maintenance. Thus, **adjacent utterances** are also used. These are utterances that occur immediately after a partner's utterance but are not related to the speaker's topic. Such utterances may be considered logical or possible elaborations of the speaker's communication.

Code switching is somewhat related to role taking. Code switching is the degree to which the individual can produce stylistic variations in the form or frequency of specific acts to meet situational requirements (Fey and Leonard, 1983) such as the ability to role play.

In an article written in 1975, Muma addressed the issue of role taking and code switching. He differentiated between two different variations in one's method of communication. One he called "dump," the other "play." Dumping pertains to the issuance of a coded message. Play involves ascertaining needed changes for appropriate recoding of a message and making necessary adjustments to achieve the message of "best fit" for a particular situation and listener. Role taking is the ability to issue a "message in the most appropriate form for conveying intended meanings to a particular person for particular efforts" (p. 299). In role taking, "both speaker and listener are active participants in formulating, perceiving and revising messages until necessary adjustments are made in form, reference or psychological distance, and acceptability in order to convey intended meanings" (p. 299). The objective of true communication is aimed at ascertaining the message most suited to achieve effective and efficient communication. (Muma [1975] tied the development of the ability to "play" with a message to cognitive development.)

Assessment in adult aphasia involves an analysis of patient ability to initiate and maintain communication in various contexts and with various partners. We ask:

1. Is the individual willing and able to accept his or her share of communicative responsibility as speaker?
2. Can and does the individual initiate various speech acts? Which ones?
3. What percentage of speech acts are initiated by the aphasic individual? By the partner?
4. What topics are selected?
5. Is topical identification appropriate to various listeners and is it interesting?
6. Is the patient able to evaluate the implicitly shared information aspect of communication?
7. Does the patient initiate conversations that contain new, relevant, and sincerely wanted information?
8. Does the patient produce contingent and adjacent utterances? To what degree?
9. Can the patient sequentially organize topics in a conversation?
10. Can the patient elaborate on a topic? To what degree?
11. Is language reduced in complexity? In quantity?
12. Is there selective reduction of elaborative material such that the most essential elements are communicated?
13. Are referential skills appropriate to the maintenance of communication?
14. Does the patient use referential gesture (i.e., gestures that communicate information about things in the world) or nonreferential gestures?
15. Are code-switching skills effective and efficient in formulating, perceiving, and revising messages until necessary adjustments are made in form, reference, and acceptability in order to ascertain the message of best fit?
16. Does the patient engage in communication that reflects that he or she has found the message most suited to achieve effective and efficient communications?
17. Can the patient produce stylistic variations in order to meet situational and partner requirements?
18. Does the patient use contextual information appropriately?
19. Does the patient attempt to actively resolve communication obstacles of form, reference, and acceptability in order to achieve the message of best fit?
20. Does the patient clarify ambiguous messages?
21. What factors affect breakdowns and repairs?
22. How effective is the patient in responding to cues to repair his or her communication?
23. Does the patient repair and/or revise communication in an attempt to maintain and regulate communication?
24. Does the patient use regulatory devises such as requests for clarification?
25. What techniques are used to repair, revise, or regulate conversation (hints, gestures, **wh**-questions, corrections, or rejections of topic or intent)?
26. What revision strategies are used (repetition, partial repetition, semantic revision, syntactic revision, phonological revision, information additions, information deletion, self-correction, unrelated)?
27. Are revision strategies successful?
28. Is the individual willing and able to accept his or her share of communicative responsibility as a listener?
29. How effective is the individual as a listener?
30. Can the individual comprehend the speaker's message? Does he or she follow changes in topic?
31. To what degree does the individual assist the speaker in conveying a message?
32. Does the individual provide appropriate feedback to the speaker concerning his or her effectiveness and acceptability?
33. Can the individual signal when he or she wishes to switch roles?
34. Does the individual pick up on the speaker's desire to relinquish his or her role as speaker?
35. Is turn taking appropriate?
36. Is transfer of the speaker's role successful?

Recently, functional assessment or the ability to perform daily living activities has taken an added importance from a public policy perspective, "providing the means to set reimbursement rates, determining eligibility for services, and measure the quality of long term rehabilitative care" (Frattali, 1992, p. 63). However, according to Frattali (1992), few tools measure functional communication in an in-depth, reliable, and valid manner. The solution to this problem, Frattali (1992) suggests, is to arrive at a fieldwide consensus of what core elements constitute multidimensional functional assessment. Further, measurements that are developed must embody the following attributes: "sensitivity to change over time; reliability of measures within and across raters, and over time; sufficient range of performance measured to prevent threshold effects; usefulness across different methods of administration; usefulness during different phases of rehabilitation and relevance to function outside the clinical setting" (Frattali, 1992, p. 79). Since functional communication is a core activity of daily living (Chapey, 1992; Frattali, 1992), this task is of the highest priority.

GOAL 9. DETERMINATION OF CANDIDACY FOR AND PROGNOSIS IN THERAPY

Formulating prognoses is one of the primary tasks facing speech-language pathologists (Tompkins et al., 1990). While relevant predictors and optimal methods of measuring prognoses are still limited, some of the prognostic indicators most commonly suggested in the literature include "*biographical variables* such as age, gender, education and premorbid intelligence, occupational history, and life situation; *medical variables* such as etiology and duration of aphasia, site and extent of brain-damage, general health, and history of previous neurological incidents; and (language) *behavioral variables* including severity of language impairment, aphasia type, . . . (and) coexisting neurologic communicative disorders" (Tompkins et al., 1990, p. 398).

Biographical Variables

Age

Age and outcome correlate significantly. Specifically, the younger the individual is, the more likely recovery will be (Darley, 1977; Sands et al., 1969). However, there are frequent exceptions, depending on other factors such as personal attitude and severity (Darley, 1977; Emerick and Hatten, 1974). In a recent article, Tompkins et al. (1990), citing Kimmel (1980), suggest that there are at least four different kinds of "age"; physiological, psychological, social, and perceived age. They note that physiological characteristics such as activity level or general health indicators and "psychosocial factors like personality, social involvement, or life satisfaction . . . are more predictive of cognitive ability, life adaptation, and morale than is chronological age" (p. 399).

Gender

Some studies show that gender and outcome correlate significantly, favoring males (Holland et al., 1989). However, future research is necessary to shed light on the exact nature of gender as a prognostic variable in language recovery (Holland et al., 1989).

Education and Premorbid Intelligence

Although many clinicians have used education level as a prognostic factor in aphasia, Tompkins et al. (1990) point out that years of formal education do not necessarily correspond to premorbid intellectual ability. Instead, these authors recommend a multifaceted estimate of premorbid intelligence developed by Wilson et al. (1979), which weights standard demographic data including age, education, gender, occupational category, and race, because they believe that this measure may have more predictive power than educational level alone.

Medical Variables

Etiology/Type of Stroke

Prognosis is more positive in traumatic than vascular etiology (Darley, 1977; Kertesz and McCabe, 1977).

Time Elapsed Since Onset

The longer the time between the onset of aphasia and the beginning of intervention, the poorer the prognosis (Sands et al., 1969).

Site and Extent of Lesion

In general, the larger the dominant-hemisphere lesion, the poorer the prognosis. Multiple small lesions also yield a poor prognosis. Lesions of the central core of the dominant-hemisphere language area, the area served by the middle cerebral artery, even when they are small, frequently result in severe aphasias (Darley, 1982). Left-side lesions generally yield a poorer prognosis for language recovery than right-side lesions (Holland et al., 1989). Bilateral damage, even when the lesions are small, also result in a poor prognosis. However, despite these generalizations, Darley (1982) suggests that some individuals with poor prognosis because of the site and extent of lesion have nevertheless recovered well.

Severity

Initial severity and outcome correlate significantly (Kertesz and McCabe, 1977; Sands et al., 1969). Specifically, initial ability to speak has a definite relationship to the person's eventual speech performance (Keenan and Brassell, 1974). Similarly, clients who are severely impaired in auditory recognition and comprehension have an unfavorable prognosis (Schuell et al., 1964; Smith, 1971). Length of hospital stay, favoring shorter stays, influences recovery (Holland et al., 1989).

Complicating Health Problems

The presence of other health problems in addition to aphasia often results in a poorer prognosis.

Medication

Certain drugs can adversely affect patient ability to respond to tasks. Therefore, the clinician needs to know what medication

each patient takes and the impact of each, separately and in combination.

Language Variables

Auditory Processing

Peripheral hearing loss such as pure-tone and speech discrimination thresholds frequently accompany advancing age and therefore aphasia. In addition, processing of auditory information is always impaired in aphasia. For example, ability to attend auditorially to incoming information as well as central auditory processing is usually impaired in aphasia. All of these aspects of auditory processing can negatively affect prognosis (Tompkins et al., 1990).

Self-Correction

Patient awareness of speech difficulty and ability to self-correct are positively related to improvement in speaking skills (Wepman, 1958).

Ability to Learn, Retain, and Generalize Language and Communication

Individual ability to learn language and communication behavior is an essential component of prognosis. Training is an integral part of assessment. Indeed, one possible way to view assessment is as an intervention-assessment process in which the emphasis is on the process of learning or functioning rather than on the product, in order to define ways in which performance can be improved. For example, the patient and the clinician could become engaged in a common quest for the mastery of a task. First, the behavior to be learned and the criteria of acquisition are determined. Then, ability to learn, retain, and transfer or generalize language-related material is assessed. We ask, Can language behavior be modified? The conditions that facilitate or retard this process are also analyzed. Some areas that are frequently assessed are discussed below.

Attention/Awareness

Can the patient attend to the task long enough to learn it? Does he or she attend to the essential components of the task? Does the patient have insight into the disorder and an awareness of the situation (van Harskamp and Visch-Brink, 1991)?

Motivation

The "kernal" of therapy is the stimulation of the individual's willingness to participate actively in the learning process and to practice (van Harskamp and Visch-Brink, 1991). "The patient's motivation is of utmost importance: patients need to exert themselves to make progress" (van Harskamp and Visch-Brink, 1991). We ask, What motivates the client to learn? Does he or she use intrinsic (self-stimulated) or extrinsic (reinforcement) motivation? Can the individual dedicate himself or herself to the task (van Harskamp and Visch-Brink, 1991)?

Materials

What materials facilitate learning? For example, does use of bright color and large size stimulate production of more relevant or correct performance?

Rate

Does the rate of presentation affect performance? Does increased duration facilitate learning?

Modality

Through which modality does the patient learn best (visual, auditory, or tactile)?

Content

What content or topics are most meaningful for the individual to learn?

Procedure

Does performance improve to a great degree when the clinician uses reauditorization, stimulation, modeling, expansion, or direct analysis of errors? Which is most effective?

Cuing

Does the use of cues increase learning? Which types of cues are successful in eliciting a correct response: the first phoneme of a word, written representation of the word, first letter of a word, synonyms, opposites, rhymes, use of the error response (Berman and Peelle, 1967)? Is there a hierarchy of cues? Can the individual learn to produce his or her own cues? Are verbal, gestural, or visual cues more effective? Do cues call attention to irrelevant rather than relevant aspects of what is to be learned?

Reinforcement

How does reinforcement affect performance? Are response patterns affected by changes in the reinforcement schedule (continuous, intermittent, immediate, delayed), type of reinforcement (verbal, gestural or token, positive or negative), or dispenser of reinforcement (self, clinician, spouse)?

Practice/Rehearsal

Did the individual have an opportunity to practice? Can he or she practice independently? Do successive uninterrupted repetitions facilitate behaviors? Do subvocal rehearsals facilitate learning? Does massed (e.g., all at one time) or distributed practice increase learning more effectively? If the individual is distracted from rehearsing the material, does he or she retain any part of it?

Patterns of Performance

Are performances random or do they reflect definite strategies that are manifested in consistent improvement and reduction of performance variability (Carson et al., 1968)? Is learning an all-or-none process or a gradual process? How rapidly does the individual learn?

Level of Learning

Can the patient learn to recognize responses that he or she cannot produce? If the patient cannot learn a specific behavior, can he or she learn an alternative or substitute form of the behavior? Can the patient learn to manipulate an alternative visual or manual communication system?

Retention and Transfer or Generalization

Can the patient learn new material, retain it over time, and integrate the knowledge gleaned into another context and with another partner? That is, is there application of what is learned to independent activities and partners thereafter (Hillis, 1989)?

Analysis of Failure

If the individual did not learn the target behavior, what was the source of difficulty? Was it because the task was too difficult or because the component skills within the behavior were not adequately defined? Were cues too weak? Were instructions adequate? Were examples provided? Were the materials meaningful to the patient?

Length, Quality and Intensity of Treatment

According to Tompkins et al. (1990), the length, quality, and intensity of treatment are crucial determinants of future communicative status. The skills of the particular clinician will also influence the course and outcome of therapy.

Personality/Social Variables

Personal Attitude

The individual's desire to improve or his or her level of motivation and aspiration influences the course and outcome of aphasia therapy (Darley, 1977). Indeed, Tompkins et al. (1990) note that personality variables and social support have been linked to health generally and to morbidity and mortality in a variety of health conditions such as stroke and to prognosis in therapy as well. These authors suggest that valid and reliable psychosocial scales that measure personality variables have the potential for enriching our understanding of individual responses to treatment and, therefore, facilitating prognoses.

Family Attitude

Family interest in the patient and their desire to see improvement in language ability will influence the progress made during intervention. Indeed, in an article assessing factors that predict optimal poststroke progress, Evans, et al. (1991) found that a patient does significantly better when the primary support person is not depressed, is married, is knowledgeable about stroke care, and is from a functional rather than dysfunctional family. These authors suggest that caregiver-related problems can have a collective effect on rehabilitation outcome and that treatment should therefore reduce caregiver depression, minimize family dysfunction, and increase the family's knowledge about stroke care. Tompkins et al. (1990) and Tompkins et al. (1987) stress the importance of developing more reliable and valid measures of social network and support resources in order to facilitate statements concerning prognosis.

In summary, it should be noted that no one factor discussed above consistently determines progress and success of therapy. Therefore, each patient should be enrolled for a period of trial therapy before a final decision is reached about termination of intervention.

Termination of Therapy

Wertz (1991) notes that we are all "handicapped by our problems in specifying what clinically significant change is" (p. 313). That is, specific and meaningful methods of measuring "clinically significant" change need to be defined in order to facilitate our decision to continue or terminate intervention. Objective criteria should be used to demonstrate that treatment is producing continued improvement in language behavior, and therapy should be terminated when the individual does not appear to be profiting from intervention. The termination decision is developed from an interaction of client characteristics, assessment and intervention data, and treatment goals (Dixon, 1980; Warren, 1976). Other factors that may influence this decision are the logistics of providing continued treatment, clinical and financial arrangements, and the aphasiologist's concern about the patient (Warren, 1976).

GOAL 10. SPECIFICATION AND PRIORITIZATION OF INTERVENTION GOALS

In an excellent chapter entitled "From Assessment to Intervention: Problems and Solutions," Snyder (1983) states that making the transition from assessment to intervention is like trying to solve a puzzle. "Success in solving puzzles seems to require that we have all of the pieces. In addition, we need to have only the correct pieces. It takes time and effort to identify and discard the wrong pieces. Further we need to be able to conceptualize how the pieces fit together and operate as a whole. The puzzle is not really solved unless it fits together and works" (p. 160). Sometimes, she notes, we solve our puzzles despite missing and/or incorrect pieces. She warns that there is no one solution to the assessment-intervention puzzle. Rather, we must remember that "individual differences of the language impaired population are such that the solution for one puzzle may not apply to another" (p. 161).

We gather the pieces of our puzzle during the data collection phase of assessment and subsequently assemble the puzzle when we attempt to organize, systematize and condense the data in a meaningful way. One possible method for condensing some of the complex and dynamic aspects of language is the checklist presented in Table 4.16. This type of checklist can sometimes help the hypothesis formation or decision-making stage of assessment, which involves sifting through all of the information obtained, delicately balancing and blending the data to arrive at a penetrating understanding of the patient's total behavior. This phase of assessment involves a sophisticated clinical judgment applied to the information collected. It is an evaluation of the type, frequency, and pattern of behaviors produced by the patient and an exploration of the interrelatedness of various behaviors in order to specify and prioritize intervention goals.

Aphasia therapy is a multidimensional process that often requires a succession of methods (van Harskamp and Visch-Brink, 1991). However, the usual focus of therapeutic activity is on auditory comprehension and verbal production, since these are the most essential components of language. Reading and writing may be used to facilitate or to cue auditory comprehension and verbal production but should rarely be the central focus of therapy. In some cases, initial intervention should be limited to auditory processing alone, since it is the foundation of all language abilities (Schuell et al., 1955). Because many patients can recognize or understand language that they cannot produce, this focus may also serve to reinforce behaviors that provide a degree of success and encouragement.

Emphasis in therapy should always be based on the comprehension and production of meaning and informational content. Language forms become the focus of therapy only when they are needed to increase the meaning of language and the functions for which language can be used. Indeed, too much attention to the formal linguistic aspects of language impedes the communicative act (van Harskamp and Visch-Brink, 1991). Although a typical session may integrate cognitive, linguistic, and communicative goals, the facilitation of meaning is viewed as the core of language therapy.

Specific remediation goals are formulated by analyzing descriptions of the patient's language and deciding the area that is most in need of intervention. Patterns of abilities and impairments are identified in order to determine behaviors that might be used as a base on which to build more complex responses. Within this area, intervention is initiated at the level where the individual begins to experience difficulty in accuracy, responsiveness, completeness, promptness, and/or efficiency of behavior. In addition, the conditions that stimulate more accurate language are defined so that they may be used to facilitate retrieval during therapy. For example, a patient may respond more accurately to a visual rather than an auditory stimuli or might find it easier to respond gesturally rather than orally. In therapy, one must always start with and build on the patient's strengths. "This means drill or stimulation confined to the most intact modalities and the reinforcement of the best communicative performance" (Rosenbeck et al., 1989, p. 138). Then, once the individual's "strengths have been enhanced, they can be used in combination with weaknesses" (Rosenbeck et al., 1989, p. 138).

Goals and strategies, then, are chosen on the basis of assessment results that show behaviors that patients can already produce either consistently or inconsistently, behaviors that they can be stimulated to produce and behaviors at the point where they begin to have difficulty. A task hierarchy is then developed (e.g., recognition, repetition, closure, confrontation naming, spontaneous production) and specific activities are chosen so that they are simple enough to ensure success and yet complex enough to stimulate learning. Thus, tasks and the criterion of performance that is expected are identified.

However, the actual type of therapy that is selected will depend on what appears to be most appropriate for a specific patient's impairment and what is compatible with a clinician's definition of aphasia. By far, the largest number of approaches and the most widely accepted approaches can be described as stimulation approaches. This concept, first suggested by Schuell et al. (1955), emphasized that the recovery process is a reorganization and retrieval of disrupted language processes rather than the relearning of highly specific language responses.

Specific examples of such stimulation approaches and other approaches are presented in subsequent chapters of this text. In many instances, an eclectic, "multidimensional" approach involving two or perhaps three of these approaches is used. This viewpoint recognizes the importance of the expertise, the competence, and the judgment of the speech pathologist in using existing knowledge and appropriate tools and in establishing a regimen for the patient.

Table 4.16.
Chapey Speech and Language Checklist

Name _____ Age _____ Date of Birth _____

Address _____ Education _____

Telephone _____

Native Language _____

Date of Examination _____

Agency _____

	Score[a]						
	1	2	3	4	5	6	7
IMITATION/PRODUCTION GROSS MOVEMENTS							
1. Protruding tongue	____	____	____	____	____	____	____
2. Touching tongue to nose/chin/corner of mouth	____	____	____	____	____	____	____
3. Puckering lips/smiling/opening mouth	____	____	____	____	____	____	____
4. Swallowing	____	____	____	____	____	____	____
COGNITION: AWARENESS/RECOGNITION/UNDERSTANDING							
1. Awareness of time and space	____	____	____	____	____	____	____
2. Awareness of speech	____	____	____	____	____	____	____
3. Awareness of emotional voice tone	____	____	____	____	____	____	____
4. Recognizing own name	____	____	____	____	____	____	____
5. Recognizing family names	____	____	____	____	____	____	____
6. Recognizing common, high frequency objects	____	____	____	____	____	____	____
7. Recognizing common, high frequency events	____	____	____	____	____	____	____
8. Recognizing common relationships named	____	____	____	____	____	____	____
9. Recognizing letter/color names	____	____	____	____	____	____	____
10. Recognizing form/number names	____	____	____	____	____	____	____
11. Recognizing phonetically similar words	____	____	____	____	____	____	____
12. Following 1 part commands/directions	____	____	____	____	____	____	____
13. Following 2 part commands/directions	____	____	____	____	____	____	____
14. Identifying items named serially	____	____	____	____	____	____	____
15. Recognizing 2 or more objects	____	____	____	____	____	____	____
16. Recognizing 2 or more events	____	____	____	____	____	____	____
17. Recognizing high frequency categories	____	____	____	____	____	____	____
18. Recognizing low frequency categories	____	____	____	____	____	____	____
19. Recognizing 2 or more categories	____	____	____	____	____	____	____
20. Recognizing objects/given their function	____	____	____	____	____	____	____
21. Recognizing 2 objects by function	____	____	____	____	____	____	____
22. Recognizing 1 event described	____	____	____	____	____	____	____
23. Recognizing 2 events described	____	____	____	____	____	____	____
24. Recognizing semantically similar objects/events/relationships	____	____	____	____	____	____	____
25. Recognizing rhyme words	____	____	____	____	____	____	____
26. Recognizing synonyms	____	____	____	____	____	____	____
27. Recognizing antonyms	____	____	____	____	____	____	____
28. Understanding simple sentences	____	____	____	____	____	____	____
29. Understanding simple conversation with 1 person	____	____	____	____	____	____	____
30. Understanding simple conversation with 2 people	____	____	____	____	____	____	____
31. Understanding concrete speech acts							
a. requesting	____	____	____	____	____	____	____
b. ordering	____	____	____	____	____	____	____
c. advising	____	____	____	____	____	____	____
d. warning	____	____	____	____	____	____	____
e. questioning	____	____	____	____	____	____	____
f. describing	____	____	____	____	____	____	____
g. greeting	____	____	____	____	____	____	____
h. repeating	____	____	____	____	____	____	____
i. protesting	____	____	____	____	____	____	____

Table 4.16.—*Continued*

	Score[a]						
	1	2	3	4	5	6	7
32. Understanding statements about objects							
a. existence	___	___	___	___	___	___	___
b. nonexistence	___	___	___	___	___	___	___
c. recurrence	___	___	___	___	___	___	___
d. rejection	___	___	___	___	___	___	___
e. denial	___	___	___	___	___	___	___
f. possession	___	___	___	___	___	___	___
g. attribution	___	___	___	___	___	___	___
h. furniture	___	___	___	___	___	___	___
i. food	___	___	___	___	___	___	___
j. clothes	___	___	___	___	___	___	___
k. personal care objects	___	___	___	___	___	___	___
l. health	___	___	___	___	___	___	___
m. kitchen utensils	___	___	___	___	___	___	___
n. family	___	___	___	___	___	___	___
o. other people	___	___	___	___	___	___	___
p. places/locations	___	___	___	___	___	___	___
q. other _____	___	___	___	___	___	___	___
33. Understanding statements about events							
a. play/entertainment	___	___	___	___	___	___	___
b. eating	___	___	___	___	___	___	___
c. activities of daily living	___	___	___	___	___	___	___
d. cooking	___	___	___	___	___	___	___
e. feelings	___	___	___	___	___	___	___
f. sports	___	___	___	___	___	___	___
g. school/work	___	___	___	___	___	___	___
h. travel	___	___	___	___	___	___	___
i. time	___	___	___	___	___	___	___
j. news	___	___	___	___	___	___	___
k. other _____	___	___	___	___	___	___	___
34. Understanding abstract speech acts							
35. Understanding complex/abstract relationships							
a. comparative relationships	___	___	___	___	___	___	___
b. possessive relationships	___	___	___	___	___	___	___
c. spatial relationships	___	___	___	___	___	___	___
d. temporal relationships	___	___	___	___	___	___	___
e. familial relationships	___	___	___	___	___	___	___
f. part-whole relationships	___	___	___	___	___	___	___
g. object-to-action relationships	___	___	___	___	___	___	___
h. agent-to-object relationships	___	___	___	___	___	___	___
i. cause-effect relationships	___	___	___	___	___	___	___
j. sequential relationships	___	___	___	___	___	___	___
k. degree relationships	___	___	___	___	___	___	___
l. inferential relationships	___	___	___	___	___	___	___
36. Understanding complex verbal directions	___	___	___	___	___	___	___
37. Holding thread of discussion in mind-identifying main ideas	___						
38. Distinguishing between relevant/irrelevant information in conversation	___		___	___	___	___	___
39. Understanding television/movies	___	___	___	___	___	___	___
40. Understanding humor	___	___	___	___	___	___	___
41. Recognizing problems	___	___	___	___	___	___	___
42. Recognizing own error responses	___	___	___	___	___	___	___
43. Comprehending pronouns							
a. personal	___	___	___	___	___	___	___
b. reflexive	___	___	___	___	___	___	___
c. indefinite	___	___	___	___	___	___	___
d. demonstrative	___	___	___	___	___	___	___
e. interrogative	___	___	___	___	___	___	___
f. negative	___	___	___	___	___	___	___
44. Comprehending adjectives							
a. color	___	___	___	___	___	___	___
b. size/shape	___	___	___	___	___	___	___

Table 4.16.—*Continued*

	Score[a]						
	1	2	3	4	5	6	7
c. length/height/width	___	___	___	___	___	___	___
d. age	___	___	___	___	___	___	___
e. taste/temperature	___	___	___	___	___	___	___
f. speed/distance	___	___	___	___	___	___	___
g. comparative/superlative	___	___	___	___	___	___	___
45. Comprehending adverbs with -ly	___	___	___	___	___	___	___
46. Comprehending conjunctions	___	___	___	___	___	___	___
47. Comprehending prepositions: locative/temporal/ directional	___	___	___	___	___	___	___
48. Comprehending articles	___	___	___	___	___	___	___
49. Comprehending morphological inflections							
a. plural /s/ /z/; possessive /s/ /z/	___	___	___	___	___	___	___
b. -ing	___	___	___	___	___	___	___
c. past /t/ and /ed/	___	___	___	___	___	___	___
50. Comprehending noun phrases	___	___	___	___	___	___	___
51. Comprehending verb phrases	___	___	___	___	___	___	___
52. Comprehending active sentences	___	___	___	___	___	___	___
53. Comprehending passive sentences	___	___	___	___	___	___	___
54. Comprehending negative sentences	___	___	___	___	___	___	___
55. Comprehending yes/no-true/false questions	___	___	___	___	___	___	___
56. Comprehending wh questions	___	___	___	___	___	___	___
MATCHING/READING							
1. Matching forms/letters/pictures	___	___	___	___	___	___	___
2. Matching words to pictures	___	___	___	___	___	___	___
3. Matching printed to spoken words	___	___	___	___	___	___	___
4. Recognizing letters	___	___	___	___	___	___	___
5. Reading letters	___	___	___	___	___	___	___
6. Reading high frequency words	___	___	___	___	___	___	___
7. Reading low frequency words	___	___	___	___	___	___	___
8. Reading concrete sentences	___	___	___	___	___	___	___
9. Reading abstract sentences	___	___	___	___	___	___	___
10. Reading and following simple directions	___	___	___	___	___	___	___
11. Reading and following complex directions	___	___	___	___	___	___	___
12. Comprehending sequences of material	___	___	___	___	___	___	___
13. Comprehending simple, short paragraphs	___	___	___	___	___	___	___
14. Comprehending longer, more complex paragraphs	___	___	___	___	___	___	___
15. Locating the main idea	___	___	___	___	___	___	___
16. Using the context to comprehend meaning	___	___	___	___	___	___	___
17. Getting the facts	___	___	___	___	___	___	___
18. Locating the answer	___	___	___	___	___	___	___
19. Drawing conclusions from reading	___	___	___	___	___	___	___
20. Seeing relationships from reading	___	___	___	___	___	___	___
21. Drawing inferences from reading	___	___	___	___	___	___	___
22. Reading street signs	___	___	___	___	___	___	___
23. Reading newspaper headlines	___	___	___	___	___	___	___
24. Reading newspaper stories	___	___	___	___	___	___	___
25. Reading newspaper ads	___	___	___	___	___	___	___
26. Comprehending movie/television schedule	___	___	___	___	___	___	___
27. Comprehending a catalog/mail order form	___	___	___	___	___	___	___
28. Comprehending labels for medication/home products	___	___	___	___	___	___	___
29. Comprehending a menu	___	___	___	___	___	___	___
30. Comprehending a table of content/index	___	___	___	___	___	___	___
31. Using a dictionary	___	___	___	___	___	___	___
32. Using a telephone directory	___	___	___	___	___	___	___
SEMANTIC MEMORY							
1. Visual linear memory							
a. remembering 1–9 letters, serially	___	___	___	___	___	___	___
b. remembering 1–9 words, serially	___	___	___	___	___	___	___
c. remembering 1–9 pictures, serially	___	___	___	___	___	___	___
2. Auditory linear memory							
a. remembering 1–9 sounds, serially	___	___	___	___	___	___	___
b. remembering 1–9 words, serially	___	___	___	___	___	___	___

Table 4.16.—*Continued*

	Score[a]						
	1	2	3	4	5	6	7
c. remembering sentences with 3–8 words	——	——	——	——	——	——	——
d. remembering objects named, serially	——	——	——	——	——	——	——
e. remembering events named, serially	——	——	——	——	——	——	——
f. remembering noun phrases	——	——	——	——	——	——	——
g. remembering verb phrases	——	——	——	——	——	——	——
3. Hierarchical/constructive memory							
a. grouping/reordering items categorically	——	——	——	——	——	——	——
b. clustering responses	——	——	——	——	——	——	——
c. remembering the meaning in sentences	——	——	——	——	——	——	——
d. remembering the meaning in short stories	——	——	——	——	——	——	——
e. remembering meaning in longer stories	——	——	——	——	——	——	——

CONVERGENT SEMANTIC BEHAVIOR

Verbal Repetition

	1	2	3	4	5	6	7
1. Repeating names of 1-syllable objects	——	——	——	——	——	——	——
2. Repeating names of 2-syllable objects	——	——	——	——	——	——	——
3. Repeating the names of 1-syllable events	——	——	——	——	——	——	——
4. Repeating the names of 2-syllable events	——	——	——	——	——	——	——
5. Repeating high probability phrases	——	——	——	——	——	——	——
6. Repeating low probability phrases	——	——	——	——	——	——	——

Automatic Speech

	1	2	3	4	5	6	7
1. Counting to 20	——	——	——	——	——	——	——
2. Naming days of the week	——	——	——	——	——	——	——

Closure Naming

	1	2	3	4	5	6	7
1. Completing high probability sentences	——	——	——	——	——	——	——
2. Completing low probability sentences	——	——	——	——	——	——	——

Spontaneous One Word Responses

	1	2	3	4	5	6	7
1. Confrontation naming, high frequency objects	——	——	——	——	——	——	——
2. Confrontation naming, low frequency objects	——	——	——	——	——	——	——
3. Confrontation naming, high frequency events	——	——	——	——	——	——	——
4. Confrontation naming, low frequency events	——	——	——	——	——	——	——
5. Confrontation naming, body parts/animals	——	——	——	——	——	——	——
6. Spontaneously producing high frequency objects	——	——	——	——	——	——	——
7. Spontaneously producing low frequency objects	——	——	——	——	——	——	——
8. Spontaneously producing events (action words)	——	——	——	——	——	——	——
9. Naming objects from description of function	——	——	——	——	——	——	——
10. Naming categories (food/clothing/furniture/transportation)	——	——	——	——	——	——	——
11. Naming objects within categories	——	——	——	——	——	——	——
12. Answering simple questions about self/family	——	——	——	——	——	——	——
13. Answering simple questions about everyday life	——	——	——	——	——	——	——

Spontaneous Longer Responses

	1	2	3	4	5	6	7
1. Describing high frequency objects	——	——	——	——	——	——	——
2. Describing high frequency events	——	——	——	——	——	——	——
3. Describing simple relationships	——	——	——	——	——	——	——
4. Telling the function of objects	——	——	——	——	——	——	——
5. Defining words	——	——	——	——	——	——	——
6. Describing pictures	——	——	——	——	——	——	——
7. Expressing simple ideas	——	——	——	——	——	——	——
8. Giving directions	——	——	——	——	——	——	——
9. Stating differences/similarities	——	——	——	——	——	——	——
10. Explaining idioms/multiple meanings/homonyms	——	——	——	——	——	——	——
11. Discussing everyday problems	——	——	——	——	——	——	——
12. Ordering ideas sequentially toward a purpose	——	——	——	——	——	——	——
13. Logically sequencing steps in a task	——	——	——	——	——	——	——
14. Expressing relationships between ideas	——	——	——	——	——	——	——
15. Predicting logical outcomes of facts	——	——	——	——	——	——	——
16. Expressing modifications in information	——	——	——	——	——	——	——
17. Making inferences/drawing conclusions	——	——	——	——	——	——	——
18. Expressing ideas clearly	——	——	——	——	——	——	——

Table 4.16.—*Continued*

	Score[a]						
	1	2	3	4	5	6	7
19. Using language to communicate specific ideas	___	___	___	___	___	___	___
20. Using language to elicit specific responses	___	___	___	___	___	___	___
21. Retelling stories (basic narrative proposition)	___	___	___	___	___	___	___
22. Retelling stories (literal details-who/when/what/where)	___	___	___	___	___	___	___
23. Producing relational words in sentences							
a. articles	___	___	___	___	___	___	___
b. prepositions	___	___	___	___	___	___	___
c. conjunctions	___	___	___	___	___	___	___
d. personal pronouns	___	___	___	___	___	___	___
24. Producing morphological inflections							
a. plural /s/ /z/; possessive /s/ /z/	___	___	___	___	___	___	___
b. -ing	___	___	___	___	___	___	___
c. past /t/ and /ed/	___	___	___	___	___	___	___
25. Producing agent-action structures	___	___	___	___	___	___	___
26. Producing action-object structures	___	___	___	___	___	___	___
27. Producing noun phrases	___	___	___	___	___	___	___
28. Producing verb phrases	___	___	___	___	___	___	___
29. Using transformational grammar							
a. passive transformations	___	___	___	___	___	___	___
b. negative transformations	___	___	___	___	___	___	___
c. question transformations	___	___	___	___	___	___	___
30. Producing complex constructions (embedding, dependent clauses)	___	___	___	___	___	___	___
31. Using self-correcting strategies							
a. delay	___	___	___	___	___	___	___
b. semantic associations	___	___	___	___	___	___	___
c. phonetic associations	___	___	___	___	___	___	___
d. descriptions	___	___	___	___	___	___	___
Copying/Writing							
1. Copying letters/words	___	___	___	___	___	___	___
2. Copying forms or shapes	___	___	___	___	___	___	___
3. Writing automatically							
a. writing own name	___	___	___	___	___	___	___
b. writing own address	___	___	___	___	___	___	___
c. writing numbers to 20	___	___	___	___	___	___	___
4. Writing to dictation							
a. letters/words	___	___	___	___	___	___	___
b. sentences/paragraphs	___	___	___	___	___	___	___
5. Spontaneously writing names/high frequency objects	___	___	___	___	___	___	___
6. Spontaneously writing low frequency objects	___	___	___	___	___	___	___
7. Spontaneously writing descriptions/object use	___	___	___	___	___	___	___
DIVERGENT SEMANTIC THINKING							
1. Producing numerous logical possibilities/perspectives/ideas where appropriate	___	___	___	___	___	___	___
2. Providing a variety of ideas where appropriate	___	___	___	___	___	___	___
3. Changing the direction of responses	___	___	___	___	___	___	___
4. Listing words beginning with a specified letter such as /s/ or /p/							
fluency	___	___	___	___	___	___	___
5. Naming objects within a group—							
fluency	___	___	___	___	___	___	___
flexibility	___	___	___	___	___	___	___
6. Listing uses for a common object—							
fluency	___	___	___	___	___	___	___
flexibility	___	___	___	___	___	___	___
7. Listing problems inherent in a common situation—							
fluency	___	___	___	___	___	___	___
flexibility	___	___	___	___	___	___	___
8. Supplying multiple possible solutions to problems—							
fluency	___	___	___	___	___	___	___
flexibility	___	___	___	___	___	___	___

Table 4.16.—*Continued*

	Score[a]						
	1	2	3	4	5	6	7

9. Suggesting ways to improve a product—
    fluency
    flexibility
10. Specifying details in planning an event/making a decision/describing a procedure—
    elaboration
11. Specifying numerous episodes or substeps in a story—
    elaboration

EVALUATIVE SEMANTIC THINKING

1. Making appraisals/comparisons/formulating evaluations re: correctness/identity/consistency
2. Judging whether a statement expresses a complete thought
3. Selecting words to form a class
4. Selecting the most unusual use of objects
5. Selecting the defining attributes of words/concepts
6. Indicating what could/could not be said in specific situations
7. Indicating what could/could not be done in specific situations
8. Interpreting events

COMPOSITE ABILITIES: PROBLEM SOLVING/DECISION MAKING/PLANNING/COMMUNICATING

1. Problem solving
2. Decision making
3. Planning
4. Having meaningful conversations
5. Keeping the meaning going in conversation
    a. initiating topics as speaker
    b. percentage of topics initiated _____
    c. sustaining topics/elaborating on topics
    d. percentage of contingent utterances _____
    e. percentage of adjacent utterances _____
6. Producing speech acts
    a. requesting/ordering
    b. informing/explaining/reporting
    c. correcting
    d. questioning
    e. agreeing
    f. disagreeing
    g. protesting/arguing
    h. asserting
    i. advising
    j. warning
    k. negotiating
    l. repeating
    m. greeting
    n. thanking
7. Discussing objects
    a. existence
    b. nonexistence
    c. recurrence
    d. rejection
    e. denial
    f. possession
    g. attribution
    h. food
    i. furniture
    j. clothing
    k. personal care objects

Table 4.16.—*Continued*

	Score[a]						
	1	2	3	4	5	6	7
l. health	___	___	___	___	___	___	___
m. kitchen utensils	___	___	___	___	___	___	___
n. family	___	___	___	___	___	___	___
o. other people	___	___	___	___	___	___	___
p. places/locations	___	___	___	___	___	___	___
q. transportation	___	___	___	___	___	___	___
r. occupations	___	___	___	___	___	___	___
s. nature	___	___	___	___	___	___	___
8. Discussing events							
a. cooking	___	___	___	___	___	___	___
b. sports	___	___	___	___	___	___	___
c. travel	___	___	___	___	___	___	___
d. work	___	___	___	___	___	___	___
e. feelings	___	___	___	___	___	___	___
f. activities of daily living	___	___	___	___	___	___	___
g. news	___	___	___	___	___	___	___
h. entertainment	___	___	___	___	___	___	___
i. other	___	___	___	___	___	___	___
9. Discussing complex/abstract relationships							
a. comparative relationships	___	___	___	___	___	___	___
b. possessive relationships	___	___	___	___	___	___	___
c. spatial relationships	___	___	___	___	___	___	___
d. temporal relationships	___	___	___	___	___	___	___
e. familial relationships	___	___	___	___	___	___	___
f. part-whole relationships	___	___	___	___	___	___	___
g. object to action relationships	___	___	___	___	___	___	___
h. cause-effect relationships	___	___	___	___	___	___	___
i. sequential relationships	___	___	___	___	___	___	___
j. degree relationships	___	___	___	___	___	___	___
k. inferential relationships	___	___	___	___	___	___	___
10. Using language to communicate specific ideas	___	___	___	___	___	___	___
11. Using language to elicit specific responses	___	___	___	___	___	___	___
12. Expressing ideas clearly and with variety	___	___	___	___	___	___	___
13. Sequentially organizing ideas in conversation	___	___	___	___	___	___	___
14. Verbalizing a variety of possibilities and perspectives	___	___	___	___	___	___	___
15. Varying language depending upon context	___	___	___	___	___	___	___
16. Producing stylistic variations to meet situational requirements	___	___	___	___	___	___	___
17. Varying language depending upon partner	___	___	___	___	___	___	___
18. Taking the role of or seeing the viewpoint of another	___	___	___	___	___	___	___
19. Overcoming obstacles in communication	___	___	___	___	___	___	___
20. Repairing/revising conversation	___	___	___	___	___	___	___
21. Responding to cues to repeat or modify message	___	___	___	___	___	___	___
22. Providing feedback to speaker (as listener)							
a. requesting message clarification/repetition/restatement	___	___	___	___	___	___	___
b. requesting that communication slow down	___	___	___	___	___	___	___
c. requesting message in alternate form (written)	___	___	___	___	___	___	___
d. indicating comprehension/agreement/disagreement with message	___	___	___	___	___	___	___
23. Using telephone directory	___	___	___	___	___	___	___
24. Speaking on telephone	___	___	___	___	___	___	___
25. Using dictionary	___	___	___	___	___	___	___
26. Using street/store signs	___	___	___	___	___	___	___
27. Using map	___	___	___	___	___	___	___
28. Following recipes	___	___	___	___	___	___	___
29. Using television schedule	___	___	___	___	___	___	___
30. Reading and following classified ads	___	___	___	___	___	___	___
BEHAVIORAL ABILITIES							
1. Understanding nonverbal attitudes, needs, moods/desires, intentions, perceptions, thoughts	___	___	___	___	___	___	___

Table 4.16.—*Continued*

	Score[a]						
	1	2	3	4	5	6	7
2. Understanding gestured directions	——	——	——	——	——	——	——
3. Understanding gestured description of object use	——	——	——	——	——	——	——
4. Using appropriate gestures	——	——	——	——	——	——	——
5. Using appropriate eye gaze	——	——	——	——	——	——	——
6. Using gestures to point out referents	——	——	——	——	——	——	——
7. Using gestures to describe	——	——	——	——	——	——	——
8. Using appropriate facial expression	——	——	——	——	——	——	——
ACTIVITIES OF DAILY LIVING							
1. Prepares own meals	——	——	——	——	——	——	——
2. Shops for food	——	——	——	——	——	——	——
3. Cares for own clothes (wash, iron, mend)	——	——	——	——	——	——	——
4. Buys own clothes	——	——	——	——	——	——	——
5. Drives car/uses public transportation	——	——	——	——	——	——	——
6. Cleans own living quarters	——	——	——	——	——	——	——

[a] 1 = correct; 2 = mildly impaired/incomplete; 3 = mildly impaired/corrected; 4 = moderately impaired/cued; 5 = moderately impaired/related; 6 = severely impaired/error; 7 = severely impaired/no response.

The main objective of verbal approaches to intervention is to increase success in using speech to exchange information and ultimately to improve communication in real life (van Harskamp and Visch-Brink, 1991). That is, the objective is to enable patients to regain as much language and communication as possible so that they can comprehend and use language as a means of conveying information about objects, events, and relationships to the fullest extent of which they are capable and to facilitate their ability to compensate in whatever way possible for the language they do not regain. The object of the rehabilitative process, then, is to increase the productive use of cognitive, linguistic, and communicative structures in spontaneous communication to the optimum level possible.

THE FUTURE

We still have a great deal to learn about assessment. We can begin this journey by developing more accurate, in-depth, and clinically relevant assessment protocols—standardized and nonstandardized, unstructured, moderately structured, and highly structured, reliable and modifiable. We need tools for quality assurance that reflect our scope of practice. These measures should contain more in-depth analyses of the cognitive and linguistic aspects of language and analyses of how these components enter into each patient's ability to communicate functionally.

There may be several reasons why the development of such measures has been seriously limited in the past. First, the development of well-conceptualized, thorough, clinically appropriate measures that have relevant service delivery implications is a highly time-consuming, extremely arduous, and very expensive task. Professionals in full-time teaching and/or clinical positions do not have the ability to allocate large amounts of time necessary for such a task, and colleges, hospitals, and clinics have been unable or unwilling to see the benefit of providing significant amounts of released time for the development of these procedures (Chapey, 1992).

Financial support through grants and other sources has also been severely limited. Few organizations fund research for adult aphasia, and the few that do typically do not have a large number of—or perhaps any—speech-language pathologists on their grant peer review committees. Further, the grant support allocated for research in the area is often given to the politically well connected and not necessarily to the conceptually well connected. However, grant money such as that proposed by a new law, PL 101-613, may provide a welcome stimulus for the development of functional, clinically relevant protocols. If one believes that creativity is the generation of a number and a variety of responses to the same task (Guilford, 1967), one would hope that such money will be used to sponsor a significant number of professionals in a variety of settings to develop different assessment techniques. Encouraging many responses from a variety of perspectives may help us to begin to formulate truly creative solutions to the assessment dilemma—solutions that will allow us to sharpen our clinical acumen (Chapey, 1992).

Subsequently, such measures could be used to compare and contrast the efficacy of various approaches to language/communicative intervention and also to determine the reliability and validity of the various assessment protocols (Chapey, 1992).

Another factor weighing against the development of therapeutically relevant quality assurance assessment measures is that many publishers appear unenthusiastic about publishing a number and variety of articles on various possible approaches to language/communication assessments and/or intervention in adult aphasia, especially when such suggestions are theoretical rather than empirical in nature or when the ideas are at variance with the conceptual status quo. Indeed, some journal publishers appear to favor articles that evaluate discrete, highly measurable, but not necessarily clinically relevant or conceptually rich behaviors. Thus, some clinicians may be reluctant to invest the time and energy into developing meaningful assessment procedures when they realize that there is little chance that they will be published (Chapey, 1992).

One of the strongest factors that has militated against the development of clinically relevant assessment techniques has been the current definition of and pressure for accountability brought about by public and insurance funding of habilitation and rehabilitation. The term "accountability" comes from the words "to account" and means "to furnish a justifying analysis or explanation" (Webster, 1977). Being accountable for one's work is laudable. However, the system of accountability that appears to have emerged is "cost accounting," which does not foster meaningful, functional communication, or reflect current definitions of language, communication and learning. Current emphasis is often on accountability and not efficacy of therapy.

Specifically, government agencies designate that the behaviors that will be produced by the individual in therapy must be specified in writing in advance. That is, such goals are usually operationally written, behavioral goals such as "By the end of this session, John will name three kinds of fruit." This leads to what Frattali (1992) calls a deficit-oriented approach to intervention. Current accountability often involves assessing whether the patient reached "criterion," or the expected level of performance. Thus, within this framework of accountability, assessment and intervention target specific language modalities that are discrete, highly measurable, surface structure behaviors that can be predicted in advance—or a "skills approach" (Frattali, 1992) to treatment—rather than targeting functional communication within a meaningful context which may be more difficult to measure.

Defining language and communication in terms of measurable surface structures seems to miss the very core of what language and communications are. Such definitions ignore the fact that meaning is the essence of language (Goodman, 1971) and that language and communication are like an iceberg—much of what is meant and communicated is below the surface, and only a small portion of the communication is spoken or written or heard or read. This view of language and communication is rooted in Chomsky's (1957) concepts of deep and surface structure. "Deep structure" specifies the basic relationship being expressed—who did what to whom. It describes the meaning relationship. "Surface structure" is the actual sentences that are spoken and written (Chapey, 1992).

Thus, within Chomsky's model, meaning is often not audible or visible. Rather, the listener or reader must identify the relationships of the concepts to the events being communicated or described. Understanding of a message depends on the memory structure of the people involved in the communication. The entire structure is not communicated if the receiver of the information can already be assumed to understand certain basic concepts. That is, some relations are assumed to be known or to be very easy to discover and therefore need not be mentioned. If I say, "Would you get me some coffee?" for example, I don't need to explain what coffee is, how it is made, that it is sold in the cafeteria or from the canteen truck, that you need money to buy it, that you must put it in a cup or some type of container, and so forth. If you know me well, I may not even have to add that I like milk and sugar; this meaning is communicated nevertheless (Chapey, 1988, 1992).

According to Chomsky, not everything we know about a sentence is revealed in the superficial string of words. That is, all information for processing speech is not present in observable behavior. Meaning is not directly expressed in the sounds we hear and the words we read. Our capacity to interpret sentences depends on our knowledge of deep structure. We do not learn a set of utterances, that is, surface structures. Rather, we learn methods of processing utterances. We have rich cognitive structures that make it possible to utter and comprehend sentences. In everyday communication, surface structure is frequently deficient, misleading, and uninformative; for example, there are many deletions, many pronouns, and ambiguous referents. Meaning structure may be communicated nevertheless. Therefore, language is an aid to communication (Chapey, 1988).

Chomsky's notion of deep and surface structure is echoed in Searle's (1969) belief that language and communication involve a *proposition*, or the words or sentences produced, and an *illocutionary force* of this proposition, or the speaker's intent in producing the utterance.

This and other current definitions of language and pragmatics focus on meaning, deep structure, and intent. They emphasize the fact that communication is the primary function of language (Muma, 1975). Communication is seen as an assertive act of coping—an active problem-solving task (Chapey, 1986). It is a constant attempt to vary the content, form, and acceptability of a message; to switch or shift sets of reference as topics change (Muma, 1975); and to be sensitive to the influence of one's communicative partner and the physical context in which communication occurs (Prutting and Kirchner, 1983) in order to achieve a message of best fit and thus effective and efficient communication (Muma, 1975).

Assessment and intervention should reflect the fact that language is communication, that it is the give and take of ideas. They must reflect the belief that meaning is the essence of language, that communication is idea oriented (not word oriented) and purpose/intent oriented. It must be recognized that the speech act involves creative and novel expression. This is the core of language. Language aids communication (Chapey, 1992).

As a field, we must answer Frattali's (1992) call to arrive at a consensus of what core elements constitute functional communication, and we must create a definition that has relevance to functioning outside clinical settings. And, as Frattali states, we must use this definition to develop a multidimensional assessment protocol that is thorough, (and therefore measures a range of performance), reliable, and sensitive to changes over time. We must also apply this definition to intervention goals and procedures. This is true accountability. We must applaud Frattali's message that functional communication is the core activity of daily living, since it is the core of what makes us human. We should be committed to make this message clear to political and fiscal policy-makers so that we can deliver the first-rate care our patients deserve.

References

Albert, M. L. (1978). Subcortical dementia. In R. Katzman, R. D. Terry, and K. L. Bick (Eds.), *Alzheimer's disease: Senile dementia and related disorders* (Aging, Vol. 7, pp. 173–180). New York: Raven Press.

Albert, M., Yamadori, A., Gardner, H., and Howes, D. (1973). Comprehension in alexia. Brain, *96*, 317–328.

ASHA. (1989, August). Guidelines for the identification of hearing impairment/handicap in adult/elderly persons. ASHA, *31*, 59–63.

Bayles, K. (1984). Language and dementia. In A. Holland (Ed.), *Language disorders in adults: Recent advances*. San Diego, CA: College Hill Press.

Berman, M., and Peelle, L. (1967). Self generated cues. *Journal of Speech and Hearing Disorders, 32*, 372–376.

Berry, M. (1969). *Language disorders in children.* New York: Appleton-Century-Crofts.

Bess, F., Lichtenstein, M., Logan, S., and Burger, M. (1989). Comparing criteria of hearing impairment in the elderly: A functional approach. *Journal of Speech and Hearing Research, 32,* 795–802.

Binder, G. M. (1984). Aphasia: A social and clinical appraisal of pragmatic and linguistic behaviors. Unpublished master's thesis, University of California, Santa Barbara, CA.

Bloom, L. (1970). *Language development: Form and function of emerging Grammars.* Cambridge, MA: MIT Press.

Bloom, L., and Lahey, M. (1978). *Language development and language disorders.* New York: John Wiley & Sons.

Borkowski, J. G., Benton, A. L., and Spreen, O. (1967). Word fluency and brain damage. *Neuropsychologia, 5,* 135–140.

Brookshire, R. (1973). *An introduction to aphasia.* Minneapolis, MN: BRK.

Brown, R. (1958). How shall things be called? *Psychological Review, 65,* 14–21.

Brown, R. (1973). *A first language: The early states.* Cambridge, MN: Harvard University Press.

Byng, S., Kay, J., Edmundson, A., and Scotts, C. (1990). Aphasia tests reconsidered. *Aphasiology, 4* one, 67–91.

Caramazza, A. (1984). The logic of neuropsychological research and the problem of patient classification in aphasia. *Brain Language, 21,* 9–20.

Carroll, J. B., Davies, P., and Richman, B. (1971). *The American heritage word frequency book.* Boston, MA: Houghton Mifflin.

Carson, D., Carson, E., and Tikofsky, R. (1968). On learning characteristics of adult aphasics. *Cortex, 4,* 92–111.

Cazden, C. B. (1976). How knowledge about language helps the classroom teacher—or does it? A personal account. *Urban Review, 9,* 74–91.

Chapey, R. (1983). Language based cognitive abilities in adult aphasia: Rationale for intervention. *Journal of Communication Disorders, 16,* 405–424.

Chapey, R. (1986). Cognitive intervention: Stimulation of cognition, memory, convergent thinking, divergent thinking, and evaluative thinking. In R. Chapey (Ed.), *Language intervention strategies in adult aphasia* (2nd ed.). Baltimore, MD: Williams & Wilkins.

Chapey, R. (1988). Aphasia therapy: Why do we say one thing and do another? In S. Gerber and G. Mencher (Eds.), *International perspectives on communication disorders,* Washington, DC: Gallaudet University Press.

Chapey, R. (1992). Functional communication assessment and intervention: Some thoughts on the state of the art. *Aphasiology 6,* 85–93.

Chomsky, N. (1957). *Syntactic structures.* The Hague, Netherlands: Mouton.

Craig, H. (1983). Applications of pragmatic language models for intervention. In T. M. Gallagher and C. A. Prutting (Eds.), *Pragmatic assessment and intervention issues in language.* San Diego, CA: College Hill Press.

Cranford, J., Boose, M., and Moore, C. (1990). Effects of aging on the precedence effect on sound localization. *Journal of Speech and Hearing Research, 33,* 654–659.

Cropley, A. (1967). *Creativity.* London: Longman.

Darley, F. (1964). *Diagnosis and appraisal of communication disorders.* Englewood Cliffs, NJ: Prentice-Hall.

Darley, F. (1977). A retrospective view: Aphasia. *Journal of Speech and Hearing Disorders, 42,* 161–169.

Darley, F. (1978). Differential diagnosis of acquired motor speech disorders. In F. Darley and D. Spiestersbach (Eds.), *Diagnostic methods in speech pathology.* New York: Harper & Row.

Darley, F. (1982). *Aphasia.* Philadelphia, PA: W. B. Saunders.

David, R. M. (1990). Aphasia assessment: The acid test. *Aphasiology, 4*(1), 103–107.

Davis, A. (1981). Incorporating parameters of natural conversation in aphasia treatment. In R. Chapey (Ed.), *Language intervention strategies in adult aphasia.* Baltimore, MD: Williams & Wilkins.

Davis, A. (1983). *A survey of adult aphasia.* Englewood Cliffs, NJ: Prentice-Hall.

De Renzi, E., and Ferrari, C. (1978). The Reporter's Test: A sensitive test to detect expressive disturbances in aphasia. *Cortex, 14,* 279–293.

Dixon, M. (1980). Terminating treatment: A round table discussion. In R. Brookshire (Ed.), *Clinical Aphasiology Conference proceedings.* Minneapolis, MN: BRK.

Dore, J. (1974). A pragmatic description of early language development. *Journal of Psycholinguistic Research, 3,* 343–350.

Dunn, L. M., and Dunn, L. M. (1981). *Peabody Picture Vocabulary Test—Revised.* Circle Pines, MN: American Guidance Service.

Emerick, L., and Hatten, J. (1974). *Diagnosis and evaluation in speech pathology.* Englewood Cliffs, NJ: Prentice-Hall.

English, H. B., and English, A. C. (1958). *A comprehensive dictionary of psychological and psychoanalytic terms.* New York: McKay.

Ernest-Baron, C., Brookshire, R., and Nicholas, L. (1987). Story structure and retelling of narratives by aphasic and non brain damaged adults. *Journal of Speech and Hearing Research, 30,* 44–49.

Evans, R., Bishop, D. and Haselkorn, J. (1991). Factors predicting satisfactory home care after stroke. *Archives of Physical Medicine and Rehabilitation, 72,* 144–147.

Fey, M., and Leonard, L. (1983). Pragmatic skills of children with specific language impairment. In T. A. Gallagher and C. A. Prutting (Eds.), *Pragmatic assessment and intervention issues.* San Diego, CA: College Hill Press.

Florence, C. (1981). Methods of communication analysis used in family interaction therapy. In R. Brookshire (Ed.), *Clinical Aphasiology Conference proceedings.* Minneapolis, MN: BRK.

Foley, J. M. (1972). Differential diagnosis of the organic mental disorders in elderly patients. In C. M. Gaitz (Ed.), *Aging and brain.* New York: Plenum Press.

Frattali, C. (1992). Functional assessment of communication: Merging public policy with clinical views. *Aphasiology, 6,* 63–83.

Gallagher, T. (1983). Pre-assessment: A procedure for accommodating language variability. In T. M. Gallagher and C. A. Prutting (Ed.), *Pragmatic assessment and intervention issues in language.* San Diego, CA: College Hill Press.

Glosser, G., Wiener, M., and Kaplan, E. (1988). Variations in aphasic language behaviors. *Journal of Speech and Hearing Disorders, 53,* 115–124.

Goldstein, K. (1948). *Language and language disturbances.* New York: Grune & Stratton.

Goodglass, H. (1968). Studies on the grammer of aphasics. In S. Rosenberg and J. Koplin (Eds.), *Developments in applied psycholinguistic research.* New York: MacMillan.

Goodglass, H., and Berko, J. (1960). Agrammatism and inflectional morphology in English. *Journal of Speech and Hearing Research, 3,* 257–267.

Goodglass, H., and Kaplan, E. (1972, rev. 1983). *The assessment of aphasia and related disorders.* Philadelphia, PA: Lea & Febiger.

Goodman, P. (1971). *Speaking and language: Defense of poetry.* New York: Random House.

Gowan, J., Demos, G., and Torrance, E. (1967). *Creativity: Its educational implications.* New York: John Wiley & Sons.

Green, E., and Boller, F. (1974). Features of auditory comprehension in severely impaired aphasics. *Cortex, 10,* 133–145.

Guilford, J. (1967). *The nature of human intelligence.* New York: McGraw-Hill.

Guilford, J., and Hoepfner, R. (1971). *The analysis of intelligence.* New York: McGraw-Hill.

Gutierrez-Clellen, V., and Iglesias, A. (1992). Clausal coherence in the oral narratives of Spanish-speaking children. *Journal of Speech and Hearing Research, 35,* 363–372.

Hagen, C. (1984). Language disorders in head trauma. In A. Holland (Ed.), *Language disorders in adults: Recent advances.* San Diego, CA: College Hill Press. Hagen, C., and Malkmus, D. (1979). *Intervention strategies for language disorders secondary to head trauma.* Short course presented at the annual convention of the American Speech-Language-Hearing Association, Atlanta, GA.

Hammons, J., and Swindell, C. (1987). Poststroke clinical depression: Neurologic, diagnostic and treatment implications. *ASHA, 29*(10), 115.

Hanna, G., Schell, L. M., and Schreiner, R. (1977). *The Nelson Reading Skills Test.* Chicago, IL: Riverside Publishing.

Harrison, R. P. (1974). *Beyond words: An introduction to nonverbal communication.* Englewood Cliffs, NJ: Prentice-Hall.

Helfer, K., and Wilber, L. (1990). Hearing loss, aging, and speech perception in reverberation and noise. *Journal of Speech and Hearing Research, 33,* 149–155.

Helm-Estabrooks, N. (1991a). *Aphasia diagnostic profiles.* Chicago, IL: Riverside Publishing.

Helm-Estabrooks, N. (1991b). *Boston Assessment of Severe Aphasia.* Chicago, IL: Riverside Publishing.

Helm-Estabrooks, N., and Nicholas, M. (1991). *Severe aphasia: New directions in assessment and treatment.* Paper presented at the annual convention of the American Speech-Language-Hearing Association, Atlanta, GA.

Helm-Estabrooks, N., Ramsberger, G., Morgan, A., and Nicholas, M. (1989). *Boston Assessment of Severe Aphasia.* Chicago, IL: Riverside Publishing.

Hillis, A. E. (1989). Efficacy and generalization of treatment for aphasic naming. *Archives of Physical Medicine and Rehabilitation, 70*(8), 632–636.

Holland, A. (1980). *Communicative abilities in daily living*. Baltimore, MD: University Park Press.

Holland, A. (1982). When is aphasia aphasia? The problem of closed head injury. In R. Brookshire (Ed.), *Clinical Aphasiology Conference proceedings*. Minneapolis, MN: BRK.

Holland, A., Fromm, D., and Swindell, C. (1986). The labeling problem in aphasia: An illustrative case. *Journal of Speech and Hearing Disorders, 51*, 176–180.

Holland, A., Greenhouse, J., Fromm, D., and Swindell, G. (1989). Predictors of language restitution following stroke: A multivariable analysis. *Journal of Speech and Hearing Research, 32*, 232–238.

Howes, D. (1964). Application of the word-frequency concept to aphasia. In A. V. S. de Reuck and M. O'Connor (Eds.), *Disorders of language*. Boston, MA: Little, Brown.

Johns, D., and Darley, F. (1970). Phonemic variability in apraxia of speech. *Journal of Speech and Hearing Research, 13*, 556–583.

Jackson, S., and Tompkins, C. (1991). Supplemental aphasia tests: Frequency of use and psychometric properties. In T. Prescott (Ed.), *Clinical Aphasiology*, (Vol. 20, pp. 91-97). Austin, TX: Pro-Ed.

Jacobs, R., and Rosenbaum, P. (1969). *English transformational grammar*. Walton, MA: Xerox College Publishers.

Johns, D. and Darley, F. (1970). Phonemic variability in apraxia of speech. *Journal of Speech and Hearing Research, 13*, 556–583.

Kay, J., Byng, S., Edmundson, A., and Scott, C. (1990). Missing the wood *and* the trees: A reply to David Kertesy, Goodglass and Weniger. *Aphasiology, 4*(1), 115–122.

Keenan, J., and Brassell, E. (1974). A study of factors related to prognosis for individual aphasic patients. *Journal of Speech and Hearing Disorders, 39*, 257–269.

Kent, R., Weismer, B., Kent, J., and Rosenbeck, J. (1989). Toward phonetic intelligibility testing in dysarthria. *Journal of Speech and Hearing Disorders, 54*(4), 482–499.

Kerlinger, F. (1964). *Foundations of behavioral research*. New York: Holt, Rinehart & Winston.

Kertesz, A. (1979). *Aphasia and associated disorders*. New York: Grune and Stratton.

Kertesz, A. (1982). *Western Aphasia Battery*. New York: Grune & Stratton.

Kertesz, A., and McCabe, P. (1977). Recovery patterns and prognosis in aphasia. *Brain, 100*, 1–18.

Kertesz, A., and Poole, E. (1974, rev. 1982). The aphasia quotient: The taxonomic approach to the measurement of aphasic disability. *Canadian Journal of Neurological Science, 1*, 7–16.

Kimmel, D. C. (1980). *Adulthood and aging* (2nd ed.). New York: John Wiley & Sons.

Kucera, H. (1967). *Computational analysis of present-day American English*. Providence, RI: Brown University Press.

Lahey, M. (1988). *Language disorders and language development*. New York: Macmillan.

LaPointe, L., and Horner, J. (1979). *Reading Comprehension Battery for aphasia*. Tigard, OR: C. C. Publications.

Lemme, M., Hedberg, N., and Bottenberg, D. (1984). Cohesion in narratives of aphasic adults. In R. Brookshire (Ed.), *Clinical Aphasiology Conference proceedings*. Minneapolis, MN: BRK.

Leonard, L., and Loeb, D. (1988). Government-binding theory and some of its applications: A tutorial. *Journal of Speech and Hearing Research, 31*, 515–524.

Levin, H. S., Grossman, R. G., Rose, J. E., and Teasdale, J. (1979). Long term neuropsychological outcome of closed head injury. *Journal of Neurosurgery, 50*, 412–422.

Lomas, J., Pickard, L., Bester, S., Elbard, H., Finlayson, A., and Zoghaib, C. (1989). The Communicative Effectiveness Index: Development and psychometric evaluation of a functional communication measure for adult aphasia. *Journal of Speech and Hearing Disorders, 54*, 113–124.

Loverso, F., Young-Charles, H., and Tonkovich, H. (1982). The application of a process evaluation form for aphasic individuals in a small group setting. In R. Brookshire (Ed.), *Clinical Aphasiology Conference proceedings*. Minneapolis, MN: BRK.

Lubinski, R. (1981). Speech, language and audiology programs in home health care agencies and nursing homes. In D. Beasley and G. A. Davis (Eds.), *Aging: Communication processes and Disorders*. New York: Grune & Stratton.

Lucas, E. (1980). *Semantic and pragmatic language disorders: Assessment and remediation*. Rockville, MD: Aspen.

Marshall, R. (1984). Greetings from CAC chairperson. In R. Brookshire (Ed.), *Clinical Aphasiology Conference proceedings*. Minneapolis, MN: BRK.

Marshall, R. (1976). Word retrieval behavior of aphasic adults. *Journal of Speech and Hearing Disorders, 41*, 444–451.

Martin, A. D. (1977). Aphasia testing: A second look at the Porch Index of Communicative Ability. *Journal of Speech and Hearing Disorders, 42*, 547–562.

Martin, A. D., and Rigrodsky, A. (1974). An investigation of phonological impairment in aphasia. *Cortex, 10*, 317–328.

McKinley, W. W. (1981). The short term outcome of severe blunt injury as reported by relatives of the injured persons. *Journal of Neurological Neurosurgical Psychiatry, 44*, 527–533.

McNeil, M. R., and Prescott, T E. (1978). *Revised Token Test*. Baltimore, MD: University Park Press.

Metter, J., Hanson, W., Riege, W., Kuhl, D., and Phelps, M. (1984). Commonality and differences in aphasia: Evidence from BDAE and PICA. In R. Brookshire (Ed.), *Clinical Aphasiology Conference proceedings*. Minneapolis, MN: BRK.

Muma, J. (1975). The communication game: Dump and play. *Journal of Speech and Hearing Disorders, 40*, 296–309.

Muma, J. (1978). Language handbook: Concepts, assessment, intervention. Englewood Cliffs, NJ: Prentice-Hall.

Muma, J. (1983). Speech-language pathology: emerging clinical expertise in language. In T. M. Gallagher and C. A. Prutting (Eds.), Pragmatic assessment and intervention issues in language. San Diego, CA: College Hill Press.

Myers, P. S. (1984). Right hemisphere impairment. In A. Holland (Ed.), *Language disorders in adults: Recent advances*. San Diego, CA: College Hill Press.

Neisser, U. (1967). *Cognitive psychology*. New York: Appleton-Century-Crofts.

Nicholas, L., and Brookshire, R. (1986). Consistency of the effects of rate of speech on brain damaged adults' comprehension of narrative discourse. *Journal of Speech and Hearing Research, 29*, 462, 470.

Obler, L. K., and Albert, M. L. (1981). Language in the elderly aphasic and dementing patient. In M. T. Sarno (Ed.), *Acquired aphasia*. New York: Academic Press.

Ochs, E., and Schieffelin, B. (Eds.). (1979). *Developmental pragmatics*. New York: Academic Press.

Odell, K., McNeil, M., Rosenbeck, J., and Hunter, L. (1990). Perceptual characteristics of consonant production by aphasic speakers. *Journal of Speech and Hearing Disorders, 55*, 345–359.

Orchik, D. (1981). Peripheral auditory problems and the aging process. In D. Beasley and G. A. Davis (Eds.), *Aging: Communication processes and disorders*. New York: Grune & Stratton.

Osgood, D., and Miron, M. (1963). *Approaches to the study of aphasia*. Urbana, IL: University of Illinois Press.

Pei, M., and Gaynor, F. (1954). *Dictionary of linguistics*. New York: Philosophical Library.

Piehler, M., and Holland, A. (1984). Cohesion in the language of aphasia. In R. Brookshire (Ed.), *Clinical Aphasiology Conference proceedings*. Minneapolis, MN: BRK.

Porch, B. (1967). *The Porch Index of Communicative Ability*. Palo Alto, CA: Consulting Psychologists Press.

Porch, B. (1971). Multidimensional scoring in aphasia testing. *Journal of Speech and Hearing Research, 14*, 776–792.

Prutting, C. A. (1979). Process/pra/,ses/n: The action of moving forward progressively from one point to another on the way to completion. *Journal of Speech and Hearing Disorders, 44*, 3–30.

Prutting, C. A., and Kirchner, D. (1983). Applied pragmatics. In T. M. Gallagher and C. A. Prutting (Eds.), *Pragmatic assessment and intervention issues in language*. San Diego, CA: College-Hill Press.

Purcell, S., and Liles, B. (1992). Cohesion repairs in the narratives of normal-language and language-disordered school-age children. *Journal of Speech and Hearing Research, 35*, 354–362.

Raven, J. C. (1965). *The Coloured Progressive Matrices*. New York: Psychological Corporation.

Research Foundation. (1990). Guide for use of the Uniform Data Set for Medical Rehabilitation. Buffalo, NY: Research Foundation, State University of New York.

Rinnert, C., and Whitaker, H. (1973). Semantic confusions by aphasic patients. *Cortex, 9*, 56–81.

Rivers, D. L., and Love, R. J. (1980). Language performance on visual processing tasks in right hemisphere lesion cases. *Brain Language, 10*, 348–366.

Rosenbeck, J., LaPointe, L., and Wertz, R. (1989). *Aphasia: A clinical approach*. Boston, MA: College Hill Press.

Rosenfeld, N. M. (1978). Conversational control function of nonverbal behavior. In A. W. Siegman and S. Feldstein (Eds.), *Nonverbal behavior and communication*. Hillsdale, NJ: Lawrence Erlbaum.

Sands, E., Sarno, M., and Shankwilder, D. (1969). Long term assessment of language function in aphasia due to stroke. *Archives of Physical Medical Rehabilitation, 50*, 202–207.

Sarno, M. T. (1969). *Functional Communication Profile Manual of Directions* (Rehabilitation Monograph 42). New York: University Medical Center.

Schuell, H. (1965). *The Minnesota Test for Differential Diagnosis of Aphasia*. Minneapolis, MN: University of Minnesota Press.

Schuell, H. E. (1970). *Aphasia in adults*. In NINDS Monograph 10, Human Communication and Its Disorders. Washington, DC: U.S. Department of Health, Education and Welfare.

Schuell, H., Carroll, V., and Street, B. (1955). Clinical treatment of aphasia. *Journal of Speech and Hearing Disorders, 20*, 43–53.

Schuell, H., Jenkins, J., and Jiminez-Paron, E. (1964). *Aphasia in Adults*. New York: Harper & Row.

Schuell, H., Shaw, R., and Brewer, W. (1969). A psycholinguistic approach to study the language deficit in aphasia. *Journal of Speech and Hearing Research, 12*, 794–806.

Schwartz, M. (1984). What the classical aphasia categories can't do for us, and why. *Brain Language, 21*, 3–8.

Searle, J. (1969). *Speech acts*. London: Cambridge University Press.

Shankweiler, D., and Harris, K. (1966). An experimental approach to the problem of articulation in aphasia. *Cortex, 2*, 277–292.

Shewan, C. M. (1979). *Auditory Comprehension Test for Sentences*. Chicago, IL: Biolinguistics Clinical Institutes.

Shewan, C. (1988a). Expressive language recovery in aphasia using the Shewan Spontaneous Language Analysis (SSLA) system. *Journal of Communications disorders, 21*, 155–169.

Shewan, C. (1988b). The Shewan Spontaneous Language Analysis (SSLA) system for aphasic adults: Description, reliability and validity. *Journal of Communication Disorders, 21*, 103–138.

Shewan, C., and Canter, G. (1971). Effects of vocabulary, syntax and sentence length on auditory comprehension in aphasic patients. *Cortex, 7*, 209–226.

Shewan, C., and Donner, A. (1988). A comparison of three methods to evaluate change in the spontaneous language of aphasic individuals. *Journal of Communication Disorders, 21*, 171–176.

Shewan, C., and Henderson, V. (1988). Analysis of spontaneous language in the older normal population. *Journal of Communication Disorders, 21*, 139–154.

Shewan, C. M., and Kertesz, A. (1980). Reliability and validity characteristics of the Western Aphasia Battery (WAB). *Journal of Speech and Hearing Disorders, 45*, 308–324.

Siegel, G. (1959). Dysphasic speech responses to visual word stimuli. *Journal of Speech and Hearing Research, 2*, 152–160.

Smith, A. (1971). Objective indices of severity of chronic aphasia in stroke patients. *Journal of Speech and Hearing Disorders, 36*, 167-207.

Snyder, L. S. (1983). From assessment to intervention: Problems and solutions. In J. Miller, D. Yoder and R. Schiefelbush (Eds.), *Contemporary issues in language intervention*. Rockville, MD: American Speech-Language-Hearing Association.

Spreen, O. (1968). Psycholinguistic aspects of aphasia. *Journal of Speech and Hearing Research, 11*, 467–480.

Spreen, O. and Benton, A. L. (1969, rev. 1977). *The Neurosensory Center Comprehensive Examination for Aphasia*. Victoria, British Columbia: Neuropsychology Laboratory, University of Victoria.

Streng, A. (1972). *Syntax, speech and hearing*. New York: Grune & Stratton.

Swindell, C., Fromm, D., and Holland, A. (1984). WAB type vs. clinical impression. In R. Brookshire (Ed.), *Clinical Aphasiology Conference proceedings*. Minneapolis, MN: BRK.

Taylor, M. (1965). A measurement of functional communication in aphasia. *Archives of Physical Medicine and Rehabilitation, 46*, 101–107.

Thornkike, E., and Lorge, I. (1944). *The teacher's book of 30,000 Words*. New York: Columbia University Press.

Tompkins, C., Jackson, S., and Schulz, R. (1990). On prognostic research in adult neurologic disorders. *Journal of Speech and Hearing Research, 33*, 398–401.

Tompkins, C., Rau, M., Schutz, R., and Rhyne, C. (1987). Post-stroke depression in primary support persons: Predicting those at risk. *ASHA, 29*(10), 79.

Trupe, E. (1984). Reliability of rating spontaneous speech in the Western Aphasia Battery: Implications for classification. In R. Brookshire (Ed.), *Clinical Aphasiology Conference proceedings*. Minneapolis, MN: BRK.

van Harskamp, F., and Visch-Brink, E. (1991). Goal recognition in aphasia therapy. *Aphasiology, 5*(6), 529–539.

Ventry, I., and Weinstein, B. (1983). Identification of elderly people with hearing problems. *ASHA, 25*, 37–42.

Wambaugh, J., Thompson, C., Doyle, P., and Camarata, S. (1991). Conversational discourse of aphasic and normal adults: An analysis of communicative function. In T. Prescott (Ed.), *Clinical aphasiology* (Vol. 20, pp.343–353). Austin, TX: Pro-Ed.

Wapner, W., Hamby, S., and Gardner, H. (1981). The role of the right hemisphere in the appreciation of complex linguistic material. *Brain Language, 14*, 15–33.

Warren, L. (1976). Termination and follow up. In R. Brookshire (Ed.), *Clinical Aphasiology Conference proceedings*. Minneapolis, MN: BRK.

Webster's New Collegiate Dictionary. (1977). Springfield, MA: Mirriam-Webster.

Weniger, D. (1990). Diagnostic tests as tools of assessment and models of information processing: A gap to bridge. *Aphasiology, 4*(1), 109–113.

Wepman, J. (1958). The relationship between self-correction and recovery from aphasia. *Journal of Speech and Hearing Disorders, 23*, 302–305.

Wepman, J., and Jones, L. (1961). *The Language Modalities Test for Aphasia*. Chicago, IL: University of Chicago Education Industry Service.

Wepman, J., and Van Pelt, D. (1955). A theory of central language disorders based on therapy. *Folia Phoniatrica* (Basel), *7*, 223–235.

Wertz, R. (1991). Aphasiology 1990: A view from the colonies. *Aphasiology, 5*(4-5), 311–322.

Whitaker, H. (1984). Two views on aphasia classification. *Brain Language, 21*, 1–2.

Wilson, R. S., Rosenbaum, G., and Brown, B. (1979). The problem of premorbid intelligence in neuropsychological assessment. *Journal of Clinical Neuropsychology, 1*, 49–53.

Yorkston, K., and Beukelman, D. (1977). A system for quantifying verbal output of high-level aphasic patients. In R. Brookshire (Ed.), *Clinical Aphasiology Conference proceedings*. Minneapolis, MN: BRK.

Zachman, L., Jorgensen, C., Huisingh, R., and Barrett, M. (1983). *Test of Problem Solving*. Moline, IL: Linguisystems.

Zraich, R. J. and Boone, D. R. (1991). Spouse attitude toward the person with aphasia. *Journal of Speech and Hearing Research, 34*,(1), 123–128.

APPENDIX 4.1

Cognitive, Linguistic, and Communicative Information Available on Selected Published Measures of Aphasia

I. The Minnesota Test for Differential Diagnosis of Aphasia

AUTHOR: H. Schuell
University of Minnesota Press
Minneapolis, MN 55455

CONTENT
Production

Visual and Reading Disturbances — Test 8—Oral reading; words

Speech and Language Disturbances — Test 3—Repeating monosyllables; Test 5—Counting to 20; Test 6—Naming the days of the week; Test 7—Completing sentences; Test 13—Naming pictures; Test 14—Defining words

Visuomotor and Writing Disturbances — Test 2—Writing numbers to 20; Test 5—Writing letters to dictation; Test 6—Written spelling; Test 7—Oral spelling

Disturbances of Numerical Relations and Arithmetic Processes — Test 1—Making change

Comprehension

Auditory Disturbances — Test 1—Recognizing common words; Test 2—Discriminating between paired words; Test 3—Recognizing letters; Test 4—Identifying items named serially

Visual and Reading Disturbances — Test 1—Matching forms; Test 2—matching letters; Test 3—Matching words to pictures; Test 4—Matching printed to spoken words

CONTENT/FORM
Production

Speech and Language Disturbances — Test 4—Repeating phrases; Test 8—Answering simple questions; Test 9—Giving biographical information; Test 10—Expressing ideas; Test 11—Producing sentences; Test 12—Describing picture; Test 15—Retelling paragraph

Visuomotor and Writing Disturbances — Test 8—Producing written sentences; Test 9—Writing sentences to dictation; Test 10—Writing a paragraph

Comprehension

Auditory Disturbances — Test 5—Understanding sentences; Test 6—Following directions; Test 7—Understanding a paragraph

Visual and Reading Disturbances — Tests 5 and 6—Reading, comprehension sentences; Test 7—Reading, comprehension, paragraph; Test 9—Oral reading, sentences

Memory

Auditory Disturbances — Test 8—Repeating digits; Test 9—Repeating sentences

Characterization of Responses: A rating scale from 0 to 6 is to quantify individual responses in the areas of comprehension, speaking, reading, and writing. Patient performance is also used to classify each individual into one of five major groups and several minor groups. The major groups are simple aphasia, aphasia with visual involvement, aphasia with sensorimotor involvement, aphasia with scattered findings compatible with generalized brain damage, and irreversible aphasic syndrome.

II. The Boston Diagnostic Aphasia Examination

AUTHORS: H. Goodglass and E. Kaplan
PUBLISHER: Lea & Febiger
600 Washington Square
Philadelphia, PA 19106

CONTENT
Production
Test II

Oral Expression: Part B—Automatized Sequences; Part D—Repetition of Words; Part E—Word Reading; Part G—Responsive Naming; Part H—Visual Confrontation Naming; Part J—Body Part Naming; Part K—Animal Naming

Test V

Writing: Part B—Recall of Written Symbols; Part C—Written Word-Finding

Comprehension
Test II

Auditory Comprehension: Part A—Word Discrimination; Part B—Body Part Identification

Test IV

Understanding Written Language: Part A—Symbol and Word Production; Part B—Phonetic Association; Part C—Word-Picture Matching

FORM
Production
Test III

Oral Expression: Part A—Oral Agility

CONTENT/FORM
Production
Test I

Conversational and Expository Speech; or

Test III

Auditory Comprehension: Part C—Commands; Part D—Complex Idential Methods

Test IV

Understanding Written Language: Part D—Reading Sentences and Paragraphs

Test V

Writing: Part A—Mechanics of Writing; Part D—Written Formulation

Comprehension
Test I

Conversational and Expository Speech; or Auditory Comprehension: Part C—Commands; Part D—Complex Idential Methods

Test IV

Understanding Written Language: Part D—Reading Sentences and Paragraphs

Characterization of Responses: Norm-referenced scores are based on the degree to which each response deviates from a normal response. Scores can be computed that allow the examiner to compare patient responses on various subtests with the performance of a standardized group of persons with aphasia. Results of testing are used to place each patient in one of four classifications of aphasia: Broca's, Wernicke's, anomic, and conduction.

III. The Porch Index of Communicative Ability
AUTHOR: Bruce Porch
PUBLISHER: Consulting Psychologists Press
55 College Avenue
Palo Alto, CA 94306

CONTENT
The same 10 common objects are used on all 18 subtests
Production
Subtest IV

Spontaneous verbal naming

Subtest IX

Verbal closure naming

Subtest XII

Verbal repetition naming

Subtest B

Graphic spontaneous naming

Subtest C

Graphic repetition naming

Subtest D

Graphic repetition spelling

Subtest E

Graphic copying

Subtest F

Graphic copying

Comprehension
Subtest X

Recognition of objects named by the examiner

Subtest VIII

Matching pictures of objects to objects

Subtest XI

Matching objects

CONTENT/FORM
Production
Subtest I

Verbal description of object use

Subtest A
Comprehension   Graphic description of object use

Subtest I   Gestural description of object use
Subtest III   Gestural description of object use
Subtest VI   Recognition of objects through a description of function
Subtest V   Reading comprehension
Subtest VII   Reading comprehension

Characterization of Responses: Norm-referenced scores are based on the degree to which each response deviates from normal response in terms of accuracy, responsiveness, completeness, promptness, and efficiency of production. In addition, percentile scores show how each patient compares with a large sample of aphasic patients on whom the test was standardized. Mean scores are then generated for each subtest and for the overall, verbal, gestural, and graphic modalities. In addition, an overall mean score is calculated.

IV. The Language Modalities Test for Aphasia
AUTHOR: J. Wepman
PUBLISHER: Education-Industry Service
                  1225 East 60 Street
                  Chicago, IL 60637

CONTENT
Production
Screening Section   Test 1 to 9 and 11
Standardized Section   Test 1 to 9 A, B and C
                                                     Test 14 to 19 A, B, C and D

Comprehension
Standardized Section   Test 1 to 9 C
                                                     Test 14 to 19 C and D

CONTENT/FORM
Production
Standardized Section   Test 10, 11, 12 A and C
                                                     Test 20 to 22 A, C and D
                                                     Test 13 and 23

Comprehension
Standardized Section   Test 10 to 12 A and C
                                                     Test 20 to 22 C and D

Characterization of Responses: Several types of norm-referenced scores are given on this test. Scores for aural and graphic responses are scored on a 6-point scale. Matching responses are scored as passed or failed. The examiner summarizes the patient's impairment in responding to spontaneous speech items 13 and 23. Results of testing are used to place each patient in one of five classifications of aphasia: syntactic, semantic, pragmatic, jargon, and global.

V. Functional Communication Profile
AUTHOR: M. T. Sarno
PUBLISHER: Institute of Rehabilitation Medicine
                  New York University Medical Center
                  400 East 34th Street
                  New York, NY 10016

CONTENT
Production
Movement   Ability to indicate ''yes'' and ''no''
Speaking   Indicating floor to elevator operator
                                                     Saying greeting
                                                     Saying own name
                                                     Saying nouns
                                                     Saying verbs
Reading   Reading single words
Comprehension
Understanding   Understanding own name
                                                     Awareness of speech
                                                     Recognition of family names
                                                     Recognition of names of familiar objects

FORM
Production

Speaking	Saying noun-verb combinations
	Saying phrases (nonautomatic)
	Saying short complete sentences (nonautomatic)
	Saying long sentences (nonautomatic)

Comprehension

Understanding	Awareness of emotional voice tone
	Understanding action verbs

CONTENT/FORM
Production

Speaking	Giving directions
	Speaking on the telephone

Comprehension

Understanding	Understanding verbal directions
	Understanding simple conversation with one person
	Understanding television
	Understanding conversation with more than one person
	Understanding movies
	Understanding complicated verbal directions
	Understanding rapid complex conversation
Reading	Reading rehabilitation program card
	Reading street signs
	Reading newspaper headlines
	Reading letters
	Reading newspaper articles
	Reading magazines
	Reading books

Characterization of Responses: Norm-referenced ratings are made on a 9-point scale indicating if a behavior is normal, good, fair, poor, or absent. A percentage score can be derived to indicate overall language ability.

VI. Communicative Abilities in Daily Living (CADL)

AUTHOR: Audrey L. Holland
PUBLISHER: University Park Press
Now available from:
Pro-Ed
5341 Industrial Oak Blvd.
Austin, TX 78735

CONTENT/FORM
Production
Writing
Social conventions and greetings
Comprehension
Reading
Social conventions and greetings
COGNITION
Thinking
Untangling cause-effect relationships
Using numbers to estimate, calculate, and judge time
Humor, absurdity and metaphor
Divergence
USE
Role playing
Speech acts: explaining
               correcting misinformation
               informing
               requesting
               negotiating
               advising
               reporting
Using verbal and nonverbal contexts to interpret verbal and nonverbal material
Deixix (movement-related or dependent communication)

Characterization of Responses: Norm-referenced ratings are made on a 3-point (0, 1, 2) scale indicating if communications fail, are somewhat successful, or are successful. The maximum score for the 68 items is 136.

APPENDIX 4.2

Parts 9 and 12 of the SSLA System for Analyzing a Language Sample[a]

Content Units (Part 9)

(a) A content unit is described as a grouping of information expressed as a unit by normal speakers. The content units for the picture are listed below with the major themes, followed by the modifiers used by normal speakers.

(b) Each content unit is counted only once, e.g.,

There is a *duck*.

The duck is *in the pond*.

(c) If two content units have the same actions, the action can be scored as one content unit for each referent, e.g.,

The girl is *watching* the boy.

The dog is *watching*.

(d) If a referent occurs only in the context of a group of information, it is scored as part of that group but not as a separate major content unit. In the following example, "tree" does not score as a separate content unit, e.g.,

The kite was stuck *in the tree*.

Content Units

boy (or equivalent)
    young man, gentleman, guy
    trying to get a kite
    flying a kite (pulling)
    looking for
    with another kite
    by his home (in front of)
    up in the tree
    climbing the tree
    wearing pants
    black
    white shirt
    in the distance
    last name
    Smith
    young (little)
    two
    both
    one (another)
    his friend (his brother)
children
    playing
    well-cared for
    clothes
    barking
    standing
    playing with the children
    at attention
kite
    out of a tree (from)
    got stuck (caught)
    some branches
    in a tree (in some)
    string
    some bows

    white
    black
    one (another)
    two
tree (trees)
    outside on the front lawn
    limb
    break very shortly
path (sidewalk, pathway)
    up to the front door (from)
    to it (house, roadway)
    leading up to the house
    little
    worn
house (home, residence)
    nearby
    out in the country (country)
    owned by J. Smith
    Smith
    four windows and a door
    two story
    shutters
    nice-looking (lovely)
    nicely cared for (nicely kept)
    normal
    nice (warm, cozy)
dog
    with him
    nearby (near his feet, beside)
    on the front lawn
    watching him
    waiting
    chasing after him (running around)
    wearing
    playing
    to the left (anything indicating direction)
    farther out in front on the house
    hand (right arm, finger)
    no
    skirt
    white
    blouse (sweater)
    black
    little
    stance
    collar
    excited (having a great time, interested)
    little
bullrushes (cattails, reeds)
    in the water
    standing straight up
scene (setting)
    country
    pretty basic (basic little)

farm (rural)
    happy
    nice, warm to raise a family
spring (fall)
    no leaves on the trees
    cool day
discontinuity
living
man (dad, father, boy)
    flying a kite
    rescuing a kite
    starting a new one
    another
    Mr. Smith
    wearing black pants
    down on the ground
girl (woman, sister)
    telling them what to do
    waving (pointing, twirling some object, using)
    watching (looking at)
    standing
        by the pond (beside, around)
    in front of the tree (by, behind)
    in the house
    in the fireplace
mailbox
    name
    with J. Smith
    people who live in the house
    out front
    at the end (roadway)
    beside the sidewalk
    rural
shrubs (bushes, shrubbery)
    few (some)
    growing
hills (mountainous)
    top
grass
_____
a Shewan, 1988.

garage (shed, porch)
    leading off from the house
    built on
    screened
fire (fireplace)
    going on
smoke (antenna, aerial)
    TV
    coming out
    of the chimney
    going straight up
    of the house
pond (fishpond, pool, water)
    little
    in front of his house (front yard)
ripples
    on the water
duck (ducks, goose)
    in the pond (around)
    swimming
    near some reeds
    floating
    little
    mallard
    only one
windy (pretty windy, windy day)
    blowing
    any direction
land (country)
    rolling and sloping
    not southern Ontario (like Vermont)
    having a good time
    somebody inside the house

Communication Efficiency (Part 12)
Communication efficiency is a measure of the efficiency of information transfer. Therefore, it reflects the rate at which information is conveyed by a speaker. It is calculated by dividing the total number of content units by the time (minutes) for the language sample.

$$CE = \frac{\text{Number of content units}}{\text{Time (minutes)}}$$

APPENDIX 4.3

Preinterview Medical History and Medical Status Form

Name _____   Birthdate _____
Address _____   Date of report _____
Phone Number _____   Information given by _____

Doctor: The following information will help us understand the above patient. Please comment on each category or answer each question as fully as possible. If you need more space, use the back of the sheet. Thank you.

PART I

1. Describe the patient's GENERAL PHYSICAL CONDITION AND STAMINA_____
_____

2. What do you feel is the patient's PROBLEM (please describe)?_____
_____

3. What is the ETIOLOGY of the problem?_____
_____

4. What is the DATE of injury (accident, stroke, illness)?_____
               MONTHS POST onset to date_____

5. What is the SITE of lesion?_____
_____

6. What is the EXTENT of the lesion?_____

7. What TYPE of lesion exists (vascular, traumatic, tumor)?_____
_____

8. HOW MANY lesions are there?_____

9. Is the lesion static or changing?_____

10. What diagnostic tests were performed to determine this information?_____
_____

11. Does the patient experience transient periods of disorientation, confusion, or loss of consciousness?_____

12. Has the patient experienced any TIAs (transient ischemic attacks)?_____
_____

13. Indicate the NUMBER OF PREVIOUS STROKES_____
               DATES OF PREVIOUS STROKES_____

14. Is the brain damage BILATERAL?_____

PART II

15. Which sensory cranial nerves are impaired?_____
    Which motor cranial nerves are impaired?_____

16. Does the patient see normally?_____ Does he wear glasses?_____
    If so, state the reason_____

17. Does the patient have any VISUAL DEFECTS?
    diplopia_____
    strabismus_____
    nystagmus_____
    visual field defects_____
    areas of blindness in the visual field_____
    right homonomous hemianopia_____
    left homonomous hemianopia_____
    total blindness in one eye_____
    other_____

18. Can he understand what he sees?_____

19. Does the patient have any problems HEARING?_____
    Has he had ear infections, running ears, ears lanced?_____
    Others?_____ Does he UNDERSTAND what he hears?_____
    Does he wear a hearing aid?_____

20. Describe the patient's SENSORY MOTOR FUNCTIONS (sensation, strength, range,
    b. upper extremities_____
    c. lower extremities_____

21. Is the patient ambulatory?_____

22. Is there:
    resistance to movement_____
    pain on movement_____
    spasticity_____
    rigidity_____

23. Do reflexes function normally?_____

24. Is there symmetry of function on both sides of the body for sensory and motor ability?_____
    a. trunk_____
    b. limbs_____

PART III

25. Describe the patient's SPEECH and LANGUAGE history_____
_____
_____

	YES	NO
Is he attempting to communicate verbally?	_____	_____
Can he tell you his name and place of birth?	_____	_____
Is his speech intelligible?	_____	_____
Can he say short sentences?	_____	_____
Can he repeat words?	_____	_____
Is there automatic speech?	_____	_____
Does he drool?	_____	_____

26. Has the patient had any speech and language therapy since the onset of aphasia?_____
    If so, give the:
    a. Name and address of the therapist_____
    _____
    b. The amount and type of therapy_____
    _____
    c. Degree of improvement as a result of therapy_____
    _____

27. Describe any impairments as a result of therapy_____
    a. thinking_____
    b. memory_____
28. Describe the patient's PSYCHOLOGICAL history_____
    _____
29. Describe the patient's FAMILY history_____
    _____

PART IV

30. Has the patient ever had SURGERY?_____ If so, give the types and dates_____
    _____
31. Does the patient take any MEDICINE?_____ If so, please state the type_____
    dosage per day_____
    schedule of use_____
    expected or realized effect on the patient's behavior including speech and language_____
32. Does the patient have other SERIOUS ILLNESSES or DISEASES (or other complicating conditions such as heart disease, endocrine or metabolic dysfunctions)?_____ If so, give type, description, and dates_____
33. Is the patient ALLERGIC?_____ If so, to what_____
    _____

APPENDIX 4.4

Preinterview Family History and Family Status Form

Name_____   Birthplace_____
Address_____   Birthdate_____
Phone Number_____   Date of Report_____

Dear Respondent: The following questions are asked to help us understand the above person. Please answer them as fully as possible. If you need more space, use the back of the sheet. Thank you.

1. What do you feel is the patient's problem? _____
   _____

2. What caused the aphasia (accident, stroke, illness)? _____
   _____

3. What is the date of the injury (accident, stroke, illness)? _____
   _____

4. If the patient had a stroke, within the months immediately preceding the appearance of the stroke, did the patient experience
   _____ severe headaches
   _____ visual disturbances
   _____ convulsions

5. Who is the patient's physician?_____
   What is the physician's address?_____
   phone number? (   )_____

6. List members of the immediate family

Name	Age	Relationship	Phone Number	Check If Living in Same Environment as Patient
_____	_____	_____	_____	_____
_____	_____	_____	_____	_____
_____	_____	_____	_____	_____

7. If the patient is living at home, are there others living in the home besides the immediate family?_____
   _____
   If the patient is not living at home, where does he live?
   _____

8. Are there relatives on the patient's side of the family who have had a similar problem with speech and language? If so, who?_____

9. What is the patient's native language?_____
   If not English, at what age did the patient learn English?_____

10. What is the patient's highest level of education?_____
    What was the name of that school?_____
    What (is/was) the patient's occupation?_____
    Who (is/was) the patient's employer?_____
    Is the patient presently working?_____
    If so, list schedule of work_____
    Describe the patient's work history (for example, kinds of employment and approximate dates)_____
    _____

11. Patient's mother's name_____ Living_____ Deceased_____
    Patient's father's name_____ Living_____ Deceased_____
    Marital status: single_____ widowed_____ separated_____
                    married_____ divorced_____ remarried_____
    (Give dates where appropriate.)

12. Does the patient have children_____ or grandchildren_____?
    If so, please complete the information below.

Children:	Name	Address	Age
	_____	_____	_____
	_____	_____	_____
	_____	_____	_____
Grandchildren:	_____	_____	_____
	_____	_____	_____
	_____	_____	_____

13. (Answer question 13 if appropriate.) What is the spouse's name?_____
    What is the spouse's highest level of education?_____
    What (is/was) the spouse's occupation?_____
    Who (is/was) the spouse's employer?_____
    Is the spouse presently working?_____ If so, list the schedule of work_____
    What is the spouse's native language?_____
    If not English, when did the spouse learn English?_____

14. Does the patient need to be taken care of at all times?_____
    If so, who performs this function?_____

15. To what extent can the patient care for himself (dress, feed, and wash himself)?_____
    _____

16. Has the patient's speech and language problem affected the family in any way?_____
    If so, how?_____
    _____

17. Describe the patient's ability to communicate_____
    _____

18. When did you first notice that the patient had difficulty talking?_____
    _____

19. How much does he talk now?_____
20. How much of this speech does the family understand?_____
    _____

21. To what degree do other adults understand the patient's communication?_____
_____
_____

22. How do you think he feels about his speech and language?_____
_____

23. Does the family do anything to help with the patient's speech?_____
If so, what?_____

	YES	NO
24. Is he attempting to communicate verbally?	_____	_____
25. Can he tell you his name and address?	_____	_____
26. Is his speech intelligible?	_____	_____
27. Can he say short sentences?	_____	_____
28. Can he say short phrases?	_____	_____
29. Can he repeat words?	_____	_____
30. Is there automatic speech?	_____	_____

31. Have you read or heard anything about aphasia?_____ If yes, what did you hear and where did you hear it?_____
_____

32. Below are words that describe a person's personality and behavior. Circle those words that you feel apply to the patient's present status.

happy	fights often	sad	enthusiastic
very friendly	warm	independent	energetic
moody	critical	dependent	prefers to be alone
jealous	authoritarian	supportive	impatient
shy	receptive	bossy	at ease
responsive	cooperative	relaxed	active
indifferent	resigned	resistant	hostile
troubled	distractible	outgoing	directive
tense	listless	cold	can't sleep
affectionate	even tempered	quarrelsome	able to focus on
vigorous	easily fatigued	curious	task
			patient

has temper tantrums	exhibits control of emotions
follows the lead of others	exhibits self help
waits for recognition	has many fears
has few fears	initiates activities
walks in sleep	seeks social relationships
demands attention	willing to try unknown
stays with an activity	

33. In general, the (spouse-patient) or (family-patient) relationship is (circle one):
comfortable   strained   hostile   indifferent

34. What are the patient's interests or favorite activities?_____
_____
_____

35. Does the patient watch TV?_____ If so, what are his favorite programs?_____

36. Has the patient been seen for:

	Dates	Agency	Address
a. speech therapy	_____	_____	_____
b. physical therapy	_____	_____	_____
c. occupational therapy	_____	_____	_____
d. psychological counseling	_____	_____	_____
e. other rehabilitation	_____	_____	_____

APPENDIX 4.5
Preinterview Patient Form

1. Do you use the phone?
   Do you answer the phone when it rings?
   Do you dial the phone yourself?
   Do you look up numbers in the phone book?
   Are you able to memorize some phone numbers?

2. Do you read a daily newspaper?
   What part of the paper do you read?
   What magazines do you read?

3. Do you watch television regularly?
   What shows do you enjoy watching most?

4. Do you go shopping?
   Do you handle your own money?

5. Do you visit with friends?
   Do you talk or listen more?

APPENDIX 4.6
Definitions of Content Categories[a]

Existence. An object exists in the environment and the individual comments on its existence. For example, the individual might say "This," "That," "What is this?" or "Look at the cup."

Nonexistence-Disappearance. Utterances are placed in this category if they refer to the disappearance of an object or the nonexistence of an object or action in a context in which its existence might somehow be expected. Terms such as "no," "gone," "no more," and "away" are used.

Recurrence. Utterances are placed in this category if they refer to the reappearance of an object or another instance of an object or event.

Rejection. If the individual opposes an action or refuses an object that is in the context or imminent within the situation and uses forms of negation, the utterances are referred to as rejection.

Denial. Comments are categorized as denial if the individual negates the identity, state, or event expressed in another's utterance or in his or her own previous utterance.

Attribution. Utterances that make reference to properties of objects with respect to (a) an inherent state of the object (for example, "broke" and "sharp"), or (b) specification of an object that distinguishes it from others in its class (for example, "red," "big," and "bread" in "bread book" are categorized as attributions).

Possession. Utterances placed in this category make reference to having or owning an object, quality, or ability.

[a] Adapted from Bloom and Lahey (1978). Other content categories are included in Bloom and Lahey's text. (Reprinted with permission from Bloom, L., and Lahey, M. (1978). *Language development and language disorders.* New York: John Wiley & Sons.)

APPENDIX 4.7

Suggested Hierarchy of Difficulty for Syntactic Constructions by Persons with Aphasia

LEVEL ONE—COMPREHENSION AND PRODUCTION OF TWO-WORD CONSTRUCTIONS

Level one is the comprehension and production of two- word constructions.
These may include structures such as:

Agent + Action	John eat
Action + Object	Eat lunch
Agent + Object	John pipe
Attribution + Object	Dirty table

LEVEL TWO—COMPREHENSION AND PRODUCTION OF MORPHOLOGICAL INFLECTIONS

Level two involves comprehension and production of morphological inflections for nouns, verbs, and adjectives. According to Goodglass and Berko (1960), the order of production difficulty for aphasic patients is based on grammatical function rather than the phonological similarity. The order is as follows:

1. plural (-z) and (-s)
2. comparative (-r)
3. superlative (-st)
4. present (-s) and (-z)
5. past (-d)
6. past (-t) and (-z)
7. possessive (-s) and (-z)

LEVEL THREE—COMPREHENSION AND PRODUCTION OF PHRASE STRUCTURE RULES

Level three involves the comprehension and production of phrase structure rules. There are two basic types of phrase structure rules: noun phrases (NP) and verb phrases (VP). Noun phrases contain an article plus a noun (NP → Art + N) such as "the man." Verb phrases contain a verb and a noun phrase such as "ate the lunch." Thus a sentence can be rewritten as a noun phrase plus a verb phrase (S → NP + VP). Subject noun phrases, object noun phrases, and verbs are produced and processed at this level

Other constructions at this stage are:

Agent + Action + Object	Girl eating the sandwich
Attribute (Modifier) + Agent + Action	Happy lady walking
Object + Relation + Object	Rain over the house
Agent + Conj + Agent + Action	John and Joe eating
Object + Prep + Object	Hat under the coat

LEVEL FOUR—COMPREHENSION AND PRODUCTION OF TRANSFORMATIONS

Ability to comprehend and produce transformed sentences characterizes level four. Transforming sentences involves rearranging parts of sentences. In order to question the statement "John can dance," for example, the auxiliary verb and the subject must be rearranged or inverted. The sentence is transformed or rearranged to 'Can John dance?' Examples of some transformations are as follows:

a. *Question transformation.* A question transformation involves the inversion of auxiliary verb and subject. For example, John can dance. → Can John dance?

b. *Do transformation.* A do transformation supplies "do" in a question transformation when there is no auxiliary verb. For example, John dances. → Does John dance?

c. *Negation transformation.* In a negation transformation, the negative element is incorporated into the sentence and is attached to the auxiliary verb. For example, John can dance. → John can't dance.

d. *Passive transformation.* A passive sentence is one in which the action denoted by the verb precedes the subject. For example, John ate lunch. → The lunch was eaten by John.

e. *Addition transformation.* The process of adding structures to an existing sentence is called an addition transformation. For example, John can read. → John can read and write.

f. *Deletion transformation.* A deletion transformation eliminates a component of a sentence that is expressed in a previous sentence or a previous part of the same sentence, or is thought to be understood by the listener. For example, John can fix the painting. → John can.

LEVEL FIVE—COMPREHENSION AND PRODUCTION OF COMPLEX SENTENCES IN WHICH TWO OR MORE CONSTRUCTIONS ARE JOINED INTO ONE SENTENCE

Level-five constructions include complex sentences in which two or more constructions are joined into one sentence. There are several types such as:

a. *Tag questions.* A tag question is a declarative sentence marked either by inflection or by an external marker (Muma, 1978); for example, It's raining outside, isn't it?

b. *Conjoined sentences.* Conjoined sentences involve the grouping of two sentences with a conjunction: for example, He ran a mile and then he ate his dinner.

c. *Relative clauses.* A relative clause is a sentence that modifies a noun phrase: for example, The man who came to dinner, stayed late.

d. *Object noun phrase complements.* An object noun phrase complement is a full sentence that takes the place of the object of a verb. It would be a noun phrase in a simple sentence: for example, I see you sit down.

e. *Wh clauses.* The *wh* clause is a very general mechanism permitting one sentence to serve virtually any role (such as subject, verb, and so forth) in another sentence: for example, Whoever did this, will pay for it.

f. *Right recursiveness.* Recursiveness means to apply a rule again and again (Muma, 1978). Right recursiveness is the production of a complex object noun phrase: for example, Fido ate a can of liver chunks and a can of spaghetti.

g. *Left recursiveness.* Left recursiveness is the production of a complex subject noun phrase: for example, The young slim and short freshman ran.

h. *Embedded sentences.* An embedded sentence is a sentence that modifies part of another sentence and is structurally within the other sentence: for example, The man who has the red and white scarf on stole the cake.

CHAPTER 5
Differential Diagnosis in Aphasia

SANDRA B. CHAPMAN and HANNA K. ULATOWSKA

Adult populations—for example, patients with a cerebral vascular insult, a dementing process, or closed head injury and even healthy elderly individuals, to mention a few—exhibit a wide range of impaired and preserved abilities that relate to language function. It is not surprising that considerable overlap of language disturbances exists across various patient populations. The commonalities across populations arise from a number of factors. The most important factors are related to (A) the way the language system is structured, (B) the neurobiological bases for language (focally organized versus diffusely organized), and (C) a common neurological basis for various processes. Intuitively, distinguishing the language impairment in cerebral vascular accidents from the language impairment in dementia, as one possible contrast, would appear to be relatively simple based on the most basic medical workup. However, making a differential diagnosis is complicated not only by the overlap of symptomatology but also by the overlap of disorders. For example, the cooccurrence of stroke and dementia is not uncommon, particularly in elderly individuals. A stroke may be the precipitating factor in the manifestation of dementia. Moreover, patients with left-hemispheric involvement often have a compromised right hemisphere (Chapman et al., 1989).

That language profiles across various clinical adult populations share common features has caused confusion regarding the appropriate use of the term ''aphasia.'' This chapter focuses on the issues related to determining when the language profile represents *aphasia*. Identifying the presence of aphasia will be guided by how one conceptualizes aphasia. The two major perspectives and their empirical bases are discussed below in the first section. As a general consensus, most agree that both viewpoints have some validity. However, aphasiologists typically take a stand that aphasia should be differentiated from the language impairment of other disorders. This position emanates from the aphasiologist's role in aphasia management. That is, the aphasiologist is charged not only with the responsibility of characterizing the language behavior but also with the goals of determining prognosis, planning rehabilitation, and implementing therapy. As a result, the differential diagnostic process for aphasiologists involves both the characterization of language abilities and the examination of the underlying mechanisms contributing to the language difficulties. This latter goal pro-

vides insight into appropriate treatment decisions. In the final part of the chapter, methodological approaches for determining when aphasia is aphasia are discussed. The utility of combining aphasia batteries with discourse tasks is presented. The addition of discourse measures may provide valuable information necessary for sorting out the critical factors that determine when the impairment is an aphasia or when it is not.

DETERMINATION OF THE PRESENCE OF APHASIA

Determining the presence of aphasia will be influenced by how one conceptualizes aphasia and by one's purpose in making the diagnosis. Adult aphasia is defined in numerous ways (See Chapter 1); however, the various definitions represent two major perspectives. One perspective conceptualizes aphasia as a primary diagnosis. From the second perspective, aphasia is viewed as a behavioral descriptor. The two viewpoints are supported by the evidence of distinct and common features in the language disruption across diverse adult clinical populations.

Primary Perspectives on Aphasia

Aphasia: Primary Diagnosis

Many aphasiologists hold the view that aphasia is a primary disorder that carries with it certain implications regarding both the etiology and the nature of the language impairment. In regard to etiology, those who perceive aphasia as a primary disorder typically contend that the term ''aphasia'' should be reserved for instances when the language impairment has an abrupt onset following a cerebral vascular accident (see Chapter 2). Traditionally, the label of aphasia implies that the patient has a circumscribed brain lesion (Holland, 1992). McNeil (1982) states that aphasia is a specific, frequently occurring pathology caused by relatively discrete central nervous system lesions to the left hemisphere from which brain-behavior relations can be inferred (excluding crossed aphasias). The brain-behavior relations are derived not only from lateralized lesions (left versus right) but also from circumscribed lesions within the left hemisphere (anterior versus posterior). That is, a relatively large number of patients can be divided into certain groups based upon similar features of language disruption. The common features of language behavior correspond with localization of lesion within the left hemisphere, dichotomized as anterior versus posterior at the most general level of categorization (see Chapters 1, 2, and 3).

In regard to the nature of the language impairment, the aphasiologists who conceptualize aphasia as a primary disorder believe that a language-processing deficit is at the root of the patient's difficulties. Those holding this viewpoint contend that the language disturbance is the primary factor that interferes with the communication process. From this perspective, patients with aphasia know what they want to say, but they have difficulty finding the words and formulating the sentences to express the message (Golper, 1988). The processing difficulties are manifested in all the modes of language function, including listening, speaking, reading, writing, and gesturing (Chapey, 1986; Darley, 1982; see Chapters 1 and 7).

The view that aphasia denotes a primary difficulty in processing language does not preclude the possibility of disturbances in other cognitive areas. However, for those who believe aphasia is a primary disorder, the diagnosis of aphasia implies that the linguistic deficit is disproportionate to impairment of other intellectual functions (Darley, 1982). This definition would argue against the language impairment associated with dementia, right-hemisphere lesions, and closed head injury being labeled as an aphasia, since cognitive deficits overshadow the more specific language disturbances.

Nonetheless, those who conceive of aphasia as a primary disorder acknowledge that cognitive processes, other than language, are likely to be compromised in aphasia. McNeil (1982) states that aphasia may affect the information-processing abilities to the degree that they rely on or are supported by symbolic deficits.

Most studies examining cognitive abilities in aphasia indicate that aphasic patients show depressed performance on cognitive tests (Darley, 1982). The performance patterns are inconsistent across cognitive tests and across patients. It is not surprising that primary language deficits disrupt or cooccur with impairment of other cognitive processes, since language and cognition are intricately related processes and the separation is artificial. Johnston (1992) eloquently stated that ''language is the tool as well as the product of cognition.'' Aphasia may impair the ability to display certain cognitive abilities by means of language (Lebrun and Hoops, 1976).

Aphasia: Behavioral Characteristics

For others, the label of aphasia is used in a more generic sense. From this perspective, the term ''aphasia,'' when applied to a patient, does not entail specific implications regarding the etiology or the nature of the language impairment, except in a broad sense. In terms of etiology, aphasia is associated with a neurogenic basis. Benson (1979) defined aphasia as the loss or impairment of language caused by brain damage. Using this more broadly based definition, aphasia is used to label a disruption to the language system across etiologies, for example, stroke, closed head injury, or dementia. Indeed, Rosenbek, et al. (1989) concede that the language deficits across the various neurogenic disorders share similar features with aphasia when defined as a primary disorder. As such, it may well be acceptable to label the language impairment as aphasia in a quick description, regardless of whether the language problem or other cognitive problems dominate the patient's behavioral profile.

Purpose in Using the Term ''Aphasia''

The issue as to whether the label of aphasia should be reserved for patients with a primary language impairment associated with a specific cerebrovascular accident or whether the term is also appropriate for patients with language impairment resulting from any brain damage remains unresolved. The two approaches arise from different perspectives on the nature of language impairment; however, both viewpoints contribute important knowledge regarding the cerebral organization of language.

The stance that one takes in determining when the language impairment is an aphasia will be influenced, to a large extent, by the underlying purpose in deriving a diagnosis. Basically, professionals share one of two purposes in using the label. For most speech-language pathologists the primary purpose of determining whether a patient has aphasia is that it provides a basis for determining prognosis and planning patient management. For others, the purpose in identifying aphasia is simply to convey the presence of a language disturbance as one aspect within a whole constellation of behaviors under consideration.

DIFFICULTIES IN MAKING A DIFFERENTIAL DIAGNOSIS

This section deals with the issue of distinguishing the language impairment in patients with the primary diagnosis of aphasia from language impairment in other adult populations, including normal elderly, demented, progressive aphasic, right-hemisphere damaged, and closed head-injured individuals. The basic concern relevant to making a differential diagnosis is whether aphasia has a characteristic profile that can be distinguished from other disorders. The process of making a differential diagnosis is complicated by three major factors. The first factor is an overlap of behavioral symptomatology in aphasia and other adult populations. The second factor is that disorders commonly cooccur, for example, aphasia and dementia. The third factor is reflected in the shared neurobiological bases across the disorders.

Commonalities in Aphasia and Related Disorders

The language profiles of aphasia and related disorders are not described here, since the profiles are described in detail in individual chapters of this book. However, selected behaviors that are shared between disorders are highlighted to illustrate some of the difficulties faced in making a differential diagnosis. Figure 5.1 summarizes the reportedly shared features of language impairment across aphasic, old elderly (OE), demented, progressive aphasic, right-hemisphere lesioned, and closed head-injured adult populations.

The Normal Elderly

Commonalities of language impairment in the normal elderly and in aphasic individuals appear primarily in production, although some aspects of comprehension are impaired for both. In production, the areas of impairment for normal elderly include naming deficits (Bowles and Poon, 1985; Obler and Albert,

OVERLAP IN LANGUAGE SYMPTOMATOLOGY

	Aph	OE	AD	Prog Aph	RH	CHI
Anomia	X	X	X	X	X	X
Paraphasic Errors	X		X	X		X
Paragrammatic Errors	X		X	X		
Fluency	X		X	X		
Syntax	X	X	X	X		X
Repetition	X		X	X		
Perseveration	X		X	X		
Verbosity	X	X	X		X	
Jargon	X		X			
Reference Errors	X	X	X	X	X	
Reduced Content	X	X	X	X	X	X
Tangentiality	X	X	X	X	X	X

Figure 5.1. Summary of literature regarding language deficits identified in aphasic (Aph), normal old elderly (OE), Alzheimer's dementia (AD), progressive aphasic (Prog Aph), right-hemisphere lesioned (RH), and closed head-injured (CHI) adult populations.

1981; Schow et al., 1978); reduction in verb forms and decreased syntactic complexity (Kemper, 1988); impairment of discourse, including disruption in reference (Ulatowska et al., 1986); increased use of vague words (North et al., 1986; Obler and Albert, 1984); and increased verbosity (Obler and Albert, 1981). Discourse differences as a function of age also include reduction of informational content and increased tangentiality (Obler and Albert, 1984; Ulatowska and Chapman, 1991). In comprehension, the difficulties involve reduced understanding of complex syntax (Kemper, 1988). All the above features are commonly found in aphasia, particularly in patients with Wernicke's aphasia.

Dementia

The following discussion on language impairment in dementia relates to patients with Alzheimer's dementia (AD), since this type represents the most widely studied dementia and has the highest incidence as compared with other dementia types. Whereas AD patients show different patterns of impairment, language disturbances are typically present (Davis, 1983). However, the pattern varies from logorrhea to mutism (Obler and Albert, 1981). As in normal elderly and aphasic individuals, anomia is a common characteristic in AD (Appell et al., 1982; Bayles and Tomoeda, 1983; Huff, et al., 1986). At a discourse level, AD patients show impairment of reference and impaired cohesion (Chapman and Ulatowska, 1992; Ripich and Terrell, 1988); perseveration, paraphasic and paragrammatic errors, and jargon (Obler, 1983); tangentiality and verbosity (Obler, 1983); circumlocution (Bayles, 1986) and diminished content (Bayles, 1982; Ulatowska and Chapman, 1991). Moreover, conversational abilities are better preserved as compared with procedural and narrative discourse in AD (Ripich and Terrell, 1988).

The language in aphasia also commonly manifests these difficulties, thus complicating a differential diagnosis. In fact, Appell and colleagues (1982) claimed that demented patients could be classified into fluent and nonfluent aphasic syndromes.

AD patients have been likened to Wernicke's and anomic aphasics in terms of fluent yet empty speech, verbal paraphasic errors, impaired naming, and impaired comprehension (Albert, 1978; Obler and Albert, 1981). Darley (1982) notes that determining whether a patient with a mild language impairment has aphasia or has a more comprehensive "thinking" problem (early dementia) may be a difficult task.

Progressive Aphasia

"Progressive aphasia" is a term used to characterize patients with a progressive disorder involving primarily the language system without the obvious intellectual and behavioral disturbances commonly seen in dementia (Mesulam, 1982). In contrast to classic aphasia, Duffy (1987) indicates that the language impairment in progressive aphasia has an insidious onset, gradual progression, and prolonged course. Although recent evidence suggests that progressive aphasia may be a precursor to the later development of a more apparent dementia (Assal, et al., 1984; Holland et al., 1985; Poeck and Luzzatti, 1988) most agree that a syndrome does exist that is characterized by a primary, progressive disruption to the language system with relative sparing of activities of daily living, judgment, and insight (at least for some period of time).

The most common features of progressive aphasia include a severe anomia, paraphasic and paragrammatical errors, and emptiness of language. The course of the disease is initially marked by fluent speech with empty and sometimes tangential language that gradually disintegrates into halting, dysfluent speech, ending in mutism (Neary and Snowden, 1991). Consequently, language is often telegraphic. Difficulties with repetition are also noted (Duffy, 1987). The features of language impairment in progressive aphasia mimic, to a large extent, those seen in the aphasia associated with acute, focal lesions to the left hemisphere.

Right-Hemisphere Damage (RH)

RH patients show difficulties on language subtests from aphasia batteries in both expressive and receptive tasks. Similar to aphasic patients, they exhibit problems on naming tasks, in following simple commands, and in reading and writing at both the word and sentential levels (Myers, 1984; see Chapters 20 and 28 in this text). Moreover, RH patients have problems at a discourse level, manifested by verbosity, tangentiality, reference errors, and reduced content (Glosser, et al., 1992; Joanette and Goulet, 1990).

Closed Head Injury (CHI)

CHI refers to brain injuries involving a trauma to the skull, excluding a penetrating brain wound (e.g., gunshot), cerebral vascular accident, or space-occupying lesion (Hagen, 1984). There has been considerable disagreement regarding the prevalence of language impairment in CHI. Frank aphasia was identified in only 2% of 750 cases (Heilman, et al., 1971) and 14% of 50 cases (Levin, et al., 1976). Sarno and colleagues (1986) suggested that most CHI patients manifest a "subclinical" aphasic pattern with shared features of language impairment to classic aphonic profiles. However, McKinely (1981) estimated that approximately 75% or more of CHI patients have a language impairment.

The language impairments identified in CHI patients include word-retrieval difficulties, reduced word fluency, paraphasic errors, and circumlocution. Conversation in CHI patients is often fragmented and tangential (Levin et al., 1976). Moreover, Glosser and Deser (1990) identified increased syntactic errors, presence of paraphasias, and impaired coherence in the discourse of CHI patients.

Despite the fact that there is no consensus over whether the language impairment in CHI is an aphasia (Braun and Baribeau, 1987; Holland, 1982; Sarno et al., 1986), many recognize that there is some overlap in the language disturbances of CHI and classic aphasia, at least superficially.

Concomitant Disorders

The likelihood that aphasia may be overlaid on another disorder or process is not surprising. Indeed, the prevalence of disease processes, such as cerebrovascular disease and degenerative brain diseases, increases with advancing age. Therefore, the possibility is great that aphasia will coexist with changes due to normal aging and to various dementing processes. Moreover, the nature of the vascular supply to the brain raises the possibility that changes to the left hemisphere may commonly be accompanied by a compromised right hemisphere (Chapman et al., 1989). Furthermore, the coexistence of aphasia and depression is a commonly reported profile (Fromm et al., 1984). The depression may be consequent to organic factors, medication side effects, or environmental factors.

Therefore, making a differential diagnosis in adult populations is complicated by the fact that various diseases as well as changes due to normal aging process may cooccur. Thus, the confounds are multiplied for elderly patients. Considerable evidence exists that language in elderly aphasic patients differs from language profiles in younger aphasic patients. The differences may result from confounding factors such as changes due to normal aging or changes due to a "threshold effect." A threshold effect is when an acute focal brain insult compromises brain function to such an extent that either an apparent or real dementia is triggered.

Below is a case study that illustrates the complexity of making a differential diagnosis in older patients. The patient is an 84-year-old stroke patient diagnosed as having both dementia and aphasia. This patient's profile dramatically illustrates the complex issues that arise in deriving a diagnosis and making treatment decisions for elderly patients. The clinical question raised is whether the primary diagnosis for this patient is aphasia, dementia, or both.

Profile of an Elderly Stroke Patient

History. Mike was an 84-year-old white male at the time of assessment, having suffered a left cerebral infarct in the temporo-parieto-occipital juncture 2 years prior to assessment. He had a history of cardiovascular disease, hypertension, and multiple strokes at the time of the diagnosed stroke. He was in the hospital for 3 months and received speech therapy for 6 to 8 weeks. He suffered a right visual field cut as a result of the stroke and had no vision in his left eye premorbidly. He was living in a retirement home and was an engineer premorbidly.

Mike's score on the Mini-Mental State Exam (MMSE) revealed marked deficits in orientation, attention, and language

that may have been confounded by both his memory impairment and his naming deficit.

Memory. Mike appeared to be disoriented because of severe memory deficits. He had limited memory of both recent and remote events (e.g., when he went to school or where he worked), daily orientation (e.g., day, month, or year), and the names and faces of supposedly familiar people (e.g., his driver or therapist). His working memory appeared to be relatively intact for a limited period of time, which enabled him to maintain a conversational topic, answer questions following a short story, or hold a sequence of letters in his mind long enough to determine the word that they spell (words from two to eight letters).

Visual Perception. Input to the visual modality appeared to be extremely limited by the left eye blindness and the visual field cut of the right eye. Mike attempted to compensate for his visual field cut by scanning the page; however, visual perception appeared to be markedly impaired. Whereas Mike was able to discriminate isolated visual symbols with some degree of success, he showed marked deficits in discriminating figures that were embedded in a figure-ground design. It is of interest to note that despite the fact that nonmeaningful figure-ground stimuli were difficult for him to decipher, his perception was enhanced using stimuli within meaningful contexts. For instance, while he showed little to no ability to identify isolated letters or words without cues, he could match a word to the appropriate picture even though he could not name the picture or read the word. His visual perception of pictures was best facilitated by the contextual surroundings (e.g., detailed Normal Rockwell paintings versus lined drawings). Similarly, orientation to the appropriate date was best aided by use of a monthly calendar rather than isolated words and/or numbers or a weekly calendar.

Expression. Mike's communication was severely limited by a severe anomic deficit on naming both pictures and objects. His conversational language also showed marked deficits in lexical access. Moreover, he rarely initiated conversation, and he was able to generate a response only if sufficient content was provided. Despite a severe reduction in verbal output, he was able to convey abstract thoughts in response to proverbs, fables, and pictures. Certain strategies that facilitated word retrieval included phonemic cues and closure stimuli. Another strategy that helped him retrieve a word was spelling the word for him or having him copy the printed word. Associational cues provided minimal help.

Mike was able to execute the mechanics of writing; however, spontaneous writing was severely reduced, even more so than his verbal language. Although most of the time he could not determine where or how to begin to write even single words to dictation, he could sometimes copy words. Copying single words seemed to cue him so that he was able to access a word and its meaning. Occasionally, Mike exhibited a spontaneous ability to write and, at times, could write a word that he could not say verbally, which suggests that this may be a strategy to aid in word retrieval. For example, when asked to write a spontaneous sentence of his choice, he did so and was then able to read it.

Sorting Out a Diagnosis

The characteristics of Mike's profile along with his medical history raise the possibility of any one or a combination of the following diagnoses: aphasia, dementia of the Alzheimer's type, multiinfarct dementia, depression, and factors related to aging. The history of previous, undetected strokes leads one to suspect multiinfarct dementia. However, the question as to how many strokes must occur before the disease is considered multiinfarct dementia rather than simply a number of strokes remains unanswered. The possibility of some form of dementia was raised in all medical and neurobehavioral evaluations. However, the evidence was inconclusive because of his preserved abilities in producing abstract responses. The clinical impression of dementia may be due to a stroke to an "older" brain, triggering confusional behavior. Another possibility is that the patient may be depressed, producing dementialike symptoms.

Based on the patient's total behavioral profile, it is our belief that the primary diagnosis is aphasia in an OE individual. Below is a summary of the diagnostic impressions.

Clinical Impression

Mike manifested a severe confrontational naming deficit, memory impairment, a visual perception deficit, and a deficit in associating meaning across modalities. It is likely that these deficits were the consequence of multiple strokes. The memory impairment included both premorbid information and new information. However, Mike showed the ability to process new information, although he did not appear to retain the information for any extended period. He used global-level strategies to fill in gaps of information. His problems are commonly seen in aphasic patients with damage to the association cortex in the temporo-parieto-occipital junction. His poor orientation to time and place, as well as a severe memory loss of remote as well as recent events, raised the possibility of a cooccurring dementia that may have been triggered by a stroke. However, his ability to abstract deep levels of meaning is not consistent with dementia. At times, there seemed to be signs of depression that may have contributed to some of his difficulties. His motivation was highly variable, and he showed flattened affect. His primary physician was consulted regarding these aspects of his behavior.

Shared Neurobiological Bases

The difficulties in making a differential diagnosis exist not only because of overlap in language behaviors across adult populations and concomitant disorders but also because many of the disorders share a common neurobiological basis. For example, the primary neurological marker of Alzheimer's disease has been bilateral posterior changes identified in structural (e.g., magnetic resonance imaging [MRI]) and functional (e.g., single photon emitted computed tomography [SPECT]) brain images. Fluent aphasics share involvement of the left posterior quadrant. This shared neurological focus may account for similarities between fluent aphasic and AD patients, to some degree.

Patients with progressive aphasia show neurological involvement primarily localized to the left perisylvian region (Duffy, 1987). Interestingly, this is the same area involved in aphasia of cerebrovascular origin. In CHI, the picture is less clear. However, recent evidence suggests that a majority of CHI patients show focal as well as diffuse injuries (Mendelsohn et al., 1992). Examining the relationship between CHI patients with frontal and extrafrontal lesions and aphasic patients with similar focality may elucidate some of the shared features in a subgroup of CHI and aphasic patients. Indeed, some parallels between CHI patients and aphasic patients with frontal lobe lesions have been described (Chapman, et al., 1992).

APHASIA VERSUS ANOTHER LANGUAGE DISORDER

Valid, logical arguments can be presented both for and against distinguishing among the classic aphasic profiles in patients with cerebrovascular accidents and the language impairment in other adult populations.

Similarities Are Important

There are differences of opinion even within the camp of those who perceive aphasia as a primary diagnosis. For example, Au and colleagues (1988) remark that the language disturbances in dementia are a variation on those seen in aphasia. These researchers suggest that viewing the language disturbances along a continuum provides insight into the dementing process and serves to elucidate brain-behavior relationships. Sarno's (1986) use of the term "subclinical aphasia" to characterize the language impairment in CHI implies that the language disturbances in CHI and aphasia may be better understood within the same framework. Duffy (1987) points out that patients with progressive aphasia share behavioral and neuroanatomical features with the classic aphasia syndrome. He proposes the possibility that the existence of progressive aphasia may justify modifying the classic definition of aphasia to take into account a progressive aspect.

Similarities Are Superficial

On the other side are those who believe that the language breakdown in other neurogenic adult populations is due to different underlying mechanisms than the language impairment in aphasia. The populations are viewed as manifesting diagnostically different syndromes with common features of language disruption representing only superficial similarities.

Indeed, there is considerable evidence that the nature of the language deficit in aphasia is different from the language deficit in other neurogenic populations. While certain isolated deficits may be similar across populations, the complete profile of symptoms characteristic of a particular population is distinct. Appreciating the differences in making a differential diagnosis has important implications for rehabilitation.

The most important difference is reflected in the relationship between language and cognition. For the most part, aphasic (and perhaps progressively aphasic until later stages) symptoms are manifested by an impairment of linguistic function that is disproportionately impaired when compared with other intellectual functions (Darley, 1979). In contrast, the language abilities in dementia, CHI, and RH patients appear to be better preserved than other cognitive abilities. Holland (1982) adamantly makes the claim that the language problems seen in CHI patients do not "look, sound, act, feel, smell, or taste" like aphasia. Consequently, traditional aphasic treatments will not be efficacious for this population. In regard to dementia, Bayles (1986) suggests that it is inappropriate to use the term "aphasia" to characterize the language impairment in dementia for three major reasons. Unlike aphasic patients, patients with dementia show insidious loss of communicative function, a greater loss of intellectual functioning, and a more chronic and diffuse neural basis. The differences between aphasia and dementia are greater than the similarities (Wertz, 1982). Similar to CHI patients, the use of the term "aphasia" in dementia has minimal value, since the language characteristics, the prognoses, and the appropriate clinical managements differ (Wertz, 1982).

Most aphasiologists do not quibble that it is important to separate the language impairment in aphasia from language impairments in other neurogenic disorders. Primarily, their stance is based on the fact that the distinction is important clinically. For example, anomic disturbances cross all populations, to some degree, as indicated in Figure 5.1. However, the populations manifest differences in accessibility of the lexicon. Holland (1992) stated that aphasic patients show difficulty in retrieving words and that cueing, either phonemic or contextual, helps the patients to recover words. For Alzheimer's patients, the actual concept appears to be compromised. Consequently, cueing is less effective in helping the AD patient access a particular word. The same pattern of lexical loss reported in AD also appears to exist in patients with progressive aphasia. The associational features are less closely related to the concept, and naming errors are qualitatively different from those seen in aphasia. Superordinate naming appears to be impaired in AD even in the early stages of the disease (Bayles et al., 1992).

Changes in syntax are also commonly reported across various adult populations. The syntactic disruptions, however, seem to reflect different underlying mechanisms. It has been suggested that certain syntactic errors in dementia as well as CHI may reflect disorganization of thought rather than the grammatical deficits common to aphasia. Syntactic changes may be manifestations of cognitive changes (e.g., attention deficits), stylistic changes (e.g., telegraphic writing style sometimes exhibited on postcard notes), or linguistic deficits (Ulatowska and Chapman, 1991).

In summary, it is important to recognize the similarities in language profiles across populations in the process of making a differential diagnosis. However, for clinical purposes, it is critical to go beyond the superficial, surface-level similarities (e.g., naming deficits, syntactic impairments), so that the diagnostic process can provide valuable information to guide rehabilitation.

METHODOLOGICAL APPROACHES FOR DETERMINING WHEN APHASIA IS APHASIA

Standardized Language Batteries

For the most part, language in adult populations has been assessed using aphasia batteries, verbal subtests from batteries of intelligence, and verbal items from screening tools of mental states. The aphasia batteries have been useful in isolating deficits and pointing out similarities across populations using similar tasks. Indeed, the comprehensive aphasia batteries (see Chapter 4) have been used to show that the language disruptions common to aphasia exist in other populations.

The major drawback in using aphasia batteries as the sole tool for assessing language function in other populations is that the tests have limitations based on their inherent design. Test construction was based on empirical evidence regarding aphasic deficits, according to modalities and severity of language (Chapman and Ulatowska, 1991). The point is that poor performance on a test of aphasia does not necessarily make one aphasic (Wertz, 1982). Aphasia batteries are limited in their

ability to discriminate aphasia-related deficits from age-related deficits (Chapman and Ulatowska, 1991; Davis and Baggs, 1985) or dementia-related deficits (Bayles et al., 1989). Despite the evidence the certain detailed and composite analysis may help to differentiate aphasia from dementia or other disorders, there is no test that can reliably place patients into the appropriate diagnostic group (Darley, 1979). According to Wertz (1982, p. 358), "To call a demented patient aphasic based on his performance on a test for aphasia is no more useful or correct than to call an aphasic patient demented on a test of intelligence." However, Wertz also remarks that the differential diagnosis process will be possible by adopting a variety of measures, probing the results and considering the patient's history and neurological data. Application of discourse measures may be particularly promising as a supplemental tool in the diagnostic process.

Discourse Measures

Aphasia batteries are clearly beneficial in diagnosing linguistic deficits. However, these tests are insufficient to distinguish between aphasia-related deficits and other potential contributing factors. Moreover, aphasia batteries have proved inadequate to assess communicative competence, even within the population of aphasic patients. Therefore, supplemental tasks should include measures of cognition as well as tasks that measure the interrelationship between language and cognition.

Importance of Cognition

As stated previously, it is useful to separate cognition from language for discussion purposes; however, the separation is highly artificial. It is more likely that language and cognition are interdependent processes. Cognitive abilities are likely to be compromised by linguistic impairments and vice versa (Bond et al., 1983; Brown, 1977; Chapman and Ulatowska, 1991; Rosenbek, 1982).

It is important to evaluate various aspects of cognition, since adult populations may manifest similar language disruptions for different reasons. Whereas aphasic, demented, and OE individuals may show comprehension deficits, these comprehension deficits may be compromised more by underlying cognitive impairments (e.g., attention, memory, or reasoning disturbances) than by primary linguistic deficits.

Discourse: A Measure of Linguistic and Cognitive Abilities

One of the most rapidly growing research areas in neurolinguistics is the study of discourse across various adult populations. This is because discourse production entails a complex interaction between linguistic and cognitive factors. Discourse formulation not only requires the understanding and manipulation of linguistic information but also involves cognitive operations essential to the organization of information (Ulatowska and Chapman, in press). Thus, discourse tasks can be designed to assess both the organization of information and facility with language. Discourse may be ideally suited for differentiating linguistically related disorders from more cognitively based disorders (Chapman and Ulatowska, 1991).

One of the most revealing constructs that has been used to evaluate the contribution of linguistic deficits and information-processing deficits to the breakdown of discourse is the construct of macrostructure. Macrostructure refers to the global semantic structure of discourse, and it is assessed through tasks that selectively reduce information while preserving the central meaning (e.g., titles, topics, themes, outlines, summaries, and morals).Discourse tasks manipulating macrostructure have revealed different patterns of performance across aphasic, old elderly, demented, RH patients and CHI populations.

In one study, mild aphasic patients showed relatively intact information structure as compared with patients with mild AD or healthy OE individuals (>80 years of age) (Ulatowska and Chapman, 1991). AD and OE individuals had difficulties producing summaries and titles and removing unimportant information. AD and OE populations produced less information yet used more language than aphasic patients or normal controls. AD and OE individuals adopted a strategy of producing a simple discourse genre (descriptive rather than narrative) and conceptually simpler information (setting with limited action or resolution information). Moreover, the gap in discourse performance for aphasic patients as compared with both AD and OE patients increased with greater memory demands, with a greater decrement in performances by the AD and OE groups. Below are discourse samples from an AD patient and an aphasic patient that reflect the discourse differences described above.

Patient with Alzheimer's Disease

Age: 58
Education: 17 years
Occupation: Accountant
Diagnosis: Probable Alzheimer's disease
Onset: 55 years
Stage: Mild
EEG: Unremarkable
Task: Tell a story using Norman Rockwell's ''The Runaway''
Discourse: Descriptive, not narrative, primarily setting information

> This picture of a uh . . . apparently at a uh . . . pardon me and uh. . . . It has a uh . . . uh . . . old time . . . uh . . . radio sitting on uh . . . on the back of this. And uh . . . there's a uh . . . uh . . . box here where pies and so forth were kept primarily and until they sell 'em and so forth. And there's a uh . . . uh . . . special today listing of uh . . . what they're, of what you could buy there for that day. And sitting that, the person that uh . . . runs this place is talking to a policeman. And they are . . . And the policeman and a small boy is sitting there at the counter. And they are talking to each other. . . . Uh . . . the uh . . . there's a uh . . . uh. . . . They have three stools shown here. . . . And uh . . . it shows uh . . . uh . . . that there's somebody probably had had some coffee because there's a cup and and and uh . . . so forth there with it. And uh . . . the uh . . . uh . . . apparently uh . . . that the person that runs this store uh . . . cafe . . . uh . . . apparently it's his son there. And uh . . . he, the son was talking to the policeman. And uh . . . it doesn't uh . . . show whether exactly what they're talking about. . . . But they are talking to each other. . . . And and the boy has and . . . the policeman are are looking to both together are looking for to each other. And uh . . . the boy his his uh . . . uh . . . coat laying over his lap while he's sitting there. And his . . . And the policeman is sitting on a stool. And he's got his uh . . . boots on the place there where they could put their feet. And the boy couldn't reach that.

Aphasic Patient

Age: 56
Education: B.A.

Occupation: District Manager for food company
Diagnosis: Nonfluent aphasia
Onset: 50 years
Severity: High/Moderate (Boston Diagnostic Aphasia Examination: 3.5)
Neurological: Lesion in left frontoparietal region
Discourse: Narrative with complete episodic structure (setting, action, resolution using direct speech). Language proportional to amount of information.

> There is a boy that is sitting in a cafe. The owner of the cafe or cook called the police officer and said, ''I have a small boy that was going to run away.'' And the policeman said, ''Talk to the boy. And I will be there in shortly.'' And the policeman sat down on the boy's chair—stool. And he said, ''Where are you going, son?'' And the boy said, ''I'm running away.'' And the policeman said, ''Why?'' And the boy said, ''I don't like home.'' And the policeman said, ''You got to be home because your mother and your dad is looking out to—looking at for you.'' And the police said, ''Where is your home?'' And the boy said, ''Where is—where is—address?'' And the police said, ''Come on. I will take you home.'' And the boy said, ''OK.'' That's my story.

There is currently considerable evidence that information structure is preserved in aphasia relative to sentential structure (Dressler and Pleh, 1988; Glosser and Deser, 1990; Huber, 1990; Ulatowska and Chapman, 1991; Ulatowska et al., 1981). AD patients show the converse pattern in that sentential structure is relatively preserved and information structure is impaired (Chapman and Ulatowska, 1992; Ulatowska and Chapman, 1991).

However, this evidence does not imply that discourse processing is unimpaired in aphasia (Chapman and Ulatowska, 1992; Huber, 1990). Indeed, more extensive investigations of macrostructure in aphasia have shown that macrostructure is impaired on tasks that require responses that generalize beyond the specific content of the stimulus (Ulatowska and Chapman, 1992). Moreover, dissociations between information structure and linguistic phenomena have also been described for RH patients (Glosser et al., 1992) and CHI patients (Hartley and Jensen, 1991).

Below are patients' responses on tasks of macrostructure including retelling a story, giving a gist, identifying the main character with a justification, and formulating the moral. Brief comparison performances appear below the responses. The story presented to each of the patients is as follows:

> Two roosters were fighting over the chicken yard. The one who was defeated hid in the corner. The other rooster flew to the top of the roost and began crowing and flapping his wings to boast of his victory. Suddenly, an eagle swooped down, grabbed the rooster, and carried him away. This was good luck for the defeated rooster. Now he could rule over the roost and have all the hens that he desired.

Aphasic Patient

Age: 71
Education: College
Occupation: Business executive
Diagnosis: Posterior stroke, fluent aphasia
Onset: 60 years
Severity: 3.5 on BDAE
Neurological information: Left posterior lesion
Two Roosters: Retell

> All right, all right, there were two roosters in the uh chicken yard. Uh they started to uh fight and finally uh one rooster uh-

uh was a-the victory and one was kind of uh cowed down on the side. And the other rooster uh start uh uh crow and everything because, ''I am number one.'' And then just a uh eagle come down and uh swoop down and got the uh rooster that was uh crowing. And then the other rooster felt that, ''Uh, uh okay, I am number one in the yard and there's a lot of other uh, hens for you.'' Gist: Well uh . . . well one is that the victory, other one was uh defeat. And then uh, and it stops again and a different one is the victory. *Main Character and Justification*: Uh before the, in the end, he was—he was number one.
Moral: Well, don't talk uh and uh crow until you're ready to (laughs) victory.

Progressive Aphasic:

Age: 52
Education: 12 years
Occupation: Stockbroker
Diagnosis: Progressive aphasia
Onset: 48 years
Severity: 4.0 on BDAE
Neurological information: MRI—left temporal atrophy, motor vehicle accident (1969), unconscious 3 to 5 days
Two Roosters: Retell

See, I've already remembered the other—I've already lost the other word. Uh, the rooster was, uh . . . he hit someone. And he hurt him he was trying to and he flew up to the top of the roost, and he was trying to—I don't know if he was trying to get something or not, but he did hurt a guy and another rooster, and the other rooster just got away and stayed away from him. And then, an eagle came in and took him away, and the other rooster was happy that he was taken away. And, uh . . . he started talking about hens. See I don't remember what it was about. The other rooster started talking about hens. . . . That's all I can remember. *Gist*: Well, the main idea was that . . . the top rooster was trying to have everything that he wanted and be the only rooster I guess with the hens. And he, uh, he was trying to get rid of some of the other roosters around and do what he wanted to do.
Main Character and Justification: The rooster that hit everybody else, and it was finally taken away. Well, he's the one that did everything. The other one stayed away and didn't even let anybody see him. Because he didn't want the rooster to kill him.
Moral: Well, I think the lesson is that you should not be trying to take everything and kill other roosters because you're going to get taken out yourself, which he finally got done.

Right-Hemisphere Lesioned Patient

Age: 82
Education: 12 years
Occupation: Book reviewer
Diagnosis: Right-hemisphere stroke
Onset: 80 years
Neurological information: right middle cerebral infarct, moderate cerebral atrophy
Two Roosters: Retell
About the two roosters who were fighting. And the bigger rooster—the smaller one had some chicken, a chicken in his mouth. I forgot whether it was just a piece of chicken or just a chicken. Of course, he finally dropped it and the other rooster immediately grabbed it and took off with the chicken and another rooster came along and picked up the first—the rooster that had picked up the chicken and flew away with him. So, I think you'd say, don't count your chickens before they hatch. It left the original rooster in possibly want. It changed his life for him.
Main Character and Justification: I'm kind of inclined to vote for the eagle. Well, because he was the stronger of the three of them and he swooped down and straightened everything out ''ker-plop'' like that.

He helped the first rooster because he defeated the second one and left him in charge. Eagles are strong, much stronger than roosters, I think. So I think he came along at the right time. But the first rooster should have realized that he could—he must have known that rooster, because he was in the same chicken yard with him. So he was too trustworthy.
Moral: Well, like I said while ago, don't count your chickens before they hatch. You see, he was all ready to boast of his victory, the second one, the one that took the chicken away was ready to boast of what he had done when the eagle arrived and he lost his bit of chicken, and also his standing—he lost a lot a lot in that day. And you have to be careful who you are going to trust, who you're going to trust.

Patient with Alzheimer's Disease

Age: 67 years
Education: 14 years
Occupation: Retired nurse
Diagnosis: Alzheimer's disease
Onset: 65 years
Stage: Moderate neurological information: Mild-moderate generalized atrophy. Mild microvascular changes, possible atrophy of the left temporal lobe

The story presented to this patient for evaluation is as follows:
The Fox and the Raven

A raven was sitting on a tree holding a piece of cheese in his beak. A fox saw him and decided he wanted the cheese. He stood under the tree and began to praise the raven. He told the raven that he was a very beautiful bird and that he should become a king. The fox said that he would like to hear the raven's voice to be sure that the raven could give orders. Then the raven decided to show off his voice. He opened his beak and the cheese fell out onto the ground. The fox grabbed the cheese and ran away.

The patient's responses are presented below:

Retell: The raven . . . uh was . . . uh holding the piece of cheese and uh, let me see if I can find some of this. Trying to . . . uh . . . talk to the fox? Was that the fox, no that's not what the fox was it? Was it? Now I've lost track . . . uh the raven was uh sitting up there with uh cheese wasn't it, cheese? And he was watching the . . . uh . . . uh . . . losing another man. (laughs) Anyway he dropped his food and the . . . the dog? It's not a dog it's a . . . whatever creature that was.
Gist: Uh, praise the raven. I don't know if this is correct or not correct. So he told the raven that he was a very beautiful bird and . . . uh . . . anyway the fox apparently was gonna try to get the—get the . . . uh . . . whatever his name was, the beautiful bird but I was the—oh the fox . . . was there. But the bird is—is the raven. The raven decided to show off his voice when the . . . fox decided he'd swing his so (laughs). And the fox grabbed the cheese and ran away with it so the . . . raven had nothing to do with it (laughs).
Moral: Well, I'm guessing that uh . . . the uh raven probably got most of the cheese. I don't really know.

Discussion of Patients' Responses
The above responses from various patient groups show different patterns of deficits, some reflecting more linguistic deficits, others more cognitive, and some obvious cognitive and linguistic disruptions. The aphasic patient showed linguistic difficulties in his story retell; however, he was able to convey most of the important information in the story. That is, the basic story structure was preserved for this patient. However,

the aphasic patient did show impairment of macrostructure as reflected in his difficulties on deriving a moral that generalized beyond the specific story content. Normal individuals typically produce generalized morals that go beyond the specific story content.

In contrast, the patient with progressive aphasia exhibited difficulty in expressing the information, because of both a severe reduction of lexicon and an impairment in the organization of the information. Disruption of reference is evident, as it is difficult to follow who is doing what in the retell. For this patient, both story structure and macrostructure are impaired. Macrostructure impairment is manifested by the patient's failure to grasp the central meaning of the story, the role reversal of the defeated rooster who became the victor. This contrast was made clear in the aphasic patient's responses.

The most obvious difference shown by the responses of the RH patient was the severe impairment of information structure but relative preservation of linguistic structure. The quantity of language is greater than the amount of information conveyed. The patient's response to the moral probe seems unexpectedly high level. However, as the patient elaborated on her response, it seemed that the central meaning of the story was not understood at all.

The responses from the demented patient showed the marked disruption to both story structure and macrostructure. The patient showed inconsistency in responding as evidenced by discourse composed of content from the story disrupted by irrelevant interjections of information. In the patient's response to the main idea probe, the patient seemed to grasp the meaning of the story momentarily but subsequently seemed to have lost it completely with the extended response.

In summary, recent neurolinguistic studies across adult populations indicate that discourse measures may provide valuable, supplemental information to that obtained by using standardized measures as part of the differential diagnostic process. Discourse measures are particularly useful in identifying similarities and differences across populations to enhance differential diagnosis. Moreover, discourse assessment provides a way of examining spared and impaired abilities. It is critical to identify losses as well as preserved abilities to establish more accurate clinical profiles of various populations. As shown earlier in this chapter, clinical populations manifest similar impairments. It is possible that these similarities are due to the fact that there are a limited number of ways in which language structure can be disturbed. However, the potential mechanisms underlying similar disruptions may be distinct and be identified through isolation of the spared abilities.

FUTURE TRENDS

Only recently has the importance been realized of sorting out not only linguistic factors but also cognitive factors that contribute to breakdown of communicative competence. This realization has come through the research and clinical experience with patient populations (e.g., dementia, CHI) with more prominent cognitive than linguistic deficits. The future diagnostic batteries may well provide a battery of in-depth interrelated tests of discourse in which the content is manipulated in different ways to tap both linguistic abilities and information-processing abilities. The framework may be comparable to that used in designing the BDAE (Goodglass and Kaplan, 1983)

and The Porch Index of Communicative Ability (Porch, 1967), in which the same content is manipulated in various ways to assess different language modalities. For the discourse tasks, the focus is more likely to be on the different processes related to communicative function and secondarily to the various language modalities.

In the future, the controversy as to when to label a language impairment in a neurogenic population as an "aphasia" will be replaced by a differential diagnostic process in which the speech-language pathologist addresses the primary question of how the linguistic impairment disrupts other cognitive systems and how the cognitive disturbances impinge on linguistic abilities.

More important, the goal will be to understand how the cognitive and linguistic disruptions hinder communicative competence. This broadened perspective will have important diagnostic and treatment implications. In terms of diagnosis, the assessment, while still concerned with classification, will no longer be restricted by certain etiologic categories (e.g., dementia, RH). Rather, assessment protocols will be global enough in scope to appreciate the fact that some aphasic patients may also have involvement of the right hemisphere, that many CHI patients have focal lesions, or that some aphasic patients may also be demented. In terms of treatment, intervention protocols for all etiologic groups can be implemented to enhance communicative competence, once the requisite spared and impaired linguistic and cognitive abilities have been identified. As health care professionals turn toward more functional concerns regarding diagnosis and treatment, the role of the speech-language pathologists will increase since communication is a basic human need. As poignantly stated by Eugene Ionesco: "Although prayer is born of silence, it is with the help of words that I scale the heavens."

Acknowledgment: This work was supported by a grant from the Texas Advanced Research Program (#009741-013) and by grant AG 09486 from the National Institute on Aging.

References

Albert, M. L. (1978). Subcortical dementia. In R. Katzmann, R. D. Terry and K. L. Bick (Eds.), *Alzheimer's disease: Senile dementia and related disorders (Aging,* Vol. 7) pp. 173–180). New York: Raven Press.

Appell, J., Kertesz, A., and Fisman, M. (1982). A study of language functioning in Alzheimer's patients. *Brain and Language, 17,* 73–91.

Assal, G., Favre, C., and Regli, F. (1984). Aphasia as a first sign of dementia. In J. Wertheimer and M. Marois (Eds.), *Senile dementia: Outlook for the future.* New York: Alan R. Liss.

Au, R., Albert, M. L., and Obler, L. K. (1988). The relationship of aphasia to dementia. *Aphasiology, 2,* 161–173.

Bayles, K. A. (1982). Language function in senile dementia. *Brain and Language. 16,* 265–280.

Bayles, K. (1986). Disorders associated with dementia. In R. Chapey (Ed.), *Language strategies in adult aphasia* (2nd ed., pp. 462–473). Baltimore, MD: Williams & Wilkins.

Bayles, K., Boone, D., Tomoeda, C., Slauson, T., and Kaszniak, A. (1989). Differentiating Alzheimer's patients from the normal elderly and stroke patients with aphasia. *Journal of Speech and Hearing Disorders, 54,* 74–87.

Bayles, K. A., and Tomoeda, C. K. (1983). Confrontation and generative naming abilities of dementia patients. In R. H. Brookshire (Ed.), *Clinical Aphasiology Conference proceedings.* Minneapolis, MN: BRK.

Bayles, K. A., Tomoeda, C. K., and Trosset, M. W. (1992). Relation of linguistic communication abilities of Alzheimer's patients to stage of disease. *Brain and Language, 42,* 454–472.

Benson, D. F. (1979). *Aphasia, alexia and agraphia.* New York: Churchill Livingstone.

Bond, S., Ulatowska, H., Haynes, S., and May, E. (1983). Discourse production in aphasia: Relationship to severity of impairment. In R. H. Brookshire (Ed.), *Clinical aphasiology* (pp. 202–210). Minneapolis, MN: BRK.

Bowles, N., and Poon, L. (1985). Aging and retrieval of words in semantic memory. *Journal of Gerontology, 40,* 71–77.

Braun, C. M. M., and Baribeau, J. M. C. (1987). Subclinical aphasia following closed head injury: A response to Sarno, Buonaguro, and Levita. In R. H. Brookshire (Ed.), *Clinical aphasiology* (pp. 326–333). Minneapolis, MN: BRK.

Brown, J. (1977). *Mind, brain, and consciousness: The neuropsychology of cognition.* New York: Academic Press. Chapey, R. (1986). The assessment of language disorders in adults. In R. Chapey (Ed.), *Language intervention strategies in adult aphasia* (2nd ed., pp. 81–180). Baltimore, MD: Williams & Wilkins.

Chapman, S. B., Culhane, K. A., Levin, H. S., Harward, H., Mendelsohn, D., Ewing-Cobbs, L., Fletcher, J., and Bruce, D. (1992). Narrative discourse after closed head injury in children and adolescents. *Brain and Language, 43,* 42–65.

Chapman, S. B., Pool, K. D., Finitzo, T., and Hong, C. (1989). Comparison of language profiles and electrocortical dysfunction in aphasia. In T. E. Prescott (Ed.), *Clinical aphasiology* (pp. 41–60). Boston: College Hill Press.

Chapman, S. B., and Ulatowska, H. K. (1991). Aphasia and aging. In D. Ripich (Ed.), *Geriatric communication disorders* (pp. 241–254). Austin, TX: Pro-Ed.

Chapman, S. B., and Ulatowska, H. K. (1992). The nature of language disruption in dementia: Is it aphasia? *Texas Journal of Audiology and Speech Pathology,* 3–9.

Darley, F. L. (1979). The differential diagnosis of aphasia. In R. H. Brookshire (Ed.), *Clinical Aphasiology Conference proceedings* (pp. 23–29). Minneapolis, MN: BRK.

Darley, F. L. (1982). *Aphasia,* Philadelphia, PA: W. B. Saunders.

Davis, A. (1983). *A survey of adult aphasia.* Englewood Cliffs, NJ: Prentice-Hall.

Davis, A., and Baggs, T. (1985). Rehabilitation of speech and language disorders. In L. Jacobs-Condit (Ed.), *Gerontology and communication disorders.* Rockville, MD: American Speech-Language-Hearing Association.

Dressler, W. U., and Pleh, C. (1988). On text disturbances in aphasia. In W. U. Dressler and J. A. Stark (Eds.), *Linguistic analyses of aphasic language* (pp. 151–178). New York: Springer-Verlag.

Duffy, J. R. (1987). Unusual aphasias: Slowly progressive aphasia. In R. H. Brookshire (Ed.), *Clinical aphasiology* (pp. 349–356). Minneapolis, MN: BRK.

Fromm, D., Holland, A., and Swindell, C. (1984). Depression following left hemisphere stroke. (Abstract). In R. H. Brookshire (Ed.), *Clinical aphasiology* (pp. 268–270). Minneapolis, MN: BRK.

Glosser, G., and Deser, T. (1990). Patterns of discourse production among neurological patients with fluent language disorders. *Brain and Language, 40,* 67–88.

Glosser, G., Deser, T., and Weisstein, C. (1992). *Structural organization of discourse production following right hemisphere damage.* Poster presented at the Twentieth Annual Meeting of the International Neuropsychological Society, San Diego, CA.

Golper, L. C. (1988). Communication and dementia: A clinical perspective. In B. B. Shadden (Ed.), *Communication behavior and aging: A sourcebook for clinicians* (pp. 279–293). Baltimore, MD: Williams & Wilkins.

Goodglass, H., and Kaplan, E. (1983). *The Boston Diagnostic Aphasia Examination.* Philadelphia, PA: Lea & Febiger.

Hagen, C. (1984). Language disorders in head trauma. In A. Holland (Ed.), *Language disorders in adults: Recent advances.* San Diego, CA: College Hill Press.

Hartley, L. L., and Jensen, P. J. (1991). Narrative and procedural discourse after closed head injury. *Brain Injury, 5,* 267–285.

Heilman, K. M., Safran, A., and Geschwind, N. (1971). Closed head trauma and aphasia. *Journal of Neurology, Neurosurgery and Psychiatry, 34,* 265–269.

Holland, A. (1982). When is aphasia aphasia? The problem of closed head injury. In R. H. Brookshire (Ed.), *Clinical Aphasiology: Conference proceedings* (pp. 345–349). Minneapolis, MN: BRK.

Holland, A. (1992, February). *What language disorders tell us about the aging brain.* Paper presented at the Aging: The Quality of Life Conference, Washington, DC.

Holland, A., McBurney, D. H., Mossy, J., and Reinmouth, O. M. (1985). The dissolution of language in Pick's disease with neurofibrillary tangles: A case study. *Brain and Language, 24,* 36–58.

Huber, W. (1990). Text comprehension and production in aphasia: Analysis in terms of micro- and macrostructure. In Y. Joanette and H. H. Brownell (Eds.), *Discourse ability and brain damage: Theoretical and empirical perspectives.* (pp. 154–179). New York: Springer-Verlag.

Huff, F. J., Corkin, S., and Growdon, J. H. (1986). Semantic impairment and anomia in Alzheimer's disease. *Brain and Language, 28,* 235–249.

Joanette, Y., and Goulet, P. (1990). Narrative discourse in right-brain-damaged right-handers. In Y. Joanette and H. H. Brownell (Eds.), *Discourse ability and brain damage: Theoretical and empirical perspectives* (pp. 131–153). New York: Springer-Verlag.

Johnston, J. (1992, June). *Cognitive abilities of language impaired children.* Paper presented at the Bruton Conference, Callier Center for Communication Disorders, University of Texas at Dallas.

Kemper, S. (1988). Aging and syntactic limitations on language. In L.L. Light and D. M. Burke (Eds.), *Language, memory and aging* (pp. 58–76). New York: Cambridge University Press.

Lebrun, Y., and Hoops, R. (1976). *Recovery in aphasics.* Atlantic Highlands, NJ: Humanities Press.

Levin, H. S., Grossman, R. G., Kelly, P. J. (1976). Aphasic disorders in patients with closed head injury. *Journal of Neurology, Neurosurgery, and Psychiatry, 39,* 1062–1070.

Mendelsohn, D., Levin, H., Bruce, D., Lilly, M., Harward, H., Culhane, K., and Eisenberg, H. (1992). Late MRI after head injury in children: relationship to clinical features and outcome. *Child's Nervous System, 8,* 533–534.

Mesulam, M. M. (1982). Slowly progressive aphasia without generalized dementia. *Annals of Neurology, 22*(4), 533–534.

McKinely, W. W. (1981). The short term outcome of severe blunt injury as reported by relatives of the injured persons. *Journal of Neurology Neurosurgery and Psychiatry, 44,* 527–533.

McNeil, M. R. (1982). The nature of aphasia in adults. In N. J. Lass, L. V. McReynolds, J. L. Northern, and D. E. Yoder (Eds.), *Speech language, and hearing: Vol. III. Pathologies of speech and language* (pp. 692–740). Philadelphia, PA: W. B. Saunders.

Myers, P. S. (1984). Right hemisphere impairment. In A. Holland (Ed.), *Language disorders in adults: Recent advances.* San Diego, CA: College Hill Press.

Neary, D., and Snowden, J. S. (1991, October). *Progressive language disorder due to lobar atrophy.* Paper presented at Academy of Aphasia, Rome, Italy.

North, A. J., Ulatowska, H. K., Macaluso-Haynes, S., and Bell, H. (1986). Discourse performance in older adults. *International Journal of Aging and Human Development, 23,* 267–283.

Obler, L. K. (1983). Language and brain dysfunction in dementia. In S. Segalowitz (Ed.), *Language functions and brain organization* (pp. 267–282). New York: Academic Press.

Obler, L. K., and Albert, M. L. (1981). *Language in the elderly aphasic and the dementing patient.* New York: Academic Press.

Obler, L. K., and Albert, M. L. (1984). Language in aging. In M. L. Albert (Ed.), *Clinical neurology of aging* (pp. 245–253). New York: Oxford University Press.

Poeck, K., and Luzzatti, C. (1988). Slowly progressive aphasia in three patients. *Brain, 111,* 151–168.

Porch, B. (1967). *The Porch Index of Communicative Ability.* Palo Alto, CA: Consulting Psychologists Press.

Ripich, D., and Terrell, B. (1988). Patterns of discourse cohesion and coherence in Alzheimer's disease. *Journal of Speech and Hearing Disorders, 53,* 8–15.

Rivers, D. L., and Love, J. J. (1980). Language performance on visual processing tasks in right hemisphere lesion cases. *Brain and Language, 10,* 348–366.

Rosenbek, J. C. (1982). When is aphasia, aphasia? In R. H. Brookshire (Ed.), *Clinical aphasiology* (pp. 360–366). Minneapolis, MN: BRK.

Rosenbek, J. C., LaPointe, L. L., and Wertz, R. T. (1989). *Aphasia: A clinical approach.* Austin, TX: Pro-Ed.

Sarno, M. T., Buonaguro, A., and Levita, E. (1986). Characteristics of verbal impairment in closed head injured patients. *Archives of Physical Medicine and Rehabilitation, 67b,* 400–405.

Schow, R. L., Christensen, J. M., Hutchinson, J. M., and Nerbonne, M. A. (1978). *Communication disorders of the aged: A guide for health professionals.* Baltimore, MD: University Park Press.

Ulatowska, H. K., and Chapman, S. B. (1992, June). *Depth of information processing for discourse in elderly populations.* Paper presented at the Clinical Aphasiology Conference, Durango, CO.

Ulatowska, H. K., and Chapman, S. B. (1991). Discourse changes in dementia. In R. Lubinski (Ed.), *Dementia and communication: Research and clinical implications* (pp. 115–130). Philadelphia, PA: B. C. Decker.

Ulatowska, H. K., and Chapman, S. B. (in press). Discourse macrostructure in aphasia. In R. L. Bloom, L. K. Obler, S. DeSanti, and J. Ehrlich (Eds.), *Discourse in adult clinical populations.*

Ulatowska, H. K., Hayashi, M. M., Cannito, M. P., and Fleming, S. G. (1986). Disruption of reference in aging. *Brain and Language, 28,* 24–41.

Ulatowska, H. K., North, A. J., and Macaluso-Haynes, S. (1981). Production of narrative and procedural discourse in aphasia. *Brain and Language, 13,* 345–371.

Wertz, R. T. (1982). Language deficit in aphasia and dementia: The same as, different from, or both. In R. H. Brookshire (Ed.), *Clinical aphasiology.* (pp. 350–359). Minneapolis, MN: BRK.

SECTION TWO
LANGUAGE AND COMMUNICATION INTERVENTION APPROACHES IN ADULT APHASIA

CHAPTER 6
Models of Aphasia Treatment

JENNIFER HORNER, FELICE L. LOVERSO, and LESLIE GONZALEZ ROTHI

INTRODUCTION

The purposes of this chapter are (A) to define the terms "theory" and "model" as they relate to treatment paradigms in the rehabilitation of neurologically impaired aphasic adults, (B) to discuss the importance of model-driven therapy, (C) to offer operational definitions of aphasia treatment models, (D) to review the prevalence of *explicit* model-driven aphasia therapy research in five major journals reporting aphasiology research, and (E) to discuss future trends in the aphasia treatment research.

What Is a Model?

A theory is "the general or abstract principles of a body of fact, a science, or an art . . . a plausible or scientifically acceptable general principle or body of principles offered to explain phenomena" (*Webster's Ninth New Collegiate Dictionary*, 1986, p. 1223). We prefer the term "model" in the present context of aphasia treatment because we think of a "theory" as a relatively more formal set of principles and a "model" as a less formal or as yet unproven set of ideas. A *model*, by definition, is "a system of postulates, data, and inferences presented as a . . . description of an entity or state of affairs" (*Webster's Ninth New Collegiate Dictionary*, 1986, p. 762). We use the term "model" in the sense of a "working theory," or "a hypothesis assumed for the sake of argument or investigation . . . an unproved assumption" (*Webster's Ninth New Collegiate Dictionary*, 1986, p. 1223). We define models of aphasia treatment operationally in terms of (A) an underlying premise about normal language, (B) a definition of aphasia, and (C) a treatment implication. All of the models to be discussed have been presented (in more or less explicit form) in the aphasia treatment literature. Therefore, for each model we also identify proponents of the model and research that is representative of that specific model.

Why Is Model-Driven Treatment Important?

Horner and Loverso (1991) suggested four major reasons for thinking about aphasia treatment in terms of explicit models. The first reason was to facilitate the translation of linguistic, psycholinguistic, neurolinguistic, and cognitive psychology literature into meaningful and rational treatment techniques. By conceptualizing aphasia similarly, we would hope to strengthen the affiliation between clinical aphasiology (whose central concern is the treatment of aphasic individuals) and our sister disciplines, whose concerns include the description of normal language development and performance (Muma, 1978), the correlation of neural substrates and language (Arbib, et al., 1982), and the description of abnormal language behaviors in order to understand the structure and function of normal language (Caramazza, 1989).

The second reason for recognizing aphasia treatment models is to articulate the rationale of treatment. To paraphrase Wilson and Patterson (1990), we assume that therapy can be effective but that its potential effectiveness is a function of its design (p. 248). We further assume that to design a therapeutic intervention that is most likely to be efficacious, a sound underlying rationale (i.e., a model) is essential. Only by designing therapeutic interventions from therapy models can we avoid trial-and-error therapy, the use of one therapy for widely diverse aphasic deficits, or the administration of ineffective therapy (Mitchum and Berndt, 1988).

The third reason for articulating models, or "working theories," is to help the clinician critique the specific therapeutic technique (Behrmann and Byng,1992). By starting with intertwined hypotheses about why the language performance is impaired and why a specific therapy technique might be helpful, we are better able to evaluate positive, negative, or equivocal therapeutic results. Clinical speech-language pathologists who adopt the perspective of model-driven therapy will move their clinical practice from the realm of "art" into the rigorous and scholarly realm of "science."

The fourth potential advantage for thinking about aphasia therapy in terms of models is that "an accumulation of model-driven scientific investigations of therapy efficacy may help us validate (or invalidate) the theoretical model in question" (Horner and Loverso, 1991, pp. 62–63).

Why Isn't Sound Methodology Enough?

Our literature review of aphasia treatment models was stimulated in part by the historical debate pertaining to the relative importance of theory, clinical relevance, and research methodology (Brookshire, 1985b; Darley 1972; Kearns and Thompson, 1991; Martin, 1975; Muma et al., 1986; Rosenbek, 1979a; Thompson and Kearns, 1991). (The reader is referred to Horner and Loverso [1991] for the full discussion.) In the formative years of clinical aphasiology, research designs were driven by the clinical relevance of the intervention. We treated the aphasic person's language deficits with relatively little attention to the methodology (the research design) or to the theoretical implications of our results. In recognition of these shortcomings, the past decade found researchers focusing more rigorously on research methodology, both in group designs (Holland and Wertz, 1988) and in single subject experimental designs (McReynolds and Kearns, 1983).

In 1991, Thompson and Kearns reviewed the "analytical and technical directions" in clinical aphasiology, and in a companion paper they identified a phenomenon they called "technical drift" (Kearns and Thompson, 1991). They defined "technical drift" as "the tendency for applied research to become a purely technical cure oriented effort with limited or declining interest in conceptual issues" (Kearns and Thompson, 1991, p. 39). In short, clinical aphasiology had drifted toward an emphasis on technical (methodological) issues, at the dual risk of minimizing clinical relevance and ignoring theory. Kearns and Thompson concluded, "Programmatic treatment research that examines and makes explicit its relationship to basic behavioral, cognitive, and linguistic principles and theories is needed to reverse our technical drift and facilitate the development and maturity of clinical aphasiology" (Kearns and Thompson, 1991, p. 40). In summary, we must embrace what we know about clinical relevance, and research methodology, while formulating our research in terms of theoretical models.

Does Aphasia Treatment Work?

A central concern to all aphasia clinicians is, Does aphasia therapy work? We contend that this question is overly broad and that it is more helpful and more scientifically manageable to ask, "What types of aphasia therapy work, for what types of aphasic deficits, at which levels of severity, and at what points in time?" We further argue that answers to these questions can be "discovered" only through scientifically rigorous approaches that are guided by theoretical models. Our literature review was motivated by these concerns.

PURPOSE

The purpose of our chapter is to review all the data-based aphasia treatment articles in five major journals typically read by speech-language pathologists. The data presented herein are an extension of Horner and Loverso's earlier report (1991), in which we reviewed Clinical Aphasiology 1972–1988. The five major journals were *Clinical Aphasiology* 1972–1991 (Brookshire, 1975–1984, 1985a, 1986, 1987; Porch, 1974; Prescott, 1989, 1991a, 1991b; Wertz and Collins, 1972); *Aphasiology* (1987–1991); *Brain and Language* (1974–1991); the *Journal of Speech and Hearing Disorders* (1971–1991); and the *Journal of Speech and Hearing Research* (1971–1991). All research articles selected for in-depth review from these journals met two criteria: They were data-based, and they addressed aphasia treatment. In our review, we asked the following questions:

1. Was the theoretical model explicit or implicit?
2. Whether explicit or implicit, what was the prevalence of six different operationally defined models?
3. What types of aphasia were treated?
4. How many patients had acute versus chronic aphasia?
5. How many patients had mild, moderate, or severe aphasia?
6. What types of resesarch designs were used to examine treatment efficacy?
7. What language performance areas were focused on in treatment?
8. Was the treatment reportedly beneficial?

METHOD

Review of Aphasia Treatment Research

The three authors were assigned the task of previewing one or more of the five journals, selecting all data-based aphasia treatment articles, and reviewing each in detail to answer the above questions. All authors hold Certificates of Clinical Competence in Speech/Language Pathology, specialize their clinical practices in neurologically impaired adults, and have over 15 years of clinical experience. Prior to the review, all authors had operational definitions of the aphasia treatment model and were knowledgeable about the representative research (Table 6.1). Responses were coded and entered onto a database along with the full citation and an abstract. Following review of each article, each reader completed a database for the specific treatment-based research work. All data were subjected to a paired comparison of independent ratings for each reviewer (Kearns and Simmons, 1988). All possible combinations among the three reviewers were calculated. These analyses reflected an agreement range among reviewers from 80% to 100%, with an overall agreement mean of 90%.

Operational Definitions

Explicit Versus Implicit Models

The model was considered *explicit* if the author formulated the research address with reference to a specific theoretical model or combination of models. The model was considered *implicit* if the authors did not state it in the article, or perhaps provided only a vague and ambivalent reference, such that it was necessary for the reader to infer the theoretical framework.

Models of Aphasia Treatment

We derived six models from models already in use in clinical aphasiology. We refer to these models as (A) the stimulation-facilitation model, (B) the modality model, (C) the linguistic model, (D) the processing model, (E) the minor hemisphere mediation model, and (F) the functional communication model. Articles that used more than one model were coded as "multitheoretic." Articles that used no model were considered to be "atheoretic." We formulated each model in terms of a premise about normal language, a definition of aphasia, and a rationale for aphasia treatment (Horner and Loverso, 1991; Rothi and Horner, 1979). Proponents of each model and representative research are shown in Table 6.1.

Aphasia Type

Seven types of aphasia were considered for this analysis (Albert, et al., 1981): (A) global, (B) Broca's (or generic "non-

Table 6.1.
Operational Definitions, Proponents, and Representative *Clinical Aphasiology* Research for Six Aphasia Treatment Models[a]

Stimulation-Facilitation Model

Premise: "Language is an integrative activity that is linked to sensory and motor modalities but cannot be considered bound to them" (Duffy, 1986; Schuell et al., 1964).
Aphasia: "A multimodality disturbance which is unidimensional in nature. . . . [A]ll modalities tend to be impaired in aphasia . . . in the same manner and to about the same degree. . . . Auditory processes are at the apex of these interacting systems which aid in the acquisition, processing, and control of language" (Duffy, 1986; Schuell et al., 1964).
Treatment: Intensive auditory stimulation; meaningful material; abundant and varied material; repetitive sensory stimulation; a response for each stimulus; elicited not forced responses; stimulation not correction; make the stimulus adequate (LaPointe, 1978; Schuell et al., 1964).
Proponents: Duffy (1986); Schuell et al. (1964); Wepman (1951, 1953).
Representative Clinical Aphasiology Research:
Cueing hierarchies and word retrieval: A therapy program (Linebaugh and Lehner, 1977). Extended comprehension training reconsidered (Marshall and Neuburger, 1984).

Modality Model

Premise: Inner language is modality bound.
Aphasia: Aphasia can be modality specific and may be characterized as a uni- or multimodality performance deficit.
Treatment: Remediate input and output modalities, singly or in combination; reorganize modalities through selective intrasystemic or intersystemic stimulation; systematically pair weak with strong modalities to "deblock" impaired performances.
Proponents: Luria (1973); Rosenbek (1979b); Weigl and Bierwisch (1970).
Representative Clinical Aphasiology Research:
Gesture as a deblocking modality in a severe aphasic patient (Rao and Horner, 1978). Gestural sign (Amer-Ind) as a facilitator of learning, generalization, and maintenance of verbs by an aphasic patient (Kearns et al., 1982).

Linguistic Model

Premise: Language is a specialized, abstract, rule-governed cognitive activity.
Aphasia: Disrupted lexical-semantic, syntactic, and/or phonologic performance.
Treatment: Restore language performance by organizing stimuli according to linguistic system and linguistic complexity.
Proponents: Goodglass and Blumstein (1973); Jakobson (1971); Lesser (1978).
Representative Clinical Aphasiology Research:
Application of verbing strategies to aphasia treatment (Loverso et al., 1979). Generative use of locatives in multiword utterances in agrammatism: A matrix training approach (Thompson et al., 1982).

Processing Model

Premise: Language reflects the operation of semiautonomous "faculties" or "modules" that carry out complex processes. The modules are highly discrete, and the relational processes are highly specific. A "central executive" governs the interaction of modules, which are probably stimulus, modality, and/or task specific.
Aphasia: Modular and relational processing deficits.
Treatment: Restore or compensate for language-specific and language-related processing deficits.
Proponents: Chapey (1986); Fodor (1983); Gardner (1985); Martin (1975); Porch (1986).
Representative Clinical Aphasiology Research:
Model-driven remediation of dysgraphia (Hills and Caramazza, 1987).
A short-term memory treatment approach to the repetition deficit in conduction aphasia (Peach, 1987).

Minor Hemisphere Mediation Model

Premise: The minor hemisphere has rudimentary linguistic, visual-spatial-holistic, affective-prosodic, and paralinguistic cognitive (organizational, interpretive) abilities.
Aphasia: A manifestation of impaired dominant-hemisphere language and spared minor-hemisphere language.
Treatment: Use minor-hemisphere abilities to mediate (facilitate) communication through the use of imagery, drawing, melody, contextually rich stimuli, novel stimuli, and humor.
Proponents: Glass et al (1973); Horner and Fedor (1983); Myers and Linebaugh (1984); Sparks et al. (1974).
Representative Clinical Aphasiology Research:
Effects of hypnosis and imagery training on naming in aphasia (Thompson et al., 1985). Back to the drawing board (BDB): A treatment program for nonverbal aphasic patients (Morgan and Helm-Estabrooks, 1987).

Functional Communication Model

Premise: Communication reflects the application of pragmatic rules, unconstrained by modality, linguistic, or neurolinguistic considerations.
Aphasia: Ineffective or inefficient language use in natural communication contexts.
Treatment: Facilitate more normal communication by emphasizing pragmatic function over linguistic form and enhancing intermodality flexibility; establish strategies for circumventing and/or repairing communication breakdowns.
Proponents: Aten (1986); Davis and Wilcox (1981); Holland (1980); Marshall (1983).
Representative Clinical Aphasiology Research:
Communicative use of signs in aphasia: Is acquisition enough? (Coehlo and Duffy, 1985). Treatment of aphasia through family member training (Simmons et al., 1987).

---

[a] From Prescott, T. E. (Ed.). (1972–1988). *Clinical aphasiology.* Austin, TX: Pro-Ed. Reprinted with permission.

fluent''), (C) Wernicke's (or generic "fluent''), (D) conduction, (E) anomic, (F) transcortical (motor, sensory, or mixed), and (G) combined aphasia and apraxia of speech. When another type of aphasia was used, we used the code "other." When no report of aphasia type was given, we used the code "no report."

Acute versus Chronic Aphasia

The total number of subjects was tallied, then subdivided into those subjects who had aphasia less than 6 months (acute aphasia) versus 6 months or more (chronic aphasia).

Aphasia Severity

As in Horner and Loverso (1991), we defined severity as mild, moderate, or severe, as described by the authors of each article. If the author did not provide a severity description, we estimated severity by using scores or percentile rankings: < 40 as severe, 41 to 79 as moderate, and 80 or better as mild. This extrapolation was possible when the Western Aphasia Battery (Kertesz, 1979), the Porch Index of Communicative Ability (Porch, 1967), or some other standardized aphasia battery was reported. When these criteria were not met, a "no report" was entered into our database.

Research Design

We considered four possible research designs: (A) single subject descriptive, (B) single subject experimental (with or without replication), (C) group, descriptive (i.e., pretest/post-test design with no control group), and (D) group experimental (i.e., pretest/posttest design with one or more comparison groups).

Language Functions Treated

The areas of treatment addressed were coded as one or more of the following: speech, comprehension, repetition, naming, reading, writing, gesturing, and pragmatics. As in other areas of analysis, a default category "other" was used when the area of interest did not fit one of our major categories.

Treatment Benefit

To complete this analysis, we used the authors' conclusions about treatment efficacy. Three categories were used: (A) yes, treatment was efficacious; (B) no, treatment was not efficacious; or (C) the treatment effect was equivocal or mixed, as described by the authors. In several recently published articles, researchers have reported beneficial treatment effects for some patients but not for others. Or, researchers have reported improvement on the treated task ("task-specific" improvement) but no improvement on select generalization measures. Generalization results fell into several categories: (A) tasks of a similar nature that were not treated, including those elicited on posttest aphasia batteries ("task-external" generalization); (B) production of novel communicative behaviors ("extended" generalization); or (C) language performance in nontherapy settings ("sociocommunicative" generalization, or "carryover"). Our main criterion for judging treatment benefit was the authors' report of task-specific improvement. When researchers qualified task-specific treat-

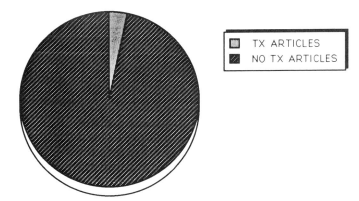

Figure 6.1. Treatment and no treatment articles. Of 4464 articles previewed from five major journals, only 3.4% reported data-based aphasia treatment (TX) articles; the remainder reported no treatment (NO TX). See text for full explanation.

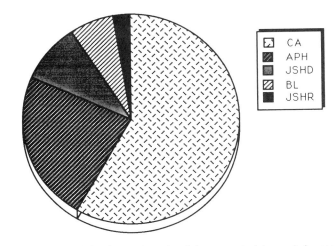

Figure 6.2. Aphasia treatment articles reported in each journal. The total number of data-based aphasia treatment articles selected for review was 152. This figures shows the relative contribution of five major journals: *Clinical Aphasiology* (CA), *Aphasiology* (APH), *Brain and Language* (BL), the *Journal of Speech and Hearing Disorders* (JSHD), and the *Journal of Speech and Hearing Research* (JSHR). See text for full explanation.

ment benefits because of lack of improvement by some patients but not others, or lack of improvement on task-external, extended, or sociocommunicative generalization, we judged the treatment benefit to be "equivocal."

RESULTS

Number of Articles

In all, we previewed 4464 articles. Of these, only 152 (3.4%) addressed data-based aphasia treatment (Figure 6.1). These 152 articles formed the basis for our analysis of models of aphasia treatment and related questions. The frequency of data-based aphasia treatment articles in the select journals is as follows (Figure 6.2). *Clinical Aphasiology* (1972–1991) published 623 articles, of which 89 (14.3%) addressed aphasia treatment in a data-based manner. *Aphasiology* (1987–1991) published 285 articles, of which 35 (12.3%) addressed aphasia treatment.

Brain and Language (1974–1991) published 1074 articles, of which 10 (0.9%) addressed aphasia treatment. The *Journal of Speech and Hearing Disorders* and the *Journal of Speech and Hearing Research* combined published 2481, of which 18 (0.7%) addressed aphasia treatment.

Number of Treated Subjects

Of the 1042 total aphasia subjects reflected in the treatment literature, *Clinical Aphasiology* reported 279 (26.8%); *Brain and Language* reported 127 (12.2%); *Aphasiology* reported 433 (41.6%); and the *Journal of Speech and Hearing Disorders* and the *Journal of Speech and Hearing Research* combined reported 203 (19.5%) (Figure 6.3).

Explicit Models

Of 152 articles, 80 of 152 (52.6%) were judged to use explicit models in the judgment of the three experienced readers (Figure 6.4). Of 89 articles in *Clinical Aphasiology*, 44 (49.4%) were explicit. Of 10 articles in *Brain and Language*, all 10 (100%) were judged to be explicit about the models used. Of 35 articles in *Aphasiology*, 19 (54.3%) were explicit. Of the 18 articles in the *Journal of Speech and Hearing Disorders* and the *Journal of Speech and Hearing Research* combined, 7 (38.9%) were explicit (Figure 6.5).

Models of Aphasia Treatment

Of 152 articles, 12 (7.9%) made reference to the "stimulation-facilitation" model of aphasia treatment, either explicitly or implicitly; 30 (19.7%), the "modality" model; 15 (9.9%), the "linguistic" model; 24 (15.8%), the "processing" model; 10 (6.6%), the "minor hemisphere mediation" model; and 12 (7.9%), the "functional communication" model. The largest number—33 (21.7%)—used a hybrid approach that we refer to as "multitheoretic," while 16 (10.5%) were classified as atheoretic or "other" (Figure 6.6).

Aphasia Type

In the 152 articles reviewed, 1042 patients were studied. Seventy-six (50.0%) of the articles contained reports of nonflu-

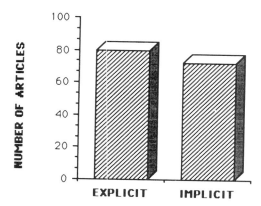

Figure 6.4. Explicit versus implicit models. Of 152 total articles, 80 used explicit models, and 72 used implicit models.

ent aphasia; 36 (23.7%), fluent aphasia; 21 (13.8%), anomic aphasia; 21 (13.8%), aphasia with apraxia of speech; 21 (13.8%), global aphasia; 13 (8.6%), conduction aphasia; and 6 (3.9%), one of the transcortical aphasias. Ten additional articles (6.6%) reported other types of aphasia, and 27 (17.8%) offered no description of aphasia type (Figure 6.7).

Aphasia Chronicity

Of the 1042 patients reported, 450 (43.2%) were acutely aphasic, while 539 (51.7%) were chronically aphasic. Of the 152 articles, 46 (30.3%) reported the effect of treatment for acutely aphasic patients, and 117 (76.9%) reported on treatment for chronically aphasic patients (Fig. 6.7). Thus, comparable *numbers* of acute and chronic patients have been reported, but a greater number of research *articles* addressed the treatment of chronic aphasia (Fig. 6.8).

Aphasia Severity

Of 152 articles reviewed, 24 (15.8%) researched the effect of therapy on mild aphasia; 89 (58.6%) on moderate aphasia; and 68 (44.7%) on severe aphasia (Fig. 6.9).

Research Design

On analysis of research design according to the number of articles, we found the following. Of 152 articles, 65 (42.8%) used a single case descriptive design; 51 (33.6%), a single case experimental design; 26 (17.1%), a group descriptive design; 6 (3.9%), a group experimental design; and 4 (2.6%), some other design (Fig. 6.10). Thus, *descriptive* designs, which qualify as bona fide research designs only by liberal criteria (Brookshire, 1985b, p. 12), accounted for 91 of 152 (59.9%) articles. In contrast, *experimental* designs accounted for 57 of 152 (37.5%) articles. The number of subjects examined within each design was as follows: single subject descriptive, 167; group descriptive, 588; single subject experimental, 112; group experimental, 165; and "other," 10 subjects.

Treatment Areas

Of 152 articles examined, the distribution of treatment areas is as follows. Some research papers addressed more than one

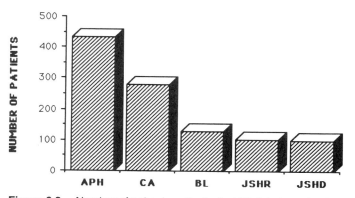

Figure 6.3. Number of aphasic patients. In 152 data-based aphasia treatment articles, 1,042 patients were reported. This figure shows the relative contribution of five major journals: *Clinical Aphasiology* (CA), *Aphasiology* (APH), *Brain and Language* (BL), the *Journal of Speech and Hearing Disorders* (JSHD), and the *Journal of Speech and Hearing Research* (JSHR). See text for full explanation.

Figure 6.5. Explicit models by journal. This figure shows the relative use of explicit models by five major journals. See text for full explanation.

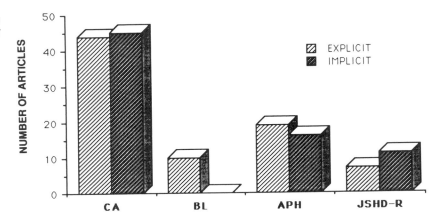

Figure 6.6. Models of aphasia treatment. The relative prevalence of operationally defined aphasia treatment models is shown in this figure: stimulation-facilitation model (STIM), modality model (MOD), linguistic model (LING), processing model (PROC), minor-hemi-sphere mediation model (MINOR), functional communication model (COMM), multitheoretic model (MULTI), or other (OTH). See text for full explanation.

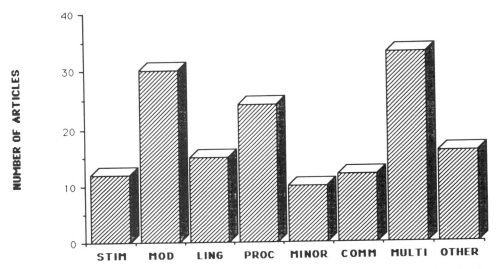

Figure 6.7. Aphasia type. This figure shows the distribution of types of aphasia, as reported in 152 articles: nonfluent (NONFL), fluent (FL), anomic aphasia (ANOM), aphasia and apraxia of speech (APHAOS), conduction (COND), global (GLOB), transcortical (TRANS), other (OTH), and no report (NR). See text for full explanation.

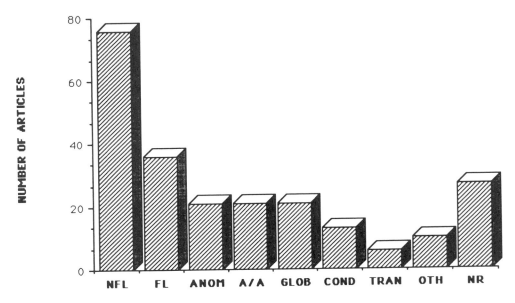

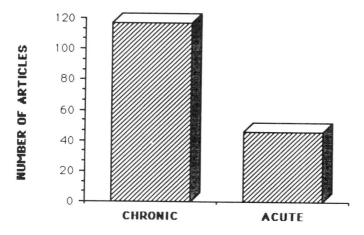

Figure 6.8. Aphasia chronicity. This figure shows the number of articles reporting treatment efficacy for chronic versus acute aphasia. See text for full explanation.

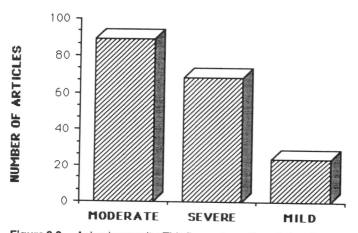

Figure 6.9. Aphasia severity. This figure shows the relative distribution of aphasia severity as reported in 152 articles. See text for full explanation.

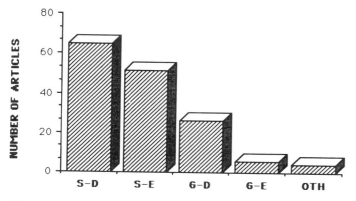

Figure 6.10. Research design. This figure shows the relative distribution of different research designs in 152 aphasia treatment studies: single subject descriptive (S-D), single subject experimental (S-E), group descriptive (G-D), group experimental (G-E), and other. See text for full explanation.

treatment area. Speech performance was treated in 62 of 152 (40.8%) articles; comprehension, in 31 (20.4%); naming, in 30 (19.7%); writing, in 23 (15.1%); gestural ability, in 19 (12.5%); reading, in 18 (11.8%); pragmatics, in 17 (11.2%); repetition, in 13 (8.6%); and other functions (e.g., computer use), in 10 (6.6%) (Fig. 6.11).

Treatment Benefit

Of 152 articles, 104 (68.4%) reported a beneficial treatment effect; 5 (3.3%) reported no benefit; and 43 (28.3%) reported equivocal results (Fig. 6.12).

DISCUSSION

To assess the state of the art regarding the use of explicit models in aphasia treatment, we reviewed 152 articles from five major journals that reported data-based aphasia treatment research. We will now summarize our results. First, the 152 data-based aphasia treatment articles represented a mere 3.4% of all articles published within the past 20 years in the five journals of interest. Second, the number of patients whose treatment was examined in a research paradigm totaled 1042 over this 20-year period. Third, only about half of the treatment research we examined used *explicit* therapeutic models. Fourth, whether implicit or explicit, the majority of papers approached their research in a "multitheoretic" fashion (33%), with the "modality" model and the "processing" model placing second and third in prevalence. Fifth, half of all studies examined nonfluent aphasia. Sixth, about half of the patients studied had acute aphasia; about half had chronic aphasia. In contrast, the number of articles reporting the effects of treatment of chronic aphasia outnumbered those for acute aphasia two to one. Seventh, articles addressing the treatment needs of moderate aphasia were in the majority. Eighth, the research design used most often was a single case descriptive approach, with single case experimental designs ranking second. Ninth, speech production was the most frequent treatment area. Tenth, the majority of articles reported a beneficial treatment effect, and just a few (3.3%) reported no benefit.

The most compelling reason for "model-driven aphasia treatment" is to test hypotheses or predictions about therapeutic outcomes (Moehle et al., 1987, p. 64). The presumed goals of model-driven treatment are to design effective therapeutic interventions, to test the validity of the underlying theoretical model, or both. With these goals in mind, we will now highlight the major problems unveiled by our literature review. The first major problem, in our opinion, was the paucity of aphasia treatment research. If one excludes from our database all descriptive studies (because these are not true research designs [Brookshire, 1985b, p. 12]), the body of experimental research literature on aphasia treatment in five major journals is reduced

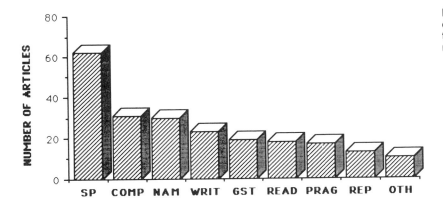

Figure 6.11.   Treatment area. This figure shows the distribution of areas of communication performance treated in 152 aphasia articles. See text for full explanation.

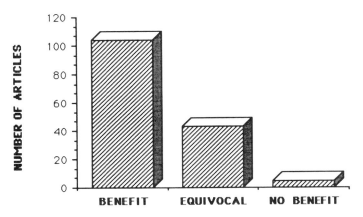

Figure 6.12.   Treatment benefit. This figure shows the benefit of aphasia treatment as reported in 152 research articles. See text for full explanation.

but with significantly lower frequency. Fifth, single case designs are in a definite majority (over group designs), with descriptive rather than experimental approaches being the most popular. We conclude, therefore, that our questions about the value of model-driven therapy are still far from answered in the present treatment literature.

FUTURE TRENDS

Three trends, already evident in the clinical research literature on aphasia, are as follows.

Aphasia Models

The first trend pertains to aphasia treatment models. Theories about language and other cognitive behaviors are in ever-growing supply. We attribute this to the dramatic advances in linguistics, cognitive psychology, neuropsychology, neurobiology, neuroimaging, and cognitive neuroscience (Arbib et al., 1982; Damasio and Damasio, 1989; Grodzinsky, 1990; Margolin, 1992; Metter et al., 1991; Naeser, et al., 1989; Osheron, and Lasnik, 1990; Seron and Deloche, 1989). Most theories in related disciplines have potential relevance to aphasia treatment, but few are formulated specifically with the goal of language remediation in mind (Cooper, 1992). In the future, researchers will, we hope, go beyond the question of ''How is language disrupted and why?'' to the question of ''How and under what conditions can language be restored, and why?'' Further, we hope that researchers will use models not only to justify a rationale for an interventional approach (i.e., ''model-driven therapy'') but also to critique the validity of the model per se (i.e., ''model-testing''). As data accumulate, we may one day have answers to the questions ''What type of treatment works, for which types of aphasic deficits, at what severity levels, and at what points in time?'' To accomplish this goal, researchers must make the theoretical underpinnings of their research explicit.

Scientific Method

The second future trend is the increasing rigor of the scientific method in clinical aphasiology research. To make valid conclusions from our data, our methodology ideally will include (A) experimental research designs (Brookshire, 1985b; McReynolds, and Kearns, 1983; Ventry and Schiavetti, 1980), (B) comprehensive subject description (Holland and Wertz, 1988),

to 57 articles of 4484 published articles (a meager 1.3%), and the number of experimentally treated aphasia subjects is reduced to 277 over the 20-year period of interest.

The second major problem was the lack of explicit models. When a model was used, or not, the typical goal of the research was to test the effect of the treatment on the aphasic behavior. In most studies, authors made reference to a theoretical model to justify the selection of the therapeutic interventional approach and only rarely used the measured treatment effect to critique (i.e., to validate or invalidate) the model. A third problem we perceived was that most studies reported a positive treatment benefit, or an equivocal treatment benefit. While these data are valuable, we contend that it is just as important for clinicians to know what does *not* work as what does work. We suggest that journal editors should encourage publication of so-called ''negative'' results, because only with both positive and negative therapeutic results can hypotheses be proved or disproved in a scientific fashion.

A fourth cluster of problems was the high frequency with which moderately or severely impaired nonfluent aphasic individuals were studied. Probably, this is the type of patient who is most available and willing to undergo our therapeutic trials. Nevertheless, the focus of researchers on this type of patient has led to an underrepresentation of the full spectrum of complex patients whom we treat in our clinics. Other language performance areas and other types of aphasic patients are being studied,

(C) random subject assignment to treatment conditions (Schoonen, 1991), (D) sophisticated knowledge of the causative lesion and its effects (Damasio and Damasio, 1989; Metter, et al., 1991); (E) the use of reliable and valid measurement techniques (Johnston et al., 1991; Kearns and Simmons, 1988); and (F) the use statistical power analyses (Schoonen, 1991).

Ecological Validity

The third future trend is the emphasis on the social or ecological validity of our behavioral interventions. Ecological validity refers to the sociocommunicative impact of our treatment by virtue of favorable changes in the individual's aphasia. Ecological concerns challenge clinicians to consider the functional outcome of aphasia treatment. This complex topic, discussed in detail elsewhere (Glosser, et al., 1988; Lyon, 1989; Simmons, 1989; Wertz 1989), has two implications.

The first implication is both ethical and humanistic. To warrant the expenditure of time, effort, and finances inherent in aphasia treatment, clinicians are advised to consider the aphasic person's communication behavior in the context of his or her needs, environment, and caretakers and loved ones. Dr. Frederick Darley reminded us of this in his keynote address at the Clinical Aphasiology Conference's 20th anniversary entitled ''I Think It Begins with an 'A.' '' He said, ''The world's scientific literature is replete with studies of aphasic patients who have been interviewed, tested, retested, overtested, stimulated, provoked, stroked, X-rayed, imaged, injected—and at times neglected as people'' (1991, p. 9). The inference to be drawn from his words is that clinicians are bound professionally and ethically to consider the whole aphasic individual. We will do this best by striving to make a difference in communication behaviors in realistic communication settings.

The second implication of the growing emphasis on ecological validity is methodological. The methodological implication pertains to generalization of treated behaviors. Several forms of generalization of interest to clinical aphasiology researchers (see Methods above) are ''task-specific,'' ''task-external,'' ''extended,'' and ''sociocommunicative.'' Despite encouraging progress in our ability to effect task-specific changes in aphasic behavior, the reasons why we observe or do not observe the various types of generalization are not fully appreciated at this time. The challenge of understanding and effecting generalization will take, we predict, an increasingly dominant place in our clinical research in the future.

In summary, the three future trends relevant to our discussion of aphasia treatment models are the description and evaluation of treatment models, the refinement of scientific methodology in aphasia research, and an emphasis on ecological validity.

References

Albert, M. L., Goodglass, H., Helm, N. A., Rubens, A. B., and Alexander, M. P. (1981). Clinical aspects of dysphasia. New York: Springer-Verlag.

Aphasiology (1987–1991). C. Code and D. Muller (Eds.). London: Taylor & Francis, Ltd.

Arbib, M. A., Caplan, D., and Marshall, J. C. (1982). Neural models of language processes. New York: Academic Press.

Aten, J. L. (1986). Functional communication treatment. In R. Chapey (Ed.), Language intervention strategies in adult aphasia (2nd ed., pp. 266–276). Baltimore, MD: Williams & Wilkins.

Behrmann, M., and Byng, S. (1992). A cognitive approach to the neurorehabilitation of acquired language disorders. In D. I. Margolin (Ed.), Cognitive neuropsychology in clinical practice (pp. 327–350). New York: Oxford University Press.

Brain and Language (1974–1991). H. Whitaker and A. R. Lecours (Eds.). Orlando: Academic Press.

Brookshire, R. H. (Ed.). (1975). Clinical aphasiology (Vol. 5). Minneapolis, MN: BRK.

Brookshire, R. H. (Ed.). (1976). Clinical aphasiology (Vol. 6). Minneapolis, MN: BRK.

Brookshire, R. H. (Ed.). (1977). Clinical aphasiology (Vol. 7). Minneapolis, MN: BRK.

Brookshire, R. H. (Ed.). (1978). Clinical aphasiology (Vol. 8). Minneapolis, MN: BRK.

Brookshire, R. H. (Ed.). (1979). Clinical aphasiology (Vol. 9). Minneapolis, MN: BRK.

Brookshire, R. H. (Ed.). (1980). Clinical aphasiology (Vol. 10). Minneapolis, MN: BRK.

Brookshire, R. H. (Ed.). (1981). Clinical aphasiology (Vol. 11). Minneapolis, MN: BRK.

Brookshire, R. H. (Ed.). (1982). Clinical aphasiology (Vol. 12). Minneapolis, MN: BRK.

Brookshire, R. H. (Ed.). (1983). Clinical aphasiology (Vol. 13). Minneapolis, MN: BRK.

Brookshire, R. H. (Ed.). (1984). Clinical aphasiology (Vol. 14). Minneapolis, MN: BRK.

Brookshire, R. H. (Ed.). (1985a). Clinical aphasiology (Vol. 15). Minneapolis, MN: BRK.

Brookshire, R. H. (1985b). Clinical research in aphasiology. In R. H. Brookshire (Ed.), Clinical aphasiology (Vol. 15, pp. 9–14). Minneapolis, MN: BRK.

Brookshire, R. H., (Ed.). (1986). Clinical aphasiology (Vol. 16). Minneapolis, MN: BRK.

Brookshire, R. H., (Ed.). (1987). Clinical aphasiology (Vol. 17). Minneapolis, MN: BRK.

Caramazza, A. (1989). Cognitive neuropsychology and rehabilitation: An unfulfilled promise? In X. Seron and G. Deloche (Eds.), Cognitive approaches in neuropsychological rehabilitation (pp. 383–398). Hillsdale, NJ: Lawrence Erlbaum.

Chapey, R. (1986). Cognitive intervention: Stimulation of cognition, memory, convergent thinking, divergent thinking and evaluative thinking. In R. Chapey (Ed.), Language intervention strategies in adult aphasia (2nd ed. pp. 215–238). Baltimore, MD: Williams & Wilkins.

Coehlo, C. A., and Duffy, R. J. (1985). Communicative use of signs in aphasia: Is acquisition enough? In R. H. Brookshire (Ed.), Clinical aphasiology (Vol. 8, pp. 222–228). Minneapolis, MN: BRK.

Cooper, J. (Ed.). (1992, October). Aphasia treatment: Current approaches and research opportunities. Bethesda, MD: U.S. Department of Health and Human Services. NIH Publication No. 93-3424.

Damasio, H., and Damasio, A. R. (1989). Lesion analysis in neuropsychology. New York: Oxford University Press.

Darley, F. L. (1972). The efficacy of language rehabilitation in aphasia. Journal of Speech and Hearing Disorders, 37, 3–21.

Darley, F. L. (1991). I think it begins with an ''A.'' In T. E. Prescott (Ed.), Clinical aphasiology (Vol. 20, pp. 9–20). Austin, TX: Pro-Ed.

Davis, G., and Wilcox, M. (1981). Incorporating parameters of natural conversation in aphasia treatment. In R. Chapey (Ed.), Language intervention strategies in adult aphasia (pp. 161–194). Baltimore, MD: Williams & Wilkins.

Duffy J. R. (1986). Schuell's stimulation approach to rehabilitation. In R. Chapey (Ed.), Language intervention strategies in adult aphasia (2nd ed. pp. 187–214). Baltimore, MD: Williams & Wilkins.

Fodor, J. A. (1983). The modularity of the mind. Cambridge, MA: MIT Press.

Gardner, H. (1985). The mind's new science: A history of the cognitive revolution. New York: Basic Books.

Glass, A. V., Gazzaniga, M., and Premack, D. (1973). Artificial language training in aphasia. Neuropsychologia, 11, 95–103.

Glosser, G., Wiener, M., and Kaplan, E. (1988). Variations in aphasic language behaviors. Journal of Speech and Hearing Disorders, 53, 115–124.

Goodglass, H., and Blumstein, S. (Eds.). (1973). Psycholinguistics and aphasia. Baltimore, MD: Johns Hopkins University Press.

Grodzinsky, Y. (1990). Theoretical perspectives on language deficits. Cambridge, MA: MIT Press.

Hillis, A. E., and Caramazza, A. (1987). In R. H. Brookshire (Ed.), Clinical aphasiology (Vol. 17, pp. 84–105). Minneapolis, MN: BRK.

Holland A. (1980). *Communicative abilities of daily living.* Baltimore, MD: University Park Press.

Holland, A. L., and Wertz, R. T. (1988). Measuring aphasia treatment effects: Large-group, small-group, and single-subject studies. In F. Plum (Ed.), *Language, communication, and the brain.* New York: Raven Press.

Horner, J., and Fedor, K. H. (1983). Minor hemisphere mediation in aphasia treatment. In H. Winitz (Ed.), *Treating language disorders: For clinicians by clinicians* (pp. 181–204). Baltimore, MD: University Park Press.

Horner, J., and Loverso, F. L. (1991). Models of aphasia treatment in *Clinical Aphasiology 1972–1988.* In T. E. Prescott (Ed.), *Clinical aphasiology* (Vol. 20, pp. 61–75). Austin, TX: Pro-Ed.

Jakobson, R. (1971). *Studies on child language and aphasia.* The Hague: Mouton.

Johnston, M. V., Findley, T. W., DeLuca, J., and Katz, R. T. (1991). Research in physical medicine and rehabilitation: XII. Measurement tools with application to brain injury. *American Journal of Physical Medicine and Rehabilitation, 70,* 40 –56.

Journal of Speech and Hearing Disorders (1971–1991). Rockville, MD: American Speech-Language-Hearing Association.

Journal of Speech and Hearing Research (1971–1991). Rockville, MD: American Speech-Language-Hearing Association.

Kearns, K. P., and Simmons, N. N. (1988). Interobserver reliability and perceptual ratings: More than meets the ear. *Journal of Speech and Hearing Research, 31,* 131–136.

Kearns, K. P. Simmons, N. N., and Sisterhen, C. (1982). Gestural sign (Amer-Ind) as a facilitator of verbalization in patients with aphasia. In R. H. Brookshire (Ed.), *Clinical aphasiology* (Vol. 12, pp. 183–191). Minneapolis, MN: BRK.

Kearns, K. P., and Thompson, C. K. (1991). Technical drift and conceptual mypopia: The Merlin effect. In T. E. Prescott (Ed.), *Clinical aphasiology* (Vol. 19, pp. 31–40). Boston, MA: College Hill/Little, Brown.

Kertesz, A. (1979). *Aphasia and associated disorders: Taxonomy, localization, and recovery.* New York: Grune & Stratton.

LaPointe, L. L. (1978). Aphasia therapy: Some principles and strategies for treatment. In D. F. Johns (Ed.), *Clinical management of neurogenic communicative disorders* (pp. 129–190). Boston, MA: Little, Brown.

Linebaugh, C. W., and Lehner, L. H. (1977). Cueing hierarchies and word retrieval: A therapy program. In R. H. Brookshire (Ed.), *Clinical aphasiology* (Vol. 7, pp. 19–31). Minneapolis, MN: BRK.

Lesser, R. (1978). *Linguistic investigations of aphasia.* London: Arnold.

Loverso, F. L., Selinger, M., and Prescott, T. E. (1979). Application of verbing strategies to aphasia treatment. In R. H. Brookshire (Ed.), *Clinical aphasiology* (Vol. 9, pp. 299–238). Minneapolis, MN: BRK.

Luria, A. R. (1973). B. Haigh (Trans.), *The working brain: An introduction to neuropsychology.* Middlesex, England: Penguin Books.

Lyon, J. G. (1989). Communicative partners: Their value in reestablishing communication with aphasic adults. In T. E. Prescott (Ed.), *Clinical aphasiology* (Vol. 18, pp. 11–17). Austin, TX: Pro-Ed.

Margolin, D. I. (Ed.). (1992). *Cognitive neuropsychology in clinical practice.* New York: Oxford University Press.

Marshall, R. C. (1983). Communication styles of fluent aphasics. In H. Winitz (Ed.), *Treating language disorders: For clinicians by clinicians* (pp. 163–179). Baltimore, MD: University Park Press.

Marshall, R. C., and Neuburger, S. (1984). Extended comprehension training reconsidered. In R. H. Brookshire (Ed.), *Clinical aphasiology* (Vol. 14, pp. 181–187). Minneapolis, MN: BRK.

Martin, A. D. (1975). A critical evaluation of therapeutic approaches to aphasia. In R. H. Brookshire (Ed.), *Clinical aphasiology* (Vol. 5, pp. 67–78). Minneapolis, MN: BRK.

McReynolds, L. V., and Kearns, K. P. (1983). *Single-subject experimental designs in communicative disorders.* Baltimore, MD: University Park Press.

Metter, E. J., Hanson, W. R., Jackson, C. A., Kempler, D., van Lancker, D., Mazziotta, J. C., and Phelps, M. E. (1991). Temporoparietal cortex in aphasia: Evidence from positron emission tomography. *Archives of Neurology, 47,* 1235–1238.

Mitchum, C. C., and Berndt, R. S. (1988). Aphasia rehabilitation: An approach to diagnosis and treatment of language production disorders. In M. G. Eisenberg and R. C. Grzesiak (Eds.), *Advances in clinical rehabilitation* (Vol. 2, pp. 160–185). New York: Springer Publishing.

Moehle, J. A., Rasmussen, J. L., and Fitzhugh-Bell, K. B. (1987). In J. M. Williams and C. J. Long (Eds.), *The rehabilitation of cognitive disabilities* (pp. 55–76). New York: Plenum Press.

Morgan, A. L. R., and Helm-Estabrooks, N. (1987). Back to the drawing board: A treatment program for nonverbal aphasic patients. In R. H. Brookshire (Ed.), *Clinical aphasiology* (Vol. 17, pp. 64–72). Minneapolis, MN: BRK.

Muma, J. R. (1978). *Language handbook: Concepts, assessment, intervention.* Englewood Cliffs, NJ: Prentice-Hall.

Muma, J. R., Hamre, C. E., and McNeil, M. R. (1986). Theoretical models applicable to intervention in adult aphasia. In R. Chapey (Ed.), *Language intervention strategies in adult aphasia* (2nd ed. pp. 277–283). Baltimore, MD: Williams & Wilkins.

Myers, P. S., and Linebaugh, C. (1984). The use of context-dependent pictures in aphasia rehabilitation. In R. H. Brookshire (Ed.), *Clinical aphasiology* (Vol. 14, pp. 145–158). Minneapolis, MN: BRK.

Naeser, M. A., Palumbo, C. L., Helm-Estabrooks, N., Stiassny-Eder, D., and Albert, M. L. (1989). Severe non-fluency in aphasia: Role of the medial subcallosal fasciculus plus other white matter pathways in recovery of spontaneous speech. *Brain, 112,* 1–38.

Osheron, D. N., and Lasnik, H. (Eds.). (1990). *Language (an invitation to cognitive science,* Vol. 1). Cambridge, MA: MIT Press.

Peach, R. K. (1987). A short-term memory treatment approach to the repetition deficit in conduction aphasia. In R. H. Brookshire (Ed.), *Clinical aphasiology* (Vol. 17, pp. 35–45). Minneapolis, MN: BRK.

Porch, B. E. (1974). *Clinical aphasiology.* Albuquerque, NM: Veterans Administration Hospital.

Porch, B. E. (1967). *Porch Index of Communicative Ability.* Palo Alto, CA: Consulting Psychologists Press.

Porch, B. E. (1986). Therapy subsequent to the Porch Index of Communicative Ability (PICA). In R. Chapey (Ed.), *Language intervention strategies in adult aphasia* (2nd ed., pp. 295–303). Baltimore, MD: Williams & Wilkins.

Prescott, T. E. (Ed.). (1989). *Clinical aphasiology* (Vol. 18). Boston, MA: College Hill/Little, Brown.

Prescott, T. E. (Ed.). (1991a). *Clinical aphasiology* (Vol. 19). Austin, TX: Pro-Ed.

Prescott, T. E. (Ed.). (1991b). *Clinical aphasiology* (Vol. 20). Austin, TX: Pro-Ed.

Rao, P. R., and Horner, J. (1978). Gesture as a deblocking modality in a severe aphasic patient. In R. H. Brookshire (Ed.), *Clinical aphasiology* (Vol. 8, pp. 180–187). Minneapolis, MN: BRK.

Rosenbek, J. C. (1979a). Wrinkled feet. In R. H. Brookshire (Ed.), *Clinical aphasiology* (Vol. 9, pp. 163–176). Minneapolis, MN: BRK.

Rosenbek, J. C. (1979b). Treating apraxia of speech. In D. F. Johns (Ed.), *Clinical management of neurogenic communicative disorders* (pp. 191–241). Boston, MA: Little, Brown.

Rothi, R. J., and Horner, J. (1979). Aphasia recovery: Theory and treatment (short course) [Abstract]. *Asha, 20,* 764.

Schoonen, R. (1991). The internal validity of efficacy studies: Design and statistical power in studies of language therapy for aphasics. *Brain and Language, 41,* 446–464.

Schuell, H., Jenkins J. J., and Jimenez-Pabon, E. (1964). *Aphasia in adults: Diagnosis, prognosis, and treatment.* New York: Hoeber Medical Division, Harper.

Seron, X., and Deloche, G. (Eds.). (1989). *Cognitive approaches in neuropsychological rehabilitation.* Hillsdale, NJ: Lawrence Erlbaum.

Simmons, N. N. (1989). A trip down easy street. In T. E. Prescott (Ed.), *Clinical aphasiology* (Vol. 18, pp. 19–30). Austin, TX: Pro-Ed.

Simmons, N. N., Kearns, K. P., Potechin, G. (1987). Treatment of aphasia through family member training. In R. H. Brookshire (Ed.), *Clinical aphasiology* (Vol. 8, pp. 106–116). Minneapolis, MN: BRK.

Sparks, R., Helm, N., and Albert, M. (1974). Aphasia rehabilitation resulting from melodic intonation therapy. *Cortex, 10,* 303–316.

Thompson, C. K., Hall, H. R., and Sison, C. E. (1985). Effects of hypnosis and imagery training on naming in aphasia. In R. H. Brookshire (Ed.), *Clinical aphasiology* (Vol. 15, pp. 301–310). Minneapolis, MN: BRK.

Thompson, C. K., and Kearns, K. (1991). Analytical and technical directions in applied aphasia analysis: The Midas touch. In T. E. Prescott (Ed.), *Clinical aphasiology* (Vol. 19, pp. 41–54). Boston, MA: College Hill/Little, Brown.

Thompson, C. K., McReynolds, L., and Vance, C. (1982). Generative use of locatives in multiword utterances in agrammatism: A matrix training approach. In R. H. Brookshire (Ed.), *Clinical aphasiology* (Vol. 8, pp. 289–297). Minneapolis, MN: BRK.

Ventry, I. M., and Schiavetti, N. (1980). *Evaluating research in speech pathology and audiology.* Reading, MA: Addison-Wesley.

Webster's ninth new collegiate dictionary. (1986, pp. 762, 1223). Springfield, MA: Merriam-Webster.

Weigl, E., and Bierwisch, M. (1970). Neuropsychology and linguistics: Topics of common research. *Language, 6*, 1–18.

Wepman, J. M. (1951). *Recovery from aphasia*. New York: Ronald Press.

Wepman, J. M. (1953). A conceptual model for the process involved in recovery from aphasia. *Journal of Speech and Hearing Disorders, 18*, 4–13.

Wertz, R. T. (1989). Utilizing trained volunteers to treat aphasia: A potential plagued with malignant misinterpretation and enigmatic evidence. In T. E. Prescott (Ed.), *Clinical aphasiology* (Vol. 18, pp. 5–10). Austin, TX: Pro-Ed.

Wertz, R. T., and Collins, M. (Eds). (1972). *Clinical aphasiology*. Madison, WI: Veterans Administration Hospital.

Wilson, B., and Patterson, K. (1990). Rehabilitation for cognitive impairment: Does cognitive psychology apply? *Applied Cognitive Psychology, 4*, 247–260.

CHAPTER 7
Schuell's Stimulation Approach to Rehabilitation

JOSEPH R. DUFFY

This chapter deals with an approach to the treatment of aphasia that places its primary emphasis on the stimulation presented to the aphasic person. Hildred Schuell was among the most lucid, scientific-minded, and insightful clinicians to propose and offer support for this approach. Because of her major role in its development, the approach described in this chapter is often referred to as "Schuell's aphasia therapy" or "Schuell's stimulation approach."

Schuell's work in aphasiology spanned two decades and included significant contributions in the areas of diagnostic testing, classification of aphasic patients, and theory development regarding the underlying nature of aphasia. It was probably this sound foundation in theory, evaluation, and methods of observing and categorizing behavior that helped develop the compelling rationale for the stimulation approach. Its sound foundation also helps to explain why the stimulation approach represents one of the main schools of thought in aphasia therapy and has been one of the most widely used treatment approaches for aphasia employed in this country for a number of years (Darley, 1975; Davis, 1983; Sarno, 1981). In this chapter, Schuell's definition, theory, and classifications of aphasia will be reviewed briefly as prerequisites for understanding the stimulation approach. The remainder of the chapter will emphasize the principles, rationale, and specific goals, procedures, and techniques associated with the stimulation approach to aphasia rehabilitation.

Before proceeding, it is necessary to delimit further the territory to be covered in this chapter. First, it is recognized that virtually all approaches used by speech-language pathologists for the treatment of aphasia necessarily must involve stimulation of some kind (Wepman, 1953); for that reason, the stimulation approach may be thought to encompass all approaches to aphasia rehabilitation. The presence of numerous other chapters in this book, however, makes it clear that this is not intended to be the case. The material presented here is conceptually related to Schuell's specific approach to treatment, and it is her name that serves to signal the scope of this chapter and distinguish it from other treatment approaches that use stimulation in more broadly or more narrowly defined ways.

The second point is intended to qualify the narrowed scope described in the previous paragraph. Although Schuell was a

"prime mover" in the development of the stimulation approach, many other clinicians and investigators have contributed to the development or refinement of its rationale, principles, design, and techniques. Wepman's (1951) contribution, for example, is particularly noteworthy, as it was the first complete elaboration of the approach (Darley, 1972). Therefore, while all current approaches to treating aphasia will not be discussed, attention will be given to the contributions of many individuals in addition to Schuell. Receiving special emphasis will be those investigations that continuously help to refine the approach by identifying stimulus factors that influence the adequacy of language performance in aphasic persons.

PREREQUISITES TO UNDERSTANDING THE STIMULATION APPROACH

Definition and Primary Symptoms of Aphasia

Systematic observation and testing of over a thousand aphasic patients led Schuell and her colleagues to define aphasia as "a general language deficit that crosses all language modalities and may or may not be complicated by other sequelae of brain damage" (Schuell et al., 1964, p. 113). The language modalities referred to in the definition include comprehension of spoken language, speech, reading, and writing. The "other sequelae"—nonphasic disturbances—most often would include modality-specific perceptual disturbances, dysarthrias, and sensorimotor deficits (including apraxia of speech). Also, other complications and secondary symptoms, such as a reduction of communication generated by depression or an altered attitude toward communication, may occur as a reaction to the primary symptoms of aphasia (Jenkins et al., 1975).

Schuell consistently viewed a reduction of available vocabulary, linguistic rules, and verbal retention span, as well as impaired comprehension and production of messages, as the primary characteristics of aphasia (Schuell, 1969, 1974a; Schuell and Jenkins, 1961a; Schuell et al., 1964). In addition, her observations indicate that not only does the impaired ability to retrieve and use the language code cross all modalities, it tends to be evident in all modalities in a similar manner. Finally, "the impairment is regular and orderly, and operates in a manner that is lawfully related to known language phenomena" (Schuell et al., 1964, p. 104). The occurrence of similar deficits across modalities within patients, and the predictable nature of those deficits are important additional characteristics, and they figure strongly in the rationale and procedures used in the stimulation approach.

Underlying Nature of Aphasia

In most scientific, clinical endeavors it is preferable that the rationale for using a particular method precede the application of the method. This is particularly important in clinical aphasiology because the efficacy of treatment continues to be debated, and we cannot always confidently, though superficially, say, "I use this approach because it works!" Until the efficacy of any approach to the rehabilitation of aphasia is unequivocally demonstrated, what we do must at least be defensible on theoretical grounds. Schuell (1974b) supported such a notion with her belief that "what you do about aphasia depends on what you think aphasia is" (p. 138). Therefore, it is important that our method(s) of treatment be linked to our beliefs about the organization of language in the brain and the nature of language breakdown that occurs when the brain is damaged. The adoption of such beliefs, however, is complicated by an abundance of choices. In fact, the existence of numerous beliefs about the underlying nature of aphasia has as one of its primary symptoms the existence of numerous approaches to treatment. Since treatment is subject to such beliefs, it is essential that we have some understanding of the model of language and beliefs about the nature of aphasia that specifically underlie the stimulation approach. If such a model and beliefs are palatable, procedures and techniques become logical extensions of the underlying rationale.

Schuell's beliefs about the organization of language and the nature of language breakdown in aphasia can be summarized as follows:

1. Language cannot be thought of as a simple sensorimotor dichotomy or a three-system cortical relay involving reception, transmission, and execution (Schuell et al., 1964). Such classical models were rejected because they ignore the complexity of perceptual and motor processes and view language as an activity bound to sensation and movement. They also allow aphasia to be thought of in terms of isolated, pure disorders reflecting disturbances at different stages of the dichotomy or relay system (for example, receptive or Wernicke's aphasia, conduction aphasia, expressive or Broca's aphasia). To many investigators, including Schuell, such notions do not correspond to modern concepts of neurophysiology and, more important, to the clinical behavior of most aphasic patients.

2. Neurophysiologically, language is the result of the dynamic interaction of complex cerebral and subcortical activities. Such complex interactions preclude the existence of simply segregated sensory and motor divisions and, in effect, place the existence of isolated sensory or motor deficits outside the realm of aphasia. Likewise, the various elements of language cannot be separated neurophysiologically. For example, the relationship between the semantic and syntactic aspects of language is so strong that their separation at the physiological level is arbitrary at best (Schuell et al., 1964).

3. The language mechanism contains a system of stored, learned elements and rules whose use and maintenance require discrimination, organization, storage, comparison, retrieval, transmission, and feedback control. Like Wepman et al., (1960), Schuell viewed language as an integrative activity that is linked to sensory and motor modalities but cannot be considered bound to them. That is, the stored elements and rules are common (central) to all input and output

modalities—speech, verbal comprehension, reading, and writing "involve the same referents and the same categorizations of individual and collective experience" (Schuell et al., 1964, p. 104). In the adult, therefore, language can exist unimpaired even in the presence of severe sensory and/or motor deficits, although it might be difficult to receive or express language through an impaired modality. Conversely, the language mechanism can be impaired in the absence of sensory or motor deficits, although in such instances the disturbance will be reflected in all modalities because the same language system is used by (or linked to) all input and output modalities through which language is channeled. Consequently, aphasia is viewed as a multimodality disturbance that is unidimensional in nature. That is, not only do all modalities tend to be impaired in aphasia, they also tend to be impaired in the same manner and to about the same degree.

It is important to recognize that Schuell's unidimensional, multimodality concept of aphasia does not require that aphasic patients vary only along a severity continuum. Schuell and Jenkins (1961b) wrote that among aphasic patients "many dimensions of impairment resulting from language deficit are identifiable, and need to be studied, in addition to the common or general dimension of language deficit" (p. 299). They also stated that "at a given level of language deficit, language tests may be arranged in subgroups which show systematic regularities in aphasic performance in various modalities as well as systematic differences in the performance of various segments of aphasic populations." The point here is that Schuell did not believe that all aphasic patients were alike. However, based on her clinical observations and objective analyses of data, she chose to emphasize the apparent universal feature of the disorder—a general disturbance of language that is reflected in a similar manner in all modalities.

4. In aphasia, the problems of most patients appear more related to performance factors than to competence factors (Schuell, 1969). That is, it appears that linguistic elements and rules are not lost or destroyed but that the language system is working with reduced efficiency or is "swamped in noise, due to faulty connections, disturbed internal signal sources, defective speech analyzers, and the general asynchronous chaos of processes whose mass action can no longer be properly coordinated" (Jenkins et al., 1975, p. 59). Schuell's belief that language is not lost or destroyed in aphasia is an important factor in determining that the stimulation approach is not one that involves the "teaching" or "reteaching" of language.

5. Although the language mechanism can exist separately from input and output modalities, our primary language processes are acquired and organized through complex, interacting sensory systems and sensorimotor processes. Notably, auditory processes are at the apex of those interacting systems that aid in the acquisition, processing, and control of language (Schuell et al., 1964). The importance of auditory processes for language and in the stimulation approach to language remediation will be discussed in more detail later.

Classification of Aphasia

Schuell's classification system for aphasia is unique when compared with most other popular systems. Her view of aphasia as a multimodality, unidimensional impairment clearly precluded categorizing patients according to modality of impairment (expressive, receptive, agraphia, alexia, etc.) or the element of language involved (semantic, syntactic, anomic, etc.). Instead, her classification system aimed at descriptive and predictive utility by classifying patients according to severity of language impairment, the presence or absence of related sensory or motor deficits, and prognosis. Originally, Schuell's system contained five categories and two minor syndromes. Later (Jenkins et al., 1975), the minor syndromes were treated as major categories. The seven categories can be summarized as follows:

1. *Simple Aphasia*. Relatively mild multimodality language impairment with no specific perceptual, sensorimotor, or dysarthric components. Prognosis for recovery is excellent.
2. *Aphasia with Visual Involvement*. Mild aphasia complicated by central impairment of visual discrimination, recognition, and recall. Prognosis for language recovery is excellent, but reading and writing recover more slowly.
3. *Aphasia with Persisting Dysfluency*. Mild aphasia with associated verbal dysfluency as an apparent result of proprioceptive disturbance (Jenkins et al., 1975). Prognosis for recovery from aphasia is excellent, but continued conscious control over speech execution remains necessary.
4. *Aphasia with Scattered Findings*. Moderate aphasia with a variety of problems compatible with generalized brain injury (for example, dysarthria, visual involvement, emotional lability). Although potential for functional language exists, prognosis is limited by the concomitant physiological and psychological problems.
5. *Aphasia with Sensorimotor Involvement*. Severe language impairment with impaired perception and production of phonemic patterns. Prognosis is for limited but functional recovery of language with persisting signs of sensorimotor impairment.
6. *Aphasia with Intermittent Auditory Imperception*. Usually severe aphasic impairment with severe involvement of auditory processes. Recovery of some language may occur, but normalcy is not achieved.
7. *Irreversible Aphasia Syndrome*. Nearly complete multimodality loss of functional language skills. Prognosis for recovery of functional language is poor.

The above classifications are useful in planning treatment with the stimulation approach in two ways. First, the various categories indicate severity of language impairment and, therefore, give some indication of the level at which stimulation should be directed. Second, the identification of associated nonaphasic deficits indicates those input avenues with the least intact access to the language system, and those output avenues through which evidence of language processing is least likely to be valid or interpretable. Such input and output problems signal a possible need to modify stimuli or restructure response demands. They also identify nonlinguistic disturbances that may require remediation.

APPROACH--GENERAL DESCRIPTION

Definition and Rationale

The stimulation approach can be defined as an approach to treatment that employs strong, controlled, and intensive auditory stimulation of the impaired symbol system as the primary tool to facilitate and maximize the patient's reorganization and recovery of language. It is an approach that recognizes that stimuli to which an intact language system can respond may be inadequate for eliciting responses from an impaired system. Because "sensory stimulation is the only method we have for making complex events happen in the brain" (Schuell et al., 1964, p. 338), the approach employs the manipulation and control of stimulus dimensions to aid the patient in making maximal responses.

Although numerous input modalities may be used, the auditory modality is at the foundation of the stimulation approach.

The use of intensive, controlled auditory stimulation is supported by the following:

1. Sensory stimulation affects brain activity. For example, sensory input alters the electrical activity of the brain; increasing stimulus strength increases the frequency of firing of neurons and the number of fibers activated; the threshold of response can be altered by repetitive stimulation (Eccles, 1973; Thompson, 1967); animals maintained in enriched environments show positive changes in brain structure and function when compared with animals in standard or deprived environments (Ansell, 1991); and structural changes in the brains of experimental animals occur in cortical areas presumably related to the behaviors they learn in response to specific stimuli (Ansell, 1991). Thus, at the neurophysiological level, stimulation can and does influence brain structure and function.
2. Many lines of research indicate that repeated sensory stimulation is essential for the acquisition, organization, storage, and retrieval of patterns in the brain. Language "patterns" appear to be no exception because language proficiency is largely the result of linguistic stimulation and experience. In addition, it is likely that language retrieval works through patterns of excitation laid down during original learning, and that appropriate stimuli are required for adequate retrieval (Schuell et al., 1964).
3. The auditory system is of prime importance in the acquisition of language, and ongoing functional language is dependent on the auditory system for processed information and control through feedback loops (Schuell et al., 1964).
4. Numerous studies indicate that nearly all aphasic people exhibit deficits in the auditory modality (Duffy and Ulrich, 1976; Schuell, 1953b; Schuell et al., 1964; Smith, 1971). It has been suggested that many of the multimodality impairments that aphasic patients experience stem from these auditory deficits (Schuell, 1953b), and that recovery of auditory functions, for many patients, is a prerequisite to recovery of other speech and language abilities (Brookshire, 1976a; Holland and Sonderman, 1974). Finally, the clinical observations of Schuell et al. (1955, 1964), and Schuell (1953a, 1969) suggest that the use of intensive, controlled auditory stimulation results in multimodality improvement that is greater than when treatment focuses on movement patterns or on each modality separately. Schuell (1974c) considered the notion of intensive auditory stimulation to be "the most important clinical discovery that we ever made" (p. 112).
5. The use of intensive auditory stimulation is consistent with the definition of aphasia as a multimodality deficit due to an underlying disturbance of language. That is, if the patient's problems in each modality are a reflection of a common underlying language disturbance, then it makes sense to channel treatment through the auditory modality because of its crucial link to language processes. In doing so, we should expect that gains made through the auditory modality will extend to all other input and output language channels.

A caveat regarding the primacy of the auditory modality in treatment is in order. Experience tells us there are some patients for whom the auditory channel is not the most appropriate avenue for stimulation. For example, there are those with disproportionately severe impairment of auditory processes who, on baseline testing, respond more favorably to written or gestural input. For such individuals, the primary stimulus channel in therapy may be visual instead of auditory. The use of intensive auditory stimulation in the stimulation approach should therefore be viewed as a rule for which there are important exceptions.

What the Stimulation Approach Is Not

The stimulation approach can be further understood by identifying some things that it is not. Wepman (1953, 1968) argued that aphasic patients do not recover because they are taught to speak. He indicated that the purpose of stimulation is not to convey new learning but rather to focus on "old learning" and stimulate the patient to produce new integrations for language. Schuell et al. (1955, 1964) emphasized that aphasia clinicians are not teachers; their role is to stimulate the adequate functioning of disrupted processes. Martin (1975), viewing the stimulation approach as conceptually related to cognitive theories of learning, indicated that the approach is an attempt "to reorganize a system already reorganized by brain damage" (p. 73). He pointed out that because the approach is based on a model that views aphasia as an interference with (not a loss of) language processes, therapy does not emphasize memory or the reproduction of stimuli as stimulus-response (S-R) learning approaches do. Instead, the approach emphasizes the action elicited within the patient by the stimuli presented. Such an approach treats the patient as an active participant in the reorganization of language and gears stimulation to maximize the ability of the patient to participate in the process.

Finally, what Taylor (1964) has called nonspecific stimulation, or the spontaneous recovery approach, is not part of the approach being discussed here. Nonspecific stimulation would include merely talking to the patient as much as possible; working to establish rapport, socialization, or interest; and reducing anxiety. Clearly, such approaches to treatment should be distinguished from the more carefully planned and controlled approach that is the focus of this chapter.

Individuals for Whom the Approach Is Appropriate

Relative to Severity

The rationale and general goals of the stimulation approach do not preclude its use with particular degrees of language impairment. However, the approach is not invariant along the severity continuum. The severity of aphasia should and does influence the nature of stimulation, specific treatment goals and procedures, and the frequency and duration of treatment. For example, severe aphasia (Schuell's irreversible aphasia syndrome) may sharply limit the use of the stimulation approach and reduce treatment to a short-term program aimed at improvement of comprehension, counseling of the patient and family, and the prevention of withdrawal and depression (Schuell, 1969). Variations of the approach as a function of severity will be discussed in more detail later.

Relative to Associated but Nonaphasic Communicative Deficits

The stimulation approach attempts to improve language or reduce the functional handicap imposed by disruption of language processes. It is not intended to remediate problems that often coexist with aphasia, such as perceptual deficits, apraxia of speech, or dysarthrias; such deficits may interfere with communication but do not disturb language per se. When present, they require treatment that differs significantly from the stimulation approach used for the treatment of the aphasia. The treatment of concomitant nonaphasic deficits may be secondary to, take precedence over, or coincide with aphasia therapy. Although the presence of nonaphasic deficits often places limits on the application of the stimulation approach and the expected outcome of aphasia therapy, their presence does not necessarily preclude the use of the stimulation approach to treat the aphasia; nor does the presence of aphasia and the use of the stimulation approach to treat it necessarily preclude the use of other approaches to treat the nonaphasic deficits.

Philosophical Underpinnings

Before discussing the general principles and design of intervention, a brief summary of the general philosophy underlying the stimulation approach is in order. This philosophy should temper any desire on the part of the reader for a rigid, universal approach to treatment.

First, Schuell et al. (1964) stated, "We believe in a general philosophy of treatment, but not an arbitrary method. There is no room for rigidity in clinical practice. . . . If the method leaves the patient behind, or if a patient outstrips the method, the method must be altered" (p. 332). Schuell believed that the main objective of treatment is to increase communication and that techniques merely assist in achieving that end. Therefore, methods should be flexible enough to be discarded if they are not working.

Second, diagnosis is a crucial part of the therapeutic process. That is, treatment must not proceed without some knowledge of the patient's assets and liabilities in each modality and some information about why performance breaks down when it does. Only with such information do we know what to work on and where to begin.

Third, treatment must be relevant. The neurological, linguistic, and social needs and interests of the patient need to be considered and used (Schuell et al., 1964; Wepman, 1953, 1968). Not only do such considerations reflect the clinician's personal sensitivity, they also help identify motivating material and pinpoint stimuli that may have very strong associational linkages in the patient's brain.

Finally, as stated earlier, treatment should be logically related to beliefs about the nature of aphasia. With the stimulation approach, there is no material to be taught and no student to learn a lost language. There is a person whose communication ability may be improved with appropriate stimulation. Such a philosophy significantly affects the principles and conduct of therapy.

GENERAL PRINCIPLES OF REMEDIATION

The design of intervention used in the stimulation approach is based on a number of general principles, many of which were articulated by Schuell et al. (1964). A number of additional, very practical principles that also apply to the stimulation approach have been presented by Brookshire (1992). It should be noted that several of these principles are indigenous to good clinical practice, regardless of the specific approach used. They are addressed here because they have grown out of observations of patients treated with a general stimulation approach. Information pertinent to the validity of the applied principles will be presented when the design of intervention is discussed. The general principles derived from those discussed by Schuell and/or Brookshire are as follows:

1. Intensive auditory stimulation should be used. As noted earlier, this is the framework of the stimulation approach and is based on the primacy of the auditory modality in language processes and the notion that the auditory modality represents a key area

of deficit in aphasia. The auditory modality need not be used exclusively. One modality may be used to reinforce another, and combined auditory and visual stimulation may be especially appropriate.

2. The stimulus must be adequate—it must get into the brain. Therefore, it needs to be controlled, perhaps along a number of dimensions. The application of this principle may be highly dependent on baseline data and may involve considerable individualized pretreatment planning. Brookshire (1992) states that tasks should be at a level of difficulty where "performance is slightly deficient, but not mostly or completely erroneous" (p. 133).

3. Repetitive sensory stimulation should be used. Auditory material that is ineffective as a single stimulus may become effective after it is repeated a number of times.

4. Each stimulus should elicit a response. This is the only way we can assess the adequacy of stimulation, and it provides important feedback that the patient and clinician may use to modify future stimuli and responses.

5. Responses should be elicited, not forced or corrected. If a stimulus is adequate, there will be a response. If a response is not elicited, the stimulus was not adequate. What the patient needs in such cases is more stimulation, not correction or information about why a response was inadequate.

6. A maximum number of responses should be elicited. A large number of adequate responses indicate that a large number of adequate stimuli have been presented. Numerous responses also provide frequent feedback and reinforcement of language and help increase confidence and language attempts outside the treatment setting.

7. Feedback about response accuracy should be provided when such feedback appears beneficial. The necessity for feedback may vary from patient to patient, but it generally is advisable. Showing patients their progress may be motivating, reinforcing, and extremely helpful in "proving" that progress is taking place or that different approaches or termination of treatment should be considered.

8. The clinician should work systematically and intensively. Treatment requires a sequenced plan of action. It should be implemented often enough to meet the patient's needs, taking into account his or her overall condition and prognosis for recovery.

9. Sessions should begin with relatively easy, familiar tasks. This allows for adjustment and "warm-up" time and enables the patient to proceed to more difficult activities after experiencing success.

10. Abundant and varied materials (Schuell et al., 1955) that are simple and relevant to the patient's deficits should be used. Treatment does not involve the learning of vocabulary or rules, so content need not be limited to "items to be learned." As Wepman (1953) indicated, the specific content of treatment is not as important as the manner in which it is conducted. A variety of material also reduces the frustration often induced by drill on a small amount of material.

11. New materials and procedures should be extensions of familiar materials and procedures. This allows the patient to concentrate on language processing and minimizes the possible disruptive effects of new material and response demands.

DESIGN OF INTERVENTION

In this section, factors that are important in the development of a treatment program will be considered. Since, by definition, the most important component of the stimulation approach is the stimulation provided to the patient, those variables that are potentially most important to structuring stimulation will receive primary emphasis. Response demands, feedback, and the sequencing of treatment steps also will be discussed. The reader is cautioned that the recommendations offered here for implementing the stimulation approach are based on rather broad generalizations derived from a potpourri of research and observation of heterogeneous groups and individual patients. Consequently, few, if any, of the recommendations can be assumed to apply effectively to all aphasic patients.

Structure of Stimulation

A great deal of information has been acquired about stimulus variables that may affect aphasic patient performance. Such data are largely the result of basic clinical and experimental research and are not derived primarily from specific treatment studies. The data are, nonetheless, invaluable to the clinician who must decide how to make stimulation adequate and effective during treatment. As Holland (1975) and Tikofsky (1968) have suggested, one strategy for designing treatment is to follow leads provided by research by turning the experimental techniques designed to isolate a particular problem into potential treatment tasks. Nowhere in the aphasiology literature are there so many "leads" as in the area related to stimulus variables that affect performance. These leads have at least three practical applications to patient management. First, knowledge about stimulus manipulations that may maximize performance can be used to ensure that a patient is working at a level where "failure" is minimized. Second, and conversely, knowledge about stimulus manipulations can be applied in the opposite direction to challenge mildly impaired patients or those who respond without difficulty to tasks designed to maximize performance. Third, many of the factors to be discussed may be useful when counseling people in the patient's environment who need information about how best to communicate with the patient in everyday interactions. The following represents a review of the variables most relevant to the structuring of stimulation.

Auditory Perceptual Clarity (Volume and Noise)

Although Schuell et al. (1964) suggested that most patients prefer to hear speech at conversational levels, they indicated that an increase in volume (not shouting!) is sometimes desirable. Only a few controlled studies have been conducted to evaluate the effects of increasing volume on auditory comprehension.

Glaser et al. (1974) found that auditory comprehension of aphasic persons under sound-field conditions at conversational level was superior to comprehension under earphones (binaurally and monaurally) at 25 dB above conversational level. Because of the interaction between volume level and earphone/sound-field methods of presentation, the results are difficult to interpret, but they do suggest that increasing volume above normal levels does not facilitate comprehension.

McNeil et al. (1979a) found no significant improvement in a group of 10 aphasic patients on a word discrimination and word sequencing task or on portions of the Revised Token Test (McNeil and Prescott, 1978) when stimuli were presented under earphones at 75, 85, and 100 dB SPL. Group data were representative of individual performance. The authors concluded that simple increases in stimulus intensity do not improve aphasic patients' auditory comprehension.

Although there is little evidence to support increasing the volume of auditory stimulation, it does appear that reducing noise or increasing the signal-to-noise ratio is beneficial. Aphasic patients often complain about the negative effects of noise on performance (Rolnick and Hoops, 1969; Skelly, 1975). Although Birch and Lee (1955) found that a binaural masking tone improved aphasic patients' naming and reading performance, other investigators have not concurred. Schuell et al. (1964), Siegenthaler and Goldstein (1967), Weinstein (1959), and Wertz and Porch (1970) either found no difference in performance accuracy in quiet versus noise or found noise to have a detrimental effect on performance on language tasks. Darley (1976) concluded from a review of such studies that "background noise apparently reduces the efficiency of the patient's performance" (p. 4).

These studies suggest that reducing noise or working in quiet generally facilitates language performance. Simply increasing loudness, on the other hand, does not appear useful, although it may enhance performance in isolated cases. Many clinicians feel confident in advising patients' families that verbal comprehension is typically better in quiet than in the presence of a variety of distracting or competing auditory stimuli (TV, radio, background conversation, etc.).

Nonlinguistic Visual Perceptual Clarity (Dimensionality, Size, Color, Context, Ambiguity, and Operativity)

Visual materials are often used as an integral part of the stimuli to which patients are asked to respond. The importance of visual stimulation, in fact, led Eisenson (1973, p. 162) to call Schuell's stimulation approach to treatment a "visual-auditory" approach. Clinical observations suggest that the properties of visual stimuli may influence responses, and the importance of the visual modality to language behavior in general has led to the investigation of visual redundancy as a potential factor influencing linguistic processing in aphasia.

In a study of 21 patients with severe verbal comprehension deficits, Helm-Estabrooks (1981) compared performance on a single-word comprehension task in which stimulus conditions consisted of line drawings, each on individual cards arranged in rows; smaller line drawings of items, all on a single page; and real objects around the room. For the group as a whole, picture-pointing was superior to identification of objects around the room, but there were no differences between the two picture conditions; however, not all patients followed the group pattern. Helm-Estabrooks concluded that auditory comprehension can be influenced by variables extrinsic to central auditory processing, such as visual search skills.

Bisiach (1966) compared the naming performance of nine aphasic subjects in response to pictures of realistic colored objects, line drawings of the same objects, and the same line drawings with superimposed curved or jagged lines. Although there were no differences among stimulus conditions for object recognition, subjects' naming of the realistic colored pictures was 15% to 18% more accurate than their naming of line drawings and distorted line drawings. The visual redundancy of the realistic colored drawings was thought to facilitate naming.

Benton et al. (1972) examined the naming performance of 18 aphasic persons in response to real objects, large line drawings, and small line drawings. Accuracy of real object naming was superior to that for small line drawings; accuracy for large line drawings fell in between. The redundancy provided by three-dimensionality was thought to enhance the conceptual associations underlying word retrieval. Because of the relatively small differences between conditions, however, the authors questioned the clinical significance of their results. The possible insignificance of three-dimensionality was supported by Corlew and Nation (1975), who found no differences in the performance of 14 aphasic persons when they named the 10 common real objects used in the Porch Index of Communicative Ability (PICA) (Porch, 1967) than when they named reduced-size line drawings of the same objects.

In a theoretically interesting study, Whitehouse and Caramazza (1978) compared the ability of 10 aphasic persons to identify line drawings of three objects (cup, bowl, glass) varying in physical features such as height and width. Stimuli consisted of prototypes (unambiguous representations) of the three objects as well as drawings in which the height-width dimensions were varied in order to make the perceptual distinction among the objects "fuzzy." In addition, some of the drawings had a handle, and some did not. Context (functional information) was also varied by presenting stimuli alone or in context with a coffee pot, cereal box, or water pitcher. Subjects "named" the pictures by selecting from multiple-choice presentations of the names of the three objects. Results were not uniform across subjects. Those with a diagnosis of Broca's aphasia performed similarly to normal control subjects in their use of context and in their ability to deal with fuzzy perceptual boundaries. Patients with a diagnosis of anomic aphasia, however, had difficulty integrating and using perceptual and functional cues (dimension and context). These findings and those of Caramazza et al. (1982) have led to the conclusion that, for some patients, naming difficulty is related to an inability to organize adequately the concepts underlying word meaning in terms of functional and perceptual information, as opposed to difficulty with retrieval of an adequately perceived/conceived lexical item. Although the implications of these findings for clinical practice are neither clear-cut nor universal, it appears that the perceptual characteristics of visual stimuli should be as unambiguous as possible for all patients. Placing a target object in a redundant conceptual setting (pairing a cup with a coffee pot) may enhance word retrieval when the target is perceptually ambiguous. When pairing a target stimulus with other visual stimuli, the additional stimuli should never introduce ambiguity about the nature of the target.

Finally, Gardner's (1973) findings suggest that the number of modalities in which associations may be evoked should be considered when selecting visual materials for treatment. He compared naming of pictures of "operative" objects (discrete, firm to the touch, and available to several modalities—for example, "rock"), with naming of "figurative" objects (not operative—for example, "cloud"), while accounting for the effects of picturability and word frequency. Most aphasic patients performed more accurately in response to the operative items, and the effects of operativity were most pronounced for patients with difficulty initiating speech. Gardner argued that operative items were superior because they aroused associations in several modalities, whereas the figurative items were limited to visual associations. The implication for treatment, therefore, is that visual stimuli that also may trigger auditory, tactile, kinesthetic, or olfactory associations are potentially more effective in aiding word retrieval than stimuli that trigger only visual associations.

To summarize, although some data suggest that some properties of visual stimuli are relatively unimportant to aphasic performance, it does seem that the clarity and redundancy of visual stimuli can influence linguistic processing (Caramazza and

Berndt, 1978). Darley (1976) recommends that we "play it safe" and use the redundant and realistic stimuli in treatment. The most potent visual stimuli appear to be characterized by three-dimensionality, color, redundant physical properties, operativity, and a lack of ambiguity in perceptual characteristics and context.

Linguistic Visual Perceptual Clarity (Size and Form)

There are little data to suggest that the size or form of reading material affects comprehension, but a few clinical observations are relevant. Rolnick and Hoops (1969) reported that aphasic patients complain about small print for word and sentence stimuli and prefer large print, even when visual-field deficits are not present. McDearmon and Potter (1975) observed varying preferences for uppercase, lowercase, or script stimuli. Schuell et al. (1955) recommended uppercase print for patients with visual impairments and thought that script should not be introduced until the reading rate for printed material is normal.

Boone and Friedman (1976) examined 30 aphasic patients' single-word reading comprehension in response to cursive versus manuscript stimuli, and Williams (1984) investigated the same factors' influence on the word and sentence comprehension of 20 patients. Neither study found significant differences between the two written forms. Williams, however, observed that two of her patients reliably responded better to one form than the other.

There is no compelling evidence to suggest that the size and form of written input are powerful stimulus factors affecting reading comprehension. When providing reading material for patients, however, the clinician should be aware of a general preference for large print, and potential idiosyncratic preferences for uppercase, lowercase, cursive, or manuscript format.

Method of Delivery of Auditory Stimulation

Many clinicians have speculated about ways to improve the delivery of auditory stimuli to patients. For example, can live-voice, binaural, free-field stimulation be improved on?

The use of earphones is intuitively attractive because of its potential for reducing extraneous noise and focusing attention. Schuell et al. (1964), however, observed that patients usually prefer direct presentation to earphones because they rely on more than auditory cues and perhaps because earphones produce distortions to which they are sensitive. The preference for free-field presentation is supported by the previously mentioned study by Glaser et al. (1974). They found that the comprehension under free-field conditions was superior to binaural and right- and left-ear monaural presentations through earphones. The superiority of the free-field condition was maintained even when the intensity of the earphone conditions was 25 dB greater than in the free-field.

It has been suggested that selective left-ear/right-hemisphere presentation of auditory stimuli may improve comprehension. Such speculation is based on the results of dichotic listening studies that have found a left-ear advantage for aphasic patients (e.g., Johnson et al., 1977; Sparks et al., 1970). LaPointe et al. (1977) examined aphasic patients' responses to portions of the Token Test (DeRenzi and Vignolo, 1962) when presented to the right ear, left ear, or binaurally, and found no significant differences among the three conditions. They concluded that selective monaural presentation of auditory stimuli is not a

useful procedure. McNeil et al. (1979b) examined the effects of selective binaural SPL variations in which stimuli were presented at 85 or 100 dB SPL to one ear, while stimuli to the other ear were presented at 70 dB SPL. Although a trend toward better comprehension on some tasks was noted when the left ear was more intensely stimulated, their general conclusion was that unilateral intensity increase is not a potent mechanism for improving auditory comprehension.

The data to date indicate that response adequacy to free-field presentation is not exceeded when earphones are used, and that selective stimulation of one ear or one hemisphere does not surpass binaural stimulation. It should also be noted that the findings of Boller et al. (1979) and Green and Boller (1974) suggest that live-voice presentation is superior to taped presentation of stimuli. Therefore, there are no compelling reasons for us not to continue to present auditory stimuli directly with live voice, binaurally, and in the free-field.

Discriminability (Semantic, Auditory, Visual)

Verbal responses of aphasic patients are often characterized by errors associated in meaning or experience. Such errors (e.g., "table" for "chair") are, in fact, the "best" errors a patient can make (Schuell and Jenkins, 1961a; Schuell et al., 1964). These characteristics suggest that response alternatives provided to patients should not promote semantic errors. This is particularly relevant for comprehension tasks that require the patient to choose from among a set of alternatives (e.g., responding to a verbally and/or visually presented word or sentence by pointing to one of several choices). Assuring that response choices are unrelated semantically often will facilitate speed and accuracy of performance. Conversely, tasks can remain unchanged in nature but often can be made more difficult by introducing semantically related response choices (Duffy and Watkins, 1984; Pizzamiglio and Appicciafuoco, 1971).

Semantic discriminability among response choices is more important than visual-perceptual discriminability. This is illustrated by the findings of Chieffi et al. (1989). Their aphasic patients made more errors on a single-word comprehension task when response choices were semantically related (e.g., banana, apple, grapes) than when they were visually related (e.g., wheel, button, lifebelt). Performance on a task in which response choices were both semantically and visually related (e.g., chair, bench, stool) was poorer than in the semantically related condition, suggesting that semantic and perceptual effects may be cumulative, although the authors argued that the semantic demands of the combined semantic and visual task were more potent than the visual ones.

Difficulty discriminating between words with minimal phonemic differences (e.g., cake/take; horse/house) is an important aspect of auditory impairment in some patients (Schuell, 1973). In addition, aphasic patients may confuse letters or words with similar visual configurations (e.g., E/F; p/b; store/stone).

An investigation by Linebaugh (1986) sheds some light on the importance of semantic, auditory, and visual discriminability in single-word reading comprehension tasks. He presented a picture-to-written-word matching task to 25 aphasic patients under two conditions. In one, all three response foils (written words) were either semantically, aurally or visually related to the target response. In the other, the three foils consisted of one semantically, one aurally, and one visually related word.

When all foils were of the same type, error rates were higher with visually than aurally related foils, with no differences among other foil comparisons. When foils contained one of each foil type, both semantic and visual errors were more frequent than auditory errors, with no differences between semantic and visual errors. There was considerable variability among subjects in their patterns and degree of susceptibility to the semantic, visual, and auditory influences, with a minority of subjects making more than 50% of their errors in one category and only two subjects doing so in both experimental conditions. These findings suggest that semantic and visual discriminability, on average, are more potent than auditory discriminability in single-word reading tasks, but the power of each factor is seldom overwhelming in individual patients.

The discriminability factor apparently is also relevant to word-retrieval tasks. The findings of Mills et al. (1979), for example, have implications for the semantic distinctiveness of visual stimuli used in naming tasks. (They also are relevant to the information discussed under nonlinguistic visual perceptual clarity.) They examined the effects of "uncertainty" on the naming performance of 10 aphasic patients, with uncertainty defined as "the number of equally probable binary choice decisions necessary to achieve a final name selection from one or several correct names available in the lexicon" (p. 75). For example, shown a picture of a cup, most control subjects respond "cup"; there are few alternative correct responses (little uncertainty). On the other hand, a picture of a country home in winter generates considerable uncertainty because "winter," "country," "cabin," "house," and other words would be reasonable responses, thus requiring a greater number of word-retrieval decisions. The aphasic patients made significantly more errors and had greater response latencies in response to high-uncertainty pictures than in response to low-uncertainty pictures, leading the authors to conclude that uncertainty affects aphasic naming performance. Their findings suggest that another way to simplify word retrieval on picture-naming tasks is to select stimuli to which there are only a few alternative responses. Similarly, reducing the number of response alternatives reduces error probability on point-to comprehension tasks.

In summary, there are compelling data to suggest that verbal comprehension tasks in which several response choices are offered can maximize performance if alternatives are semantically unrelated to the target response. The auditory and visual-perceptual "distinctiveness" of the target from response alternatives may also be important, with visual similarity generally being more important than auditory similarity on written word comprehension tasks. Although there is considerable variability among patients in their responsiveness to these semantic, auditory, and visual influences, reducing the number of response choices on point-to tasks will usually lead to improved performance.

Combining Sensory Modalities

Although the auditory modality is paramount in the stimulation approach, the use of several modalities in combination is often recommended. Schuell (1974b) indicated that various modalities should be used to reinforce one another and, in fact, thought that patients often do better when auditory and visual stimuli are combined. Schuell and Jenkins (1961a) reported that patients do better on single-word comprehension tasks when written and auditory stimuli are used instead of auditory stimuli alone.

Goodglass et al. (1968) examined the naming performance of 27 patients in response to auditory (characteristic sound associated with the target item), tactile, olfactory, and picture stimuli. They found a uniformity in performance across all modalities for the great majority of patients, although reaction times were fastest to visual stimuli. By extension, the work of Mills (1977) and Smithpeter (1976) suggest that combining some of those stimuli may enhance performance. Mills found that pairing an environmental sound (e.g., whinny) with a picture to be named (e.g., horse) facilitated naming performance over time, generalized to nondrilled words, and resulted in posttherapy improvement in naming without the auditory stimulus. Smithpeter (1976) reported that olfaction was effective in stimulating accurate language responses in some aphasic patients when it preceded or accompanied other stimuli.

Caramazza and Berndt (1978) cite the work of North (1971), who found that aphasic patients' word recall improved when information was available through several sense modalities. North argued that various senses may contribute additively to word recall. Gardner's (1973) previously discussed findings regarding operativity suggest that such additivity of multisensory stimulation need not be overt. That is, performance may be enhanced if visual stimuli, for example, are capable of "arousing" multisensory associations.

Combining the auditory and visual modalities is the most widely used form of multisensory stimulation, and a number of studies support the practice, although with some qualifications. Gardner and Brookshire (1972) found naming and single-word reading performance of eight aphasic patients to be better during combined auditory and visual stimulation than during auditory or visual stimulation alone. By varying the order in which the stimulus conditions were presented, they also determined that combined stimulation facilitated performance during subsequent unisensory stimulus conditions. While analysis of single-subject profiles indicated that combined stimulation may not be best for all patients, their results generally supported the conclusion that combined stimulation is better than unisensory stimulation. They also suggest that combined auditory-visual stimulation should generally precede auditory or visual stimulation alone, at least on treatment tasks requiring naming responses. Halpern (1965a, 1965b), reporting similar results, supported the concept of multisensory stimulation but noted that a multisensory approach sometimes can be distracting.

Auditory stimulation often involves some potentially useful visual input as well; for example, the patient's visual contact with the examiner may provide a number of facilitory verbal or paralinguistic cues. Green and Boller (1974) found that the comprehension of severely impaired aphasic patients was not as accurate or appropriate when stimuli were presented by tape or with the examiner behind the patient as when stimuli were presented face to face. Boller et al. (1979) confirmed the superiority of face-to-face presentation over the use of taped stimuli, and Lambrecht and Marshall (1983) showed that the comprehension of severely impaired patients was better when they looked and listened than when stimuli were just heard. Whether the performance differences in these studies were due to situational, extralinguistic cues or to additional visual verbal input through lipreading is not clear. It does seem, though, that having the visual and auditory attention of the patient during the presentation of verbal material is important.

To summarize, providing multimodality stimulation can improve response adequacy for many aphasic patients, and combining auditory and visual stimulation may be the best and most practical way of doing so. Combined auditory-visual stimulation may facilitate responses to subsequent unisensory stimuli and, therefore, may be employed first when responses to unisensory stimulation are deficient to a significant degree. Other modalities, such as the tactile, also may be helpful. It seems that the effectiveness of multimodality stimulation stems from the redundancy of information it provides and the additional associations that it may help to trigger. This appears desirable for many patients, although the clinician needs to be sure that such multiple inputs improve performance and that they do not somehow overload or exceed the capacity of the patient to use them effectively.

Stimulus Repetition

Repetitive sensory stimulation is a principle of treatment espoused by Schuell et al. (1964). They recommended, for example, that on word recognition or repetition tasks, as many as 20 repetitions of a stimulus word might be appropriate/necessary before eliciting a response. Few studies, however, have directly examined the effects of repetitive stimulation on language comprehension or expression in aphasic patients.

Helmick and Wipplinger (1975) examined naming behavior in one aphasic patient under a nontreatment and two treatment conditions, each condition containing different target words. In a minimal stimulus condition, six "stimulations" (including verbal identification, contextual cue, picture identification/discrimination, tracing, and copying) were provided before eliciting a naming response. In the maximum stimulus condition, the six stimulations were repeated four times for each word. Both conditions were more effective than the nontreatment condition, but there were no differences between the results obtained from minimum and maximum stimulation. The authors concluded that a relatively small amount of stimulation can be as effective as a great deal of stimulation.

LaPointe et al. (1978) evaluated the effects of two methods of repetition of Token Test commands on the auditory comprehension of 12 aphasic patients. In one condition, stimulus repetitions of commands preceded responses. In the other, repetition occurred only following incorrect responses. When items were repeated following failure (to a ceiling of four repetitions of the original stimulus), significant improvement occurred in response to the first and second repetitions; further but nonsignificant gains were noted for the third and fourth repetitions. In numeric terms, while accuracy was 24% without repetition, it rose to 58% after repetition to ceiling level. Degree of language impairment was negatively correlated with gains from repetition. In contrast, when items were presented twice or four times prior to a response, no significant group gains over the no-repetition condition were noted. However, there were some individual subject differences; one subject did "remarkably poorer" when commands were repeated prior to responses and another apparently benefited from the prerepsonse repetition.

Considering the lack of experimental support, the use of numerous repetitions prior to eliciting a response cannot be considered a verified, generally applicable principle of aphasia treatment. Some individuals may respond differently to prerepsonse repetitive stimulation, however, with some benefiting and others deteriorating. In contrast, repetition of stimuli subsequent to errors generally does appear to increase adequate responses, with maximum benefits derived from the first or second repetition.

Rate and Pause

It has been suggested that slowing speech rate may aid auditory comprehension (Schuell et al., 1964), and this is something experienced clinicians apparently are aware of subconsciously. Salvatore et al. (1978) reported that experienced clinicians give Token Test commands more slowly than their inexperienced colleagues by inserting more pause time within commands. They also found that experienced clinicians tend to slow their presentation rate when repeating commands that previously had generated error responses. Such clinician behavior obviously is not desirable during standardized diagnostic testing and some baseline procedures, but it does offer indirect support for the facilitating effect of rate reduction on verbal comprehension.

Gardner et al. (1975) examined sentence comprehension in 46 aphasic patients with comprehension problems ranging from mild to severe. They reported improvement in comprehension—independent of form of aphasia—when sentences were spoken at a rate of one word per second. They recommended that, when proceeding from single-word to sentence stimuli, words initially should be "slowly enunciated."

Weidner and Lasky (1976) found improved performance in a group of 20 aphasic patients on four measures of auditory comprehension when presentation rate was reduced from 150 words per minute (wpm) to 110 wpm. Differences between the two rate conditions were greatest for patients scoring above the 50th percentile on the PICA. Similarly, Poeck and Pietron (1981) induced an 11 to 12% improvement in Token Test scores of a group of 42 aphasic patients by electronically expanding speech rate by 25%. Pashek and Brookshire (1982) extended these findings by showing that reducing the rate from 150 to 120 wpm facilitated paragraph comprehension in a group of 20 patients; performance was facilitated in those with poor as well as those with good sentence level comprehension.

The facilitative effect of reduced rate also has been demonstrated for a patient with aphasia and severe auditory imperception (Albert and Bear, 1974). The authors found that their patient's comprehension improved dramatically when rate was slowed to "one-third or less of normal."

Liles and Brookshire (1975) examined the comprehension of 20 patients when 5-second pauses were inserted into various portions of Token Test commands. The insertion of pauses facilitated comprehension for many of their patients. Patterns of patient performance led them to hypothesize that the pauses aided the processing of strings of lexical items but not the processing of syntactic components. In contrast, Hageman and Lewis (1983) inserted 2-second pauses at major within-sentence breaks of the Revised Token Test and failed to find qualitative or quantitative performance differences when compared with a no-pause condition. They suggested that a 2-second pause may not be long enough to facilitate performance.

Salvatore (1976) reported a facilitation of comprehension for an aphasic patient when 4-second pauses were inserted into

Token Test commands. By gradually fading pause duration, it was also possible to maintain improved comprehension with 2- and sometimes only 1-second pauses. Although there was no generalization to nonpause stimulation, the results do suggest that pause time can be faded, to some degree, while maintaining high levels of comprehension.

Are the effects of rate reduction and pause insertion cumulative? Lasky et al. (1976) examined the effects of rate reduction (120 versus 150 wpm) and the insertion of 1-second interphrase pauses on the sentence comprehension of 15 aphasic persons. Comprehension improved when rate was slowed or when pauses were inserted, and combining reduced rate and interphrase pauses resulted in the best performance.

In an effort to examine how slowing the rate facilitates comprehension, Blumstein et al. (1985) compared aphasic patients' comprehension of sentences spoken at normal rates to (A) a vowel condition, in which vowel duration in each word was increased (140 wpm); (B) a word condition, in which silences were added between words (110 wpm); (C) a syntactic condition, in which silences were added at constituent phrase boundaries (90 wpm); and (D) a natural condition, in which sentences were read at a naturally slowed rate (110 wpm). In general, reducing rate had a relatively small facilitory effect and was significant only for the syntactic condition and only for patients with Wernicke's aphasia. The authors concluded that it may not be slowed rate per se that facilitated comprehension but rather the effect of a syntactically well-placed pause on the processing of preceding syntactic and semantic elements. Although this may be the case, the fact that the rate of the syntactic condition (90 wpm) was slower than any other slowed condition confounds the interpretation and leaves open the possibility that slowing the rate to a comparable degree in other ways might also facilitate comprehension.

The positive effects of slowed rate may not be as robust for narrative discourse. Nicholas and Brookshire (1986a) examined narrative comprehension across two test sessions in aphasic patients with relatively good and relatively poor comprehension; narratives were spoken at fast (190 to 210 wpm) versus slow (110 to 130 wpm) rates. Only the group with relatively poor comprehension benefited from rate reduction, and this held only for the first of the two test sessions. In addition, the facilitory effect of slow rate was not present for all patients in the poor comprehension group. The authors concluded that the effect of slow rate was undependable and transitory, and they noted that variables with strong effects on comprehension at the sentence level may have only weak effects at the discourse level.

To summarize, it appears that slowing the rate and lengthening pauses at phrase boundaries can have a facilitory effect on sentence comprehension. This effect is neither always present nor generally dramatic, and there are no consistent indications across studies that the ability to benefit from rate and pause modifications is tied to either type or severity of aphasia. The positive effects of slowing rate may be less consistent and pervasive at the discourse level than at the sentence level. From the practical standpoint, however, it is reasonable to accept Nicholas and Brookshire's (1986a) advice that "it seems reasonable to counsel those who speak with brain-damaged listeners to speak slowly, because slow speech rate does not affect most brain-damaged listeners negatively, and for some it may be beneficial, at least on some occasions" (p. 469).

Length and Redundancy

As previously stated, Schuell believed that reduced verbal retention span is a near universal feature of aphasia. Although this feature is pervasive, she reported that retention deficits are highly reversible with the use of carefully controlled intensive auditory stimulation characterized by gradual increases in stimulus length (Schuell, 1953a; Schuell et al., 1955).

The importance of stimulus length receives additional support from a number of sources, including patients themselves. Rolnick and Hoops (1969), in interviews with several mild aphasic patients, found numerous complaints about the processing and retention demands imposed by lengthy messages. Patients thought that reduced message length facilitated comprehension and retention.

In addition, numerous studies have demonstrated that, with other factors held constant, sentence comprehension tends to decrease as length increases (e.g., Curtiss et al., 1986; Shewan and Canter, 1971; Weidner and Lasky, 1976).

Although Goodglass et al. (1970) found that 52 patients with different classical forms of aphasia had varying degrees of success on a verbally presented retention span test, all were deficient to some degree. Albert (1976) examined the ability of 28 aphasic patients on a short-term memory task in which they pointed to objects named serially by the examiner. They were inferior to control subjects and nonaphasic brain-injured patients on total item retention and in retention of the accurate sequence of presentation. Response patterns indicated that sequencing problems increased as information load increased. Information load and sequencing deficits were both present regardless of clinical type of aphasia. The findings of Martin and Feher (1990) suggest that degree of short-term memory limitation in aphasia affects semantic processing (i.e., sentences with a large number of content words) but is not strongly related to processing of syntactic complexity. Finally, Gardner et al. (1975) found poorer comprehension when length increased from single words to nonredundant sentences containing the same single words.

Length appears to be an important factor in the visual as well as the auditory modality. Siegel's (1959) 31 aphasic patients had more difficulty reading words of two or more syllables (six or more letters) than single-syllable words of less than five letters. Halpern (1965a, 1965b) compared verbal responses of 33 patients on tasks involving single-word repetition, reading single words, and reading single words with simultaneous auditory and visual stimulation. Stimuli in each task were either long (two or more syllables or six letters) or short (one syllable or less than four letters), and also varied as a function of abstraction level and part of speech. Results showed that long words resulted in more verbal errors—including perseveration—than short words, regardless of modality of presentation. Differences between errors on long and short words were greatest for the visual modality. On the basis of his findings, Halpern (1965a, 1965b) recommended that, for such tasks, auditory or auditory-visual stimulation usually should precede visual stimulation alone.

Going beyond the word level, Webb and Love (1983) examined the reading abilities of 35 aphasic patients and found more errors on sentence recognition than letter or word recognition; more errors on oral reading of sentences and paragraphs than letters or words; and more errors on paragraph comprehension than sentence comprehension.

Friederici et al. (1981) have shown that word length also influences writing. In their group of 12 aphasic patients, written accuracy was reduced by more than 50% as word length increased from one to three syllables.

Wepman and Jones (1961) found that verbal responses to words are easier than verbal responses to sentences whether stimuli are presented aurally or visually. At the word level, verbal responses to written stimuli were better for one-syllable than two-syllable words. On the other hand, verbal responses to aurally presented words did not differ between one- and two-syllable words. In contrast to Halpern's (1965a, 1965b) findings, they indicated that the length factor for sentence material is most pronounced for the auditory, not the visual, modality. It is possible that the different results are due to the fact that Halpern dealt with variations of length within single words, while Wepman and Jones were referring to differences between words and sentences. If so, this highlights the fact that differences in the processing and/or retention of words between modalities are not identical to differences in the processing and/or retention of sentences (and discourse) between modalities.

It is important to note that the detrimental effects of increasing message length may vary as a function of message redundancy. For example, the findings of Gardner et al. (1975) support the notion that aphasic patients comprehend redundant sentences better than nonredundant sentences of equal length. Clark and Flowers (1987) demonstrated that increasing sentence redundancy facilitated comprehension even when redundant sentences were longer and syntactically more complex than nonredundant ones (e.g., sentences like "Which one is the book you read?" were easier than "Which one is the book?"). Also, the remarkable sensitivity of the Token Test to subtle comprehension deficits is at least partially due to the nonredundant properties of its verbal stimuli. Clearly, the potent effect of length strongly interacts with redundancy; the two factors can seldom, if ever, be considered separately. Further discussion of this interaction can be found in the section on grammar and syntax.

To summarize, there can be little doubt that controlling length at the word and sentence levels is a potent stimulus factor for most or all aphasic patients, and most clinicians discuss this factor when counseling families about their verbal input to the aphasic person. Length is an influential factor regardless of whether stimuli are auditory, visual, or auditory-visual. In the visual modality, reducing length at both the word and sentence levels can be expected to facilitate comprehension. For auditory input, length may be relatively unimportant at the word level; but it becomes highly important when proceeding from the word to phrase to sentence level. When controlling length, it seems that nonredundant components are the most crucial elements to control, since increases in message redundancy may limit or even overcome the generally negative effects of increases in message length. This may be particularly true at the paragraph and narrative discourse levels (to be discussed in the section on context).

Cues, Prompts, and Prestimulation

It is well recognized that, under the right circumstances, the skillful clinician can employ a variety of techniques—often referred to as cues, prompts, or prestimulation—that will facilitate patients' word retrieval or comprehension. Such techniques are often used following an inadequate response to a less powerful stimulus. However, when less powerful stimuli consistently are incapable of generating a high proportion of adequate responses, the cue (prompt or prestimulus) may become a distinct treatment condition to which acceptable responses must be generated prior to proceeding to the less powerful stimuli. In this section, a number of potentially useful cues that have not been identified already under other headings will be discussed.

McDearmon and Potter (1975) offered a number of suggestions regarding representational prompts, which they defined as symbolic or realistic cues that directly suggest the concept referred to in a response. Prompts are strongly related to the concepts of stimulus redundancy and multimodality stimulation. They suggest that more than one representation of the response be presented and that one representation—the prompt—gradually be faded. For example, on naming tasks, pictures and their written names may be presented with resultant adequate responses; the written prompts may then be faded gradually by blocking out increasing portions of the word until it is entirely eliminated. Some other suggested prompts, not already implied under other headings, include tracing letters to facilitate letter recognition, writing words to aid word retrieval, using pantomime or Amerind sign to facilitate word retrieval, and using pictures in conjunction with corresponding written words to facilitate reading.

Barton et al. (1969) examined word retrieval of 36 patients under three conditions: picture naming, sentence completion (e.g., "You clean teeth with a _____"), and object description. In order, the most powerful cues were sentence completion, picture naming, and object description. It is important to note, however, that 44% of the subjects in their study did not follow the group's ordering of responses to the three naming conditions. This highlights the importance of examining the individual patient's responsiveness to stimulus cues; a powerful cue for one patient may not be powerful for another. Along these lines, Marshall and Tompkins (1982) and Golper and Rau (1983) point out that careful analysis of individual patient strategies may provide clues about the best cues for the clinician to give during therapy. Such information may also be used to increase the patient's own use of successful cues.

Linebaugh and Lehner (1977) have described a cuing program for word retrieval that is based on two principles: (A) that recovery is best served by eliciting the desired response with a minimal cue, and (B) that when a cue is successful, continued elicitation of the appropriate response with less powerful cues is reinforcing and conducive to stimulating the processes underlying word retrieval. When a patient is unable to name a pictured object, the following cues, in order, are given until an adequate response is elicited: directions to state the object's function, clinician states the function, clinician states and demonstrates function, sentence completion, sentence completion plus the silently articulated first phoneme of the response, sentence completion plus the vocalized first sound, sentence completion plus the first two phonemes vocalized, and, finally, word repetition. When an adequate response is elicited, the order of cues is reversed until the patient names the picture without a cue. Linebaugh and Lehner presented data for several patients that demonstrate improved word retrieval and generalization to nontreatment words. Importantly, they indicate that cuing hierarchies must be individually determined.

A facilitory effect of semantic cues also seems to exist for on-line tasks (tasks in which the cues are not necessarily obvious to the patient). Chenery et al. (1990) studied patients' ability to recognize whether the second word in a pair of verbally presented words was real or nonsense when the first word was functionally related to the target (e.g., eat-knife), superordinally associated (e.g., cutlery-knife), unrelated (door-knife), or nonsense (e.g., lamiel-knife). Subjects were told to ignore the first word. All aphasic subjects, including a subgroup with severe comprehension and naming deficits, more accurately identified words as real in response to the functional and superordinate semantic primes than in the other priming conditions. This led to a conclusion that information is preserved in semantic memory in aphasia. (This on-line facilitation of semantic processing may partially explain why redundancy can facilitate sentence comprehension.)

Podraza and Darley (1977) investigated the effects of three types of prestimulation on picture naming in five aphasic patients. The prestimulus conditions (cues presented prior to picture presentation) included the first phoneme of the target word; an open-ended sentence; three words, one of which was the target word; and three semantically related words. Naming was generally facilitated by the phoneme, open-ended sentences, and three-words-containing-the-target-word cues, while performance decrements occurred for the three semantically related words cues. The facilitative failure of the semantically related word cues is in disagreement with the findings by Blumstein et al. (1982) and Weigl (1968) that such cues may serve a "deblocking function" and facilitate retrieval. Podraza and Darley (1977) suggest that their own patients may already have been operating in the appropriate "semantic field" (Goodglass and Baker, 1976) and that additional stimuli in that field may have served to confuse the selection of an appropriate response. Similarly, patients with Wernicke's aphasia, who frequently make phonemic errors, benefit less from phonemic cues than patients with other types of aphasia (Kohn and Goodglass, 1985).

Stimley and Noll (1991) examined naming accuracy in a group of aphasic patients when pictures were accompanied by a semantic cue (e.g., "this is something you wear on your foot," for "sock") or a phonemic cue (e.g., "This is something that starts with /s/," for "sock"). Compared with a no-cue condition, the semantic and phonemic cues both facilitated naming, although the average effect was only about 9%–10%. The authors thought the small effect may have been because cues were presented for all items, not just following failure to name without a cue. They also observed (as have others) that semantic errors were more frequent in the semantic cue condition and that phonemic errors were more frequent in the phonemic cue condition. (Li and Canter [1991] have made similar observations.) Thus, while semantic and phonemic cues are generally facilitory, they also tend to "move" errors toward the cuing category.

Some recent efforts have attempted to tailor the type of cue to the level at which naming tends to break down. Thompson et al. (1991) examined the effects of a phonemic cuing treatment program on two patients with Broca's aphasia whose naming deficits appeared to be related to phonological breakdowns (e.g., they had naming difficulties in spite of being able to

match spoken words to pictures and perform conceptual matching tasks; in other words, they appeared to have access to word meaning but not the phonological form of words). The program consisted primarily of providing a rhyming cue (e.g., "It sounds like mat," for the target "bat") or, if that failed, the first phoneme, whenever the patient failed to name without a cue. Both subjects improved in oral naming, and there was some generalization to untrained items and to oral reading tasks. Li and Williams (1989) examined the effect of semantic and phonemic cues on noun and verb naming after failure to name on picture confrontation. Patients with Broca's and conduction aphasia responded better to phonemic than semantic cues, and the opposite pattern occurred for patients with anomic aphasia. In general, phonemic cues were more effective than semantic cues for nouns, and the two cue types did not differ for verbs. This suggests that cue type effectiveness may vary as a function of both the source of naming failure (semantic versus phonological, presumably related to aphasia type) and word category (nouns versus verbs).

Are cues presented in combination more effective than single cues? Weidner and Jinks's (1983) findings say yes. They examined the naming performance of 24 patients who were presented with single cues (e.g., sentence completion, written words, first phoneme) or cues in combination. Combined cues were more facilitative than were single cues or single cues presented in succession. They suggest that if one cue fails, a combination of cues may help.

Finally, cuing also may facilitate sentence production. Roberts and Wertz (1986) used a contrastive task paradigm to facilitate sentence production in two chronic aphasic patients. After demonstrating comprehension of sentence meaning, patients imitated the clinician production of a sentence (e.g., "The bed is made") and then spontaneously produced a minimally contrasting sentence in response to a picture stimulus (e.g., "The bed is not made"). Imitation was then faded over additional steps to a point where patients had to produce on their own both contrasting sentences in response to picture stimuli. Both patients' sentence production improved, and there was evidence of some carryover to spontaneous sentence production.

It is reasonable to conclude that there are a large number of cues, prompts, and preparatory stimuli that may facilitate language processing in aphasia. Care must be taken to demonstrate the utility of cues in each case because even the most widely used facilitators may not be effective for every patient. Careful analysis of the level at which language tends to break down (e.g., semantic versus phonological) and the types of successful cues that patients adopt spontaneously can help identify the type of cuing likely to be most successful.

Frequency and Meaningfulness

It has been established repeatedly that the reduction of available vocabulary in aphasia is related to the frequency of occurrence of words in the language. Schuell (1969, 1974d) also predicted a reduction of available linguistic rules and a hierarchy for their recovery, and speculated that the hierarchy is related to the frequency of occurrence of those structures in general or individual language usage.

Schuell et al. (1961) tested the auditory comprehension of 48 aphasic patients in response to four word lists varying in frequency of occurrence. Decrements in performance as a function of decreasing word frequency were found, supporting the conclusion that word frequency is an important factor in comprehension. They also reported that single-word comprehension improves in an orderly and predictable manner that is strongly related to word frequency. Relatedly, Gerratt and Jones (1987), in a reaction time task, have shown that aphasic, like nonaphasic, individuals recognize words as real (versus nonsense) more rapidly when they have multiple meanings and high frequency of occurrence than when they have few meanings and low frequency of occurrence.

Word frequency remains a factor at the sentence level. Shewan and Canter (1971) found that increasing vocabulary difficulty (reducing word frequency) reduced the accuracy and promptness of sentence comprehension in aphasic patients. In addition, frequency of occurrence also applies to phrases and sentences as they occur as familiar units. For example, Van Lancker and Kempler (1987) have shown that aphasic patients comprehend familiar phrases (idiomatic expressions such as ''While the cat's away the mice will play'') more readily than novel sentences matched for word frequency, length, and structure.

Word frequency effects are also apparent in verbal output, reading, and writing. For example, Gardner (1973), Schuell et al. (1964), and Williams and Canter (1982) have reported negative correlations between errors on naming tests and frequency of occurrence; Siegel (1959) found that less frequently occurring words were more difficult to read than frequently occurring words; Bricker et al. (1964) reported that word frequency (and length) accounted for almost all aphasic spelling errors; and San Pietro and Rigrodsky (1982) found that verbal perseveration on naming and reading tasks increased as word frequency decreased.

Although word frequency is certainly positively correlated among speakers of the language, we need to bear in mind that word frequency for individuals is determined by their unique experiences, needs, occupation, culture, and numerous other factors (the word ''aphasia'' is certainly more available to the speech-language pathologist than it is to the political scientist!). Although word lists such as Thorndike and Lorge's (1944) are useful in selecting stimulus material, it is also important that we identify verbal stimuli that are meaningful, relevant, and personally significant to the individual (Schuell, 1969; Schuell et al., 1955; Wepman, 1953).

The importance of this was demonstrated by Wallace and Canter (1985), who examined severely impaired aphasic patients' responses to personally relevant versus nonpersonal stimuli on verbal and reading comprehension tasks (e.g., ''Is your birthday in ____?'' versus ''Is Christmas in February?''); repetition tasks (e.g., patient repeats his or her name versus another name); and naming tasks (e.g., television versus giraffe). Performance was better in response to personally relevant materials on all tasks, although the authors pointed out that personally relevant stimuli had a generally higher frequency of occurrence than nonpersonal material. Relatedly, Correia et al. (1989) asked if gender bias in pictures used to elicit narrative responses from male aphasic patients affects what they say about them. After having nonaphasic subjects identify picture stimuli as male or female biased (e.g., men working out in a gym versus women in a beauty salon), they used them to obtain narratives from aphasic and non-brain-damaged subjects. Subjects produced more words in response to male-biased stimuli,

but there were no differences in measures of efficiency or amount of information conveyed. The authors concluded that gender bias in picture stimuli is not of great concern (at least for males) unless the number of words in responses is important. Thus, some dimensions of personal relevance may or may not affect all dimensions of performance to the same or to an important degree.

The concept of meaningfulness is also tied to emotion and expectations. Reuterskiöld (1991) has demonstrated that patients with significant verbal comprehension deficits perform more adequately on single-word comprehension tasks when stimuli consist of objects and actions with emotional connotations (e.g., casket, kissing) than when they have no obvious emotional connotations (e.g., paper, typing). Graham et al. (1987) examined aphasic patients' comprehension in response to contextually relevant commands (e.g., ring the bell), contextually neutral commands (e.g., touch the bell), and contextually inappropriate commands (e.g., roll the bell). Contextually related tasks were easier than neutral or inappropriate ones, leading the authors to state that ''if we pair objects with actions that are most expected both in terms of meaning and structure, we facilitate comprehension'' (p. 183). Finally, Deloche and Seron (1981) and Kudo (1984) have established that comprehension is better when sentence meaning does not violate our knowledge of the world (e.g., ''The policeman arrests the thief'') than when meaning is implausible or unlikely (e.g., ''The thief arrests the policeman'').

Abstractness

It has been suggested that aphasic individuals have more difficulty with abstract than concrete words (Goldstein, 1948) and that they categorize words in a relatively concrete-emotional manner when compared with nonaphasic individuals (Zurif et al., 1974).

Two problems present themselves when the concept of abstractness arises. First, abstractness is strongly tied to—and difficult to separate from—frequency of occurrence (concrete words occur more frequently than abstract words). Spreen (1968), however, has pointed out that words scaled as abstract are not perceived or recalled as readily as words scaled as concrete even when frequency of occurrence is controlled. Halpern (1965a), controlling for frequency of occurrence, found that aphasic patients made more verbal errors in response to written words of high or medium abstractness than in response to words of low abstractness. Abstractness did not play a role in repetition of verbally presented stimuli, however.

The second problem is more relevant to stimulus selection and is related to the fact that abstractness is a difficult concept to define. Words, however, are scalable on an abstractness dimension (Darley et al., 1959), and Spreen (1968) has suggested that degree of abstractness can be related tangibly to sense experience (''book'' is more concrete than ''hope'' because it presumably generates more multimodality associations).

The performance of aphasic patients suggests that we should be aware of the abstractness factor when selecting and ordering stimulus material. Problems related to isolating and defining abstractness, however, present practical clinical problems. Fortunately, we probably account for most of the effects of abstractness when we account for the more easily defined concepts of word frequency and intersensory redundancy or operativity.

Part of Speech and Semantic Word Category

When word-retrieval and comprehension abilities are examined or treated at the single-word level, there is a marked tendency for clinicians to focus on nouns, particularly object-nouns. However, evidence makes it clear that all parts of speech and word categories are typically affected in aphasia. This speaks against an object-noun orientation to treatment.

Because different parts of speech (e.g., nouns versus verbs) serve different linguistic functions, it seems possible that, for some patients or under some circumstances, they may present differing levels of difficulty. For example, it has been fairly common for groups of aphasic patients to have less difficulty with objects (nouns) than actions (verbs) on picture-naming tasks (e.g., Williams and Canter, 1987; Zingeser and Berndt, 1990). In addition, where there is a discrepancy between nouns and verbs on synonym-generating and sentence generation tasks, the difference favors nouns over verbs (Kohn et al., 1989). Finally, that the processing of nouns versus verbs can differ is also supported by the finding of Li and Canter (1991) that aphasic patients responded better to phonemic than semantic cues for noun naming but that there was no difference between the cue types for verb naming; the authors thought that the greater concreteness, static nature, and imagability of nouns than verbs might explain some of the differences between them.

Differences may also exist for other word categories and tasks. Halpern (1965a) found that aphasic patients made more errors when repeating or reading adjectives and verbs than nouns. Siegel (1959) and Marshall and Newcombe (1966) reported similar findings for reading tasks. In contrast, Noll and Hoops (1967) did not find selective spelling difficulty among nouns, verbs, adjectives, and adverbs for a group of 25 patients, but did find that pronouns, prepositions, and conjunctions were more difficult than other parts of speech. Finally, Goodglass et al. (1970) found different comprehension patterns among Broca's, Wernicke's, and anomic patients across measures of receptive vocabulary (nouns and verbs) and measures of comprehension of directional and grammatical prepositions.

It appears that stimulus selection should consider possible differences among substantive word categories—such as nouns, verbs, and adjectives—with nouns likely to be easiest when word frequency is controlled. In general, the literature suggests that grammatical words—such as prepositions, conjunctions, and articles—are more difficult to comprehend for aphasic patients than substantive words (Lesser, 1978). Such differences should also be considered in stimulus selection.

The possibility that specific semantic word categories may be selectively impaired in aphasia is a matter of debate (see Lesser, 1978, pp. 97–107), but some studies suggest that semantic word categories should be considered for some patients. For example, Goodglass et al. (1966) assessed the naming and comprehension of objects, actions, letters, numbers, and colors in aphasic patients. Objects and actions were the easiest to comprehend and letters the most difficult, but objects were the most difficult to name and letters the easiest. This not only suggests differences among word categories but also implies that the difficulty of a particular category may vary between input and output tasks.

Although many investigators and clinicians argue convincingly against common or marked differences among semantic word categories, it does appear that stimuli restricted to a single semantic category (e.g., objects) occasionally may yield misleading diagnostic and treatment results; also, consideration of semantic category may lead to the identification of treatment stimuli with varying degrees of difficulty.

Grammar and Syntax

As noted earlier, Schuell hypothesized that there is a hierarchically based reduction of available linguistic rules in aphasia. While her idea that such a hierarchy is based on the frequency of occurrence of grammatical structures in general language usage is untested and perhaps overly simplistic in light of current linguistic theory, there is ample evidence that grammatical complexity is an important factor in language activities. In other words, as is true for intact language users, there is a grammatical hierarchy of difficulty for aphasic patients; some grammatical structures are more difficult to comprehend and produce than others. Grammar and syntax, therefore, are important variables to consider when devising language stimuli. Following is a sampling of the numerous studies that have examined the relationship between grammatical variations and performance in aphasia. For more information on these factors, see Chapters 9, 10 and 22 in this volume.

The importance of grammar is illustrated by the fact that, even when lexical comprehension is quite good, sentence interpretation may be impaired because of grammatical processing deficits. Caramazza and Zurif (1976), for example, have shown that some patients have problems when sentence comprehension is dependent on syntax rather than on the logical relations expressed by individual semantic elements. To illustrate, the meaning of the semantically constrained sentence, "The apple that the boy is eating is red," can be derived from an understanding of the meaning of its critical elements and the limited logical relationships that exist among them. That is, our knowledge of the world tells us it must be the boy who is eating and not the apple, and it must be the apple that is red. On the other hand, consider the requirements for accurate comprehension of the reversible sentence, "The girl that the boy is hitting is tall." Here, either the boy or the girl logically can do the hitting and either can be tall. Correct interpretation requires the appropriate pairing of boy with hitting and girl with tall, an interpretation arrived at only through adequate syntactic processing. Several studies have found that some patients have considerably more difficulty comprehending reversible sentences than semantically constrained ones, implying the presence of significant deficits in grammatical processing (Caramazza and Zurif, 1976; Kolk and Friederici, 1985; Sherman and Schweikert, 1989; Wulfeck, 1988).

There is ample additional evidence that sentences requiring structural-syntactic analysis are generally difficult for aphasic patients (usually regardless of aphasia type), and that sentence comprehension probably is maximized when interpretation can be based on world knowledge and the understanding of critical individual elements (e.g., see Ansell and Flowers, 1982a, 1982b; Blumstein et al., 1983; Caplan and Evans, 1990; Curtiss et al., 1986; Friederici, 1983; Gallaher, 1981; Gallaher and Canter, 1982; Mack, 1982; Parisi and Pizzamiglio, 1970; Peach et al., 1988). Constructing sentence stimuli with this in mind is of practical import for another reason; Gallaher and Canter (1982) suggest that the syntactic impact on comprehension in *real life* may be minimal because much of what is said in everyday communication can be interpreted on the basis of real-world knowledge and comprehension of lexical items, with grammar and syntax providing largely redundant information.

It is apparent that demands for processing of grammar and syntax should not and cannot be avoided entirely. There are a number of studies that provide very useful information about the relative processing ease or difficulty of a variety of grammatical and syntactic devices for aphasic patients. The following represent a sampling of these findings:

1. Present-tense sentences are easier than past- or future-tense sentences (Naeser et al., 1987; Parisi and Pizzamiglio, 1970; Pierce, 1981). When tense changes, the use of an additional tense marker tends to facilitate tense comprehension (e.g., "The man has caught the ball" should be easier than "The man caught the ball"; "The man has already combed his hair" should be easier than "the man has combed his hair"). Words like "yesterday" and "tomorrow" also help to mark tense (Ansell and Flowers, 1982b; Pierce, 1981, 1982, 1983).
   The distinction discussed in the preceding paragraph is one example of what seems to be a fairly consistent hierarchy of syntactic difficulty that can affect comprehension. For example, gender, negative/affirmative, and singular/plural distinctions tend to be easier than past/present, subject/object, and past, future/present distinctions. Within distinctions, the marked features tend to be more difficult; for example, negative is more difficult than affirmative, plural more difficult than singular, and future and past more difficult than present tense (Lesser, 1974; Naeser et al., 1987; Parisi and Pizzamiglio, 1970).

2. Other morphological distinctions can also affect comprehension. For example, Goodglass and Hunt (1958) examined the ability of aphasic patients to comprehend and express noun plurals and possessives that are represented by identical phonological forms (e.g., horses-horse's). Expressively, patients made many more errors on possessive endings than on plurals. Receptively, the same pattern was noted with the additional observation that third-person singular verbs also generated more errors than plurals. Goodglass and Berko (1960) have reported similar error patterns. Goodglass (1968) indicated that such patterns of deficit are independent of form of aphasia (nonfluent versus fluent) and, therefore, are not just specific to patients who are labeled "agrammatical." At the same time, it is important to keep in mind that syntactic deficits in aphasia are not an all-or-none phenomenon. The deficits typically encountered are relative, not absolute, and aphasic patients (even "agrammatical" ones) are often able to process a good deal of syntactic information (Baum, 1989).

3. Aphasic patients tend to use an active subject-verb-object (SVO) strategy for processing sentences and find active sentences easier to comprehend than other forms. In general, this means that sentences in which the order of mention reflects the agent-action-object relationship (e.g., "The mother kissed the baby") are easier than when word order does not reflect that relationship (e.g., "The policeman was punched by the robber") (Ansell and Flowers, 1982b; Brookshire and Nicholas, 1980, 1981; Friederici and Graetz, 1987; Grossman and Haberman, 1982; Lasky et al., 1976; Pierce, 1983; Shewan and Canter, 1971). As mentioned above, SVO sentences that are nonreversible are easier than reversible sentences.

4. Aphasic patients tend to have more difficulty processing grammatically encoded (compact) sentences (e.g., "The man greeted by his wife was smoking a pipe" or "The woman was taller than the man") than sentences that are simplified syntactically by expansion into a series of propositions (e.g., "The man was greated by his wife and he was smoking a pipe" or "The woman was tall and the man was short") (Goodglass et al., 1970; Nicholas and Brookshire, 1983). These findings demonstrate that sentence comprehension is not simply a function of amount of information and length, because compact and expanded sentences can contain the same amount of information and easier-to-comprehend sentences can be longer than compact ones. Results like these also highlight the complexity of the interactions among stimulus factors and show that maximizing the facilitory effect of one factor may increase the difficulty imposed by another; for example, the generally desirable strategy of reducing sentence length may necessitate a generally undesirable increase in syntactic complexity. In addition, it has become evident that factors influencing sentence comprehension do not have the same effects on discourse comprehension and that performance on sentence-level material does not always predict discourse comprehension (Brookshire and Nicholas, 1984) (for further discussion, see section on context).

5. Syntactic context, or the form in which sentence-level tasks are expressed, can influence response appropriateness, if not accuracy. For example, Green and Boller (1974) evaluated auditory comprehension in severe aphasia by testing differences in response to commands, yes/no questions, and information questions when such tasks were directly worded (e.g., "Point to the ceiling"), indirectly worded (e.g., "I would like you to point to the ceiling"), or directly worded but preceded by an introductory sentence (e.g., "Here's something. Point to the ceiling"). Commands constituted the easiest task, followed by yes/no questions and the information questions. The various syntactic contexts did not affect response accuracy, but directly worded items were associated with a greater number of appropriate (relevant, although incorrect) responses than were indirectly worded items. Directly worded items preceded by an introductory sentence were easier than indirectly worded items.

It is clear that a number of syntactic and grammatical factors may influence comprehension, repetition, and verbal formulation performance. It also appears that the hierarchy of difficulty for a number of syntactic and grammatical tasks is fairly stable across patients with different types of aphasia. Because variations in the grammatical and syntactic complexity of language have such effects, they should be accounted for when structuring stimulation for treatment purposes.

Context

In recent years, there has been a surge of interest in aphasic patients' discourse comprehension and expression, the factors that influence discourse comprehension and expression, and the relationship of discourse to word- and sentence-level abilities. Findings indicate that word and sentence comprehension do not predict very well the comprehension of discourse (Brookshire and Nicholas, 1984; Hough, 1990; Hough et al., 1989; Pashek and Brookshire, 1982; Stachowiak et al., 1977; Waller and Darley, 1978) and that discourse comprehension is often better than single-sentence comprehension. Brookshire (1992) points out that because communication in daily life usually occurs more in the form of connected speech than as single sentences, it may be that measures of sentence comprehension underestimate daily life comprehension competence.

It appears that context, redundancy, predictability, and extralinguistic cues within discourse and conversation facilitate communication for aphasic patients. The following summary represents a sampling of findings from studies of aphasic patients' comprehension and expression of language in discourse or natural communicative contexts. They provide clues for the design of intervention tasks that, for some patients, may be easier than shorter and apparently simpler word- and single-sentence-level activities:

1. Comprehension of syntactically complex sentences (e.g., reversible passive sentences) is facilitated when preceded or followed by contextually relevant sentences containing semantic or syntactic information that predicts the relationship expressed in the target sentence (Boyle and Canter, 1986; Cannito et al., 1989; Pierce, 1988; Waller and Darley, 1978). (An example of a prior facilitative context task is, "The girl is on the ground. The girl was tripped by the boy. Who was tripped?" An example of a subsequent facilitative context task is, "The woman went to the library. She returned a book. Where did the woman go?" [Pierce, 1988].) Some studies also show that the context that precedes or follows a target sentence may not have to predict specific information as long as it facilitates the processing of the target information by, for example, identifying the topic, setting, or theme (Cannito et al., 1986; Hough et al., 1989). (But Cannito et al. [1989] found that nonpredictive context did not facilitate comprehension of target sentences.) Extralinguistic context, in the form of a picture depicting target sentence information, also facilitates comprehension (Pierce and Beekman, 1985), although Waller and Darley (1978) found that the facilitory effect of a contextual picture was less powerful than verbal context. Pierce (1991) has pointed out that these facilitory effects are most apparent for patients with relatively poor comprehension. The benefits of this kind of contextual cue seem to derive from redundancy or the fact that certain events or relationships are made more plausible than others.

2. Predictability provided by discourse may explain why it is comprehended better than sentences. Armus et al. (1989) found that mild-moderate aphasic patients' knowledge of scripts is not significantly compromised (scripts are used to organize common situations; for example, after repeatedly eating in restaurants we "know" the events that usually occur). Thus, if a patient has an internalized script for a discourse event, it may allow him or her to predict what will happen next, infer what is not stated, and organize it for recall. The authors suggest that scripts may be used in treatment to facilitate comprehension, with fading of the degree to which discourse follows a script when comprehension improves.

3. Aphasic patients comprehend implied meanings quite well, especially in situations aided by extralinguistic context. In fact, Foldi (1987) reported that aphasic individuals, like non-brain-injured people, tend to prefer the pragmatic interpretation of indirect requests over the literal interpretation. Wilcox et al. (1978) presented videotaped "natural" situations to patients in which the correct interpretation of an utterance was the meaning conveyed by the request in a particular context; for example, while the literal interpretation of "Can you move the table?" simply requires a yes/no response, the indirect, conveyed/contextual meaning is a request that the table be moved. Aphasic patients generally performed similarly to normal controls in their ability to use extralinguistic cues to comprehend the intent conveyed in many indirect requests. These results suggest that the use of natural communicative contexts in treatment may raise communicative performance over and above that derived from more traditional, relatively pure linguistic tasks that often intentionally minimize extralinguistic cues.
   It also appears that linguistic information may help some patients appreciate the meaning of extralinguistic information. For example, Tompkins (1991) found that increased semantic redundancy facilitated the interpretation of emotions that were conveyed linguistically or prosodically to aphasic patients.

4. Aphasic patients have been shown to comprehend main ideas expressed in discourse—the most salient information—better than details, and information that is expressed directly better than information that must be inferred (Katsuki-Nakamura et al., 1988; Nicholas and Brookshire, 1986a). Of interest, increasing directness and salience (through repetition or elaboration) seems to be a more reliable way to improve discourse comprehension than decreasing speech rate. Nicholas and Brookshire (1986b) have also shown that

the advantage of directly expressed information over that requiring inference is maintained in multiple-sentence-reading tests.

5. Context can facilitate performance in certain word-retrieval tasks. Hough (1989) and Hough and Pierce (1989) have shown this effect for tasks requiring generation of words in ad hoc categories, categories that are constructed for use in specialized contexts (e.g., things not to eat on a diet). Significantly, more items were generated when contextual vignettes preceded ad hoc category tasks (e.g., before listing things to take on a picnic, the patient heard "Sam wanted to spend time outdoors. It was a beautiful day so he packed up some items and went to a nearby park") than when they did not. The facilitative effect of context was not found for common categories (e.g., foods). Hough and Pierce (1989) suggest that ad hoc category tasks may be useful for aphasic patients because they are more divergent in nature and allow reliance on experience and world knowledge to a greater extent than do common category tasks.

6. Methods used to elicit narrative discourse from aphasic patients have variable effects. For example, picture sequences representing stories generally lead to a greater number of words in narratives than do single pictured scenes, but the two types of stimuli generally do not affect other measures of production differently (Bottenberg et al., 1987). Gender bias of pictures (e.g., men in a gym versus women in a beauty salon) may result in differences in number of words and information but does not affect words per minute or efficiency, at least in males (Correia et al., 1990).

7. Main ideas are expressed to a proportionately greater degree than are details when stories are retold (Ernest-Baron et al., 1987). This may explain why patients get along reasonably well in daily life; it is usually main ideas that must be recalled rather than details.

8. Situational context may affect the manner in which aphasic patients respond. Glosser et al. (1988) reported that, in spite of their linguistic deficits, aphasic patients showed appropriate and predictable changes in response to nonlinguistic social contextual variables (e.g., face-to-face conversation versus telephone versus conversation over video monitors). In contrast, Brenneise-Sarshad et al. (1991) found few meaningful differences in the verbal output of aphasic patients when they narrated a sequenced picture story for a listener known to them who looked at the pictures as the story was being told versus a newly introduced person who could not see the picture stimuli. The authors thought that it may not be important to create treatment situations in which the patient believes the listener is naive to the information in order to obtain valid measures of communicative effectiveness.

In summary, the contextual information provided within discourse and natural communicative contexts can exert significant facilitative effects on language and communication for patients with aphasia. These effects not only occur for the processing of the main ideas and intents expressed in discourse but also extend "backward" to the comprehension and expression of semantic and syntactic relationships expressed within the context of discourse. It is clear that discourse tasks, particularly comprehension tasks, need not await recovery of word and sentence comprehension ability to become a focus of treatment. In fact, in some instances it appears that discourse should precede word- and sentence-level tasks in the treatment hierarchy.

Stress

In spite of some evidence that aphasic patients may be deficient in their ability to derive meaning from information provided by vocal stress (Baum et al., 1982), it appears that stress can influence response adequacy in a positive way. For example, Swinney et al. (1980) have shown that aphasic patients respond more rapidly to stressed than unstressed words. More important, Kimelman and McNeil (1987) and Pashek and Brookshire (1982) found improved paragraph comprehension when exaggerated stress on critical words was employed. Pashek and Brookshire observed that improved comprehension in response to exaggerated stress was independent of improvement induced by slow rate, suggesting that slowed rate and exaggerated stress may be additive facilitators of auditory comprehension. More recently, Kimelman and McNeil (1989) showed that aphasic patients' comprehension of normally stressed target words in paragraphs is better when preceded by stressed as opposed to normally stressed context. The magnitude of the facilitative effect was greater for more severely impaired patients, those individuals most likely to need extralinguistic cues for comprehension. Finally, Kimelman (1991) has presented data that suggest that the facilitative effect of stressing target words may actually derive from changes in duration and fundamental frequency in the context preceding the target word. Thus, it may be contextual stress modifications that alert the listener to the salience of the target word.

Eliminating consideration of information strongly associated with melodic intonation therapy (MIT) (see Chapter 19 in this volume), the most representative study on stress and speech output in aphasia has been conducted by Goodglass et al. (1967). They found that fluent and nonfluent patients omitted initial unstressed function words much more frequently than initial stressed words in a sentence repetition task. The omission of unstressed words occurred more frequently for nonfluent patients. They also found that the stress pattern /-/ was easier to repeat than any other three-word pattern tested, when a function word was in the first or second position. Moreover, the facilitative effect of this stress pattern seemed to override grammatical complexity. For example, the negative interrogative "Can't you swim?" (/-/) was easier to repeat than the grammatically simpler "Can you swim?" (-//). The authors thought that nonfluent (and, therefore, usually apraxic) patients, in particular, may depend on stress features in order to initiate and maintain a flow of speech. Goodglass (1968) interpreted these and similar findings as supportive of the importance of "saliency" in the initiation of speech. That is, for many patients there is a need for a salient word in order to initiate speech, saliency being characterized by stress and phonological prominence, as well as other factors, already discussed, such as informational and personal significance.

The clinical implications of these findings are obvious. The selection of sentence and paragraph material for comprehension and repetition tasks should consider stress-saliency as a variable capable of affecting the verbal comprehension and verbal production of aphasic patients.

Order of Difficulty

Within a given treatment task, stimuli probably should be ordered so that more difficult items are presented last. This recommendation is based on evidence that suggests that success tends to breed success and failure breeds failure for patients with aphasia.

Brookshire (1972) studied the effects of task difficulty on naming behavior in nine patients. A group of easy-to-name and a group of hard-to-name pictures were derived from baseline measures for each patient and were subsequently presented in different orders. When easy pictures preceded hard pictures, responses to hard pictures were better than predicted by baseline measures. When easy pictures followed hard pictures, performance on easy pictures was poorer than expected on the basis of baseline measures. Brookshire speculated that when a patient experiences a high proportion of failures, emotional responses may be generated that disrupt subsequent responses. Although such negative effects tended to decay over time, he suggested that treatment should keep error rates low and that easy items should precede difficult ones. Brookshire (1976b) subsequently demonstrated very similar task difficulty effects for a sentence comprehension task in a group of 22 patients. The results differed from the study on naming only in that easy items facilitated comprehension on subsequent hard items for only a small number of patients.

Support for an order effect can be found in several other studies. Gardner and Brookshire (1972) found that naming performance under unisensory conditions often is facilitated when preceded by a generally easier auditory-visual stimulus condition, and that responses to auditory-visual stimuli are reduced when preceded by a generally more difficult visual stimulus condition. Similarly, Brookshire (1971b) found that forcing subjects to respond at rapid rates depresses performance on subsequent items in which they are given more time to respond. Finally, Brookshire and Lommel (1974) reported on the disruptive effects of failure on aphasic and nonaphasic brain-injured subjects' performance on a nonverbal sequencing task.

Dumond et al. (1978) questioned (or qualified) the significance of the order effect. They readministered the PICA to 20 patients in split-half form, with the 18 subtests rearranged in two orders of difficulty—one ascending and one descending. No performance differences were found between the two orders of difficulty. In contrasting their results with those of Brookshire (1972), they pointed out that he examined a single task containing items of varying difficulty, while they examined differences across tasks containing items of equal difficulty. They also indicated that "the changes in difficulty level between subtests were apparently less extensive than the changes in difficulty level within Brookshire's experiment" (p. 358) and that this may have reduced subjects' perception of their performance adequacy. They concluded that presenting PICA-like tasks in order of increasing difficulty is not likely to adversely affect performance on nonevaluative tasks whose difficulty levels do not vary extensively.

The available data appear to warrant the following generalizations regarding order of presentation during treatment: Error rates should be kept low; stimulus presentation generally should proceed from easiest to hardest, particularly within a given task and on tasks in which the patient is likely to be most sensitive to performance inadequacies; if error rates are kept low, potential across-task order effects should be minimized. (In line with these generalizations, Crosky and Adams [1969] present some practical procedures for selecting and ordering vocabulary stimulus materials for individual patients.) Finally, it is reasonable to follow Brookshire's (1992) suggestion that sessions begin with familiar, easy tasks; proceed to less familiar and more difficult ones; and end with tasks that result in a great deal of success.

Psychological and Physical Factors

In addition to stimuli that are directly intended to stimulate language, factors that affect the psychological and physical "set" of patients can influence response adequacy.

Skelly's (1975) interviews with aphasic patients indicate that even relatively subtle signs of disinterest or impatience on the part of the clinician "bothers" patients. Stoicheff (1960) found that the overt attitudes expressed during instructions to patients can significantly affect responses. Using three groups of aphasic patients, she examined the effects of encouraging, discouraging, and neutral instructions and comments during performance on naming, reading, and self-evaluation tasks. After 3 days of exposure to one of the conditions, the self-evaluation, naming, and reading performance of the group receiving the discouraging instructions was lower than the performance of the groups receiving neutral or encouraging instructions. No differences were found between the encouraging and neutral conditions. Obviously, the performance differences were attributed to the negative effects of discouraging instructions. Finally, the previously discussed findings of Brookshire and his colleagues on the effects of order of stimulus difficulty suggest that failure, or stress induced by failure, may produce emotional responses that disrupt subsequent responses. It seems, therefore, that disruptive psychological effects may result from negative attitudes expressed by the clinician during instructions and performance, or from the failures that the patient may experience during the course of a treatment session.

The effects of physical fatigue on language performance have been examined by Marshall and King (1973). Subjects were given the PICA following a period of isokinetic exercise and, on another day, following rest. PICA scores were significantly lower following exercise than following rest for verbal, graphic, and overall PICA measures. Fatigue had its most pronounced effect on speaking and writing tasks. The authors suggested that language therapy be scheduled prior to physical exertion, such as physical or occupational therapy. In another study that probably reflects the cumulative effects of fatigue over the course of a day, Marshall et al. (1980) found that aphasic patients did better on assessment measures administered in the morning than in the afternoon.

It seems that psychological and physical factors facilitate performance best when treatment is conducted in a positive, encouraging, success-producing milieu and at a time when the patient's physical status during the treatment day is optimal.

Pattern of Auditory Deficit

Auditory impairments are not uniform and may reflect a number of different underlying problems. As a result, to ignore differences in the auditory deficits of aphasic patients is to ignore a factor that may bear on the way we structure auditory stimulation in treatment. Consideration of such differences may help identify stimulus factors that are especially important for a given patient and, in some cases, may serve to qualify or alter the generalizations and recommendations that have been made about those factors thus far.

Brookshire (1974) summarized and discussed five kinds of auditory deficits whose characteristics may have an important bearing on treatment planning. They reflect the need to avoid considering auditory deficits in aphasia as a unitary problem.

These deficits and implications for stimulus selection are discussed in the following sections.

Slow Rise Time. Patients whose auditory systems are characterized by slow rise time tend to miss the initial portion of incoming messages. They may be able to repeat or comprehend only the last part of sentences, may miss short messages entirely, or may do better on the final items of a subtest or treatment activity than on initial items. Brookshire suggests that the use of warning signals prior to presenting auditory stimuli may facilitate processing for these patients. Loverso and Prescott (1981) provide some indirect support for this. They found response times of aphasic subjects on a same-different visual judgment task to be reduced when the visual stimuli were preceded by a half-second warning tone; maximum benefit was derived when the tone preceded the stimulus by 1.5 seconds. Presenting items with gradually increasing intervals between successive items may also help the patient keep his or her "processor" active over longer intervals or help activate the processor more quickly.

Patients with slow rise time illustrate the fact that generalizations about a number of stimulus factors do not always hold. For example, contrary to "average" performance, the patient with slow rise time may respond better to redundant sentences than to single words, or may respond more appropriately to directly worded input preceded by an introductory sentence than to a directly worded sentence alone.

Noise Buildup. Patients with noise buildup tend to respond more accurately to the initial portion of auditory messages than to following portions. More complex material tends to produce noise more rapidly than less complex material. Such patients may not be able to repeat or comprehend the final portion of sentences, may make more errors on complex than simple materials, and may deteriorate progressively across items on a particular task. Brookshire suggests that they may benefit from a program with messages of gradually increasing length and complexity, with gradually decreasing silent intervals between successive items.

Retention Deficit. Patients with retention deficits also deteriorate as length increases, but they are not as susceptible to complexity factors as are those with noise buildup. Performance breakdown tends to occur at the same point in all messages regardless of complexity. The important treatment consideration here is to increase message length gradually.

Information Capacity Deficit. Patients with information capacity deficit do not seem able to receive and process information at the same time (see Wepman [1972] for a discussion of the "shutter principle"). In such cases, performance may be alternately good or poor within a message—good for information that is received and can be acted on, and poor for information directed at the system while processing of prior stimuli is taking place. Such patients may, for example, be able to repeat the beginning and end of a sequence of words but not the middle elements. Brookshire suggests that these patients may benefit from the insertion of pauses within messages. Such pauses may initially be frequent and of relatively long duration, with fading of their frequency and duration as processing ability improves.

Intermittent Auditory Imperception. Patients with this problem constitute a separate category in Schuell's system of classification. Their auditory-processing ability appears to fade in and out randomly, leading to sporadic and unpredictable performance. Because we do not understand the controlling factors in such a problem, Brookshire recommends that treatment be directed to other areas of deficit.

Brookshire points out that the above categories may be simplistic and incomplete, although the existence of several of them appears to have been verified by other investigators (McNeil and Hageman, 1979; Porch, 1967; Schuell et al., 1964). It is quite probable, however, that they exist in varying combinations within many patients and are seen atypically in pure form. Regardless, the ability to recognize them when they occur has direct implications for the selection of potent stimulus factors when planning treatment.

Response Considerations

Although the emphasis of the stimulation approach is on input to the patient, it is obvious that the effectiveness of such stimulation can be assessed only if responses are elicited. Regardless of the form of response, three of the general principles of remediation stated earlier are relevant to response considerations: (a) there should be a response to each stimulus, (b) responses should not be forced, and (c) a maximum number of responses should be elicited. To those we can add one additional principle—response demands generally should proceed from short to long. Just as length is a potent stimulus factor, it is also a potent response factor for most patients, with short responses nearly always easier than long ones. In addition to these principles, certain other response considerations must be addressed when planning treatment.

Response Mode

Decisions regarding the mode of response are based on specific goals and baseline data. For example, if we wish to improve auditory comprehension or retention, we should place minimal demands on output and let baseline data aid us in selecting the most intact mode of response. If the goal is to improve spoken language ability, then the response mode has already been determined by the chosen goal.

Sometimes response adequacy in a particular modality can be facilitated by a simultaneous response in another modality. For example, Hanlon et al. (1990) found that patients with anterior lesions, hemiparesis, and Broca's aphasia named pictures more adequately when they simultaneously attempted to point to the picture with their hemiparetic right arm. (Note that this may represent facilitation of problems more related to apraxia of speech than to language per se.)

Output modes usually include pointing, nodding, object or picture manipulation, pantomime, other gestures, speech, and writing. "Point-to" tasks are used frequently when treatment focuses on auditory processes because the motor control of simple pointing responses usually is unimpaired. However, Brookshire (1992) observes that such tasks can be relatively difficult for some patients. Such observations reinforce the need for letting the individual patient's abilities determine the mode of response.

Temporal Relationship

The temporal relationship between stimulus and response should be considered. Responses may be elicited in unison with a stimulus, immediately following a stimulus, or after a delay. Patients also may be asked to repeat a response consecutively.

Unison responses may be especially appropriate for severely impaired patients because they give simultaneous auditory and visual feedback and are a step down the response hierarchy from repetition (Schuell et al., 1955; Wertz, 1978). Although immediate responses represent the most frequent and desirable temporal relationship, they may impose unreasonable demands on some patients; requiring rapid responses may depress performance adequacy for some patients. In such cases, allowing a delay for processing may be very useful. Marshall (1976), for example, found that delay was the most effective response "strategy" employed by aphasic patients for word retrieval.

How much delay? Schuell et al. (1964) suggested 60 seconds for some tasks. Brookshire (1971b) found that 30 seconds were better than 0, 5, or 10 seconds on an object-naming task but noted that when patients were able to name objects they usually did so within 10 seconds. It seems that delays allowed for processing rarely should have to exceed 30 seconds, and probably should not, considering the principle that treatment should elicit a large number of responses.

On comprehension tasks the effect of imposing delays between stimulus and response may not be predictable. Schulte (1986) examined 10 aphasic patients' comprehension on a Token Test type of task in which 0-, 5-, 10-, and 20-second delays were imposed before patients were allowed to look at response choices and respond. No consistent effects on comprehension were found among the delay conditions for the group as a whole, but performance within subjects varied by nearly 20% between some conditions, and a few of the more severely impaired patients benefited from brief delays in some conditions. Schulte suggested that, for some patients, imposed delay may facilitate full processing before a response but that it may be detrimental for others because of poor rehearsal mechanisms or reduced retention capacity. It therefore appears that imposing a delay between stimulus presentation and response has no generally predictable influence on sentence comprehension accuracy, but that it may be a useful response parameter if its effects are predictable for individual patients.

In addition to using delay as an aid to comprehension or formulation, imposing delays before allowing the patient to respond may be a useful strategy for improving retention span. Imposing a delay between a patient's response and the next stimulus also may be an effective strategy for reducing perseveration in some patients. San Pietro and Rigrodsky (1982) found that the frequency of perseveration on sentence completion, naming, and reading tasks decreased as the time between a response and subsequent stimulus increased from 1 second to 10 seconds.

Delay sometimes can be used actively by patients to improve response adequacy (this point could also be considered under the section dealing with consequences/feedback). Berstein-Ellis et al. (1987) taught a mildly impaired aphasic patient with reduced conversational fluency (because of hesitation, revisions, and paraphasias) to use a pacing board (Helm, 1979) to slow speech rate. This reduced syntactic and paraphasic errors and permitted the same or more information to be conveyed with fewer verbalizations. Whitney and Goldstein (1989) used a different technique and achieved the same result for three mildly aphasic patients whose discourse was dysfluent because of revisions, repetitions, and audible pauses. After learning to recognize and identify their dysfluencies from audiorecorded samples of their speech, the patients were trained to monitor/identify their dysfluencies during picture description tasks. This resulted in reduced speech rate, a dramatic reduction of dysfluencies, and increased efficiency in the form of increased length of uninterrupted utterances.

Finally, there are some subtle uses of temporal relationships in stimulus presentation that may influence processing demands and response adequacy. Brookshire and Nicholas (1980) have shown that aphasic patients tend to use a find-and-compare strategy on sentence verification tasks in which the truth value of a sentence is based on a comparison with a simultaneously presented picture stimulus; that is, instead of processing the full meaning of the sentence, they may simply match key words to elements in the picture. To force the patient to deal with the fuller meaning of the sentence, they suggest that the spoken sentence and the picture stimulus presentations be staggered (e.g., present sentence and then present picture) rather than simultaneous. It is quite possible that this more challenging approach to stimulus presentation in a verification task would also apply to point-to comprehension tasks (i.e., present sentence and then present picture choices).

Response Characteristics

Although accuracy is certainly the most commonly expected response characteristic, it is not the only relevant one. Green and Boller (1974) found that severely impaired patients, unable to respond very accurately to auditory tasks, often are able to respond appropriately; that is, they show signs of rudimentary comprehension by, for example, looking around the room when asked to point to the door, or nodding when asked yes/no questions. In such cases, appropriateness of response may be the most appropriate initial response expectation. At the other end of the continuum, when a patient can respond with a relatively high degree of accuracy, it may be appropriate to expect a reduction of self-corrections and of incomplete, delayed, or distorted responses. (Such response characteristics are reflected in Porch's multidimensional scoring scale and are discussed in Chapter 18 in this volume.) The important point is that response expectations need not be geared solely to accuracy. For some patients, a high degree of accuracy may not be possible and expectations may have to be lowered; for others, a high proportion of accurate responses may still leave considerable room for response refinement along a number of other response dimensions.

Consequences (Feedback)

The stimulation approach presumes that the stimulus (antecedent event) is that part of the treatment sequence that facilitates, or is largely responsible for, the ability of the patient to respond adequately. This is in contrast to operant approaches, in which increased adequacy of responses is attributed primarily to the controlling influence of consequences on subsequent behavior. Because antecedents are theoretically the crucial modifier of language processing in the stimulation approach, however, does not mean that we should not respond to patient behavior.

It has already been stated that feedback about response accuracy and appropriateness should be given when appropriate. Boone (1967) suggests that any specific response-contingent

feedback may be trivial or unnecessary when patients are motivated (as is usually the case), know the target response, and can assess their response in relation to the target. Support for this comes from the finding that mild to moderately impaired aphasic patients modify their picture descriptions in response to failure in a referential communication task in the same way nonaphasic speakers do. In the relatively rare case where a patient is not motivated, response contingent rewards or punishment may be necessary; but, in general, reinforcement or punishment has little effect on speech and language performance in aphasia (Brookshire, 1977). When patients are motivated but give deficient responses, it may be most appropriate to confirm response adequacy or give information about the closeness of a response to the target. Whether feedback is in the form of reward, punishment, confirmation, or information, Brookshire's (1971a) finding that markedly-to-severely impaired patients were sensitive to the effects of short delays between responses and their consequences on a nonlanguage learning task implies that feedback, when appropriate, should be immediate.

What information should be given to patients when their responses are inadequate? First, in most instances, such information should not be negative. Stoicheff's (1960) findings suggest that discouraging comments during performance, such as "That's wrong," at least when combined with discouraging instructions, have a detrimental effect on performance. Second, Schuell et al. (1964) thought that one of the most common errors made by clinicians was overcorrection or overexplanation of errors, and that the proper contingency for an inadequate response is usually more stimulation. In support of this, Holland and Sonderman (1974), in their evaluation of an auditory comprehension program, thought that explaining errors to patients confused rather than aided subsequent performance. Brookshire and Nicholas' (1978) analysis of clinical interactions in aphasia treatment indicated that patients tend to make errors following corrective explanations of previous errors. It seems that confirmation of adequate performance may be helpful and encouraging and generally represents good clinical practice. Explanation and correction, on the other hand, should be carefully controlled and concise, bearing in mind that such feedback may be of little value, may waste time, and may be counterproductive.

In addition to response-dependent feedback, general encouragement and reassurance during a treatment session is always desirable. Brookshire (1992) supports the value of showing patients their progress over time, with graphs often being an effective format for doing so. Such feedback—aside from being information the patient has a right to know about—has motivational and reinforcement functions and provides a framework for discussing and/or supporting the continuation, alteration, or termination of certain treatment activities.

Sequencing Steps in the Treatment Program

Where to Start

Schuell et al. (1964) indicated that treatment should begin where language breaks down and should proceed through gradually increasing levels of difficulty. Bollinger and Stout (1976), arguing for the critical importance of stimulation in treatment, suggested that treatment should progress from highly clinician-cued antecedent events to low cued events in which the patient carries most of the processing load. Brookshire (1992) offers some more specific suggestions regarding starting points, which can be summarized as follows.

1. Treatment should begin at levels where slight deficiencies exist and never where performance is completely inadequate. This assures that patients are not pushed beyond their capacity but forces them to work near capacity.
2. Tasks where 60–80% of responses are correct and immediate represent good starting points. That is, not more than 20%–40% of responses should be self-corrected or delayed.
3. Tasks should not be too easy. Difficulty should be increased when 90% or more of responses are completely adequate in the dimensions that are the focus of treatment.

The selection of appropriate starting points should be based on adequate baseline data, for without such information, treatment begins without knowing if tasks or stimuli are appropriate. Baseline data may be established through standardized tests, systematic sampling of patients' responses to their environment (this is critical for the establishment of relevant, practical tasks and stimuli) or selected stimuli, or probing of variations in stimuli to see how changes influence speech and language behavior (Hendrick et al., 1973). For example, standardized testing may indicate that the ability to identify objects named from among 10 choices is very adequate (e.g., 90% immediate, accurate responses) but that identifying objects by function from among 10 choices is below the level at which treatment would be appropriate (e.g., 50% inaccurate responses). Subsequent assessment of responses to functional items might confirm standardized results, but probing might establish that identifying those same objects by function from among only four choices generates response characteristics at a level appropriate for treatment (e.g., 80% accurate with 20% delayed or self-corrected responses). Such baseline data identify a starting point for stimulating auditory abilities, specify the stimulus conditions and response expectations to be employed during treatment, and give direction about the organization of succeeding steps. No less important is the fact that baseline data provide a pretreatment measure of ability against which the results of treatment can be compared.

Criteria for Determining Success

Once tasks and stimuli have been established and target behaviors or response characteristics have been identified, we must determine the criterion for acceptable performance for each task. When this criterion is reached, it is assumed that the specific task is no longer necessary and that the patient is ready to move on to tasks with greater demands. Experienced clinicians agree that a target behavior criterion of 90% is generally appropriate (Brookshire, 1992; LaPointe, 1977). LaPointe also suggests that the criterion be maintained for three consecutive sessions before terminating the task to ensure that the behavior is stable. When a patient's performance plateaus at a level below the criterion for a number of sessions, he suggests that the task be terminated or modified to make it slightly easier.

Compatibility of the Stimulation Approach and Programming

The discussion of the design of intervention has included information about stimulus and response considerations, contin-

gencies, the selection of starting points, and progression of activities. The acquisition of baseline data and the setting of criterion levels also have been highlighted. All of these considerations can be strongly associated with programmed approaches to treatment. This may be somewhat surprising because the appearance of information about the stimulation approach and programmed approach to treatment in the same discussion has been typically in the form of contrast (e.g., see Darley [1975], and Sarno [1974]). Although operant-programmed approaches are dissimilar to the stimulation approach because of their emphasis on consequences as the primary modifiers of behavior, it is inappropriate to consider the stimulation approach and the application of general programming principles as mutually exclusive treatment strategies (LaPointe, 1978b). A careful reading of Schuell's work shows that her principles and suggestions regarding treatment are compatible with the rigor and systematic nature of programming. Her admonitions to choose realistic goals, know where performance breaks down, elicit large numbers of responses, work systematically, and discard techniques when they aren't working are things that a systematic, behavioral approach to programming is highly capable of assisting. It seems most appropriate, in this context, to consider programming as a tool for systematically implementing the stimulation approach. Programming is particularly desirable because of its commitment to accountability and its capacity for making treatment replicable and accessible to analysis (Holland, 1975; LaPointe, 1983). LaPointe's (1977) "Base-10 Programmed Stimulation" and Bollinger and Stout's (1976) "Response-Contingent Small-Step Treatment" are excellent, clinically applicable examples of the compatibility of the stimulation approach and structured behavioral methods.

EXAMPLES OF THERAPY TASKS

The preceding discussion of the design of intervention included numerous implied suggestions about tasks and techniques that may be appropriate for therapy. In this section a number of specific tasks will be listed. They are offered as examples of activities that are considered appropriate for aphasic patients and have enjoyed varying or undefined degrees of success. They are not offered as prescriptions or even as recommendations, for given our current state of knowledge we have no way of predicting reliably which tasks and techniques work best with individual patients.

The focus of the examples will be on tasks that emphasize auditory processes, because that is consistent with the stimulation approach. A number of examples of tasks requiring verbal output, many of which also involve auditory input, also will be given. It should be understood that nearly all auditory and verbal tasks are readily adaptable to the reading and writing modes. However, a few examples of tasks unique to reading and writing also will be given.

The examples offered here cover a range of difficulty so as to include suggestions that are appropriate for mildly to severely impaired patients. The tasks are ordered from the anticipated easiest to hardest, but the reader is cautioned that the order provided is not empirically derived and probably cannot be because of patient variability. It is also important to note that difficulty level can be altered not only by switching tasks but also merely by altering certain stimulus factors or stimulus-response relationships associated with a given task. For example, increasing the number of response choices in a point-to auditory comprehension task may significantly increase task difficulty.

Many of the examples given below have been derived from suggestions offered in the following sources: Brookshire (1992); Darley (1982); Kearns and Hubbard (1977); LaPointe (1978a); Rosenbek et al. (1989); Schuell (1953a); Schuell et al. (1955, 1964). Many other examples are of such universal, long-standing use that they defy or make trivial accurate referencing.

Tasks Emphasizing Auditory Abilities

Point-to Tasks

These activities involve the presentation of information auditorily and require a simple identification-by-pointing response. The ease of the motor response allows patients to focus primarily on the reception, processing, and retention of the auditory message. Difficulty level on these and many other auditory tasks can be altered by variations of many of the stimulus factors discussed earlier in the chapter (rate, pause, stress, similarity and number of response choices, visual cues, syntactic complexity, etc.). Many of these tasks can be employed as speech activities by requiring verbal instead of gestural responses. Some examples follow:

1. Point to an item (picture or object) named.
2. Point to an item described by function ("Point to the one used for writing").
3. Point to an item in order to complete a sentence ("Please pass the bread and ____").
4. Point to an item in response to questions ("What do you find in the kitchen?"—stove). A more complex but analogous task might involve responses to questions based on preceding sentence or paragraph material.
5. Point to two (or more) items named ("Point to the book and point to the pen" or "Point to book and point to the comb").
6. Point to two (or more) items described by function.
7. Point to an item best described by a sentence ("Those people are very busy"—represented by people building a house).
8. Point to an item whose name is spelled.
9. Point to an item described by a varying number of descriptors ("Point to the large white circle," "Point to the one that is long, silver, and sharp"—knife).

Following Directions

These tasks allow for greater flexibility and complexity in the auditory demands placed on the patient.

1. Follow one-verb instructions ("Pick up the pen").
2. Follow two-object location instructions ("Put the pencil in front of the cup").
3. Follow two-verb instructions ("Point to the cup. Pick up the eraser").
4. Follow two-verb instructions with time constraint ("Before touching the penny, pick up the spoon").

Yes/No Questions and Sentence Verification

These formats also increase flexibility, can reduce the possible effects of visual deficits on performance, and often allow for the extension of stimulus material beyond the immediate environment. Only a simple verbal or nonverbal response is required.

1. Questions dealing with general information ("Was Kennedy president in 1861?").
2. Questions requiring phonemic discrimination ("Do people wear shoes and blocks on their feet?").
3. Questions requiring semantic discrimination ("Do you start a car with a tire?").
4. Questions about picture material ("Is the boy walking?"—picture of boy running).
5. Questions involving verbal retention ("Are cows, horses, dogs, trees, and lions all animals?").
6. Questions about preceding sentences or paragraph material ("I like to swim, play tennis, and go to the ballpark. Did I say I like to play football?").
7. The above question examples may be converted to sentence or paragraph verifications tasks, in which the patient is asked to verify the truth of various statements ("Kennedy was president in 1861," "Cows, horses, dogs, trees, and lions are all animals," etc.).

Response Switching

These tasks require the patient to switch responses from item to item and, therefore, require close attention to the nature of the task on each trial. Such activities may simply combine the auditory tasks previously discussed or also may include items requiring speech, reading, or writing abilities. For example, a response-switching activity might include the following successive items:

1. Point to the door.
2. Give me the cup.
3. Is the floor lower than the ceiling?
4. Spell your name.
5. How are you feeling today?
6. Have I asked you to give me the cup?
7. Read this and do what it says to do.

Tasks Emphasizing Verbal and Auditory Abilities

Repetition Tasks

These require reception and retention of auditory information and the ability to repeat the information verbally. Auditory comprehension is not necessary, although it may facilitate performance. Minimal demands are placed on word retrieval.

1. Repeat spoken words.
2. Repeat phrases ("in the house"; "on the beach"; "to the store"; "black and white"; "shoes and socks").
3. Repeat series of items ("book-table"; "penny-key-knife"; "long-under-baby-pencil").
4. Repeat stereotypical or functional phrases ("Where are you going?"; "What time is it?"; "Please pass the salt"; "How are you?").
5. Repeat sentences with or without corresponding picture stimuli ("The girl is chasing the boy"; "The cat is up in the tree").

Sentence or Phrase Completion

These tasks typically place more demand on auditory comprehension and word-retrieval processes and less demand on auditory retention than do repetition tasks. For most patients, they are more difficult than single word repetition tasks but less difficult than single-word recall tasks without auditory input.

1. Complete sentences with nouns with varying degrees of predictability ("Please pass the salt and ____"; "Throw me the ____"; "Read a ____"; "Buy me some ____").
2. Complete sentences with verbs ("I use a fork for ____"; "I use a paint brush for ____").

3. Complete paired associates ("black and ____"; "hot and ____"; "salt and ____").

Verbal Association

These tasks require verbal comprehension but minimal retention. Verbal retrieval processes are taxed.

1. Oral opposites (e.g., hot-cold; night-day; early-late).
2. Rhyming—clinician says word and patient rhymes (e.g., hot-pot).
3. Word fluency/rapid word retrieval—clinician provides a letter of the alphabet, a common category (e.g., clothes, sports), or a concept (e.g., things to do on vacation, things that can roll) and patient generates as many words, categories, or concepts as possible.
4. Synonyms (e.g., "Think of a word that means the same as 'car' ").

Answering Wh- questions

These tasks always place some demand on auditory comprehension and may require significant retention as well. Word retrieval and sentence formulation may be taxed to varying degrees.

1. Answering questions after imitative cues and a question prompt (clinician—"Answer the phone"; patient imitates; clinician—"What should I do?"; patient—"Answer the phone").
2. Answering questions after a model (clinician—"The boy went to the movies. What did the boy do?").
3. Answering familiar conversational questions (How old are you?; "How do you feel?").
4. Answering questions about preceding sentence or paragraph material (e.g., "John was on the ground. John was tripped by Mary. Who was on the ground?")
5. Answering general questions ("What do you do when you're hungry?"; "Who is the president of the United States?"; "How did you get here today?"). High-level patients may be asked questions requiring lengthy responses ("How do you change a flat tire?"; "Exactly how do you get from here to ____?").

Connected Utterances in Response to Single Words

Minimal demands are placed on auditory input processes. Maximal demands are on word retrieval and on sentences formulation.

1. Use selected words of varying parts of speech, word class, tense, and so on, in sentences (put, how, television, red, running, bigger, given).
2. Define words.
3. Use sentences beginning (or ending) with selected words or phrases (I eat, when, if, she).

Retelling

These tasks can place relatively heavy demands on comprehension and retention and always tax word retrieval and sentence formulation.

1. Listen to paragraph material and retell.
2. Listen to radio or television broadcast and retell.
3. Retell a familiar story.

"Self-Initiated" or Conversational Verbal Tasks

These tasks are not dependent on preselected auditory input to the patient, with the exception of directions about the general nature of the task. Other stimuli may be used to focus content

and aid retrieval, but the primary demands are placed on the patient's verbal retrieval and formulation abilities, and often on the ability to follow naturally occurring auditory and situational cues.

1. Name pictures.
2. Describe the function of objects.
3. Describe activities in pictures.
4. Tell everything possible about pictured objects or activities (urge patient to describe all possible uses of objects, objects' physical properties, associated situations, people, etc.).
5. Describe activity of the clinician (clinician points to two pictures—patient describes; clinician touches an object, places another object near it, and then places an object on top of another—patient describes the activity when completed).
6. General conversation about a selected topic with one or more individuals.
7. Open-ended conversation on unrestricted topics with one or more individuals.

Tasks Involving Reading and Writing Abilities

Reading

Nearly all of the tasks previously described involving auditory input can be adapted easily for reading tasks simply by using written input. Following are some additional tasks that are associated more uniquely with reading:

1. Match written words, phrases, or sentences to pictures (gradually reducing stimulus exposure time may be employed in an effort to increase reading rate).
2. Identify letters named by the clinician among a number of written choices.
3. Name letters.
4. Read in unison with the clinician with gradual increase in rate and/or fading of the clinician's input.
5. Fill in missing words in sentences from among written choices (e.g., "They went to the movies last [day, night, show, fight]"; "John is [to, went, going, come] in a little while").
6. Read sentences or paragraphs silently, followed by questions about content.
7. Read aloud a paragraph or story and then retell.

Writing

Most of the examples offered under the sections dealing with auditory and verbal activities also can be adapted readily to the writing mode merely by requiring written instead of gestural or verbal responses. Following are some additional tasks that are associated more uniquely with writing modality activities:

1. Copy forms, letters, and words.
2. Write letters to dictation.
3. Write words dictated letter by letter.
4. Write overlearned materials such as name, the alphabet, numbers 1 to 10 and so on.
5. Fill in missing letters or words in written stimuli, with or without associated picture stimuli (e.g., "He is reading a ____; He is reading a b-ok").
6. Clinician reads paragraph material, and the patient writes down the essential facts. Have the patient rewrite the paragraph based on those notes.

EFFICACY OF THE STIMULATION APPROACH

It is impossible to make a single, empirically based statement about the efficacy of the stimulation approach. Nor would it be appropriate or particularly enlightening, within the context of this chapter, to review all of the group and single-subject studies that might bear on the issue of treatment efficacy (the reader is referred to Darley's [1972, 1975, 1982] review, and the comprehensive reviews by Rosenbek et al. [1989] of such studies and issues related to assessing the effectiveness of treatment). However, a number of general statements about the effectiveness of treatment, particularly the stimulation approach, may help to put the current state of the art in perspective.

While no single study can conclusively "prove" the efficacy of treatment (Holland, 1975), reviews and observations by well-respected, active clinical aphasiologists and some neurologists generally have yielded cautious-to-confident conclusions that therapy helps aphasic patients (see, for example, Benson [1979], Darley [1977, 1979, 1882], Helm-Estabrooks [1984] and Wertz [1983, 1991]). Today, the evidence accumulated from many group and single-subject treatment studies, at the least, justifies a general conclusion that "there is ample evidence that what we do for some aphasic patients does some good" (Wertz, 1991, p. 318).

Do we know something about the effectiveness of the stimulation approach that we do not know about therapy for aphasia in general? We do know that Schuell and her colleagues believed in and reported observations of the effectiveness of the stimulation approach, excluding patients with an irreversible (severe) aphasic syndrome. Many other users of the approach also report measurable progress (for more recent, relatively unambiguous examples of studies supporting the efficacy of the stimulation approach, see Basso et al. [1979]; Marshall et al. [1989]; Poeck et al. [1989]; Shewan and Kertesz [1984]; Wertz et al. [1981]; and Wertz et al. [1986]).

Because of the widespread use of the stimulation approach, it probably has been studied more extensively than any other approach to treatment (although the interpretation of most efficacy studies requires this conclusion to be inferred, since treatment approaches rarely have been well specified). Therefore, conclusions that therapy is generally effective are based on studies that have used, or probably have used, a stimulation approach. More pessimistically, we can say that much of our inconclusive evidence about treatment efficacy is derived from studies of the stimulation approach. However, it is very possible that such inconclusiveness is due more to the study of the treatment than to the treatment itself. Taken as a whole, treatment studies employing the stimulation approach are more conclusive than inconclusive, and the conclusion they generate is that it has a significant positive effect on the communication ability of many patients with aphasia.

FUTURE TRENDS

What does the future hold for the stimulation approach? Answering this question is risky business, subject to the predictor's biases and misperceptions, new fads and fashions, major advances in other therapy approaches, altered availability of funding for continued investigation, and so on. With these pitfalls in mind, we can address three questions about the future: (a) Will we increase our understanding of the efficacy and dynamics of the stimulation approach? (b) Is the approach likely to change? (c) How will we understand and use it in relation to other therapy approaches?

Will we increase our understanding of the efficacy of the stimulation approach and the dynamics that explain its success?

There are a number of reasons to anticipate that this will happen. First, clinical aphasiologists have made a commitment to accountability—a commitment to providing "proof" of the effectiveness, or lack thereof, of treatment for aphasia. Second, we have identified many of the flaws in our previous attempts, as well as those variables that must be accounted for in any study of treatment efficacy. Third, our measuring instruments have become more sensitive and reliable (e.g., the PICA). Fourth, we have begun to specify and study the dynamics of treatment more precisely (especially in single-subject studies) so that we know better what is effective and under what circumstances. Fifth, although we have acquired a substantial body of data about stimulus factors that affect the performance of aphasic patients in nontreatment conditions, we know very little about the specific effects of using such stimulus manipulation in ongoing treatment. That is, the simple observation of improved performance under a certain stimulus condition in a single-trial nontreatment study does not constitute proof that use of that stimulus factor in treatment will be responsible for short- or long-term language gains within or beyond the specific language task. This gap in our knowledge is true for many of the stimulus factors reviewed in this chapter, and it is close to the heart of questions about whether stimulation in general and/or specific stimulation is important to inducing language gains with the stimulation approach. We are in a position to test the effects of many stimulus factors in treatment, and it is likely that this will be pursued in the future. Finally, the effect of stimulus factors and other variables that affect communication in discourse, conversation, and natural communicative settings is receiving increased attention. These efforts should help identify the components of stimulation likely to have the greatest impact on communication in daily life and, thus, stimulus factors that are most meaningful to the patients we treat.

Is the stimulation approach likely to change? Probably not in any fundamental way. Major change is unlikely because the stimulation approach is an old and established one whose major principles and techniques have been reasonably well articulated and, in principle, consistently employed. It is likely that any major departures from the basic approach will be considered new approaches, given new names, and studied and employed separately. Several chapters in this volume reflect this trend and demonstrate divergence from the stimulation approach along many different lines.

The change that can be expected for the stimulation approach is refinement of our understanding of stimulus factors that do and do not influence performance and, as mentioned previously, an increase in our ability to selectively and effectively employ that knowledge in treatment. It is hoped that these changes will be rapid and numerous and significantly improve overall treatment efficacy. Probably they will be slow and painstakingly acquired. Certainly, they will require the efforts of many investigators who are interested in the increased understanding of the essence of aphasia as well as its effective management.

Finally, how will we understand and use the stimulation approach in relation to other therapy approaches? There is no way to answer this because so little has been done to compare the effects of different treatment approaches. This is at least partly due to the enormous past efforts expended to establish that treatment, in general, is effective, and to develop new approaches and preliminary efficacy data for them. Another reason, really not to be confronted until more comparative studies are attempted, has been perceived by Sarno (1981). She said, "It is probably appropriate that there have been few studies comparing treatment methods in view of the seemingly insurmountable methodological problems associated with such research and our present state of knowledge" (p. 512). In spite of these past priorities and ever-present methodological challenges, it can be argued that unless comparative studies are done, we will not learn what works best and with whom, and either we will become complacent in our use of a single "old and familiar" approach or, out of boredom, frustration, or faddism, we will move randomly from one approach to another. There are numerous comparative questions that should be addressed: How do various treatment approaches differ in terms of ultimate level of recovery, time demands, cost-effectiveness, professional and family requirements, and so on? What is the best approach to use for patients with particular severity levels and forms of aphasia? Are some approaches more effective early postonset or late postonset? Is there a best sequence of approaches to use over the course of treatment? Is language recovery enhanced if certain approaches are used in combination? Do some approaches have to be used in isolation for them to be effective?

It is likely that some of the above questions will be addressed in the next 5 to 10 years. The number of approaches now in use make this increasingly necessary for rational, data-based clinical decision making. In addition, because more appears to be known about the efficacy of the stimulation approach than almost any other, it is likely that it will frequently be among the approaches compared; in fact, we might anticipate that it will be the standard against which the effectiveness of other approaches will be measured.

References

Albert, M. L. (1976). Short-term memory and aphasia. *Brain and Language*, *3*, 28–33.

Albert, M. L., and Bear, D. (1974). Time to understand: A case study of word deafness with reference to the role of time in auditory comprehension. *Brain*, *97*, 373–384.

Ansell, B. J. (1991). Slow-to-recover brain-injured patients: Rationale for treatment. *Journal of Speech and Hearing Research*, *34*, 1017–1022.

Ansell, B. J., and Flowers, C. R. (1982a). Aphasic adults' understanding of complex adverbial sentences. *Brain and Language*, *15*, 82–91.

Ansell, B. J., and Flowers, C. R. (1982b). Aphasic adults' use of heuristic and structural linguistic cues for sentence analysis. *Brain and Language*, *16*, 61–72.

Armus, S. R., Brookshire, R. H., and Nicholas, L. E. (1989). Aphasic and non-brain-damaged adults' knowledge of scripts for common situations. *Brain and Language*, *36*, 518–528.

Barton, M., Maruszewski, M., and Urrea, D. (1969). Variation of stimulus context and its effect on word finding ability in aphasics. *Cortex*, *5*, 351–365.

Basso, A., Capitani, E., and Vignolo, L. A. (1979). Influence of rehabilitation on language skills in aphasic patients: A controlled study. *Archives of Neurology*, *36*, 190–196.

Baum, S. R. (1989). On-line sensitivity to local and long-distance syntactic dependencies in Broca's aphasia. *Brain and Language*, *37*, 327–338.

Baum, S. R., Daniloff, J. K., Daniloff, R., and Lewis, J. (1982). Sentence comprehension by Broca's aphasics: Effects of some suprasegmental variables. *Brain and Language*, *17*, 261–271.

Benson, D. F. (1979). Aphasia rehabilitation (editorial). *Archives of Neurology*, *36*, 187–189.

Benton, A. L., Smith, K. C., and Lang, M. (1972). Stimulus characteristics and object naming in aphasic patients. *Journal of Communication Disorders*, *5*, 19–24.

Berstein-Ellis, E., Wertz, R. T., and Shubitowski, Y. (1987). More pace, less fillers: A verbal strategy for a high-level aphasic patient. In R. H. Brookshire (Ed.), *Clinical aphasiology*, (Vol. 17, pp. 12–22). Minneapolis, MN: BRK.

Birch, H. G., and Lee, M. (1955). Cortical inhibition in expressive aphasia. *A.M.A. Archives of Neurology and Psychiatry*, *74*, 514–517.

Bisiach, E. (1966). Perceptual factors in the pathogenesis of anomia. *Cortex*, *2*, 90–95.

Blumstein, S. E., Goodglass, H., Statlender, S., and Biber, C. (1983). Comprehension strategies determining reference in aphasia: A study of reflexivization. *Brain and Language*, *18*, 115–127.

Blumstein, S. E., Katz, B., Goodglass, H., Shrier, R., and Dworetsky, B. (1985). The effects of slowed speech on auditory comprehension in aphasia. *Brain and Language*, *24*, 246–265.

Blumstein, S. E., Milberg, W., and Shrier, R. (1982). Semantic processing in aphasia: Evidence from an auditory lexical decision task. *Brain and Language*, *17*, 301–315.

Boller, F., Vrtunski, B., Patterson, M., and Kim, Y. (1979). Paralinguistic aspects of auditory comprehension in aphasia. *Brain and Language*, *7*, 164–174.

Bollinger, R. L., and Stout, C. E. (1976). Response-contingent small-step treatment: Performance-based communication intervention. *Journal of Speech and Hearing Disorders*, *41*, 40–51.

Boone, D. R. (1967). A plan for the rehabilitation of aphasic patients. *Archives of Physical Medicine and Rehabilitation*, *48*, 410–414.

Boone, D. R., and Friedman, H. M. (1976). Writing in aphasia rehabilitation: Cursive vs. manuscript. *Journal of Speech and Hearing Disorders*, *41*, 523–529.

Bottenberg, D., Lemme, M., and Hedberg, N. (1987). Effect of story on narrative discourse of aphasic adults. In R. H. Brookshire (Ed.), *Clinical Aphasiology*, (Vol. 17, pp. 202–209). Minneapolis, MN: BRK.

Boyle, M., and Canter, G. J. (1986). Verbal context and comprehension of difficult sentences by aphasic adults: A methodological problem. In R. H. Brookshire (Ed.), *Clinical aphasiology* (Vol. 16, pp. 38–44). Minneapolis, MN: BRK.

Brenneise-Sarshad, R., Nicholas, L., and Brookshire, R. H. (1991). Effects of apparent listener knowledge and picture stimuli on aphasic and non-brain-damaged speakers' narrative discourse. *Journal of Speech and Hearing Research*, *34*, 168–176.

Bricker, A. L., Schuell, H., and Jenkins, J. J. (1964). Effect of word frequency and word length on aphasic spelling errors. *Journal of Speech and Hearing Research*, *7*, 183–192.

Brookshire, R. H. (1971a). Effects of delay of reinforcement on probability learning by aphasic subjects. *Journal of Speech and Hearing Research*, *14*, 92–105.

Brookshire, R. H. (1971b). Effects of trial time and inter-trial interval on naming by aphasic subjects. *Journal of Communication Disorders*, *3*, 289–301.

Brookshire, R. H. (1972). Effects of task difficulty on the naming performance of aphasic subjects. *Journal of Speech and Hearing Research*, *15*, 551–558.

Brookshire, R. H. (1974). Differences in responding to auditory materials among aphasic patients. *Acta Symbolica*, *5*, 1–18.

Brookshire, R. H. (1976a). The role of auditory functions in rehabilitation of aphasic individuals. In R. T. Wertz and M. Collins (Eds.), *Clinical Aphasiology Conference proceedings 1972*. Madison, WI: Clinical Aphasiology Conference.

Brookshire, R. H. (1976b). Effects of task difficulty on sentence comprehension performance of aphasic subjects. *Journal of Communication Disorders*, *9*, 167–173.

Brookshire, R. H. (1977). A system for coding and recording events in patient-clinician interactions during aphasia treatment sessions. In M. Sullivan and M. S. Kommers (Eds.), *Rationale for adult aphasia therapy*. Omaha, NE: University of Nebraska Medical Center.

Brookshire, R. H. (1992). *An introduction to neurogenic communication disorders* (4th ed.). St. Louis, MO: Mosby Year Book.

Brookshire, R. H., and Lommel, M. (1974). Perception of sequences of visual temporal and auditory spatial stimuli by aphasic, right hemisphere damaged, and non-brain-damaged subjects. *Journal of Communication Disorders*, *7*, 155–169.

Brookshire, R. H., and Nicholas, L. E. (1978). Effects of clinician request and feedback behavior on responses of aphasic individuals in speech and language treatment sessions. In R. H. Brookshire (Ed.), *Clinical Aphasiology Conference proceedings*. Minneapolis, MN: BRK.

Brookshire, R. H., and Nicholas, L. E. (1980). Sentence verification and language comprehension of aphasic persons. In R. H. Brookshire (Ed.), *Clinical Aphasiology Conference proceedings*, Minneapolis, MN: BRK.

Brookshire, R. H., and Nicholas, L. E. (1981). Verification of active and passive sentences by aphasic and monoaphasic subjects. *Journal of Speech and Hearing Disorders, 23*, 878–893.

Brookshire, R. H., and Nicholas, L. E. (1984). Comprehension of directly and indirectly stated ideas and details in discourse by brain-damaged and non-brain-damaged listeners. *Brain and Language, 21*, 21–36.

Cannito, M. P., Jarecki, J. M., and Pierce, R. S. (1986). Effects of thematic structure on syntactic comprehension in aphasia. *Brain and Language, 27*, 38–49.

Cannito, M. P., Vogel, D., and Pierce, R. S. (1989). Sentence comprehension in context: Influence of proper visual stimulation? In T. E. Prescott (Ed.), *Clinical aphasiology*, (Vol. 18, pp. 433–446). Boston, MA: Little, Brown.

Caplan, D., and Evans, K. L. (1990). The effects of syntactic structure on discourse comprehension in patients with parsing impairments. *Brain and Language, 39*, 206–234.

Caramazza, A., and Berndt, R. S. (1978). Semantic and syntactic processes in aphasia: A review of the literature. *Psychological Review, 85*, 898–918.

Caramazza, A., Berndt, R. S., and Brownell, H. H. (1982). The semantic deficit hypothesis: Perceptual parsing and object classification by aphasic patients. *Brain and Language, 15*, 161–189.

Caramazza, A., and Zurif, E. B. (1976). Dissociation of algorithmic and heuristic processes in language comprehension: Evidence from aphasia. *Brain and Language, 3*, 572–582.

Chenery, H. J., Ingram, J. C. L., and Murdoch, B. E. (1990). Automatic and volitional semantic processing in aphasia. *Brain and Language, 38*, 215–232.

Chieffi, S., Carlomagno, S., Silveri, M. C., and Gainotti, G. (1989). The influence of semantic and perceptual factors on lexical comprehension in aphasic and right brain-damaged patients. *Cortex, 25*, 592–598.

Clark, A. E., and Flowers, C. R. (1987). The effect of semantic redundancy on auditory comprehension in aphasia. In R. H. Brookshire (Ed.), *Clinical aphasiology*, (Vol. 17, pp. 174–179). Minneapolis, MN: BRK.

Corlew, M. M., and Nation, J. E. (1975). Characteristics of visual stimuli and naming performance in aphasic adults. *Cortex, 11*, 186–191.

Correia, L., Brookshire, R. H., and Nicholas, L. E. (1989). The effects of picture content on descriptions by aphasic and non-brain-damaged speakers. In R. H. Brookshire (Ed.), *Clinical aphasiology* (Vol.18, pp. 447–462). Boston, MA: Little, Brown.

Correia, L., Brookshire, R. H., and Nicholas, L. E. (1990). Aphasic and non-brain-damaged adults' descriptions of aphasia test pictures and gender-based pictures. *Journal of Speech and Hearing Disorders, 55*, 713–720.

Crosky, C.S., & Adams, M.R. (1969). A rationale and clinical methodology for selecting vocabulary stimulus material for individual aphasic patients. *Journal of Communication Disorders, 2*, 340–343.

Curtiss, S., Jackson, C. A., Kempler, D., Hanson, W. R., and Metter, E. J. (1986). Length vs. structural complexity in sentence comprehension in aphasia. In R. H. Brookshire (Ed.), *Clinical aphasiology* (Vol. 16, pp. 45–53). Minneapolis, MN: BRK.

Darley, F. L. (1972). The efficacy of language rehabilitation in aphasia. *Journal of Speech and Hearing Disorders, 37*, 3–21.

Darley, F. L. (1975). Treatment of acquired aphasia. In W. J. Friedlander (Ed.), *Advances in neurology* (Vol. 7). New York: Raven Press.

Darley, F. L. (1976). Maximizing input to the aphasic patient. In R. H. Brookshire (Ed.), *Clinical Aphasiology Conference proceedings*. Minneapolis, MN: BRK.

Darley, F. L. (1977). A retrospective view: Aphasia. *Journal of Speech and Hearing Disorders, 42*, 161–169.

Darley, F. L. (1979). Treat or neglect. *ASHA, 21*, 628–631.

Darley, F. L. (1982). *Aphasia*. Philadelphia, PA: W.B. Saunders.

Darley, F. L., Sherman, D., and Siegal, G. M. (1959). Scaling of abstraction level of single words. *Journal of Speech and Hearing Disorders, 2*, 161–167.

Davis, G. A. (1983). *A survey of adult aphasia*. Englewood Cliffs, NJ: Prentice-Hall.

Deloche, G., and Seron, X. (1981). Sentence understanding and knowledge of the world: Evidence from a sentence-picture matching task performed by aphasic patients. *Brain and Language, 14*, 57–69.

DeRenzi, E., and Vignolo, L. A. (1962). The Token Test: a sensitive test to detect receptive disturbances in aphasics. *Brain, 85*, 665–678.

Duffy, J. R., and Watkins, L. B. (1984). The effect of response choice relatedness on pantomime and verbal recognition ability in aphasic patients. *Brain and Language, 21*, 291–306.

Duffy, R. J., and Ulrich, S. R. (1976). A comparison of impairments in verbal comprehension, speech, reading, and writing in adult aphasics. *Journal of Speech and Hearing Disorders, 41*, 110–119.

Dumond, D. L., Hardy, J. C., and Van Demark, A. A. (1978). Presentation by order of difficulty of test tasks to persons with aphasia. *Journal of Speech and Hearing Research, 21*, 350–360.

Eccles, J. C. (1973). *The understanding of the brain*. New York: McGraw-Hill.

Eisenson, J. (1973). *Adult aphasia: assessment and treatment*. Englewood Cliffs, NJ: Prentice-Hall.

Ernest-Baron, C. R., Brookshire, R. H., and Nicholas, L. E. (1987). Story structure and retelling of narratives by aphasic and non-brain-damaged adults. *Journal of Speech and Hearing Research, 30*, 44–49.

Foldi, N. S. (1987). Appreciation of pragmatic interpretations of indirect commands: Comparison of right and left hemisphere brain-damaged patients. *Brain and Language, 31*, 88–108.

Friederici, A. D. (1983). Aphasics' perception of words in sentential context: Some real time processing evidence. *Neuropsychologia, 21*, 351–358.

Friederici, A. D., and Graetz, P. A. M. (1987). Processing passive sentences in aphasia: Deficits and strategies. *Brain and Language, 30*, 93–105.

Friederici, A. D., Schoenle, P. W., and Goodglass, H. (1981). Mechanisms underlying writing and speech in aphasia. *Brain and Language, 13*, 212–222.

Gallaher, A. J. (1981). Syntactic versus semantic performances of agrammatic Broca's aphasics on tests of constituent-element-ordering. *Journal of Speech and Hearing Research, 2*, 217–223.

Gallaher, A. J., and Canter, G. J. (1982). Reading and lexical comprehension in Broca's apahsia: Lexical versus syntactical errors. *Brain and Language, 17*, 183–192.

Gardner, B., and Brookshire, R. H. (1972). Effects of unisensory and multisensory presentation of stimuli upon naming by aphasic patients. *Language and Speech, 15*, 342–357.

Gardner, H. (1973). The contribution of operativity to naming capacity in aphasic patients. *Neuropsychologia, 11*, 213–220.

Gardner, H., Albert, M. L., and Weintraub, S. (1975). Comprehending a word: The influence of speed and redundance on auditory comprehension in aphasia. *Cortex, 11*, 155–162.

Gerratt, B. R., and Jones, D. (1987). Aphasic performance on a lexical decision task: Multiple meanings and word frequency. *Brain and Language, 30*, 106–115.

Glaser, R., Stoioff, M., and Weidner, W. E. (1974). The effect of controlled auditory stimulation on the auditory recognition of adult aphasic subjects. *Acta Symbolica, 5*, 57–68.

Glosser, G., Wiener, M., and Kaplan, E. (1988). Variations in aphasic language behaviors. *Journal of Speech and Hearing Disorders, 53*, 115–124.

Goldstein, K. (1948). *Language and language disturbances*. New York: Grune & Stratton.

Golper, L., and Rau, M. T. (1983). Systematic analysis of cuing strategies in aphasia: Taking your "cue" from the patient. In R. H. Brookshire (Ed.), *Clinical Aphasiology Conference proceedings*. Minneapolis, MN: BRK.

Goodglass, H. (1968). Studies on the grammar of aphasics. In S. Rosenberg and J. Koplin (Eds.), *Developments in applied psycholinguistic research*. New York: Macmillan.

Goodglass, H., and Baker, E. (1976). Semantic field, naming, and auditory comprehension in aphasia. *Brain and Language, 3*, 359–374.

Goodglass, H., Barton, M. I., and Kaplan, E. F. (1968). Sensory modality and object naming in aphasia. *Journal of Speech and Hearing Research, 11*, 488–496.

Goodglass, H., and Berko, J. (1960). Agrammatism and inflectional morphology in English. *Journal of Speech and Hearing Research, 3*, 257–267.

Goodglass, H., Fodor, I. G., and Schuloff, C. (1967). Prosodic factors in grammar: Evidence from aphasia. *Journal of Speech and Hearing Research, 10*, 5–20.

Goodglass, H., Gleason, J. B., and Hyde, M. R. (1970). Some dimensions of auditory language comprehension in aphasia. *Journal of Speech and Hearing Research, 13*, 595–606.

Goodglass, H., and Hunt, J. (1958). Grammatical complexity and aphasic speech. *Word, 14*, 197–207.

Goodglass, H., Klein, B., Carey, P. W., and Jones, K. J. (1966). Specific semantic word categories in aphasia. *Cortex, 2*, 74–89.

Graham, L. F., Holtzapple, P., and LaPointe, L. L. (1987). Does contextually related action facilitate auditory comprehension? Performance across three conditions by high and low comprehenders. In R. H. Brookshire (Ed.), *Clinical aphasiology* (Vol. 17, pp. 180–187). Minneapolis, MN: BRK.

Green, E., and Boller, F. (1974). Features of auditory comprehension in severely impaired aphasics. *Cortex*, 10, 133–145.

Grossman, M., and Haberman, S. (1982). Aphasics' selected deficits in appreciating grammatical agreements. *Brain and Language*, 16, 109–120.

Hageman, C. F., and Lewis, D. L. (1983). The effects of intrastimulus pause on the quality of auditory comprehension in aphasia. In R. H. Brookshire (Ed.). *Clinical Aphasiology Conference proceedings*. Minneapolis, MN: BRK.

Halpern, H. (1965a). Effect of stimulus variables on dysphasic verbal errors. *Perceptual and Motor Skills*, 21, 291–298.

Halpern, H. (1965b). Effect of stimulus variables on verbal perseveration of dysphasic subjects. *Perceptual and Motor Skills*, 20, 421–429.

Hanlon, R. E., Brown, J. W., and Gerstman, L. J. (1990). Enhancement of naming in nonfluent aphasia through gesture. *Brain and Language*, 38, 298–314.

Helm, N. (1979). Management of palilalia with a pacing board. *Journal of Speech and Hearing Disorders*, 44, 350–353.

Helm-Estabrooks, N. (1981). ''Show me the . . . whatever'': Some variables affecting auditory comprehension scores of aphasic patients. In R. H. Brookshire (Ed.), *Clinical Aphasiology Conference proceedings*. Minneapolis, MN: BRK.

Helm-Estabrooks, N. (1984). Treatment of the aphasias. *Seminars in Neurology*, 4, 196–202.

Helmick, J. W., and Wipplinger, M. (1975). Effects of stimulus repetition on the naming behavior of an aphasic adult: A clinical report. *Journal of Communication Disorders*, 8, 23–29.

Hendrick, D. L., Christman, M. A., and Augustine, L. (1973). Programming for the antecedent event in therapy. *Journal of Speech and Hearing Disorders*, 38, 339–344.

Holland, A. L. (1975). The effectiveness of treatment in aphasia. In R. H. Brookshire (Ed.), *Clinical Aphasiology Conference proceedings*, Minneapolis, MN: BRK.

Holland, A. L., and Sonderman, J. C. (1974). Effects of a program based on the Token Test for teaching comprehension skills to aphasics. *Journal of Speech and Hearing Research*, 17, 589–598.

Hough, M. S. (1989). Category concept generation in aphasia: The influence of context. *Aphasiology*, 3, 553–568.

Hough, M. S. (1990). Narrative comprehension in adults with right and left hemisphere brain-damage: Theme organization. *Brain and Language*, 38, 253–277.

Hough, M. S., and Pierce, R. S. (1989). Contextual influences on category concept generation in aphasia. In T. E. Prescott (Ed.), *Clinical aphasiology* (Vol. 18, pp. 507–519). Boston, MA: Little, Brown.

Hough, M. S., Pierce, R. S., and Cannito, M. D. (1989). Contextual influences in aphasia: Effects of predictive versus nonpredictive narratives. *Brain and Language*, 36, 325–334.

Jenkins, J., Jimnez-Pabn, E., Shaw, R., and Sefer, J. (1975). *Schuell's aphasia in adults* (2nd ed.). New York: Harper & Row.

Johnson, J., Sommers, R., and Weidner, W. (1977). Dichotic ear preference in aphasia. *Journal of Speech and Hearing Research*, 20, 116–129.

Katsuki-Nakamura, J., Brookshire, R. H., and Nicholas, L. E. (1988). Comprehension of monologues and dialogues by aphasic listeners. *Journal of Speech and Hearing Disorders*, 53, 408–415.

Kearns, K., and Hubbard, D. J. (1977). A comparison of auditory comprehension tasks in aphasia. In R. H. Brookshire (Ed.), *Clinical Aphasiology Conference proceedings*. Minneapolis, MN: BRK.

Kimelman, M. D. Z. (1991). The role of target word stress in auditory comprehension by aphasic listeners. *Journal of Speech and Hearing Research*, 34, 334–339.

Kimelman, M. D. Z. and McNeil, M. R. (1987). Emphatic stress comprehension on adult aphasia: A successful constructive replication. *Journal of Speech and Hearing Research*, 30, 295–300.

Kimelman, M. D. Z., and McNeil, M. R. (1989). Contextual influences on the auditory comprehension of normally stressed targets by aphasic listeners. In T. E. Prescott (Ed.), *Clinical aphasiology* (Vol. 18, pp. 407–420). Boston, MA: Little, Brown.

Kohn, S. E., and Goodglass, H. (1985). Picture-naming in aphasia. *Brain and Language*, 24, 266–283.

Kohn, S. E., Lorch, M. P., and Pearson, D. M. (1989). Verb finding in aphasia. *Cortex*, 25, 57–69.

Kolk, H. H. J., and Friederici, A. D. (1985). Strategy and impairment in sentence understanding by Broca's and Wernicke's aphasics. *Cortex*, 21, 47–67.

Kudo, T. (1984). The effect of semantic plausibility on sentence comprehension in aphasia. *Brain and Language*, 21, 208–218.

Lambrecht, K. J., and Marshall, R. C. (1983). Comprehension in severe aphasia: A second look. In R. H. Brookshire (Ed.), *Clinical Aphasiology Conference proceedings*. Minneapolis, MN: BRK.

LaPointe, L. L. (1977). Base-10 programmed stimulation: Task specification, scoring, and plotting performance in aphasia therapy. *Journal of Speech and Hearing Disorders*, 42, 90–105.

LaPointe, L. L. (1978a). Aphasia therapy: Some principles and strategies for treatment. In D. F. Johns (Ed.), *Clinical management of neurogenic communicative disorders*. Boston, MA: Little, Brown.

LaPointe, L. L. (1978b). Multiple baseline designs. In R. H. Brookshire (Ed.), *Clinical Aphasiology Conference proceedings*. Minneapolis, MN: BRK.

LaPointe, L. L. (1983). Aphasic intervention in adults: Historical, present, and future approaches. In J. Miller, D. E. Yoder, and R. Schiefelbusch (Eds.), *Contemporary issues in language intervention* (ASHA Reports No. 12). Rockville, MD: American Speech-Language-Hearing Association.

LaPointe, L. L., Horner, J., and Lieberman, R. (1977). Effects of ear presentation and delayed response on the processing of Token Test commands. In R. H. Brookshire (Ed.), *Clinical Aphasiology Conference proceedings*. Minneapolis, MN: BRK.

Lapointe, L. L., Rothi, L. J., and Campanella, D. J. (1978). The effects of repetition of Token Test commands on auditory comprehension. In R. H. Brookshire (Ed.), *Clinical Aphasiology Conference proceedings*, Minneapolis, MN: BRK.

Lasky, E. Z., Weidner, W. E., and Johnson, J. P. (1976). Influence of linguistic complexity, rate of presentation, and interphrase pause time on auditory verbal comprehension of adult aphasic patients. *Brain and Language*, 3, 386–396.

Lesser, R. (1974). Verbal comprehension in aphasia: An English version of three Italian tests. *Cortex*, 10, 247–263.

Lesser, R. (1978). *Linguistic investigations of aphasia*. New York: Elsevier.

Li, E. C., and Canter, G. J. (1991). Varieties of errors produced by aphasic patients in phonemic cueing. *Aphasiology*, 5, 51–61.

Li, E. C., and Williams, S. E. (1989). The efficacy of two types of cues in aphasic patients. *Aphasiology*, 3(7), 619–626.

Liles, B. Z., and Brookshire, R. H. (1975). The effects of pause time on auditory comprehension of aphasic subjects. *Journal of Communication Disorders*, 8, 221–235.

Linebaugh, C. W. (1986). Variability of error patterns on two formats of picture-to-word matching. In R. H. Brookshire (Ed.), *Clinical aphasiology* (Vol. 16, pp. 181–189). Minneapolis, MN: BRK.

Linebaugh, C., and Lehner, L. (1977). Cueing hierarchies and word retrieval: A therapy program. In R. H. Brookshire (Ed.), *Clinical Aphasiology Conference proceedings*, Minneapolis, MN: BRK.

Loverso, F. L., and Prescott, T. E. (1981). The effect of alerting signals on left brain damaged (aphasic) and normal subjects' accuracy and response time to visual stimuli. In R. H. Brookshire (Ed.), *Clinical Aphasiology Conference proceedings*. Minneapolis, MN: BRK.

Mack, J. L. (1982). The comprehension of locative prepositions in nonfluent and fluent aphasia. *Brain and Language*, 14, 18–92.

Marshall, J. C., and Newcombe, F. (1966). Syntactic and semantic errors in paralexia. *Neuropsychologia*, 4, 169–176.

Marshall, R. C. (1976). Word retrieval behavior of aphasic adults. *Journal of Speech and Hearing Disorders*, 41, 444–451.

Marshall, R. C., and King, P. S. (1973). Effects of fatigue produced by isokinetic exercise on the communication ability of aphasic adults. *Journal of Speech and Hearing Research*, 16, 222–230.

Marshall, R. C., and Tompkins, C. A. (1982). Verbal self-correction behaviors of fluent and nonfluent aphasic subjects. *Brain and Language*, 15, 292–306.

Marshall, R. C., Tompkins, C. A., and Phillips, D. S. (1980). Effects of scheduling on the communication assessment of aphasic patients. *Journal of Communication Disorders*, 13, 105–114.

Marshall, R. C., Wertz, R. T., Weiss, D. G., Aten, J. L., Brookshire, R. H., Garcia-Bunuel, L., Holland, W. L., Kurtzke, J. F., LaPointe, L. L., Milianti, F. J., Brannegan, R., Greenbaum, H., Voge, D., Carter, J., Barnes, N. S., Goodman, R. (1989). Home treatment for aphasia patients by trained nonprofessionals. *Journal of Speech and Hearing Disorders*, 54, 462–470.

Martin, A. D. (1975). A critical evaluation of therapeutic approaches to aphasia. In R. H. Brookshire (Ed.), *Clinical Aphasiology Conference proceedings*. Minneapolis, MN: BRK.

Martin, R. C., and Feher, E. (1990). The consequences of reduced memory span for the comprehension of semantic versus syntactic information. *Brain and Language, 38,* 1–20.

McDearmon, J. R., and Potter, R. E. (1975). The use of representational prompts in aphasia therapy. *Journal of Communication Disorders, 8,* 199–206.

McNeil, M., Darley, F. L., Rose D. E., and Olsen, W. O. (1979a, June). *Effects of diotic intensity increments on auditory processing deficits in aphasia.* Paper presented to the Ninth Annual Clinical Aphasiology Conference, Phoenix, AZ.

McNeil, M., Darley, F. L., Rose, D. E., and Olsen, W. O. (1979b, June). *Effects of selective binaural intensity variations on auditory processing in aphasia.* Paper presented to the Ninth Annual Clinical Aphasiology Conference, Phoenix, AZ.

McNeil, M., and Hageman, C. (1979). Prediction and pattern of auditory processing deficits on the Revised Token Test. In R. H. Brookshire (Ed.), *Clinical Aphasiology Conference proceedings.* Minneapolis, MN: BRK.

McNeil, M., and Prescott, T. E. (1978). *Revised Token Test.* Baltimore, MD: University Park Press.

Mills, R. (1977). The effects of environmental sound on the naming performance of aphasic subjects. In R. H. Brookshire (Ed.), *Clinical Aphasiology Conference proceedings.* Minneapolis, MN: BRK.

Mills, R. H., Knox, A. W., Juola, J. F., and Salmon, S. J. (1979). Cognitive loci of impairments in picture naming by aphasic subjects. *Journal of Speech and Hearing Research, 22,* 73–87.

Naeser, M. A., Mazurski, P., Goodglass, H., Peraino, M., Laughlin, S., and Leaper, W. C. (1987). Auditory syntactic comprehension in nine aphasia groups (with CT scans) and children: Differences in degree but not order of difficulty observed. *Cortex, 23,* 359–380.

Nicholas, L., and Brookshire, R. H. (1983). Syntactic simplification and context: Effects on sentence comprehension by aphasic adults. In R. H. Brookshire (Ed.), *Clinical Aphasiology Conference proceedings,* Minneapolis, MN: BRK.

Nicholas, L. E., and Brookshire, R. H. (1986a). Consistency of the effects of rate of speech on brain-damaged adults' comprehension of narrative discourse. *Journal of Speech and Hearing Research, 29,* 462–470.

Nicholas, L. E., and Brookshire, R. H. (1986b). Types of errors in multiple-sentence reading comprehension of aphasic adults. In R. H. Brookshire (Ed.), *Clinical aphasiology* (Vol. 16, pp. 190–195). Minneapolis, MN: BRK.

Noll, J. D., and Hoops, H. R. (1967). Aphasic grammatical involvement as indicated by spelling ability. *Cortex, 3,* 419–432.

North, B. (1971). *Effects of stimulus redundancy on naming disorders in aphasia.* Unpublished doctoral dissertation, Boston University.

Parisi, D., and Pizzamiglio, L. (1970). Syntactic comprehension in aphasia. *Cortex, 6,* 204–215.

Pashek, G. V., and Brookshire, R. H. (1982). Effect of rate and stress on auditory paragraph comprehension in aphasic individuals. *Journal of Speech and Hearing Research, 25,* 377–383.

Peach, R. K., Canter, G. J., and Gallaher, A. J. (1988). Comprehension of sentence structure in anomic and conduction aphasia. *Brain and Language, 35,* 119–137.

Pierce, R. S. (1981). Facilitating the comprehension of tense related sentences in aphasia. *Journal of Speech and Hearing Disorders, 46,* 364–368.

Pierce, R. S. (1982). Facilitating the comprehension of syntax in aphasia. *Journal of Speech and Hearing Research, 25,* 408–413.

Pierce, R. S. (1983). Decoding syntax during reading in aphasia. *Journal of Communication Disorders, 16,* 181–188.

Pierce, R. S. (1988). Influence of prior and subsequent context on comprehension in aphasia. *Aphasiology, 2,* 577–582.

Pierce, R. S. (1991). Short report: Contextual influences during comprehension in aphasia. *Aphasiology, 5,* 379–381.

Pierce, R. S., and Beekman, L. A. (1985). Effects of linguistic and extralinguistic context on semantic and syntactic processing in aphasia. *Journal of Speech and Hearing Research, 28,* 250–254.

Pizzamiglio, L., and Appicciafuoco, A. (1971). Semantic comprehension in aphasia. *Journal of Communication Disorders, 3,* 280–288.

Podraza, B. L., and Darley, F. L. (1977). Effect of auditory prestimulation on naming in aphasia. *Journal of Speech and Hearing Research, 20,* 669–683.

Poeck, K., Huber, W., and Willmes, K. (1989). Outcome of intensive language treatment in aphasia. *Journal of Speech and Hearing Disorders, 54,* 471–479.

Poeck, K., and Pietron, H. (1981). The influence of stretched speech presentation on Token Test performance of aphasic and right brain damaged patients. *Neuropsychologia, 19,* 135–136.

Porch, B. E. (1967). *Porch Index of Communicative Ability.* Palo Alto, CA: Consulting Psychologists Press.

Reuterskild, C. (1991). The effects of emotionality on auditory comprehension in aphasia. *Cortex, 27,* 595–604.

Roberts, J. A., and Wertz, R. T. (1986). TACS: A contrastic-language treatment for aphasic adults. In R. H. Brookshire (Ed.), *Clinical aphasiology* (Vol. 16, pp. 207–212. Minneapolis. MN: BRK.

Rolnick, M., and Hoops, H. R. (1969). Aphasia as seen by the aphasic. *Journal of Speech and Hearing Disorders, 34,* 48–53.

Rosenbek, J., LaPointe, L. L., and Wertz, R. T. (1989). *Aphasia: A clinical approach.* Boston, MA: College Hill.

Salvatore, A. P. (1976). Training an aphasic adult to respond appropriately to spoken commands by fading pause duration within commands. In R. H. Brookshire (Ed.), *Clinical Aphasiology Conference proceedings,* Minneapolis, MN: BRK.

Salvatore, A. P., Strait, M., and Brookshire, R. H. (1978). Effects of patient characteristics on delivery of Token Test commands by experienced and inexperienced examiners. *Journal of Communication Disorders, 11,* 325–333.

San Pietro, M. J., and Rigrodsky, S. (1982). The effects of temporal and semantic conditions of the occurrence of the error response of perseveration in adult aphasics. *Journal of Speech and Hearing Research, 25,* 184–192.

Sarno, M. T. (1974). Aphasia rehabilitation. In S. Dickson (Ed.), *Communication disorders: Remedial principles and practices.* Glenview, IL: Scott Foresman.

Sarno, M. T. (1981). Recovery and rehabilitation in aphasia. In M. T. Sarno (Ed.), Acquired aphasia. New York: Academic Press.

Schuell, H. (1953a). Auditory impairment in aphasia: Significance and retraining techniques. *Journal of Speech and Hearing Disorders, 18,* 14–21.

Schuell, H. (1953b). Aphasic difficulties understanding spoken language. *Neurology, 3,* 176–184.

Schuell, H. (1969). *Aphasia in adults.* (NINDS, Monograph No. 10). *Human communication and its disorders.* Washington, DC: Department of Health, Education and Welfare, National Institutes of Health.

Schuell, H. (1973). (Revised by J. W. Sefer). *Differential diagnosis of aphasia with the Minnesota test.* Minneapolis, MN: University of Minnesota Press.

Schuell, H. (1974a). Clinical symptoms of aphasia. In L. F. Sies (Ed.), *Aphasia theory and therapy: Selected lectures and papers of Hildred Schuell.* Baltimore, MD: University Park Press.

Schuell, H. (1974b). The treatment of aphasia. In L. F. Sies (Ed.), *Aphasia theory and therapy: Selected lectures and papers of Hildred Schuell.* Baltimore, MD: University Park Press.

Schuell, H. (1974c). The development of a research program in aphasia. In L. F. Sies (Ed.), *Aphasia theory and therapy: Selected lectures and papers of Hildred Schuell.* Baltimore: University Park Press.

Schuell, H. (1974d). A theoretical framework for aphasia. In L. F. Sies (Ed.), *Aphasia theory and therapy: Selected lectures and papers of Hildred Schuell.* Baltimore: University Park Press.

Schuell, H., Carroll, V., and Street, B. (1955). Clinical treatment of aphasia. *Journal of Speech and Hearing Disorders, 20,* 43–53.

Schuell, H., and Jenkins, J. J. (1961a). Reduction of vocabulary in aphasia. *Brain, 84,* 243–261.

Schuell, H., and Jenkins, J. J. (1961b). Comment on "dimensions of language performance in aphasia." *Journal of Speech and Hearing Research, 4,* 295–299.

Schuell, H., Jenkins, J. J., and Jimnez-Pabn, E. (1964). *Aphasia in adults.* New York: Harper & Row.

Schuell, H., Jenkins, J. J., and Landis, L. (1961). Relationship between auditory comprehension and word frequency in aphasia. *Journal of Speech and Hearing Research, 4,* 30–36.

Schulte, E. (1986). Effects of imposed delay of response and item complexity on auditory comprehension by aphasics. *Brain and Language, 29,* 358–371.

Sherman, J. C., and Schweickert, J. (1989). Syntactic and semantic contributions to sentence comprehension in agrammatism. *Brain and Language, 37,* 419–439.

Shewan, C. M., and Canter, G. J. (1971). Effects of vocabulary, syntax, and sentence length on auditory comprehension in aphasic adults. *Cortex, 7,* 209–226.

Shewan, C. M. and Kertesz, A. (1984). Effects of speech and language treatment on recovery from aphasia. *Brain and Language, 23,* 272–299.

Siegel, G. M. (1959). Dysphasic speech responses to visual word stimuli. *Journal of Speech and Hearing Research, 2,* 152–167.

Siegenthaler, B. M., and Goldstein, J. (1967). Auditory and visual figure-background perception by adult aphasics. *Journal of Communication Disorders, 1*, 152–158.

Skelly, M. (1975). Aphasic patients talk back. *American Journal of Nursing, 75*, 1140–1142.

Smith, A. (1971). Objective indices of severity of chronic aphasia in stroke patients. *Journal of Speech and Hearing Disorders, 36*, 167–207.

Smithpeter, J. V. (1976). A clinical study of responses to olfactory stimuli in aphasic adults. In R. H. Brookshire (Ed.), *Clinical Aphasiology Conference proceedings*. Minneapolis, MN: BRK.

Sparks, R., Goodglass, H., and Nickel, D. (1970). Ipsilateral versus contralateral extinction in dichotic listening resulting from hemisphere lesions. *Cortex, 8*, 249–260.

Spreen, O. (1968). Psycholinguistic aspects of aphasia. *Journal of Speech and Hearing Research, 11*, 467–480.

Stachowiak, F. K., Huber, W., Poeck, K., and Kerschensteiner, M. (1977). Text comprehension in aphasia. *Brain and Language, 4*, 177–195.

Stimley, M. A., and Noll, J. D. (1991). The effects of semantic and phonemic prestimulation cues on picture naming in aphasia. *Brain and Language, 41*, 496–509.

Stoicheff, M. L. (1960). Motivating instructions and language performance of dysphasic subjects. *Journal of Speech and Hearing Research, 3*, 75–85.

Swinney, D. A., Zurif, E. B., and Cutler, A. (1980). Effects of sentential stress and word class upon comprehension in Broca's aphasics. *Brain and Language, 10*, 132–144.

Taylor, M. T. (1964). Language therapy. In H. G. Burr (Ed.), *The aphasic adult: Evaluation and rehabilitation*. Charlottesville, VA: Wayside Press.

Thompson, C. K., Raymer, A., and Le Grand, H. (1991). Effects of phonologically based treatment on aphasic naming deficits: A model-driven approach. In T. E. Prescott (Ed.), *Clinical aphasiology* (Vol. 20, pp. 239–261). Austin, TX: Pro-Ed.

Thompson, R. F. (1967). *Foundations of physiological psychology*. New York: Harper & Row.

Thorndike, E. L., and Lorge, I. (1944). *The teacher's word book of 30,000 words*. New York: Columbia University.

Tikofsky, R. (1968). Basic research in aphasic behavior: could it and should it contribute to rehabilitation? In J. Black and E. Jancosek (Eds.), *Proceedings of the Conference on Language Retraining for Aphasics*. Washington, DC: Social and Rehabilitation Service, Department of Health, Education and Welfare.

Tompkins, C. A. (1991). Redundancy enhances emotional inferencing by right- and left-hemisphere-damaged adults. *Journal of Speech and Hearing Research, 34*, 1142–1149.

Van Lancker, D. R., and Kempler, D. (1987). Comprehension of familiar phrases by left- but not by right-hemisphere damaged patients. *Brain and Language, 32*, 265–277.

Wallace, G. L., and Canter, G. J. (1985). Effects of personally relevant language materials on the performance of severely aphasic individuals. *Journal of Speech and Hearing Research, 50*, 385–390.

Waller, M. R., and Darley, F. L. (1978). The influence of context on the auditory comprehension of paragraphs by aphasic subjects. *Journal of Speech and Hearing Research, 21*, 732–745.

Webb, W. G., and Love, R. J. (1983). Reading problems in chronic aphasia. *Journal of Speech and Hearing Disorders, 48*, 164–171.

Weidner, W. E., and Jinks, A. F. G. (1983). The effects of single versus combined cue presentations on picture naming by aphasic adults. *Journal of Communication Disorders, 16*, 111–121.

Weidner, W. E., and Lasky, E. Z. (1976). The interaction of rate and complexity of stimulus on the performance of adult aphasic subjects. *Brain and Language, 3*, 34–40.

Weigl, E. (1968). On the problem of cortical syndromes: Experimental studies. In M. L. Simmel (Ed.), *The reach of the mind: essays in memory of Kurt Goldstein*. New York: Springer.

Weinstein, S. (1959). Experimental analysis of an attempt to improve speech in cases of expressive aphasia. *Neurology, 9*, 632–635.

Wepman, J. M. (1951). *Recovery from aphasia*. New York: Ronald Press.

Wepman, J. M. (1953). A conceptual model for the process involved in recovery from aphasia. *Journal of Speech and Hearing Disorders, 18*, 4-13.

Wepman, J. M. (1968). Aphasia therapy: Some relative comments and some purely personal prejudices. In J. Black and E. Jancosek (Eds.), *Proceedings of the Conference on Language Retraining for Aphasics*, Washington, DC: Social and Rehabilitation Service, Department of Health, Education and Welfare.

Wepman, J. M. (1972). Aphasia therapy: A new look. *Journal of Speech and Hearing Disorders, 37*, 203–214.

Wepman, J. M., and Jones, L. V. (1961). *Studies in aphasia: An approach to testing*. Chicago: University of Chicago Education Industry Service.

Wepman, J. M., Jones, L. V., Bock, R. D., and Van Pelt, D. (1960). Studies in aphasia: Background and theoretical formulations. *Journal of Speech and Hearing Disorders, 25*, 323–332.

Wertz, R. T. (1978). Neuropathologies of speech and language: An introduction to patient management. In D. F. Johns (Ed.), *Clinical management of neurogenic communicative disorders*. Boston, MA: Little, Brown.

Wertz, R. T. (1983). Language intervention context and setting for the aphasic adult: When? In J. Miller, D. E. Yoder, and R. Schiefelbusch (Eds.), *Contemporary issues in language intervention* (ASHA Report No. 12). Rockville, MD: American Speech- Language-Hearing Association.

Wertz, R. T. (1991). Keynote paper: Aphasiology 1990: A view from the colonies. *Aphasiology, 5*, 311–322.

Wertz, R. T., Collins, M. J., Weiss, D., Kurtzke, J. F., Friden, T., Brookshire, R. H., Pierce, J., Holtzapple, P., Hubbard, D. J., Porch, B. E., West, J. A., Davis, L., Matovitch, V., Morley, G. K., and Ressureccion, E. (1981). Veterans Administration cooperative study on aphasia. *Journal of Speech and Hearing Research, 24*, 580–594.

Wertz, R. T., and Porch, B. E. (1970). Effects of masking noise on the verbal performance of adult aphasics. *Cortex, 6*, 399–409.

Wertz, R. T., Weiss, D. G., Aten, J. L., Brookshire, R. H., Garcia-Bunuel, L., Holland, A. L., Kurtzke, J. F., LaPointe, L. L., Milianti, F. J., Brannegan, R., Greenbaum, H., Marshall, R. C., Vogel, D., Carter, J., Barnes, N. S., and Goodman, R. (1986). Comparison of clinic, home, and deferred language treatment for aphasia: A Veterans Administration cooperative study. *Archives of Neurology, 43*, 653–658.

Whitehouse, P., and Caramazza, A. (1978). Naming in aphasia: Interacting effects of form and function. *Brain and Language, 6*, 63–74.

Whitney, J. L., and Goldstein, H. (1989). Using self-monitoring to reduce dysfluencies in speakers with mild aphasia. *Journal of Speech and Hearing Disorders, 54*, 576–586.

Wilcox, J. M., Davis, G. A., and Leonard, L. B. (1978). Aphasics' comprehension of contextually conveyed meaning. *Brain and Language, 6*, 362–377.

Williams, S. E. (1984). Influence of written form on reading comprehension in aphasia. *Journal of Communication Disorders, 17*, 165–174.

Williams, S. E., and Canter, G. J. (1982). The influence of situational context on naming performance in aphasic syndromes. *Brain and Language, 17*, 92–106.

Williams, S. E., and Canter, G. J. (1987). Action-naming performance in four syndromes of aphasia. *Brain and Language, 32*, 124–136.

Wulfeck, B. B. (1988). Grammaticality judgments and sentence comprehension in agrammatic aphasia. *Journal of Speech and Hearing Research, 31*, 72–81.

Zingeser, L. B., and Berndt, R. S. (1990). Retrieval of nouns and verbs in agrammatism and anomia. *Brain and Language, 39*, 14–32.

Zurif, E. B., Caramazza, A., Myerson, R., and Calvin, J. (1974). Semantic feature representation for normal and aphasic language. *Brain and Language, 1*, 167–187.

CHAPTER 8

Treatment of Aphasia Subsequent to the Porch Index of Communicative Ability (PICA)

BRUCE E. PORCH

Before initiating treatment, and at various critical points during the therapeutic process, the clinician must answer a series of critical questions about the conduct of that treatment. The issues of major concern are how the brain lesion has affected the communicative ability of the patient; whether those deficits are treatable; what modalities, tasks, and stimuli should be used in treatment; what behavior should be reinforced; and when should treatment be terminated. Traditionally, answers to these problems are evolved empirically during treatment through trial-and-error methods or are arbitrarily decided on because of the clinician's bias for certain techniques and methods. In recent years, there is a growing tendency among clinicians who use the Porch Index of Communicative Ability (PICA) (Porch, 1981) to rely on the test results to help with the therapeutic decision making.

The discussion that follows will consider some of these treatment issues and will illustrate how PICA test results and PICA theory can assist the clinician in therapy planning. Much of this material is drawn from basic and advanced training courses that are designed to prepare the clinician for the use of the test. Therefore, although it is hoped that the concepts presented here are useful to a general audience, the full application of some of these methods will necessarily be limited to PICA-trained people who have demonstrated accuracy in the use of the multidimensional scoring system.

APHASIA VIEWED AS A PROCESSING PROBLEM

A cerebral insult results in a reduction in the capacity of the brain to process. In cybernetic terms, the patient has a reduced capacity to store, switch, and monitor, and to do the many other steps necessary for the brain to receive, assimilate, and send information. Since these processes cannot be observed directly, they must be assessed by exposing the patient to standard tasks, stimuli, and test conditions, and then the clinician, by carefully noting the response characteristics of the patient, can make inferences about the relative efficiency of various "brain circuits." Once the types and severity of processing dysfunctions are revealed, a suitable treatment plan may be developed.

The PICA is well suited to document and measure processing problems and to quantify behavior. The psychometric character-

istics of this test battery have been fully described elsewhere (McNeil, 1979; Porch, 1981, 1971) and are beyond the scope of the present discussion. However, some of the psychometric strengths of the PICA are equally potent in the treatment situation.

Multidimensional Scoring

The PICA's multidimensional scoring system offers several advantages over plus-minus scoring. During the treatment sessions the clinician must be sensitive to small changes in behavior and to response characteristics that indicate that the patient's communicative system is not yet fully operational. It is not sufficient simply to note that the patient got a response right or wrong during treatment. Subtle gradations of accuracy and inaccuracy must be perceived and quantified so that they can be better understood and manipulated. During successful treatment, the patient should get all responses correct if he is to improve his processing. After quantifying accuracy, the clinician should be sensitive to the patient's level of responsiveness, that is, whether the patient needs the stimulus repeated or if he needs additional cues before he can respond accurately. Another type of reduced responsiveness in the system is the self-correction that indicates that the patient is unable to compare and monitor his responses prior to expressing them, and, therefore, he must actually perform the response and evaluate it externally rather than internally.

In addition to *accuracy* and *responsiveness,* the PICA scoring system documents *completeness,* the degree to which the patient carries out the task in its entirety and follows the rules and restrictions of the task; *promptness,* the amount of processing time that the patient requires to complete the item; and *efficiency,* the motoric skill and coordination the patient demonstrates in carrying out the task. Each of these dimensions of behavior is quantified through the use of a binary choice scoring system shown in Figure 8.1. Using this system, the clinician can arrive at a single number that describes each response multidimensionally. This system not only provides a useful shorthand method for quantifying the nature of the response, but it also forces the clinician to be sensitive to small changes in behavior.

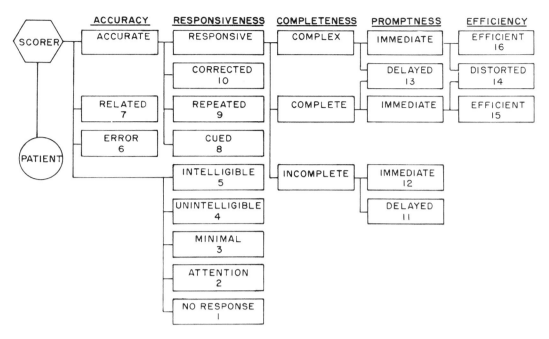

Figure 8.1. The multidimensional binary choice scoring system.

Table 8.1.
Examples of Patterns of Response

Stimuli	Patient		
	A	B	C
Cat	5	15	11
Dog	8	15	11
Boy	9	15	11
Apple	10	15	11
Cup	13	15	11
Shoe	15	13	11
Car	15	10	11
Soup	15	9	11
Ball	15	8	11
Pie	15	5	11
Mean score	11.0	11.0	11.0

Internal Consistency of Tasks

The PICA is designed so that all of the subtests revolve around 10 common objects. This has the psychometric advantage of holding content constant across subtests and therefore making it possible to compare the patient's skill across modalities and tasks. It also produces subtests that have very high internal consistency, with all of the items on a subtest being relatively equally difficult for the patient. Under these conditions, it is possible to detect patterns of response that are normally obscured by conventional aphasia tests that begin with easy items and get progressively more difficult. Table 8.1 shows how having stimuli that are relatively equally difficult will reveal various types of processing problems during testing or treatment.

In this simple example we see the scores for three different patients on a task involving 10 relatively equally difficult items.

Patient A rejects the first item but is able to respond to the next few items after the stimulus is repeated or cued or after a significant delay. Eventually he begins to respond at normal levels and receives scores of 15s. With Patient A it is apparent that he had trouble tuning into the task and adjusting his system to perform adequately during the first part of the task, but he eventually reached fully operational levels. Patient B starts out with no difficulty but gradually has decreasing scores and tunes out on the task, suggesting that he lacks the ability to keep his system locked into the task or to handle cumulative noise that might build up during the task. Patient C has a performance that is very homogeneous and shows no variation from item to item.

We see in the bottom row of Table 8.1 that all three patients got a mean score of 11.0, indicting that they are all functioning at about the same communicative level on this task. However, it is clear that the type of processing difficulties that each manifests is quite different. In addition, Patients A and B demonstrate several fully operational responses, suggesting that their circuits have the capacity to carry out the task once the processing problems are resolved. Patient C, although he got all of the 10 items correct on a plus-minus basis, shows no ability to do the task at operational levels, and his system is indicating that, at least at this point in time, it is performing the task as well as it can.

Because the PICA has high internal consistency, it is able to give some indication about these types of processing problems, and it indicates potential levels of ability that a patient may have on a given task. These same principles can be employed in treatment if the clinician will take the time to ensure that the stimulus items used on the task are relatively equally difficult.

DESIGNING A PLAN OF TREATMENT

Once the clinician has gained a thorough familiarity with the patient and his or her history, has completed comprehensive testing, and has found that the patient's condition is no longer changing dramatically from day to day, treatment planning can be initiated. The usual sequence of considerations at this point is to determine if the patient is a suitable candidate for treatment, to choose the tasks and stimuli to be used during treatment, to decide on which types of behavior will be reinforced on each task and, finally, to determine when treatment should be terminated.

Selecting Patients for Treatment

Determining whether a patient is treatable is a relatively new concern, arising in recent years as treatment became more expensive and available funding for treatment became more scarce. During the 1960s, Schuell and coworkers (1964) did some work on prognosis that assigned postrecovery, stabilized patients to one of five major or two minor prognostic groups. More recently, in an effort to develop earlier predictions, Porch and coworkers (1974, 1980) have described other prognostic studies that attempted to develop more accurate predictions of eventual recovery levels; however, these studies employing multiple discriminate analysis have not yet been validated for clinical use.

Perhaps the most widely used clinical method currently is the high-overall prediction (HOAP) method (Porch, 1970) that was developed during the late 1960s as an interim approach to prediction but that proved to be reasonably accurate and simple to use and therefore has persisted for a decade. In this method, it was theorized that the capacity of the patient's total communicative system was indicated by the highest scores or peak abilities. Therefore, the clinician could estimate the maximum potential for communication by using the average of the nine highest subtest scores achieved on the PICA or by using the highest modality score, whichever was the greatest. Appropriate tables or graphs enable the clinician to convert these scores into an estimate of the eventual outcome level and thereby make appropriate plans regarding treatment of the patient. Because this HOAP method may be applied as early as 1 month postonset in most cases, and because it takes into consideration the normal recovery stages, the clinician is in a better position to select the patients who are most treatable and to counsel families and physicians regarding the eventual recovery levels (Porch and Callaghan, 1981).

Estimating treatment potential is equally important later in the course of recovery. Eventually, the patient's condition seems to stabilize and the clinician must decide whether to continue treatment. Once again PICA scores are helpful in several ways in making this decision. First, discrepancies between the patient's overall score and the high modality score indicate the amount of potential change that remains. Second, after the patient is past the acute stage, it is expected that when he is at maximum recovery his subtest percentiles will be approximately equal and, therefore, differences between the nine highest subtest percentiles and the nine lowest subtest percentiles will also suggest a range of possible change or the lack of it.

These same principles hold true within subtests. The PICA scoring system provides 16 scores for any given response, and it is therefore possible for a patient to obtain a wide range of item scores. As a patient undergoes treatment for aphasia, the intrasubtest variability of scores gradually reduces until all of the item scores within the subtests are quite homogeneous, indicating that there are no peaks or depressions of ability on the task. This homogeneity suggests that the patient, at least at that point in time, is functioning at near maximum ability on that particular task. The circuits necessary to carry that task are consistently performing at their highest, current, potential levels of efficiency; there are no low responses that might be brought up to the patient's average level, and there are no higher scores that might serve as a target level toward which to strive. When the patient demonstrates homogeneity in all modalities on the PICA, his brain is indicating that it is performing communicatively and cybernetically near its maximum potential level of functioning and that further treatment of the processing problems may not be fruitful. At that point, the clinician may evolve new treatment goals of maximizing the patient's use of his functional systems, of modifying the patient's environment to facilitate his communication, and to educate the people in his environment as to the status of the patient's abilities and deficits and how to assist him in communicating.

In summary, an ideal treatment candidate is a cooperative patient whose medical condition is stable, who has a predicted overall percentile significantly above his or her present overall score, and who exhibits variation on item scores within subtests in some modalities.

Selecting Treatment Tasks

Before the discussion on treatment can continue, it is necessary to introduce some concepts and terminology related to PICA theory. As we see in Figure 8.2, we may visualize a continuum of communicative tasks ranging from the most simple vegetative communicative processes to the most complex learned processes. The ordinate represents the response continuum ranging at the top from the most complex levels of responses to the bottom of the continuum where the patient fails to attend or give any type of response.

The PICA samples a test field somewhere in the middle of the task continuum. The tasks sampled range from relatively simple ones with which only the most involved patients have difficulty to moderately challenging tasks on which even mild patients demonstrate some processing problems. The standard PICA test battery samples 18 points in the test field and establishes the subject's capacity to carry out tasks of varying difficulty.

The PICA tests have demonstrated that the interaction between the task and the response continua is best depicted by a sigmoidal function curve. If one were to test a normal subject longitudinally from infancy to adult levels of communication, this sigmoidal function curve would move from right to left on the task continuum and finally stabilize at some fairly high level of communicative ability. When a normal brain is damaged, that sigmoidal function curve shifts negatively to the right. The PICA locates the position of that response curve on the task continuum and, as indicated above, predicts how far positively that curve can be shifted with treatment.

Returning to our premise that aphasia represents a reduction in the processing efficiency of the brain, we can see that the sigmoidal function curve depicts the individual's processing abilities on a series of tasks ranked according to their difficulty level. The highest part of the curve on the right represents processing ability that is fully operational, and so the patient

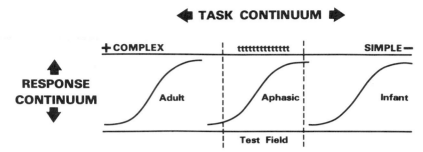

Figure 8.2. The task and response continua.

carries out these tasks accurately, immediately, efficiently, and without requiring additional information in order to understand the task. The middle or fulcrum of the curve shows those tasks on which the patient is responding accurately, but only if he receives additional information in the form of repeats, cues, or self-corrections, or if he takes additional processing time to carry out the task. The bottom of the curve represents those tasks on which the patient is responding inaccurately, demonstrating that the processing necessary to carry out those tasks is beyond his capacity at that time.

Using this schema, the problem of task and modality selection is greatly simplified for the clinician, since the patient's system indicates precisely those tasks that need immediate attention. Once the PICA has been administered and the results plotted to indicate the patient's response curve, it is quite apparent which tasks are already operational and do not require treatment, which tasks are on the fulcrum of the curve and should be treated, and which tasks are beyond the capacity of the patient's system at this time and should be excluded from the treatment format.

The reader should not confuse the concept of the fulcrum of the curve with the earlier suggestion that tasks on which the patient has the greatest item variability have the most potential for change and, therefore, that these tasks should be chosen for treatment. While it is true that tasks on which the patient has a large variety of scores, including high target scores and low scores that may be improved, have good potential for *eventual* change, such a task is too far down the curve. Attempts at treating it produce some errors, suggesting that the circuits involved are getting insufficient information to perform the task or that more efficiency in the circuit needs to be developed by using tasks more within the capacity of the circuits, that is, farther up the curve. In general, errors during treatment usually suggest that the task selected is too difficult at this point in time, or that the stimuli have been poorly chosen.

Selecting Treatment Stimuli

After the tasks in various modalities have been selected from the fulcrum of the curve, it is then necessary to select appropriate treatment stimuli to serve as vehicles for resolving the patient's processing problems on those tasks. Although it is common practice for clinicians to select stimuli on some a priori basis and then proceed with treatment, expecting the patient to do as well as he or she can with whatever stimuli selected, this is a dangerous practice because it does not take into consideration the specific type of processing problem the

patient has. Stimuli that are too difficult and overdrive the patient's system, or those that are too "noisy" and interfere with processing, not only may reduce the amount of positive results from treatment but may actually produce problems rather than resolve them.

The danger of using inappropriate stimuli can be obviated by testing their appropriateness on the tasks selected. The PICA score sheet may have already indicated to the clinician that the patient has more difficulty on certain types of stimuli such as polysyllabic words, words with consonant blends, or words that are too short to provide adequate clues for decoding. This type of information might be used in assisting in the selection of the repertoire of stimuli that the clinician plans to use for the treatment tasks. However, it is still important to verify the selected stimuli under the actual treatment conditions.

Stimulus verification is done through the use of PICA scoring, since the classic plus-minus is relatively insensitive to processing disorders. Having selected 20 or 30 stimuli that seem appropriate for the task, the clinician then explains to the patient what the task is and what he or she is expected to do. It is also useful to explain to the patient that the clinician will be scoring the responses so as to determine which stimuli will be the best to use in subsequent treatment sessions. Each stimulus, which has been listed on a treatment score sheet, is presented in order and the patient's responses are scored for later analysis. After all of the stimuli have been presented once, it is usually informative to present them again after a brief rest period to see how consistent the patient's processing is on each stimulus.

Table 8.2 shows how a few stimuli might be scored during a stimulus verification session. The clinician has selected some common nouns for treatment stimuli and has presented the list twice. In addition to the specific item scores the patient received, some other more general observations may be made about these two trials. First, the patient tends to improve slightly on the second trial, demonstrating that he has a good potential for improving after repeated trials. Second, it appears that the patient does somewhat better on polysyllabic words, thus suggesting that his auditory system may not be able to decode short stimuli rapidly enough and that the longer duration and increased information in longer words makes it easier to process them. Finally, it does not appear that there are any orderly changes as one scans down the column of scores on either trial. It is not unusual to find some patients whose scores gradually increase during a trial, suggesting that it takes several items for them to make the necessary adjustments to carry out the

Table 8.2.
Verification of Treatment Stimuli

Stimuli	Trial	
	First	Second
Apple	8	9
Hammer	13	15
Shoe	10	13
Cup	6	6
Baseball	15	15
Hat	9	9
Bicycle	15	15
Car	7	10
Window	13	13
Bus	9	10

task. Other patients may start out a given trial with high scores and then suddenly have decreasing scores as the trial proceeds, indicating that they are unable to lock their system into the task and they gradually tune out on the succeeding stimuli. In the example in Table 8.2, these types of trends are not seen, and therefore the variation in scores is probably attributable to the stimuli themselves.

Having made these general observations, the clinician is now ready to decide on which stimuli he or she will use in subsequent treatment sessions. The first rule here is to drop out any stimuli on which the patient received errors, scores 7 or below. The fact that the patient got error scores on one of the trials on those stimuli indicates that they are either too noisy or too difficult to be used in treatment and can only interfere with processing and progress. Too often the inexperienced clinician will attempt to "teach" these words to the patient but instead ends up putting more noise into his or her system and practice errors. A second consequence of using error type responses is that not only do you prohibit the facilitation of good switching on these stimuli, but the effect spreads to other stimuli on the list and it creates a spread of poor processing to other stimuli in the treatment trial. When a clinician is treating the processing problems of the patient, no given stimulus can be considered as sacred, and whenever one presents a problem it should be dropped out of the program.

This concept of dropping error items or stimuli should also be incorporated into the stimulus verification process, since items that are too difficult may have an interaction effect on other items. It is generally a good policy when running such trials to eliminate any error items from second and third trials to rule out possible interactions. In addition, the items that produce errors should be carefully analyzed for characteristics that are in contrast with items that invariably elicit 15-level responses. Such an analysis will give the clinician important information about what variables affect the circuits involved and what type of stimuli should be avoided in treatment.

It should be apparent that plus-minus scoring is too gross to yield meaningful information about the patient's system and that PICA scoring should be used if possible. However, clinicians who are not trained in PICA methods may achieve similar results by sorting stimuli into three categories: "easy" items that the patient has responded to accurately, without effort

or delay in a manner that might be referred to as "normal"; "medium" items that are responded to accurately but only after processing delays, self-corrections, or repeats of the stimuli, or after cues or additional information are given; and "hard" items that yield error responses. When using this system it is customary to designate the type of response as E, M, or H, or 3, 2, and 1, or the stimuli may be sorted into three separate piles if card-type stimuli are used.

At this point, after all of the sorting and analyzing of stimuli is complete, it would seem that the selection of tasks and stimuli is complete and the actual treatment might begin, but one more preliminary step is quite informative. Having selected a treatment task on which the patient gets 9- to 15-type scores (easy and medium responses), the clinician, instead of simply presenting the task multiple times in an effort to eventually achieve all easy responses, should manipulate some single variable of the task in a way that will immediately produce higher scores. If a particular manipulation does in fact improve responses, the clinician has discovered an important factor about the patient's system and what helps it to function successfully. By the same token, if the manipulation produces lower scores, evidence is obtained as to what variables have negative effects on the system. No change in responses as a result of the manipulation signifies that that variable is not a relevant factor in the patient's performance of the task.

A simple auditory task might illustrate how one carries out this probe technique. The clinician has selected a task that involves placing six pictures of common things in front of the patient and having him point to the one named. The clinician on the initial presentation obtained three easy responses (15s), a correct response after a repeat of the stimulus (9), a self-correction, and a delayed response (13). The question now is how may the task be modified to produce all easy-type responses immediately? There are several possibilities—reduce the number of items from six to four to simplify the task and reduce visual loading; use a carrier phrase before the noun ("Point to the __") to negate rise-time problems; add the printed word for the noun ("Car") to the picture to add visual information to assist the auditory system; give an arousal signal ("Ready? . . .Car") for system activation or attention problems; and so on.

Gradually, as various modifications of the task succeed, the patient is able to come to all easy responses until he or she finally achieves all 15s. During the process the clinician learns what factors make the patient's processing more or less efficient, information that will assist on this and future therapy tasks. In addition, possible tasks for subsequent treatment have also been documented. As the original probe task that started out down the curve was manipulated, it gradually moved up the curve until it reach the all 15-level. With each change the clinician documented the location of the various modifications of the task on the curve during this upward movement. Therefore, the clinician may, by working in reverse order down the curve, move from one task to the next in that sequence documented during the probe. As each task is raised to the all-easy level, the circuits under treatment become available for assisting the processing of other tasks down the curve and the entire response curve moves toward the more complex end of the task continuum.

Treatment Format

Once the tasks and the stimuli have been selected for treatment, the clinician is now ready to organize them into a treatment format that is designed to present a consistent presentation of tasks that will facilitate the patient responding at the all-15 level. That is, it is the goal of the clinician and the patient working as a team to have the patient eventually respond to every stimulus on the task without requiring cues, repeats, self-corrections, or significant delays. Not only is this type of treatment designed to be error-free, but as much as possible it tries to facilitate the patient's responses so that they are produced easily and without any processing difficulty.

All of these principles discussed thus far are roughly what is meant by "treating on the fulcrum of the curve." Processes on which the patient demonstrates delays and self-corrections are tentative processes that break down when used in more complex tasks used farther down the curve. If these minor processing problems are cleared up and the patient reaches the all-15 level in carrying out the processes, then these become available farther down the curve and all of the more complex processes can take advantage of the now normal, simpler processes. This phenomenon may, in part, explain why so many times we see tasks improving in the clinic that have not been treated directly during the therapeutic process. This schema also makes it clear why it is so inappropriate to treat tasks too far down the response curve because we are expecting the patient to carry out complex processes that require other basic processes that are not yet available to him or her.

When setting up the sequence of presentation of treatment activities, it must be realized that the goal of treatment is to assist the patient in mastering noisy, inadequate circuits and switching. Because sudden changes in tasks, target behavior, or methods of reinforcement invariably produce distraction and noise in the patient's communicative system, it is advisable to establish an orderly and fairly fixed format of treatment. If patients can anticipate the treatment events and if they have time to make leisurely transitions from task to task, they will maintain a more efficient, quieter system.

A useful format for ensuring adequate stimulation of the patient's system without producing noise or overload might be summarized as follows:

Module 1 {
1. Adjustment period (clearing out)
2. General activation (warmer upper)
3. Consolidation (old stuff)
4. Modification (new stuff)

Module 2 {
5. Consolidation (old stuff)
6. Modification (new stuff)
7. Conclusion (winder upper)

Adjustment Period

The adjustment period that initiates the treatment session is a brief but important time. After the patient enters the room and sits down at the treatment table, the clinician greets him and simply asks a broad, nondirective question such as "How's everything?" or "What's new?" This is designed to give the patient the opportunity to clear out his system and to tell the clinician about any special occurrences, problems, or questions that may have arisen since the last session. It also gives him an opportunity to try out in a free-speech situation some of the processes that he has been working on previously. The clinician, on the other hand, is trying to observe several things about the patient. First, it should be noted if there is a significant difference between the patient as he now appears compared with previous sessions. If he is markedly improved, it may be necessary to redesign the treatment session or to retest the patient to determine his new level of functioning. If he is functioning poorly compared with previous sessions, it may be necessary to probe into the cause of the problem or to discuss the matter with the family to see if there has been an exacerbation of the patient's medical problem. Sometimes the patient has less serious problems such as headache, shoulder pain, or some psychological or social issue that produces a depression in his ability and may make it necessary to be somewhat less adventurous in the treatment session on that day. Finally, while the patient is gradually adjusting his system to the room and to the clinician and is getting prepared for more difficult treatment tasks, the clinician is carefully noting the quality of the patient's communication and observing how much carryover there is from those processes that are being attacked during treatment to a spontaneous speech situation.

General Activation

Once it is certain that the patient is functioning adequately and that he has cleared his storage systems in preparation for treatment, the clinician can begin to focus the patient's attention on treatment-type tasks. For this purpose, a task is selected from the highest or consolidated part of the patient's response curve. This fairly easy, all-15-type task is for activating the patient's communicative systems and warming them up and for furnishing the patient with a gradual transition into the more difficult tasks. This activation period also will provide the clinician with a second check on the patient's general level of functioning on that day, and it gets the patient off to a successful start in his treatment session.

When initiating treatment with a new patient, information about what might be suitable warm-up tasks might be obtained from the PICA score sheet if one looks at the all-15 items on the easiest subtests. In the case of the patient who has been treated for a period of time, the clinician may elect tasks that at one time were on the fulcrum of the curve but that eventually became fully operational. Selecting these old tasks serves to verify that the patient is maintaining skills that were worked on formerly.

If, after a short period of general activation, the patient seems to be responding easily to simpler processing tasks, the clinician is ready to move on to the next step in treatment.

Just as in testing, where making a definite and clear transition in between tasks is important, the change between one step in treatment to the next should be made obvious to the patient so that he can clear out his system and make the necessary switching adjustments for the new task. This is done by giving the patient a general positive reinforcement for his efforts on the previous task and then suggesting that the patient just relax for a moment while the clinician makes notes about what has occurred in the session to that point. Then the clinician announces to the patient that they are going to be doing something different. The clinician should explain what the task will be and what the patient is expected to do, and then the first item of that task should be demonstrated for the patient. When it is apparent that the patient understands the task, the task should then be started with the demonstration item so that the patient's system is gently eased into the task. Generally, following this type of transition will minimize the amount of noise in the patient's system and greatly reduce his anxiety and fatigue.

Consolidation

Having moved through the adjustment and activation steps, the patient and clinician now are ready to begin the first of several treatment modules. A treatment module is a series of tasks directed at a given modality or process. Depending on how many steps there are in each module and how much time the total program takes, there may be two or three modules in a 1-hour treatment session. For instance, the first module might be devoted to consolidating and modifying auditory processing, and the clinician may then move on to the second module for consolidating and modifying verbal processing and, finally, turn to work on reading or writing as a third module.

A module is usually begun with a task that the clinician is trying to consolidate and make fully operational. This is a task quite high on the fulcrum of the curve, which on the first presentation has occasional delays in it but by the second or third presentation is all 15s. If, in a given session, it is found that this task is done at the all-15 level on the first presentation, the clinician might consider using that task as a warm-up in the future. If, on the other hand, the patient has continuing difficulty and cannot get to the all-15 level even after several presentations, it generally means that he is not ready to go on to new tasks in that module. If, after a few presentations, the patient is able to get all 15s, the clinician should do the task several times to consolidate those 15s and then prepare to move on to the next step in the module.

Modification

As the patient approaches the point where he or she is fully operational on a given task, it is then appropriate to think about modifying that task slightly so that it involves some new aspect of switching or storage. For instance, if, on an auditory task that requires the patient to point to one of four pictures after the clinician says the noun, the task might be modified by using six pictures, by having the patient point to two pictures instead of one, or by not allowing the patient to see the pictures while the clinician is saying the noun. Any of these changes probably would produce an increase in the number of delays or self-corrections that the patient might have on the task. The goal then would be to increase his performance until he achieves all 15s on the new task. If the clinician makes what is considered a small modification in the task and the patient begins to make errors or requires multiple repeats and cues before he gets a correct response, then it is apparent that the modification has been larger than expected and the task should be moved more in the direction of the consolidation task.

If the patient does fairly well with the new material and seems to understand it after several trials, he should be given a brief rest period in preparation for the next module. Usually shifting to a new modality means a shifting to new stimuli and treatment materials, but, once again, the transition should be verbalized to help the patient readjust his system for the new task. This same general procedure is then followed beginning with old material in the modality that needs to be consolidated

and then, if appropriate, moving on to some new modifications of the task to increase the patient's processing capabilities.

Conclusion

The final step in the treatment format should involve a fairly easy task at the all-15 level. The patient and the clinician have moved through a variety of fairly arduous tasks during the previous hour and have just completed a relatively new modification task that has been somewhat difficult, and concluding the treatment session on that note would be psychologically undesirable. Therefore, the clinician should select a task from the easy, consolidated part of the curve, which will assure winding up the session on a successful note. The clinician may also use this final step as a verification that the patient is maintaining his skills on one of the earlier treated processes. It is also a nice technique to use wind-up tasks from one day's session for a warm-up task on the next day's session. This helps the patient get back to the same point that he was at during the previous session, and it reduces intersession regression.

To summarize this section on the treatment format, the tasks are selected and sequenced in such a way as to maximize the efficiency of the patient's communicative systems and to minimize noise. Treatment of a given process or modality is begun with tasks selected from the consolidated, all-15 part of the curve to prepare those circuits for the more difficult tasks. Next, slightly more difficult tasks are selected from the fulcrum of the curve, and these are worked on until the patient eventually reaches the all-15 level. At that point, these newly consolidated processes are available for use on other tasks and, therefore, the patient's response curve moves positively toward the predicted target level.

TREATMENT PRINCIPLES
Patient-Clinician Team

Implicit in the treatment method being described here is the involvement of the patient in the conduct of the treatment process. The patient should understand that the clinician is not trying to teach the patient words but rather is attempting to return him to "easy" processing, free of self-corrections, repeats, and delays. The patient must be taught what "15" behavior feels like. It is sometimes helpful in teaching what is meant by "easy" processing to present the task using all "medium" items first, and then to repeat the task with all "easy" items so that the patient can get the feel of the contrast between the two levels of performance. Once this distinction is clear to the patient, he must also be taught to advise the clinician when a response is tentative or slightly off target so that it can be consolidated. In this sense the two people become a team in which the patient relies on the clinician to assist in selecting the tasks and stimuli and the patient keeps the clinician informed as to the impact of those items on his system.

Setting Treatment Priorities

The establishment of the specific modalities and processes to be treated is facilitated by careful examination of the PICA score sheet. All-15 tasks are selected for warm-up and wind-up tasks, the 13–15 level tasks should be treated, and the 9–13 level tasks, when slightly simplified, may soon be appropriate as modification tasks in the format.

In general, it is best to first treat processing problems that are not stimulus related. This includes difficulty in shifting tasks, tuning in, cumulative noise, and tuning out. These problems are diagnosed when a series of homogeneous items are presented on a task and the patient always has trouble (repeats, self-corrections, or delays) with the first few items or tunes out the last few, regardless of the order of stimulus presentation. When these temporal problems occur, a specific program may be designed to overcome them. For instance, the goal of eliminating tuning out might be achieved by discussing the problem with the patient and then presenting stimuli that generally elicit 15-type responses. At first, only a few stimuli are used, and these are worked on until the patient achieves all 15s. The number is then gradually increased until the patient can keep his system locked in to the task for a full complement of stimuli.

If the patient has problems that are more random or are stimulus related, those problems are overcome by getting the circuits necessary for the task to the 15 level and then processing multiple times at that level. The circuits for the task are facilitated and they will store processing information once the 15 level is achieved. Therefore, as treatment proceeds, those items on which the patient scored below 15 should be repeated until 15 is achieved and then repeated some more so that the circuit can sense what 15 processing entails and store that information.

Very often clinicians move through a series of stimuli and score responses without repeating items enough for success to occur. This is essentially testing rather than treating because the patient's circuits never have the opportunity to experience the target behavior and achieve fully operational circuits. It is probably more beneficial to move lower scores to 15s and practice the 15s if stable improvement is desired.

Criteria for Shifting Tasks

It should be very apparent by this point in the discussion that plus-minus scoring is completely inadequate for carrying out this type of treatment and that a more detailed type of scoring such as a PICA scoring system must be used. Second, the clinician must mentally score every response of every task in order to decide whether he or she should repeat the item or move on to the next one. Some clinicians like to write down every score for every response during the session so that they have a running account of exactly what happened in the patient's system. In that way they can make the correct adjustments in the program, and they can document the patient's change very precisely over time. Another approach is to record the scores on the first presentation of the task to establish a baseline and then to work on the task for a period of time and then rescore to measure change. Still other clinicians, who plan their treatment for a longer period of time and change the format less frequently, prefer to score the response at the beginning of the treatment week and then rescore them at the end of the week to see what changes have taken place. Specific application of PICA scoring has been described by Bollinger and Stout (1974) in their discussion on response contingent small step treatment; by LaPointe (1974), who gives examples of PICA scoring as used in Base 10 Program Stimulation; and by Brookshire (1973) in his general consideration of aphasia treatment.

Some of the major differences between these types of programs and the PICA program described here are the criteria for selecting tasks and stimuli and the criteria for shifting to new tasks or terminating tasks. Many programs suggest an 80% or 90% correct criterion, which is undoubtedly too low, since this would allow the patient to have repeats, self-corrections, or delays on every item and still meet the criterion. Even a standard of 95%, 13s (delays), or better allows the patient to have significant problems with 5% of the items. When this amount of interference in processing occurs, the information being processed is probably considered by the system as being tentative, and, therefore, it is not stored for long-term use. This in turn means that the process being treated is not fully consolidated and is not available for use on tasks farther down the curve.

PICA theory, therefore, suggests that the target for changing or terminating tasks is all-15 responses. This may seem overly idealistic, but it is in fact realistic and essential. Such a goal is attainable because the tasks and the stimuli used have been carefully chosen and verified through the patient's system.

The second reason that all-15 responses are an appropriate treatment goal is that this type of processing seems to transfer better and is more resistant to regression. Unless a task is fully consolidated, it will tend to deteriorate in a normal life situation or in a more difficult treatment task. Cued (8) to self-corrected (10) responses often become errors, and delayed responses (13) shift to lower, more tentative scores. For this reason, transfer of these skills rarely occurs because they are not operational. Conversely, if the patient develops a good awareness of what "easy" responses are and achieves them on all of the items on the task, transfer can be maximized and regression can be prevented.

FUTURE TRENDS

The treatment methods based on PICA test results and multidimensional scoring described in this chapter offer several advantages over less structured approaches. In starting treatment, the clinician and the patient are offered a specific target level of overall communicative ability to work toward, and this can be computed quite early in the course of recovery. The treatment, once initiated, focuses on modalities and processes that the patient's own communicative systems have indicated are appropriate to modify at that point in time; and the exact difficulty levels of the tasks, the stimuli, and the target behavior are prescribed and verified by the level of multidimensional scores the patient achieves. All of this evolves naturally out of a treatment format that maximizes the patient's processing efficiency while minimizing the possibility that the clinician is misdesigning the treatment. Finally, the predictive formulas and the measures of intrasubtest variability indicate when the patient is at last functioning at his or her highest possible levels so that plans for terminating treatment may be made.

In contrast to these advantages, the PICA approach to treatment has disadvantages in that it requires special training to see the behavior in detail and to convert that behavior into scores; it requires a great deal of preparation and planning at every stage of treatment; it necessitates a considerable amount of book work to record and analyze all of the response scores; and, because of its emphasis on cybernetics rather than content, it is quite structured and, therefore, gives the clinician less freedom to experiment during the treatment session.

References

Bollinger, R., and Stout, C. E. (1974). Response contingent small step treatment. In B. E. Porch (Ed.), *Clinical Asphasiology Conference proceedings*. Albuquerque, NM: VA Hospital.

Brookshire, R. H. (1973). *An introduction to aphasia*. Minneapolis, MN: BRK.

LaPointe, L. L. (1974). Base 10 "programmed-stimulation": Task specification, scoring, and plotting performance in aphasia therapy. In B. E. Porch (Ed.), *Clinical Aphasiology Conference proceedings*. Albuquerque, NM: VA Hospital.

McNeil, M. R. (1979). The porch index of communicative ability. In F. L. Darley (Ed.), *Evaluation of appraisal techniques in speech and language pathology*. Cambridge, MA: Addison-Wesley.

Porch, B. E. (1981). *The Porch Index of Communicative Ability*. Palo Alto, CA: Consulting Psychologists Press.

Porch, B. E. (1970). PICA interpretation: Recovery and treatment (video training tape). Albuquerque, NM: VA Hospital.

Porch, B. E. (1971). Multidimensional scoring in aphasia testing. *Journal of Speech and Hearing Research* 14, 777–792.

Porch, B. E., and Callaghan, S. (1981). Making predictions about recovery: Is there HOAP? In R. H. Brookshire (Ed.), *Clinical Aphasiology Conference proceedings*. Minneapolis, MN BRK.

Porch, B. E., Wertz, R. T., and Collins, M. (1974). Statistical and clinical procedures for predicting recovery from aphasia. In B. E. Porch (Ed.), *Clinical Aphasiology Conference proceedings*. Albuquerque, NM: VA Hospital.

Porch, B. E., Collins, M., Wertz, R. T., and Friden, T. P. (1980). Statistical prediction of change in aphasia. *Journal of Speech and Hearing Research* 23, 312–321.

Schuell, H., Jenkins, J., and Jiminez-Pabon, E. (1964). *Aphasia in adults*. New York, Harper & Row.

CHAPTER 9
Language-Oriented Treatment: A Psycholinguistic Approach To Aphasia

CYNTHIA M. SHEWAN and DONNA L. BANDUR

HISTORY OF APHASIA TREATMENT

Little in the way of what we now know as orthodox treatment for aphasia appeared before the beginning of the 20th century. In the early 1900s, the literature reported a few studies describing treatment (Franz, 1906, 1924; Frazier and Ingham, 1920; Mills, 1904; Weisenburg and McBride, 1935), and even as far back as this, questions were raised, although not answered, relative to the efficacy of treatment.

After World War II, there was a surge of interest in aphasia treatment because of the number of war veterans with aphasia as a result of trauma. The focus of these rehabilitation efforts was on reeducation, the approach developed for treatment. Because of the effects of trauma on the personality of these individuals, many psychotherapy groups became a part of rehabilitation efforts (Backus, 1952; Blackman, 1950). Reportedly, these groups provided support and positively influenced both communication and personality adjustment (Aronson et al. 1956; Blackman and Tureen, 1948). Questions of treatment efficacy were raised, but few answers were given. Data, however, with the exceptions of Eisenson (1949) and Wepman (1951), were primarily anecdotal and not statistically supported. In addition, the data available focused on trauma rather than stroke.

In the 1950s, aphasia treatment shifted to dealing with individuals who became aphasic as a result of cerebrovascular accident (CVA). Schuell's work in this era and in the 1960s dominated the scene (Schuell et al., 1964). The data published about treatment were controversial, and whether aphasia treatment was efficacious remained an issue. On the one hand, Vignolo's study (1964) reported the significantly positive effects of treatment, while the study by Sarno et al. (1970) failed to show the positive effects of language treatment.

The 1970s and early 1980s witnessed the publication of several studies, some with and some without control groups, that supported the efficacy of language treatment with aphasic individuals (Basso et al., 1979; Basso et al., 1975; Broida, 1977; Dabul and Hanson, 1975; Deal and Deal, 1978; Hagen, 1973; Prins et al., 1978; Sefer, 1973; Shewan and Kertesz, 1984; Smith, et al., 1972; Wertz et al., 1978; Wertz et al., 1981). The ideal study, using a randomized no-treatment control group, was not done, and some believed that only this study

would lay to rest their doubts about the efficacy of aphasia treatment. Despite some studies that disputed the efficaciousness of language treatment (David et al., 1982; Meikle et al., 1979), enough evidence had been gathered by 1982 for Darley (1982) to conclude that "the foregoing collage of studies . . . collectively provides a series of answers and together lays our doubt about efficacy to rest" (p. 175).

However, Darley's proclamation did not convince everyone, and efficacy studies continued throughout the 1980s and into this decade, with the majority favoring the significant and positive effects of treatment (Brindley et al., 1989; Holland and Wertz, 1988; Poeck et al., 1989; Schönle, 1988; Springer et al., 1991; Wertz et al., 1986; Whitney and Goldstein, 1989). One of the most interesting additions of these more recent studies has been the use of single-subject designs as a methodological approach to studying efficacy. A second interesting feature has been the breadth of different types of treatment used.

EVOLUTION OF LANGUAGE-ORIENTED TREATMENT

Language-oriented treatment (LOT) developed from a need to provide the best possible clinical services to individuals with aphasia. At the time of its conception in the 1970s, several conditions produced a fertile climate for development of such an approach. The aphasia literature contained few descriptions of treatment that were sufficiently detailed to permit clinicians to use them, confident that they were using them as designed. Few treatments had been demonstrated to be efficacious, and the efficacy questions were still prevalent. While the predominant treatment approach among clinicians was stimulation therapy, research data were accumulating about how aphasic patients* processed language. Also, as clinicians, we were finding that some patients did not seem to improve with a stimulation approach in which the content of treatment was not controlled. Therefore, an approach with a structured methodology in which

---

*The terminology used to refer to persons with aphasia who are being treated differs according to treatment facility, author preference, etc. In this chapter, such individuals are referred to as patients.

a subject progressed through steps of increasing difficulty, combined with content based on research data of how aphasics process language, seemed to be promising, at least conceptually.

Over a period of 2 years, Shewan evolved the LOT method (Shewan, 1977) and pilot-tested it with a small group of patients. The data were promising, and a full-scale clinical trial was later undertaken. The results of that trial form the efficacy data reported later in this chapter. A decade passed from ideational conception to publication of a book fully describing LOT, complete with treatment guidelines, treatment materials, and efficacy data (Shewan and Bandur, 1986).

Philosophy and Rationale

Many aphasia treatments derive from theories of what aphasia is. This is also true for LOT. Defined here, aphasia represents an impairment in the language system and potentially in the access to the language system. In addition, aphasia involves an impairment to the processes for understanding and producing language. This theoretical view of aphasia derives from the work of Zurif and his colleagues (Zurif and Caramazza, 1976; Zurif et al., 1972; Zurif et al., 1976).

The content of language treatment is important in the LOT method. LOT does not represent indiscriminant stimulation of the language system, with the hope that something takes and improvement occurs. LOT's goal is to provide a patient with a language-processing system that operates at its maximum functional level. This is accomplished by applying neurolinguistic findings to treatment. Unfortunately, technology does not yet exist whereby we can determine whether the brain accomplishes this by increasing the efficiency of the language-processing system, by reorganizing it, and/or by establishing language functions in homologous brain areas.

The content of LOT is based on language materials that are arranged in hierarchies of difficulty that, in turn, reflect research information about how adults, normal and aphasic, process language. Consequently, LOT is psycholinguistic in nature and may be categorized as a psycholinguistic approach to aphasia treatment. Because it is based on neurolinguistic theory and applies neurolinguistic research findings to treatment, Helm-Estabrooks (1988) has categorized LOT as a neurolinguistic approach to treatment.

The content of treatment is distinguished from methodology. Content is the "what" of treatment, while methodology is the "how." Treatment is individualized and tailored to each aphasic individual's pattern of language difficulties and interests. LOT provides guidelines, not prescriptions, about how to organize treatment. The method is flexible enough so that each aphasic person has an individualized plan, but structured enough so that the approach is replicable across clients and clinicians.

Content of Language-Oriented Treatment

To provide a system whereby the content of language could be described comprehensively and to facilitate data collection, LOT divided the communication system into five modalities, which are nonoverlapping and mutually exclusive (Fig. 9.1). The five modalities are auditory processing, visual processing, gestural and combined gestural-verbal communication, oral expression, and graphic expression.

Each modality is subdivided into mutually exclusive areas that collectively encompass that entire modality. With each modality segmented into component parts, a clinician can specify clearly the content of treatment being provided. Although many segmentations of the communication system are possible, the particular segmentation used in LOT seemed reasonable and descriptive. Rather than advocating a particular division of the communication system, the division was intended to facilitate specifying the content of treatment and to permit its replication.

Within each area of a modality—for example, comprehension of sentences within auditory processing—treatment materials are organized according to difficulty level, based on the research literature describing how aphasic individuals process language. The goal of language treatment, then, is to improve a patient's language deficits by presenting material that increases in difficulty level at a pace that the patient can accommodate.

Methodology of Language-Oriented Treatment

Methodology refers to the "how" of treatment. LOT methodology adopted a paradigm in which the major components are stimulus, response, and reinforcement. However, the goal of LOT, in contrast to operant conditioning, is not to learn specific stimulus-response connections, that is, to learn specific words in a word-retrieval task or specific sentences in a sentence formulation task. Rather, the paradigm of presenting stimuli, followed by responses with appropriate feedback, is to provide opportunities for aphasic patients to process language at levels appropriate to their current abilities. Feedback provides information regarding the adequacy of performance. Aphasic patients are not always aware of the accuracy of their performance or the improvements they make over time.

The advantages of approaching the delivery of treatment in this way are many. It permits a clinician to collect data about each patient's performance. It allows a clinician to evaluate the treatment provided: Is the patient improving or not? It also allows the replication of procedures across patients, clinicians, and treatment centers.

Difficulty Levels

In LOT, materials are presented to the aphasic patient in order of increasing difficulty. How is this order ascertained for each patient? Sources of information include the results of any standardized testing administered, a patient's case history, or the determination that a patient is following an already established hierarchy reported in the literature. If a clinician does not have a hierarchy to follow, one can be created by collecting baseline data and constructing a criterion-based test. If establishment of a hierarchy for sentence comprehension is needed, several examples each of several sentence types can be constructed and presented to the aphasic patient. For example, combining the work of Caramazza and Zurif (1978), Levy and Taylor (1968), Parisi and Pizzamiglio (1970), and Shewan and Canter (1971) would produce a sentence-type hierarchy as shown in Table 9.1. The sentences are listed, top to bottom, from easiest to most difficult. Results of this test demonstrate the order of difficulty for the patient. This order of difficulty would then constitute the hierarchy to be followed in treatment.

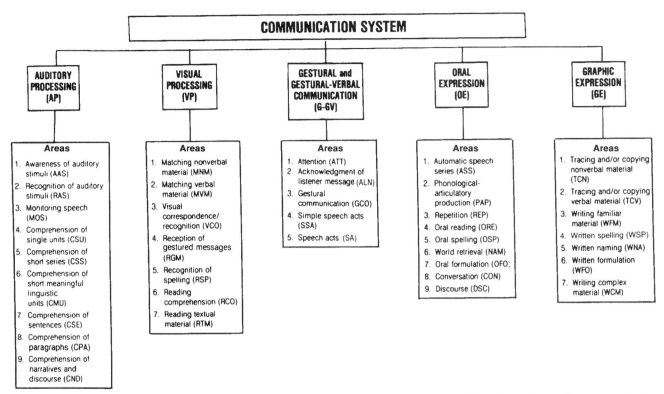

Figure 9.1. A schematic model of the language modalities and areas within these modalities that make up the communication system.

Table 9.1.
Difficulty Hierarchy for Sentence Types Ordered According to Difficulty[a]

Sentence Type	Example
Simple active affirmative Declarative	The dog is chasing the cat.
Negative	The dog is not chasing the cat.
Passive	
Nonreversible	The ball is being caught by the dog.
Reversible	The cat is being chased by the dog.
Negative-passive	The cat is not being chased by the dog.
Center-embedded	
Nonreversible	The cat that the dog is chasing is meowing.
Reversible	The cat that the dog is chasing is black.

[a] Adapted from Shewan, C. M., and Bandur, D. L. (1986). *Treatment of aphasia: A language-oriented approach* (p. 47). Austin, TX: Pro-Ed.

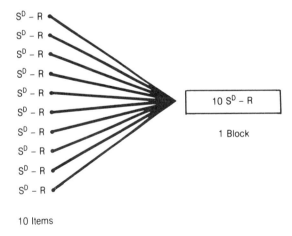

Figure 9.2. Ten stimulus items (S^D) and their responses (R) constitute one block.

Increasing Difficulty Level. The stimuli and their responses in treatment are presented in blocks of 10 items each (Fig. 9.2). As shown in Figure 9.3, to advance the difficulty level of a task, a patient must achieve 70% or more correct on two consecutive blocks of items at the same difficulty level. When this criterion is achieved, the difficulty level of the task is increased to the next level in the hierarchy. If the 70% correct criterion is not achieved, the block of 10 stimulus items is repeated. If 70% correct is still not achieved, the level of diffi-

culty of the task is decreased. If, even with a decrease in the task difficulty, the 70% correct criterion is not obtained, the task is discontinued. The patient obviously cannot perform that language task.

A criterion of 70% correct was chosen to allow flexibility in response performance and to tolerate some error without unduly delaying progress in treatment. The small number of items in a block (10) means that one error reduces performance 10%. If a particular patient demonstrates the need for a higher criterion, one can be used. It is important to remember, however, that the efficacy data reported in this chapter used the 70% criterion.

A discussion of difficulty level raises three related topics: cuing, criterion response, and branching.

Cuing

If a patient cannot generate an independent response, a clinician may accept a cued response as correct. The goal in using a cuing system is to determine which cues are effective, to develop the patient's awareness of those helpful cues, to transfer the responsibility for initiating and providing cues from the clinician to the patient, and to increase the patient's use of independent responses, using self-cuing as necessary.

Criterion Response

To determine whether to increase the difficulty level of a task requires assessing whether a client's responses are correct or incorrect. Therefore, it is very important for the clinician to define what response will meet the criterion of "correct." In most tasks, many different levels of response are possible, and what is accepted as correct may change with time and as improvement occurs. However, for each task, a clinician must decide what target response will meet criterion. For example, early in treatment a clinician may decide that in a naming task, a recognizable production meets criterion. Later, a phonetically correct production may be required to score the response as meeting criterion.

Branching

When the difference between two adjacent levels of difficulty proves to be too great for a patient to master, a clinician can create levels of intermediate difficulty (branching). This will create a bridge between the initial tasks and help the patient to reach the next level. Branching is easy to signify on the LOT data record forms. Another situation requiring branching may arise when a clinician wants to divide a large group of equally difficult material into two subgroups in order to provide language-processing opportunities with each subgroup and to avoid omitting some materials.

Scoring Responses

Patient responses in LOT are scored as correct or incorrect. The clinician decides what constitutes a correct response, as described earlier. Because the clinician has flexibility in establishing this decision, the definition of a correct response differs for each task. Just as increasing the difficulty of the stimuli presented increases the difficulty level of a task, so does increasing the complexity of the response required.

Feedback

Feedback is an important part of the LOT methodology and refers to information provided to a patient about his or her performance. The ultimate goal is for the patient to self-monitor performance in daily living communication situations, but clini-

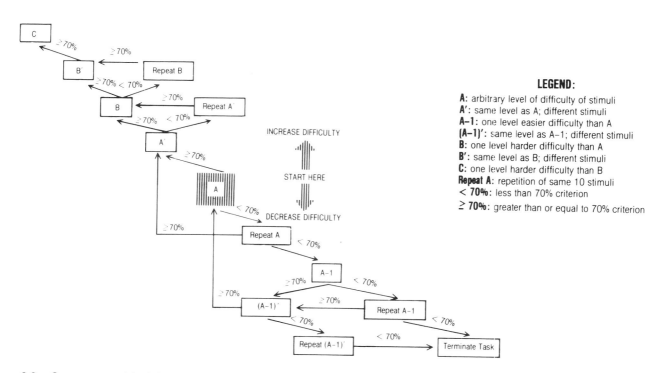

LEGEND:

A: arbitrary level of difficulty of stimuli
A': same level as A; different stimuli
A-1: one level easier difficulty than A
(A-1)': same level as A-1; different stimuli
B: one level harder difficulty than A
B': same level as B; different stimuli
C: one level harder difficulty than B
Repeat A: repetition of same 10 stimuli
< 70%: less than 70% criterion
≥ 70%: greater than or equal to 70% criterion

Figure 9.3. Summary model of the administration of LOT. The starting point is A. A block of 10 items is presented to the aphasic patient. If the patient achieves 70% or more, the level of difficulty is increased and the clinician proceeds to B to initiate another cycle. If the patient achieves less than 70% correct responses at A, the clinician repeats A. If the patient achieves 70% or more, the clinician proceeds to A'; if not, the level of difficulty is reduced and the clinician regresses to A-1. If the level of difficulty is reduced one level and repeated with less than 70% success, the task is terminated.

cian feedback is important during treatment activities. This feedback points out progress and provides encouragement. Our experience is that it also helps the patient better understand treatment and its goals as well as making the patient a more active participant in the clinical process. However, it is important to be honest with the patient. Telling a patient everything is fine when it obviously is not will undermine trust and credibility, both important ingredients in a therapeutic relationship.

Sequence of Treatment Activities

Sequencing of activities in LOT occurs along several dimensions. Already discussed is the sequence whereby the difficulty level of materials is increased as the client progresses through the treatment hierarchies. Sequencing also refers to the selection sequence of the modalities to be included in treatment, that is, which to choose first. Some rehabilitation data report that auditory comprehension recovers first and most (Basso et al., 1979; Henri, 1973). Because understanding is crucial to the treatment process and to so much of life, it is important to include auditory comprehension early if it is impaired to any great extent. Because comprehending and speaking are the most frequent communication activities, the auditory-processing and oral expression modalities are often included early in treatment. LOT is flexible, and the appropriate selections can be made by the patient and clinician.

Activities are also sequenced within any given treatment session. With an awareness of proactive and retroactive facilitation and inhibition, a clinician can sequence activities to take as much advantage of facilitation as possible. It is desirable to initiate a treatment session with an activity on which the patient performs well. The initial success will lead to increased motivation. Generally, the difficulty of activities is increased as the session progresses. If perseveration occurs, the best strategy is to change the task. It is also desirable to end the session on a positive note, with an activity that is successful and enjoyable for the patient.

Recording Data

Recording data is very important in LOT because it is the patient's performance that dictates when tasks should be increased or decreased in difficulty. Two forms (Appendices 9.1 and 9.2) have been helpful in this respect. An LOT Goals Form, if used for each area in each modality, can chart the course of treatment. The difficulty level, the stimuli, the presentation method, cuing, criterion for a correct response, and response method are all recorded. Additional responses are also noted. Using this form, a clinician can show how treatment is changing over time. An LOT Data Record Form specifies the amount of time spent in each session for each area and modality, the difficulty level of the task, the number of items presented, the data collected, and any comments a clinician wishes to record. Glancing at this form indicates what transpired in each session and tells a clinician when the task level should be increased. Again, it seems easiest to record data for each area and each modality using a separate form.

Patient-Clinician Interaction

In any treatment approach to aphasia, it is paramount to remember that you are dealing first with a person, a person who has experienced a tremendous loss, certainly in communication abilities, and perhaps in physical, psychological, and social areas as well. LOT, although structured in content and methodology, is carried out within a caring and positive interpersonal environment. The person is not ignored or diminished by structuring the content of treatment.

The following sections will provide a brief overview of the structure and implementation of LOT, while addressing problems in the modalities of auditory processing, visual processing, gestural and gestural-verbal communication, oral expression, and graphic expression. Variables to consider in establishing goals and developing treatment activities are discussed, although inclusion of detailed treatment hierarchies is not possible, given the scope of this chapter. The reader is referred to *Treatment of Aphasia: A Language-Oriented Approach* (Shewan and Bandur, 1986) for an in-depth description of specific treatment procedures, methodology, and treatment materials. Case examples, highlighting implementation of LOT, will be discussed. These patients, although not participants in the efficacy study, serve to illustrate the continued applicability of this treatment approach.

AUDITORY PROCESSING PROBLEMS

General Considerations

Various types of auditory-processing problems occur in aphasic patients, including auditory imperception, pure-word deafness, and auditory agnosia. The most prominent difficulties, however, are generally associated with auditory comprehension, and these have, thus, received the most attention in designing treatment strategies. In LOT, auditory processing has been divided into two major categories: Auditory Perceptual Processing Deficits and Auditory Comprehension Deficits. Generally, auditory perceptual activities are introduced only if success cannot be attained with auditory comprehension activities. By developing auditory perceptual skills, the patient may learn to tune into the auditory modality and prepare this mechanism for comprehension activities.

Auditory Perception

Auditory perceptual deficits are addressed in three areas: Awareness of Nonspeech and Speech Stimuli, Recognition of Nonspeech and Speech Stimuli, and Monitoring Speech.

In establishing awareness of nonspeech and speech stimuli, the patient is required only to respond differentially, but not necessarily to demonstrate recognition of the stimuli. Environmental sounds, music, familiar and unfamiliar speakers, and foreign languages may be used. In Area 2, however, the patient must attach meaning to the stimuli presented, such as matching a telephone ring to its corresponding referent.

In the final area, Monitoring Speech, activities are incorporated to develop the patient's ability to monitor the accuracy and/or meaningfulness of speech stimuli, whether they are his or her own productions or those of others.

This particular area may be one that is addressed throughout the course of the patient's treatment in conjunction with activities of other areas, within this modality, and from other modalities.

	Broca's	Wernicke's	Anomic
Easy	Body parts	Body parts	Body parts
	Actions	Actions	Objects
	Objects	Objects	Actions
	Numbers	Numbers	Numbers
	Colors	Letters	Colors
	Letters	Colors	Letters
Difficult	Geometric forms	Forms	Forms

Figure 9.4. Hierarchies in difficulty levels showing differences according to semantic categories.

Auditory Comprehension

Auditory comprehension is influenced by a number of factors. Particularly with sentences, stress as a suprasegmental cue has been found to influence performance (Goodglass, 1975, 1976; Kellar, 1978; Pashek and Brookshire, 1980). Patients with severe comprehension problems may obtain information from intonational contour to differentiate between questions, statements, and commands (Boller and Green, 1972; Green and Boller, 1974). Word frequency has been shown to affect comprehension, both in isolation and in sentences, with common, more frequently occurring vocabulary items being more easily understood. Sentences that are longer and reflect more complex syntax also tend to be more difficult (Shewan, 1979). Sentence comprehension may be influenced not only by vocabulary and syntax but also by grammatical contrasts. Aphasic patients have been shown to perform better on language tasks, including comprehension of yes/no questions (Wallace and Canter, 1985) when personally relevant material is used. Additional factors to be considered include situational context, speech rate, emotional content, and topic familiarity.

Treatment for auditory comprehension has been divided into six areas. Comprehension of Single Units deals with stimuli at the single-word level. In designing activities, important variables related to vocabulary selection are frequency of occurrence, grammatical class, and semantic category. Altering response variables, such as picture relatedness and number of response choices, may also contribute to task difficulty (Pierce et al., 1990). Depending on the type of aphasia, various hierarchies may be established through systematic alteration of both stimuli and response variables. The hierarchies shown in Figure 9.4 reflect alterations in semantic categories for various aphasia types (Goodglass et al., 1966).

Comprehension of Short Series is typically used when memory variables need to be stressed, as the word series themselves do not form a syntactic unit. For example, when presenting a group of numbers, the patient must attend to each item in order to identify the series corrrectly. Syntactic units are introduced in Comprehension of Short Meaningful Linguistic Units, where variables such as word frequency and topic familiarity are important to consider.

In developing a hierarchy for the following area, Comprehension of Sentences, syntax, grammatical contrasts and word frequency are altered. Patients may benefit from the use of context in sentence comprehension activities (Pierce, 1988), such that reducing contextual information may increase task difficulty.

Comprehension of Paragraphs requires the clinician to address sentence length, syntax, word frequency, cohesion among sentences, number of facts, topic familiarity, and patient interest. Of course, only those variables that affect the particular patient being treated are altered in the treatment program.

Less specific information from the literature is available for developing stimuli in the area of Comprehension of Narratives and Discourse. Variables similar to those in the last area affect performance, as does overall length. Some patients may also experience difficulty in comprehending referents from contextual information (Chapman and Ulatowska, 1989) and may therefore require specific assistance with processing referents. Patients tend to experience more errors in recalling details of high-ratio dialogues (i.e., ones in which the amount of speaking between the participants is significantly disproportionate). Greater difficulty may also be found in recalling implied information as opposed to information that is directly stated (Katsuki-Nakamura et al., 1988). Mode of presentation may affect performance such that audiotape, videotape, and live presentations can have varying impacts, depending on the individual patient. As with many other aspects of the treatment program, the patient may be the most valuable source of information by reflecting on his or her own day-to-day experiences in processing auditory information.

Case Example

S.K. is a 24-year-old university student. Following excision of a left temporal occipital arteriovenous malformation, he demonstrated a fluent aphasia, characterized by moderate anomia, auditory- and visual-processing problems, and a mild agraphia. Formalized testing included administration of the Boston Diagnostic Aphasia Evaluation, the Auditory Comprehension Test for Sentences, the Revised Token Test, and the Boston Naming Test.

Auditory comprehension problems were initially found in S.K.'s comprehension of material at the paragraph level and in his processing of linguistically complex, lengthy instructions. The first treatment area selected was comprehension of paragraphs. Further probing revealed that S.K. experienced increased difficulty when required to make inferences and when the number of facts included within a paragraph was substantially increased.

S.K. was an active participant in developing treatment goals and hierarchies. He provided detailed feedback on the variables that he found affected his performance, and he reported on specific situational problems.

For the first level of difficulty, the clinician aurally provided short paragraphs consisting of a high degree of redundancy, with S.K. required to answer inferential questions. When a 70% success rate was achieved at this level, difficulty was increased by including more facts in the paragraphs. As treatment progressed, difficulty levels were further adjusted by altering topic familiarity. More complex responses on the part of the patient were gradually introduced, so that prior to questioning by the clinician, S.K. was asked to recall as many details as possible from the paragraph. Further information was then extracted through use of either factual or inferential questions.

Comprehension of Narratives and Discourse was next developed. Short radio broadcasts were presented, followed by videotaped news segments and lengthier documentaries. Task difficulty was again increased by increasing the complexity of the response and varying the degree of topic familiarity.

Sample Activities

Level 1

Stimuli: Paragraphs 60 to 80 syllables in length; high degree of redundancy; high degree of topic familiarity.

Procedure: The paragraph is read aloud by the clinician, followed by inferential questions, requiring a yes/no response.

Level 2

Stimuli: Paragraphs 60 to 80 syllables in length; low degree of redundancy; high degree of topic familiarity.

Procedure: The paragraph is read aloud by the clinician, followed by inferential questions, requiring a yes/no response.

Level 3

Stimuli: Paragraphs 60 to 80 syllables in length; low degree of redundancy; low degree of topic familiarity.

Procedure: The paragraph is read aloud by the clinician, followed by inferential questions, requiring a yes/no response.

VISUAL PROCESSING PROBLEMS

General Considerations

Visual processing refers to the processing of information presented in pictorial, gestural, and/or written forms. As with the auditory modality, this area can be subdivided into visual perception and reading comprehension problems. Aphasic patients demonstrate reading problems to varying degrees. Those with the most severe language impairments experience limitations with visual recognition, such that even matching objects, drawings, forms, colors, letters, and words may be compromised. Visual acuity and field defects can also affect performance, resulting in visual attention, scanning, and tracking problems.

Inability to comprehend written material due to cerebral injury is also referred to as alexia. When applied to the aphasic population, this term is used only when particular patterns are observed. Posterior alexia consists of reading problems with preserved writing. Patients may have difficulty recognizing words, although letter recognition may be better. Words are comprehended by using a letter-by-letter spelling approach, making longer and more complex reading difficult to impossible.

Central alexia is characterized by a severe reading impairment, often along with problems in reading musical notes and numbers, and a calculation deficit. Patients are unable to recognize spelled words and are unable to spell words orally. A severe writing disorder typically coexists.

Some patients may experience difficulty in recognizing letters but are still able to read some substantive words. Problems tend to arise with less frequently occurring letters, structurally more complex ones, and phonetically and visually similar letters (Hecaen and Kremin, 1976; Lecours et al., 1983). This profile

is called frontal alexia. Written output is usually severely impaired, with poorly formed letters and incorrect spelling.

Another recognized syndrome, although rare, is visual agnosia. Patients experience difficulty recognizing material presented visually (Benson and Geschwind, 1969; Eisenson, 1984), but presentation through another modality meets with success. Breakdown occurs for both verbal and nonverbal material (forms, objects). Writing is generally well preserved.

Many factors—such as the patient's educational level, occupation, and avocational interests—are considered in determining the extent to which the visual modality is addressed in treatment. In addition, with severely impaired aphasic patients, this modality may be better preserved than others (Helm and Barresi, 1980; Helm-Estabrooks, 1983) and may serve as an appropriate starting point in treatment.

Visual Perception

Treatment for visual processing is divided into six areas, with the first area dealing specifically with visual perceptual deficits. Area 1, Matching Nonverbal Material, requires the patient to match objects, pictures, and geometric forms. In developing a hierarchy of difficulty, picture complexity and degree of stylization can be adjusted, in addition to altering the stimulus category. The task may then be made more difficult by requiring category recognition. For example, using the category "chair," the patient is asked to match two types of chairs.

Area 2 incorporates Matching of Verbal Material such as numbers, letters, and words. Individual hierarchies are again established considering variables such as length, visual similarity, and size of the stimulus. To tax memory and attention span, a series of these items may be introduced.

Area 3, Visual Correspondence-Recognition, demands that the patient recognize different visual forms of the same stimulus. For example, the task may require matching a printed word to a corresponding object or matching trademarks to referents. Other activities in this area might also address semantic categories through having the patient make decisions about subordinate-superordinate relationships. Aphasic patients may experience even more difficulty in performing categorization tasks that involve functional relationships (e.g., "things that write") as opposed to those consisting of superordinate relations (McCleary and Hirst, 1986).

Visual Comprehension

Area 4 focuses on Reception of Gestured Messages. Although gesture recognition may be a less impaired modality (Porch, 1967), aphasic patients, as a group, tend to perform more poorly in interpreting pantomimes than do normal persons. Gestural communication abilities also tend to correlate with reading comprehension skills (Varney, 1978, 1982).

One hierarchy that has been suggested, in increasing order of difficulty, is associating object, action picture, object picture, and line drawing to corresponding gestures (Daniloff et al., 1982; Netsu and Marguardt, 1984).

Recognition of Spelling is addressed in Area 5. Tasks may involve proofreading activities that include presentation of the patient's written production or those of others, for correction. This activity might be considered a form of monitoring for those who rely heavily on written communication. Also, individuals with Surface Dyslexia may benefit from sentence judgment tasks requiring homophone recognition (e.g., "We took our/hour car") (Scott and Byng, 1989).

Reading Comprehension

Reading Comprehension Activities are initiated in Area 6, where stimuli may consist of single words, phrases, sentences, or paragraphs. Variables affecting vocabulary selection include word length, frequency, operativity, figurativity, abstractness, and grammatical form class. Task difficulty may be altered by varying the response choices to include auditory, semantic, or visual confusions (Gardner and Zurif, 1976; Van Demark et al., 1982).

When phrases and sentences are introduced, other factors such as syntax and number of content words relevant to the overall length may be considered.

At the paragraph level, overall length can be systematically adjusted, while varying individual sentence length, complexity, vocabulary difficulty, and thematic content. Requiring the patient to respond to inferential versus factual questions may increase difficulty. Area 7 completes this modality with Reading Textual Material. As empirical data are lacking, individual hierarchies must be developed, considering factors such as overall length, readability level, vocabulary, redundancy, grammatical complexity, amount of cohesion, use of anaphoric reference, and familiarity (Shewan and Bandur, 1986).

Case Example

N.H. is a 69-year-old homemaker who suffered from multiple strokes resulting in left frontal and right parietal occipital lobe infarcts. Administration of the Western Aphasia Battery, the Auditory Comprehension Test for Sentences, and the Boston Naming Test revealed a mild auditory-processing problem, a mild verbal dyspraxia, anomia, and moderate visual-processing and graphic expression difficulties. Because the patient reported being an avid reader up until the time of her most recent stroke, visual-processing activities were introduced simultaneously with activities from other modalities.

Language testing suggested good single-word reading comprehension and ability to read short, simple paragraphs. Additional probing demonstrated reading comprehension to be compromised above a Grade 3 readability level. Degree of abstractness also significantly affected performance. The first difficulty level involved presentation of short paragraphs with a readability level of Grade 3 to Grade 4. The patient was required to read the paragraphs and to reformulate them orally using printed "who, what, when, where, why/how" prompts. Once N.H. was successful in recounting the significant points from the paragraphs at this level, the same length of paragraph was used but the grade level was increased to Grade 5. Over time, paragraph length, abstractness, and grade level were all systematically increased. Newspaper articles and short stories were gradually introduced, with the patient eventually reporting success in reading romance novels for enjoyment.

Sample Activities

Level 1

Stimuli: Paragraphs 75 to 100 syllables in length; Grade 3

to Grade 4 readability; printed "who, what, when, where, why/how" cards.

Procedure: The patient reads the paragraph and orally provides responses to the "who, what, when, where, why/how" prompts.

Level 2

Stimuli: Paragraphs 75 to 100 syllables in length; Grade 5 readability; printed "who, what, when, where, why/how" cards.

Procedure: The patient reads the paragraph and orally responds to the "who, what, when, where, why/how" prompts.

Level 3

Stimuli: Paragraphs 75 to 100 syllables in length; Grade 5 readability; no printed cues.

Procedure: The patient reads the paragraph and orally provides the relevant information.

GESTURAL AND GESTURAL-VERBAL COMMUNICATION

General Considerations

Gestural communication may prove to be an alternative for some severely impaired aphasic patients or may be used to augment verbal expression attempts. For some, this modality may serve as a starting point in treatment with gradual transition to oral expression activities. For others, this may ultimately be the only feasible method of communication.

As noted in the previous section, the gestural modality tends to be less affected than others in the aphasic population (Porch, 1967), although more severely impaired aphasic individuals have been shown to use fewer complex gestural forms spontaneously in their communication attempts, with gestures becoming nonspecific and unclear (Glosser et al., 1986). Differing views regarding the nature of gestural impairment, classification of gestures, and the effects of treatment have been cited in the literature. Some positive effects on the reception and production of gestures through pantomime training have been described (Schlanger and Freeman, 1979). The Amer-Ind Sign System (Skelly, 1979) has been used with varying reports of success. Severely impaired patients may be able to acquire some single signs, with less involved patients perhaps capable of acquiring and generalizing simple grammars (Coelho, 1990). Ability to generalize signs has been inversely related to severity of aphasia (Coelho and Duffy, 1987). Aphasia severity may, in fact, be the most significant determinant of successful sign use (Coelho and Duffy, 1986).

Successful outcomes have been described with Visual Action Therapy (VAT) in improving both apraxia and gestural communication abilities (Helm-Estabrooks et al., 1982). In this nonvocal, visual/gestural program, a hierarchy of activities is used, ranging from activities such as requiring the patient to match objects and pictures to gesturing the use of items hidden from view. Modifications to VAT have been based on the finding that patients experience less difficulty using gestures representing objects involving proximal movements than those involving distal movements (Helm-Estabrooks et al., 1989b). With severely impaired patients, VAT may serve as the initial phase in treatment, advancing to the incorporation of LOT activities to refine the gestural communication system further.

LOT treatment areas tend to form a natural progression of activities, although some areas may not require attention, depending on the particular individual. Because of the inconsistent success reported in the literature regarding gestural communication training, LOT provides only tentative treatment hierarchies, with customization needed for individual patients. With the wide variety of patients seen, greater success may be obtained by tailoring communication systems to what the individual uses naturally in his or her environment (Kraat, 1990).

Social Signals

Area 1, Attention, is an elementary step in gestural communication. The patient obtains the attention of a communication partner through eye contact, touch, vocalization, gesture, or a combination of these.

With Area 2, Acknowledgment of the Message Received, some form of gesture, such as a head nod, is used to indicate that a message has been received, although not necessarily understood.

Gestures

Single gestures and combinations of gestures are used in Area 3, Gestural Communication. Some investigators have found propositional gestures to be more difficult to acquire than nonpropositional ones (Buck and Duffy, 1980). A possible hierarchy might consist of appropriate facial expression, conventional gestures, and propositional gestures.

Communicative importance or personal relevancy is another factor that may affect the ease of sign acquisition (Coelho and Duffy, 1986). There is also a tendency for patients to experience less difficulty in learning signs that have a high degree of iconicity, that is, those whose meanings are evident, based on their physical or structural characteristics (Coelho and Duffy, 1986). Other important variables to consider are the stimuli selected to teach the gestures. Objects and action pictures have been found to evoke superior gestural performance to line drawings (Netsu and Marguardt, 1984).

Speech Acts

Area 5, Simple Speech Acts, incorporates both message content (proposition) and intent of the speaker (elocutionary force). Elocutionary force is communicated with gestures and/or vocalization to signal a command, statement, or question. Simple pointing gestures may be used to communicate content, such as indicating the action, agent, or object. Area 5, Speech Acts, includes a combination of verbal and nonverbal communication. Gestures continue, however, to carry the burden of communication, although some verbalization may be produced.

Case Example

A.G. is a 62-year-old retired political consultant who suffered a stroke, with a large left middle cerebral artery infarct, resulting in Global Aphasia and a right hemiplegia. Initially, the Boston Assessment of Severe Aphasia was administered. Relative strengths were found in the areas of oral-gestural expression, gesture recognition, and visuospatial tasks. A variety of treatment strategies were used to develop oral expression skills, including VAT and Melodic Intonation Therapy (MIT), as well as LOT naming and sentence formulation activities. Functional oral communication skills, however, remained severely limited.

The Amer-Ind Sign System (Skelly, 1979) was next introduced. Because this treatment approach focuses on new learning as opposed to stimulation of previously learned material, a strict LOT paradigm could not apply. Ten common agents and actions were chosen for training. Initially, the clinician provided a gesture, along with an array of four action pictures from which the patient was to select the one associated with the gesture. Once recognition was established, A.G. was required to produce the gesture in response to an action picture. In the next treatment phase, situations were simulated in which A.G. provided the gesture in the absence of the action picture.

The subsequent difficulty level involved encouraging the use of trained gestures in conversational attempts. A.G. consistently progressed through his treatment program, successfully producing gestures that had not even been trained. Continuous encouragement and counseling were needed, however, as A.G. was reluctant to use gestural communication as a substitute for oral speech, even several months poststroke.

Sample Activities

Level 1

Stimuli:	Ten pictured actions, along with 20 foils.
Procedure:	The clinician presents an array of four pictures to the patient and produces a gesture corresponding to one of the actions depicted. The patient points to the appropriate picture.

Level 2

Stimuli:	The 10 action pictures used in Level 1 for identification.
Procedure:	The pictures are presented one at a time and the patient is required to produce the associated gesture.

Level 3

Stimuli:	The 10 action pictures used in Levels 1 and 2.
Procedure:	A sentence or brief story is aurally presented, and the patient is required to complete the sentence with the appropriate gesture (e.g., ''When you are hungry, you'' ____).

ORAL EXPRESSION PROBLEMS

General Considerations

Oral expression problems vary with respect to both type and severity among aphasic patients. Although various oral expression patterns are observed in different types of aphasia, many patients share common areas of difficulty.

Problems may be encountered with highly overlearned or automatic speech, with phonological-articulatory skills, repetition, oral reading, naming, sentence formulation, and discourse planning. Because these areas are not mutually exclusive, limitations involving one area may directly affect another. Treatment may, therefore, simultaneously incorporate two or more areas. In developing a treatment plan, the areas of deficit, along with their nature and severity, are carefully examined.

Automatic Speech

Area 1 addresses development of Automatic Speech Series. Activities are designed to facilitate oral speech in those with very limited verbal output. Stimuli such as greetings, number sequences, poems, days of the week, months of the year, and letters of the alphabet may be incorporated.

Voluntary Control of Involuntary Utterances (VCIU) is a treatment approach that has successfully used patients' own stereotypic expressions as a step to develop meaningful propositional speech (Helm and Barresi, 1980). VCIU incorporates a progression through oral reading, confrontation naming, and conversational use of the stereotypic words and phrases.

Phonological-Articulatory Production

Misarticulations that occur with aphasia may be the result of phonological problems, articulatory problems, or a combination of both. Phonological-articulatory impairment resulting from an anterior left-hemisphere lesion, in and surrounding Broca's area, is most often termed verbal dyspraxia. Posterior left-hemisphere lesions may also result in sound production errors, generally in the form of literal or phonemic paraphasias.

LOT activities in Area 2, Phonological-Articulatory Production, are based on Shewan's Content Network (1980) for treating verbal dyspraxia. Separate hierarchies for presentation method, stimulus characteristics, type of response, and facilitation of response variables have been constructed according to difficulty levels. These hierarchies are based on data provided by a variety of researchers.

A step-by-step progression toward the goal of achieving spontaneous production of propositional speech is used, as the patient can accommodate. Support provided by the clinician is gradually reduced to ensure that the patient develops more independence in his or her oral speech.

In selecting treatment stimuli, several variables may be critical. At the phoneme level, vowels are easier to produce than consonants, and highly frequent consonants are less difficult than those of low frequency. Distinctive feature characteristics also play a role in ease of production, with nasality and voicing features being less problematic than manner and place. In phoneme selection, the clinician can, therefore, establish a hierarchy incorporating all of these parameters.

When introducing single words, concrete, functional words tend to influence performance positively. Additional variables that may be important to control are word frequency and length. Beyond single words, phrase/sentence length, stress pattern, and linguistic complexity may be systematically varied to increase the difficulty levels in treatment.

Altering presentation methods can also be incorporated into a hierarchy. Combined auditory-visual presentation may facilitate correct speech production better than either auditory or visual presentation in isolation.

The clinician may vary the type of response required, such as production following a model, unison production, or production requiring a number of consecutive responses. Facilitating response variables can also be manipulated to elicit more accurate productions. For example, associated movements, such as finger tapping, may accompany speech. Inserting a schwa (/a/) between consonants in a consonant cluster may also enhance performance. Facilitating responses may be used, temporarily, by some, and be required as long-term strategies by others.

As the patient advances within the treatment hierarchy, additional response complexity can be required, while maintaining constant the presentation method, stimuli, and facilitating response variables. More spontaneous productions are incorporated, and the clinician gradually withdraws assistance.

Repetition

Although the ability to repeat is not an end goal in treatment, this skill is described in Area 3 to facilitate performance of other related speech-language behaviors. For example, repetition tasks may be used in treating verbal dyspraxia and are an important component of MIT. MIT, which was suggested as a branch step in gestural and gestural-verbal communication, may also be used here with patients meeting suggested candidacy criteria (Helm-Estabrooks et al., 1989).

When preparing stimuli for repetition activities, many variables can influence performance. High probability (Goodglass and Kaplan, 1972, 1983) and personally relevant material (Wallace and Canter, 1985) are easier to repeat, as are shorter items (Gardner and Winner, 1978). When sentence-level material is introduced, a hierarchy that varies sentence forms (Goodglass 1968, 1976) can be used, as patients demonstrate difficulty with increasing syntactic complexity.

Altering response variables may also affect accuracy and/or ease of production. For some individuals, use of a delay prior to initiation of a response can facilitate performance, although for others this strategy may have a negative impact (Gardner and Winner, 1978). It is, therefore, important for the clinician to determine the direction of this effect prior to implementing it in the patient's treatment program.

Oral Reading and Spelling

As in the previous area, Oral Reading, Area 4, is most often used as a vehicle for improving other aspects of speech-language skills and is rarely a goal in and of itself. Improvements in language functioning, such as reading comprehension, oral expression, auditory comprehension, and written expression have been described (Cherney et al., 1986; Tuomainen and Laine, 1991). Oral reading of sentences and paragraphs, in unison and independently, have resulted in improved language skills of both fluent and nonfluent aphasics.

Some forms of dyslexia have been characterized by differences in oral reading performance. As such, pure alexia, phonological dyslexia, surface dyslexia, and deep dyslexia have been clearly documented (Coltheart, 1982). Based on the particular oral reading profile exhibited, treatment hierarchies can be developed, taking into account those variables affecting performance in each type of alexia. With deep dyslexia, content words may be easier to read than function words. Some individuals may misread words for which little semantic information can be accessed (Hillis and Caramazza, 1991). Word frequency, concreteness, imageability, and grammatical form class are potential factors to consider in developing a treatment plan. Use of nonwords and irregularly spelled stimuli may increase difficulty for those with surface dyslexia. Word length is an important variable to consider when designing stimuli for those with pure alexia. As word length increases, accuracy and latency of

Most Effective	Cue	Description
	Repetition	The target word is presented as a model for the subject.
	Delay	The subject delays before responding with a name.
	Phonemic	The initial phoneme or syllable is provided by the clinician.
	Sentence completion	A sentence is presented by the examiner with a blank for the subject to complete with the target word. The fewer the number of possible words that can complete the sentence the more efficient the cueing.
	Semantic association	A word that is semantically associated with the target word is presented by the clinician.
	Printed word	The printed target word is presented.
	Description	A description of the item is provided by the clinician.
	Rhyming word	A word that rhymes with the target is presented by the clinician.
	Situational context	A situation in which the item would be found is provided.
	Spelled word	The target word is spelled orally for the subject.
	Functional description	The function of the target item is given by the clinician.
Least Effective	Superordinate	A superordinate term is provided by the clinician.
	Generalization	A general statement that provides little specific information is given by the clinician.

Figure 9.5. Hierarchy of cues according to effectiveness level.

responding are affected (Benson et al., 1971; Coltheart, 1982; Gardner and Zurif, 1975).

Beyond the single-word level, the clinician may advance to the use of phrases, sentences, and paragraphs. Grade level, topic familiarity, and overall length are additional variables that may be altered.

Area 5, Oral Spelling, may be used as an activity to enhance written spelling skills. Individuals, such as those with pure alexia, who find oral spelling easier, may learn to use this strategy to associate meaning with the printed word. Stimuli may be altered along the parameters of length, frequency, and regularity of spelling.

Word Retrieval

Word-finding problems are associated with all types of aphasia and may also occur in nonaphasic disorders. Benson (1979) has outlined five varieties of anomia associated with aphasia and four nonaphasic types. In developing activities in Area 6, for aphasic patients, the goal is to facilitate the actual word-retrieval process rather than to teach specific vocabulary items. The clinician first establishes the vocabulary level at which the patient experiences errors and determines whether patterns of performance vary when picture description, confrontation naming, or conversational activities are used.

Treatment activities are developed to facilitate word retrieval by first selecting an appropriate hierarchy of stimuli. Some stimulus variables that may be altered are word length, frequency, concreteness, operativeness, and semantic category. Semantic and grammatical categories may be differentially affected, depending on the type of aphasia (Goodglass et al., 1966). Items may also be easier to name if the label is of low uncertainty. Uncertainty refers to the consistency with which an item is given a particular label. Some aphasic patients may be sensitive to prototypicality, or the degree to which an item is characteristic of its class.

Once stimuli have been selected, effective cuing strategies can be determined for each patient. Overall, phonemic cues prove to be the most facilitative for the various aphasia types (Li and Williams, 1989). Anomic patients, however, seem to demonstrate a preference for semantic cues (Li and Williams, 1990) when verbs are presented. Some findings (Stimley and Noll, 1991) suggest that presentation of semantic cues increases the number of semantic paraphasias, with a decrease in unrelated word errors. Phonemic cue presentation, on the other hand, may increase the number of phonemic paraphasias. Another factor to consider in cue presentation is the use of simultaneous cues (e.g., initial syllable combined with sentence completion format). Particularly with severely impaired patients, combined presentation may be most effective (Huntley et al., 1986).

The hierarchy shown in Figure 9.5 is based on the findings of various researchers.

A number of activities may be employed to assist the patient in developing an understanding of the effectiveness and use of cues. Differing findings regarding use of real objects, colored photos, or line drawings have been cited, so the clinician may need to alter this presentation variable on an individual basis (Benton et al., 1972; Bisiach, 1966). Ultimately, tasks should be implemented that allow practice to occur in meaningful, natural situations. For example, application of PACE (Promoting Aphasics' Communicative Effectiveness) (Davis and Wilcox, 1981), which encourages patients to use multiple channels to communicate, has met with some success in developing effective cuing strategies (Li et al., 1988).

As patients advance along a hierarchy, using increasingly difficult levels of vocabulary and cue presentation, responsibility for cuing is shifted from the clinician to the patient.

Sentence Formulation

Area 7 focuses on the generation of meaningful units at the phrase and sentence levels. A hierarchy of sentence types may be established, such as that found in the Helm Elicited Language Program for Syntax Stimulation (HELPSS) (Helm-Estabrooks, 1981). This approach was developed for use with nonfluent aphasic patients to improve their use of syntax by training 11 sentence types with a story completion format. Sentence types range from the imperative intransitive to use of the future verb tense.

A hierarchy of sentence types for training might also be created based on order of reappearance in aphasics' language samples (Ludlow, 1973). Difficulty levels can be developed by varying the uses of morphological markers (Goodglass and Berko, 1960) and by varying phrase/sentence length. The stress pattern of a sentence may influence performance of some individuals. Broca's aphasic patients, for example, tend to initiate utterances with stressed words. Use of stress in these cases would be an important variable to include in the treatment hierarchy.

Contextual variables, such as use of pictured stimuli or conversation, may affect the nature of the responses. Some patients produce a greater number of major utterances (subject-predicate) in response to pictures than in conversation (Easterbrook et al., 1982); others may produce more words, depending on the gender bias of the picture (Correia et al., 1990).

Conversation and Discourse

Less research data are available for developing hierarchies in treatment Area 8, Conversation. The natural communication style of the patient should be considered when planning treatment. Activity variables to be considered in developing hierarchies include length of utterances, sentence complexity, topic familiarity, and the number of familiar communication partners.

Increased verbal complexity may result when face-to-face conversation is restricted, such as during telephone exchanges (Glosser et al., 1989). The communicative intent of the speaker may be another important factor to consider in planning a treatment hierarchy for conversation. Specific opportunities may be needed to develop use of requests, comments, instructions, and so forth.

In Area 9, Discourse, the patient retells or relates experiences or events. Several types of discourse may be developed, including narratives (e.g., using anecdotes), procedures (e.g., explaining how to do something), and expositions (e.g., providing a lecture on a particular topic). Increased levels of difficulty can be introduced by altering the length and complexity of the responses required.

Case Example

L.P. is a 44-year-old engineer who underwent a craniotomy with resection of a left frontal glioma. The Western Aphasia Battery, the Auditory Comprehension Test for Sentences, and the Boston Naming Test were administered. A nonfluent aphasia was exhibited, with oral speech limited to sentence fragments and frequent word retrieval problems. Auditory and reading comprehension were both mildly impaired. Written output paralleled spoken speech.

Along with activities targeting other areas, word retrieval was chosen for treatment. Probing revealed that L.P. was 80% successful in naming pictured objects characterized by monosyllabic word forms, using Grade 1 and Grade 2 vocabulary levels. Polysyllabic nouns were named spontaneously, with only 50% accuracy at these grade levels. No successful responses were elicited when pictured actions were presented.

Subsequent testing determined that the most effective cues for L.P. were presentation of the initial phoneme, description of physical and/or functional properties, and provision of the situational context (that is, the situation in which the item may be found). Because the clinician believed that phonemic cuing might be a difficult process to transfer from the clinician to the patient, use of description and situational contexts was emphasized.

In the first stage of the treatment hierarchy, specific training in the area of providing physical and functional descriptions and identifying situational contexts for pictured polysyllabic objects at a Grade 1 to a Grade 3 level was provided. Written prompts were used on individual cards to remind the patient of the various physical and functional attributes. For example, the phrases, "What color?" "What size?" "What shape?" and "What material?" were printed on one card, and on another, the question "What is it used for?" was printed. Once L.P. achieved a 70% success rate in providing the required information, another series of stimuli at the same difficulty level was presented. In this activity, the patient, by providing descriptions and situational contexts, was required to help the clinician name pictured objects hidden from her view.

When the provision of the cues became more automatic for L.P., confrontation naming tasks were used, in which he provided needed cues only when naming was not spontaneous. To limit the patient's reliance on the clinician, the pictured items were again seen only by L.P. Difficulty levels were also systematically increased by introducing advanced vocabulary grade levels and other grammatical form classes (e.g., verbs, adjectives). Practice with implementing self-cuing strategies was also provided, using various conversational activities. When treatment was discontinued, L.P. was a highly functional communicator, encountering word-finding problems primarily beyond a Grade 6 vocabulary level. His self-cuing strategies usually proved successful in helping him to retrieve the desired word.

Sample Activities

Level 1

Stimuli:	Grades 1 to 3 polysyllabic pictured objects; printed cue cards: "What color?" "What size?" "What shape?" "What material?" and "What is it used for?"
Procedure:	The patient is required to provide oral responses to information requested on the cue cards.

Level 2

Stimuli:	Grades 1 to 3 polysyllabic pictured objects; printed cue cards: "What color?" "What size?" "What shape?" "What material?" and "What is it used for?"
Procedure:	The pictures are hidden from the clinician's view. The patient provides information prompted by the cue cards to enable the clinician to guess the identity of the pictures.

Level 3

Stimuli:	Grades 1 to 3 polysyllabic pictured objects; printed

Procedure: cue cards: ''What color?'' ''What size?'' ''What shape?'' ''What material?'' and ''What is it used for?''

The pictures are hidden from the clinician's view. The patient first attempts to name the object spontaneously. If unsuccessful, he or she provides the information prompted by the cue cards to facilitate self-retrieval or identification by the clinician.

GRAPHIC EXPRESSION

General Considerations

Graphic Expression refers to the written output of communication through the use of graphemes (letters) or drawing. Writing is frequently the most severely affected modality in aphasic patients. Varying patterns of writing problems or agraphia have been described in the literature, along with a variety of classification systems (Benson, 1979; Ellis, 1982; Margolin, 1984).

Some patients may experience writing abnormalities because of motor problems related to hand paresis/paralysis. Their writing is characterized by poorly formed letters, sometimes severe enough to make writing illegible. With apractic agraphia, difficulty in selecting the appropriate grapheme motor pattern is observed. Disconnection between the physical letter code and the graphic motor pattern has been termed transitional agraphia (Margolin, 1984).

Phonological agraphia has been described as a disorder in which phoneme to grapheme conversion is disrupted, with patients experiencing difficulty writing nonwords (Margolin, 1984; Shallice, 1981). Derivational (e.g., historian/historical) and structural (e.g., sanity/sanitation) errors, when the patient is spelling, are also noted. These symptoms, in concert with increased difficulty in spelling abstract and functor words and production of more errors on verbs than on nouns, constitute deep agraphia. In lexical or semantic agraphia, the semantic root to spelling is impaired, with the patient attempting to spell words phonetically, producing more errors on irregularly spelled items.

Nonaphasic agraphias have been cited, such as pure agraphia, which occurs in the absence of other language impairments. Also, right-hemisphere lesions may result in disrupted spatial organization of writing. These problems tend to be mechanical in nature, as opposed to linguistically based.

LOT focuses on areas that require the recall and production of graphic and graphemic patterns, spelling and retrieval of individual words, and semantic-syntactic linguistic processing. At the semantic-syntactic levels of graphic expression, performance differences exist among aphasic types and most often reflect patterns of oral language formulation.

Physical Letter Code

Areas 1 and 2 focus on establishing graphic and graphemic motor patterns, with Area 3 stressing the recall of highly overlearned grapheme motor patterns. In Area 1, Tracing and/or Copying Nonverbal Material, two- and three-dimensional representations of nonverbal material are used. Task difficulty may be increased by altering the complexity of the designs in producing geometric forms and objects. Letters, numbers, and words are introduced in Area 2, Tracing and/or Copying Verbal Material. Activities are designed to address such problems as incorrect letter elements, inappropriate spatial positioning, rotation of letters/elements, and repetition of elements/letters. Single items may be practiced followed by those in a series, for example, letters and numbers. In Area 3, Writing Familiar Material, highly overlearned stimuli are incorporated, such as the patient's name, address, and telephone number.

Phoneme-Grapheme Conversion and Lexical Processing

Area 4, Written Spelling, may include such activities as writing to dictation, orally spelling words, or producing a letter series. Variables may be controlled along several dimensions. Word length, frequency, imageability, concreteness, emotionality, and grammatical class may influence the accuracy of the patient's performance.

Although order of difficulty varies among patients and among the types of aphasia observed, use of double vowels, double consonants, words with homonyms, and regular versus irregular spelling may be incorporated into a treatment hierarchy. In addition, words containing suffixes may prove more difficult for aphasic patients (Langmore and Canter, 1983), while words that can be spelled only one way (e.g., cup) tend to be easier.

Success in improving written performance has been described using two different approaches (Carlomagno et al., 1991). In one method, semantic and visual cues are used to stimulate writing through the lexical route, and in the other, nonword writing from dictation, along with presentation of phonological cues, is employed to enhance the nonlexical phoneme-grapheme correspondence. Both methods may be useful in improving written skills, although patients tend to respond preferentially to one approach over the other, depending on the type of agraphia that they display.

In Area 5, Written Naming, the emphasis shifts toward word selection. Some of the same factors as those cited in Area 4 will influence performance. Objects may be easier to name than pictures (Bub and Kertesz, 1982), and shorter words occasion fewer errors than longer ones (Friederici et al., 1981). Words containing the most regular expression of phoneme-grapheme correspondence rules are less difficult than those in which letter combinations are a less frequent realization of sounds (e.g., /f/ in telephone) (Friederici et al., 1981). A possible treatment hierarchy may therefore be established by altering word length, frequency, and degree of phoneme-grapheme regularity.

Semantic-Syntactic Linguistic Processing

Grammatical structures are first introduced in Area 6, Written Formulation, where material at the phrase, sentence, and paragraph levels may be used. Sentence complexity and length may be altered, along with topic familiarity. Many of the same variables found to influence oral expression can be incorporated into this area. At the paragraph level, a hierarchy can be established dealing with the structure of discourse (Labov, cited in Freedman-Stern et al., 1984), such that task requirements might include mention of time, place, participants, complicating action, and result/resolution. Once the patient is successful in including these obligatory elements, optional ones—for example, coda/moral of the story—may be required. Use of cohesive devices, such as anaphoric reference, relative clauses, temporal ordering, and so forth, may also be systematically introduced.

Writing Complex Material, Area 7, concludes this section. Variables to consider are the structure of the discourse, length, complexity of the grammatical structures, and use of cohesive devices. In addition, a response hierarchy, which addresses the complexity of the discourse, can be established. A possible progression from easy to difficult is narrative, letter, and expository (Freedman-Stern et al., 1984).

Again, the degree of emphasis placed on treatment of this modality depends on a number of factors, including the patient's premorbid functioning, occupation, avocational interests, and current priorities.

Case Example

B.C. is a 64-year-old self-employed business consultant. A left-hemisphere stroke resulted in an infarct involving the white matter in the region of the superior temporal lobe and angular gyrus, with extension into the white matter in the left corona radiata. The Western Aphasia Battery, the Auditory Comprehension Test for Sentences, and the Boston Naming Test were administered. A fluent aphasia, characterized by moderately impaired auditory comprehension, with paraphasic speech production, anomia, mildly impaired reading comprehension, and agraphia were revealed.

At the time of initial testing, B.C. successfully wrote his name, but not his address. Only a portion of the alphabet and numbers to 20 were correctly written. Writing single words to dictation resulted in no correct responses. Letter substitutions and additions made words, for the most part, unidentifiable. Over the course of the next 2 weeks, however, spontaneous improvement was noted, such that short sentence formulation was possible, with word-finding problems identical to those in oral speech.

Spelling errors were found mainly at the ends of words, where letter substitutions were noted. Irregularly spelled words occasioned the most errors. Further probing revealed that written naming was 50% successful, using Grades 7 and 8 polysyllabic irregularly spelled words. Oral naming, followed by oral spelling, proved to be effective cues for B.C. to write the word correctly.

B.C. identified graphic expression to be an important focus in treatment. His day-to-day work activities relied heavily on written skills, particularly related to correspondence.

As oral naming activities were being used in treatment, Area 5, Written Naming, was simultaneously developed. Once B.C. was able to write stimuli at the Grades 7 and 8 levels successfully, including polysyllabic, regularly spelled nouns, the difficulty level was increased by using nouns with irregular spelling, followed by other word classes, such as adjectives and verbs. Eventually, the vocabulary level was altered, along with grammatical form class, word length, and degree of imageability. Written naming activities were later incorporated into Area 7, Writing Complex Material, in preparation for the patient's eventual return to work.

Sample Activities

Level 1

Stimuli: Grades 7 and 8 polysyllabic, regularly spelled nouns.

Procedure: A written sentence is presented with the stimulus word omitted. The patient orally provides the word, spells it aloud, and finally writes it.

Level 2

Stimuli: Grades 7 and 8 polysyllabic, irregularly spelled nouns.

Procedure: A written sentence is presented with the stimulus word omitted. The patient orally provides the word, spells it aloud, and finally writes it.

Level 3

Stimuli: Grades 7 and 8 polysyllabic, regularly spelled verbs.

Procedure: A written sentence is presented with the stimulus word omitted. The patient orally provides the word, spells it aloud, and finally writes it.

EFFICACY

The LOT subjects for whom the efficacy data are reported here were part of a larger project designed to study the efficacy of three different types of aphasia treatment. LOT subjects were drawn from a population in London, Ontario, and the surrounding southwestern Ontario region in Canada. Table 9.2 shows the entry criteria met by all subjects. Only adult subjects were included, that is, individuals between the ages of 18 and 85 years. The upper cutoff of 85 years was used to eliminate subjects who were at high risk of not being available for a 1-year treatment period, the treatment duration provided in the study. Only literate subjects and those with a single, unilateral CVA, whose symptoms had lasted at least 5 days, were included in the sample.

Subjects who had a medical condition that interfered with testing or survival were eliminated, as were subjects with hearing impairment or blindness. Subjects were included if they were referred and tested within 2 to 4 weeks post-CVA. Native speakers of English and competent bilinguals for whom treatment in English was appropriate were included. Subjects who achieved an initial Western Aphasia Battery (WAB) Aphasia Quotient (AQ) score of less than 93.8, the cutoff score defining normal performance, were included in the study.

Random assignment to treatment type resulted in 28 subjects being assigned to LOT. To avoid an imbalance for severity or type of aphasia, assignment was stratified for these variables. Because hemorrhagic patients appeared to behave differently from those with an etiology of CVA, the hemorrhagic subject was excluded from data analysis.

Demographic Data of LOT Subjects

Age of the aphasic subjects ranged from 28 to 82 years, with a mean age of 62.3 years (Table 9.3). Education ranged from 4 to 21 years of formal education, with a mean of 9.85 years. (In Ontario, 9 years represents completion of the first year of high school.) Socioeconomic status was measured using the Blishen Scale (Blishen and McRoberts, 1976), which rates 500 occupations based on income and education. The mean rating of 38.92 was similar to the mean for a group of 60 older normal subjects gathered in the area (Shewan and Henderson, 1988). This suggested that the socioeconomic status of the LOT

Table 9.2.
Entry and Exit Criteria for Aphasic Subjects[a]

Criterion Variable	
	Entry Criteria
Age	18 to 85 yr
Education	Literacy by history
Etiology	Infarcts
	Stable intracerebral hemorrhages
	Excluded hemorrhages due to AV malformation
	Subarachnoid hemorrhage
	Aneurysm
	Single unilateral strokes
	TIAs (5 days or less) excluded
Medical status	Excluded unstable medical illnesses interfering with testing or survival
Sensory status	Passed hearing screening for age appropriateness
	Blind patients (defined clinically) excluded
	Tactile dysfunction not excluded
Time postonset	2 to 4 weeks poststroke
Language severity	Native speakers of English or competent bilinguals for whom treatment in English was appropriate
	Severe language barrier or accent excluded
	Exit Criteria
Language recovery	WAB LQ of 94.0 or above
Death	Subject died
Second stroke	Neurological deficit persisting longer than 5 days
Prolonged illness	Absence or illness longer than 3 weeks' duration
Geographical relocation	Subject moved
Voluntary withdrawal	Subject did not wish further treatment and/or tests
Termination of project	Data collection terminated at end of funding period

[a] From Shewan, C. M., and Bandur, D L. (1986). *Treatment of aphasia: A language-oriented approach* (p. 246). Austin, TX: Pro-Ed.

Table 9.3.
Demographic Data for 27 LOT Subjects[a]

Age (Years)	
Mean	62.33
Median	63.0
Range	28–82
Education (Years)	
Mean	9.85
Median	9.0
Range	4–21
Socioeconomic Status	
Mean	38.92
Sex	
Male	17
Female	10
Handedness	
Right	25
Left	1
Ambidextrous	1
Language	
English	22
Polyglot	5
Etiology	
Infarction	27

[a] From Shewan, C. M., and Bandur, D. L. (1986). *Treatment of aphasia: A language-oriented approach* (p. 249). Austin, TX: Pro-Ed.

tors who were independent of the clinicians providing treatment in the study. Tests occurred 2 to 4 weeks post-CVA (Entry Test) and at 3 months, 6 months, and 12 months after the first test. A follow-up test at 6 months after termination of treatment was also completed for as many subjects as possible.

The test battery included the Western Aphasia Battery (Kertesz and Poole, 1974), the Auditory Comprehension Test for Sentences (ACTS) (Shewan, 1979), Raven's Coloured Progressive Matrices (RCPM) (Raven, 1956), and a neurological examination, with site and side of lesion confirmed by computerized tomographic (CT) scan or isotope brain scan. Twenty-six subjects had left-sided lesions, and one had a right-sided lesion. Seventeen subjects showed some hemiplegia, 8 were hemianopsic, and 11 demonstrated some hemisensory loss.

Speech and language treatment was initiated as soon after administration of the Entry Test as possible and always within 7 weeks postonset of aphasia. Treatment was controlled for both duration and intensity. Subjects received treatment for 1 year unless they exited from the study prior to that time (for exit criteria, see Table 9.2). Intensity of treatment was controlled by providing three 1-hour sessions weekly. LOT subjects received a mean of 55.3 sessions, with a range of 1 to 118 sessions. Only subjects who received at least 3 months of treatment were included in the efficacy evaluation. Six subjects were lost to follow-up: One died, two relocated geographically, and three withdrew voluntarily.

Treatment was provided by trained speech-language pathologists. Each clinician was trained by C. M. Shewan, the developer of LOT. Prior to providing LOT in the study, each clinician demonstrated the competence to plan LOT. Competence was assessed by having each clinician design a 1-month LOT patient treatment plan, which passed evaluation by CMS and an inde-

group was similar to that of the general older population. The LOT group was composed of 17 male subjects and 10 female subjects. This ratio of 1.7:1.0 was similar to ratios in other literature reports (Abu-Zeid et al., 1975; Kurtzke, 1976). Most subjects were right-handed, with one left-handed and one ambidextrous person in the group. All subjects received treatment in English. For 22 subjects, English was their only language; 5 subjects spoke two or more languages, one of which was English.

Methods and Procedures

All LOT subjects met entry criteria (Table 9.2) and were tested at periodic intervals by trained, reliable test administra-

pendent, external evaluator. At 6-month intervals, each clinician was evaluated by a second independent, external evaluator to ensure that LOT was the treatment type being provided.

Efficacy Data

The efficacy of LOT was demonstrated by comparing the LOT subjects with a no-treatment control (NTC) group. The NTC group contained 22 aphasic subjects who did not wish to or could not attend treatment. The NTC group was comparable with the LOT group for age, education, socioeconomic status, handedness, language, and etiology. Unlike the LOT group, however, the NTC group contained an equal number of men (n = 11) and women (n = 11).

Whether LOT resulted in significantly greater language gains than no treatment was examined using analysis of covariance, controlling for initial severity of language impairment. The dependent variable in the comparison was the final test Language Quotient (LQ) score (LQLAST) on the WAB for each subject. The LQ score is a composite of the WAB oral and written language tests (Shewan, 1986). Initial severity was controlled through covarying for initial WAB LQ score (LQEN-TRY), because the LQ score was designed to be a measure of severity of language impairment, which, in turn, is known to affect language outcome. LOT had significant positive effects compared with no treatment ($p \leq .02$) (Table 9.4) when the Entry Test and the Last Test were compared. The estimate of the difference between LOT and NTC group means, after adjusting for entry score and educational level, was 11.50, with a standard error of 4.71. When age and sex, variables that could possibly influence outcome results, were added as concomitant variables in the analysis of covariance, the results remained essentially the same.

To control for the effects of spontaneous recovery, additional analyses of covariance were performed comparing LQTEST 2 (3 months after the Entry Test) with LQLAST. Again, controlling for initial severity, the analysis of covariance indicated the gains for the LOT group were significantly greater than those for the NTC group ($p \leq .02$) (Table 9.4).

The number of subjects within each aphasia type was too small to permit statistical comparisons among groups. However, tracking the LQ scores over the course of treatment and through follow-up showed some interesting recovery curves. Because

the number of subjects who contributed to the mean LQ score at each test could be different, as a result of subjects exiting from the group, the subjects were grouped according to the number of tests they received and were followed accordingly in streams (Fig. 9.6). When the entire LOT group was considered, gains in the streams were greatest within the first 3 months of treatment, although substantial gains were noted at each test thereafter, and the gains were maintained for the most part for 6 months following treatment. The LQ mean at Test 5 (follow-up) was only 1.4 points lower than at Test 4 (treatment termination).

Type of Aphasia

For global aphasics, gains were greatest in the first 3 months, although gains were substantial in the second 3 months as well. After this time, LQ scores plateaued. For the three subjects with follow-up tests, the gains from treatment were maintained. As seen in Figure 9.6, although global subjects did make notable gains, they both started and ended with lower LQ scores than the other types of aphasia.

The Broca's subjects made gains throughout the treatment period. As with other groups, the largest gains were in the first 3 months. At follow-up, scores were slightly lower than at the end of treatment (2.4 points).

The Wernicke's aphasic group contained only four subjects, who made substantial gains in the first 3 months of treatment. Because scores for only one subject were available beyond that point, no generalizations can be made. This subject did make gains in all treatment periods and showed a slight decline during the 6-month follow-up period.

Anomic aphasics, as other groups, made their greatest gains in the first 3 months, although gains were also substantial during the next 3-month treatment period. The single subject remaining beyond that time made additional gains in the 6- to 12-month period, although no scores at follow-up were available. Overall, gains for the anomic aphasics were nearly 20 LQ points, and, in general, they were less severely impaired than the Broca's, Wernicke's, or global subjects.

Conduction aphasic individuals were among the less severely impaired subjects, as might be expected. In concert with other groups, they made the greatest gains in the first 3 months of treatment. The two subjects remaining at Test 3 (6-month test) were approaching complete recovery (LQ >94). No scores were available beyond this point.

Severity of Aphasia

The aphasic subjects were separated into mild, moderate, and severe groups on the basis of the initial test battery, and subjects in these groups were followed in streams, similar to the analysis for type of aphasia (Fig. 9.7). The mild aphasic group made visible gains throughout the treatment period, averaging 24.8 LQ points. The greatest gains occurred in the first 3 months of treatment. The single aphasic subject remaining for the follow-up test showed only a slight decline from the termination of treatment.

Moderate subjects showed the greatest LQ gains in the first 3-month period (at least 20 LQ points on average). Scores stabilized for the next 3 months and increased again for the 6- to 12-month treatment period. The mean overall gain for the group was 33.8 LQ points. The one subject available at follow-

Table 9.4.
Summary of Analyses of Covariance for LQ Outcome Measure for LOT and NTC Groups[a]

	LQ	
p	Estimate of Adjusted Mean Difference	Standard Error
	Entry–Last Test	
≤.02	11.50	4.75
	Entry—Test 2	
≤.43	3.93	4.90
	Test 2–Last Test	
≤.02	5.86	2.19

[a] Adapted from Shewan, C. M., and Bandur, D. L. (1986). *Treatment of aphasia: A language-oriented approach* (p. 254). Austin, TX: Pro-Ed.

Figure 9.6. Mean LQ scores at Tests 1, 2, 3, 4, and 5 for the total LOT group and the five types of aphasia: global, Broca's, Wernicke's, anomic, and conduction. Patients have been grouped into streams according to the number of tests received. The numbers in parentheses refer to the number of patients included at each test. Termination of treatment (Rx termination) is represented with a dashed line. Test 5 is a follow-up test 6 months after treatment terminated.

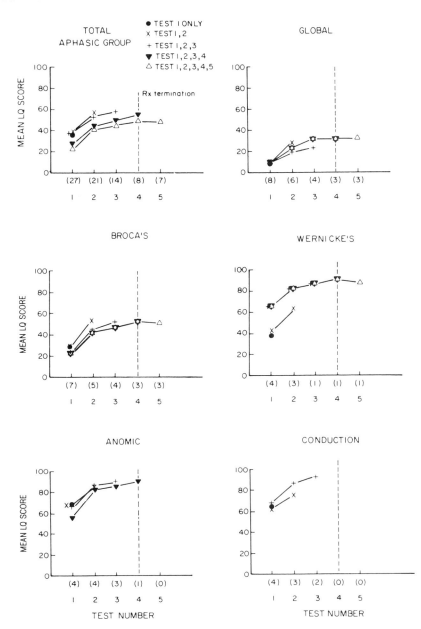

up showed a moderate decline in the LQ score from the termination of treatment.

The severe group, despite obtaining the lowest scores overall, did improve an average of 24.8 points on the LQ. Although greatest in the first 3 months, gains were also seen in the second 3-month treatment period, after which scores leveled off. These gains were maintained at the follow-up test.

QUALITATIVE BENEFITS

In addition to the objective quantitative treatment results associated with LOT, as discussed in the section on efficacy, other positive aspects have been cited by patients, clinicians, and supervisors. In selecting treatment areas and establishing hierarchies, the clinician is challenged to develop a detailed conceptual framework regarding the many facets of the patient's communication problem. As this information is translated into treatment activities and is communicated to the patient, he or she acquires an appreciation for the variables that affect performance. When stimuli and tasks are selected on a more random basis, as when using a general stimulation approach, increased variability in performance tends to occur, which can lead to confusion and discouragement on the part of both the patient and the clinician.

The LOT paradigm provides a clear and effective vehicle for regular feedback to the patient, family, and other members of the health care team regarding treatment progress. Given the goal-directed nature of LOT, daily changes in performance can be readily observed, where changes may not be substantial enough to quantify through standardized testing or informal observation. This feedback can be particularly motivating and can serve to legitimize provision of ongoing treatment when doubts are raised.

Conversely, LOT can assist the clinician in coming to a decision with the patient and family regarding the termination of treatment. Because a carefully planned, systematic approach has been implemented, the clinician is better able to review records and determine if, in fact, all possible avenues for language improvement have been explored.

Supervisors have reported positive effects to the supervisory process when LOT is being implemented. Treatment plans are more easily evaluated and readily reflect when goals and activities are inappropriate. Supervisees have found that in providing LOT, they are better prepared to make changes during their treatment sessions, when planned strategies prove unsuccessful.

In summary, LOT can foster greater understanding of an individual aphasic patient's language behavior by encouraging the clinician to examine and control the myriad of variables influencing performance. As this understanding grows and is shared with the patient, greater opportunities for success are realized.

FUTURE TRENDS

LOT has evolved over the last 15 years as new research developments have contributed additional information to our knowledge of aphasia. Given the theoretical foundations of LOT, it has been, and will continue to be, essential to take into account the effects of new treatment procedures as they emerge and to update continually the approaches that have already been outlined. Where up to date empirical evidence has been lacking, new treatment hierarchies will require development, and existing treatment will require modifications to reflect the growing body of research data.

With increased attention in the literature on functional outcomes, greater emphasis will be placed on extending activities

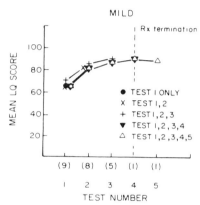

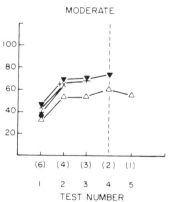

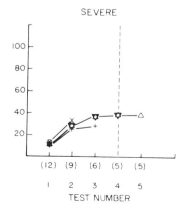

Figure 9.7. Mean LQ scores at Tests 1, 2, 3, 4, and 5 for the mild, moderate, and severe groups. Patients have been grouped into streams according to the number of tests received. The numbers in parentheses refer to the number of patients included at each test. Termination of treatment (Rx termination) is represented with a dashed line. Test 5 is a follow-up test 6 months after treatment terminated.

to more functional or naturalistic settings. In addition to examining which treatment areas are the most effective in promoting functional communication, multiple baseline studies designed to examine the effects of treatment on untreated areas could also be undertaken.

For highly functioning aphasic patients, LOT may continue to offer the most promise. Clinicians who feel unable to provide opportunities to challenge these individuals effectively can obtain direction through the LOT process. Because the ultimate goal for highly functioning patients is to return to a work force that requires good command of written as well as oral communication, a greater emphasis on developing reading and writing skills is required. It will be important to address further the patterns of symptoms exhibited by those with specific alexic or agraphic syndromes.

Ultimately, however, the most significant achievement for the clinician will be to recognize which LOT strategies are the most beneficial for a given set of aphasic patients. While various treatments, including LOT, have been demonstrated to be efficacious for patients of different types and severities of aphasia, we do not yet know the optimum sequence for treatment or what methods are most effective at various points along the recovery process. All of these areas offer abundant research opportunities for those intrigued with exploring aphasia and finding creative solutions to this complex human condition.

APPENDIX 9.1

This LOT Goals Form is used to record goals for each area within each modality. It records the level of difficulty, the stimuli and their presentation method, any cuing that is provided, the criterion for a correct response, the response method, and any additional responses. The clinician can use this form to record training both within and across sessions.

MODALITY: _____

AREA: _____

GOAL: _____

LOT GOALS

CLIENT: _____

CLINICIAN: _____

Level	Stimulus	Presentation Method	Cuing Provided	Criterion For Correct Response	Response Method	Additional Responses

APPENDIX 9.2

Language-Oriented Treatment Data Record Form

This form records identifying information and patient performances for training in an area for the language modality specified.

MODALITY: _____

AREA: _____

LOT DATA RECORD

CLIENT: _____

CLINICIAN: _____

Session No.	Date	Time Spent (minutes)	Difficulty Level	No. of Items	DATA and COMMENTS

References

Abu-Zeid, H. A. H., Choi, N. W., and Nelson, N. A. (1975). Epidemiologic features of cerebrovascular disease in Manitoba: Incidence by age, sex and residence, with etiologic implications. *Canadian Medical Association Journal, 113*, 379–384.

Aronson, M., Shatin, L., and Cook, J. (1956). Sociopsychotherapeutic approach to the treatment of aphasia. *Journal of Speech and Hearing Disorders, 21*, 325–364.

Backus, O. (1952). The use of a group structure in speech therapy. *Journal of Speech and Hearing Disorders, 17*, 116–122.

Basso, A., Capitani, E., and Vignolo, L. A. (1979). Influence of rehabilitation on language skills in aphasia patients: A controlled study. *Archives of Neurology, 36*, 190–196.

Basso, A., Faglioni, P., and Vignolo, L. A. (1975). Étudée controlée de la reeducation du language dans l'aphasie: Comparaison entre aphasiques traités et nontraités. *Révue Neurologique, 131*, 607–614.

Benson, D. F. (1979). *Aphasia, alexia, and agraphia.* New York: Churchill Livingstone.

Benson, D. F., Brown, J., and Tomlinson, E. B. (1971). Varieties of alexia. *Neurology, 21*, 951–957.

Benson, D. F., and Geschwind, N. (1969). The alexias. In P. J. Vinken and G. Bruyn (Eds.), *Handbook of clinical neurology* (Vol. 4). Amsterdam: North Holland Publishing.

Benton, A. L., Smith, K. C., and Lang, M. (1972). Stimulus characteristics and object naming in aphasic patients. *Journal of Communication Disorders, 5*, 19–24.

Bisiach, E. (1966). Perceptual factors in the pathogenesis of anomia. *Cortex, 2*, 90–95.

Blackman, N. (1950). Group psychotherapy with aphasics. *Journal of Nervous and Mental Disorders, 111*, 154–163.

Blackman, N., and Tureen, L. L. (1948). Aphasia—psychosomatic approach in rehabilitation. *Transactions of the American Neurology Association, 73*, 193–196.

Blishen, B. R., and McRoberts, H. A. (1976). A revised socioeconomic index for occupations in Canada. *Canadian Review of Sociology and Anthropology, 13*, 71–73.

Boller, F., and Green, E. (1972). Comprehension in severe aphasia. *Cortex, 8*, 382–394.

Brindley, P., Copeland, M., Demain, C., and Martyn, P. (1989). A comparison of the speech of ten chronic Broca's aphasics following intensive and nonintensive periods of therapy. *Aphasiology, 3*, 695–707.

Broida, H. (1977). Language therapy effects in long term aphasia. *Archives of Physical Medicine and Rehabilitation, 58*, 248–253.

Bub, D., & Kertesz, A. (1982). Evidence for lexicographic processing in a patient with preserved written over oral single word naming. *Brain, 105*, 697–717.

Buck, R., and Duffy, R. J. (1980). Nonverbal communication of affect in brain-damaged patients. *Cortex, 16*, 351–362.

Caramazza, A., and Zurif, E. B. (1978). Comprehension of complex sentences in children and aphasics: A test of the regression hypothesis. In A. Caramazza and E. B. Zurif (Eds.), *Language acquisition and language breakdown* (pp. 145–161). Baltimore, MD: Johns Hopkins Press.

Carlomagno, S., Colombo, A., Casadio, P., Emanuella, S., and Rassano, C. (1991). Cognitive approaches to writing rehabilitation in aphasics: Evaluation of two treatment strategies. *Aphasiology, 5*(4–5), 355–360.

Chapman, S. B., and Ulatowska, H. K. (1989). Discourse in aphasia: Integration deficits in processing reference. *Brain and Language, 36*, 651–669.

Cherney, L. R., Merbitz, C. T., and Grip, J. C. (1986). Efficacy of oral reading in aphasia treatment outcome. *Rehabilitation Literature, 47*(5–6), 112–118.

Coelho, C. A. (1990). Acquisition and generalization of simple manual sign grammars by aphasic subjects. *Journal of Communication Disorders, 23*, 383–400.

Coelho, C. A., and Duffy, R. J. (1986). Effects on iconicity, motoric complexity, and linguistic function on sign acquisition in severe aphasia. *Perceptual and Motor Skills, 63*, 519–530.

Coelho, C. A., and Duffy, R. J. (1987). The relationship of the acquisition of manual signs to severity of aphasias: A training study. *Brain and Language, 31*, 328–345.

Coltheart, M. (1982, October). *The alexias.* Paper presented at the 20th annual meeting of the Academy of Aphasia. Lake Mohonk, N.Y.

Correia, L., Brookshire, R. H., and Nicholas, L. E. (1990). Aphasic and non-brain-damaged adults' descriptions of aphasic test pictures and gender biased pictures. *Journal of Speech and Hearing Disorders, 55*, 713–720.

Dabul, B., and Hanson, W. R. (1975, October). *The amount of language improvement in adult aphasics related to early and late treatment.* Paper presented at the annual convention of the American Speech Language and Hearing Association, Washington, DC.

Daniloff, J. K., Noll, J. D., Fristoe, M., and Lloyd, L. L. (1982). Gestural recognition in patients with aphasia. *Journal of Speech and Hearing Disorders, 47*, 43–49.

Darley, F. L. (1982). *Aphasia.* Philadelphia, PA: W. B. Saunders.

David, R., Enderby, P., and Bainton, D. (1982). Treatment of acquired aphasia: Speech therapists and volunteers compared. *Journal of Neurology, Neurosurgery, and Psychiatry, 45*, 957–961.

Davis, G. A., and Wilcox, M. J. (1981). Incorporating parameters of natural conversation in aphasia treatment. In R. Chapey (Ed.), *Language intervention strategies in adult aphasia.* Baltimore, MD: Williams & Wilkins.

Deal, J. L., and Deal, L. A. (1978). Efficacy of aphasia rehabilitation: Preliminary results. In R. H. Brookshire (Ed.), *Clinical Aphasiology Conference proceedings* (pp. 66–77). Minneapolis, MN: BRK.

Easterbrook, A., Brown, B. B., and Perera, K. (1982). A comparison of the speech of adult aphasic subjects in spontaneous and structured interactions. *British Journal of Disorders of Communication, 17*, 93–107.

Eisenson, J. (1949). Prognostic factors related to language rehabilitation in aphasic patients. *Journal of Speech Disorders, 14*, 262–264.

Eisenson, J. (1984). *Adult aphasia* (2nd ed.). Englewood Cliffs, NJ: Prentice-Hall.

Ellis, A. W. (1982). Spelling and writing (and reading and speaking). In A. W. Ellis (Ed.), *Normality and pathology in cognitive functions.* London: Academic Press.

Franz, S. I. (1906). The reeducation of an aphasic. *Journal of Philosophy, Psychology and Scientific Methods, 2*, 589–597.

Franz, S. I. (1924). Studies in re-education: The aphasics. *Journal of Comparative Psychology, 4*, 349–429.

Frazier, C. H., and Ingham, D. (1920). A review of the effects of gun-shot wounds of the head. *Archives of Neurology and Psychiatry, 3*, 17–40.

Freedman-Stern R., Ulatowska, H. K., Baker, T., and Delacoste, C. (1984). Description of written language in aphasia: A case study. *Brain and Language, 22*, 181–205.

Friederici, A. D., Schönle, P. W., and Goodglass, H. (1981). Mechanisms underlying writing and speech in aphasia. *Brain and Language, 13*, 212–222.

Gardner, H., and Winner, E. (1978). A study of repetition in aphasic patients. *Brain and Language, 6*, 168–178.

Gardner, H., and Zurif, E. (1975). Bee but not be: Oral reading of single words in aphasia and alexia. *Neuropsychologia, 13*, 181–190.

Gardner, H., and Zurif, E. (1976). Critical reading of words and phrases in aphasia. *Brain and Language, 3*, 173–190.

Glosser, G., Wiener, M., and Kaplan, E. (1986). Communicative gestures in aphasia. *Brain and Language, 27*, 345–359.

Glosser, G., Wiener, M., and Kaplan, E. (1989). Variations in aphasic language behaviours. *Journal of Speech and Hearing Disorders, 53*, 115–124.

Goodglass, H. (1968). Studies on the grammar of aphasics. In S. Rosenberg and J. Koplin (Eds.), *Developments in applied psycholinguistic research* (pp. 177–208). New York: Macmillan.

Goodglass, H. (1975). Phonological factors in aphasia. In R. H. Brookshire (Ed.), *Clinical Aphasiology Conference proceedings* (pp. 132–144). Minneapolis, MN: BRK.

Goodglass, H. (1976). Agrammatism. In H. Whitaker and H. A. Whitaker (Eds.), *Studies in neurolinguistics* (Vol. 1, pp. 237–260). New York: Academic Press.

Goodglass, H. and Berko, J. (1960). Aphasia and inflectional morphology in English. *Journal of Speech and Hearing Research, 10*, 257–262.

Goodglass, H., and Kaplan, E. (1972). *The assessment of aphasia and related disorders.* Philadelphia, PA: Lea & Febiger.

Goodglass, H. and Kaplan, E. (1983). *The assessment of aphasia and related disorders* (2nd ed.). Philadelphia, PA: Lea & Febiger.

Goodglass, H., Klein, B., Carey, P.W., and Jones, K. J. (1966). Specific semantic word categories in aphasia. *Cortex, 2*, 74–89.

Green, E., and Boller, F. (1974). Features of auditory comprehension in severely impaired aphasics. *Cortex, 10*, 133–145.

Hagen, C. (1973). Communication abilities in hemiplegia: Effect of speech therapy. *Archives of Physical Medicine and Rehabilitation, 54*, 454–463.

Hécaen, H., and Kremin, H. (1976). Neurolinguistic research on reading disorders resulting from left hemisphere lesions: Aphasia and ''pure'' alexias. In H. Whitaker and H. A. Whitaker (Eds.), *Studies in neurolinguistics* (Vol. 2, pp. 269–329). New York: Academic Press.

Helm, N. A., and Barresi, B. (1980). Voluntary control of involuntary utterances: A treatment approach for severe aphasia. In R. Brookshire (Ed.), *Clinical Aphasiology: Conference proceedings.* Minneapolis, MN: BRK.

Helm-Estabrooks, N. (1981). *Helm elicited language program for syntax simulation.* Austin, TX: Exceptional Resources Inc.

Helm-Estabrooks, N. (1983). Approaches to treating subcortical aphasias. In W. Perkins (Ed.), *Current therapy of communication disorders* (pp. 97–103). New York: Thieme-Stratton.

Helm-Estabrooks, N. (1988). The application of neurobehavioral research to aphasia rehabilitation. *Aphasiology, 2,* 303–308.

Helm-Estabrooks, N., Fitzpatrick, P., and Barresi, B. (1982). Visual action therapy for global aphasia. *Journal of Speech and Hearing Disorders, 44,* 385–389.

Helm-Estabrooks, N., Nicholas, M., and Morgan, A. (1989a). *Melodic intonation therapy program.* San Antonio, TX: Special Press.

Helm-Estabrooks, N., Ramsberger, G., Brownell, H., and Albert, M. (1989b). Distal versus proximal movement in limb apraxia (Abstract). *Journal of Clinical and Experimental Neuropsychology, 7,* 608.

Henri, B. (1973). *A longitudinal investigation of patterns of language recovery in eight aphasic patients.* Unpublished doctoral dissertation, Northwestern University, Evanston, IL.

Hillis, A. E., and Caramazza, A. (1991). Mechanisms for accessing lexical representations for output: Evidence from a category-specific semantic deficit. *Brain and Language, 40,* 106–144.

Holland, A. L., and Wertz, R. T. (1988). Measuring aphasia treatment effects: Large-group, small-group, and single-subject designs. In F. Plum (Ed.), *Language, communication, and the brain.* New York: Raven Press.

Huntley, R. A., Pindzola, R., and Werdner, W. (1986). The effectiveness of simultaneous cues on naming disturbance in aphasia. *Journal of Communication Disorders, 19,* 261–270.

Katsuki-Nakamura, J., Brookshire, R. H., and Nicholas, L. E. (1988). Comprehension of monologues and dialogues by aphasic listeners. *Journal of Speech and Hearing Disorders, 53,* 408–415.

Kellar, L. A. (1978). *Stress and syntax in aphasia.* Paper presented at the Academy of Aphasia, Chicago, IL.

Kertesz, A., and Poole, E. (1974). The aphasia quotient: The taxonomic approach to measurement of aphasic disability. *Canadian Journal of Neurological Sciences, 1,* 7–16.

Kraat, A. W. (1990). Augmentative and alternative communication: Does it have a future in aphasia rehabilitation? *Aphasiology, 4*(4), 321–338.

Kurtzke, J. F. (1976). An introduction to the epidemiology of cerebrovascular disease. In P. Scheinberg (Ed.), *Cerebrovascular diseases: Tenth Princeton Conference.* New York: Raven Press.

Langmore, S. E., and Canter, G. J. (1983). Written spelling deficit of Broca's aphasics. *Brain and Language, 18,* 293–314.

Lecours, A. R., L'hermitte, F., and Bryans, B. (1983). *Aphasiology.* London: Bailliere Tindall.

Levy, C. B., and Taylor, O. L. (1968). *Transformational complexity and comprehension in adult aphasics.* Paper presented at the annual convention of the American Speech-Language-Hearing Association, Denver, Co.

Li, E. C., Kitselman, K., Dusatko, D., and Spinelli, C. (1988). The efficacy of PACE in remediation of naming deficits. *Journal of Communication Disorders, 21,* 491–503.

Li, E. C., and Williams, S. E. (1989). The efficacy of two types of cues in aphasic patients. *Aphasiology, 3* (7), 619–626.

Li, E. C., and Williams, S. E. (1990). The effects of grammatic class and cue type on cueing responsiveness in aphasia. *Brain and Language, 38,* 48–60.

Ludlow, C. L. (1973). *The recovery of syntax in aphasia: An analysis of syntactic structures used in connected speech during the initial recovery period.* Unpublished doctoral dissertation, New York University.

Margolin, D. I. (1984). The neuropsychology of writing and spelling: Semantic, phonological, motor and perceptual processes. *Quarterly Journal of Experimental Psychology, 36A,* 459–489.

McCleary, C., and Hirst, W. (1986). Semantic classification in aphasia: A study of basic superordinate and functional relations. *Brain and Language, 27,* 199–209.

Meikle, M., Wechsler, E., Tupper, A., Benenson, M., Butler, J., Mulhally, D., and Stern, G. (1979). Comparative trial of volunteer and professional treatments of dysphasia after stroke. *British Medical Journal, 2,* 87–89.

Mills, C. K. (1904). Treatment of aphasia by training. *Journal of American Medical Association, 43,* 1940–1949.

Netsu, R., and Marguardt, T. P. (1984). Pantomime in aphasia: Effects of stimulus characteristics. *Journal of Communication Disorders, 17,* 37–46.

Parisi, P., and Pizzamiglio, L. (1970). Syntactic comprehension in aphasia. *Cortex, 6,* 204–215.

Pashek, G. V., and Brookshire, R. H. (1980). Effects of rate of speech and linguistic stress on auditory paragraph comprehension of aphasic individuals. In R. H. Brookshire (Ed.), *Clinical Aphasiology Conference proceedings* (pp. 64–65, Abstract). Minneapolis, MN: BRK.

Pierce, R. S. (1988). Influence of prior and subsequent context on comprehension in aphasia. *Aphasiology, 2*(6), 577–582.

Pierce, R. S., Jarecki, J., and Cannito, M. (1990). Single word comprehension in aphasia: Influence of array size, picture relatedness and situational context. *Aphasiology, 4*(2), 155–156.

Pöeck, K, Huber, W., and Willmes, K. (1989). Outcome of intensive language treatment in aphasia. *Journal of Speech and Hearing Disorders, 54,* 471–478.

Porch, B. E. (1967). *Porch Index of Communicative Ability.* Palo Alto, CA: Consulting Psychologists Press.

Prins, R. S., Snow, C. E., and Wagenaar, E. (1978). Recovery from aphasia: Spontaneous speech versus language comprehension. *Brain and Language, 6,* 192–211.

Raven, J. (1956). *Coloured Progressive Matrices: Sets A, A_B, B* (Revised Order). London: Lewis and Company Limited.

Sarno, M. T., Silverman, M., and Sands, E. S. (1970). Speech therapy and language recovery in severe aphasia. *Journal of Speech and Hearing Research, 13,* 607–623.

Schlanger, P. H., and Freemann, R. (1979). Pantomime therapy with aphasics. *Aphasia-Apraxia-Agnosia, 1,* 34–39.

Schönle, P. W. (1988). Compound noun stimulation: An intensive treatment approach to severe aphasia. *Aphasiology, 2*(3–4), 401–404.

Schuell, H., Jenkins, J. J., and Jiménez-Pabón, E. (1964). *Aphasia in adults: Diagnosis, prognosis, and treatment.* New York: Harper & Row.

Scott, C., and Byng, S. (1989). Computer assisted remediation of homophone comprehension disorder in surface dyslexia. *Aphasiology, 3*(3), 301–320.

Sefer, J. W. (1973). A case study demonstrating the value of aphasia therapy. *British Journal of Disorders of Communication, 8,* 99–104.

Shallice, T. (1981). Phonological agraphia and the lexical route in writing. *Brain, 104,* 413–429.

Shewan, C. M. (1977). *Procedures manual for speech and language training: Language-Oriented Therapy (LOT).* Unpublished manuscript. The University of Western Ontario, London, Ontario.

Shewan, C. M. (1979). *Auditory Comprehension Test for Sentences (ACTS).* Menomonee, WI: Biolinguistics Clinical Institutes.

Shewan, C. M. (1980). Verbal dyspraxia and its treatment. *Human Communication, 5,* 3–12.

Shewan, C. M. (1986). The Language Quotient (LQ): A new measure for the Western Aphasia Battery. *Journal of Communication Disorders, 19,* 427–439.

Shewan, C. M., and Bandur, D. L. (1986). *Treatment of aphasia: A language-oriented approach.* Austin, TX: Pro-Ed.

Shewan, C. M., and Canter, G. J. (1971). Effects of vocabulary, syntax, and sentence length on auditory comprehension of aphasic patients. *Cortex, 7,* 209–226.

Shewan, C. M., and Henderson, V. L. (1988). Analysis of spontaneous language in the older normal population. *Journal of Communication Disorders, 21,* 139–154.

Shewan, C. M., and Kertesz, A. (1984). Effects of speech and language treatment on recovery from aphasia. *Brain and Language, 23,* 272–299.

Skelly, M. (1979). *Amer-Ind gestural code.* New York: Elsevier.

Smith, A., Champoux, R., Leri, J., London, R., & Muraski, A. (1972). Diagnosis, intelligence and rehabilitation of chronic aphasics. University of Michigan, Department of Physical Medicine and Rehabilitation. Social and Rehabilitation Service (Grant No. 14-P-55198/5-01).

Springer, L., Glindemann, R., Huber, W., and Willmes, K. (1991). How efficacious is PACE-therapy when ''Language Systematic Training'' is incorporated? *Aphasiology, 5,* 391–399.

Stimley, M. A., and Noll, J. D. (1991). The effects of semantic and phonemic prestimulation cues in picture naming in aphasia. *Brain and Language, 41,* 496–509.

Tuomainen, J., and Laine, M. (1991). Multiple oral reading technique in rehabilitation of pure alexia. *Aphasiology, 5*(4–5), 401–409.

Van Demark, A. A., Lemmer, E. C. J., and Drake, M. L. (1982). Measurement of reading comprehension in aphasia with the RCBA. *Journal of Speech and Hearing Disorders, 47,* 288–291.

Varney, N. R. (1978). Linguistic correlates of pantomime recognition in aphasic patients. *Journal of Neurology, Neurosurgery, and Psychiatry, 41,* 564–568.

Varney, N. R. (1982). Pantomime recognition defect in aphasia: Implications for the concept of asymbolia. *Brain and Language, 15,* 32–39.

Vignolo, L. A. (1964). Evolution of aphasia and language rehabilitation: A retrospective exploratory study. *Cortex, 1,* 344–367.

Wallace, G. L., and Canter, G. J. (1985). Effects of personally relevant language materials on the performance of severely aphasic individuals. *Journal of Speech and Hearing Disorders, 50,* 385–390.

Weisenburg, T., and McBride, K. E. (1935). *Aphasia.* New York: Hafner Publishing Company.

Wepman, J. M. (1951). *Recovery from aphasia.* New York: Ronald Press Company.

Wertz, R. T., Collins, M., Weiss, D., Brookshire, R. H., Friden, T., Kurtzke, J. F., and Pierce, J. (1978). *Preliminary report on a comparison of individual and group treatment.* Paper presented at the annual meeting of the American Association for the Advancement of Science, Washington, DC.

Wertz, R. T., Collins, M., Weiss, D., Kurtzke, J. F., Frident, T., Brookshire, R. H., Pierce, J., Holtzapple, P., Hubbard, D. J., Porch, B. E., West, J. A.,

Davis, L., Matovitch, V., Morley, G. K., and Resurrection, E. (1981). Veterans Administration cooperative study on aphasia: A comparison of individual and group treatment. *Journal of Speech and Hearing Research, 24,* 580–594.

Wertz, R. T., Weiss, D. G., Aten, J. L., Brookshire, R. H., Garcia-Buñuel, Holland, A. H., Kurtzke, J. F., LaPointe, L. L., Milianti, F. J., Brannegan, R., Greenbaum, H., Marshall, P. C., Vogel, D., Carter, J., Barnes, N. S. and Goodman, R. (1986). Comparison of clinic, home, and deferred language treatment for aphasia. *Archives of Neurology, 43,* 653–658.

Whitney, J. L., and Goldstein, H. (1989). Using self-monitoring to reduce disfluencies in speakers with mild aphasia. *Journal of Speech and Hearing Disorders, 54,* 576–586.

Zurif, E. B., and Caramazza, A. (1976). Psycholinguistic structures in aphasia. In H. Whitaker and H. A. Whitaker (Eds.), *Studies in neurolinguistics* (Vol. 1). New York: Academic Press.

Zurif, E. B., Caramazza, A., and Myerson, R. (1972). Grammatical judgments of agrammatic aphasics. *Neuropsychologia, 10,* 405–417.

Zurif, E. B., Green, E., Caramazza, A., and Goodenough, C. (1976). Grammatical intuitions of aphasic patients: Sensitivity to functors. *Cortex, 12,* 183–186.

CHAPTER 10
Contributions from Cognitive Analyses

ARGYE ELIZABETH HILLIS

MODELS OF COGNITIVE PROCESSES UNDERLYING LANGUAGE TASKS

Imagine that an aphasic patient looks at a picture of a chair and says, "table." Now imagine that the same patient looks at the pictured chair and writes, *table*. A different patient also verbally names the pictured chair as "table," but writes *chair*. How are we to understand the types of errors made by these patients? Do we want to treat the naming problems of these two patients in the same manner? First, we might want to know if the naming errors in these patients are symptoms of the same underlying problem in the two cases. In this chapter it will be argued that the identical errors in naming might arise from different cognitive deficits, and that the different deficits can often be identified by detailed analyses of the patients' performance on a variety of tasks other than naming (in addition to naming performance). The discussion will focus on the cognitive processes underlying naming, and disorders that result from breakdown in these processes, as an illustration of a general approach to understanding language and its disorders.

We can begin by assuming that naming is a complex process, requiring a number of mental processes. If we can delineate what mental processes the task of picture naming normally entails, then perhaps we can identify which of these normal processes have been disrupted in a particular patient. To develop an understanding of the cognitive processes involved in naming, we might start by considering what problems must be solved by the cognitive system in order to produce a correct word in response to a picture. That is, we would want to identify the computational problems encountered in picture naming. We would want to specify how pronunciations are computed in response to a combination of lines, shadings, and dots that make up a picture. Such cognitive operations must allow recognition of objects from all angles, such as a picture of a chair that is turned over, so that only the bottom of the chair is seen. Additionally, there must be mechanisms that are responsible for recognition of relative sizes, so that, for example, a speaker assigns "toy chair" to a dollhouse chair, but "chair" to a miniature picture of a full-sized chair. We must also be able to access information about what makes a chair a chair (e.g., information that allows us to know that a metal chair and a wooden chair have the same name). In other words, these mechanisms must support recognition of a picture as representing a set of objects with a specific name (e.g., recognition of a picture of a chair never before encountered as an instance of chair). And, finally, we must be able to access the stored information about how the name "chair" is to be pronounced. Consideration of these computational problems leads to the proposal of the major processes involved in picture naming.

One approach to understanding language, and its breakdown as a consequence of brain damage, in terms of these sorts of computations, has been the articulation of information-processing models of specific language tasks (a major thrust of cognitive neuropsychology). A model of this type specifies the mechanisms for solving the necessary computational problems of a particular task, such as naming, as a sequenced set of representations (i.e., stored visual, orthographic, semantic, or phonological information) and the processes required to compute each representation from the preceding one. So, for example, we might propose that picture naming involves, at the very least, the following: discrimination of the lines, edges, and shadings of the picture to develop a representation of the visual image; matching the computed visual representation to a stored representation of the physical structure of the object (i.e., accessing "the structural/visual description"); accessing stored information about the set of instances with a particular name (i.e., accessing a "semantic representation"); accessing the stored pronunciation (the "phonological representation") of the word to which it corresponds; and activating representations of the motor programs involved in articulating the word.

One such information-processing model of the lexical system is schematically depicted in Figure 10.1. This figure depicts some of the principal cognitive processes underlying reading, spelling, and naming, understood as a series of transformations of mental representations. It is important to note that although each component is dedicated to a particular aspect of lexical processing, some of the components are involved in more than one lexical "task." For example, both reading and naming involve computing the phonological representation of a word for output from a semantic representation. Hence, if computation of the phonological representation were to be disrupted by brain damage, it should be manifest as impairment in both

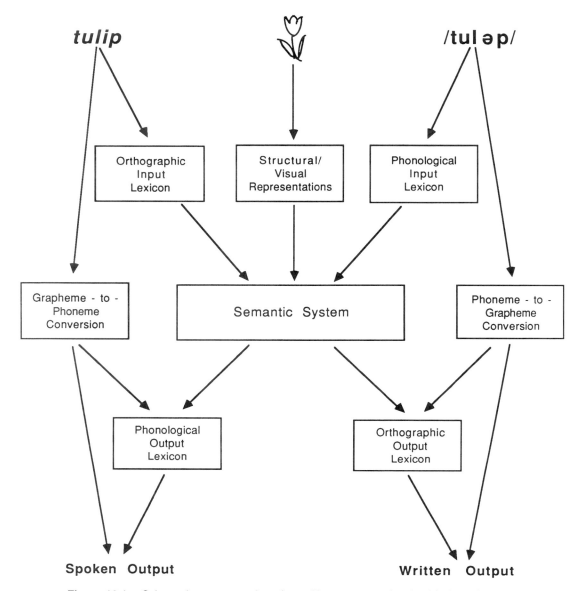

Figure 10.1.   Schematic representation of cognitive processes involved in lexical tasks.

reading and naming, although the consequences for output may be somewhat different in the two tasks. In the case of reading, additional information about the pronunciation of the name is available from the printed word. Therefore, if the patient is unable to compute ''chair'' from the semantic representation of CHAIR, he or she will be unable to name the pictured chair but may yet be able to correctly read *chair* on the basis of orthography-to-phonology (print-to-sound) correspondence mechanisms.

Motivation for proposing specific representations and processes comes from considering the computational requirements of the cognitive task, and the proposals are supported by empirical evidence from studies of normal subjects and from single case studies of brain-damaged subjects. To illustrate, evidence for proposing separate mechanisms for computing phonological and orthographic representations of words from a semantic

representation comes from patients who show good comprehension of printed and spoken words (indicating adequate access to the semantic representation) and are able to write the corresponding written word (in dictation or picture-naming tasks), but are not able to access the pronunciation of the same word. Such a pattern of performance (reported in Caramazza and Hillis, 1990; Ellis et al., 1983; Hier and Mohr, 1977) is inconsistent with an alternative proposal that computation of the orthographic representation first requires computation of the phonological representation. Thus, such models are constrained by patterns of performance of brain-damaged patients that cannot be otherwise explained by proposing specific loci of damage to the existing model. This chapter will cite cases that provide evidence for proposing those components of lexical processing that are involved in picture naming; other recent reviews focus on evidence for postulating components that are involved in writing (Ellis, 1982; Goodman and Caramazza, 1986) and those involved in reading (papers in Coltheart, et al., 1980; Hillis and Caramazza, 1992; Patterson et al., 1985).

In turn, the models serve to guide our understanding of patterns of performance by aphasic individuals; that is, language disorders resulting from brain damage that disrupts previously normal language can be characterized by proposing particular deformations of one or more of the constituent mental representations or cognitive processes underlying language production and comprehension. For example, imagine a patient who understands spoken and written words and writes the names of pictures adequately but is unable to say the correct names, despite unimpaired motor skills for articulating the correct name. We might propose in this case that the patient is unable to retrieve the accurate pronunciation of the word from among the stored pronunciations of all words he or she knows (''the phonological output lexicon''). Thus, a pattern of performance consistent with a proposed locus of disruption in the lexical system at the level of the phonological output lexicon would include demonstrated access to the semantic system from printed and spoken words (i.e., intact reading and auditory comprehension) and from pictures, *and* access to printed words from semantics (i.e., intact written expression of names and of self-generated ideas), but failure to access the phonological representation from written words (impaired oral reading). This example illustrates that the data crucial to proposing a specific locus of damage include the patient's profile of performance across lexical tasks in all modalities. To understand a patient's writing, for example, we need to know about his or her reading, comprehension, and speech, as well as performance on various spelling tasks. In addition, an analysis of the types of errors made in the affected task(s) and the stimulus parameters that influence performance (e.g., word frequency, part of speech, word length, and so on) may be required, as illustrated in several cases to follow.

The contributions of this approach in research and clinical aphasiology will be illustrated in this chapter by reviewing an information-processing model of naming, the evidence for various components of the model obtained from studies of aphasic individuals, and the results from a number of treatment studies that can be understood in light of the model. The cases described in detail are those from our own laboratory (the Johns Hopkins Cognitive Neuropsychology laboratory), in order to provide a comparison of the profile of performance across the same tasks and stimuli for all of the patients. The treatment cases are described not to recommend specific treatment strategies but to illustrate some general conclusions about the applications and limitations of this approach in the management of aphasic individuals.

AN EXAMPLE: A MODEL OF THE COGNITIVE PROCESSES UNDERLYING NAMING

A functional model of the major cognitive processes underlying verbal object naming consists of a subset of the components of the lexical system depicted in Figure 10.1: access to structural/visual representations, semantic representations, and phonological representations (stored pronunciations of words). For example, naming a picture of a dog would involve (*a*) developing a visual representation of the picture that would activate a stored representation of the ''structure'' of a dog (that it has four legs, fur, and so on); (*b*) activating a semantic representation—stored information about what makes a dog a dog (which would distinguish dogs from cats and from all other nondogs); (*c*) activating a stored phonological representation—the pronunciation /dog/—in the phonological output lexicon; and (*d*) activating motor programs for verbally producing /dog/. Empirical evidence for proposing each of the components is briefly described below.

Structural/Visual Representations

Marr (1982) has described visual recognition as a process that entails computation of successive representations with increasing abstraction from the physical stimulus, beginning with an early representation composed of bars, blobs, and dots with retinal coordinates and culminating in an abstract, canonical representation with object-centered coordinates—the three-dimensional (3-D) sketch—which in turn serves to access a stored, structural representation for object ''recognition.'' Information such as the distance and orientation of the object with respect to the viewer is not represented in the 3-D sketch, so that recognition of objects does not require viewing the object from a particular angle.

Evidence for proposing that a computed structural/visual representation of a visual stimulus is used to access a stored representation comes from patients who are able to demonstrate intact visual acuity (e.g., by copying) in the face of severely impaired recognition of objects. This so-called ''visual agnosia'' may take a variety of forms, depending on the level of disruption in computing visual representations. At a very peripheral level, visual analysis can be disrupted by isolated impairments in the appreciation of shape, color, or location, each occurring independently of impaired acuity (Hecaen and Albert, 1978; Warrington, 1986). Deriving a 3-D representation of an object might also require a number of separable processes, such as identifying local distinctive features of objects and extracting information about the object's principal axis, volume, and shape (Humphreys and Riddoch, 1984).

Another level of disruption may involve access to the semantic system from the stored structural/visual description. What sort of pattern of performance might be expected to result from such a disruption in the transformation of a structural/visual description to a semantic representation? In keeping with the model of the process underlying naming presented in Figure 10.1 and assuming that the semantic system itself is unimpaired, we would expect accurate written and spoken naming in response to definitions, in response to orthographic stimuli (reading), and perhaps in response to tactile presentation, but not in response to visual objects or pictures. Furthermore, with an intact structural description of the object, the patient should have some rudimentary information about the structure of the object (e.g., about its components). In some cases, the individual components of the stimuli may even access semantic information (see Hillis et al., 1990, for discussion). For example, perception of the seat of a chair may provide information that the object is for ''sitting.'' The availability of such ''partial information'' might support certain responses, such as miming the use of objects (say, sitting in response to a pictured chair) and might allow selection of responses within the correct category (in this example, naming a chair as any object used for sitting, such as chair, sofa, or stool). Thus, we might expect in the case of

Table 10.1.
A.G.'s Performance as a Function of Input Modality (given in percentage of total responses; N = 47)

	Total Errors	Structural Errors	Semantic Errors	Suffix Errors or Elaboration
Naming to:				
Visual input				
Picture naming	54.7	0	46.8	2.1
Object naming	57.4	0	46.8	4.2
Graphic input (oral reading)	10.7	0	0	10.7
Auditory input (naming to definition)	6.4	0	0	0
Tactile input (object naming)	19.1	10.7	4.3	4.2
Comprehension:				
Gestures use of pictured objects	4.3	0	0	n.a.
Definition–printed word matching	12.8	0	2.1	0

impaired access to semantics from the structural/visual description that in picture-naming tasks the patient would produce words that share visual and/or semantic features with the stimulus.

Riddoch and Humphreys (1987) described a patient, J.B., who showed this profile of performance. He demonstrated intact naming of objects from tactile presentation, but not from visual presentation. The authors argued that J.B.'s disruption in the naming process did not occur prior to accessing a stored structural description, however, because he could produce adequate gestures corresponding to the pictures he was unable to name. Other aspects of his performance indicated failure to compute a complete semantic representation from vision; thus, with picture stimuli he made errors in distinguishing close versus far semantic associates (e.g., that an orange is more closely related to a lemon than to a pear).

Similarly, our patient, A.G., a 64-year-old woman 5 months postonset of a left frontotemporal stroke, was able to name most objects presented for tactile exploration or described (orally or in print) and was able to read the names of the same objects, but was unable to name more than half of the pictures of the very same objects, as shown in Table 10.1. The 47 stimuli used in this task were presented in blocks across tasks (oral naming, word/picture matching, tactile naming, etc.), such that every item was presented each session, but in only one task. On a larger set of 144 object pictures, hereafter called the "semantic battery," nearly all of A.G.'s errors again were on tasks that involved picture stimuli: picture naming, auditory word/picture matching, and printed word/picture matching (Table 10.2). These stimuli were presented in the same manner described for the smaller set (of 47)[a].

Table 10.2.
A.G.'s Performance Across Lexical Tasks (given in percentage of total responses; N = 144)

	Total Errors	Semantic Errors	Suffix Errors or Elaboration
Repetition	2.8	0	2.8
Oral reading	10.4	0	7.6
Oral picture naming	54.2	50.7	2.1
Auditory word/picture matching	43.8	43.8	n.a.
Printed word/picture matching	54.2	52.8	n.a.

It was not only A.G.'s profile of performance across tasks but also the nature of her errors that was consistent with the hypothesis of a disruption in the proposed model of naming in accessing the semantic representation from a structural/visual representation. Nearly all of her errors on tasks with picture stimuli were semantically related to the target (e.g., PAPERCLIP→"stapler"; CARROT→"spinach"), whereas her uncommon errors on other tasks such as tactile naming and oral reading were morphological errors (e.g., MITTEN→"mittens") or other expansions of the target word (e.g., RAZOR→"razorblade"; *screw*→"screwdriver"[b]). Like J.B., A.G. was able to produce gestures in response to pictures that she could not name, indicating at least that some kind of stored representation (perhaps corresponding to one or more of the individual components of the visual stimulus) was accessed. Examples of her gestures and names given in response to pictures are given in Table 10.3. Computation of a complete semantic representation in nonvisual tasks was indicated by her accurate oral naming in response to tactile presentation or definitions; her contrasting failure to access the complete semantic representation from vision was indicated by her semantic errors in all tasks

---

[a] This set of tasks, using the set of 144 items, was administered in the same way to each of the patients reported from our laboratory. Word/picture matching tasks were presented as follows: All word stimuli to be presented for spoken word/picture matching that day were presented three times, once with a semantically related picture, once with an unrelated picture, and once with the correct picture. The patient's task was to verify or reject correspondence between the word and the picture; a word was scored as correct in word/picture matching only if she correctly verified the corresponding picture and correctly rejected both foils. The order in which the foils were presented across the three stimulus presentations was determined randomly (the whole word list was repeated three times; each stimulus was presented once during a given presentation, not repeatedly presented in succession).

[b] Here and in all later examples, the word preceding an arrow is the stimulus word, and the word following the arrow is the response. Written word stimuli and written word responses are given in italics, and spoken words are given in quotations. Capital letters indicate picture or object stimuli.

with picture or visual object stimuli for the same items that elicited correct names in nonvisual tasks (Tables 10.1 and 10.2) and an inability to sort pictures of related items into sets of items that would have the same name. For the latter task, pictures of various types of chairs were to be placed in one group, pictures of various types of sofas in another group, and so on; neither verbal stimuli nor verbal responses were needed. The accuracy of A.G.'s performance was 65% for distinguishing types of furniture (chairs/sofas/stools) and 69% for distinguishing types of birds (ducks/geese/turkeys). A.G.'s relatively spared oral reading and ability to trace and copy figures indicated that more peripheral visual processing was spared. Thus, her pattern of errors across a variety of tasks is consistent with the proposal of a disruption in accessing a complete semantic representation from a visual representation of the object that was computed adequately, at least to an early level of representation.

Semantic Processing

Words, of course, correspond to meaning. The nature of the representations of meaning is a matter of long and considerable debate, beyond the scope of this chapter (see Caramazza et al., 1990; Humphreys and Riddoch, 1988; Shallice, 1988a, and 1988b, for recent discussions in the domain of cognitive neuropsychology). The crucial aspects of the semantic system for the present purpose are that it both represents the culmination of those processes known as "comprehension" and serves to activate phonological and orthographic representations for output. That is, in its multiple roles in the lexical process, the semantic representation is the final representation activated in word comprehension tasks, and the initial representation activated in self-generated ideas. Furthermore, in the model under consideration, a unitary semantic representation is the single, common mediator of all lexical tasks. An alternative proposal is that there are separate semantic systems that are activated by different input modalities (e.g., a semantic system accessed through written words, another accessed from pictures).

What sort of evidence would favor the proposal that there is a single semantic system that is activated in all lexical tasks? We would predict from the model of the lexical system depicted in Figure 10.1 that damage to the semantic system would result in equal impairments of the following transformations: phonological input lexicon to semantics (auditory word comprehension); orthographic input lexicon to semantics (written word comprehension); semantics to phonological output lexicon (oral naming); and semantics to orthographic output lexicon (written naming). In addition, if there were also damage to nonlexical mechanisms for converting print to sound (orthography-to-phonology conversion, hereafter OPC processes) and mechanisms for converting sound to print (phonology-to-orthography conversion, hereafter POC mechanisms), damage to the semantic system should also affect, to the same degree and in the same manner, oral reading of words and writing words to dictation. This pattern of performance was shown by K.E. (reported by Hillis et al., 1990).

K.E., a 49-year-old executive, suffered a stroke that rendered him severely aphasic and hemiplegic. K.E. was given the tasks and stimuli described for A.G. However, K.E. showed a very different pattern of naming and comprehension performance. His rates of total errors and semantic errors (given as proportion of stimuli presented) were essentially identical across the various modalities of input and output (Tables 10.4 and 10.5). Furthermore, the semantic categories that were most impaired in one task (e.g., oral naming) were also the most impaired categories in other tasks (written naming, spelling-to-dictation, oral reading, and printed and spoken word/picture matching). These results could not be attributed to the varying degrees of "difficulty" of words in different categories, since the categories were matched for frequency and word length in letters and syllables—the dimensions that are generally considered to reflect degree of general difficulty across subjects, at least in reading and spelling. Hence, K.E.'s similar pattern of semantic errors across all lexical tasks provides evidence favoring the hypothesis that there is a single semantic system that is activated in all lexical tasks.

However, it was not the case that K.E. was completely unable to activate the semantic system; he not only showed

Table 10.3.
Examples of A.G.'s Correct Gestures Following Inaccurate Names

Stimulus	Oral Name	Gesture
Stapler	"Typewriter"	Pressed down with palm of hand, just above table top
Glove	"Sock"	Held out hand and wiggled fingers
Tie	"Glove"	Circled hand around neck, then showed 2-inch width from neck to just above waist
Sponge	"Dustpan"	Squeezed out imaginary sponge, then wiped table
Belt	"Collar"	Circled hand around waist
Fork	"Can opener"	Pretended to eat

Table 10.4.
K.E.'s Performance as a Function of Input Modality (given in percentage of total responses; *N* = 47)

	Total Errors	Semantic Errors	"Don't Know" or Other Error
Oral naming to:			
Visual input (picture naming)	40.4	38.3	2.1
Graphic input (oral reading)	42.6	42.6	0
Tactile input (object naming)	46.8	44.7	2.1
Written naming to:			
Visual input (picture naming)	38.3	34.0	4.2
Tactile input (object naming)	40.4	34.0	6.3
Auditory word/picture matching	40.4	40.4	0
Printed word/picture matching	31.9	31.9	0

relatively good performance in some semantic categories, but he also showed access to some semantic information even in the most affected categories of words. For example, his errors in comprehension and production tasks were essentially always within-category semantic errors, such as chair/table. One explanation for these findings is that the semantic representations of related words are somehow ''linked'' such that increased ''noise'' in the system results in activation of a linked word rather than the target. Another potential explanation, favored in the report on K.E., is that a semantic representation is decomposable into a set of features, of which some become unavailable as a result of brain damage. For example, the semantic representation of CHAIR might consist of a set of features such as <movable> <object> <seat> and <backrest> (see Miller and Johnson-Laird, 1976, and Jackendoff, 1983, for detailed descriptions of this sort of semantic theory). In this example, if neurological damage resulted in impaired activation of one or more features, say <backrest>, the spared subset of features would be consistent with a number of related objects (stool, ottoman, etc.). This hypothesis would account for the observation that for any given stimulus picture, K.E. inconsistently responded with the correct word or any of several semantically related words. Furthermore, for any given word, K.E. accepted either the correct picture or any related picture as its referent, but rejected unrelated pictures. Thus, K.E.'s impairment can be understood as damage at the levels of (a) the semantic system in which there is failure in computation of a complete semantic representation, such that the impaired semantic representation is consistent with a number of related items; and (b) nonlexical, OPC and POC mechanisms. The latter deficit, demonstrated by his inability to ''sound out'' nonwords or nonsense syllables (e.g., gib) in reading or to produce any kind of plausible spelling for such stimuli in dictation, prevented K.E. from accomplishing oral reading and spelling of words through these mechanisms.

This case indicates that one of the organizational principles of the semantic component reflects ''semantic category'' or relatedness among words. Additional support for this proposal comes from ''category-specific'' semantic impairments, in which performance on tasks that involve semantic processing is intact for items in some semantic categories and impaired for items in other semantic categories. Cases have been reported of selective damage to living things or to nonliving things (Warrington and McCarthy, 1983, 1987), fruits and vegetables (Hart et al., 1985), and so on. It has been argued that such

category-specific impairments merely reflect that members of some semantic categories are more visually/structurally similar to each other than are the members of other semantic categories, making distinctions between them more difficult (and thus, semantic errors more probable (Humphreys and Riddoch, 1987). In particular, such an account would explain why selective impairment in the category of ''animals'' is among the most frequently reported category-specific naming deficit (Basso et al., 1988; McCarthy and Warrington, 1985; Warrington, 1981; Warrington and Shallice, 1984). However, this account of the category influence is undermined by the pattern of performance by our patient, J.J. (Hillis and Caramazza, 1991a; see also Sartori, et al., in press).

J.J., a 67-year-old retired executive, suffered a left temporal and basal ganglia stroke that resulted in impaired comprehension and reduced meaningful content of speech, with no compromise of speech fluency. On our ''semantic battery'' at 13 months poststroke, J.J.'s naming and comprehension performance was best for the category of animals—the category with the highest degree of structural overlap among members (Table 10.6). He was most impaired in the categories of foods and body parts. A second patient, P.S., showed a pattern of performance in naming tasks with the very same stimuli that was the opposite of J.J.'s with respect to categories—most impaired for animals and least impaired for foods and body parts (Table 10.7). Therefore, category distinctions cannot be solely attributed to greater degree of ''general difficulty'' of some categories, nor to greater visual similarity among members of some semantic categories.

Another aspect of J.J.'s pattern of performance is worth noting. The data in Table 10.6 show that J.J.'s category-specific deficit was reflected only in naming and comprehension tasks, not in oral reading. How can we accommodate this result within the hypothesis that J.J.'s performance can be explained by a category-specific deficit to a modality-independent semantic system shared by all lexical tasks? In accord with our model in Figure 10.1, this pattern of performance can be explained by assuming selective damage to the semantic system if J.J., unlike K.E., is able to use OPC procedures to support relatively good oral reading. In fact, J.J.'s spared use of these sublexical mechanisms was demonstrated by his impressive ability to read nonwords (e.g., mushrame) plausibly, as well as his relatively more accurate reading of regular over irregular words (Hillis and Caramazza, 1991b)[c].

Phonological Output Lexicon

To produce a spoken word to represent a meaning (whether from a self-generated thought or computed from a lexical or visual representation), one must have access to a stored representation of the correct pronunciation of the word. It is not enough to have access to the stored orthographic representation, for example, since an orthographic representation would not guide us to say ''cow'' rather than /ko/ (rhyming with know) to indicate the meaning of cow. What is the empirical evidence for proposing that access to the stored phonological representa-

Table 10.5.
K.E.'s Performance Across Lexical Tasks (given in percentage of total responses; N = 144)

	Total Errors	Semantic Errors
Oral reading	41.7	36.1
Oral picture naming	44.4	41.0
Written picture naming	46.5	34.7
Spelling-to-dictation	41.7	27.8
Auditory word/picture matching	42.4	42.4
Printed word/picture matching	36.8	36.1

---

[c] J.J.'s accurate reading of some irregular words that he failed to understand was attributed to a combined activation of the phonological representation from partial semantic representation together with partial phonological information. Similar mechanisms, involving a summation of information from POC procedures and impoverished semantic information, were proposed to account for J.J.'s relatively accurate spelling-to-dictation of words he failed to understand completely.

Table 10.6.
J.J.'s Accuracy Rates Across Categories in Various Tasks (given in percentage correct of total responses)

	N	Oral Naming	Auditory Word/Picture	Printed Word/Picture	Oral Reading
Land animals	20	95.0	90.0	100.0	100.0
Birds	13	76.9	92.3	92.3	100.0
Water animals	13	100.0	92.3	100.0	100.0
Vegetables	12	8.3	33.3	33.3	91.7
Fruits	10	30.0	70.0	60.0	90.0
Transportation	12	58.3	58.3	66.6	91.7
Furniture	19	21.1	78.9	31.6	89.5
Body parts	20	5.0	55.0	30.0	95.0
Food	11	9.1	36.4	45.5	100.0
Clothing	14	21.4	78.6	50.0	85.7

Table 10.7.
P.S.'s Accuracy Rates Across Categories in Various Tasks (given in percentage correct of total responses)

	N	Oral Naming	Auditory Word/Picture	Printed Word/Picture	Oral Reading
Land animals	20	40.0	95.0	100.0	100.0
Birds	13	46.2	92.3	76.9	85.0
Water animals	13	30.8	92.3	84.6	84.6
Vegetables	12	25.0	91.7	83.3	75.0
Fruits	10	70.0	100.0	90.0	100.0
Transportation	12	91.7	100.0	100.0	91.7
Furniture	19	84.2	100.0	73.7	84.2
Body parts	20	100.0	100.0	80.0	65.0
Food	11	100.0	100.0	90.9	81.8
Clothing	14	85.7	100.0	78.6	57.1

tion for output is a process independent of both access to the phonological representation during input (i.e., in response to the aurally received word) and access to the orthographic representation for output? One source of evidence of the functional independence[d] of these mechanisms comes from the dissociation of impairment to one of these mechanisms, with sparing of the other two. Another look at the model of the lexical system in Figure 10.1 allows us to predict the following consequences of selective damage at the level of the phonological output lexicon (in the presence of unimpaired functioning at the levels of the phonological input lexicon and orthographic output lexicon): (*a*) access to the semantic system from the phonological and orthographic input lexicons should be unhindered (reflected in intact spoken and printed word comprehension); (*b*) activation of an orthographic representation—an entry in the orthographic output lexicon—from the semantic representation should be spared (reflected in intact written naming); but (*c*) activation of the phonological representation—an entry in the phonological output lexicon—from the semantic representation should be disrupted, as reflected in impaired oral naming and impaired oral reading. (Although, if sublexical OPC mechanisms for converting print to sound are not damaged, the

patient should be able to correctly read regular words like *bike*, as well as nonwords like *fike*, but not irregular words like *heir*.)

However, the model as articulated thus far does not allow us to predict the types of errors that are likely to be made in oral naming and oral reading. Several types of errors might be produced, depending on how phonological representations are accessed and further processed. For example, one hypothesis about the phonological output lexicon is that stored representations of the pronunciations of words have some resting threshold of activation; only activation from the semantic system (and/or the OPC mechanisms) that reaches this "threshold" will allow the entry to be selected for further processing. Words that occur with low frequency are assumed to have higher resting thresholds of activation. Furthermore, some cases of brain damage affecting this level of lexical processing could result in elevated thresholds of all or some of the representations. In these cases, activation from the semantic system may yet be sufficient to reach threshold for high-frequency words, but not for low-frequency words, resulting in (*a*) higher accuracy in oral reading and naming of high-frequency compared to low-frequency words; and (*b*) production of high-frequency, semantically related words in place of low-frequency target responses. The latter hypothesis is based on the further assumption that whenever a phonological representation is activated by the semantic representation, those phonological representations that are semantically related to the target are also activated to some degree. Recall that one hypothesis about the semantic representations is that they consist of a set of semantic features.

---

[d] The hypothesis of functional independence of these mechanisms is silent with respect to where and how such representations are computed in the brain. That is, this proposal does not undermine the possibility that information about a word's pronunciation is stored in only one area of brain, and that information is accessed for output and for input. But if the input and output processes can be disrupted independently of each other, we can assume that there are separate dissociable means of activating the stored information.

Table 10.8.
Accuracy Rates Across Lexical Tasks by H.W. (given in percentage of total responses)

	Lexically Accurate Responses[a]	Semantic Errors
Oral reading	66.7	26.4
Oral naming	65.3	25.7
Written naming	90.0	0
Writing to dictation	93.7	0
Auditory word/picture matching	100	0
Printed word/picture matching	100	0

[a] Includes all responses recognizable as the correct word.

Thus, each individual feature of the semantic representation might activate all those phonological representations to which it corresponds. For example, in the representation of sofa, <seat> would activate phonological representations of chair, sofa, swing, bench, bicycle, and so on; <backrest> would activate phonological representations of chair, sofa, bench, and so on; and <for more than one> would activate sofa, bench, bus, airplane, meeting, and so on. Only the phonological representation of sofa would receive maximal activation, from all of the component features of the semantic representation of sofa, so it alone would normally be selected in oral naming or oral reading of *sofa*. However, in the presence of brain damage that elevates the resting threshold of words, this "maximal activation" might not be sufficient to reach the elevated threshold level for sofa, so that a related but higher frequency representation, say chair, that received enough activation to meet its threshold would be selected instead for further processing. In this way, semantically related words might be produced as a consequence of damage at the level of the phonological output lexicon.

Evidence consistent with this set of hypotheses about the phonological output lexicon comes from patient H.W., who had fluent aphasia secondary to a left-hemisphere stroke more than 2 years prior to testing (Caramazza and Hillis, 1990). Her performance on lexical tasks is presented in Table 10.8. Her oral naming performance is not unlike that reported for A.G. or for K.E. However, in sharp contrast to A.G. and K.E., H.W. was entirely accurate in word/picture matching (and a variety of other word comprehension tasks administered) and did not make semantic errors in written naming or writing to dictation. Her written responses were recognizable as the target response even though she made some spelling errors (e.g., *cha-r* or *chaer* for *chair*). The spared comprehension and written naming performance contraindicate any difficulty at the level of the semantic system. But consistent with our hypotheses about how phonological representations are activated, she made errors in oral reading, oral naming, and spontaneous speech that could all be loosely classified as a semantic errors: semantically related word substitutions (e.g., *vegetables*→"fruit"); definitions of the target word or circumlocution (e.g., *frog*→"the thing that jumps"), and morphological errors (*pea*→"peas"). Further evidence that she understood words that she misread was provided by her consistently accurate definitions of words elicited immediately following each oral reading response. For example, H.W. read *pirate* as "money" and then defined the word as follows: "Has a thing over its eye . . . I would say

they don't have any anymore, but they do in business. He wants your money and your gold."

H.W. was unable to demonstrate accurate use of OPC or POC procedures to aid in oral reading or in writing to dictation, as indicated by her complete failure to read nonwords plausibly. For example, the patient could not even begin to read *hannee* or even to say whether or not *hannee* would begin with /h/. But in patients with spared use of such sublexical mechanisms, we would expect that oral reading would be substantially better than oral naming (see, for example, Miceli et al., in press).

Other types of errors may also occur as a result of damage at the level of the phonological output lexicon. For example, damage or impaired access to phonological representations might be the source of some phonemic errors (literal paraphasias) in oral naming and oral reading tasks. Alternatively, phonemic errors might occur in further processing of the phonological representation after it is correctly activated in the output lexicon (Butterworth, 1979) or in motor planning/execution for articulating the word (see Wertz et al., 1984, for discussion of output processes).

POTENTIAL CLINICAL USEFULNESS OF COGNITIVE MODELS

Understanding the Deficit

The most straightforward clinical application of the types of cognitive analyses of patient performance that have been described in this chapter is in obtaining a more thorough understanding of each patient's impairments. Reasonable clinical management of an aphasic individual cannot even begin until the clinician has an idea of what is "wrong" with the patient's language. Of course, treatment can be effective even in the absence of a complete understanding of the deficit, but we assume that focusing on specific cognitive functions—and knowing which are impaired and which are preserved—is preferable to a "hit and miss" approach. Making a "diagnosis" of the level of disruption in a certain language task requires evaluation of (*a*) the profile of performance across tasks; (*b*) the types of errors made by the patient; and (*c*) the stimulus dimensions that influence performance. Since these aspects of performance are not readily apparent from most standard aphasia tests, some ideas for how to evaluate them are given below.

With respect to the profile of performance, the examples cited above illustrate that performance on lexical tasks that involve all cognitive processes, as well as spontaneous language, need to be considered in order to understand the locus of impairment within a single cognitive task. For example, analysis of performance in oral reading, written naming, and comprehension tasks is crucial to identifying the locus of the problem in oral naming. It is preferable to use the same stimuli in each of the tasks, so that direct comparison across modalities is possible, since damage can be restricted to certain categories or types of words both at the level of the semantic system (as described for J.J.) and at the level of the phonological output lexicon (H.W.'s performance was much more impaired for verbs than for nouns, as described in Caramazza and Hillis, 1991a). However, the number of items given first in oral naming must be equal to the number given first in comprehension tasks, to assure that differences between tasks cannot be attributed to an "order" effect, learning, or some degree of recovery or improvement between sessions. Therefore, an ABBA blocked presentation of two subsets would be appropriate if two tasks are to be evaluated. Finally, assessment of naming and comprehension should be equivalent in difficulty, that is, in the level of demands on the semantic system. To appreciate the importance of this requirement, consider K.E., whose frequent semantic errors could be explained by proposing that he activated "impoverished" semantic representations that were equally compatible with the target item and a number of related items. His oral naming errors were attributed to a semantic deficit, even though he was able to respond errorlessly on a forced choice test of word/picture matching with unrelated foils. Even if related foils are used, such a task would only be as demanding as oral naming for K.E. if foils included *all* items that were compatible with his impaired semantic information. Our verification task, in which he was required to both accept the correct word/picture match and reject a closely related picture as a match for the word, seemed to be a closer approximation to the naming task in level of demands on the semantic system. In summary, oral naming performance that is less accurate than comprehension provides evidence for an output deficit as the basis of naming errors only if (*a*) comprehension and naming are assessed for the same items; (*b*) a learning or time effect is avoided by controlling the order of presentation; (*c*) the tasks are comparable in level of semantic processing required for correct performance. Similar controls are necessary to draw conclusions about oral versus written naming (e.g., as evidence for selective damage to the phonological output lexicon) and oral naming versus oral reading (e.g., as evidence for selective damage to a component specific to reading, such as the orthographic input lexicon).

Along with the profile of accuracy across tasks, an analysis of error types can also be informative as to the nature of the problem. However, the cases reported earlier show that no single error type is pathognomonic of a single locus of impairment in lexical processing. For instance, semantic errors in naming can occur as a result of impaired access to the semantic representation from the structural representation (as proposed for A.G.), or as a result of damage to the semantic component (as in K.E.), or as a consequence of damage at the level of the phonological output lexicon (as in H.W.). Phonemic errors may occur as a result of damage at the phonological output lexicon, or to more peripheral mechanisms of motor planning or execution. Similarly, "regularization errors" in oral reading (e.g., reading *one* as "own") may occur whenever the patient is using exclusively OPC mechanisms to compute a pronunciation as a result of damage to lexical mechanisms at any level of the reading process (orthographic input lexicon, semantic system, or phonological output lexicon).

In the same way, analysis of the stimulus parameters that influence performance is useful only in conjunction with the other aspects of the patient's performance. That is, word frequency should be an important factor in successful performance when naming and reading are disrupted at the level of the phonological output lexicon (as for H.W.) or when reading is is disrupted at the level of the orthographic input lexicon (see Gordon, 1983). Word frequency may also play a role in performance that follows damage to the semantic system, since impaired activation from the damaged semantic system will more likely be sufficient to activate high-frequency phonological representations than to activate low-frequency representations in the output lexicon. There may even be role of frequency,

and/or related dimensions such as familiarity, in early visual processing of pictures. Dimensions of semantic category and concreteness are important in processing, at least at the level of the semantic system, and word class is important at the levels of the semantic system and the phonological output lexicon in the naming process.

Focusing Treatment

The clinician's primary goal in understanding the patient's deficit is to focus treatment on just those levels of processing that are impaired or to identify methods that will allow the patient to process language successfully by "getting around" the deficit. The types of cognitive analyses described in the earlier sections have been used by a number of investigators to focus treatment on specific levels of processing (although, as discussed below, there are serious limitations in our ability to determine which cognitive mechanisms are actually affected by a given treatment). Some notable examples of studies in which cognitive analyses have been used to focus intervention include the following: focusing treatment on mapping of syntactic functions to thematic roles to improve sentence comprehension (Byng and Coltheart, 1986); focusing therapy on verb retrieval and verb morphology in the domain of tense/aspect markers to improve sentence production (Mitchum and Berndt, in press); training use of orthography-to-phonology assembly to improve oral reading (Berndt and Mitchum, in press; de Partz, 1986); facilitating use of POC skills to improve spelling (Carlomagno, et al., in press; Hillis Trupe, 1986); and pairing words and their meanings to improve lexical spelling (Behrmann, 1987; Behrmann and Herdan, 1987).

Like these methods used to improve reading, writing, and sentence processing, therapy to improve naming ability might be reasonably focused on the particular component of the naming process found to be impaired. In fact, J.J., whose pattern of performance across lexical tasks indicated a disruption at the level of semantic system, did show more improvement in naming performance when treatment tasks explicitly required semantic processing (printed word/picture matching) than when treatment tasks did not overtly require semantic processing (oral reading with phonological cues). In contrast, H.W., whose naming impairment could be localized to the phonological output lexicon, showed greater improvement in naming performance as a consequence of the facilitated oral reading treatment (see Hillis and Hillis, 1992, for details and discussion). Thompson et al., (1991) also reported that phonological strategies to facilitate naming (e.g., using rhyming word cues) improved naming performance of patients whose impairment was localized to the phonological output lexicon. Additional reports of treatment focused on specific components of the naming process are reported by Raymer et al. (1993). However, many types of naming treatment described in the literature—including those that directly facilitate production of the name in response to the picture—might improve naming at either (or both) the level of the semantic system and/or the level of the phonological output lexicon (e.g., Hillis, 1989; Howard et al., 1985; Linebaugh, 1983; Thompson and Kearns, 1981).

Predictions About Generalization

Localization of a patient's impairment within the cognitive process underlying a particular language task also leads to some specific expectations about what aspects of performance should change if treatment successfully modifies processing at that level. There are two types of "generalization" of improvement one might look for following treatment directed to a specific component of processing: generalization across behaviors and generalization across stimuli.

First, consider changes in performance across "treated" and "untreated" behaviors. Here we would expect that if processing at a given level of representation improves, then performance on all tasks that involve that level of representation should improve. An illustration of such changes comes from the case of H.G., a 24-year-old female several years after left fronto-temporal-parietal damage from blunt head trauma (see Hillis, 1991, for details). H.G. exhibited a semantic impairment comparable to that of K.E., which homogeneously affected all lexical tasks. But in addition, she had a profound impairment at the level of the phonological output lexicon. Since access to information in the orthographic output lexicon was relatively spared, H.G. spontaneously wrote words in naming tasks and conversation. As she relearned (or regained access to) sublexical OPC procedures for converting print to sound, she began to pronounce the entries she activated in the orthographic output lexicon. Essentially all of these "verbal" responses in oral naming as well as oral reading reflected consistent use of OPC procedures that could be called "regularization" errors. For example, she named SUGAR as /sugar/ ("sue–gar"). HG's performance on lexical tasks could be accounted for by proposing two separate loci of impairment in the naming process: (a) at the level of the semantic system, resulting in frequent semantic errors in spoken and written word comprehension, naming, writing to dictation, and repetition (she was unable to use sublexical mechanisms to repeat words or nonwords); and (b) at the level of the phonological output lexicon, reflected in impaired access to the correct pronunciation of words in oral reading, repetition, and oral naming. Treatment that focused on the semantic component, which involved reestablishing access to, or relearning of, the meanings of words, using only written naming tasks resulted in a reduction of semantic errors not only in written naming but also in oral naming, dictation, repetition, and comprehension tasks. A subsequent treatment that focused on relearning/reestablishing the pronunciation of words in the oral reading task resulted in improved accuracy of her oral responses in oral reading, oral naming, and repetition, but not of her written or comprehension responses (see Hillis, 1991). The latter intervention was associated with improved reading only of treated items, indicating that perhaps processing of specific phonological representations in the output lexicon was influenced. Furthermore, H.G.'s improvement in naming and comprehension tasks associated with the "semantic" treatment of written naming (teaching semantic distinctions between her response and the target) was observed for the 50 items that were treated and semantically related words, but not for unrelated words. The semantically related words, in fact, might have been inadvertently "treated," since the intervention focused on distinctions between the treated words (target responses) and her incorrect responses, which were semantically related words.

Behrmann and Lieberthal (1989) reported comparable generalization results—improvement in categorization of untreated items within treated categories—of a therapy strategy that also focused on teaching semantic distinctions among related items.

Their patient, like H.G., showed a pattern of performance consistent with damage to the semantic system, as indicated in particular by his category-specific impairment in comprehension (but unlike H.G. he showed some improvement of items in one of the untrained categories). Additional reports in the literature of item-specific treatment include treating reading of functors using association with visually/phonologically similar content words (Hatfield, 1983) and improving printed word recognition by reinforcing correct word/nonword, semantic, phonological decisions about the "treated" set of words (Hillis, 1993). These reports are consistent with the hypothesis that if treatment influences specific representations (or access to them), performance involving the target representations (treated stimuli) should improve across tasks, but performance would not be expected to improve for other representations (of untreated words).

A different type of generalization concerns changes in performance *across* treated and untreated stimuli. Here, we would expect that if treatment influences a general processing mechanism (say, holding representations in a short-term memory system), processing should improve across all stimuli that are subject to that mechanism. Many examples of therapy that influenced both treated and untreated stimuli have been reported, such as improving reading speed by reinforcing rapid semantic decisions about printed words ("gestalt processing") (Gonzales-Rothi and Moss, 1989), improving comprehension of sentences (Byng and Coltheart, 1986); improving use of a self-correction strategy in spelling (Hillis and Caramazza, 1987), and improving use of sublexical OPC mechanisms or "phonological assembly" to improve oral reading (Berndt and Mitchum, in press; de Partz, 1986; Hillis, 1993) or POC mechanisms to improve spelling (Carlomagno et al., in press; Hillis Trupe, 1986). The problem in making predictions as to whether or not to expect improvement across stimuli is that we have no way of knowing, a priori, how treatment affects processing— a point we turn to in the following discussion. Indeed, we might instead use treatment results to propose whether a general mechanism or specific representations were affected by our treatment (see Goodman-Schulman et al., 1990, for discussion and illustration).

Limitations of the Models for Developing Strategies

One criticism that has been made of treatment specifically focused on improving a single cognitive mechanism of a complex language task is that improved functioning of the single targeted aspect of language will not always improve use of language in everyday situations. This limitation of treatment arises in the case frequently confronted in the clinic of a patient with multiple loci of damage in the cognitive processes underlying any given language task. For example, improving processing at the level of the phonological output lexicon will not especially help the patient produce words in conversation if the patient also has a severe articulatory (motor) deficit or severe semantic deficit. A more subtle example was reported by Mitchum and Berndt (in press); their patient, M.L., had an impairment in naming verbs that seemed to interfere with his sentence production. Treatment that focused on improving naming of verbs (in response to pictures) did not alone improve his sentence production, however. It was only when additional therapy targeted verb tense/aspect morphology that M.L. improved in producing grammatical sentences.

A related limitation of this approach is that many of the specific treatment strategies described are "item-specific"; that is, they seem to influence the processing of specific lexical or semantic representations. This "gain" will obviously benefit the patient in conversation only if treatment has involved those words the patient wishes to say. But this limitation does not necessarily undermine the utility of the treatment. Particularly in the case of patients with severe difficulties, a limited vocabulary of successfully produced words, developed over the course of therapy using carefully selected sets of words that will be useful to the patient, can result in substantially more functional communication skills in everyday situations. Consider again the case of H.G. (see Hillis, 1991, for details).

Before initiation of the item-specific "semantic" treatment described earlier, at 7 years postonset of her brain damage, H.G.'s spontaneous speech was limited to low-volume jargon. No content words were recognizable, although repetitive "empty" strings of words were noted (e.g., "You know you mean, please understand, what you know?"). Furthermore, her comprehension of words in the absence of contextual cues (which often constrain meaning to one target of all the words related to the target) was nonfunctional. Treatment focused on the semantic distinctions between related words involved sets of words that HG required in daily living situations (foods, names of people, clothing), and those that she would need in specific job settings (e.g., numbers, stationery and office items for clerical work, and vocationally related vocabulary like "application," "salary," "time card," "punch in," "break"). Once she obtained competitive employment, continued therapy was coordinated with her employers and job counselor and was designed to meet her expanding communication needs. H.G. consistently demonstrated spontaneous use (and comprehension) of words that had been used in therapy tasks on the job, at home, and in restaurants (both by report and direct observation by the clinician). For example, her parents knew what words she had been trained recently in therapy. Later in the course of therapy, H.G. chose sets of words that she wanted to work on (e.g., names of drinks for social settings).

Similarly, H.W.'s "phonological" (cued oral reading) treatment seemed to involve improved access to specific phonological representations in the output lexicon. Like H.G., she produced mostly fluent speech with few content words before this item-specific therapy was initiated more than 5 years poststroke. However, her improvements in using trained sets of words were sufficiently rapid that she was able to receive treatment for many sets of words she selected. She was also observed to use "trained" words in conversation at home, in restaurants, and over the telephone in follow-up calls. In describing the "Cookie Theft" picture from the Boston Diagnostic Aphasia Examination, H.W. improved in the number of accurate content units produced, from 5 before the phonological treatment to 12 after treatment (cf Yorkston and Buekelman, 1977, for description of content units). Furthermore, not only were her gains maintained more than a year after treatment, but additional gains were achieved: She produced 15 content units. The further progress was probably achieved in part through H.W.'s oral reading practice with her husband's cues.

Perhaps a more important limitation of conclusions reached about the results of a given treatment for an individual patient is that it is not possible to determine, a priori, which other patients will respond to the same treatment in the same way.

Ideally, we would like to be able to conclude that treatment of a specific component of cognitive processing would help all patients with damage to that component. Unfortunately, such conclusions are not possible in light of our current levels of theory. As noted previously, we have no way of knowing how any specific mechanisms are actually modified by our interventions (see Caramazza and Hillis, in press, for discussion). Thus, the observation that a "semantic" approach was associated with improved naming in a patient with a semantic deficit does not directly imply that all patients with semantic deficits will show improved naming with that treatment. Earlier studies have shown that sometimes patients with putatively "the same" locus of impairment fail to respond to the same treatment approach, but different approaches have been beneficial for the individuals; and sometimes patients with different loci of damage in the lexical system respond to the same treatment (Hillis, 1993; Hillis and Caramazza, in press). This finding is not unexpected, since the characteristics of the patient and the form of impairment at any given level of processing that may influence treatment outcomes have yet to be precisely defined. Although studies have identified recovery as a function of a variety of individual factors, these studies have not been integrated with the (a) the specific cognitive mechanisms that are impaired in the patient, and (b) the cognitive mechanisms that might be influenced by the treatment.

It should be noted that this inability to predict whether a particular patient will benefit from a given treatment strategy is certainly not specific to the approach described in this chapter, which relies on a cognitive analysis of patient performance but applies equally to other "schools" of treatment.

The final, and perhaps the most important, limitation is that the current models of cognitive processing provide no direct motivation for specific treatment strategies. For example, knowing the patient's level of disruption in the naming process does not guide the clinician as to *how* to treat the problem (see Caramazza, 1989, and Wilson and Patterson, in press, for discussion). In fact, such knowledge does not even guide the clinician as to *what* to treat. Should we "treat" the damaged component of processing, or should we try to exploit the preserved components in the hopes for more functional, but not normal, language processing? The models alone do not help us in this regard, because they do not specify which components are subject to remediation, nor how the system might be reorganized following damage to circumscribed parts. Hence, choices of treatment must rely on the clinician's intuitions about what might help, and ongoing evaluation of treatment effects. Empirical reports of improvement in functioning associated with specific treatment approaches in well-described cases of damage to selective components of language processing might give the clinician hope that a particular component is "treatable," but valid predictions about improvement in a different case of damage to the same component would also require evidence as to the patient characteristics that influence outcome and nature of damage to the impaired component (see Hillis and Caramazza, in press, for detailed discussion).

In summary, information-processing models of specific language tasks are useful for understanding the nature of impairment consequent to brain damage in individual patients but do not constitute a theory of language rehabilitation. The latter would require motivated hypotheses about how mental representations or transformations are modified, how particular interventions bring about these modifications, and how particular patient characteristics influence response to treatment. Moreover, a theory of rehabilitation would need to specify the interactions among these variables, in order to make predictions about results of a given treatment approach for an individual aphasic patient.

FUTURE TRENDS

The recent emergence of the discipline of cognitive science, which brings together research in neuroscience, cognitive neuropsychology, linguistics, and artificial intelligence, has paved the way for the development of models of recovery of cognitive function after brain damage. We can be hopeful that the convergence of experimental results from these various branches of cognitive science will lead to more detailed models of both normal cognitive processing and mind/brain relationships. In turn, coordination of research in cognitive science and neurological rehabilitation should lead to models of neurological plasticity and theories of intervention (what specific treatments do to the damaged cognitive system to bring about improved performance). Toward this goal, research in all of the individual fields, as well as integration of new information from each, should be encouraged. A crucial stepping stone in this process is the interaction among investigators from various branches of cognitive science and language rehabilitation.

Acknowledgments

The author is grateful to Lisa Benzing, Brenda Rapp, and Alfonso Caramazza for helpful comments on an earlier version of this chapter. This research was supported in part by NIH Grant (NINCD) RO1 19330-01 to Johns Hopkins University.

References

Basso, A., Capitani, E., and Laiacona, M. (1988). Progressive language impairment without dementia: A case with isolated category-specific naming defect. *Journal of Neurology, Neurosurgery, and Psychiatry, 51*, 1201–1207.

Behrmann, M. (1987). The rites of righting writing: Homophone remediation in acquired dysgraphia. *Cognitive Neuropsychology, 4*, 365–384.

Behrmann, M. and Herdan, S. (1987). The case for cognitive neuropsychological remediation. *South African Journal of Communication Disorders, 34*, 3–9.

Behrmann, M. and Lieberthal, T. (1989). Category-specific treatment of a lexical-semantic deficit: A single case study of global aphasia. *British Journal of Communication Disorders, 24*, 281–299.

Berndt, R., and Mitchum, C. (in press). Approaches to the rehabilitation of "phonological assembly": Elaborating the model of non-lexical reading. In M. J. Riddoch and G. W. Humphreys, (Eds.), *Cognitive neuropsychology and cognitive rehabilitation*. London: Lawrence Erlbaum Associates.

Butterworth, B. (1979). Hesitation and the production of verbal paraphasia and neologisms in jargon aphasia. *Brain and Language, 8*, 133–161.

Byng, S., and Coltheart, M. (1986). Aphasia therapy research: Methodological requirements and illustrative results. In E. Hjelmquist and L.-G. Nilsson (Eds.), *Communication handicap: Aspects of psychological compensation and technical aids*. North-Holland: Elsevier Science Publishers B.V.

Caramazza, A. (1989). Cognitive neuropsychology and rehabilitation: An unfulfilled promise? In T. Seron and G. DeLoche (Eds.), *Cognitive approaches in rehabilitation*. (pp. 383–398). Hillsdale, NJ: LEA.

Caramazza, A., and Hillis, A. E. (1990). Where do semantic errors come from? *Cortex, 26*, 95–122.

Caramazza, A., and Hillis, A. E. (1991a). Lexical organization of nouns and verbs in the brain. *Nature, 349*, 788–790.

Caramazza, A., and Hillis, A. E. (in press). For a theory of rehabilitation. *Neuropsychological Rehabilitation*.

Caramazza, A., Hillis, A. E., Rapp, B. C. and Romani, C. (1990). Multiple semantic or multiple confusions? *Cognitive Neuropsychology, 7*, 161–168.

Carlomagno, S., Iavarone, A. and Colombo, A. (in press). Cognitive approaches to writing rehabilitation. In M. J. Riddoch and G. Humphreys (Eds.), *Cognitive neuropsychology and cognitive rehabilitation*. London: Lawrence Erlbaum Associates.

Coltheart, M., Patterson, K., and Marshall, J. C. (Eds.) (1980). *Deep dyslexia*. London: Routeledge & Kegan Paul.

de Partz, M. P. (1986). Re-education of a deep dyslexic patient: Rationale of the method and results. *Cognitive Neuropsychology, 3*, 149–177.

Ellis, A. W. (1982). Spelling and writing (and reading and speaking). In A. W. Ellis (Ed.), *Normality and pathology in cognitive functions*. London: Academic Press.

Ellis, A. W., Miller, D., and Sin, G. (1983). Wernicke's aphasia and normal language processing: A case study in cognitive neuropsychology. *Cognition, 15*, 111–114.

Gonzales-Rothi, L., and Moss, S. (1989). *Alexia without agraphia: A model-driven therapy*. Paper presented at Academy of Aphasia, Santa Fe, NM.

Goodman, R. A., and Caramazza, A. (1986). Aspects of the spelling process: Evidence from a case of acquired dysgraphia. *Language and Cognitive Processes, 1*, 263–296.

Goodman-Schulman, R. A., Sokol, S., Aliminosa, D., and McCloskey, M. (1990). *Remediation of acquired dysgraphia as a technique for evaluating models of spelling*. Paper presented at the Academy of Aphasia, Baltimore, MD.

Gordon, B. (1983). Lexical access and lexical decision: Mechanisms of frequency sensitivity. *Journal of Verbal Learning and Verbal Behavior, 22*, 146–160.

Hart, J., Berndt, R., and Caramazza, A. (1985). Category-specific naming deficit following cerebral infarction. *Nature, 316*, 338.

Hatfield, M. F. (1983). Aspects of acquired dysgraphia and implications for re-education. In C. Code and D. J. Muller (Eds.), *Aphasia therapy* (pp. 157–169). London: Edward Arnold Ltd.

Hecaen, H., and Albert, M. L. (1978). *Human neuropsychology*, New York: Wiley.

Hier, D. B. and Mohr, J. P. (1977). Incongruous oral and written naming. *Brain and Language, 4*, 115–126.

Hillis, A. E. (1989). Efficacy and generalization of treatment for aphasic naming errors. *Archives of Physical Medicine and Rehabilitation, 70*, 632-636.

Hillis, A. E. (1991). Effects of separate treatments for distinct impairments within the naming process. In T. Prescott (Ed.), *Clinical aphasiology, 1989*. (pp. 255–265). Austin, TX: Pro-Ed.

Hillis, A. E. (1992). Facilitating written language. In R. Peach (Ed.), *Clinics in Communication Disorders: Approaches to treatment of aphasia*, 19–33.

Hillis, A. E. (1993). The role of models of language processing in rehabilitation of language impairments. *Aphasiology, 7*, 5–26.

Hillis, A. E., and Caramazza, A. (1987). Model-driven treatment of dysgraphia. In R. H. Brookshire (Ed.), *Clinical aphasiology, 1987* (pp. 84–105). Minneapolis, MN: BRK.

Hillis, A. E., and Caramazza, A. (1991a). Category-specific naming and comprehension impairment: Theoretical and clinical implications. In T. Prescott (Ed.), *Clinical aphasiology* (Vol. 20, pp. 191–200). Austin, TX: Pro-Ed.

Hillis, A. E., and Caramazza, A. (1991b). Mechanisms for accessing lexical representations for output: Evidence from a category-specific semantic deficit. *Brain and Language, 40*, 106–144.

Hillis, A. E., and Caramazza, A. (1992). The reading process and its disorders. In D. Margolin (Ed.), *Cognitive neuropsychology in clinical practice* (pp. 229–261). New York: Oxford University Press.

Hillis, A. E., and Caramazza, A. (in press). Theories of lexical processing and theories of rehabilitation. In M.J. Riddoch & G. Humphreys (Eds.), *Cognitive neuropsychology and cognitive rehabilitation*.

Hillis, A. E., and Hillis, A. M. (1992). *A method for comparing the effectiveness of two treatments exemplified in single subject studies of naming treatment*. Paper presented at the Clinical Aphasiology Conference, Durango, CO.

Hillis, A. E., Rapp, B., Romani, C., and Caramazza, A. (1990). Selective impairments of semantics in lexical processing. *Cognitive Neuropsychology, 7*, 191–243.

Hillis Trupe, A. E. (1986). Effectiveness of retraining phoneme to grapheme conversion. In R. H. Brookshire (Ed.), *Clinical aphasiology, 1986*. (pp. 163–171). Minneapolis, MN: BRK Publishers.

Howard, D., Patterson, K., Franklin, S., Orchard-Lisle, V., and Morton, J. (1985). The facilitation of picture naming in aphasia. *Cognitive Neuropsychology, 2*, 42–80.

Humphreys, G. W., and Riddoch, M. J. (1984). Routes to object constancy. *Quarterly Journal of Experimental Psychology, 36A*, 385–415.

Humphreys, G. W., and Riddoch, M. J. (1987). On telling your fruits from your vegetables: A consideration of category-specific deficits after brain damage. *Trends in Neurosciences, 10*, 145–148.

Humphreys, G. W., and Riddoch, M. J. (1988). On the case for multiple semantic systems: A reply to Shallice. *Cognitive Neuropsychology, 5*, 143–150.

Jackendoff, R. (1983). *Semantics and cognition.* Cambridge, MA: MIT Press.

Linebaugh, C. (1983). Treatment of anomic aphasia. In C. Perkins (Ed.), *Current therapies for communication disorders: Language handicaps in adults.* New York: Thieme-Stratton.

Marr, D. (1982). *Vision.* New York: W.H. Freeman and Co.

McCarthy, R. A., and Warrington, E. K. (1985). Category specificity in an agrammatic patient: The relative impairment of verbal retrieval and comprehension. *Neuropsychologia, 23*, 709–723.

Miceli, G., Giustolisi, L., and Caramazza, A. (1991). The interaction of lexical and nonlexical mechanisms: Evidence from anomia. *Cortex, 27*, 57–80.

Miller, G. A., and Johnson-Laird, P. N. (1976). *Language and perception.* Cambridge, MA: Harvard University Press.

Mitchum, C., and Berndt, R. (in press). Verb retrieval and sentence construction: Effects of targeted intervention. In M.J. Riddoch and G.W. Humphreys (Eds.) *Cognitive neuropsychology and cognitive rehabilitation.*

Patterson, K. E., Coltheart, M., and Marshall, J. C. (1985). *Surface dyslexia.* London: Lawrence Erlbaum Associates.

Raymer, A., Thompson, C., Jacobs, B., and le Grand, H. (1993). Phonological treatment of naming deficits in aphasia: Model-based generalization analysis. *Aphasiology*, 27–53.

Riddoch, M. J., and Humphreys, G. W. (1987). Visual optic processing in optic aphasia: A case of semantic access agnosia. *Cognitive Neuropsychology, 4*, 131–185.

Sartori, G., Miozzo, M., and Job, R. (in press). Category-specific naming impairments? Yes. *Cognitive Neuropsychology.*

Shallice, T. (1988a). Specialisation within the semantic system. *Cognitive Neuropsychology, 5*, 133–142.

Shallice, T. (1988b). *From neuropsychology to mental structure.* Cambridge: Cambridge University Press.

Thompson, C., and Kearns, K. (1981). Experimental analysis of acquisition and generalization of naming behaviors in a patient with anomia. In R. H. Brookshire (Ed.), *Clinical Aphasiology Conference* (Vol. 10, pp. 35–45). Minneapolis, MN: BRK.

Thompson, C. K., Raymer, A., and leGrand, H. (1991). Effects of phonologically based treatment on aphasic naming deficits: A model-driven approach. In T. Prescott (Ed.), *Clinical aphasiology* (Vol. 20, pp. 239–259). Austin, TX: Pro-Ed.

Warrington, E. K. (1981). Neuropsychological studies of verbal semantic systems. *Philosophical transactions of the Royal Society of London, B295*, 411–423.

Warrington, E. K., (1986). Visual deficits associated with occipital lobe lesions in man. *Experimental Brain Research Supplementum, 11*, 247–251.

Warrington, E. K., and McCarthy, R. A. (1983). Category-specific access dysphasia. *Brain, 106*, 859–878.

Warrington, E. K., and McCarthy, R. A. (1987). Categories of knowledge: Further fractionations and an attempted explanation. *Brain, 110*, 1273–1296.

Warrington, E.K., and Shallice, T. (1984). Category specific semantic impairments. *Brain, 107*, 829–853.

Wertz, R., LaPoint, L., and Rosenbek, J. (1984). *Apraxia of speech in adults: The disorder and its management.* Orlando, FL: Grune & Stratton.

Wilson, B., and Patterson, K. (in press). Rehabilitation for cognitive impairment: Does cognitive psychology apply? *Applied Cognitive Psychology.*

Yorkston, K., and Buekelman, D. (1977). A system for assessing grammatically connected speech for mildly aphasic individuals. In R. Brookshire (Ed.), *Clinical Aphasiology Conference proceedings.* Minneapolic, MN: BRK.

CHAPTER 11

Cognitive Intervention: Stimulation of Cognition, Memory, Convergent Thinking, Divergent Thinking, and Evaluative Thinking

ROBERTA CHAPEY

The stimulation approaches to therapy form the cornerstone of language intervention strategies used with adult aphasic patients (Chapey, 1981a). None of these approaches attempts to teach naming or other specific responses to particular stimuli. Rather, each emphasizes the reorganization of language through stimulation or increased cortical activity through problem solving (Duffy, 1981). The stimulation approach, first articulated and later developed and refined by Schuell et al. (1955, 1964), places its primary emphasis on the stimulation presented to the aphasic individual. The stimulation approach is grounded in the observation that the patient has not lost linguistic elements or rules but, rather, that the language system is working with reduced efficiency. This approach, therefore, employs strong, controlled, and intensive auditory stimuli as the primary tool to facilitate and maximize the patient's reorganization and recovery of language. It emphasizes the action elicited within the patient by the stimuli presented, since "sensory stimulation is the only method we have for making complex events happen in the brain" (Schuell et al., 1964, p. 338). Some proponents of the stimulation approach encourage us to stimulate patient ability to solve problems (Jennings and Lubinski, 1981; Zachman et al., 1982), to predict outcomes, to determine causes of events (Zachman et al., 1982), and to think (Chapey, 1977a, 1981b; Chapey and Lubinski, 1979; Chapey et al., 1976, 1977).

In light of the current emphasis on cognition, one might ask, What are the types of cortical activity that are increased through problem solving, predicting outcomes, and/or determining causes of events? What complex events happen in the brain when one stimulates a patient? What are cognition, intelligence, and information processing, and how do they relate to these complex events in the brain? Are problem solving and decision making unitary or composite abilities? What is the difference between cognitive processes and products? What language-based cognitive abilities elicit action within the patient and make complex events happen in the brain in order to stimulate the comprehension and production of language?

Answers to these questions and operational definitions of these abilities are crucial if we are to develop a coherent and generative rationale for intervention, as opposed to the listing of tasks that should be presented to patients. We need a better understanding and specification of the processes we are stimulating in the brain, and an operational definition of the action elicited within the patient and the complex events that happen in the brain. We need to concretize the cognitive processes and the processes involved in problem solving and decision making. Specification of the underlying targets of our stimulation therapy may increase the effectiveness of our intervention efforts.

The following discussion represents one possible way to answer the above questions.

DEFINITIONS OF COGNITION IN THE APHASIA LITERATURE

A review of the literature in the area of adult aphasia suggests that definitions of cognition vary greatly. For example, Ulatowska et al. (1980) measure cognition in terms of responses to "standard tests to evaluate cognitive functioning," such as the Knox Cube Test, the Associated Learning Test from the Wechsler Memory Scale (Wechsler, 1973), and the Block Design and the Picture Arrangement subtests of the Wechsler Adult Intelligence Scale (WAIS; Wechsler, 1955). Salvatore et al. (1981) define cognitive behavior in terms of responses to the (WAIS) (Wechsler, 1955), the Purdue Peg Board (Tiffin, 1968), and the Halstead Reitan Battery (Reitan, n.d.). Wolfe et al. (1981) similarly suggest that cognitive behavior involves responses to the WAIS (Wechsler, 1955) and the Wechsler Memory Scale (WMS) (Wechsler, 1973). These authors, thus, define cognition in terms of patient responses to specific tasks.

According to Rosenbek (1982) most traditional aphasiologists would like to separate cognition and language and leave cognitive deficit out of the definition of aphasia. He notes, however, that both Martin (1981) and Brown (1972, 1977) define cognition in ways that inextricably tie it to language, thereby suggesting cognitive deficits as central to aphasia. According to Rosenbek (1982), these authors define cognition differently from traditional aphasiologists, who seem to assume that cognition is only that which goes awry in dementia.

In a 1975 article, Martin cites Neisser's (1967) definition: "Cognition refers to all the processes by which sensory input is transformed, reduced, elaborated, stored, recovered and used." Martin (1975) further suggested that cognitive learning involves the use of memory, problem solving, and/or reorganization.

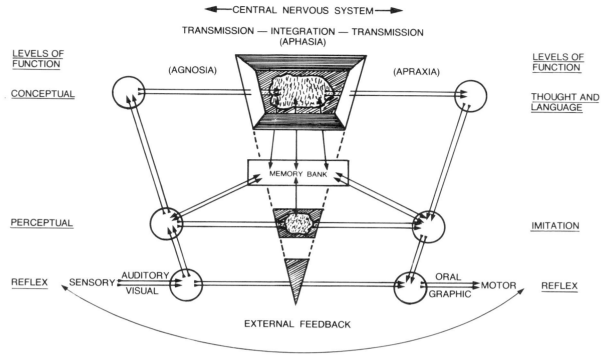

Figure 11.1. Wepman's revised model: an operational diagram of levels of function in CNS

Thus, both Martin and Brown define cognition in terms of the processes involved in responding to tasks rather than by listing tasks that necessitate the use of "cognition."

DEFINITIONS OF INFORMATION PROCESSING IN THE APHASIA LITERATURE

The model developed by Wepman et al. in 1960 (Fig. 11.1) is one of the most popular theoretical models used to explain function in the central nervous system (CNS). Indeed, it was cited by both Darley (1982) and Davis (1983) in their texts on aphasia.

Several other authors, such as Haaland (1979), have supported the need for utility of an information-processing model/ approach in aphasia in order to help aphasiologists understand how tasks are solved and information is processed. Haaland (1979) suggests, "In the context of aphasia, the goal is to understand what is happening between the stimulus and the response. Very simply, there is an attempt to separate tasks into input, processing and output components" (p. 1). This author also notes that the "processing aspect of the information processing model which is the most difficult to operationally define also has significant implications for language evaluation" (p. 3). She encourages aphasiologists to explore how information is organized, remembered, and used.

At a Clinical Aphasiology Conference, Martin (1979) encouraged us to "turn to the work of cognitive psychologists for further identification of the subsystems whose interaction is necessary for processing." Luria (1973) also suggests that a more complete understanding of aphasia is more likely to be found in the study of the psychological structures underlying cognitive process.

DEFINITIONS OF COGNITION IN THE PSYCHOLOGY LITERATURE

The study of cognition represents the work of numerous psychologists with a variety of related approaches. Thus, there is no single comprehensive theory of cognition. Rather, cognitive psychologists are viewed as "information-processing" theorists who seek to determine what "functional mental events transpire while a person actually behaves" (Rosenthal and Zimmerman, 1978). Their focus is not on observable behavior but, rather, on examining the characteristics of internal, central brain processing or mental events such as perception, recognition, reasoning, thinking, evaluation, concept formation, abstraction, generalization, decision making, and problem solving.

Cognition, then, is a generic term for any process whereby an organism becomes aware of or obtains knowledge of an object (English and English, 1958). It "refers to all the processes by which sensory input is transformed, reduced, elaborated, stored, recovered, and used" (Neisser, 1967, p. 4). It is a group of processes by which we achieve knowledge and command of our world, that is a method of processing information. It is "the activity of knowing; the acquisition, organization, and use of knowledge" (Neisser, 1967, p. 1)—knowledge that will, in turn, influence or instigate and guide subsequent and more overt behavior (Rosenthal and Zimmerman, 1978).

It should be noted that cognitive psychologists do not interpret the above mental processes as occurring in stages or in

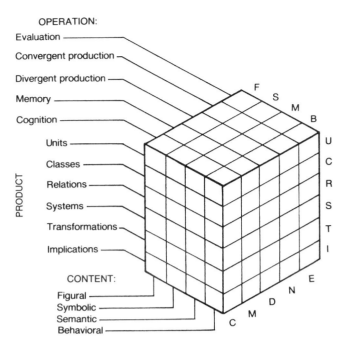

Figure 11.2. Guilford's Structure of Intellect model.

isolation but, rather, they are seen as dynamic and interacting variables.

INTELLIGENCE AS DEFINED IN THE PSYCHOLOGY LITERATURE

The most widely accepted definition of intelligence is that "intelligence is what the intelligence tests test." Another definition, that specified in the Structure of Intellect model (Fig. 11.2), was developed by J. P. Guilford (1967) during his 20 years as the director of the Aptitudes Research Project at the University of Southern California from 1949 to 1969. This project, funded by the Personnel and Training Branch of the Psychological Sciences Division of the U.S. Office of Naval Research, was designed to define various intellectual abilities in order to match the native skills of navy personnel to specific job requirements. For example, he sought to determine which subjects were best suited for officer status, for pilot training, and so on.

In an attempt to define the numerous intellectual abilities available to individuals and, thereby, achieve a taxonomy of intellectual functioning, Guilford and his colleagues (1967, 1971) developed numerous tests, each of which was thought to tap a specific intellectual ability. The validity of each test and ability was then assessed by performing numerous factor analytic studies of responses to the tests and determining which tests loaded on specific statistical factors. Results to this research suggest that there are 120 factors in humans (Fig. 11.2). These 120 factors are divided into three parameters: mental operations, contents, and products. The five **mental operations** are cognition, memory, convergent thinking, divergent thinking, and evaluation or judgment. The four **content areas** are figural, symbolic, semantic, and behavioral. The six **products** of this model are units, classes, relations, systems, transformations, and implications (5 × 4 × 6 = 120). An **ability** is a combination of one kind of operation, one kind of content, and one kind of product (e.g., convergent symbolic units, divergent semantic classes).

Mental Operations

The five mental operations are cognition, memory, convergent thinking, divergent thinking, and evaluative thinking or judgment.

Cognition

The mental operation of cognition is basic to all other operations, hence, it is first. "If no cognition, no memory; if no memory, no production, for the things produced come largely from memory storage. If neither cognition nor production, then no evaluation" (Guilford, 1967, p. 63).

Cognition involves knowing, awareness, immediate discovery (or rediscovery), and recognition of information in various forms (comprehension or understanding). Recognition involves acknowledgment that something has been seen or perceived previously. For example, cognition of semantic material might be tested by using a multiple-choice vocabulary test in which the correct alternative is a synonym of the word to be defined and the others are not. Tests of cognition determine how much the examinee knows or can readily discover on the basis of what is known. (The term "cognition" has been used to refer to all mental operations by most cognitive psychologists. Guilford used the term to refer to one specific mental operation. This can be confusing.)

Memory

Memory is the power, act, or process of fixing newly gained information in storage. It involves the ability to insert new information into memory and to retain the new information. According to Guilford (1967), good memory tests require that subjects, essentially, have a full comprehension of the studied information. Therefore, test material is not difficult. Otherwise, tests may load on cognition, convergent thinking, and/or divergent thinking. The operation of memory, then, is the fixation and retention of new information.

Convergent Thinking

Convergent thinking is the generation of logical conclusions from given information, where emphasis is on achieving conventionally best outcomes. Usually, the information given fully determines the outcome, as in mathematics and logic. In accordance with the information given them, examinees must converge on the one right answer (Guilford, 1967; Guilford and Hoepfner, 1971).

Convergent production is in the area of logical deductions or compelling inferences. It involves the generation of logical necessities. An example of a convergent semantic test would be verbal analogies completion, in which the subject has to supply his or her own answers, or picture group naming, in which the individual writes a class name for each group of five pictured objects.

Divergent Thinking

Divergent production involves the generation of logical alternatives from given information, where emphasis is on variety, quantity, and relevance of output from the same source. It is concerned with the generation of logical possibilities, with the ready flow of ideas and with the readiness to change the direction of one's responses (Guilford, 1967). It involves providing ideas in situations where a proliferation of ideas on a specific topic is required. Such behavior necessitates the use of a broad search of memory storage, and the production of multiple possible solutions to a problem. It is the ability to extend previous experience and knowledge or to widen existing concepts (Cropley, 1967). Divergent behavior is directed toward new responses—new in the sense that the thinker was not aware of the response before beginning the particular line of thought (Gowan et al., 1967).

Divergent questions are open-ended and do not have a single correct answer. For example, the individual might be asked to list numerous things that are soft and fluffy, to think of problems that anyone might have in eating lunch, or to list what might happen if people no longer needed or wanted sleep. Responses can be grouped according to the number of ideas produced (fluency) and the variety of ideas suggested (flexibility). If an individual was asked to list objects that can roll, and responded with, "a baseball, a football, a basketball, a nickel, a dime, a quarter, a car, and a truck," this person would receive a fluency score of eight and a flexibility score of three (balls, money, transportation). Guilford also used originality and elaboration scores to measure divergent ability. Originality relates to the unusualness of the response. Elaboration is the ability to specify numerous critical details in planning an event or making a decision. Responses are also evaluated for relevance. Answers that are not relevant to the specific questions are not scored. Thus, if the above individual had responded, "Isn't that an interesting question?" or "I like to eat lunch," these responses would not be scored because they do not answer the question (see Appendices 11.1 and 11.2).

Evaluative Thinking or Judgment

According to Guilford (1967), judgment involves the ability of the individual to use knowledge to make appraisals or comparisons, or to formulate evaluations in terms of known specifications or criterion, such as correctness, completeness, identity, relevance, adequacy, utility, safety, consistency, logical feasibility, practical feasibility, or social custom. Although judgment behavior is based on the individual's previous experience and knowledge of the subject involved, it is always an extension of what is known. It is an appraisal or evaluation based on knowledge.

Guilford (1967) developed a number of tests to study judgment or evaluation skills. These tests require that the individual keep specific criteria in mind and select one best answer or solution from among several alternatives. In one test, for example, the individual must choose the best word for the sentence, "A sandwich always has (a) bread, (b) butter, (c) lettuce, (d) meat. Which one *must* it have in order to be a sandwich?" In another, the subject must judge whether a sentence expresses a complete thought. For example, "Is 'Milk comes from' a sentence?" In yet another test, the individual is given specific classifications and asked to determine if new information can be assigned to the previously established class. For example, "Should the word *chair* be put with the words *cow* and *horse* or with the words *table* and *lamp*?" Each judgment task has a

predetermined best response or solution (Chapey and Lubinski, 1979).

Content

There are four broad, substantive, basic kinds (or areas) of information, material, or content that the organism discriminates. They are figural, symbolic, semantic, and behavioral.

Figural

Figural content pertains to "information in concrete form, as perceived or as recalled in the form of images. The term 'figural' minimally implies figure-ground perceptual organization" (Guilford and Hoepfner, 1971).

Symbolic

Symbolic content pertains to "information in the form of denotative signs having no significance in and of themselves, such as letters, numbers, musical notations (and) codes" (Guilford and Hoepfner, 1971).

Semantic

Semantic content pertains to "information in the form of conceptions or mental constructs to which words are often applied. Therefore, it involves thinking and verbal communication. However, it need not necessarily be dependent on words. For example, meaningful pictures also convey semantic information" (Guilford and Hoepfner, 1971).

Behavioral

Behavioral content pertains to psychological information—that is, to essentially nonfigural and nonverbal aspects of human interactions, where the attitudes, needs, desires, moods, intentions, perceptions, and thoughts of others and of ourselves are involved. Some of the cues that the human organism obtains about the attention, perception, thinking, feeling, emotions, and intentions of others come indirectly through nonverbal means. For example, this might involve matching two faces that are similar in terms of the mental state conveyed. This ability enables us to keep aware of what behavior is going on and enables us to interpret it. It is important for coping with other individuals in face-to-face encounters, in solving interpersonal problems, in detecting and analyzing problems, and in generating information that is needed toward solutions. This type of content is sometimes called social intelligence (Guilford and Hoepfner, 1971).

Products

The six types of products are units, classes, relations, systems, transformations, and implications. These products are thought to replace the time-honored concept of association. That is, products represent the way in which things are associated. The present writer believes that the products represent a possible continuum from simple (units) to complex (implications).

Units

Units are relatively "segregated or circumscribed items or 'chunks' of information having 'thing' character" (Guilford and Hoepfner, 1971). Units are things to which nouns are often applied. Units may be synonymous with Gestalt psychology's "figure-on-ground." An example of a semantic units test might be a multiple-choice vocabulary test in which the correct alternative is a synonym of the word to be defined, and the others are not. Semantic units are meanings, ideas, or thoughts in the form of particular wholes. "Of the products, units are regarded as basic, hence they appear at the top. Units enter into classes, relations, systems and also transformations and implications" (Guilford, 1967).

Classes

Classes are "conceptions underlying sets of items of information grouped by virtue of their common properties" (Guilford and Hoepfner, 1971). That is, they involve common properties within sets. For example, semantic classes can involve choosing the class name that best describes a given set of words or objects. Semantic classes involve class ideas or concepts.

Relations

Relations are meaningful connections or "connections between items of information based upon variables or points of contact that apply to them" (Guilford and Hoepfner, 1971). For example, a semantic relation can be a test of logical relations in the form of a syllogism that presents two premises and four alternative conclusions, only one of which is correct. It might also involve an analogy task, in which case the individual must grasp the relations between the initial pair of words and apply it to the second.

Systems

Systems are organized patterns or "structured aggregates of items of information; complexes of interrelated or interacting parts" (Guilford and Hoepfner, 1971). For example, a semantic system can be a "sentence—a complex of relationships among ideas, an organized thought—a sequence of events, or a common situation" (Guilford and Hoepfner, 1971). It might involve double meanings, puns, homonyms, and redefinitions or shifts in meaning.

Transformations

Transformations are changes of various kinds (such as redefinitions, shifts, transitions, or modifications) in existing information.

Implications

Implications are "circumstantial connections between items of information, as by virtue of contiguity, or any condition that promotes 'belongingness'" (Guilford and Hoepfner, 1971). Implications involve information expected, anticipated, suggested, or predicted by other information. For example, a semantic implication can be sensitivity to problems such as stating two things seen wrong with a common appliance or problems that might arise in the use of each given object.

Composite Abilities

According to Guilford and Hoepfner (1971):

> It must not be supposed that, although the abilities are separate and distinct logically and they can be segregated by factor analysis, they function in isolation in mental activities of the individual. Two or more of the abilities are ordinarily involved in solving the same problem. The fact that they habitually operate together in various mixtures in ordinary mental functioning has been the reason for the difficulty of recognizing them by direct observation or even by ordinary laboratory procedures (pp. 19–20).

Indeed, it was largely through the construction of special tests, each one aimed at a specific ability, and the sensitive and searching procedures of factor analysis that Guilford and his colleagues clearly demonstrated the separateness of the various mental operations, contents, and products.

The following sections will explore the composite or unified notions of problem solving, decision making, and information processing.

PROBLEM SOLVING

According to Guilford and Hoepfner (1971), problem solving is a complex composite ability. A problem is presented whenever a situation calls for the individual doing anything novel in order to cope with something that is different from the past behavior. Problem solving involves the use of all five mental operations, all types of content or information, and any kind of product, depending on the context in which the problem arises and the kinds of products required in order to reach a solution.

Initially, the individual must become aware that a problem exists. This is a matter of cognition, often involving implications. Next, the problem must be analyzed or structured, which usually involves cognition of systems. After the problem is structured:

> [the] individual generates a variety of alternative solutions, which is divergent production. If sufficient basis for a solution is cognized and then produced, there is convergent production (Guilford and Hoepfner, 1971, p. 31).

At each stage in the problem-solving process there is evaluation:

> in the form of accepting or rejecting cognitions of the problem and generated solutions. At any step what happens may become fixated and retained for possible later use, so that memory is involved. When evaluation leads to rejections, there may be new starts, with revised cognitions and productions (Guilford and Hoepfner, 1971, p. 31).

Thus, problem solving can be said to have five steps: preparation (recognition of a problem, cognition); analysis (cognition); production (divergent and convergent); verification (evaluation); and reapplication.

The problem-solving factors found in factor analyses were as follows:

Cognition	CMU		
	CMC		
	CMR	inductive	Therefore, there are
	CMS		eight factors involved

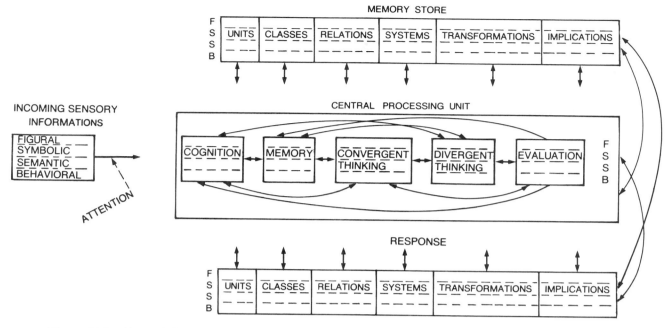

Figure 11.3.   Human Information processing model based upon the Guilford Structure of Intellect model by Chapey.

	CMI[a]	in reasoning (five cognition, three convergent).
Divergent	DMU	
	DMR	
	DMT	
Convergent	NMC	
	NMR	deductive
	MNI	
Evaluation	EMI[a]	

DECISION MAKING

Decision making and planning ability both belong in the category of problem solving and usually entail all of the steps described above.

Guilford (1967) notes that the more a problem, decision, or plan involves the generation of numerous responses or novelty, or the more creative the solution to the problem, the more it involves divergent production abilities—especially divergent transformation abilities—or possibly all transformation abilities.

INFORMATION PROCESSING

The present writer suggests that Guilford's (1967) Structure of Intellect (SOI) model can also be viewed as an information-processing model (Fig. 11.3). Within this information-processing model, incoming sensory information is figural, symbolic, semantic, and/or behavioral. An attention mechanism selects a small portion of sensory information to be held for several seconds for further processing. This further processing takes place in the central processing unit. The processes of

this central processing unit are cognition, memory convergent thinking, divergent thinking, and evaluative thinking or judgment. It is suggested that these are the functional mental events that transpire while a person actually behaves. These are the mental events or processes by which sensory information is transformed, reduced, elaborated, stored, recovered, and used. This is the group of mental processes that are used to acquire, organize, store, and use knowledge; the processes whereby an organism becomes aware of or obtains knowledge of an object, event, or relationship.

Within this information-processing model, then, incoming figural, symbolic, semantic, and/or behavioral sensory information is attended to and processed in the central processing unit by one or more of the five SOI mental operations. If the information is immediately recognized, known, comprehended, or understood, then the mental operation of cognition has occurred. When situations call for the individual to generate logical conclusions from given information, where emphasis is on achieving conventionally best outcomes, convergent thinking occurs. When a novel response is required, the divergent operation is generated. Inserting newly gained information into storage involves memory. Judging the appropriateness, acceptability, relevance, and/or correctness of information requires evaluation.

When the mental operations are used and new information or knowledge is produced, these new discriminations come about in the form of new products: units, classes, relations, systems, transformations, and implications. Products are the basic forms that figural, symbolic, semantic, and behavioral information take as a result of being processed by one or all of the organism's mental operations. These new associations are usually produced as responses and/or may also be processed by the mental operation of memory and inserted into memory storage.

---

[a]CMI, EMI = sensitivity to problems.

Memory

It is important to differentiate between memory as an operation and long-term memory or memory storage. The operation of memory is the act or process of fixing newly gained information in storage. In contrast, long-term memory is a storage area that contains everything that is retained for more than a few minutes, such as all learned experience, including language and the rules of language. It retains the products generated by the various mental operations as they process or act on experience.

Thus, each individual has his or her own summary of past experiences, or a memory structure of the world in long-term memory. It has been shown that the capacity of this storage is not static or fixed; it is dynamic. Indeed, "the more you know, the more you can know, the more you remember, the more you can remember" (Muma, 1978). This "theory of the world in our heads serves as the foundation for learning." Indeed, what we know makes our experience meaningful.

One of the characteristics of long-term memory is that what is recalled is often not simply what was seen or heard but a modification of the original learning. That is, external stimuli cannot enter into the organism. According to Guilford (1967), "organisms react not directly to the real world but rather to their representations of that world, which means reacting to information that they themselves construct" (p. 6). An individual's representation of reality as internal symbols and the interrelations among these symbols are what is called "information."

When the amount of memory we need to process is large, the operation of memory is capable of collapsing the data it receives (or "chunking" it) in more efficient ways and treating it in groups, such as classes. Through chunking, we can successfully deal with larger amounts of information with minimal difficulty in storage and retrieval. Chunking provides a way of representing information so that it conforms with one's conceptual organization (Muma, 1978), that is, one's previously stored associations or products.

When the individual is faced with a meaningful problem and uses all of the cognitive processes to solve a problem, the results of this information processing frequently are inserted into long-term memory. Rote memory, on the other hand, uses only one mental operation: memory. The use of more numerous operations during problem solving and the establishment of numerous associations, or products, during the process may be one reason why meaningful memory is longer lasting.

All of the mental operations depend on memory storage; all operations retrieve information from this store (Fig. 11.3). That is, all of the mental operations search long-term memory in order to recall information that has been stored. Thus, there is cognitive retrieval, memory retrieval, convergent retrieval, divergent retrieval, and evaluative retrieval.

Perception

Where, one may ask, is perception in all this? In the literature, perception is defined as knowing and comprehending the nature of the stimulus (Muma, 1978). To perceive is to know. Therefore, within this model, perception is viewed as part of cognition.

LEARNING

According to cognitive psychologists, learning is an active process of problem solving (Lazerson, 1975). A learning situation arises whenever our present cognitive structures prove inadequate for making sense of the world, when something in our experience is unfamiliar or unpredictable (Smith, 1975). Thus, learning is an interaction between the world around us and the theory of the world in our heads. In this view, the learner is seen as a scientist who constructs theories or forms hypotheses about the world and conducts experiments to test these hypotheses.

A distinguishing feature of the "cognitive" approach to learning is the assumption that what is learned are concepts or schema and conceptual associations about the relationships between and among objects, events, and relationships. This process of concept formation involves identifying common features and grouping together all things that have a common feature (i.e., forming classes). Concept learning involves the acquisition of a common response to dissimilar stimuli (Saltz, 1971). It is regarded as the process of making differentiations and discriminations, a process of recognizing similarities and differences or reorganizing material into new patterns or products. It involves the generation of lists of specific characteristics to differentiate membership into particular categories.

Concept formation enables us to transform the world of infinite appearances into finite essences (Saltz, 1971) and to organize past learning in such a way that it is no longer bound to the specific situation in which the learning occurred. Thus, instead of having to react to each object as something unique, we learn to make generalized responses to classes of objects. The generalized responses function as principles or laws. When we learn something in this type of generic manner, we are able to benefit from analogy when we deal with a new problem. When this occurs, one of the major objectives of learning has been accomplished: We are able to adapt to our environment in more satisfactory ways, and we are saved from subsequent learning (Bruner, 1968).

According to Bruner (1968), all of human beings' interactions with the world must involve classifying input in relation to classes or categories that they have already established. It is Bruner's (1968) contention that to perceive is to categorize; to conceptualize is to categorize; to learn is to form categories; to make decisions is to categorize.

In SOI theory, learning is "the acquisition of information which comes about in the form of new discriminations in terms of new products" (Guilford and Hoepfner, 1971, p. 30). Learning and concept formation employ the five operations of the SOI theory. According to Guilford and Hoepfner (1971):

> . . . (no) item of information has been learned until it has been cognized. That which is learned cannot have any future effects unless it is fixated and retained (memory). Items of information produced (divergent and convergent) in response to new cues may also be fixated and remembered. In attempting to learn, the individual makes errors and he must discriminate between errors and correct information. This involves evaluation. Evaluation is conceived as playing an important role in reinforcement (p. 30).

Concept formations, the largest product of cognitive processing, are products of SOI operations and are called units, classes, relations, systems, transformations, and implications. Thus, the SOI model is also a model of learning.

Results of factor analyses led Guilford and his colleagues (1967 , 1971) to redefine some of the terminology traditionally used in reference to learning. For example:

Serial learning is essentially dealing with systems, since learned order is a system.

Reasoning, redefined as relational thinking, involves mostly cognition and convergent production—but especially cognition of semantic systems (CMS).

Induction is thought to be in the area of cognition because of its discovery properties.

Deduction is primarily in the area of convergent production because it has to do with drawing firm conclusions.

Classifying objects involves cognition of semantic classes.

Sensitivity to problems his primarily cognition of meaningful implications.

Analysis and *synthesis* were not coherent SOI factors.

Abstraction, Generalization, and Transfer

Abstraction occurs when the person selectively picks "abstract dimensions of the object" and reacts to those dimensions and no others. With transfer, "he is obviously adding some personal component to his original learning experience. Thus, more than the literal, external properties of stimuli guide the individual's behavior" (Rosenthal and Zimmerman, 1978).

Abstraction is apparent during concept development: "Concepts are developed by abstracting the common stimulus elements in a series of stimulus objects" (Staats, 1968). After having experience with the common stimulus elements of the concept, the individual will then be able to pick this common component from a new set containing the same element.

Abstraction and transfer are apparent during rule learning.

> By a rule, we mean that two or more objects or events are related to one another in a systematic way. For example, we learn that a flashing red light signifies stopping before crossing an intersection. Later, we exhibit transfer of this rule by stopping when we unexpectedly see a flashing red light beside a stalled car on the highway (Rosenthal and Zimmerman, 1978).

Abstraction and transfer are involved in a judgment of class inclusion. For example, a baby concludes that certain objects are movable. Understanding the "abstract dimension" of movability the child transfers this by adding some personal component to his or her original learning experience: The child knows that one way of moving something is to pull it; another way is to kick it; and yet another is to get a parent to pull it (Boden, 1980). This is analogous to the child who knows that the class of beads includes the subclass of green beads (Boden, 1980).

The transfer of learning to new stimuli means that the individual will add quite dissimilar response elements that were not directly related to his or her original learning (Rosenthal and Zimmerman, 1978).

Transfer is an additional concept used in problem solving. It is when an individual uses something he or she learned previously and transfers it to a new situation. Positive transfer is when what was learned for one situation helps solve a problem in a new situation. Negative transfer is when what was learned for one situation makes it harder to solve a problem in a new situation. When an individual is continuously exposed to similar sorts of problems he or she learns strategies for solving them. A skill that can be transferred to solve problems in new situations is a strategy. Harry Harlow (1949) calls this "learning to learn."

Strategies can be transferred from one situation to another. A strategy can also be divided into its components, and then the components can be recombined in new ways (transforma-tions). A transfer in which the components are recombined to "suddenly" solve a problem is called insight. It is when a problem is solved with "aha! reaction" (Lazerson, 1975).

The intellectual ability to generalize is a significant component of the definition of "cognition." To incorporate specific knowledge and generalize it into everyday experiences is "cognition" well defined and developed (Scott et al., 1979).

Why We Solve Problems or Learn

According to cognitive psychologists, the mind possesses an innate order-generating capacity—a built-in drive to learn. We carry out that drive by acting on our environment. Thus, the individual must act on and interact with the physical, emotional, social, language, and thinking world in order for cognitive processing to occur. When something is unfamiliar or unpredictable, or when we do not understand, we are motivated to learn (Smith, 1975). According to Smith (1975):

> We learn because we do not understand, cannot relate, cannot predict. Everything we know, then, is a consequence of all our previous attempts to make sense of the world. Our present knowledge arises out of a history of problem solving or of predicting the consequences of potential actions (p. 161).

We learn by relating new information to previous information and by seeing relationships among various bits of information.

For cognitive psychologists, learning is an active process that is significantly influenced by motivation, especially intrinsic motivation (Bruner, 1968), and by curiosity (Yardley, 1974). Bruner (1968) explains this intrinsic motivation in terms of curiosity drive, a drive to achieve competence, and a need to work cooperatively with others, which he termed reciprocity.

Leon Festinger conceived of cognitive dissonance, the motivating effect of possessing simultaneously compatible items of information. "It is assumed that dissonance leads to behavior designed to reduce conflict" (Lefrancois, 1982, p. 71). An individual remembers more distinctly and for longer periods of time material that is somewhat different from what is already known. If it is completely new and unrelated to anything in his or her cognitive structure, according to Ausubel (Lefrancois, 1982, p. 225), rote learning rather than meaningful learning will occur. If it is too similar, it is rapidly forgotten.

Other variables that intervene between the stimuli and the response are the individual learner's purpose, aspirations, beliefs, and ideals (Marx, 1970). In addition, the learning potential of an individual includes the requisite intellectual capacities, the ideational context, and the existing store of knowledge as it is currently organized (Ausubel, 1965). It is on this basis that the potential meaningfulness of learning material varies with factors such as age, intelligence, occupation, and cultural membership.

Two people, therefore, are likely to respond differently to the very same stimuli because of what they have already learned, what they feel they are capable of achieving, differences in the ways their minds work, or other differences that distinguish one person from another (Dember and Jenkins, 1979). Smith (1975) observes there are two other crucial conditions for the individual to exercise a capacity to learn. One is that the individual have the expectation that there is something to learn; second, the learner must have some reasonable expectation of a positive outcome.

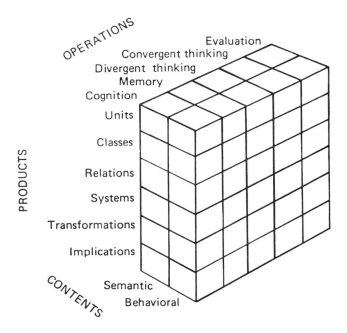

Figure 11.4. Model of Language

COGNITION

Cognition, then, can be operationally defined as the use of the five mental operations: cognition (recognition/understanding/comprehension), memory, convergent thinking, divergent thinking, and evaluative thinking or judgment. These are the mental events or processes by which we learn or obtain knowledge of our world, by which we organize, store, recover and use that knowledge. Knowledge is a product of cognition and is associated or organized into units, classes, relations, systems, transformations, and implications.

LANGUAGE DEFINED

Psycholinguistics is the study of the mental processes underlying the acquisition and use of language (Slobin, 1971). Within the context of the Guilford model, incoming information or language experience is semantic and behavioral (Fig. 11.4). This information is then processed by one or more of the five cognitive operations: cognition, memory, convergent thinking, divergent thinking, and evaluative thinking. These are the mental processes underlying the acquisition and use of language.

Language is something *we know* (Slobin, 1971). It is a body of knowledge represented in the brains of speakers of a language, whose content is inferred from overt behavior (Slobin, 1971). According to Bloom and Lahey (1978), language can be defined as "a knowledge of a code for *representing ideas about the world* through a conventional system of arbitrary signals for *communication*" (p. 23). Specifically, there are three types of language knowledge: content, form, and use. Thus, "language consists of some aspect of *content* or meaning that is coded or represented by linguistic form for some purpose or *use* in a particular context" (p. 23). These three types of language knowledge come together in both understanding and saying messages and indeed linguistic competence can be defined as the interaction of content, form, and use (Bloom and Lahey, 1978; Lahey, 1988).

Content: Language Represents Ideas About the World

Psycholinguistic research suggests that our

> . . . code or means of representing information can operate only in relation to what (we) the speaker and hearer of the language *know* about objects and events in the world. Speakers of a language need to know about objects and actions in order to know the names for objects and actions [O]ne cannot know about sentences and the relations between the parts of a sentence unless one also knows about relations between persons and objects in different kinds of events. . . . It is the knowledge that individuals have about objects, events and relations in the world that is coded by language—ideas about events are coded, not events themselves (Bloom and Lahey, 1978, p. 5).

It is this knowledge, these ideas, that are the meaning, topic or subject matter involved in conversation. For example, an individual might comment about a specific *object*, such as a pipe, a particular *action*, such as eating lunch, or a specific *relation*, such as between Harry and his pipe. Or, meaning could relate to a content category such as *possession*, or having or owning an object, quality, or ability; *recurrence*, or the reappearance of an object or event; or *rejection* the opposition to an action or object.

An individual learns to understand and use language in relation to the ideas or mental concepts that have been formed through experience (Bloom and Lahey, 1978). The experience of many different objects—some of which are more alike than others—is "an active process whereby persons perceive patterns of structure and invariance in the environment" (Bloom and Lahey, 1978, p. 7), such as similarities among different chairs and the movability of certain objects and not others. The ability to perceive the similarities in repeated encounters with physical and social events involves the ability to process and analyze experience using the five cognitive processes. Words and categories represent regularities that the individual notes in his or her environment. Individuals learn new words and categories gradually, by testing hypotheses of what a word means in different situations in which they think one or another word might fit (Bloom and Lahey, 1978; Lahey, 1988). This results in the organization or association of information—or the formation of schema into *units* (or chunks of information having "thing" character; things to which words are often applied; meaning, ideas, or thoughts in the form of particular wholes—such as a cookie); *classes* (or conceptions underlying sets of items such as cookies); *relations* (or meaningful connections between items of information—such as all desserts); *systems* (or complexes of interrelated or interacting relationships among objects, ideas and events; double meanings, puns, homonyms, and redefinitions or shifts in meaning—such as "This is what I call cheesecake"); *transformations* (or various types of changes such as redefinitions, shifts, transitions, or modifications in existing information—such as when baking a cake, if a recipe calls for two eggs and there is only one, one might open one egg, put it into a measuring cup, and then double the volume by adding water or milk); and *implications* (or the formation of hypotheses of what is expected, anticipated, suggested, or predicted by other information—such as "Desserts are sweet, fattening, and taste good; are sold in a bakery; are frequently chocolate; can often become stale or spoil"; and so forth).

New experiences may cause the brain to place the experience into an existing unit or class; to create a new concept; to reprocess existing information and reformulate the structure of individual units or to group units together into classes, systems, and/or relations; to transform the information; and/or to see the implications of such information.

Language content is developed and used within the context of the speech act (see under language "Use"). Communication, which is a problem-solving task, is usually initiated and/or maintained in order to convey meaning about certain topics or ideas or to convey an intent. For example, during communication, an individual may become aware that it is necessary to describe something (an intent) that he or she knows (cognition). The individual may sort through all the possible ways to express this intent (divergent thinking) and may make a judgment, based on past experience, that certain content would be inappropriate (evaluation) for his or her purpose, intent, or listener. The individual therefore comes to a logical conclusion about the conventionally best content for his or her intent (convergent thinking), and then conveys the content to the listener.

Form: Language Is a System

The rules of language specify how to arrange symbols to express ideas (McCormick and Schiefelbush, 1984). Specifically, a system of rules determines the "ways in which sounds combine to form words and words combine to form sentences for representing knowledge" (Bloom and Lahey, 1978, p. 7). For words, a limited number of rules specify which sounds can and cannot combine. For sentences, a limited number of rules specify how linguistic elements (words and morphemes) are combined to code meaning (Bloom and Lahey, 1978; Lahey, 1988). According to Slobin (1971), syntax is a device that relates sound and meaning. Thus, the form of language or system of rules "is the means for connecting sounds or signs with meaning" (Bloom and Lahey, 1978, p. 15). Linguistic competence is a system of rules that relates semantic interpretations of a sentence to their acoustic phonetic representations (Slobin, 1971). It is a set or system of rules for processing utterances (Slobin, 1971).

Two rule systems in English are word order and markers. **Word order** tells us about the subject-object relationship. There are two types of **markers**: function words (the, a, with) and suffixes (-s, -ing).

> The markers do such things as identify classes (for example, *the* identifies a noun), specify relations (*with* relates girl to eyes), or signal meanings (-ing), signals ongoing activity, -s signals plurality) and so on (Slobin, 1971, p. 2).

Chomsky (1957) postulated that there are two basic sorts of rules or two levels of sentence interpretation. **Phrase structure rules** generate deep structures, which are directly related to the meaning of the sentence. The semantic component of grammar "relates deep structures to meanings" (Slobin, 1971, p. 19). **Transformational rules** convert deep structures into surface structures. The surface level of a sentence is directly related to the sentence as it is heard. The phonological component of grammar "converts surface structures into sound patterns of spoken utterances" (Slobin, 1971, p. 19).

According to Chomsky (1972), the surface structure is often misleading and uninformative: "Our knowledge of language involves properties of a much more abstract nature, not directly

in the surface structure" (p. 32). Since the meaning of utterances are not always directly expressed in the sounds we hear, we must have rich inner mental structures that make it possible to utter and comprehend sentences (Slobin, 1971). We cannnot explain language learning on the basis of "observable 'stimuli' and 'responses' alone, because all of the information for the processing of speech is not present in observable behavior" (Slobin, 1971, p. 19). Rather, the individual is biologically predisposed to learn a set or system of rules for processing utterances.

Grammar then is

> . . . a device for pairing phonetically represented signals [into a] system of abstract structures generated by the syntactic component. Thus, the syntactic component must provide for each sentence (actually for each interpretation of each sentence) a semantically interpretable *deep structure* and a phonetically interpretable *surface structure*, and in the event that these are distinct, a statement of the relation between these structures (Chomsky, 1964, p. 52).

Abstract structural patterns underlie grammatical sentences. Understanding a sentence is based on knowledge of this structure. Indeed, "you can only make sense of the string of words you hear if you 'know' . . . the grammar of your language" (Slobin, 1971). This syntactic knowledge or finite system of rules makes it possible for us to comprehend and generate an infinite number of sentences and connect sounds or signs with meaning.

These rules of language that allow us to process and/or generate utterances and connect sounds or signs with meaning are learned by "listening to the language of the environment and abstracting from it the rules that are used to generate it" (Naremore, 1980). Individuals do not learn language form and then apply this to meaning. Rather, they focus on what they see and hear and "use their conceptual capacity for linguistic inductions" (Bloom and Lahey, 1978, p. 72) to develop a knowledge of language content, form, and use in order to communicate meaning. Meaning is the essence of language (Goodman, 1971).

Developing a language system is a problem-solving task. It involves, among other things, hypothesis formation, abstraction, transfer, judgment of class inclusion, and generalization. As individuals process and use semantic and behavioral information, they become aware that the system of rules they now possess is not adequate for expressing meaning or what they would like to say. Becoming aware that a problem exists is a matter of cognition, often involving implications. Next, the problem in the rule system is analyzed or structured, which usually involves cognition of systems. After the problem is structured, the individual generates a variety of possible ways to code what he or she wishes, which is divergent production. If sufficient basis for a solution to the rule system is cognized and then produced, there is convergent production. At each stage in the process, there is evaluation or judgment in the form of accepting or rejecting cognitions of the problem and generated solutions. At any step, what happens may become fixated and retained for possible later use, so that memory is involved. When evaluation leads to rejections, there may be new starts, with revised cognitions and productions.

Thus, we learn new forms of language when our present system of rules proves inadequate for expressing meaning. The acquisition of new rules comes about in the form of new dis-

Table 11.1.
Discourse Structures

1. Physical context variables
2. Communicative partner variables
3. Communication of intent

Label	Greeting	Attention
Response	Repeating	Protesting (Dore, 1974)
Request	Description	
Request	Order	Warn (Searle, 1969)
Assert	Argue	
Question	Advise	

4. Turn taking
   A. Initiation of speech act
   B. Maintenance of communication
      (i) Role switching/turn taking
      (ii) Sustaining a topic
         a. Contingent utterances
         b. Adjacent utterances
         c. Feedback to speaker
         d. Repair/revision
         e. Code switching

criminations in terms of new products. Individuals learn rules gradually by testing hypotheses of what a form can express in different situations where they think the rule might be appropriate for the expression of meaning.

Use: Language Is Used for Communication

Communication is an assertive act of coping—an active problem-solving task. It is a constant attempt to vary the content, form, and acceptability of a message; to switch or shift sets of reference as topics change (Muma, 1975); and to be sensitive to the influence of one's communicative partner and the physical context in which communication occurs (Prutting and Kirchner, 1983) in order to achieve a message of best fit and thus effective and efficient communication (Muma, 1975).

Therefore, communicative competence implies a knowledge of how to converse with different partners and in different contexts (Craig, 1983) and a knowledge of the rights, obligations, and expectations underlying the maintenance of discourse (Ochs and Schieffelin, 1979). It is a knowledge of who can say what to whom, in what way, where and when, and by what means (Prutting, 1979).

Pragmatics involves the acquisition and use of such conversational knowledge and of the semantic rules necessary to communicate an intent in order to affect the hearer's attitudes, beliefs, or behaviors (Lucas, 1980). This semantic knowledge develops and is "used within the context of a speech act, a theoretical unit of communication between a speaker and a hearer" (Lucas, 1980). According to Searle (1969), the speech act includes "what the speaker means, what the sentence (or other linguistic elements) uttered means, what the speaker intends, what the hearer intends, what the hearer understands, and what the rules governing linguistic utterances are" (p. 12). Speech acts include making promises, statements, requests, assertions, and so on. (Table 11.1). In Searle's (1969) theory, the proposition is the words or sentences produced, and the elocutionary force of this proposition is the speaker's intent in producing the utterance.

Thus, pragmatics involves the interactional aspects of communication including sensitivity to various aspects of social contexts (Prutting and Kirchner, 1983). It is an analysis of the use of language for communication. The emphasis is not on sentence structure but on how meaning is communicated—how units of language function in discourse (Prutting and Kirchner, 1983).

Pragmatics is inextricably related to cognition, and indeed the conversational knowledge or discourse structures that are derived by an individual are the products of one or all of the five SOI cognitive processes or operations (Table 11.1). This incoming semantic and/or behavioral information is processed by cognition, memory, convergent thinking, divergent thinking, and/or evaluative thinking in order to generate pragmatic (semantic and/or behavioral) units, classes, relations, systems, transformations, and implications. Communication, and therefore pragmatics or language use, is an active process of problem solving. We learn new pragmatic rules when our present pragmatic knowledge proves inadequate for a situation or when something in our experience is unfamiliar or unpredictable. The acquisition of new pragmatic information comes about in the form of new discourse structures, as a result of the use of one or all of the five mental operations of the SOI model.

Discourse Structures

A number of cognitive/pragmatic products or discourse structures are discussed in the literature. They relate to physical context variables, communicative partner variables, communication of intent, and turn-taking rules (including topic selections, maintenance and change, code switching, and referential skills) (Table 11.1).

Physical Context Variables. A pragmatic view of language assumes that language will vary with each context, that contexts are dynamic, and that any language sample will therefore be the interactive product of contextual variables and the individual's structural linguistic knowledge (Gallagher, 1983). Various conversational settings may affect the number and variety of utterances produced by a speaker (Gallagher, 1983). For example, one may have a rule that says, "Don't talk in church"; one that says, "Don't talk loudly in an elegant restaurant"; and yet another that says, "Cheer loudly for your team at a football game."

As individuals encounter various contexts or settings, they categorize or classify these contexts and simultaneously or subsequently develop rules for interacting in specific types of contexts. The individual tries to determine if he or she knows or recognizes the context; may perhaps try to think of all of the other possible responses or behaviors that might be appropriate to this context; may make judgments about certain variables within the context; may try to hypothesize what is expected, anticipated or suggested for this or for analogous situations; and so on.

Communicative Partner Variables. Specific communicative partners may affect the length, complexity, redundancy, fluency, and responsiveness (such as elaborations of comments), semantic relatedness of comments, and the amount of eye contact during an utterance (Gallagher, 1983). Indeed, partner characteristics such as age, sex, familiarity, and status frequently affect communication. Again, the individual categorizes and classifies partners and develops rules for interacting with specific partners, types of partners, and groups of partners.

When a person first encounters a potential communicative partner, he may determine if he knows or recognizes the partner or type of partner. He may sort through all the possible topics or intents that would be appropriate for this partner and subsequently judges or evaluates the form, reference and acceptability of various possible communications and the implications of such communication.

Communication of Intent. Language is used to communicate a variety of intentions. For example, Dore (1974) specified the following intents: to label, to respond, to request, to greet, to protest, to repeat, to describe, and to call attention to something. The intents specified by Searle (1969) are to request, to assert, to question, to order, to argue, to advise, and to warn.

Language intent may be communicated and comprehended through semantic-syntactic utterances and/or by previous or subsequent utterances. In addition, intent may be expressed (and comprehended) through facial expression or accompanying actions, gestures, or tone of voice. What is not said may also communicate intent. One can also say one thing and mean another. Individuals frequently use their knowledge of the physical context variables and the communication partner to help them decipher between what is said and what is meant. Thus, the communication of intent involves the use of semantic content (what is said) as well as behavioral content, or the nonfigural and nonverbal information that communicates the attitudes, needs, desires, moods, intentions, perceptions, and thoughts of others and ourselves. It may even involve the use of symbolic content when symbolic gestures are used.

Individual intents are semantic and/or behavioral units—that is, items or "chunks" of information. These units are developed when the brain processes semantic and behavioral experiences using the five cognitive operations. New experiences may cause the brain to place the experience into an existing unit or class; to create a new concept; to reprocess existing information and reformulate the structure of individual units or to group units together into classes, systems, and/or relations; and/or to see implications of such information. The way in which the individual chooses to communicate an intent at any particular point in time will reflect his or her knowledge of physical context variables and his or her communicative partner(s). Thus, the individual evaluates group membership, ability of the listener to interpret the various levels of complexity, receptiveness to various intents, and so on. Comprehension of the intent will be based on the units, classes, systems, relations, transformations, and implications that the listener has already established, as well as the information, associations, or products that he or she has constructed with respect to this specific partner or class of partner, this type of context, this type of topic, and so on. According to Haviland and Clark (1974), comprehension of an utterance in context also involves relating new information to assumed information. Thus, the individual makes a judgment based on past experience, as to what is new information and what he or she can assume this particular partner knows.

Turn Taking Rules. The reciprocal nature of communication involves a number of aspects, including the initiation of the speech act and the maintenance of communication. Initiation of the speech act (as speaker) includes topic selection and introduction and/or change of topic. Usually, the communicative act should contain new, relevant, and what is judged to be sincerely wanted information. It is important to evaluate the implicitly shared information aspect of the communication act. Thus, topical or referential identification involves searching one's long-term memory for information that is judged to be relevant to this partner, wanted by this partner, and perhaps interesting.

Maintenance of communication involves a number of variables. First, role taking involves the establishment and variation of roles with respect to the speaker and the listener and the reciprocal roles of speaker-initiator and listener-respondent.

The listener's role is to comprehend the speaker's message, which involves cognition. He maintains his role with nonverbal (behavioral) responses that are "characterized by visual orientation rather than gaze avoidance" (Davis and Wilcox, 1981, p. 172), a head nod, or leaning forward. He may also respond with a short and usually affirmative verbal response such as "yes."

Feedback to the speaker is also essential. This involves the listener's ability to monitor and evaluate the speaker's message and ability/willingness to indicate whether he believes it is effective and acceptable. Listener feedback will depend on the listener's previously established concepts of effectiveness and acceptability in general and his or her concepts relevant to this speaker and this context. Occasionally, the listener will assist the speaker in conveying the message, which involves cognition, judgment, and possibly convergent and divergent thinking.

Role switching may occur as the result of the speaker's desire to relinquish the role. This can be communicated and/or comprehended semantically and/or behaviorally. In many instances, nonverbal (behavioral) cues are used by partners to signal a wish to maintain or change roles (Harrison, 1974; Rosenfeld, 1978). The speaker usually retains his or her role by gaze avoidance and a hand gesture that is not maintained or not returned to a resting state through a phonetic clause juncture (Rosenfeld, 1978). When a speaker wants a listener's reaction, he or she signals "with a pause between clauses" or "with a rising or falling pitch at the end of a phonemic clause" (Davis and Wilcox, 1981, p. 171). Thus, the listener needs to use knowledge as such cues as well as the cues themselves in order to formulate a judgment concerning the speaker's willingness to switch roles. However, when role switching occurs in the absence of the speaker's readiness to switch, it may be accompanied by overloudness and a shift of the head away from the speaker (Davis and Wilcox, 1981), which would be behavioral content.

Maintenance of communication may also involve a response that sustains a topic (the listener becomes the speaker)–one that involves a specific response to the speech act. For example, *contingent utterances* are utterances that share the same topic with the preceding utterance and that add information to the prior communication act. A contingent utterance is an elaboration of the speaker's topic. Production of contingent utterances would usually involve semantic and behavioral cognition in order to understand or comprehend an utterance and its intent; convergent production, or a logical and sequentially ordered response; and divergent thinking, or an elaboration of a topic and judgment as to the relevance, accuracy, and appropriateness of a response in this context to this communicative partner.

Maintenance of communication also involves a sequential organization of topics. Thus, *adjacent utterances* are also used. These are utterances that occur immediately after a partner's utterance but are not related to the speaker's topic. Such utterances are considered logical or possible elaborations of communication and therefore involve convergent and divergent semantic thinking.

Repair and revision are also part of discourse maintenance and regulation. This involves the speaker's sensitivity to cues provided by the listener, which involves semantic and behavioral cognition and judgment, and the ability to respond to such cues by repeating and/or modifying the message when necessary. This is the speaker's use of convergent production, divergent production, and judgment. Moves by the speaker and the listener to repair sequences and respond to such regulatory devices as requests for clarification are essential to the maintenance of communication (Fey and Leonard, 1983).

Code switching is the degree to which the individual can produce stylistic variations in the form or frequency of specific acts to meet situational requirements (Fey and Leonard, 1983) such as the ability to role play. Judgment is essential.

In an article written in 1975, John Muma addressed the issue of role/code switching. In this article, he differentiated between two different variations in one's method of communication. One he called ''dump'' and the other ''play.'' Dumping pertains to the issuance of a coded message. Play involves ascertaining needed changes for appropriate recoding of a message and making necessary adjustments in order to achieve the message of best fit.

According to Muma (1975), role-taking attitudes involve the active resolution of communicative obstacles of form, reference, and acceptability in an effort to achieve the message of best fit for a particular situation and listener. It is the ability to issue a ''message in the most appropriate form for conveying intended meanings to a particular person for particular efforts'' (p. 299). In role taking, ''both speaker and listener are active participants in formulating, perceiving and revising messages until necessary adjustments are made in form, reference or psychological distance, and acceptability in order to convey intended meanings'' (p. 299). The objective of true communication is aimed at ascertaining or judging the message most suited to achieve effective and efficient communication.

Content, Form, and Use

Language learning and use, then, are problem-solving tasks. A problem is presented whenever a situation calls for the individual doing anything novel in order to cope with something that is different from his or her past behavior. A problem is a question or a proposition that necessitates consideration and a solution (Webster, 1977). Problem solving involves the use of all five mental operations, all types of content or information, and any kind of product, depending on the context in which the problem arises and the kinds of products required in order to reach a solution.

If the information is immediately recognized, known, comprehended, or understood, the mental operation of cognition has occurred. When situations call for the individual to generate logical conclusions from given information where emphasis is on achieving conventionally best outcomes, convergent thinking occurs. When a novel response is required, the divergent operation is generated. Inserting newly gained information into storage involves the operation of memory. Judging the appropriateness, acceptability, relevance, and/or correctness of information requires evaluation.

The three types of language knowledge that develop and are used (content, form, and use) are products of these five mental operations. Normal language functioning, then, requires the efficient action and interaction of all five cognitive processes in order for effective decoding (cognition, memory) and encoding (convergent thinking, divergent thinking, evaluative thinking) to occur.

ASSESSMENT OF COGNITIVE OPERATIONS

Guilford and Hoepfner (1971) developed a number of tests to assess each of the five mental operations. Some of these tests are listed below.

Semantic Awareness/Recognition Tests

Verbal Comprehension. Choose a word that means about the same as the given word.

Reading Comprehension. Answer questions about a short passage.

Verbal Opposites. Give a word that is opposite in meaning to the given word.

Sentence Synthesis. Rearrange scrambled words to make a meaningful sentence.

Vocabulary. Choose the alternative word that has the same meaning as a word that completes a sentence.

Semantic Memory Tests

Picture Memory. Recall names of common objects pictured on a previously studied page.

Recalled Words. Recall words presented on a study page.

Word Recognition. Recognize whether given words were on a previously studied page.

Memory for Facts. Answer questions regarding information previously given in two sentences.

Convergent Semantic Tests

Picture Group Naming. Write a class name for each group of five pictured objects.

Associations 1. Write a word that is associated with each of two given words.

Largest Class. Form the largest class possible from a given list of words so that the remaining words also make a class.

Attribute Listing. List attributes of objects needed to serve a specific function.

Divergent Semantic Tests

Common Situations. List problems that are inherent in a common situation.

Brick Uses. List many different uses for a common object.

Product Improvement. Suggest ways to improve a particular object.

Consequences. List the effect of a new and unusual event.

Object Naming. List objects that belong to a broad class of objects.

Differences. Suggest ways in which two objects are different.

Similarities. Produce ways in which two objects are alike.

Word Fluency. List words that contain a specified word or letter.

Planning Elaboration. List many detailed steps needed to make a briefly outlined plan work.

Semantic Evaluation Tests

Word Checking 1. Choose one of four words that fits a single criterion.

Double Descriptions. Select the one object of four that best fits two given descriptions or adjectives.

Class Name Selection. Select a class name that most precisely fits a group of four given words.

Commonsense Judgment 1. Select the two best of five given reasons why a briefly described plan is faulty.

Behavioral Tests

Alternate Expressional Groups. Group pictured expressions in different ways so that each group expresses a common thought, feeling, or intention.

Cartoon Predictions. Choose one of three alternative cartoon frames that can be most reasonably predicted from the given frame.

Expression Grouping. Choose one of four expressions that belongs with a given group by virtue of common psychological dispositions.

Expressions. Choose one of four expressions that indicates the same psychological state as another given expression.

In addition, Torrance (1966) adapted Guilford and Hoepfner's (1971) work on divergent thinking and developed the *Torrance Test of Creative Thinking* (Torrance, 1966). (Norms are available only for children.) Parts of this test along with other tests from Guilford and Hoepfner (1971) have been used with aphasic, right brain damaged, closed head injured, and elderly individuals (Braverman, 1990; Chapey, 1974, 1983; Chapey and Lubinski, 1979; Chapey et al., 1976, 1977; Diggs and Basili 1987; Law and Newton 1991; Schwartz-Crowley and Gruen, 1986) in order to assess abilities and impairments of specific mental operations in these groups. The tests, scoring instructions, and flexibility categories used by Chapey to measure divergent semantic ability in aphasic and normal adults are presented in Appendices 11.1, 11.2, and 11.3.

The Test of Problem Solving (Zachman et al., 1983), developed to measure reasoning abilities in children, can also be used with adults to assess specific cognitive semantic abilities such as explaining inferences, determining causes, answering negative *wh* questions, determining solutions, and avoiding problems.

Other techniques for assessing cognitive semantic abilities can be obtained through the Educational Testing Services' Microfiche Test Collection Department, which has a number of unpublished research instruments measuring aptitude and cognition. Several of these measures target Guilford and Hoepfner's (1971) mental operations.

Clinicians who use the cognitive semantic approach to intervention should also evaluate the specific language assets and liabilities of each patient so that the therapeutic effort is individualized to fit the needs, interests, and abilities of each person who receives such therapy.

For example, clinicians will want to explore the nature of each patient's language impairment—including performance on appropriate tasks, types(s) of errors made, and the manner in which each patient goes about tasks (Byng et al., 1990).

Clinicians will also need to break tasks (such as comprehending sentences reading aloud single words, gesturing, hailing a bus, filling in a check, turn taking) down into their component processes and examine the functioning of each of those processes in detail (Byng et al., 1990, p. 82) in order to derive hypotheses about the nature of the underlying processing problems in the language deficits in specific patients. A more in-depth discussion of assessment techniques can be found in Chapter 4.

INTERVENTION

The present writer agrees with Martin (1979):

> *Normal functioning* is the "efficient action and interaction of the cognitive processes which support language behavior within and by the organism."
> The *disorder* is "(a) reduction of the efficiency of action and interaction of the cognitive processes which support language behavior."
> *Therapy* is "the attempt to manipulate and to excite the action and interaction of the cognitive processes which support language behavior within and by the organism so as to maximize their effective usage. . . . Therapy [is] directed toward the subsystems which process language" (pp. 157–158).

Within the context of the present paper, the cognitive processes or subsystems that process language are cognition, memory, convergent thinking, divergent thinking, and evaluation. Aphasia is a reduction in the efficient action and interaction of these processes. Therapy is an attempt to manipulate and excite the action and interaction of these processes. We employ strong, controlled, and intensive figural, symbolic, semantic, and behavioral stimuli—most frequently, semantic stimuli—in order to elicit the action of cognition, memory, convergent thinking, divergent thinking, and evaluation. These are the cognitive processes or the complex events that happen in the brain.

What is happening between the stimulus and the response is that the individual is using one or all of his or her mental operations. **Task input** is defined as figural, symbolic, semantic, and/or behavioral. **Processing** occurs through the use of cognition, memory, convergent thinking, divergent thinking, and evaluative thinking. **Output** is generated in units, classes (or categories), relations, transformations, systems, and implications. This holds true for problem solving, decision making, learning, and language tasks.

Rationale

A cognitive approach to therapy is based on the belief that propositional language (H. Jackson, cited in Head, 1915), or functional communication, is an active problem-solving task that necessitates the use of all five cognitive processes. These operations are the intervening mediating variables or constructs responsible for language comprehension and production. Thus, cognitive semantic therapy advocates the stimulation of all five mental operations, since this type of processing is required for the comprehension and production of spontaneous language. Indeed, most definitions of language and communication have components that are highly suggestive of all five operations. For example, Hughy and Johnson (1975) state that language is used primarily for information getting and giving, problem solving, and persuasion. Another definition, that proposed by

Muma (1975), notes that communication entails the ability to switch or shift sets of reference as topics change, to initiate such shifts, and to overcome obstacles to communication flow. Both definitions reflect the fact that language and communication require the use of all five cognitive processes.

Ability to produce functional communication or spontaneous speech also involves what Noam Chomsky (1957, 1964) refers to as *deep structure* and *surface structure*. Deep structure specifies the basic relationship being expressed—who did what to whom. It tells the meaning relationship. The surface structure is the actual sentences that are spoken and written. Meaning is often not audible or visible. Rather, the listener or reader must identify the relationships of the concepts to the events being communicated or described. Understanding a message depends on the memory structure of the people involved in the communication. The entire structure is not communicated if the receiver of the information can already be assumed to understand certain basic concepts. That is, some relations are assumed to be known or to be very easy to discover and therefore not necessary to mention.

According to Chomsky (1957, 1964), not everything we know about a sentence is revealed in the superficial string of words. That is, all information for processing speech is not present in observable behavior. Meaning is not directly expressed in the sounds we hear and the words we read. Our capacity to interpret sentences depends on our knowledge of deep structure. We don't learn a set of utterances (surface structures). Rather, we learn methods of processing utterances. We have rich cognitive structures that make it possible to utter and comprehend sentences.

In everyday communication, surface structure is frequently very deficient, misleading, and uninformative. For example, there are extensive deletions, extensive use of pronouns, and ambiguous referents. But meaning structure may be communicated nevertheless. Therefore, language is an aid to communication.

Production of spontaneous, functional language and therefore deep and surface requires the use of all five mental operations. These are the methods for processing utterances. These are the rich cognitive structures that make it possible to comprehend and produce sentences. Cognitive therapy therefore targets all five mental operations for the production of meaningful ideas and the elaboration of those ideas.

A third rationale is based on the observation that aphasic patients are unable to produce the highest level central nervous system integrations (Wepman, 1951). Research by Bolwinick (1967) indicates that the highest level cognitive integrations are thinking—such as convergent thinking, divergent thinking, and evaluative thinking; problem solving—all five cognitive operations are viewed as essential components of problem solving; and creativity—divergent thinking is used as a synonym for creativity. Tasks using all five mental operations will focus on the essence of the aphasic impairment: inability to produce the higher level cognitive integrations.

Cognitive therapy is also rooted in the observation that aphasia is a problem in language retrieval (Schuell et al., 1964) or in the searching and scanning mechanism that selects among many possibilities. Schuell and coworkers (1964) noted that the search mechanism is controlled by instructions, directing it to go to a specific address and bring out information. They suggest that appropriate stimuli are required to activate or reacti-

vate patterns. The information-processing model presented in this chapter hypothesizes that divergent production and evaluative production involve the use of a broad search of memory storage, while cognition and convergent production involve a narrow search of long-term memory. Tasks that stimulate retrieval under a variety of cognitive operations appear to facilitate the patient's reorganization and retrieval of language. Specifically, the stimuli presented foster the action of a broad and narrow search of memory within the individual. The clinician attempts to manipulate the patient's retrieval strategy in order to aid the patient in making maximal responses.

ACCOUNTABILITY[b]

Despite the wide acceptance of the cognitive and pragmatic approaches to therapy in our literature, and the acceptance of the distinction between deep structure and surface structure, many intervention agencies and many government agencies mandate that each therapy session have an operationally written, behavioral goal. Many clinicians also use such goals. For example, at a recent workshop, the audience (all ASHA certified speech-language pathologists) was asked to write short-term goals for a moderately language-impaired patient. More than half wrote goals such as "By the end of this session, X will say the name of five common objects."

Behavioral, operationally written objectives are counterproductive to the development of language. They are unacceptable within both a cognitive model and a pragmatic model of intervention. Behavioral objectives target surface structures. Cognitive and pragmatic intervention focus on meaning or deep structure. In cognitive-pragmatic intervention, we attempt to increase the patient's viability as a communicative partner (Lubinski, 1986).

Behavioral, operationally written objectives are inappropriate because they ignore the fact that meaning is the essence of language and that meaning is not an observable behavior. They ignore the fact that a conversation is like a game. It involves a series of moves by participants. Every conversation is altogether new for the participants. Therefore we continually communicate creativity (Lindfors, 1980). (Lindfors's text concerns language intervention in children.)

Behavioral, operationally written objectives ignore the fact that content and form are developed and used within the context of a speech act. The individual develops communicative competence "through discerning rules underlying the diverse interaction contexts which she observes and in which she participates" (Lindfors, 1980, p. 311).

Behavioral, operationally written objectives ignore the fact that the speaker's intent in producing an utterance and a hearer's intent in hearing an utterance are the essence of communication and meaning. The intent of the message is the reason we communicate. The intent is the function that language serves. We use verbal utterances to express an intention or function. We use language to question, to request, and to inform. Our attention as speakers and listeners is on the meaning, the intention of what someone is trying to say (Cazden, 1976). Language forms are heard through the meaning intended (Cazden, 1976).

Thus, communication is idea oriented, not word oriented. Language is rooted in meaning, not in surface structures. Lan-

---

[b] Adapted from Chapey (1988, 1992).

guage is used for communication. It is a tool, not an end in itself. Language is an aid to communication.

Clinical aphasiologists must encourage regulating agencies to realize that language is facilitated by an environment that focuses on meaning rather than on form. Getting the message across is more important for individuals than the form they use to do so.

These agencies should realize that "language is not labeling or matching pictures to words or repeating what someone else said" (Holland, 1975, p. 518). (Holland's article concerns language intervention in children.) Instead, language is "an active, dynamic interpersonal interchange" (Holland, 1975, p. 518). If we focus on tasks like labeling, matching pictures to words, or repeating what someone else said, "we run the risk of inadvertently teaching the erroneous principle that language is a skill on the order of playing the piano. This helps the (individual) . . . miss the point of communicating" (Holland, 1975, p. 518).

> Language training must be to some very significant extent concerned with helping (the individual) . . . discover his potential as a verbal communicator. Without this discovery, language will remain something akin to a well practiced talent, a recital, not a . . . part of him (p. 519).

Verbalizations must not replace language. Drill is *not* language. According to Lindfors (1987), "there is no language apart from meaning" (p. 217). Language "is communicating—the back and forth, the give and take of ideas, not . . . the mindless parroting of rigid, fixed forms" (Lindfors, 1980, p. 218). Where in a language drill is the meaning that we know to be the very base of language (Lindfors, 1980)? Where is the creativity, the novel expression, that is the core of language? Where is the communicating—the interacting with someone, about something, for some reason (Lindfors, 1987)?

Drill is opposed to language in its meaninglessness, in its rigidity, in its purposelessness (Lindfors, 1987). Drill may make clients very good at doing drills but not at using language and communication. Indeed, according to Lindfors, drill may adversely affect language growth and retrieval. She maintains that problem solving, planning, discussing ideas, brainstorming, recording ideas, presenting ideas, and selecting the best ideas involve listening, speaking, reading, and writing with a purpose. The real question is, Is the individual a more effective user of language after completing an exercise or drill? The answer is no. We become more effective communicators as a result of using language in communication with others. According to Lindfors (1980):

> labeling syntactic (or semantic) items simply makes you a better "syntactic item labeler" (at least for a few days). Talking about forms doesn't help you express meaning more effectively (p. 220).

Lindfors apparently believes that it is inappropriate to structure a simple-to-complex sequence of forms. Rather, the communication itself will determine the language forms the individual uses and responds to. She believes that we need to focus on language use for effective communication. When we do so, our clients may then use the language forms that help them accomplish effective communication.

Individuals, Lindfors (1987) claims, become effective interactants as they have more opportunities to interact. Language intervention should reflect the individual's interests and concerns. Natural shaping of semantics and syntax happens not through sequenced curriculum but through feedback as to whether one has been understood and whether one has achieved the purpose of the communication.

New meanings find expression as individuals wonder, question, inform, argue, and reason through language in real-life situations rather than contrived situations (Lindfors, 1987). Language lives in shared experience, in decision making, and in planning. Language is stimulated and facilitated by an environment rich in diverse verbal and nonverbal experiences. Language lives and grows in rich experiences.

As human beings, we develop a theory of the world in our head (Smith, 1975). This theory shapes the way we look at past experience (recall and interpret it) and the way we look at new experience. We comprehend or interpret the world by relating new experience to the already known—by placing new experiences in our existing cognitive structure or "theory" (Smith, 1975). To learn is to alter our existing cognitive structure when experience does not conform to our theory (Lindfors, 1987).

Language helps us to comprehend and learn—especially as language is used in questioning (curiosity and procedural or social-interactional questioning), focusing attention, making understandings more precise, making understandings more retrievable, reinterpreting past experience, and going beyond present personal experiences (Lindfors, 1987). Interaction is essential to both comprehension and learning. In real gut-level, meaningful learning, what is to be learned cannot be specified in advance. Such learning is characterized by curiosity, exploration, problem solving, planning, decision making, discussion of ideas, brainstorming, and evaluative thinking (Chapey, 1988, 1992; Guilford, 1967; Lindfors, 1980, 1987).

The present pressure to establish accountability has actively discouraged exploration, curiosity, and problem solving. Skills, drills, rules, and facts become ends in themselves (Lindfors, 1987). We have packaged clinical programs with a renewed emphasis on memorizing words, on defining words, on identifying parts of speech in sentences that no one ever said or ever will say, so that individuals can get higher standardized test scores and move on to the next highest level of memorization, definition, and identification (Lindfors, 1987).

As a profession, we must, as Frattali (1992) has indicated, first and foremost become concerned that our clients become competent communicators. Emphasis on learning rote skills and specified sets of behaviors means increased emphasis on the use of lower-level cognitive processes (Lindfors, 1987). Lower-level cognitive behavior means that clients can give back the same information they received (recalling, memorization), but to display **higher-level** cognitive behavior, they must go beyond the given information some way—relating it to something else, reorganizing it, inferring from it, and using it as a springboard for creatively solving new problems. It involves applying, analyzing, synthesizing, and evaluating. Questioning is the individual's most important tool for learning—especially curiosity questioning (Lindfors, 1987). Conversation should be the locus, process, and goal of language intervention (Warren and Rogers-Warren, 1985). Content-centered discussion therapy and embellishment of ideas within a topic (Wepman, 1972, 1976) should be our focus.

THERAPY OBJECTIVES

Therefore, the objective of a cognitive approach to rehabilitation is to stimulate the five cognitive processes—cognition (awareness, immediate discovery, recognition, comprehension), memory, convergent thinking, divergent thinking, and evaluative thinking—in order to improve overall functional communication. Whenever possible, the focus should be on the stimulation of these abilities within the context of conversational discourse. That is, conventional discourse is seen as the procedural plan for intervention. Whenever possible, turn taking, cuing, modeling, and reinforcement are essential components of therapy.

General Objectives

The general objectives are:

1. To stimulate ability to recognize and comprehend language
2. To stimulate ability to fix new information in memory in order to improve communication
3. To stimulate ability to generate logical information or conclusions during communication
4. To stimulate ability to generate logical alternatives to given information, to produce a quantity and variety of responses during communication, and to be able to elaborate on ideas and plans during communication
5. To stimulate ability to make judgments or appraisals or to formulate evaluations in terms of criteria such as correctness, completeness, identity, relevance, adequacy, utility, safety, consistency, feasibility, social custom, and so forth in order to communicate more effectively and efficiently
6. To stimulate the integration of all cognitive operations through the use of problem solving, decision making, and planning tasks and through conversational discourse in order to communicate more effectively and efficiently

There are four levels of specific objectives within this approach. However, this model of therapy suggests that, regardless of the level at which the patient is functioning, the initial stage of intervention should focus on language-related cognition: knowing, awareness, immediate discovery, recognition, comprehension, and understanding. This suggestion is based on the rationale that individuals with aphasia should be provided with an opportunity to hear and grasp the language behavior of others over and over again. That is, auditory stimulation is seen as an essential component of language retrieval in aphasic patients (Schuell et al., 1955). Thus, for example, the clinician might videotape a group of normal adults responding to a divergent task such as, ''Can you think of a problem that anyone might have in eating lunch?'' Concomitantly, the patient could be reinforced for all listening and attending behavior. Specifically, movements of the eye that result in a better visual stimulus for the patient or movements of the ear that result in a better auditory stimulus (Staats, 1968) of the videotape would be reinforced. Although no verbal responses would be required during this phase of therapy, all verbal responses that relate to the task at hand could be highly reinforced.

Exposure to the videotaped responses of others may prove to be a vicarious learning experience (Bandura and Walters, 1963; Harris and Evans, 1974) for the individual with aphasia. This suggestion appears to be in consonance with Cooper and Rigrodsky's (1979) finding that persons with aphasia are able to model the verbal behavior of normal subjects and improve

their explanations of material that is presented. If modeling is to occur, however, it may be helpful to consider several facts. First, it may be beneficial if the subjects on the videotape are of comparable age and sex as the individual with aphasia, so that the patient will identify with the person who is producing the divergent responses. Second, the clinician could attempt to choose tasks that are interesting and relevant to the particular subject. Third, since Pieres and Morgan (1973) empirically determined that a relaxed, receptive, and uncritical environment increased the divergent behavior of normal subjects, it may be important to provide this type of climate for persons with aphasia. This exposure to the divergent semantic behavior of others, perhaps filed in competitive ''game show'' style (Torrance, 1974), can continue to be a component of the intervention strategy throughout the process of therapy.

Principles

Intervention should be oriented toward the following traditional therapeutic principles:

1. Begin with the tangible (here and now) and move toward the representational.
2. Begin with the concrete and move toward the abstract.
3. Begin with the simple and move toward the complex.
4. Begin with the real and move toward the complex.
5. Begin with actions on objects and move toward verbalizations concerning these actions.
6. Begin with simple classifications and move toward reclassifications and multiple classifications.
7. Begin with exaggerated sensory stimulation—for example, talking through a microphone or using a variety of inflectional patterns (McConnell et al., 1974)—and gradually decrease this exaggeration.
8. Begin with short stimuli/responses and move toward longer stimuli/responses.
9. Begin with continuous reinforcement and move toward intermittent reinforcement (Grant et al., 1951; Jensen and Cotton, 1960).
10. Begin with clinician reinforcement and move toward self-reinforcement (Staats, 1968).

During the course of both diagnosis and therapy, the aphasiologist will attempt to isolate specific conditions under which language retrieval is maximized and to increase the number and variety of these conditions. That is, with whom and under what conditions does language behavior increase? The clinician may wish to manipulate some of the following variables and observe their effect on patient behavior: the listener, referent, intent, situation, cuing devices, repetition and reauditorization, intonation, level of abstraction, cognitive complexity, linguistic complexity, length of stimuli, and frequency of occurrence of word stimuli. The conditions that augment semantic retrieval for each cognitive operation should become an integral component of all subsequent sessions.

Examples of specific objectives at each of the four levels of therapy are presented below.

Level I. Specific Objectives

To stimulate ability

Cognition

To be aware of time/space/speech/emotional voice tone
To recognize stimulus equivalence such as matching Letters/matching objects to objects/matching objects to pictures/matching words to pictures/matching words to objects

To recognize very high-frequency, concrete objects/events/relationships named
To recognize own name/family names
To follow one-part, simple commands
To understand simple greetings/requests/questions

Memory

To remember one to two letters/words/pictures
To remember one to two high-frequency, concrete objects/events named

Convergent Thinking

To repeat one syllable, high-frequency objects/events/relationships
To produce automatic language
To complete high probability closure tasks

Level II. Specific Objectives

To stimulate ability

Cognition

To recognize concrete, high-frequency, familiar objects/events/relationships
To recognize family names/body parts/community helper occupations
To recognize high-frequency objects given their function
To recognize high-frequency events described
To recognize concrete, brief ideas
To comprehend simple conversation with one person
To understand concrete, high-frequency statements about objects such as existence/nonexistence/recurrence/rejection/denial/possession/food/clothing/personal care objects
To understand concrete, high-frequency, brief statements about events such as playing/eating/activities of daily living
To comprehend concrete agent-action and action-object constructions
To comprehend concrete yes/no questions
To comprehend concrete active and negative phrases/sentences
To comprehend articles
To comprehend morphological inflections such as plural /s/, /z/, possessive /s/, /z/, past /t/, /ed/
To comprehend concrete noun phrases and verb phrases
To recognize forms/letters/pictures
To recognize high frequency printed words and pictures
To match high frequency printed words to spoken words
To recognize printed letters

Memory

To remember one to three concrete, high-frequency objects/events/relationship, serially
To execute one- to two-step commands, serially
To remember one to four pictures, serially
To group items to facilitate ability to recall

Convergent Thinking

To produce automatic language
To complete high-probability phrases/closure tasks
To name high-frequency objects/events/relationships
To comment on objects noting their existence, nonexistence, recurrence, location, possession, and so forth
To talk about common objects such as food, clothing, furniture, transportation
To comment on events such as cooking, eating, activities of daily living
To produce agent-action and action-object constructions

To produce concrete speech acts such as requesting, informing, greeting, questioning
To name members of categories
To list many words that start with a specific letter
To generate numerous and varied objects within a class
To list numerous possible topics of conversation

Level III. Specific Objectives

To stimulate ability

Cognition

To recognize high- and low-frequency objects/events/relationships
To recognize high- and low-frequency objects/events/relationships described by function
To recognize letter/color/form/number names, and rhyme words
To recognize phonetically similar words
To recognize categories
To comprehend concrete ideas/sentences
To understand relationships between words
To understand statements about objects such as existence/nonexistence/recurrence/rejection/denial/possession/attribution/food/furniture/clothes/personal care objects/health/kitchen utensils, family/other people/places/locations
To understand statements about events such as play/entertainment/eating/activities of daily living/cooking/feelings/sports/school/work/travel/time/news
To understand concrete speech acts such as requesting/ordering/advising/warning/questioning/describing/greeting/repeating/protesting
To hold the thread of discussion in mind, identifying main ideas
To distinguish between relevant and irrelevant information
To understand television/movies
To comprehend inferences
To comprehend short paragraphs
To recognize the existence of problems
To recognize own errors and errors of others
To comprehend simple, concrete analogies
To comprehend active and negative sentences
To comprehend pronouns such as personal, reflexive, indefinite, demonstrative, interrogative, negative
To comprehend adjectives such as color, size, shape, length, height, width, age, taste, temperature, speed, distance, comparative, superlative
To comprehend adverbs with -ly
To comprehend conjunctions
To comprehend prepositions such as locative/temporal/directional
To read concrete, high-frequency and low-frequency sentences
To read and comprehend sequences of material
To read and comprehend short paragraphs
To read and identify main ideas
To read and obtain facts
To read and locate answers
To read and draw conclusions
To read and grasp relationships
To read and grasp inferences
To read street signs
To read newspaper headlines/newspaper stories/newspaper ads

Memory

To identify one to five names serially
To follow one- to five-part directions and commands
To remember one to five ideas/facts just presented
To group items to facilitate recall
To remember meaning in sentences/short paragraphs/stories/songs

Convergent Thinking

To answer questions about self, family, everyday life
To name high- and low-frequency objects/events/relationships
To name categories
To name objects/events/relationships within categories
To describe objects/events/relationships
To tell the function of objects, the purpose of events
To define words
To judge the suitability of class inclusion
To judge the similarity of relationships
To judge the suitability of class properties
To identify absurdities
To evaluate implications
To express simple ideas with specificity
To sequentially order ideas or topics toward a purpose
To retell stories—both the literal (who, when, what, where) details and the inferential implications
To describe procedures
To state the relationship between objects/events such as similarities/differences
To predict possible outcomes
To make inferences and draw conclusions
To answer true/false, yes/no and *wh*-questions
To write letters and numbers
To write own name and address
To write sentences with high-frequency, concrete words

Divergent Thinking

To produce numerous logical possibilities/perspectives/ideas where appropriate
To provide a variety of ideas where appropriate
To change the direction of one's responses
To generate categories of objects/events/relationships/ideas
To predict many different possible outcomes of situations
To generate many different solutions to problems
To list many different problems inherent in situations
To generate numerous steps in a plan
To elaborate on a topic

Evaluative Thinking

To judge the correctness, completeness, identity, relevance, adequacy, utility, safety, consistency, logical feasibility, and social acceptability of facts
To judge the suitability of words to a topic

Level IV. Specific Objectives

To stimulate ability

Cognition

To comprehend high- and low-frequency objects/events/relationships
To recognize concrete and more abstract classes/concepts
To understand relationships among objects/events/ideas
To comprehend analogies
To recognize problems
To recognize own errors and errors of others
To comprehend concrete and more abstract speech acts in conversation with one to five partners
To follow changes in the topic of conversation
To hold the thread of discussion in mind and identify main ideas
To understand changes in interpretation
To comprehend TV/movies
To comprehend more rapid, complex conversations
To comprehend longer sentences/directions/commands

To comprehend more complex/abstract relationships such as comparative, possessive, spatial, temporal, inferential, familial, part-whole, object-action, action-object, cause-effect, sequential, degree, and antonym and synonym relationships
To comprehend negative, passive, and question transformations
To read both short, concrete and longer, more abstract sentences/paragraphs
To read and identify main ideas
To read and obtain facts
To read and locate answers
To read and draw conclusions
To read and grasp relationships
To read and draw inferences
To comprehend newspaper stories/ads
To comprehend catalog/mail order forms
To comprehend a menu
To comprehend a table of contents/index
To use a dictionary/telephone directory

Memory

To remember one to nine high- and low-frequency objects/events/relationships/categories
To remember facts and commands of increasing length and complexity
To remember meaning in sentences and paragraphs
To use hierarchical organization to facilitate recall
To cluster information in order to facilitate recall

Convergent Thinking

To describe high- and low-frequency objects/events/relationships
To indicate the function of high- and low-frequency objects/events/relationships
To specify attributes of objects
To specify the defining attributes of concepts
To define words
To express ideas clearly and with variety
To use language to communicate specific ideas
To use language to elicit specific responses
To express relationships between and among objects/events/relationships and ideas such as similarities and differences
To produce analogies
To sequentially order ideas toward a purpose
To use language to request, inform, explain, question, greet, advise, thank, order, negotiate
To keep meaning going in conversation
To produce class names for groups of words/pictures
To logically deduce the most predictable outcome of a set of facts
To tell the literal (who, what, when, where) details of a story
To make inferences and draw conclusions
To write high- and low-frequency words, sentences, and paragraphs

Divergent Thinking

To produce numerous logical possibilities and perspectives where appropriate
To provide a variety of ideas where appropriate
To change the direction of one's responses
To stimulate ability to generate many different uses for common and uncommon objects
To predict many possible outcomes of a situation
To list many different problems inherent in a common situation
To think of many different ways to initiate a conversation
To think of many different ways to maintain a conversation
To define many possible rules for communicative partners and communicative contexts
To think of many different ways to repair conversation

To elaborate on topics
To elaborate on or list many different steps needed to do a particular task

Evaluative Thinking

To make appraisals, comparisons, and formulate evaluations regarding correctness, completeness, relevance, adequacy, utility, safety, consistency, logical feasibility, and social acceptability
To judge the intent of messages
To judge the coherence of a conversation
To judge what can and cannot be said in different contexts, to different partners
To use context and partner variables to decipher between what is said and what is meant
To determine the meaning of proverbs
To judge a situation in which a proverb could be used
To select the word that best fits a single criterion
To select the best of given reasons why a briefly described plan is faulty

INTEGRATION OF THE FIVE COGNITIVE PROCESSES

The present therapeutic approach suggests that all five mental operations should be integrated in therapy by requiring responses that involve composite abilities. Problem solving, planning, decision-making tasks, and conversational interaction are excellent for this purpose, since they are composite operations or processes depending on the content of the problem, decision, or conversation and on how the problem/decision/conversation is worded or phrased. Thus, while conversational interaction such as the use of speech acts is sometimes convergent in nature, it will also often involve the use of other mental operations and become problem solving, planning, and decision making in nature depending on the listener, the context and the intent. Individuals can be stimulated to use language to question, to request, to inform, to wonder, to argue, to reason, and to comprehend such speech acts.

In addition, formulating solutions to problems posed in the "Dear Abby" or "Dear Meg" column in the local newspaper can be used to stimulate all five cognitive operations. If carefully chosen, such tasks reflect "real-life" situations that patients face—or can allow them to increase their self-concept, since their opinion is being sought and valued. The use of such tasks is conversational in nature and frequently allows for reciprocal role reversal. These tasks can therefore be used to stimulate brainstorming, discussing, recording and presenting ideas, and selecting best outcomes. They can also be used to stimulate individuals to question (curiosity, procedural, and social-interactional), to focus attention, to make understanding more precise, to reinterpret past experience, and to go beyond present personal experience. Conversational management, conversational turn taking, topic manipulation, and conversational repair management can also be targeted using these tasks.

Thus, whenever possible, intervention should involve the stimulation of two or three or more mental operations. For example, the clinician might begin a session by asking the client, "Can you list all of the things that can be folded?" After the patient has produced some responses, the clinician summarizes these responses and asks, "Can you think of any more?" (Table 11.2). When the client has finished responding, the clinician then uses convergent techniques such as those described by Aurelia (1974), Butfield and Zangwill (1946),

Goldstein (1948), Keenan (1975), Sarno et al., (1970), Schuell et al., (1955), Vignolo (1964), and Wepman (1953) to stimulate retrieval of appropriate and desired responses that the patient had not produced. Such techniques might involve confrontation naming, recognition naming, oral spelling, reading, categorizing similar responses, creating sentences with a word, and so forth (Table 11.2). In an attempt to develop each patient's ability to correct his or her own errors, the clinician may use cuing techniques such as those suggested by Berman and Peelle (1967). For example, the initial letter of a word could be used as a cue technique. Alternative stimuli for self-cuing might include (*a*) the first phoneme of a word, (*b*) the association of a word with a gesture, or (*c*) the use of an incorrect associational response to cue the correct verbal response. Subsequently, the aphasiologist attempts to transfer the semantic material retrieved in the convergent context and integrate this information into a divergent one. For example, the clinician might ask another divergent question that would call for some of the responses that the patient has been able to retrieve, such as "Can you think of all of the things that we could pull over our heads?" (Table 11.2). Progress is evaluated by keeping a record of the number and variety of responses produced by the patient (Table 11.2).

Spontaneous language tasks that have divergent, convergent, and/or evaluative components can also be used in therapy. For example, the clinician might present a picture description task such as the "Cookie Thief" picture from the Boston Diagnostic Aphasia Examination (Goodglass and Kaplan, 1972) and encourage the client to produce as many responses as possible. (A list of possible responses to this task are presented by Yorkston and Beukelman [1977] [see Chapter 4.].) Clients can also be encouraged to produce functional spontaneous communication related to a specific theme (Wepman, 1976) such as food, nutrition, food service, restaurants, great parks, interesting sights, vacation destinations, health and diet, sexual issues, social security, legal and money issues, current events, and pharmaceutical issues (AARP's *Modern Maturity* magazine provides interesting and timely topics for the 50+ audience). In each instance, the clinician records the number and variety of ideas produced by the client.

Levels III and IV. Specific Objectives to Stimulate Use of Composite Abilities

To stimulate ability

To use language to explain, request, correct information, report, advise, question, greet, thank, argue, negotiate
To comprehend speech acts produced by another
To overcome obstacles in communication
To keep meaning going in conversation
To role play (especially to take the viewpoint of someone else) during communication
To select, introduce, maintain, and change the topic of conversation
To initiate and maintain conversation
To use language to discuss objects, events, relationships
To use language to communicate specific ideas
To use language to elicit specific responses
To use language to verbalize a variety of possibilities and perspectives such as the pros and cons of ideas and issues, the advantages and disadvantages of certain actions, ideas
To vary language depending on the context
To vary language depending on the partner

Table 11.2.
Sample Therapy Plan That Includes Both Divergent and Convergent Tasks

Objective	Tasks[a]	Cue	Evaluation
General—to stimulate the communication of ideas *Specific*—to stimulate language related to a holiday, Christmas, through divergent and convergent thinking	Greeting *Divergent Tasks* 1. We're coming close to Christmas. What are all of the things that you think of when you think of Christmas?	After 2 minutes summarize responses given and ask, "Can you think of anymore?"	1.(a) List responses: ———— ———— Total fluency: ———— 1.(b) List categories: ———— ———— Total flexibility: ————
	2. Someone mentioned that Santa carries a sack. Can you think of all of the things that could fit into Santa's sack?	Same as above	2. Score as in number one
	3. What are all of the things we might get for Christmas that: could be folded? couldn't be folded? that might break if it were dropped? that wouldn't break if it were dropped? that we could wash? that could be hauled in a truck? that we could pull over our head? that might have buttons? that could be worn in summer (winter)? that could be made of paper? that could come in a box? that could be round (square)? that are made of glass (plastic, rubber)? that someone could drink? that someone could eat? that has handles? that has a neck? that moves?	Same as above	3. Score as in number one
	4. List all of the things that you could possibly use a Christmas box for (or bells, string, ribbon).	Same as above	4. Score as in number one
	5. How could you improve a ⎯ so that it would be more useful (better, more fun)?	Same as above	5. Score as in number one
	6. If Santa didn't have a sack, he could use ⎯. If Santa lost his belt, he could use ⎯.	Same as above	6. Score as in number one
	7. Imagine you are in a department store (church, living room) at Christmas time. What are all of the things that you might possibly see?	Same as above	7. Score as in number one
	8. Let's make up a story about Christmas.	Same as above	8. Score as in number one
	9. The word *Christmas* begins with the sound "k." What other words can you think of that start with "k"? The word *bell* begins with the sound "b." What other words can you think of that start with "b"?	Same as above	9. Score as in number one

Table 11.2.—*continued*

Objective	Tasks[a]	Cue	Evaluation
	10. What are all of the possible questions that you could ask about this Christmas picture?	Same as above	10. Score as in number one
	11. List all of the different parts of Santa's suit. How could we change each one to make it better?	Same as above	11. Score as in number one
	12. Suppose that we did not celebrate Christmas anymore. What do you think might happen? Can you guess	Same as above	12. Score as in number one
	13. List all of the problems that someone might have in shopping for a Christmas present.	Same as above	13. Score as in number one
	14. Someone mentioned a cymbal and a drum. They make noise. Can you list all of the things that could be used to make noise?	Same as above	14. Score as in number one
	15. Santa's suit is red. What are all of the other things that could be red?	Same as above	15. Score as in number one
	16. Tomorrow we will have a Christmas party. What are all the different things we'll need to do before the party? *Convergent Tasks* Present responses given to question number one. Oral and/or visual representation of responses can be used. (Later, responses to question two, then three, etc., can be presented.)	Same as above	16. Score as in number one
	Responses that might be appropriate to this question but that were not given by the patient are now presented.	Give first sound of a word	Use Porch's (1971) multidimensional scoring system to evaluate responses
	Convergent techniques that might be used to stimulate retrieval of items not produced are as follows: a) confrontation naming b) definition naming c) closure naming d) recognition naming e) repetition naming f) following oral and/or printed directions or commands g) yes/no comprehension h) word associations: antonyms, synonyms i) rhyming j) description k) recognition spelling l) oral spelling m) analogies n) recognition of categories o) spontaneous generation of categories p) concept learning q) reading r) writing s) copying t) creating sentences with words u) creating sentences telling the function of an object v) memory tasks w) read a story—ask questions x) read a story and retell a story y) role play	Give first letter of a word Give semantic association	

[a] Turn taking, cuing, modeling, and reinforcement are essential components of therapy.

To comprehend various speech acts and intents in relationship to various partners and contexts
To produce stylistic variations to meet situational requirements
To overcome obstacles in communication
To repair and revise communication
To use cues as a signal to repeat or modify messages
To provide feedback to the speaker, as listener, such as requesting message clarification/repetition/restatement, requesting that the message slow down, requesting the message in alternate form, indicating agreement/disagreement with message
To define the problems and solutions inherent in certain objects, events, and relationships
To use a telephone
To use a telephone directory, a dictionary, and a television schedule
To use street and store signs and maps

THERAPY TASKS AND MATERIALS

Guilford and Hoepfner (1971) developed a number of tasks for each of the five mental operations. Some of these tests are listed above under "Assessment." All of these tasks can be readily used to stimulate specific mental (cognitive) operations during therapy.

In addition, most traditional workbooks in the field of aphasia have presented tasks that stimulate cognition (recognition/comprehension) and convergent thinking. However, within the last few years, a number of workbooks have been published that focus on the stimulation of divergent thinking, evaluative thinking, problem solving, and decision making. They include:

Brubaker, S. H. (1983). *Workbook for reasoning skills: Exercises for Cognitive Facilitation.* Detroit, MI: Wayne State University.
Fawcus, M. (1988). *Working with aphasic clients: A practical guide to therapy for aphasia.* Tucson, AZ: Communication Skill Builders.
Harndek, A. (1979). *Inductive thinking skills: Cause and effect.* Pacific Grove, CA: Critical Thinking Press & Software.
Holloran, S., and Bressler, E. (1983). *Cognitive reorganization: A stimulus handbook.* Tigard, OR: C. C. Publications.
Karnes, M. (1986). *Primary thinking skills Al.* Pacific Grove, CA: Critical Thinking Press & Software.
Kazzari, A., and Peters, P. M.(1987–1991). *Handbook of exercises for language processing (Help)* (Vols. 1, 2, 3, 4, 5). Moline, IL: LinguiSystems.
Kilpatrick, K. (1979). *Therapy guide for the adult with language and speech Disorders, Vol. 2: Advanced Stimulus Materials.* Akron, OH: Visiting Nurse Service.
Lazzari, A. (1990). *Just for adults.* East Moline, IL: LinguiSystems.
Main, J., and Eggen P. (1991). *Developing critical thinking through science, I.* Pacific Grove, CA: Critical Thinking Press & Software.
O'Connor, M., and Voice, P. (1990). *Cognitive connection.* East Moline, IL: LinguiSystems.
Tomlin, K. (1984). *Workbook for adult language and cognition.* East Moline, IL: LinquiSystems.
Tomlin, K. (1986). *Advanced communication exercises.* East Moline, IL: LinguiSystems.
Wiig, E. (1982). *Let's talk,* Columbus, OH: Charles E. Merrill.
Zachman, L., Jorgensen, C., Barrett, M., Huisingh, R., and Snedden, M. (1983). *Manual of exercises for expressive reasoning (MEER).* East Moline, IL: LinguiSystems.

RELATIONSHIP OF COGNITIVE INTERVENTION TO WEPMAN'S THOUGHT PROCESS THERAPY

Wepman (1972) noted that the aphasic patient frequently substitutes a word that is associated with a word he or she is attempting to produce, and that the remainder of the individual's communicative effort often relates to the approximated rather than to the intended word. In addition, the aphasic person's inaccurate verbal formulation may feed back an altered message

to the thought process and change the thought process so that it is in consonance with the utterance. For example, if the patient is trying to say "circle" and instead utters "square," his or concept of circle may change so that it agrees with the utterance, and the patient will begin to think of a circle as a square. Wepman (1972) suggested that aphasia may be a thought process disorder in which impairment of semantic expression is the result of an impairment of thought processes that "serve as the catalyst for verbal expression" (p. 207).

Individuals who cannot retrieve the most appropriate lexical symbol for a context are impaired in their ability to communicate a number and variety of specific propositional ideas. When the remainder of the aphasic's communication relates to the approximated rather than the intended word, spontaneous language will be even more impaired, since, in this instance, the aphasic patient becomes incapable of using the learned code to communicate his or her true feelings and thoughts.

For Wepman (1972, 1976) the first stage of therapy is content-centered, discussion therapy in which the patient is stimulated to remain on a topic. Similarly, cognitive therapy is content centered and idea oriented; the individual is encouraged to generate functional communication and to produce a variety of ideas related to topics.

During Wepman's (1972, 1976) second stage of therapy, individuals are encouraged to elaborate on various topics. The ability to elaborate on a topic is a divergent ability. Thus, Wepman's thought process therapy involves stimulating convergent, divergent, and evaluative thinking as well as recognition/comprehension and memory.

RELATIONSHIP OF COGNITIVE INTERVENTION TO RESPONSE ELABORATION TRAINING

Response elaboration training (RET) is a program developed by Kearns (1985, 1990; Gaddie et al., 1991; Kearns and Potechin, 1988; and Kearns and Yedor, 1991) to increase the length and information content of verbal responses of nonfluent aphasic patients. RET is a "loose training" program that attempts to loosen control over stimuli and response during therapy by using client-initiated responses as the primary content of therapy. The emphasis is on shaping and chaining client-initiated responses. Patients are encouraged to elaborate on "whatever they are reminded of" when they are responding to picture stimuli of everyday activities and sports. Naming and describing are discouraged. Informational content rather than linguistic form is reinforced.

Specifically, according to Kearns (1990),

> The basic RET sequence entails (1) eliciting spontaneous responses to minimally contextual picture stimuli, (2) modeling and reinforcing initial responses, (3) providing "wh" cues to prompt clients to elaborate on their initial responses, (4) reinforcing attempted elaborations and then modeling sentences that combine initial and all subsequent responses to a given stimulus picture, (5) providing a second model of sentences that combine previous responses and then requesting a repetition of the sentence, (6) reinforcing repetitions of combined sentences and providing a final model of the sentence. Throughout this sequence clients' responses are not directly corrected by the clinician. Instead, naturalistic feedback is provided during the structured interactions through conversational modeling.

Progress during RET is measured by counting the number of content words per stimulus picture (fluency) and the variety of responses to the same stimulus picture (flexibility). Novel and varied responses are encouraged. Thus, RET stimulates fluency, flexibility, originality, and elaboration—or divergent semantic thinking as well as functional spontaneous speech, which necessitates all five mental operations.

Kearns' (1990) data demonstrate that RET procedures facilitate an increase in the amount of information (i.e., number of content words) generated by aphasic individuals. Further, a moderate degree of generalization across stimuli, people, and settings was reported (see Chapter 15).

CONCLUSION

Most of the literature on cognition specifies *what* is learned, or the products of cognition. Similarly, the literature in language intervention specifies therapy objectives or *what* is to be learned. Therapy objectives emphasize the types of tasks used. The goal of therapy is the appropriate accomplishment of these tasks. The criterion of success is based on the percentage of appropriate versus inappropriate responses.

Today, however, speech-language pathologists are shifting from an orientation of simplistic listing of tasks used in therapy, which define them as technicians, to a comprehensive understanding of the rationale behind the selection of these tasks and a description of why these tasks stimulate complex events to happen in the brain; this defines them as true clinicians.

An attempt to separate tasks into input, processing, and output components and, more important, the identification of the subsystems whose interaction is necessary for processing and specification of the complex events that happen in the brain, may save us from performing therapy tasks backward. That is, we recognize that what we are attempting to stimulate in therapy is the patient's mental operations or processes, since these are the complex events that happen in the brain. We also stimulate these mental operations because functional language requires the use of these mental processes. Thus, language therapy must reflect the fact that language is communicating—that it is the give and take of ideas. It must reflect the belief that meaning is the essence of language; that communication is idea oriented, not word oriented; that it is purpose/intent oriented. It must be recognized that the speech act involves creativity and novelty of expression. This is the core of language. Language is an aid to communication.

There are several other advantages to applying the Guilford model to adult aphasia. Most important, it enables us to identify and operationally define the action elicited within the patient by the stimuli presented, the complex events that happen in the brain, and/or the cognitive processes that are used in generating language products, such as words, classes, rules of languages, and semantic implications. It enables us to make use of an empirical statistically documented model or taxonomy of behaviors, in order to give the concepts of cognition, information processing, and problem solving a firm, comprehensive, and systematic theoretical and yet operationally defined foundation. Guilford supported the separate and distinct existence of each of the 120 abilities in normal individuals through the use of factor analysis. Some of these abilities, such as memory, divergent thinking, convergent thinking, evaluative thinking or judgment, and semantic and behavioral content, also have been documented in persons with adult aphasia, right brain damaged, closed head injured and aged (Braverman, 1990; Chapey,

1977b; Chapey and Lubinski, 1979; Chapey et al. 1976; Diggs and Basili, 1987; Law & Newton 1991; Lubinski and Chapey, 1978; Schwartz-Crowley and Gruen, 1986). In addition, this model provides a set of tests whose validity and reliability have been established. These tests can be used in therapy to stimulate specific parameters of the model and also to assess, evaluate, and describe patient behavior. Use of these tests may help us to someday make a statement about the efficacy of treatment based on this model.

FUTURE TRENDS IN COGNITIVE SEMANTIC INTERVENTION

Recovery today is too documentation oriented—too focused on cost containment. This orientation has generated a "pricing by activity" mentality in which government and insurance agencies emphasize unimportant but measurable goals, activities, and abilities. Many of these do not help the patient to regain as much functional, meaningful propositional language as possible or to increase their ability to become better adept at the back and forth—the give and take of ideas.

The current emphasis on measurable, operationally written, behavioral goals should be reconsidered. In the future, we need therapy goals and procedures that are based on rich and shared experiences that encourage individuals to apply, analyze, synthesize, and evaluate such experience; relate it to something else; reorganize it; infer from it; and use it as a springboard to solve new problems creatively.

A cognitive approach to recovery appears to meet this need. In addition, it has the added advantage that stimulating thinking and cognitive processing stimulates aphasic individuals' natural acquisition ability, or their ability to acquire language independently.

A cognitive approach also stimulates generalization. Therefore, there is a strong need to develop additional therapy materials appropriate for this approach. In addition, there is a strong need to develop assessment protocols that will measure these cognitive-semantic processes separately and within the context of functional, meaningful communication. Such a measure may help clinicians to assess progress in therapy and generalization and therefore sharpen our quality assurance systems.

References

Aten, J. L. (1986). Functional communication treatment. In R. Chapey (Ed.), *Language intervention strategies in adult aphasia*, (2nd ed.). Baltimore, MD: Williams & Wilkins.

Aurelia, J. (1974). *Aphasia therapy manual.* Danville, IL: Interstate.

Ausubel, D. (1965). Introduction. In R. Anderson and D. Ausubel (Eds.), *Readings in the psychology of cognition.* New York: Holt, Rinehart & Winston.

Bandura, A., and Walters, R. (1963). *Social learning and personality development.* New York: Holt, Rinehart & Winston.

Berman, M., and Peelle, L. (1967). Self-generated cues: A method for aiding aphasic and apractic patients. *Journal of Speech and Hearing Disorders, 32*, 372–376.

Bloom, L., and Lahey, M. (1978). *Language development and language disorders.* New York: John Wiley & Sons.

Boden, M. (1980). *Jean Piaget.* New York: Viking Press.

Bolwinick, J. (1967). *Cognitive processes in maturity and old age.* New York: Springer.

Braverman, K. M. (1990). *Divergent semantic and behavioral production skills in aphasia and right-hemisphere communication impairment.* Unpublished doctoral dissertation. University of Cincinnati, Cincinnati, OH.

Brown, J. (1972). *Aphasia, apraxia and agnosia: Clinical and theoretical aspects.* Springfield, IL: Charles C Thomas.

Brown, J. (1977). *Mind brain and consciousness: The neuropsychology of cognition.* New York: Academic Press.

Bruner, J. (1968). *Processes of cognitive growth: Infancy.* Worcester, MA: Clark University Press.

Butfield, E., and Zangwill, O. (1946). Reeducation in aphasia: A review of 70 cases. *Journal of Neurology, Neurosurgery and Psychiatry, 9,* 75–79.

Byng, S., Kay, J., Edmundson, A., and Scott, C. (1990). Aphasia tests reconsidered. *Aphasiology, 4*(1), 67–92.

Cazden, C. B. (1976). How knowledge about language helps the classroom teacher—or does it? A personal account. *Urban Review, 9,* 74–91.

Chapey, R. (1974). *Divergent semantic behavior in aphasia.* Unpublished doctoral dissertation, Columbia University, New York.

Chapey, R. (1977a). A divergent semantic model of intervention in adult aphasia. In R. Brookshire (Ed.), *Clinical aphasiology: conference proceedings.* Minneapolis, MN: BRK.

Chapey, R. (1977b). The relationship between divergent and convergent semantic behavior in adult aphasia. *Archives of Physical Medicine and Rehabilitation, 58,* 357–362.

Chapey, R. (Ed.). (1981a). *Language intervention strategies in adult aphasia.* Baltimore, MD: Williams & Wilkins.

Chapey, R. (1981b). Divergent semantic intervention. In R. Chapey (Ed.), *Language intervention strategies in adult aphasia.* Baltimore, MD: Williams & Wilkins.

Chapey, R. (1983). Language-based cognitive abilities in adult aphasia: Rationale for intervention. *Journal of Communication Disorders, 16,* 405–424.

Chapey, R. (1988). Aphasia therapy: Why do we say one thing and do another? In S. Gerber and G. Mencher (Eds.), *International perspectives on communication disorders.* Washington, DC: Gallaudet University.

Chapey, R. (1992). Functional communication assessment and intervention: Some thoughts on the state of the art. *Aphasiology, 6*(1), 85–93.

Chapey, R., and Lubinski, R. (1979). Semantic judgment ability in adult aphasia. *Cortex, 14,* 247–255.

Chapey, R., Rigrodsky, S., and Morrison, E. (1976). The measurement of divergent semantic behavior in aphasia. *Journal of Speech and Hearing Research, 19,* 664–677.

Chapey, R., Rigrodsky, S., and Morrison, E. (1977). Aphasia: A divergent semantic interpretation. *Journal of Speech and Hearing Disorders, 42,* 287–295.

Chomsky, N. (1957). *Syntactic structures.* The Hague: Mouton.

Chomsky, N. (1964). *Current issues in linguistic theory.* The Hague: Mouton.

Chomsky, N. (1972). *Language and mind.* New York: Harcourt, Brace, Jovanovich.

Cooper, L., and Rigrodsky, S. (1979). Verbal training to improve explanations of conservation with aphasic adults. *Journal of Speech and Hearing Research, 33,* 818–828.

Craig, H. (1983). Application of pragmatic language models for intervention. In T.M. Gallagher and C. A. Prutting (Eds.), *Pragmatic assessment and intervention issues in language.* San Diego, CA: College Hill Press.

Cropley, A. (1967). *Creativity.* London: Longman.

Darley, F. L. (1982). *Aphasia.* Philadelphia, PA: W. B. Saunders.

Davis, G. A. (1983). *A survey of adult aphasia.* Englewood Cliffs, NJ: Prentice-Hall.

Davis, G. A., and Wilcox, M. J. (1981). Incorporating parameters of natural conversation in aphasia treatment. In R. Chapey (Ed.), *Language intervention strategies in adult aphasia.* Baltimore, MD: Williams & Wilkins.

Dember, W., and Jenkins, J. (1979). *General psychology: Modeling behavior and experience.* Englewood Cliffs, NJ: Prentice-Hall.

Diggs, C., and Basili, A. (1987). Verbal expression of right cerebrovascular accident patients: Convergent and divergent language. *Brain and Language, 30,* 130–146.

Dore, J. (1974). A pragmatic description of early language development. *Journal of Psycholinguistic Research, 3,* 343–350.

Duffy, J. R. (1981). Schuell's stimulation approach to rehabilitation. In R. Chapey (Ed.), *Language intervention strategies in adult aphasia.* Baltimore, MD: Williams & Wilkins.

English, H. B., and English, A. C. (1958). *A comprehensive dictionary of psychological and psychoanalytic terms.* New York: McKay.

Fey, M., and Leonard, L. B. (1983). Pragmatic skills of children with specific language impairments. In T. Gallagher and C. A. Prutting (Eds.), *Pragmatic assessment and intervention issues in language.* San Diego, CA: College Hill Press.

Frattali, C. (1992). Functional assessment of communication: Merging public policy with clinical view. *Aphasiology, 6*(1), 63–83.

Gaddie, A., Kearns, K., and Yedor, K. (1991). A qualitative analysis of response elaboration training effects. In T. Prescott (Ed.), *Clinical Aphasiology: Conference Proceedings, 21,* 171-184.

Gallagher, T. (1983). Pre-assessment: A procedure for accommodating language use variability. In T. Gallagher and C. A. Prutting (Eds.), *Pragmatic assessment and intervention issues in language.* San Diego, CA: College Hill Press.

Goldstein, K. (1948). *Language and language disturbances.* New York: Grune & Stratton.

Goodglass, H., and Kaplan, E. (1972). *The assessment of aphasia and related disorders.* Philadelphia, PA: Lea & Febiger.

Goodman, P. (1971). *Speaking and language: Defense of poetry.* New York: Random House.

Gowan, J. Demos, G. and Torrance, E. (1967). *Creativity: Its educational implications.* New York: John Wiley & Sons.

Grant, D., Hake, H., and Hornseth, J. (1951). Acquisition and extinction of verbally conditioned response with different percentages of reinforcement. *Journal of Experimental Psychology, 42,* 1–5.

Guilford, J. P. (1967). *The nature of human intelligence.* New York: McGraw-Hill.

Guilford, J. P., and Hoepfner, R. (1971). *The analysis of intelligence.* New York: McGraw-Hill.

Haaland, K. Y. (1979). The utility of an information processing approach in speech and language evaluations. In R. Brookshire (Ed.), *Clinical aphasiology: Conference proceedings.* Minneapolis, MN: BRK.

Harlow, H. (1949). The formation of learning sets. *Psychological Review, 56,* 51–56.

Harris, M., and Evans, R. (1974). The effects of modeling and instruction on creative responses. *Journal of Psychology, 86,* 123–130.

Harrison, R. P. (1974). *Beyond words: An introduction to nonverbal communication.* Englewood Cliffs, NJ: Prentice-Hall.

Haviland, S. E., and Clark, H. H. (1974). What's new? Acquiring new information as a process in comprehension. *Journal of Verbal Learning and Verbal Behavior, 13,* 512–521.

Head, H. (1915). Hughlings Jackson on aphasia and kindred affections of speech. *Brain, 38,* 1–27.

Holland, A. (1975). Language therapy for children: Some thoughts on context and content. *Journal of Speech and Hearing Disorders, 40,* 514–523.

Hughy, J., and Johnson, A. (1975). *Speech communication: Foundations and challenges.* New York: Macmillan.

Jennings, E., and Lubinski, R. (1981). Strategies for improving productive thinking in the language impaired adult. *Journal of Communication Disorders, 14,* 255–271.

Jensen, G., and Cotton, J. (1960). Successive acquisitions and extinctions as related to differing percentages of reinforcement. *Journal of Experimental Psychology, 60,* 41–49.

Kearns, K. P. (1985). Response elaboration training for patient initiated utterances. In R. Brookshire (Ed.), *Clinical aphasiology: Conference proceedings* (pp. 196–204). Minneapolis, MN.: BRK.

Kearns, K. P. (1990). Broca's aphasia. In L. La Pointe (Ed.), *Aphasia and related neurogenic language disorders.* New York: Thieme Medical Publishers.

Kearns, K. P., Potechin, G. (1988). The generalization of response elaboration training effects. In T. Prescott (Ed.), *Clinical aphasiology.* Boston, MA: College Hill Press.

Kearns, K., and Yedor, K. (1991). An alternating treatments comparison of loose training and a convergent treatment strategy. In T. Prescott (Ed.), *Clinical aphasiology, 20,* 223–238.

Keenan, J. A. (1975). *A procedure manual in speech pathology with brain-damaged adults.* Danville, IL: Interstate.

Lahey, M. (1988). *Language disorders and language development.* New York: Macmillan.

Law, P., and Newton, M. (1991). Divergent semantic behavior in aged persons. Atlanta, GA: American Speech Language Hearing Association Convention.

Lazerson, A. (Ed.). (1975). *Psychology today.* New York: Random House.

Lefrancois, G. (1982). *Psychological theories of human learning* (2nd ed.). Belmont, CA: Brooks-Cole.

Lindfors, J. W. (1980; rev. 1987). *Children's language and learning.* Englewood Cliffs, NJ: Prentice-Hall.

Lubinski, R. (1986). A social communication approach to treatment in aphasia in an institutional setting. In R. Marshall (Ed.), *Case studies in aphasia rehabilitation.* Austin, TX: Pro-Ed.

Lubinski, R., and Chapey, R. (1978). Constructive recall strategies in adult aphasia. In R. Brookshire (Ed.), *Clinical aphasiology: Conference proceedings.* Minneapolis, MN: BRK.

Lucas, E. (1980). *Semantic and pragmatic language disorders: Assessment and remediation.* Rockville, MD: Aspen.

Luria, A. R. (1973). *The working brain.* New York: Basic Books.

Martin, A. D. (1975). A critical evaluation of therapeutic approaches to aphasia. In R. Brookshire (Ed.), *Clinical aphasiology: Conference proceedings.* Minneapolis, MN: BRK.

Martin, A. D. (1979). Levels of reference for aphasia therapy. In R. Brookshire (Ed.), *Clinical aphasiology: Conference proceedings.* Minneapolis, MN: BRK.

Martin, A. D. (1981). Therapy with a jargonaphasic. In J. W. Brown (Ed.), *Jargonaphasia.* New York: Academic Press.

Marx, M. (1970). *Learning theories.* London: Macmillan.

McConnell, F., Love, R., and Smith, B. (1974). Language remediation in children. In S. Dickson (Ed.), *Communication disorders: Remedial principles and practices.* Glenview, IL: Scott Foresman.

McCormick, L., and Schiefelbush, R. (1984). *Early language intervention: An introduction.* Columbus, OH: Charles E. Merrill.

Muma, J. (1975). The communication game: Dump and play. *Journal of Speech and Hearing Disorders, 40,* 296–309.

Muma, J. R. (1978). *Language handbook: Concepts, assessment and intervention.* Englewood Cliffs, NJ: Prentice-Hall.

Naremore, R. (1980). Language disorders in children. In T. Hixon, L. Shriberg, and J. Saxman (Eds.), *Introduction to communication disorders.* Englewood Cliffs, NJ: Prentice-Hall.

Neisser, U. (1967). *Cognitive psychology.* New York: Appleton-Century-Crofts.

Ochs, E., and Schieffelin, B. (Ed.). (1979). *Developmental pragmatics.* New York: Academic Press.

Pieres, E., and Morgan, F. (1973). Effects of free associative training on children's ideational fluency. *Journal of Personality, 41,* 42–49.

Porch, B. (1971). Multidimensional scoring in aphasia testing. *Journal of Speech and Hearing Research, 14,* 776–792.

Prutting, C. (1979). Process/pra/,ses/n: The action of moving forward progressively from one point to another on the way to completion. *Journal of Speech and Hearing Disorders, 44,* 3–30.

Prutting, C., and Kirchner, D. (1983). Applied pragmatics. In R. M. Gallagher and C. A. Prutting (Eds.), *Pragmatic assessment and intervention issues in language.* San Diego, CA: College Hill Press.

Reitan, R. M. (n. d.). *Manual for the administration of neuropsychological test batteries for adults and children.* Tucson Neuropsychological Laboratory: University of Arizona.

Rosenbek, J. (1982). When is aphasia aphasia? In R. Brookshire (Ed.), *Clinical aphasiology: Conference proceedings.* Minneapolis, MN: BRK.

Rosenfeld, N. M. (1978). Conversational control function of nonverbal behavior. In A. W. Siegman and S. Felstein (Eds.), *Nonverbal behavior and communication.* Hillsdale, NJ: Lawrence Erlbaum.

Rosenthal, T., and Zimmerman, B. (1978). *Social learning and cognition.* New York: Academic Press.

Saltz, E. (1971). *The cognitive bases of human learning.* Homewood, IL: Dorsey Press.

Salvatore, A. P., Blackwood, D., and Sachdev, J. (1981). The effects of dexamethasone on cognitive, speech and language behavior: A model for the study of recovery of function. In R. Brookshire (Ed.), *Clinical aphasiology: Conference proceedings.* Minneapolis, MN: BRK.

Sarno, M., Silverman, M., and Sands, E. (1970). Speech therapy and language recovery in severe aphasia. *Journal of Speech and Hearing Research, 13,* 607–623.

Schuell, H., Carroll, V., and Street, B. (1955). Clinical treatment of aphasia *Journal of Speech and Hearing Disorders, 20,* 43–53.

Schuell, H., Jenkins, J., and Jiminez-Pabon, E. (1964). *Aphasia in adults.* New York: Harper & Row.

Schwartz-Crowley, R., and Gruen, A. (1986). Rehabilitation assessment of communicative, cognitive-linguistic, and swallowing functions. *Trauma Quarterly, 3*(1), 63–75.

Scott, W., Osgood, W., and Peterson, C. (1979). *Cognitive structure, theory and measurement of individual differences.* New York: Halstead Press.

Searle, J. (1969). *Speech acts.* London: Cambridge University Press.

Slobin, D. (1971). *Psycholinguistics.* Glenview, IL: Scott Foresman.

Smith, F. (1975). *Comprehension and learning.* New York: Holt, Rinehart and Winston.

Staats, A. (1968). *Learning, language and cognition.* New York: Holt, Rinehart and Winston.

Tiffin, J. (1968). *The Purdue Pegboard examiner manual.* Chicago, IL: Science Research Associates.

Torrance, E. P. (1966). *Torrance Test of Creative Thinking.* Princeton, NJ: Personnel Press, Inc.

Torrance, E. P. (1974). Interscholastic brainstorming and creative problem solving competition for creatively gifted. *Gifted Child Quarterly, 18,* 3–7.

Ulatowska, H., Macaluso-Haynes, A., and North, J. (1980). Production of narrative and procedural discourse in aphasia. In R. Brookshire (Ed.), *Clinical aphasiology; Conference proceedings.* Minneapolis, MN: BRK.

Vignolo, L. (1964). Evolution of aphasia and language rehabilitation: Retrospective exploratory study. *Cortex, 1,* 344–367.

Warren, S., and Rogers-Warren, A. K. (Eds.). (1985). *Teaching functional language.* Austin, TX: Pro-Ed.

Webster's new collegiate dictionary (1977). Springfield, MA: G. and C. Merriam Co.

Wechsler, D. (1955). *Manual for the Wechsler Adult Intelligence Scale.* New York: Psychological Corp.

Wechsler, D. (1973). *Wechsler Memory Scale.* New York: Psychological Corp.

Wepman, J. (1951). *Recovery from aphasia.* New York: Ronald Press.

Wepman, J. (1953). A conceptual model for the processes involved in recovery from aphasia. *Journal of Speech and Hearing Disorders, 18,* 4–13.

Wepman, J. (1972). Aphasia therapy: A new look. *Journal of Speech and Hearing Disorders, 37,* 203–214.

Wepman, J. (1976). Aphasia: Language without thought or thought without language. *ASHA, 18,* 131–136.

Wepman, J. M., Jones, L. U., Bock, R. D., and Van Pelt, D. (1960). Studies in aphasia: Background and theoretical formulations. *Journal of Speech and Hearing Disorders, 25,* 323–332.

Wolfe, U., Florance, C. L., Mendelowitz, D., and Evans, W. (1981). Cognitive changes post carotid endarterectomy. In R. Brookshire (Ed.), *Clinical aphasiology: Conference proceedings.* Minneapolis, MN: BRK.

Yardley, A. (1974). *Structure in early learning.* New York: Citation Press.

Yorkston, K., and Beukelman, D. (1977). A system for quantifying verbal output of high level aphasia patients. In R. Brookshire (Ed.), *Clinical aphasiology: Conference proceedings.* Minneapolis, MN: BRK.

Zachman, L., Jorgensen, C., Barrett, M., et al. (1982). *Manual of exercises for expressive reasoning.* Moline, IL: LinguiSystems.

Zachman, L., Jorgensen, C., Huisingh, R., and Barrett, M. (1983). *Test of Problem Solving.* Moline, IL: LinguiSystems.

CHAPTER 12
Pragmatics and Treatment

MONICA STRAUSS HOUGH and ROBERT S. PIERCE

Pragmatics has been referred to as the interaction between language behavior and the specific contexts in which language occurs. In essence, pragmatics guides how language is normally used in context (Coggins, 1991; Davis, 1986, 1989; Davis and Wilcox, 1985; Newhoff and Apel, 1990; Prutting, 1982; Prutting and Kirchner, 1983). Context provides knowledge regarding the conditions and situations that determine how language is used for communicative purposes (Coggins, 1991; Prutting, 1982). Thus, pragmatics includes the intentions and attitudes that are conveyed while speaking as well as the prosodic or paralinguistic and gestural features that accompany speech (Newhoff and Apel, 1990; Weylman et al., 1988). Pragmatics can be considered the study of communication or, more specifically, the study of the functions of language.

Pragmatic rehabilitation for aphasia focuses on more than the patient's environment and nonverbal behavior; treatment is aimed at improvement of language function. Intervention strategies that are pragmatically oriented are based on the relationships between language processing in general and the contexts in which language is used. More specifically, aphasia pragmatic treatment involves traditional stimulation approaches as well as the manipulation of particular contexts in which these techniques are presented. That is, treatment addresses how these clinical procedures can be conducted in a more pragmatic fashion (Davis and Wilcox, 1981, 1985). From the standpoint of the patient, pragmatic approaches focus on the individual's communicative assets as well as the role of other communicative participants in the individual's environment. The emphasis is on dialogue rather than monologue, considering situational context rather than language processing in the traditional sense (Davis and Wilcox, 1981; Holland, 1977; Lesser, 1991).

Although aphasiologists did not originally refer to the behaviors constituting the area of pragmatics as such, since the late 1960s there has been concern with the functional and communicative aspects of language impairment (Aten et al., 1982; Holland, 1991; Newhoff and Apel, 1990). Assessment and treatment methods were and have been introduced under the guise of the functional approach to aphasia rehabilitation (Aten, 1986; see Chapter 14 in this volume). Procedures have included tasks emphasizing (*a*) the comprehension and production of words,

phrases, and sentences in more naturalistic settings; (*b*) practice on the mores of conversation; and (*c*) the improvement of nonverbal skills as a means to increasing communicative efficiency. Appraisal and treatment of the overall communicative abilities of brain-damaged adults and aphasic individuals in particular have led to the conclusion that communication is intrinsically interactive in nature. This realization has yielded more systematic examination of the reception and expression of language in various contexts, thus expanding the boundaries of the functional approach to a pragmatic treatment framework. Consequently, researchers and clinicians are beginning to view pragmatic assessment and intervention of overall communicative skills as a science of language function (Davis, 1986, 1989).

Pragmatic approaches to aphasia treatment are frequently quite comprehensive in nature; however, this type of rehabilitation should not preclude intensive intervention on more traditionally defined aspects of language (Davis, 1989; Holland, 1991). Emphasis on pragmatic issues to the exclusion of remediating other aspects of disordered language is a disservice to our aphasic patients. Although pragmatic strategies should always be a consideration in treatment, reliance on these techniques needs to be constrained by clinicians' knowledge about aphasia and by their basic intuition and common sense.

The purpose of this chapter is to provide a comprehensive overview of pragmatics and aphasia including consideration of various evaluative and treatment systems. An in-depth discussion of pragmatic functioning in aphasia is presented. Comprehension and expressive skills are discussed separately in regard to aphasic adults' pragmatic abilities. Both modalities are addressed in relation to three major areas. One area examined for both comprehension and expression involves the specific contexts in which language is used; these consist of linguistic, extralinguistic, and paralinguistic contexts. A second major area involves the interaction of these contexts with language, referred to as conversational and prosocial context. In regard to comprehension, this section addresses sensitivity to speaker meaning, conversational moves, and speaker strategies to improve communication. For production, use of conversational devices, strategies to repair conversational breakdowns, and polite forms in conversation and social contexts is explored. The third major area addressed in comprehension involves world knowledge influences. For expression, the third area focuses on the use of gesture. Variables that contribute to the facilitating effects of context with aphasic adults also are considered. References to relevant studies on normal language processing and aphasia are included in each section.

Although the view of pragmatics presented here is currently supported by most clinicians and researchers, organization of a pragmatic framework may differ among professionals. The present structure is somewhat different from the frameworks provided by James (1990), Smith (1988), or Weylman et al. (1988). Smith (1988) divides pragmatics into eight categories: function, context, paralinguistic features, the given and the new, deixis, speech acts, temporal integration/discourse, and metacommunication. Weylman et al. (1988) consider five pragmatic aspects: following indirect requests, understanding attitudes expressed using figurative language, appreciating and conveying humor, drawing inferences, and interpreting figurative language. James's (1990) organization encompasses three major areas: use of language for various communicative intents, rules for conversational interactions, and rules for the use of different speech styles in different communicative situations. Of key importance is that the phenomena identified in each descriptive framework are the same. Structural differences in the organization of pragmatics as an area of study will continue to exist as we learn how to implement pragmatic considerations in assessment and treatment more effectively.

PRAGMATIC FUNCTIONING IN APHASIA: COMPREHENSION

A major component of pragmatic functioning in comprehension relates to the influence of context. Listening/reading seldom occurs in isolation, and the information provided by the situational context affects the derivation of meaning. This information can be linguistic, extralinguistic, and/or paralinguistic in form. However, the organization of this section evolves primarily around the type of processing that the context affects, that is, how well aphasic patients derive meaning from syntax, semantics, and discourse structure when context is present compared with when it is absent.

Syntax

Most aphasic patients have difficulty deriving meaning from the syntax of a sentence (Naeser et al., 1987; Parisi and Pizzamiglio, 1970; Peach et al., 1988), including those who demonstrate relatively good comprehension skills as determined by formal assessments and/or informal conversational interaction. While different syntactic structures present with varying degrees of difficulty, some of the most challenging are those that contain potentially reversible thematic roles for the target nouns, such as reversible active/passive sentences and relative clauses (Butler-Hinz et al., 1990; Caramazza and Zurif, 1976; Parisi and Pizzamiglio, 1970). However, the surrounding context can significantly influence aphasic patients' ability to comprehend these kinds of sentences in several ways.

One manner is for the context to allow aphasic patients to change the processing mechanism that they use to derive the sentence's meaning. This occurs when the thematic roles of the nouns are identifiable based on semantic/pragmatic constraints associated with world knowledge. For example, the sentence "The flower was picked by the girl" is relatively easy for

aphasic patients to comprehend because their world knowledge dictates only one possible thematic role for the two nouns. The patients no longer need to rely on a syntactic parsing of the sentence to derive its meaning (Caplan and Evans, 1990; Caramazza and Zurif, 1976). A similar facilitation can occur when world knowledge makes certain thematic roles more plausible or probable than others even though the sentences remain technically reversible (Deloche and Seron, 1981; Kudo, 1984).

The application of semantic/pragmatic processing strategies in lieu of syntactic parsing can also be based on the surrounding linguistic and extralinguistic information (Cannito et al., 1988, 1990; Germani and Pierce, 1992; Hough et al., 1989; Pierce, 1988, a, b; Pierce, 1991; Pierce and Beekman, 1985; Pierce and Wagner, 1985). In this case, comprehension of a reversible sentence is enhanced when knowledge derived from an adjacent sentence or narrative or from a picture predicts a particular thematic role for the nouns in the target sentence. The potential generalization of these findings to real-life situations is straightforward. Imagine seeing a man coming toward you with a bloody nose and a bruise around his eye. On inquiring as to what happened, you hear ''John was hit by Bill.'' The extralinguistic environment surrounding this utterance provides enough information for the listener to determine who was hit without having to parse the sentence syntactically. Contrast this to a traditional aphasia treatment setting where the patient is told ''John was hit by Bill'' and then asked ''Who was hit?'' Reliance on pragmatic approaches to decoding language has also been reported by Juncos-Rabadan (1992) and Schnitzer (1989).

A concern has been raised about whether these predictive contexts actually facilitate aphasic patients' processing of target syntactic structures or whether the targets can simply be ignored and responses made based only on the predictive contextual information (Brookshire, 1987; Huber, 1990). Results from Germani and Pierce (1992) showed that aphasic listeners responded as accurately when only predictive narrative contexts were provided as when only the reversible passive target sentences were provided. However, their comprehension was significantly better when both the context and target sentences were presented together. This suggests that context improves comprehension by interacting with target information, not by replacing it.

A second manner in which context can influence comprehension of syntactic structures is through redundancy. Not all contexts are predictive of thematic roles. Some provide a setting in which certain actions occur but do not restrict which noun serves as the subject of that action. Aphasic patients can benefit from this type of nonpredictive narrative context in both listening (Cannito et al., 1986; Hough et al., 1989) and reading (Germani and Pierce, 1992). Although the mechanism underlying this type of contextual facilitation is unclear, one can speculate that it works by altering the allocation of the aphasic patients' processing resources during comprehension. For example, when presented with a reversible passive sentence in isolation (e.g., The boy is hit by the girl), the aphasic listener must decode the meaning of the nouns and the verb, parse the syntactic structure, and identify the thematic roles of the nouns (Caramazza and Miceli, 1991). A preceding narrative context, although not predictive of the thematic roles within the target sentence, familiarizes the listener with the nouns and the probable forthcoming action. Accordingly, less processing attention needs to be devoted to determining these things from the target sentence and more attention can be devoted to identifying the thematic roles. For a fuller discussion of the role of resource allocation in aphasia, the reader is referred to McNeil et al. (1990).

The potential generalization of these results to real life is equally straightforward. When one hears "Bill was hit by John" one probably knows who Bill and John are and what they were doing. Accordingly, most of one's effort can be put into determining the thematic roles in the sentence.

Redundancy may not be as pervasive of a facilitating mechanism for aphasic patients as is prediction. First, in contrast to narrative contexts, single-sentence nonpredictive contexts have not been found to significantly facilitate aphasic patients' comprehension of reversible passive sentences (Pierce and Wagner, 1985). Similarly, simply repeating a target sentence also does not lead to significantly improved comprehension. It may be that single sentences do not provide sufficient exposure to the key nouns to alleviate processing demands during the target sentences. Second, aphasic patients do not always benefit from nonpredictive narrative contexts (Cannito et al., 1990). Those patients who have shorter times postonset and/or more impaired comprehension skills benefit from predictive but not nonpredictive narrative contexts (Cannito et al., 1991).

The extent to which context enhances aphasic patients' comprehension of syntactic structures depends on the degree of difficulty the patients have with the syntax in isolation. The more difficulty they have, the more context is of benefit (Cannito et al., 1988, 1990; Pierce and Beekman, 1985; Pierce and Wagner, 1985; Sherman and Schweickert, 1989). However, this relationship has not been found for reading comprehension (Grogan, 1993). In contrast, aphasia type as measured by fluency does not relate to contextual benefit (Hough et al., 1989; Pierce and Beekman, 1985).

Semantics

Context influences semantic processing at the levels of both word identification and word meanings. Word identification occurs when a particular word is activated in a person's mental lexicon. The information that is needed to cause this activation varies along a continuum from strictly data driven (i.e., based on the acoustic/printed signal, as when unpredictable words are presented in isolation) to strictly knowledge based (i.e., based on contextual information only, such as completing the sentence "The bank called and indicated that my wife bounced yet another . . ."). More typically, a combination of data-driven and knowledge-based information is used to activate a word, and the percentage of each depends on the situation. The more context that is available, the less a listener/reader must rely on the acoustic/printed signal. Conversely, with little context available, the incoming signal becomes more important (Balota et al., 1991; Bard et al., 1988; Oden et al., 1991; Rueckl and Oden, 1986). Aphasic patients are often successful at using context to compensate for degraded acoustic signals (Pierce and DeStefano, 1987) and perceptual problems (Miceli et al., 1980).

An emerging view in psycholinguistics is that word meanings consist of a flexible set of features that become activated in particular groups depending on the situational demands (Balota et al., 1991; Kellas et al., 1991; Tabossi, 1991; Van Petten and Kutas, 1991). While some of these features tend to be activated consistently regardless of the context (Barsalou, 1982; Greenspan, 1986), others are activated primarily when the context emphasizes or highlights them. For example, the concept of "piano" can be very different for the accomplished musician than for the company movers (Barclay et al., 1974). Accordingly, the particular set of activated features that make up the meaning of a word presented in isolation may be different from the meaning for that word provided in some context (Kellas et al., 1991). This may be particularly pertinent for aphasic patients because they appear to have impoverished semantic representations of words presented in isolation (Chenery et al., 1990; Germani, 1992; Goodglass and Baker, 1976; Silveri et al., 1989). For example, using words on which aphasic patients demonstrated accurate comprehension by selecting an appropriate picture from an array of unrelated foils, Germani (1992) found that the aphasic patients identified high-importance features correctly but were impaired in their identification of low-importance features. The extent of low-importance feature knowledge correlated significantly with overall comprehension level, suggesting that those patients with better comprehension skills had not only knowledge of more words but fuller semantic knowledge of those words they did know.

Context influences word meanings by priming a smaller or larger set of relevant features (Schwanenflugel, 1991). Contexts that predict a small set of words highlight a large set of features that can be satisfied by only those few words. Conversely, less predictive contexts place fewer restrictions on the semantic features that a word must match and, thus, can be satisfied by a greater number of words. Aphasic patients are responsive to this variation in contextual predictiveness (Clark and Flowers, 1987; Grogan, 1993; Pierce, 1988b; Pierce and Beekman, 1985). That is, their comprehension of specific words is significantly better when the context is more predictive of those words than when it is less predictive. This facilitation may occur because the more predictive contexts enhance the activation of specific semantic features that may not have been sufficiently activated by the less predictive contexts. It is interesting to note that context is of greater benefit to those patients with poorer auditory comprehension skills (Pierce and Beekman, 1985). It is also these patients who have impoverished semantic knowledge for words presented in isolation (Germani, 1992).

More specifically, the effect of prediction on semantic processing may depend on the extent to which the target word is the one that the context leads the listener to expect (Schwanenflugel and Shoben, 1985). For example, "I drive a . . ." leads the listener to expect the word "car." However, other completions such as "truck," "lorry," or "taxi" are also possible. Puskaric and Pierce (1991) found that aphasic readers were more accurate comprehending unexpected target words when the sentence contexts were more predictive rather than less predictive. A similar distinction was not found for expected target words, although a ceiling effect may have influenced performance.

While considerably more research is needed, these results suggest that aphasic patients' knowledge of word meanings may not be accurately reflected by traditional "point to the picture" comprehension tasks. First, the depth of semantic knowledge is not assessed. Second, aphasic patients' comprehension of specific words may be better in more natural communication environments where the context might enhance the appreciation of semantic features that were not realized when the context was absent.

Discourse

Perhaps the greatest influence of pragmatics and context is captured at the level of discourse comprehension, as this most closely resembles the normal structure of natural communication interactions. While this section will review pertinent aspects of these processes, particularly as they relate to the comprehension of narrative discourse, the interested reader is referred to Pierce and Grogan (1992) for a more detailed discussion of these issues.

Similarly, to the process of word identification discussed previously, the development of a mental representation of the meaning of a narrative is a flexible process that uses varying amounts of data-driven and knowledge-based sources of information (Whitney and Waring, 1991). One reason that narrative comprehension is so sensitive to pragmatic and contextual influences is that the listener's knowledge plays an important role at all levels of the process. At the microstructural level, the listener identifies propositions contained in the narrative and organizes them into a hierarchical representation (Mross, 1990). Among other factors, success at this level relates to the coherence of the narrative, that is, the listeners' ability to identify relationships among the propositions. While coherence is certainly a function of the way a narrative is constructed, it also depends on the listener's ability to infer these relationships, and this ability depends on the listener's knowledge of the topic. Increased knowledge makes inferencing easier, which leads to greater coherence and better comprehension (Morrow et al., 1990; Yekovich et al., 1990).

Aphasic patients' ability to make inferences is poorly understood. They comprehended indirectly stated information about details in a narrative as accurately as they comprehended directly stated information when the required inferences were minimal (Brookshire and Nicholas, 1984), but comprehension was less accurate when the inferences were more difficult (Nicholas and Brookshire, 1986). In contrast, Rosenthal and Bisiacchi (submitted) found that aphasic patients readily made inferences based on causal relationships even when specifically asked not to. More information about the influence of inference type and complexity on aphasic patients' narrative comprehension is needed. The ability to identify relationships among propositions is facilitated by knowledge of the central topic or theme of the narrative. Waller and Darley (1978) found aphasic patients comprehended less cohesive narratives more accurately when a topic theme was provided than when it was not. Patterson and Pierce (1991) found that delayed recall of narratives by aphasic patients was more accurate when the topic theme was provided as a cue than when it was not. Furthermore, in contrast to individuals with right-hemisphere brain damage, aphasic patients can use topic themes that are provided either at the beginning or at the end of a narrative (Hough, 1990). This result resembles Pierce's (1988a) findings, which demonstrated successful use of predictive linguistic context that occurred before or after either semantic or syntactic target information.

At the macrostructural level, listeners form the gist or main idea of the narrative. This ability seems to be fairly intact for all but the most severely aphasic patients (Huber, 1990). Comprehension of main ideas is significantly better than for

details in narratives (Brookshire and Nicholas, 1984; Nicholas and Brookshire, 1986; Wegner et al., 1984) and in monologues and conversational dialogues (Katsuki-Nakamura et al., 1988).

The development of broader components of meaning from narratives, or macropropositions, is directed by knowledge sources such as schemata or superstructures. Schemata consist of knowledge about particular events and appear to be relatively intact in aphasic patients, at least for common scripts such as going to a restaurant (Armus et al., 1989). Superstructures are schemata for conventional narrative forms such as stories or articles. They are also relatively intact for patients with mild or moderate levels of aphasia (Ulatowska and Chapman, 1989).

The ability to form successful macrostructures can exist despite limitations at the micropropositional level (Huber, 1990). For example, violations in the temporal ordering of given/new information did not affect aphasic patients' comprehension (Cannito et al., 1986). Similarly, aphasic patients were able to comprehend cohesive and noncohesive narratives equally well (Huber, 1990).

Although it is beneficial that aphasic patients' knowledge plays a crucial role in narrative comprehension, there is a cautionary note. It is sometimes difficult to determine whether a patient's understanding of a narrative comes from information contained in the narrative or from his or her prior knowledge. For example, responses to questions about a narrative may be based solely on prior knowledge and may not reflect narrative comprehension at all (Nicholas et al., 1986). The notion that knowledge contributes to the comprehension of narratives has pragmatic implications. The most direct implication is that aphasic patients' comprehension will probably be better for discourse topics that they have knowledge about than for those they do not. Thus, if discourse occurs as part of the normal events of daily life and relates to topics that aphasic patients have knowledge about, then comprehension may be more successful than for more esoteric topics introduced in treatment sessions.

Comprehension of Nonliteral Meanings

All of the previous discussion has concerned the comprehension of literal meanings where the speaker's intent is directly represented by the semantics and syntax of a sentence. However, there are many instances in normal communication where the speaker's intent does not match the literal meaning of his or her utterance. These include idioms, metaphors, expressions, and indirect requests/commands. What makes these utterances different is that they must be interpreted with respect to the situational context. For example, "They shot the bull" can be understood literally and probably would be if farmers were discussing an injured animal. However, in most instances, the listener interprets this to mean something completely different. The comment "It's cold in here" can be simply a statement of opinion. However, it often is a request for an action. For the most part, aphasic patients retain the ability to understand these kinds of nonliteral meanings (Foldi, 1987; Huber, 1990; Myers and Linebaugh, 1981; Van Lancker and Kempler, 1987; Wilcox et al., 1978). This retained ability in aphasic patients, coupled with impairments in this skill in patients with right-hemisphere brain damage, suggests that these nonliteral interpretations are supported by the right hemisphere.

Another skill that appears to be supported by the right hemisphere and is retained in globally aphasic patients is the comprehension of personally relevant information or of famous people and landmarks (Van Lancker and Nicklay, 1992). However, a similar benefit was not found for personally relevant objects such as shoes.

Paralinguistic Factors in Comprehension

Anyone who speaks a foreign language or listens to a foreign individual speak English knows how important stress and intonation can be to comprehension. One can say all of the correct sounds in a word but be unintelligible simply because the stress pattern is wrong. Although not perfect, aphasic patients are often able to use this type of information to assist in comprehension. Emphatic stress on target words in a paragraph can lead to improved comprehension of those words (Pashek and Brookshire, 1982), although this effect appears to be more related to the prosodic changes occurring before the target word than to the stress placed on the target word (Kimelman, 1991). Although not necessarily understanding the meaning of a sentence, severely impaired patients can identify whether an utterance is a statement, question, or command (Green and Boller, 1974). This judgment becomes more difficult, however, when the semantic content is removed and only the prosodic features remain (Heilman et al., 1984). Stress and juncture help differentiate utterances such as "She is homesick" from "She is home sick" and "convict," the noun, from "convict," the verb. Aphasic patients have been found to be fairly good at this type of task (Blumstein and Goodglass, 1972); however, sometimes performance is not very good (Baum et al., 1982). Aphasic patients seldom have to rely only on these paralinguistic cues, as other sources of contextual information are typically present (Davis and Wilcox, 1985).

Prosody can also convey information about the speaker's emotional state. Aphasic patients' ability to interpret emotional state from the prosodic characteristics of utterances is relatively good, although it may fluctuate with the severity of aphasia (Heilman et al., 1984; Schlanger et al., 1976; Seron et al., 1982).

Rate of speech can also influence comprehension. Aphasic patients' comprehension is more accurate when sentences or narratives are presented at a slower rate, although this fluctuates across patients and listening events (Nicholas and Brookshire, 1986).

Conversational Interactions

When communication occurs within a conversational context, other aspects of aphasic patients' comprehension skills become important. One of these is recognizing the signals that guide turn taking. Schienberg and Holland (1980) reported on two patients with Wernicke's aphasia who respected turn-taking rules. However, Penn (1988) noted a patient with Wernicke's aphasia who did not. No one has questioned this skill in patients with other types of aphasia. Another aspect is whether aphasic patients recognize when they do not understand something. Apel et al. (1982) found that aphasic patients do make contingent queries when they are faced with speaker ambiguity.

PRAGMATIC FUNCTIONING IN APHASIA: EXPRESSION

Contexts of Language Function

As mentioned previously, the contexts of language function include the linguistic, paralinguistic, and extralinguistic contexts. In expression, these variables influence the social appropriateness of a message uttered by a speaker. Conversational tasks and discourse, particularly narratives, have been used to investigate the influence of these contexts in aphasia.

Linguistic Context

Linguistic context refers to the verbal information that is presented before and/or after a target linguistic unit (Davis, 1986, 1989; Pierce, 1988). The study of linguistic context in expression primarily involves the production of discourse or text. Discourse is a series of connected sentences that conveys a message; it is an expression of ideas (Davis, 1989; Dennis and Lovett, 1990; Ulatowska et al., 1990). Ulatowska et al. (1990) suggest that discourse may be as short as a phrase or sentence, the length of which is determined by the communicative function of the message. Text refers to written rather than spoken language.

Discourse or text production can be examined within (intrasentential) and between (intersentential) sentences or at a global level. Kintsch and van Dijk (1978) refer to the sentential structures as the microstructure, or the local level of discourse. The global or thematic features that characterize the discourse as a whole are considered the macrostructure. Both structural levels contribute to the coherence of discourse (Davis, 1986; Hough and Pierce, 1987). Coherence refers to the plausibility of content as well as the conceptual organization of discourse (Agar and Hobbs, 1982; Glosser and Deser, 1990). Coherence depends on a speaker's ability to maintain a unified theme within a language unit (Agar and Hobbs; Hough, 1990). Microstructural (local) and macrostructural (global) features or devices to maintain coherence usually are examined separately (Agar and Hobbs, 1982; Glosser and Deser, 1990; Kintsch and van Dijk, 1978; Tracy, 1984; Ulatowska and Bond, 1983).

Microstructure.   At the microstructural level, local coherence involves the conceptual links between sentences and/or propositions. These links or connections are devices that establish meaning in a discourse (Glosser and Deser, 1990). Several devices have been identified as useful in maintaining coherence in a conversation. A particular device, referential coherence, refers to the relationships between propositions or sentences that share the same semantic construct (Hough and Pierce, 1987); that is, there is an overlap of elements among sentences (Kintsch and van Dijk, 1978). Referential coherence can be observed, as in the following: "The boy rushed across the street. He was nearly hit by a car." This example illustrates referential coherence using the pronoun "he" to refer to the semantic element, "the boy."

Ulatowska and Bond (1983) and colleagues (Ulatowska et al., 1983b; Ulatowska et al., 1981b) observed that mildly and moderately impaired aphasic adults committed linguistic errors in discourse production, particularly in the area of referencing. Errors consisted primarily of ambiguous use of pronouns, possibly contributing to lack of clarity in the aphasic subjects' discourse. Berko-Gleason et al. (1980) also observed frequent use of pronouns without referents in the narrative productions of moderate to severely impaired Broca's and Wernicke's aphasic adults. This violation in the use of discourse rules was observed despite similar total output for the Wernicke's aphasic and non-brain-damaged subjects. Kimbarow and Brookshire (1983) studied aphasic adults' rule knowledge for referent activation and pronominalization. Nonfluent and fluent aphasic and non-brain-damaged subjects described one- and two-person video-taped vignettes. In the two-person vignettes, the degree of shared information regarding pronoun referents varied between speaker and listener. The aphasic subjects produced better descriptions for the two-person vignettes than they did for the one-person vignettes. Although neither aphasic group performed as well as the non-brain-damaged subjects, the results suggest that aphasic communicators are aware as well as tuned into the responsibility of ensuring that their listeners can identify participants when the referent is possibly ambiguous. Contrastive findings between this investigation and Ulatowska and Bond (1983; Ulatowska et al., 1983a; Ulatowska et al. 1981a) and Berko-Gleason et al. (1980) are probably the result of differential demands of the experimental tasks as well as differences in severity of linguistic impairment of the aphasic participants.

Kimbarow and Brookshire's (1983) findings suggest that fluent and nonfluent aphasic adults can maintain referential coherence, at least when discourse production demands are minimal. Furthermore, the results reflect aphasic speakers' sensitivity to distinguishing given and new information for listeners. The given/new contract (Clark and Haviland, 1977; Haviland and Clark, 1974) or distinction purports that *given* information is already known by the speaker and listener whereas *new* information should be unknown or novel to the listener. A speaker indicates this presupposition through the use of various referential or syntactic devices that aid the listener in identifying the given and new information.

Referential coherence also is exemplified at the sentence level through the use of articles and ellipsis or lexicalization (production). Articles establish clear referential links between sentences by indicating to a listener or reader specifically what the speaker or writer is referring to or communicating. Ellipsis refers to a construction that is incomplete in a literal sense; however, the absent linguistic unit is comprehended (MacWhinney and Bates, 1978). This phenomenon can be illustrated in the following sequence: Mother says, ''Clean your room.'' Child responds, ''I will'' (clean my room). In this example, ''clean my room'' is understood even though it is missing or not produced. Bates et al. (1983) examined Broca's and Wernicke's aphasic adults' abilities to topicalize and focus information in their utterances when describing pictures. The given/new premise (Clark and Haviland, 1977; Haviland and Clark, 1974) was investigated, specifically examining aphasic subjects' use of certain referential devices, including manipulation of definite and indefinite articles, pronominalization, and omission/commission of information (ellipsis/lexicalization). Subject groups described picture triplets with one varying element (object or action) and the other elements remaining constant. Both aphasic groups were sensitive to lexicalization, producing more variable referents than constant referents. For example, when the subjects were shown a sequence of three different people, each eating an apple, they lexicalized the agent in each instance (man, woman, girl); however, they mentioned the common activity of eating an apple only once (ellipsis).

These results provide additional support for aphasic speakers' sensitivity to shared information between speakers and listeners.

Early and Van Demark (1985) also investigated the given/new distinction by examining the use of indefinite and definite markers in descriptions of sequential picture cards by mildly aphasic and non-brain-damaged speakers. The non-brain-damaged adults substituted one type of marker for another with equal frequency, whereas the aphasic subjects substituted a significantly higher frequency of definite for indefinite markers than indefinite for definite markers. The results suggest that even mildly aphasic individuals have some difficulty in signaling new information by misusing articles. It is possible that definite and indefinite markers place differential demands on the word-retrieval process itself. Specifically, definite articles may be easier to retrieve because they are more concrete or salient.

Another variable that contributes to referential coherence among sentences is cohesion. ''Cohesion'' is a term that refers to the specific meaning relations between elements within discourse (Glosser and Deser, 1990). Coherence is linguistically expressed through specific cohesive devices, such as coreference and anaphora, thereby providing clarity in text or discourse. Coreference is a device in which the meaning of one linguistic element, such as a word or phrase, is dependent on previous linguistic context or another linguistic unit. For example, ''A bluejay was squawking loudly. *The bird* was hit by a rock.'' Anaphora is referencing by use of a pronoun produced in close proximity to the noun to which it refers and was mentioned previously in a particular sentence, as in the following: ''He brought the letter and lost *it*.'' Both of these linguistic conventions produce cohesive ties between sentences. Cohesive ties are linguistic devices that connect propositions in a meaningful manner. In ''John plays the piano. He plays it every day,'' there are two ties, each consisting of two parts. The first tie consists of the referring item ''it'' and the item to which it refers, ''John.'' The second tie consists of the referring item ''it'' and the item to which it refers, ''piano.''

Both Piehler and Holland (1984) and Lemme et al. (1984) employed Halliday and Hasan's (1976) system for analyzing cohesive ties in their investigations of aphasic adults' use of linguistic context in verbal output. Piehler and Holland (1984) evaluated changes in the language of two acute stroke patients, one with Broca's and one with Wernicke's aphasia, using cohesion analysis. Both individuals' use of cohesive ties changed, with the Wernicke's patient using fewer ties over time, whereas the Broca's patient increased the use of ties. Although individual patterns were different, both subjects increased their use of lexical ties. It has been suggested that increased use of this particular type of cohesive tie frequently accompanies improved mastery of spoken language. Lemme et al. (1984) examined mildly aphasic adults' use of cohesive ties in narratives by increasing the structure of the visual stimuli used to elicit oral productions. Increased stimuli structure did not influence the number of cohesive ties, percentage of total words used in cohesive ties (Bottenberg et al., 1987), or the use of logical connectives in narrative production (Bottenberg et al., 1985). Logical connectives are devices that indicate cause-effect relations among sentences in narratives. Ulatowska and Bond (1983) found that mildly and moderately impaired aphasic adults used a restricted range of connectors, thereby disrupting direct interpretation of the relationships between clauses.

The degree of stimuli structure has been found to affect cohesive harmony in narrative discourse productions of mildly impaired aphasic adults (Bottenberg et al., 1985). Cohesive harmony is a measure of grammatical and lexical relationships in narratives, reflecting how the percentage of cohesive ties in a discourse form a coherent whole. Armstrong (1987) examined the relationship between using Hasan's (1985) 50% criterion index to measure cohesive harmony in fluent aphasic speakers' discourse and listeners' perception of coherence. Listeners' ratings of coherence were significantly correlated with the cohesive harmony index. More important, the aphasic subjects were rated as being relatively incoherent and displayed a below-criterion percentage of cohesive harmony. Glosser and Deser (1990) reported no significant differences between fluent aphasic and non-brain-damaged adults in local coherence ratings of expository and narrative discourse productions. Contrastive findings on coherence ratings between this investigation and Armstrong (1987) may have been the result of listener familiarity with the subject, listener expertise, and task differences. Glosser and Deser (1990), however, did find that fluent aphasic subjects produced significantly more instances of incomplete cohesion than normal control subjects. Bottenberg and Lemme (1989) also observed that mild and moderately impaired aphasic adults produced significantly more cohesion errors than non-brain-damaged adults in narratives, regardless of the amount of shared listener knowledge. These results confirm the notion that aphasic speakers have difficulty producing cohesive discourse, resulting in productions that lack clarity.

Macrostructure.   At the macrostructural level, discourse or text is evaluated in regard to its global coherence. This type of coherence pertains to overall comprehensibility as well as the manner in which discourse is organized. Macrolinguistic devices, such as theme, gist, topic, plan, main idea, or goal, contribute to global coherence, with identification of the particular device depending on the specific type or form of discourse. In general, four types of discourse have been identified: (*a*) conversation, in which speaker and listener take turns exchanging information; (*b*) expository, which is centered on a particular topic; (*c*) procedural, which involves telling how something is done; and (*d*) narrative, which is a description of a happening expressed as a sequence of events or episodes. Each type of discourse has its own characteristic macrostructure in conjunction with the particular macrolinguistic device(s) that provides global meaning for the discourse. Narrative discourse has been studied most frequently in both normal and aphasic populations. In narratives, the essential discourse components include (*a*) setting, which provides information related to identification of the participants, time of occurrence, and place; (*b*) a complicating action that relates the events of the story; and (*c*) a resolution that provides the outcome of the actions (Ulatowska and Bond, 1983).

Linguistic context in aphasia at the macrostructural level has been extensively investigated by Ulatowska and her colleagues (Bond et al., 1983; Ulatowska et al., 1990; Ulatowska and Bond, 1983; Ulatowska et al., 1983a; Ulatowska et al., 1983b; Ulatowska et al., 1980; Ulatowska et al., 1981a, 1981b). In these investigations, mildly, moderately, or severely impaired aphasic subjects were presented with picture-story sequences and story retelling tasks to elicit narrative discourse. Mildly

and moderately impaired subjects preserved all the necessary elements of the discourse superstructure, including the setting, complicating action, and story resolution. However, the amount and complexity of language expressing settings and resolutions were selectively reduced. This *selective* reduction may have been the result of using cognitive and linguistic strategies to deal with the exchange of information in communication. As mentioned previously, referencing and connector errors contributed to reduced clarity in the narrative productions, as compared with non-brain-damaged subjects. Severely impaired aphasic adults displayed communicative intent, but attempts to produce narratives were unsuccessful, resulting in discourse structure that was not intact. Similar patterns of performance were observed for procedural discourse. Mildly and moderately impaired subjects were able to produce the essential elements of instruction on how to perform an activity. However, because of their reduced language ability, severely impaired subjects were unable to specify the steps on how to do something. Bottenberg et al. (1987) also observed that mildly and moderately impaired aphasic adults were able to produce a complete story with setting, complicating action, and resolution for picture-story sequences, regardless of length and structure of the stimuli.

Rivers and Love (1980) reported that aphasic adults produced significantly fewer complete stories than non-brain-damaged subjects using picture-story sequences. Nonfluent aphasic adults, in particular, had some difficulty producing the theme of the story. Using the Picture Story Test, Berko-Gleason et al. (1980) investigated the ability of moderately severe Broca's and Wernicke's aphasic subjects to retell narratives. Both groups produced significantly fewer meaningful themes than did non-brain-damaged subjects. Although the aphasic subjects often produced salient themes, it is unclear whether they specified the elements that were essential for preservation of narrative structure. Hough (1990) found that fluent and nonfluent aphasic adults produced significantly fewer central themes than non-brain-damaged controls on a narrative retelling task. Interestingly, nonfluent subjects produced significantly more central themes than did the fluent group. Reduction in linguistic ability probably accounts for the limited production of themes at the macrostructural level in aphasic adults. That is, aphasic adults are able to produce the essential elements of a narrative, but they have some difficulty in conveying the discourse theme. However, although Ernest-Baron et al. (1987) reported that mildly and moderately impaired aphasic adults consistently produced less information than did non-brain-damaged subjects on story retelling, aphasic subjects were as sensitive to the saliency of information in stories as non-brain-damaged subjects. Both groups produced a greater proportion of information units that were central rather than peripheral to the story structure. These latter contrastive findings may have been the result of differences in severity of the aphasic subjects' language impairment.

Ulatowska et al. (1981a, 1981b; Ulatowska and Bond, 1983) also rated the global coherence of narratives produced by mildly and moderately impaired aphasic adults. The aphasic subjects were rated consistently lower than the non-brain-damaged controls. Glosser and Deser (1990), however, found no significant differences between fluent aphasic and non-brain-damaged subjects in ratings of global coherence of discourse. Different findings may have been due to speaker familiarity with the specific narrative activity; Ulatowska et al. (1981b) used story-retelling tasks, whereas Glosser and Deser (1990) had subjects produce narratives about personally familiar events and topics. Other researchers also have suggested that equivocal findings among investigations may be partly due to sampling methodology (Shadden et al., 1990; Wambaugh et al., 1990).

Aside from the specific manner of eliciting discourse, the particular type of discourse examined may influence linguistic output. Roberts and Wertz (1988) found that expository discourse, in the form of picture description, elicited more productive syntax than conversation in a group of aphasic adults. However, there were no differences in clause type or complexity. Shadden et al. (1990) demonstrated differences between narrative, procedural, and expository discourse production for a variety of linguistic measures with a group of normal elderly adults and two aphasic adults (one fluent, one nonfluent) over time. As Ulatowska and Chapman (1989) indicate, "The distinct structural organization and content of each discourse type places different cognitive and linguistic demands on the communicator" (p. 299) and therefore needs to be taken into consideration.

Paralinguistic Context

Paralinguistic context is an inherent feature of verbal output that includes the prosody, intonation, and suprasegmental features of language. Prosodic and suprasegmental devices refer to variables such as rhythm, tone, and stress patterns of speech, vocal quality, juncture/pauses, speaking rate and duration, and pitch and intensity variations.

Prosody and Intonation.   Prosodic and intonational variations are used to convey emotional states, to identify novel material, to indicate the meaning of a word, and to convey certain types of syntactic information (Davis, 1989; Feyereisen, 1988). These factors have not been investigated very often in regard to the expressive abilities of aphasic adults. Global and Broca's aphasic individuals have been observed to display impaired prosody with monotonic output (Goodglass and Kaplan, 1963; Ryalls, 1982). Danly and Shapiro (1982), however, have reported that Broca's aphasic subjects exhibit appropriate contour manipulations, characteristic of simple sentences produced by normal speakers. Normal listeners may be unable to perceive this contour because of the long pauses separating words as well as Broca's patients' generally lengthened speech patterns. Although fluent aphasias, specifically Wernicke's patients, have been associated with normal prosody, these individuals may present with a hypermelodic speech quality in which they produce higher peaks of intonation in regard to contour than do normal speakers (Danly et al., 1983; De Bleser and Poeck, 1985; Ryalls, 1984). Foldi et al. (1983) have suggested that individuals' inaccurate perception of Wernicke's aphasic adults' prosody may be related to the tendency to listen to the entire sentence pattern, thereby overlooking subtle inappropriate prosodic alterations. Bryan (1989) found that aphasic adults were rated consistently lower than non-brain-damaged subjects on a general measure of prosody during conversational discourse. Additionally, aphasic patients were found to have significant difficulty repeating appropriate lexical stress patterns as well as using emphatic stress to distinguish new from given information to a listener as compared with normal subjects.

Emotion.   In general, aphasic adults are characterized as having a normal range of emotional capability. Gainotti (1972)

reported that individuals with severe aphasia display a dramatic but relatively appropriate depressive reaction when experiencing failure. Buck and Duffy (1980) observed that aphasic adults maintained normal expression of emotions through facial gestures.

Very few researchers have examined the vocal expression of emotion through prosody in aphasia. Speedie et al. (1984) found that two adults with transcortical aphasia could repeat the content but not the emotional tone of sentences. Interestingly, spontaneous display of emotion was normal in these subjects, suggesting a dissociation of the control mechanisms for speech production and vocal expression. These results also indicate possible contribution of the left hemisphere in controlling emotional prosody. Data on the ability of aphasic adults to express emotion are conflicting and appear to depend on how the behavior is evaluated. Impairments have been identified when expressive behavior is analyzed objectively, whereas behavior is judged to be normal when the communicative value of facial or vocal expression is assessed (Feyereisen, 1988).

Extralinguistic Context

As mentioned previously, extralinguistic contexts are separate from the utterances themselves, being either external or internal to an individual in a monologue or conversation. External contexts are those outside of the person, pertaining to influences of setting or situation and the participant(s) in communication. Internal contexts are those influences within the individual, consisting of world knowledge and emotional state.

Influence of Setting.   The setting or situation of communication provides the structure or rules for speaking. It includes knowledge of place, environment, time, and other individuals. Awareness of these factors contributes to an individual's communicative style and to what Prutting (1982) referred to as "social competence" (p. 123).

Clinical reports generally have indicated that aphasic adults are oriented to person, time, and place and are sensitive to their surroundings (Davis, 1989). However, setting has been examined formally in a very limited manner. Potechin et al. (1987) examined the effect of length of picture sequence stimuli on the discourse production of fluent and nonfluent aphasic adults. They found that stimuli length had no significant influence on the efficiency of eliciting accurate information or in the amount of anumeration for either aphasic group. These results are consistent with Bottenberg et al. (1987), who observed similar findings for mildly and moderately impaired aphasic adults. Correia et al. (1990) also examined influences of specific picture stimuli on aphasic and non-brain-damaged adults' verbal descriptions. For both groups, the speech elicitation picture from the Western Aphasia Battery yielded significantly more information than Boston Diagnostic Aphasia Exam (BDAE) (Goodglass and Kaplan, 1983) and Minnesota Test for Differential Diagnosis of Aphasia (MTDDA) (Schuell, 1965) pictures. In a more extensive investigation of setting, Glosser et al. (1988) examined the effect of changes in communicative context on linguistic errors produced by mildly and moderately impaired aphasic adults in discourse. Aphasic but not non-brain-damaged adults' performance was influenced by specific communicative context in that aphasic adults increased the syntactic and semantic complexity of their verbalizations and decreased their use of gesture when visual access between the speaker and listener was restricted. This study supports the hypothesis that aphasic adults retain pragmatic competence despite an impaired linguistic system. Pragmatic skills enhance the interactive quality of aphasic adults' language production.

Participant Influences. Participant influences include factors such as sensitivity to shared knowledge, the actual role of participants in communicative interactions, and speech act production.

As mentioned previously, shared knowledge addresses awareness of specific information that is between participants in a communicative activity. Shared knowledge between individuals is quite variable, depending on the topic of discussion and the particular individual(s) in the interaction. The success of communication is dependent on the degree to which participating persons share information. Aphasic adults may have difficulty sharing knowledge and, therefore, be unsuccessful in their communicative efforts with a clinician because of limited linguistic abilities. That is, the client may have problems in providing a common knowledge base regarding a particular topic so that the clinician can follow the conversation. However, it is important to note that the particular topic will have a significant impact on the successfulness of communication between client and clinician. With certain topics, the amount of shared knowledge naturally is greater or more established than for other topics.

For aphasic and non-brain-damaged adults, Bottenberg and Lemme (1989) found that the effects of shared versus unshared listener knowledge did not influence findings for several linguistic variables (cohesion, story grammar, productivity) in narrative production. Brenneise-Sarshad et al. (1991) also examined the effects of listener knowledge on aphasic and non-brain-damaged speakers' narrative discourse production. Although the non-brain-damaged group was significantly more productive for most of the linguistic measures examined, listener knowledge had a minimal effect on the stories produced by either group. In both of these studies, it is possible that the variables investigated were not sensitive to the adjustments made by participants when shared knowledge in communication is altered. However, in Brenneise-Sarshad et al. (1991), both the aphasic and non-brain-damaged groups produced significantly more words and content information units during a naive listener condition than during a knowledgeable listener condition, suggesting that aphasic individuals are as sensitive as non-brain-damaged adults to the amount of shared information between conversants in a communicative interaction.

The role of the participant in communication pertains to variables that differentiate individuals from one another, such as occupation or social/cultural group. Role also is defined by the relationship between individuals in an interaction. Role has been studied in aphasia primarily through examining aphasic adults' communicative skills with different participants. Yorkston et al. (1980) presented a system of quantifying efficiency of information exchange when aphasic adults were paired with different communicative partners (experienced and inexperienced speech-language clinicians). Lubinski et al. (1980) analyzed conversational breakdowns and repairs in an aphasic woman with different communicative partners (spouse and clinician) and in interactions with different purposes (treatment and conversation). These variables appeared to affect breakdowns in communication as well as repair of these miscommunications. Shared knowledge between communication partners may play a role in repair of miscommunications; that is, in conversation, the different knowledge base between the spouse and subject and between the clinician and subject affected the agenda as well as the manner in which breakdowns were repaired. In a related study, Gurland et al. (1982) examined the use of communicative and conversational acts of two aphasic subjects with different communication partners. Both subjects demonstrated an awareness of turn taking as well as knowledge that they maintained a conversational role with each of the partners. However, it was the subjects' communicative style and shared knowledge between participants that differentiated responses of nonaphasic communication partners.

Speech act theory, based on the adaptations by Searle (1969), distinguishes between the literal meaning and the conveyed meaning of an utterance or proposition. The speech act indicates how the utterance is used in an interactive situation, such as asserting, requesting, or questioning. Wilcox and Davis (1977) used speech act analysis to compare the communicative effectiveness of aphasic subjects in two different settings: individual therapy and an unstructured social group. Speech act usage was limited and relatively unchanged across settings for both aphasic subjects and clinicians. The clinicians appeared to retain their therapeutic role in the social setting, with subjects responding accordingly. Treatment sessions, however, also did not provide situations for the subjects to demonstrate an intent to communicate; therefore, subjects did not have opportunities to relearn how to use speech acts. Wambaugh et al. (1990) reported that speech act usage may be related to severity of aphasic involvement, particularly severity of verbal impairment. However, Prinz (1980) examined the production of speech acts in aphasic adults by constructing the environment so as to provide a situation for eliciting requests. Although the aphasic subjects' proposition often lacked clarity, their actions consistently were identified as requests, regardless of aphasia type or severity. Guilford and O'Connor (1982) also observed intact ability to express varied intentions in aphasic adults. Recently, Ulatowska et al. (1992) also observed preservation in the range of speech acts used by a group of aphasic adults as compared with normals in conversational discourse.

Gesture

Gestural movements may be used to accompany verbal behavior or may be used as a substitute for verbal output, as a mode of communication. Gestural abilities often are retained in aphasia to some degree; however, the nature of gestural impairment and the use of gesture as a means of communication in aphasia have been topics of controversy (Feyereisen and Seron 1982; Petersen and Kirshner, 1981). Roy (1982, as cited by Feyereisen, 1988) identified four theories of gestural impairment in aphasia: (*a*) conceptual deficit hypothesis, indicating a general cognitive impairment underlying both gesture and verbal behavior; (*b*) motor deficit hypothesis, suggesting the existence of ideomotor apraxia for the gestural impairment; (*c*) perceptual deficit hypothesis, suggesting an impairment of mental representation of the body as the basis for gestural impairment; and (*d*) disconnectional hypothesis, in which the speech area and the motor cortex of the right hemisphere are disconnected because of callosal lesion, preventing execution of left-hand gestures.

Gesture Accompanying Linguistic Contexts

A primary means of examining gesture has been through the exchange of information in context. Cicone et al. (1979) compared Broca's and Wernicke's aphasic adults on the physical parameters of gestural production and the points where gestures occurred in conversation. Gestures paralleled the verbal output of the aphasic speakers. Wernicke's subjects resembled normals in regard to the number of semantically meaningful and nonmeaningful gestures produced; however, the relationship between gestural units lacked clarity. Broca's subjects' gestural output was sparse but demonstrated clarity. These results suggest that aphasic individuals do not compensate for linguistic impairments through use of gesture, providing support for the conceptual hypothesis theory. The findings of Glosser et al. (1986) are consistent with these observations in which moderately impaired aphasic adults produced fewer complex communicative gestures and more nonspecific unclear gestures than mildly impaired subjects. For the aphasic adults, gestural complexity was negatively correlated with severity of linguistic impairment. However, Feyereisen (1983) found no significant differences in movement duration or frequency of gesture between fluent and nonfluent aphasic adults, refuting the hypothesis that gestural behaviors mirror verbal output because of a general conceptual deficit.

Herrmann et al. (1988) observed that severely nonfluent aphasic adults used gestures with significantly more frequency and for significantly longer periods of time than their non-brain-damaged partners in conversation. The aphasic subjects used gestures as substitutes for speech more frequently than their non-brain-damaged partners, indicating that gestural abilities may be retained in this particular aphasic subgroup. These findings are consistent with those of Behrmann and Penn (1984), who reported that nonfluent aphasic adults use more gestures that substitute for speech, frequently relying on partners' verbalizations as a catalyst for gestural productions. Fluent aphasic adults use more accompaniment gestures. These results indicate that the communicative functions of gesture are related to the content of verbal utterances; therefore, gesture may provide an alternative means of communication if language is impaired, but this remains a controversial issue.

Larkins and Webster (1981) studied gestural use in dyads involving an aphasic and a non-brain-damaged adult. A nonfluent subject increased gestural use with strangers but not with his or her spouse, and a fluent subject showed no differences between these communication partners. Nonaphasic participants used gesture with speech more frequently with an aphasic than with a non-brain-damaged partner. As the nonfluent subject had been instructed in using a gestural system in therapy, he or she may have subsequently used gestures more frequently in any situation in which there was a limited amount of shared knowledge between communication partners (i.e., strangers). The nonaphasic participants may have assumed that aphasic individuals have difficulty comprehending verbal output; therefore, they supplemented speech with gesture to improve chances of communicative success.

Pantomime and Imitation

Gestural production also has been examined in regard to pantomime and imitative skills. Pantomime is a descriptive symbolic gesture that is not arbitrary in nature. Duffy et al.

(1984) observed that a Broca's aphasic and a Wernicke's aphasic patient differed in the number of movements per pantomime, with their performance paralleling their verbal output skills. These results are consistent with Duffy and Duffy (1981), who found parallels between pantomime recognition and expression in a group of aphasic adults. Daniloff et al. (1986) reported that aphasic subjects, regardless of severity of linguistic impairment, were unable to imitate gestures as well as non-brain-damaged controls were. Severity of aphasic involvement influenced gestural performance, with severely impaired subjects displaying the poorest performance relative to all other subjects. These findings provide additional support for the conceptual deficit hypothesis.

Conversation and Social Context

The contexts of language function (linguistic, paralinguistic, extralinguistic) and gesture have been presented separately in the previous sections to illustrate the *controlled* manipulation of these variables. Naturally, these contexts interact with each other and influence the production of utterances or propositions in conversation. This section addresses the dynamic blending of the various contexts in conversational dyads, particularly examining the pragmatic adequacy of communicative interactions and general awareness of social skills in conversation.

Conversation is considered a cooperative endeavor in that each participant is aware of the specific nature of the communicative interaction. Grice (1975) identified the cooperative principle, delineating four maxims that should be followed to achieve cooperation in conversation. These are (a) be informative, providing no less or no more information than is needed; (b) be truthful, reporting what you believe; (c) be relevant to the purpose or topic of conversation; and (d) be orderly, so as to enable understanding of the conversation. The cooperative principle is a social agreement between participants in a conversation, as the speaker considers the shared knowledge between speaker and listener while he or she formulates the verbal productions.

Pragmatic Adequacy

Pragmatic adequacy refers to use of specific conversational devices as well as strategies to improve or repair conversational breakdowns. Conversational devices have been referred to as "moves" in a conversation. Turn taking is an example of a device that directs organization of the conversation. Gesture and termination of a speaker turn in expressing an utterance are used to take turns in conversation, aiding in the identification of boundaries for speaker/listener roles. As mentioned previously, turn-taking awareness has been observed between Wernicke's aphasic partners (Schienberg and Holland, 1980). Ulatowska et al. (1992) also observed adequate turn-taking skills in a group of aphasic adults paired with both aphasic and normal partners in conversation.

Another conversational device, contingent query, is used when there is a need for clarification of information, such as "What do you mean?" Contingent queries also can be nonverbal indications for additional information. Apel et al. (1982) found that aphasic adults were able to use contingent queries appropriately in conversation as frequently as were non-brain-damaged adults. Differences were revealed only with respect to mode of production with non-brain-damaged subjects using more verbal queries. These results are consistent with Linebaugh et al. (1985), who found that aphasic adults employed contingent queries appropriately, using a variety of queries similar to their most frequent communication partner.

Strategies to repair miscommunication in a conversation have been investigated in aphasia, as communication breakdowns are common when one partner has aphasia. Lubinski et al. (1980) found that when conversational breakdowns occurred between an aphasic adult and a nonaphasic partner, attempts were made to revise communication most of the time, with the majority of repairs being successful. The most commonly used strategy was guessing. This finding was consistent with Flowers and Peizer (1984), who also investigated strategies employed by communication partners when aphasic individuals were unsuccessful in conveying messages. Newhoff et al. (1985) also examined revision strategies used by aphasic and non-brain-damaged adults. Differences in strategies between the two groups were apparent only in regard to the specific revisions used. Aphasic patients made consistent attempts to revise communication breakdowns; these attempts were constrained only by their linguistic impairments. In a referential communication task, Busch et al. (1988) found that fluent and nonfluent aphasic individuals revised communication breakdowns in a manner consistent with non-brain-damaged adults. In repair attempts, all groups produced fewer words and information units, possibly attempting to be more concise and efficient in their productions. These results indicate that most aphasic adults are successful in revising communicative attempts within the limits of their language impairment.

Linebaugh et al. (1982) examined the relationship between communicative burden and aphasic individuals' functional communication level on the Communicative Abilities In Daily Living (CADL) (Holland, 1980). Communicative burden was defined as "the share of responsibility each participant in a conversation must bear to ensure the adequate transfer of information" (p. 4). Partners of subjects with poorer functional communication abilities consistently felt that they needed to assume a greater share of the communicative burden.

Social Skills

Social skills analysis usually addresses evaluation of an individual's use of polite forms and his or her prosocial awareness. Polite form use is basically an appraisal of an individual's ability to preserve social relations through appropriate verbal forms ("please," "thank you," etc., and indirect requests) and nonverbal manners such as appropriateness of eye contact, smiling, and so on (DeMarco and Hough, 1991). Little research has formally addressed aphasic adults' ability to display politeness verbally. Clinical observation indicates that most fluent aphasic adults, particularly those with Wernicke's, anomic, or conduction aphasia, generally are able to produce polite forms verbally, including indirect requests. Nonfluent aphasic individuals appear to have greater difficulty, primarily because of their limited verbal output and the need to focus on producing the most salient linguistic information for communication to be successful.

Some researchers have addressed use of nonverbal manners and coverbal movements in aphasia. Katz et al. (1978) found no significant differences between aphasic and non-brain-damaged adults in the rate and duration of coverbal behaviors (head nod,

head tilt, head shake, eye contact, eyebrow raising, and smiling) during conversation on selected topics. Feyereisen and Lignian (1981, as cited by Feyereisen, 1988) reported a reduction in duration of eye contact in nonfluent aphasic adults during the central part of speaking turns when turn duration was longer than 15 seconds. This phenomenon, however, also has been observed in non-brain-damaged subjects, possibly signaling turn-taking regulation in conversation. These coverbal behaviors may be an attempt or a means of maintaining social competence in conversation when there is linguistic impairment.

Prosocial awareness addresses *how* an individual uses pragmatic skills in order to function adequately in everyday communicative situations. It is the basis of true socialization, focusing on how a person responds to specific common social situations, such as dealing with embarrassment, apologizing, giving criticism, and dealing with accusation. Prosocial awareness is a difficult variable to study in the laboratory setting; to date, it has been evaluated only anecdotally in aphasic adults. As with verbal production of polite forms, one constraint on expression of prosocial awareness in aphasic adults is their limited linguistic abilities. However, because of the abstractness as well as the encompassing nature of prosocial skills, it is of paramount importance to examine the simultaneous interaction of all modes, aspects, and contexts of communication in aphasic adults in order to determine their sensitivity to social situations.

EVALUATION OF PRAGMATIC SKILLS

Language Sampling

Because pragmatics is the study of language use in context, the assessment of pragmatic skills should be conducted within a context that is as natural as possible. However, since contexts vary considerably, aphasic patients' performance may also vary, making generalizations across assessment materials, times, and settings tenuous. Knowledge about the effect of these contextual variables is beginning to accumulate.

As previously reviewed, aphasic patients' comprehension is influenced by several variables within the contextual environment. Although it would be possible to systematically evaluate the influence of these variables for any given patient using structured tasks, assessing their influence during more natural communication interactions, such as conversations, is very difficult. Not only would it be necessary to identify when comprehension of specific messages was successful, but the contextual environment would have to be scrutinized to see how supportive it was of those messages.

Expressively, performance can vary as a function of the type of discourse elicited. As mentioned previously, Shadden et al. (1990) found significant differences in a variety of measures of syntactic complexity and cohesion on narrative versus procedural tasks. Certainly, additional differences could occur during conversational discourse because of the opportunities for other pragmatic behaviors such as turn taking, topic initiation, and topic maintenance. Within conversational discourse, Wambaugh et al. (1990) reported significant differences on 17 of 26 communicative functions between two elicited conversational tasks (referential and planning). Differences also may occur with variations in the extent to which conversational topics are of interest to aphasic patients and the extent to which knowledge about the topics is shared between speakers and listeners. However, as previously indicated, the presence of shared versus unshared knowledge did not influence aphasic patients' performance during narrative tasks involving the verbal description of pictured stories (Bottenberg and Lemme, 1989; Brenneise-Sarshad et al. 1989). Similarly, Hinckley and Craig (1992) found that aphasic patients' successive remarks were similar on measures of cohesion when made in response to comments by the examiner either to picture stimuli or during spontaneous conversation. The nature of the aphasic patients' communication partners may also influence performance, depending on the extent to which they are familiar or unfamiliar to the patients. In addition to these differences among task variables, aphasic patients' performance can also vary across different stimuli used within a particular task (Bottenberg and Lemme, 1989; Brenneise-Sarshad et al., 1989; Shadden et al., 1990). While the length of a language sample for narrative and procedural tasks is generally dictated by the stimulus, it is more flexible for conversational tasks. The most common length is approximately 15 minutes.

Formal Assessment Tools

Sarno's (1972) Functional Communication Profile (FCP) is credited as ushering in a new era in the assessment of aphasia. Rather than emphasizing strictly linguistic analyses, the FCP looks at how well aphasic patients function in more natural communication settings. The FCP rates 45 behaviors in five areas (movement, speaking, understanding, reading, and other) using a nine-point scale reflecting normal, good, fair, or poor performance. While the notion of evaluating aphasic patients in more natural communication interactions is certainly pragmatic in purpose, the content assessed in the FCP is more functional than pragmatic in nature (Gerber and Gurland, 1989).

The Communicative Abilities of Daily Living (CADL) (Holland, 1980) remains the sole "test" that evaluates functional and pragmatic skills in aphasic patients. It uses a structured set of speaker/listener interactions that include natural discourse, question-answer sequences, responses to picture stimuli, and role-playing situations to evaluate patients' ability to communicate in a variety of more natural situations. Many of the 68 test items are pragmatic in nature, including speech acts, use of context, social conventions, deixis, and humor/absurdity/metaphors. However, because of the structured nature of the test, much of the aphasic patients' behavior is responsive in nature rather than self-initiating. Accordingly, observation of the patients' ability to play an active role in conversational exchanges is limited (Gerber and Gurland, 1989). The CADL's scoring system marks a radical departure from traditional systems. It has three points and reflects whether a message is communicated successfully, regardless of the manner in which it is communicated (e.g., communication channel or structural integrity). The CADL has extensive norms with cutoff scores to differentiate aphasic from normal performance that reflect such variables as age, gender, and living arrangement.

More recent tools for assessing pragmatic behaviors have relied on profiles or protocols. The Pragmatic Protocol (PP) (Prutting and Kirchner, 1987) directs the examiner to score patients on 30 parameters after observing their participation in a 15-minute unstructured conversation with familiar communication partners (family, friends, or speech-language pathologists). The 30 parameters are divided into seven areas and are outlined in Table 12.1. These parameters include verbal aspects

(i.e., speech acts, topic, turn taking, lexical selection/use, and stylistic variations), paralinguistic aspects (intelligibility and prosodics), and nonverbal acts (kinesics and proxemics). Each parameter is scored as appropriate, inappropriate, or no opportunity to observe. A parameter is marked as inappropriate if there is one instance in which the patient was inappropriate and this appeared to penalize the interaction. Appropriateness is viewed with respect to the sociolinguistic background of the patient. The authors reported good interscorer reliability (90.9% to 100% agreement) when examiners had 8 to 10 hours of training and met a criteria of 90% reliability before completing training. Less acceptable reliability (70%) was reported by Ball et al. (1991) when using two examiners who did not have training and the patients retold the Cinderella story rather than participating in unstructured conversation.

Using the PP with 11 aphasic patients, Prutting and Kirchner (1987) found that 82% of their pragmatic behaviors were appropriate. Inappropriate behaviors occurred most frequently in the areas of specificity/accuracy, quantity/conciseness, pause time, variety of speech acts, and fluency. The authors indicated that the inappropriate behavior profiles varied among patients (perhaps as a function of aphasia type) and were related to linguistic constraints.

The Profile of Communicative Appropriateness (PCA) (Penn, 1988) directs the examiner to score 51 parameters within six main areas/scales (response to interlocutor, control of semantic content, cohesion, fluency, sociolinguistic sensitivity, and nonverbal communication) (see Table 12.2). Scoring is based on a 20-minute interaction with the patient's therapist that contains conversational (topics of shared interest and reference), narrative (description of the patient's onset of aphasia), and procedural components (how to change a tire or make a cup of tea). A six-point scale is used containing judgments of inappropriate, mostly inappropriate, some appropriate, mostly appropriate, appropriate, and could not evaluate. The author reported adequate interscorer reliability (weighted Kappa values of 0.73 to 0.82), using examiners who had received between 20 and 30 minutes of training on each of the six scales. Ball et al. (1991) reported lower reliability values of 31% agreement for the six-point scale and 64% agreement when the scale was condensed into three points (appropriate, inappropriate, no observation). These authors indicated that their two examiners preferred the six-point scale over the three-point scale on the PP, despite its reduced reliability.

Penn (1988) applied the PCA to language samples from 14 aphasic patients. She found that the number of inappropriate ratings related to the patients' severity of aphasia. In addition, scores on the scales of response to interlocutor and cohesion correlated significantly with scores on the FCP and the CADL. Performance on the control of semantic content scale also correlated significantly with performance on the FCP. Penn suggested that the majority of behaviors were a direct result of patients readapting to their linguistic difficulty and that structural and pragmatic aspects of language are interrelated.

In the Discourse Abilities Profile (DAP), Terrell and Ripich (1989) stress the importance of sampling discourse in the three areas of conversation, narratives, and procedures. Accordingly, DAP has a section for each of these discourse types as well as a fourth section for general discourse features, including paralinguistic behaviors, nonlinguistic behaviors, and coherence. As can be seen in Table 12.3, narrative and procedural

Table 12.1.
Pragmatic Protocol[a]

Verbal Aspects	*Paralinguistic Aspects*
Speech acts	Intelligibility and prosodics
1. Speech act pair analysis	19. Intelligibility
2. Variety of speech acts	20. Vocal intensity
Topic	21. Vocal quality
3. Selection	22. Prosody
4. Introduction	23. Fluency
5. Maintenance	*Nonverbal aspects*
6. Change	Kinesics and proxemics
Turn taking	24. Physical proximity
7. Initiation	25. Physical contact
8. Response	26. Body posture
9. Repair/revision	27. Foot/leg, hand/arm movements
10. Pause time	28. Gestures
11. Interruption/overlap	29. Facial expression
12. Feedback to speakers	30. Eye gaze
13. Adjacency	
14. Contingency	
15. Quantity/conciseness	
Lexical selection/use across speech acts	
16. Specificity/accuracy	
17. Cohesion	
Stylistic variations	
18. The varying of communicative style	

[a] From Prutting, C. A., and Kirchner, D. M. (1987). A clinical appraisal of the pragmatic aspects of language. *Journal of Speech and Hearing Disorders, 52,* 105–119.

discourse are scored for the presence or absence of content units, while the conversational discourse is scored for 11 features in the areas of turn-taking skills, topic skills, conversational repair, and speech acts. Each feature is scored as present or absent. However, no guidelines are provided for what constitutes "present." Presumably, if a feature occurs once in the sample, it is scored as present. In addition, no scoring reliability data are presented. A second component of the scoring procedure is that each of the first three sections receives an overall rating that is based on the examiner's subjective judgment of the adequacy of that behavior independent of the number of specific features present. Overall administration takes from 10 to 15 minutes, with the conversation lasting from 3 to 5 minutes. The conversation should be about topics of probable interest to the patients. The DAP can be applied to interactions between patients and spouses or other persons. It can also be applied to patients' interaction with their therapist. In this case, rapport should be established before generating the discourse to be evaluated. Terrell and Ripich (1989) provide guidelines for interpreting DAP results and planning treatment based on the interaction between the number of features present and the overall adequacy ratings for each discourse genre.

Other efforts at pragmatic analyses have concentrated on breakdown-repair sequences in aphasic discourse (Gerber and Gurland, 1989; Milroy and Perkins, 1992). Gerber and Gurland (1989) recommend that the unit of analysis should be conversational turns occurring during conversation between the aphasic patient and two partners (one familiar and one unfamiliar to the patient). An utterance is considered to be unsuccessful when the partner signals for a repair. At this point, the Assessment

Protocol of Pragmatic Linguistic Skills (APPLS) can be used to analyze the interaction from the point of breakdown until the point of the repair. In Part I (see Table 12.4), the breakdown is rated both linguistically (as a phonological, word-retrieval, or semantic-syntactic problem) and pragmatically (as contextually irrelevant or a problem in presupposition-referencing, topic maintenance, topic shift, or turn taking). In Part II, the breakdown-repair sequence is analyzed by noting the patient's strategies for revision and the partner's strategies for signaling the need for repair. Part III describes the linguistic structures and pragmatic functions that lead to successful conversational turns. Part IV provides for both quantitative and qualitative summaries of the behaviors. Gerber and Gurland (1989) stress the need to look at the interaction between pragmatic and linguistic functioning, and they note that the APPLS can be used to highlight linguistic-pragmatic strengths as well as limitations.

A more detailed approach to the analysis of cohesion in aphasic discourse is provided by Armstrong (1991). This procedure looks at lexical chains and chain interactions as a measure of the extent to which content/lexical entities are interrelated in a unit of discourse. The cohesive harmony index, discussed previously, is calculated to measure a discourse's coherence. These measures can be used to identify both strengths and weaknesses in aphasic patients' discourse and can suggest specific treatment goals.

Functional Communication and Prosocial Rating Scales/Checklists

The Revised Edinburgh Functional Communication Profile (Wirz et al., 1990) is a means of organizing the observation and analysis of an individual's functional communication. The profile is based on speech act theory (Searle, 1969) and provides information on two specific aspects of functioning: interaction and communicative performance. Interaction analysis evaluates the individual's ability to participate in and maintain an interaction on a six-point rating scale. Communicative performance analysis identifies the modalities used to communicate. The Edinburgh was designed to *supplement* traditional aphasia assessment by providing pragmatic information about an individual's ability to use language in context.

A broader measure, the Checklist of Adaptive Living Skills (CALS) (Morreau and Bruininks, 1991), is a criterion-referenced measure of adaptive living skills. It is used to identify specific abilities individuals have in their repertoire and what skills they need to master for adequate functioning in specific environments. The CALS is organized into four major categories of skills, including personal living, home living, community living, and employment. Skills are evaluated with respect to whether the individual can perform them independently. The checklist can be used with a variety of populations and age groups.

The Communicative Effectiveness Index (CETI) (Lomas et al., 1989) is a functional communication measure for examining change in performance over time in the pragmatic skills of aphasic adults (see Chapter 4). Sixteen daily living situations are rated on a visual analogue scale through direct observation of the aphasic individual by a significant other (e.g., spouse, relative, neighbor, friend). The scale allows an evaluation of performance relative to premorbid ability of the individual. The value in the instrument is to enable clinicians to evaluate an individual patient's progress in therapy, particularly in regard to everyday life situations. Another measure geared to assess change in performance over time is the Conversation Assessment developed by Copeland (1989). This instrument evaluates the use of speech functions and global interaction in conversation, which are rated separately. Global interaction addresses mode of communication, ability to assume the burden of conversation and successfulness in conveying messages.

The Adult Social Communication Rating Scale (Hough, 1991, as cited by DeMarco and Hough, 1991) is a measure of prosocial awareness, adapted from work by Goldstein et al. (1980) for use with adults. It examines a variety of communicative behaviors in specific conversational situations. These behaviors are divided into clusters or groups of skills that include (*a*) skills for initiating and maintaining conversation; (*b*) advanced social conversation skills; (*c*) skills for dealing with feelings; (*d*) skill alternatives to aggression; (*e*) skills for dealing with stress; and (*f*) planning skills. There are approximately 6

Table 12.2.
Profile of Communicative Appropriateness[a]

Response to interlocutor	Sociolinguistic sensitivity
Request	Polite forms
Reply	Reference to interlocutor
Clarification request	Placeholders, filers, stereotypes
Acknowledgment	Acknowledgments
Teaching probe	Self-correction
Others	Comment clauses
Control of semantic content	Sarcasm/humor
Topic initiation	Control of direct speech
Topic adherence	Indirect speech acts
Topic shift	Others
Lexical choice	Nonverbal communication
Idea completion	Vocal aspects
Idea sequencing	Intensity
Others	Pitch
Cohesion	Rate
Ellipsis	Intonation
Tense use	Quality
Reference	Nonverbal aspects
Lexical substitution forms	Facial expression
Relative clauses	Head movement
Prenominal adjectives	Body posture
Conjunctions	Breathing
Others	Social distance
Fluency	Gesture/pantomime
Interjections	Others
Repetitions	
Revisions	
Incomplete phrases	
False starts	
Pauses	
Word-finding difficulties	
Others	

[a] From Penn, C. (1988). The profiling of syntax and pragmatics in aphasia. *Clinical Linguistics and Phonetics, 2,* 179–208.

Table 12.3.
Discourse Abilities Profile[a]

Narrative Discourse	Spontaneous Conversation
Abstract	Turn-taking skills
Setting	Takes turns
Episode	Relinquishes turn
Initiating event	Appropriate turn
Initiating response	Topic skills
Plan	Initiation
Attempt	Maintenance
Consequence	Shift/transitions
Reaction	Conversational repair
Procedural Discourse	Requests clarification
(how to fix toast and jelly)	Clarifies
Essential steps	Speech acts
Get bread	Responses
Get jelly	Requests
Get toaster	Assertions
Toast bread	
Target step: Put jelly on	
Optional steps	

General Discourse Rating
1. Paralinguistic behavior: e.g., stress, intonation, rate
2. Nonlinguistic behavior: e.g., eye contact, gestures
3. Coherence: e.g., appropriate use of pronouns, articles, or ellipses

[a] From Terrell, B., and Ripich, D. (1989). Discourse competence as a variable in intervention. *Seminars in Speech and Language: Aphasia and Pragmatics, 10,* 282–297.

to 10 behaviors that are rated within each cluster of skills. Each behavior is rated on a five-point scale, in conjunction with a ''never-seldom-sometimes-often-always'' rating. The scale attempts to address the variable of conversational style as it can be completed by a variety of participants who interact with the individual (e.g., spouse, friend, clinician, child, employer). Furthermore, the behavioral rating can be conducted in a variety of settings (e.g., home, work, school, hospital) by the significant people who are in the individual's environment. The protocol was developed to provide an *additional* perspective for examining communication in context. Many of the pragmatic checklists/rating scales available that are appropriate for use with aphasic adults emphasize evaluation of the mechanics of conversation and/or linguistic adequacy, rather than addressing the skills involved in active socialization.

Several rating scale measures have been developed specifically for examining functional communication and pragmatic skills in severely impaired aphasic individuals. These include the Communicative Competence Evaluation Instrument (CCEI) (Houghton et al., 1982), Rating of Functional Performance (Wertz et al., 1981), and Assessment of Communicative Skills Interview (Herrmann et al., 1989).

Other Evaluative Approaches

Role-playing probes (Davis and Wilcox, 1981; Wilcox, 1983) are a means of assessing communicative effectiveness using a set of common situations. The situations are representative of everyday activities that are acted out with an aphasic patient. Scoring is multidimensional, based on the number of prompts required to communicate a message effectively. The mode of communication is not considered in the successfulness of conveying messages.

Efficiency of information exchange (Yorkston et al., 1980) is an observational system examining the accuracy and duration of time spent in conveying messages in conversation between aphasic adults and communication partners. Efficiency is scored based on the completeness and relevancy of the information exchanged. Davis and Wilcox (1981) developed a similar system for rating communicative adequacy.

Duration of communicative interaction (Wilcox, 1983) is another means of evaluating communicative effectiveness in conversation or role playing. The number of turns exchanged between an aphasic adult and his or her communication partner are tallied during a given communicative encounter. Communication is considered to be reduced in efficiency if there is a large number of turns.

Dembowski et al. (1989) have developed an evaluation system of discourse for use with aphasic adults. The analysis includes an assessment of narrative and procedural superstructure and content as well as a rating scale of pragmatic behaviors for narrative, procedural, and conversational discourse.

PRAGMATIC TREATMENT IN APHASIA

Treatment: Improving Weakness and Capitalizing on Strengths

The primary goal of aphasia treatment is to assist patients to communicate better in a variety of settings. Advances in our knowledge of pragmatics have influenced how this treatment is conducted. Treatment goals, procedures, and the control of stimuli have all benefited from pragmatic influences. One of the primary contributions has been an increased recognition of aphasic patients' communication strengths as well as their deficits. Those things that patients do well can be used in treatment both to enhance those things with which they have trouble and to support successful communication despite those things with which they have trouble. The following three sections discuss this notion in more depth.

Pragmatic and Linguistic Behavior

Many of the pragmatic deficits seen in aphasic patients can be traced to linguistic problems and/or their attempts to compensate for linguistic problems (Newhoff and Apel, 1990; Penn, 1988; Prutting and Kirchner, 1987). Communication breakdowns occur when patients cannot retrieve the specific words they need to convey a message, cannot formulate sufficient syntactic frames, or fail to comprehend the meaning of what they hear or read. Accordingly, the traditional treatment emphasis on basic linguistic skills remains an important component of aphasia treatment. However, pragmatic aspects of communication can affect how treatment on linguistic skills is accomplished.

In the area of comprehension, evidence is accumulating that some aphasic patients comprehend word meanings better in supportive contexts than without those contexts. For example, contexts may stimulate awareness of relevant semantic features that are not activated in isolation. Accordingly, the training of semantic knowledge might incorporate appropriate contexts that increase the depth of knowledge patients have about words. Improving this knowledge capitalizes on aphasic patients' strengths in that they often use semantic/pragmatic strategies to replace syntactic parsing during sentence comprehension. Accordingly, comprehension becomes more successful despite limitations in syntactic decoding skills. At discourse levels, comprehension could be improved through the systematic ma-

nipulation of variables such as the patient's knowledge of the topic, saliency of the information, and inferencing demands (Armus et al., 1989; Pierce and Grogan, 1992).

When treating expression, discourse demands can be reduced in order to emphasize linguistic skills while maintaining a contextual framework (Terrell and Ripich, 1989; Ulatowska and Chapman, 1989). Protocols such as the DAP can be used to identify which discourse genre is most successful for a patient. Using familiar partners, discussing topics with extensive shared knowledge, and emphasizing only essential components of discourse content can simplify the communication task such that linguistic skills can be highlighted. These skills might include word selection, marking given versus new information, appropriate referencing, use of connectors, and morphological and syntactic accuracy. As linguistic skills improve, discourse components and genres can be expanded to increase task difficulty and to resemble more typical communication settings.

Successful and Unsuccessful Communication

A major contribution of pragmatics to aphasia treatment is the emphasis on communication and whether it is successful, regardless of form. Analyses such as the APPLS highlight when communication breaks down. The reasons for the breakdown can be analyzed in terms of both linguistic and pragmatic functioning, which can then be targeted in treatment. Equally important, however, is the ability of pragmatic profiles and tests like the CADL to highlight successful communication so that patients' strengths can be used in treatment. Patients may successfully convey information through nonverbal means such as gestures or a communication board. Alternatively, patients may use circumlocutions or verbal descriptions to compensate suc-

Table 12.4.
Assessment Profile of Pragmatic Linguistic Skills

Part I: Breakdowns	
Linguistic problems	Pragmatic problems
Phonological problem	Contextually irrelevant
Word-retrieval problem	Presuppositional-referencing problem
Semantic-syntactic problem	Topic maintenance problem
	Topic shift problem
	Turn-taking problem
	Other
Part II: Breakdown-Repair Sequence	
Client strategies (revisions)	Partner strategies (signals to repair)
Acknowledgment	Nonspecific request
Repetition of partner's utterance	Bid for more specific information
Paraphrase	Conversational directive
Adding information	Other
Semantic-syntactic revision	
Gesture	
Other	
Part III: Successful Conversational Turns	
Linguistic structures	
Pragmatic functions	
Part IV: Quantitative and Qualitative Summaries	

cessfully for word-finding lapses. Careful analyses of patients' use of cohesive ties may reveal particular ones that are successful (Armstrong, 1991).

It is also important to look at how aphasic patients' communication partners handle communication failures (Gerber and Gurland, 1989; Newhoff and Apel, 1989). Partners can be trained to provide better or more focused repair signals that may be more successful in helping patients through communication breakdowns. In addition, the larger communication environment can be analyzed to make it more receptive to communication attempts by aphasic patients (Lubinski, 1981).

Pragmatic Goals

Pragmatic aspects of communication are sometimes viable treatment goals themselves (Terrell and Ripich, 1989; Ulatowska and Chapman, 1989). Working within the limitation of their linguistic system, patients can attempt to develop a variety of speech acts such as topic initiation and maintenance. They can also expand their ability to express components of discourse content through elaboration and contingent queries.

Treatment Procedures

Role-Playing Activities and Script Development

Role-playing activities (Green, 1982, 1984; Hand and Tonkovich, 1979; Newhoff and Apel, 1990) have several purposes: (*a*) The patient has the opportunity to practice communicating in contexts of daily life within the clinical environment; (*b*) the clinician can work with the patient to develop and employ strategies that can be used outside of the therapeutic setting; and (*c*) role playing focuses on the functions of language, as the emphasis is on communicative interaction. Role-playing situations should entail specific contextual activities in which language can be used actively depending on the specific pragmatic goal of treatment.

In a role-playing activity, the aphasic individual and the clinician should initially discuss the script of the situation, including the specific events in the activity. Particular responses and behaviors within the script can be identified, especially those functions targeted for remediation. This is consistent with therapeutic considerations for discourse management discussed by Ulatowska and Bond (1983; Chapman and Ulatowska, 1992) in which patients are aided in outlining the essential elements of a particular discourse. In the actual role playing of the situation, spontaneity of the conversational interaction should be maintained. This will provide the most accurate representation of the activity for the client to demonstrate target responses or behaviors. If possible, videotaping or, minimally, audiotaping of the role play should be conducted. This will aid in the review and evaluation of the communicative interaction by the client and the clinician. Strengths and weaknesses in the exchange should be identified in terms of adequacy of the specific messages conveyed and the overall successfulness of communication.

Promoting Aphasics' Communicative Effectiveness (PACE)

PACE (Davis, 1986, 1989; Davis and Wilcox, 1981, 1985; Wilcox, 1983) has been discussed extensively as a means of organizing the interaction between an aphasic patient and the clinician so as to simulate the essential features of conversation within the realm of a therapeutic task. The focus in this approach is on the conveyance of ideas rather than on linguistic adequacy of the message.

PACE is based on four principles: (*a*) The clinician and the patient participate equally as senders and receivers of information. As sender, this provides the clinician an opportunity to model pragmatic behaviors appropriately and use communication modes that may aid the client in more successful communication. (*b*) There is an exchange of new information between the clinician and the patient. This enables the patient to experience communication failures and practice strategies for overcoming them. (*c*) The sender has free choice as to the modes of communication used in sending information. The clinician does not direct the patient to use a particular strategy. (*d*) The receiver provides feedback as to the successful transmission of the message. The patient's success is partly dependent on the clinician's ability to understand the message.

Use of PACE in aphasia treatment has focused frequently on picture description between the patient and the clinician. The patient and the clinician take turns describing contents of pictures unknown to each other. However, the PACE approach can be extended to a variety of other activities, such as event description or story completion (Gibbs, 1981). The important issue is to maintain the four principles of sending and receiving information in relation to the pragmatic treatment goals of an individual patient.

Use of Simulated Situations

Simulated situations can involve (*a*) barrier activities (Newhoff and Apel, 1990), which incorporate some of the principles of PACE; or (*b*) conducting traditional treatment tasks and/or conversational activities while simulating naturally occurring extralinguistic variables, such as background noise or other people in the environment (Green, 1984).

Barrier activities involve placement of a visual barrier between patient and clinician, thereby focusing the communicative partners primarily on verbal conveyance of messages. Frequently, participants will have similar materials on their side of the barrier, with the task usually requiring communication regarding alterations or movement of the materials and/or asking for clarification of conveyed information. Hence, the barrier activity can simulate procedural discourse, when communicating directions on how to change materials, or expository discourse, when describing the current status of materials. Regardless of the task, the barrier encourages a communicative interaction between the participants, with each partner playing an equal role in this exchange.

The introduction of simulated extralinguistic variables in the therapeutic setting should be carefully manipulated. The therapeutic task and the specific "natural" variables to be presented require clear identification. It also may be valuable to conduct the therapeutic activity initially in the more traditional clinical environment without introduction of the specific contextual variable(s). This control may be useful in aiding the patient's adjustment to the "new" task demands and to naturally occurring distractions in communicative interactions, in general. Furthermore, it may help the clinician identify any spontaneous compensations that the patient makes in response to the extralinguistic variables. The clinician and the patient may want to discuss the general nature of most communicative interactions, emphasizing that in many situations, redundancy and misunderstanding are normal encounters and exchanges are frequently conducted with minimal verbal output.

Training Use of Speech Acts

Possible training of the use of speech acts has been discussed by Wilcox (1983; Wilcox and Davis, 1977). Doyle et al. (1989a) presented a behavioral methodology for training speech acts—specifically, requesting—in conversation with Broca's aphasic adults. The training procedure was designed specifically to facilitate generalization. The approach involved training the aphasic adults with multiple trainers on several conversational topics with a list of prompts available to be used by the trainer. Prompts were employed to introduce and facilitate topics so that aphasic individuals could request information and maintain the topic. Requests were required to be intelligible and had to be related to the specified topic, but grammatical accuracy was not necessary. Weekly probes revealed increased requesting behavior, resulting in comparable performance to non-brain-damaged adults. Social validation of the treatment effects revealed significant improvement in the variables of talkativeness, inquisitiveness, and conversational success. More frequent requests for information were observed with both familiar and unfamiliar conversational partners; however, this finding was more robust for the familiar participants. Doyle et al. (1989b) replicated these findings with a more severely involved aphasic patient. This approach is structured yet provides the aphasic adult with opportunities for practice of basic communicative acts.

Conversational Strategy Development

Conversational strategies are devices that aid the aphasic patient in conveying messages or increase his or her ability to comprehend what others are saying. They can be verbal or nonverbal, ranging from circulocution to signaling non-brain-damaged speakers to speak more slowly. Holland (1991) suggests that when aiding an aphasic adult in developing useful strategies, the patient should be observed in interaction with the clinician and with significant others, including his or her most frequent communication partner (videotaped). Strategies used are identified, including those employed both by the patient and by the significant others with whom the patient communicates. Each strategy's effectiveness is determined. Observations are reported to the aphasic patient as well as to his or her significant other(s). Any possible compensations available to the patient should be discussed. If the patient and significant other require specific instruction in the use and/or development of conversational strategies, specific strategies are identified and targeted initially in constrained drill contexts. Contexts that require the patient to employ the particular strategy are then introduced, gradually moving to using the strategy in a more natural communicative context.

Conversational Coaching

Conversational coaching is a pragmatic approach developed by Holland (1991) as a means of transferring strategy usage to patient-generated conversation, approximating communication

beyond the clinical setting. The aphasic patient is required to produce a short monologue or script prepared by the clinician. The script should be a bit too difficult for the patient to produce, thereby encouraging the patient to use strategies he or she has practiced previously. The clinician and the patient practice the script, focusing on the use of strategies to convey the message of the monologue. The patient is then required to communicate the monologue to significant others while being coached by the clinician. Significant others also are coached by the clinician to practice strategies identified previously. Coaching sessions are videotaped for later review and discussion by the patient, clinician, and significant other. The process also should be conducted with an unfamiliar communication partner, providing an opportunity to generalize the approach. Scripts should vary in their information value and familiarity to the listener.

Enhancement of Standard Language Treatment

The premise of enhancing traditional language treatment from a pragmatic standpoint is to conduct standard clinical procedures in a more pragmatic fashion (Davis, 1989; Davis and Wilcox, 1985). This basically involves incorporating stimuli that are useful to patients and are consistent with their knowledge of the world. Clinicians should obtain as much information as possible about a patient's environment to establish sources of semantic content, thereby providing conditions that maximize shared knowledge between patient and clinician. Emotionally arousing content, in particular, may have a facilitative effect on verbal output (Davis, 1989). Hence, pragmatic treatment is conducted within the therapeutic setting, but features of the patient's outside environment interact with language treatment in typical stimulation activities. Davis and Wilcox (1985) suggest incorporating information from both horizontal and vertical contexts. Horizontal contexts are those representing current persons and settings, whereas vertical contexts represent settings and people from the individual's past.

Communication Partner Training

The value of training aphasic adults' communication partners has been identified (Garcia and Terrell, 1991; Linebaugh et al., 1984; Lyons, 1988, 1992; Newhoff et al., 1981; Simmons, et al., 1987; Towey and Pettit, 1980). In Lyons's (1988, 1992) approach, communicative partners are instructed on employing communication strategies that are effective in exchanging information. Subsequently, partners use the strategies with the aphasic adult in simulated situations, similar to role playing or PACE. The communicative partners are volunteers who are not obligated to meet the needs and desires of the patient. When the aphasic adult and partner are comfortable and competent in exchanging information, treatment is conducted in natural settings. The patient is encouraged to select an afternoon activity within the community in which he or she would like to engage but has avoided since the stroke. This activity is undertaken with the communication partner. Lyons views this process as a means of integrated both psychosocial and communication concerns into treatment, providing aphasic adults with the opportunity to view themselves as a viable companion with individuals who are not committed to them.

Summary of Pragmatic Treatment

As mentioned previously, the general aim of pragmatics treatment is to improve language function. Elements of natural communication are applied to traditional clinical procedures by modifying the contexts in which these approaches are conducted. Therefore, overall goals of aphasia treatment are not dramatically revised by incorporating the principles of pragmatics. That is, objectives continue to be geared toward altering behaviors/situations that limit aphasic adults' communication.

The procedures presented here demonstrate an application of pragmatics by either manipulating features of the aphasic individual's natural communicative contexts or creating interactional situations that are typical of natural conversation, within the therapeutic setting.

FUTURE TRENDS

Pragmatics is currently viewed as the interaction between language behavior and the specific contexts in which it is used. In the last few years, cognitive psychology and psycholinguistic practices of exploring these language-context interactions have been applied to the study of brain-damaged populations, particularly those individuals with aphasia. This trend appears to be continuing, with future emphasis on improving the methodology for examining natural contexts, developing valid and convenient tools for the clinical assessment of pragmatic skills, and using efficacious treatment techniques to remediate the functions of language. In identifying pragmatic therapeutic approaches that are reliable and effective, clinical aphasiologists will continue to grapple with the apportioning of clinical time among the pragmatic and the more traditionally defined linguistic aspects of aphasia treatment. However, concern for the overall communicative abilities of aphasic adults should lead clinicians to the realization that pragmatic considerations should always be a factor in treatment. This is because the primary goal of therapeutic remediation with aphasic adults should be to converse about whatever that individual wants to discuss.

The study of pragmatics as the science of language functions has validated treatment of language-contextual interactions as relevant to stimulating language behavior. Some researchers have begun to identify particular contextual settings and situations that result in increased language processing for the aphasic adult. The nature and specific features of these facilitating contexts require clear delineation, however, so that clinicians can use this information consistently and appropriately with other aphasic adults. Furthermore, attention should be devoted to exploring aphasic adults' prosocial awareness systematically. *How* an individual specifically responds within common social situations is the basis of true socialization. It is hoped that expanding the study of pragmatics to the investigation of this sociolinguistic phenomenon will enhance clinical aphasiologists' understanding of the simultaneous interaction of various components of communication.

Recently, neurogenic research has addressed the pragmatic abilities of other brain-damaged populations, including adults who have suffered right-hemisphere damage as the result of a cerebrovascular accident and diffuse damage as the result of a closed head injury. This trend will probably continue, focusing on the specific cues and contexts with which these populations have difficulty. In addition, further emphasis should be placed on identifying the underlying bases for the significant pragmatic deficits observed in both populations. The speech-language pathologist has been responsible for intervention with these individuals. However, assessment and treatment of these prag-

matic communication problems has been relatively incomplete. Development and implementation of tools for evaluating and remediating the pragmatic abilities of adults with right-hemisphere damage and/or closed head injuries should continue to be an area of study.

References

Agar, M., and Hobbs, J. R. (1982). Interpreting discourse: Coherence and the analysis of ethnographic interview. *Discourse Processes, 5,* 1–32.

Apel, K., Newhoff, M., and Browning-Hall, J. (1982, November). *Contingent queries in Broca's aphasia.* Paper presented at the American Speech-Language-Hearing Association convention, Toronto.

Armstrong, E. (1987). Cohesive harmony in aphasic discourse and its significance in listener perception of coherence. In R. H. Brookshire (Ed.), *Clinical Ahasiology Conference proceedings.* Minneapolis, MN: BRK.

Armstrong, E. (1991). The potential of cohesion analysis in the analysis and treatment of aphasic discourse. *Clinical Linguistics and Phonetics, 5,* 39–52.

Armus, S., Brookshire, R., and Nicholas, L. (1989). Aphasic and non-brain-damaged adults' knowledge of scripts for common situations. *Brain and Language, 36,* 518–528.

Aten, J. L. (1986). Functional communication treatment. In R. Chapey (Ed.), *Language intervention strategies in adult aphasia.* Baltimore, MD: Williams & Wilkins.

Aten, J., Caligiuri, M., and Holland, A. (1982). The efficacy of functional communication therapy for chronic aphasic patients. *Journal of Speech and Hearing Disorders, 47,* 93–96.

Ball, M., Davies, E., Duckworth, M., and Middlehurst, R. (1991). Assessing the assessments: A comparison of two clinical pragmatic profiles. *Journal of Communication Disorders, 24,* 367–379.

Balota, D., Ferraro, R., and Connor, L. (1991). On the early influence of meaning in word recognition: A review of the literature. In P. Schwanenflugel (Ed.), *The psychology of word meaning.* Hillsdale, NJ: Lawrence Erlbaum.

Barclay, J., Bransford, J., Franks, J., McCarrell, N., and Nitsch, K. (1974). Comprehension and semantic flexibility. *Journal of Verbal Learning and Verbal Behavior, 13,* 471–481.

Bard, E., Shillcock, R., and Altmann, G. (1988). The recognition of words after their acoustic offsets in spontaneous speech: Effects of subsequent context. *Perception and Psychophysics, 44,* 395–408.

Barsalou, L. (1982). Context-independent and context-dependent information in concepts. *Memory and Cognition, 10,* 82–93.

Bates, E., Hamby, S., and Zurif, E. (1983). The effects of focal brain-damage on pragmatic expression. *Canadian Journal of Psychology, 37,* 59–84.

Baum, S., Daniloff, J., Daniloff, R., and Lewis, J. (1982). Sentence comprehension by Broca's aphasics: Effects of some suprasegmental variables. *Brain and Language, 17,* 261–271.

Behrmann, M., and Penn, C. (1984). Non-verbal communication of aphasic patients. *British Journal of Disorders of Communication, 19,* 155–168.

Berko-Gleason, J., Goodglass, H., Obler, L., Green, E., Hyde, M., and Weintraub, S. (1980). Narrative strategies of aphasic and normal speaking subjects. *Journal of Speech and Hearing Research, 23,* 370–382.

Blumstein, S., and Goodglass, H. (1972). The perception of stress as a semantic cue in aphasia. *Journal of Speech and Hearing Research, 15,* 800–806.

Bond, S., Ulatowska, H., Macaluso-Haynes, S., and May, E. (1983). Discourse production in aphasia: Relationship to severity of impairment. In R. Brookshire (Ed.), *Clinical Aphasiology Conference proceedings.* Minneapolis, MN: BRK.

Bottenberg, D., and Lemme, M. L. (1989). Effect of shared and unshared listener knowledge on narratives of normal and aphasic adults. In T. Prescott (Ed.), *Clinical aphasiology* (Vol. 19, pp. 109–116). Austin, TX: Pro-Ed.

Bottenberg, D., Lemme, M., and Hedberg, N. (1985). Analysis of oral narratives of normal and aphasic adults. In R. Brookshire (Ed.), *Clinical Aphasiology Conference proceedings.* Minneapolis, MN: BRK.

Bottenberg, D., Lemme, M., and Hedberg, N. (1987). Effect of story content on narrative discourse of aphasic adults. In R. H. Brookshire (Ed.), *Clinical Aphasiology Conference proceedings.* Minneapolis, MN: BRK.

Brenneise-Sarshad, R., Brookshire, R., and Nicholas, L. (1989). Effects of listener knowledge on stories told by aphasic and non-brain-damaged subjects. In T. Prescott (Ed.), *Clinical aphasiology* (Vol. 19). Austin, TX: Pro-Ed.

Brenneise-Sarshad, R., Nicholas, L. E., and Brookshire, R. H. (1991). Effects of apparent listener knowledge and picture stimuli on aphasic and non-brain-damaged speakers' narrative discourse. *Journal of Speech and Hearing Research, 34,* 168–176.

Brookshire, R. (1987). Auditory language comprehension disorders in aphasia. *Topics in Language Disorders, 8,* 11–23.

Brookshire, R., and Nicholas, L. (1984). Comprehension of directly and indirectly stated main ideas and details in discourse by brain-damaged and non-brain-damaged listeners. *Brain and Language, 21,* 21–36.

Bryan, K. L. (1989). Language prosody and the right hemisphere. *Aphasiology, 3,* 285–300.

Buck, R., and Duffy, R. J. (1980). Nonverbal communication of affect in brain-damaged patients. *Cortex, 16,* 351–362.

Busch, C. R., Brookshire, R. H., and Nicholas, L. E. (1988). Referential communication by aphasic and nonaphasic adults. *Journal of Speech and Hearing Disorders, 53,* 475–482.

Butler-Hinz, S., Waters, G., and Caplan, D. (1990). Characteristics of syntactic comprehension deficits following closed head injury versus left cerebrovascular accident. *Journal of Speech and Hearing Research, 33,* 269–280.

Cannito, M., Jarecki, J., and Pierce, R. (1986). Effects of thematic structure on syntactic processing in aphasia. *Brain and Language, 27,* 38–49.

Cannito, M., Vogel, D., and Pierce, R. (1988). Sentence comprehension in context: Influence of prior visual stimulation. In T. Prescott (Ed.), *Clinical aphasiology* (Vol. 18). Boston, MA: College Hill Press.

Cannito, M., Vogel, D., and Pierce, R. (1990). Contextualized sentence comprehension in nonfluent aphasia: Predictiveness and severity of comprehension impairment. In T. Prescott (Ed.), *Clinical aphasiology* (Vol. 20). Austin, TX: Pro-Ed.

Cannito, M., Vogel, D., Pierce, R., and Hough, M. (1991). Time post-onset and contextualized sentence comprehension in nonfluent aphasia. In M. Lemme (Ed.), *Clinical aphasiology* (Vol. 21). Austin, TX: Pro-Ed.

Caplan, D., and Evans, K. (1990). The effects of syntactic structure on discourse comprehension in patients with parsing impairments. *Brain and Language, 39,* 206–234.

Caramazza, A., and Miceli, G. (1991). Selective impairment of thematic role assignment in sentence processing. *Brain and Language, 41,* 402–436.

Caramazza, A., and Zurif, E. (1976). Dissociation of algorithmic and heuristic processes in language comprehension: Evidence from aphasia. *Brain and Language, 3,* 572–582.

Chapman, S. B., and Ulatowska, H. K. (1992). Methodology for discourse management in the treatment of aphasia. *Clinics in Communication Disorders, 2,* 64–81.

Chenery, H., Ingram, J., and Murdock, B. (1990). Automatic and volitional processing in aphasia. *Brain and Language, 38,* 215–232.

Cicone, M., Wapner, W., Foldi, N., Zurif, E., and Gardner, H. (1979). The relationship between gesture and language in aphasic communication. *Brain and Language, 8,* 324–349.

Clark, A., and Flowers, C. (1987). The effect of semantic redundancy on auditory comprehension in aphasia. In R. K. Brookshire (Ed.), *Clinical Aphasiology Conference proceedings.* Minneapolis, MN: BRK.

Clark, H. H., and Haviland, S. E. (1977). Comprehension and the given-new contract. In R. O. Freedle (Ed.), *Discourse production and comprehension.* Norwood, NJ: Ablex.

Coggins, T. E. (1991). Bringing context back in assessment. *Topics in Language Disorders, 11,* 43–54.

Copeland, M. (1989). An assessment of natural conversation with Broca's aphasics. *Aphasiology, 3,* 301–306.

Correia, L., Brookshire, R. H., and Nicholas, L. E. (1990). Aphasic and non-brain-damaged adults' descriptions of aphasia test pictures and gender-biased pictures. *Journal of Speech and Hearing Disorders, 4,* 713–720.

Daniloff, J. K., Fritelli, G., Buckingham, H. W., Hoffman, P. R., and Daniloff, R. G. (1986). Amer-Ind versus ASL: Recognition and imitation in aphasic subjects. *Brain and Language, 28,* 95–113.

Danly, M., Cooper, W., and Shapiro, B. (1983). Fundamental frequency, language processing, and linguistic structure in Wernicke's aphasia. *Brain and Language, 19,* 1–24.

Danly, M., and Shapiro, B. (1982). Speech prosody in Broca's aphasia. *Brain and Language, 16,* 171–190.

Davis, G. A. (1986). Pragmatics and treatment. In R. Chapey (Ed.), *Language intervention strategies in adult aphasia* (2nd ed.). Baltimore, MD: Williams & Wilkins.

Davis, G. A. (1989). Pragmatics and cognition in treatment of language disorders. In X. Seron and G. Deloche (Eds.), *Cognitive approaches in neuropsychological rehabilitation.* Hillsdale, NJ: Lawrence Erlbaum.

Davis, G. A., and Wilcox, M. J. (1981). Incorporating parameters of natural conversation in aphasia treatment. In R. Chapey (Ed.), *Language intervention strategies in adult aphasia.* Baltimore, MD: Williams & Wilkins.

Davis, G. A., and Wilcox, M. J. (1985). *Adult aphasia rehabilitation: Applied pragmatics.* San Diego, CA: College Hill Press.

De Bleser, R., and Poeck, K. (1985). Analysis of prosody in the spontaneous speech of patients with CV-recurring utterances. *Cortex, 21,* 405–416.

Deloche, G., and Seron, X. (1981). Sentence understanding and knowledge of the world: Evidence from a sentence-picture matching task performed by aphasic patients. *Brain and Language, 14,* 57–69.

DeMarco, S., and Hough, M. S. (1991, April). *Conversational skills in children and adults with right hemisphere dysfunction.* Miniseminar presented at the annual North Carolina Speech-Hearing-Language Association convention, Raleigh, NC.

Dembowski, J., Ulatowska, H. K., and Haynes, S. M. (1989, November). *Clinical evaluation of aphasic discourse.* Paper presented at the annual American Speech-Language-Hearing Association convention, St. Louis, MO.

Dennis, M., and Lovett, M. W. (1990). Discourse ability in children after brain damage. In Y. Joanette and H. H. Brownell (Eds.), *Discourse ability and brain damage.* New York: Springer-Verlag.

Doyle, P. J. Goldstein, H., Bourgeois, M. S., and Nakles, K. O. (1989a). Facilitating generalized requesting behavior in Broca's aphasia: An experimental analysis of a generalization training procedure. *Journal of Applied Behavior Analysis, 22,* 157–170.

Doyle, P. J., Oleyar, K. S., and Goldstein, H. (1989b). Facilitating functional conversational skills in aphasia: An experimental analysis of a generalization training procedure. In T. Prescott (Ed.), *Clinical aphasiology* (Vol. 19 pp. 229–242). Austin, TX: Pro-Ed.

Duffy, R. J., and Duffy, J. R. (1981). Three studies of deficits in pantomimic recognition in aphasia. *Journal of Speech and Hearing Research, 24,* 70–84.

Duffy, R. J., Duffy, J. R., and Mercaitis, P. A. (1984). Comparison of the performances of a fluent and a nonfluent aphasic on a pantomimic referential task. *Brain and Language, 21,* 260–273.

Early, E. A., and Van Demark, A. A. (1985). Aphasic speakers' use of definite and indefinite articles to mark given and new information in discourse. In R. Brookshire (Ed.), *Clinical Aphasiology Conference proceedings.* Minneapolis, MN: BRK.

Ernest-Baron, C. R., Brookshire, R. H., and Nicholas, L. E. (1987). Story structure and retelling of narratives by aphasic and non-brain-damaged adults. *Journal of Speech and Hearing Research, 30,* 44–49.

Feyereisen, P. (1983). Manual activity during speaking in aphasic subjects. *International Journal of Psychology, 18,* 545–556.

Feyereisen, P. (1988). Non-verbal communication. In F. C. Rose, R. Whurr, and M. A. Wyke, (Eds.), *Aphasia.* London: Whurr Publishers.

Feyereisen, P., and Seron, X. (1982). Nonverbal communication and aphasia: A review II. Expression. *Brain and Language, 16,* 213–236.

Flowers, C., and Peizer, E. (1984). Strategies for obtaining information from aphasic persons. In R. Brookshire (Ed.), *Clinical Aphasiology Conference proceedings.* Minneapolis, MN: BRK.

Foldi, N. (1987). Appreciation of pragmatic interpretations of indirect commands: Comparison of right and left hemisphere brain-damaged patients. *Brain and Language, 31,* 88–108.

Foldi, N. S., Cicone, M., and Gardner, H. (1983). Pragmatic aspects of communication in brain-damaged patients. In S. Segalowitz (Ed.), *Language functions and brain organization.* New York: Academic Press.

Gainotti, G. (1972). Emotional behavior and hemispheric side of lesion. *Cortex, 8,* 41–55.

Garcia, J. M., and Terrell, P. (1991, November). *Communication competence: including partner training in treatment for Broca's aphasia.* Paper presented at the American Speech-Language-Hearing annual convention, Atlanta, GA.

Gerber, S., and Gurland, G. (1989). Applied pragmatics in the assessment of aphasia. *Seminars in Speech and Language: Aphasia and Pragmatics, 10,* 263–281.

Germani, M. (1992). *Semantic attribute knowledge in adults with right and left hemisphere damage.* Unpublished doctoral dissertation, Kent State University, Kent, OH.

Germani, M., and Pierce, R. (1992). Contextual influences in reading comprehension in aphasia. *Brain and Language, 42,* 308–319.

Gibbs, R. W., Jr. (1981). Your wish is my command: Convention and context in interpreting indirect requests. *Journal of Verbal Learning and Verbal Behavior, 20,* 431–444.

Glosser, G., and Deser, T. (1990). Patterns of discourse production among neurological patients with fluent language disorders. *Brain and Language, 40,* 67–88.

Glosser, G., Weiner, M., and Kaplan, E. (1986). Communicative gestures in aphasia. *Brain and Language, 27,* 345–359.

Glosser, G., Weiner, M., and Kaplan, E. (1988). Variations in aphasic language behaviors. *Journal of Speech and Hearing Disorders, 53,* 115–124.

Goldstein, A. P., Sprafkin, R. P., Gershaw, N. J., and Klein, P. (1980). *Skill-streaming the adolescent: A structured approach to teaching prosocial skills.* Champaign, IL: Research Press Company.

Goodglass, H., and Baker, E. (1976). Semantic field, naming, and auditory comprehension in aphasia. *Brain and Language, 3,* 359–374.

Goodglass, H., and Kaplan, E. (1963). Disturbance of gesture and pantomime in aphasia. *Brain, 86,* 703–720.

Goodglass, H., and Kaplan, E. (1983). *The assessment of aphasia and related disorders.* Philadelphia, PA: Lea & Febiger.

Green, E., and Boller, F. (1974). Features of auditory comprehension in severely impaired aphasics. *Cortex, 10,* 133–145.

Green, G. (1982). Assessment and treatment of the adult with severe aphasia: Aiming for functional generalization. *Australian Journal of Human Communication Disorders, 10,* 11–23.

Green, G. (1984). Communication in aphasia therapy: Some of the procedures and issues involved. *British Journal of Disorders of Communication, 19,* 35–46.

Greenspan, S. (1986). Semantic flexibility and referential specificity of concrete nouns. *Journal of Memory and Language, 25,* 539–557.

Grice, H. (1975). Logic and conversation. In P. Cole and J. Morgan (Eds.), *Syntax and semantics.* New York: Academic Press.

Grogan, S. (1993). *An assessment of reading comprehension for adults with aphasia.* Unpublished doctoral dissertation, Kent State University, Kent, OH.

Guilford, A., and O'Connor, J. (1982). Pragmatic functions in aphasia. *Journal of Communication Disorder, 15,* 337–346.

Gurland, G., Chwat, S., and Wollner, S. (1982). Establishing a communication profile in adult aphasia: Analysis of communicative acts and conversational sequences. In R. Brookshire (Ed.), *Clinical Aphasiology Conference proceedings.* Minneapolis, MN: BRK.

Halliday, M., and Hasan, R. (1976). *Cohesion in English.* London: Longman.

Hand, R., and Tonkovich, J. (1979). *Language pragmatics: Implications for the diagnosis and treatment of aphasia.* Paper presented at the Kansas Symposium on Speech, Language and Auditory Pathology, Overland Park, KS.

Hasan, R. (1985). The texture of a text. In M. A. K. Halliday and R. Hasan (Eds.), *Language, context and text: Aspects of language in a social-semiotic perspective.* Victoria, Canada: Deakin University Press.

Haviland, S., and Clark, H. (1974). What's new? Acquiring new information as a process in comprehension. *Journal of Verbal Learning and Verbal Behavior, 13,* 512–521.

Heilman, K., Bowers, D., Speedie, L., and Coslett, H. (1984). Comprehension of affective and nonaffective prosody. *Neurology, 34,* 917–921.

Herrmann, M., Koch, U., Johannsen-Horbach, H., and Wallesch, C. W. (1989). Communicative skills in chronic and severe nonfluent aphasia. *Brain and Language, 37,* 339–352.

Herrmann, M., Reichle, T., Lucius-Hoene, G., Wallesch, C. W., and Johannsen-Horbach, H. (1988). Nonverbal communication as a compensatory strategy for severely nonfluent aphasics—a quantitative approach. *Brain and Language, 33,* 41–54.

Hinckley, J., and Craig, H. (1992). A comparison of picture-stimulus and conversational elicitation contexts: Responses to comments by adults with aphasia. *Aphasiology, 6,* 257–272.

Holland, A. (1977). Some practical considerations in aphasia rehabilitation. In M. Sullivan and M. Kommers (Eds.), *Rationale for adult aphasia therapy.* Omaha, NE: University of Nebraska Press.

Holland, A. (1980). *Communicative abilities in daily living: A test of functional communication for aphasic adults.* Baltimore, MD: University Park Press.

Holland, A. L. (1991). Pragmatic aspects of intervention in aphasia. *Journal of Neurolinguistics. 6,* 197–211.

Hough, M. S. (1990). Narrative comprehension in adults with right and left hemisphere brain-damage: Theme organization. *Brain and Language, 38,* 253–277.

Hough, M., Pierce, R. S. (1987, Spring). Pragmatic functioning in adult aphasia. *HEARSAY—Journal of the Ohio Speech and Hearing Association,* pp. 46–53.

Hough, M., Pierce, R., and Cannito, M. (1989). Contextual influences in aphasia: Effects of predictive versus nonpredictive narratives. *Brain and Language, 36,* 325–334.

Houghton, P., Pettit, J., and Towey, M. (1982). Measuring communication competence in global aphasia. In R. Brookshire (Ed.), *Clinical Aphasiology Conference proceedings.* Minneapolis, MN: BRK.

Huber, W. (1990). Text comprehension and production in aphasia: Analysis in terms of micro- and macrostructure. In Y. Joanette and H. Brownell (Eds.), *Discourse ability and brain damage: Theoretical and empirical perspectives.* New York: Springer-Verlag.

James, S. (1990). *Normal language acquisition.* Boston, MA: College Hill Press.

Juncos-Rabadán, O. (1992). The processing of negative sentences in fluent aphasics: Semantic and pragmatic aspects. *Brain and Language, 43,* 96–106.

Katsuki-Nakamura, J., Brookshire, R., and Nicholas, L. (1988). Comprehension of monologues and dialogues by aphasic listeners. *Journal of Speech and Hearing Disorders, 53,* 408–415.

Katz, R. C., LaPointe, L. L., and Markel, N. N. (1978). Coverbal behavior and aphasic speakers. In R. Brookshire (Ed.), *Clinical Aphasiology Conference proceedings.* Minneapolis, MN: BRK.

Kellas, G., Paul, S., Martin, M., and Simpson, G. (1991). Contextual feature activation and meaning access. In G. Simpson (Ed.), *Understanding word and sentence.* New York: North-Holland.

Kimbarow, M., and Brookshire, R. (1983). The influence of communicative context on aphasic speakers' use of pronouns. In R. Brookshire (Ed.), *Clinical Aphasiology Conference proceedings.* Minneapolis, MN: BRK.

Kimelman, M. (1991). The role of target word stress in auditory comprehension by aphasic listeners. *Journal of Speech and Hearing Research, 34,* 334–339.

Kintsch, W., and van Dijk, T. (1978). Toward a model of text comprehension and production. *Psychological Review, 85,* 363–394.

Kudo, T. (1984). The effect of semantic plausibility on sentence comprehension in aphasia. *Brain and Language, 21,* 208–218.

Larkins, P., and Webster, E. (1981). The use of gestures in dyads consisting of an aphasic and nonaphasic adult. In R. Brookshire (Ed.), *Clinical Aphasiology Conference proceedings.* Minneapolis, MN: BRK.

Lemme, M., Hedberg, N., and Bottenberg, D. (1984). Cohesion in narratives of aphasic adults. In R. Brookshire (Ed.), *Clinical Aphasiology Conference proceedings.* Minneapolis, MN: BRK.

Lesser, R. (1991). Three developments in aphasiology: Cognitive neuropsychology, computers in therapy, pragmatic-ethnological approach. *Journal of Neurolinguistics, 6,* 71–77.

Linebaugh, C., Kryzer, K., Oden, S., and Myers, P. (1982). Reapportionment of communicative burden in aphasia: A study of narrative instructions. In R. Brookshire (Ed.), *Clinical Aphasiology Conference proceedings.* Minneapolis, MN: BRK.

Linebaugh, C. W., Marguiles, C. P., and Mackisack, E. L. (1985). Contingent queries and revisions used by aphasic individuals and their most frequent communication partners. In R. Brookshire (Ed.), *Clinical Aphasiology Conference proceedings.* Minneapolis, MN: BRK.

Linebaugh, C. W., Marguiles, C. P., and Mackisack-Morin, E. L. (1984). The effectiveness of comprehension-enhancing strategies employed by spouses of aphasic patients. In R. Brookshire (Ed.), *Clinical Aphasiology Conference proceedings.* Minneapolis, MN: BRK.

Lomas, J., Pickard, L., Bester, S., Elbard, H., Finlayson, A., and Zoghaib, C. (1989). The Communicative Effectiveness Index: Development and psychometric evaluation of a functional communication measure for adult aphasia. *Journal of Speech and Hearing Disorders, 54,* 113–124.

Lubinski, R. (1981). Environmental language intervention. In R. Chapey (Ed.), *Language intervention strategies in adult aphasia.* Baltimore, MD: Williams & Wilkins.

Lubinski, R., Duchan, J., and Weitzner-Lin, B. (1980). Analysis of breakdowns and repairs in aphasic adult communication. In R. Brookshire (Ed.), *Clinical Aphasiology Conference proceedings.* Minneapolis, MN: BRK.

Lyons, J. G. (1988). Communicative partners: Their value in reestablishing communication with aphasic adults. In T. Prescott (Ed.), *Clinical aphasiology* (Vol. 18, pp. 11–18). Austin, TX: Pro-Ed.

Lyons, J. G. (1992). Communication use and participation in life for adults with aphasia in natural settings: The scope of the problem. *American Journal of Speech-Language Pathology, 1,*(3), 7–14.

MacWhinney, B., and Bates, E. (1978). Sentential devices for conveying giveness and newness: A cross-cultural developmental study. *Journal of Verbal Learning and Verbal Behavior, 17,* 539–558.

McNeil, M., Odell, K., and Tseng, C. (1990). Toward the integration of resource allocation into a general theory of aphasia. In T. Prescott (Ed.), *Clinical aphasiology* (Vol. 20). Austin, TX: Pro-Ed.

Miceli, G., Gainotti, G., Caltagirnone, C., and Masullo, C. (1980). Some aspects of phonological impairment in aphasia. *Brain and Language, 11,* 159–169.

Milroy, L., and Perkins, L. (1992). Repair strategies in aphasic discourse: Towards a collaborative model. *Clinical Linguistics and Phonetics, 6,* 27–40.

Morreau, L. E., and Bruininks, R. H. (1991). *Checklist of Adaptive Living Skills.* Allen, TX: DLM.

Morrow, D., Bower, G., and Greenspan, S. (1990). Situation-based inferences during narrative comprehension. In A. Graesser and G. Bower (Eds.), *Inferences and text comprehension.* New York: Academic Press.

Mross, E. (1990). Text analysis: Macro- and microstructural aspects of discourse processing. In Y. Joanette and H. Brownell (Eds.), *Discourse ability and brain-damage: Theoretical and empirical perspectives.* New York: Springer-Verlag.

Myers, P., and Linebaugh, C. (1981). Comprehension of idiomatic expressions by right-hemisphere-damaged adults. In R. Brookshire (Ed.), *Clinical Aphasiology Conference proceedings.* Minneapolis, MN: BRK.

Naeser, M., Mazurski, P., Goodglass, H., Peraino, M., Laughlin, S., and Leaper, W. (1987). Auditory syntactic comprehension in nine aphasia groups (with CT scans) and children: Differences in degree but not order of difficulty observed. *Cortex, 23,* 359–380.

Newhoff, M., and Apel, K. (1989). Environmental communication programming with aphasic persons. *Seminars in Speech and Language: Aphasia and Pragmatics, 10,* 315–328.

Newhoff, M., and Apel, K. (1990). Impairments in pragmatics. In L. LaPointe (Ed.), *Aphasia and related neurogenic language disorders.* New York: Thieme Medical Publishers, Inc.

Newhoff, M., Bugbee, J. K., and Ferreira, A. (1981). A change of PACE: Spouses as treatment targets. In R. Brookshire (Ed.), *Clinical Aphasiology Conference proceedings.* Minneapolis, MN: BRK.

Newhoff, M., Tonkovich, J. D., Schwartz, S. L., and Burgess, E. K. (1985). Revision strategies in aphasia. *Journal of Neurological Communication Disorders, 2,* 2–7.

Nicholas, L., and Brookshire, R. (1986). Consistency of the effects of rate of speech on brain-damaged adults' comprehension of narrative discourse. *Journal of Speech and Hearing Research, 29,* 462–470.

Nicholas, L., MacLennan, D., and Brookshire, R. (1986). Validity of multiple-sentence reading comprehension tests for aphasic adults. *Journal of Speech and Hearing Disorders, 51,* 82–87.

Oden, G., Rueckl, J., and Sanocki, T. (1991). Making sentences make sense, or words to that effect. In G. Simpson (Ed.), *Understanding word and sentence.* New York: North-Holland.

Parisi, D., and Pizzamiglio, L. (1970). Syntactic comprehension in aphasia. *Cortex, 6,* 204–215.

Pashek, G., and Brookshire, R. (1982). Effects of rate of speech and linguistic stress on auditory paragraph comprehension of aphasic individuals. *Journal of Speech and Hearing Research, 25,* 377–383.

Patterson, J., and Pierce, R. (1991, November). *Memory for narrative discourse in adults with mild language impairment following left or right cerebrovascular accident.* Paper presented at the American Speech-Language-Hearing Association annual convention, Atlanta, GA.

Peach, R., Canter, G., and Gallaher, A. (1988). Comprehension of sentence structure in anomic and conduction aphasia. *Brain and Language, 35,* 119–137.

Penn, C. (1988). The profiling of syntax and pragmatics in aphasia. *Clinical Linguistics and Phonetics, 2,* 179–208.

Petersen, L. N., and Kirshner, H. S. (1981). Gestural impairment and gestural ability in aphasia: A review. *Brain and Language, 14,* 333–348.

Piehler, M., and Holland, A. (1984). Cohesion in aphasic language. In R. H. Brookshire (Ed.), *Clinical Aphasiology Conference proceedings.* Minneapolis, MN: BRK.

Pierce, R. (1988a). Influence of prior and subsequent context on comprehension in aphasia. *Aphasiology, 2,* 577–582.

Pierce, R. (1988b). Language processing and the effects of context in aphasia. In M. J. Ball (Ed.), *Theoretical linguistics and disordered language.* San Diego, CA: College Hill Press.

Pierce, R. (1991). Contextual influences during comprehension in aphasia. *Aphasiology, 5,* 1–36.

Pierce, R., and Beekman, L. (1985). Effects of linguistic and extralinguistic context on semantic and syntactic processing in aphasia. *Journal of Speech and Hearing Research, 28,* 250–254.

Pierce, R., and DeStefano, C. (1987). The interactive nature of auditory comprehension in aphasia. *Journal of Communication Disorders, 18,* 203–214.

Pierce, R., and Grogan, S. (1992). Improving listening comprehension of narratives. *Clinics in Communication Disorders: Aphasia, 2,* 54–63.

Pierce, R., and Wagner, C. (1985). The role of context in facilitating syntactic decoding in aphasia. *Journal of Communication Disorders, 18,* 203–214.

Potechin, G. C., Nicholas, L. E., and Brookshire, R. H. (1987). Effects of picture stimuli on discourse production by aphasia. In R. H. Brookshire (Ed.), *Clinical Aphasiology Conference proceedings.* Minneapolis, MN: BRK.

Prinz, P. (1980). A note on requesting strategies in adult aphasics. *Journal of Communication Disorders, 13,* 65–73.

Prutting, C. A. (1982). Pragmatics as social competence. *Journal of Speech and Hearing Disorders, 47,* 123–134.

Prutting, C. A., and Kirchner, D. M. (1983). Applied pragmatics. In T. Gallagher and C. A. Prutting (Eds.), *Pragmatic assessment and intervention issues in language.* San Diego, CA: College Hill Press.

Prutting, C. A., and Kirchner, D. M. (1987). A clinical appraisal of the pragmatic aspects of language. *Journal of Speech and Hearing Disorders, 52,* 105–119.

Puskaric, N., and Pierce, R. (1991, November). Reading comprehension in aphasia: Effects of prediction and expectation. Paper presented at the American Speech-Language-Hearing Association annual convention, Atlanta, GA.

Rivers, D. L., and Love, R. J. (1980). Language performance on visual processing tasks in right hemisphere lesion cases. *Brain and Language, 10,* 348–366.

Roberts, J. A., and Wertz, R. T. (1988). Comparison of spontaneous and elicited oral-expressive language in aphasia. In T. Prescott (Ed.), *Clinical aphasiology* (Vol. 18, pp. 479–488). Austin, TX: Pro-Ed.

Rosenthal, V., and Bisiacchi, P. (submitted). Tacit integration and referential structure in the language comprehension of aphasics and normals.

Rueckl, J., and Oden, G. (1985). The integration of contextual and featural information during word identification. *Journal of Memory and Language, 25,* 445–460.

Ryalls, J. H. (1982). Intonation in Broca's aphasias. *Neuropsychologia, 20,* 355–360.

Ryalls, J. H. (1984). Some acoustic aspects of fundamental frequency of CVC utterances in aphasia. *Phonetica, 41,* 103–111.

Sarno, M. (1972). A measurement of functional communication in aphasia. In M. Sarno (Ed.), *Aphasia: Selected readings.* New York: Appleton-Century-Crofts.

Schienberg, S., and Holland, A. (1980). Conversational turn-taking in Wernicke's aphasia. In R. H. Brookshire (Ed.), *Clinical Aphasiology Conference proceedings.* Minneapolis, MN: BRK.

Schlanger, B., Schlanger, P., and Gerstman, L. (1976). The perception of emotionally toned sentences by right hemisphere-damaged and aphasic subjects. *Brain and Language, 3,* 396–403.

Schnitzer, M. (1989). *The pragmatic basis of aphasia: A neurolinguistics study of morphosyntaxis among bilinguals.* Hillsdale, NJ: Lawrence Erlbaum.

Schuell, H. (1965). *The Minnesota Test for Differential Diagnosis of Aphasia.* Minneapolis, MN: University of Minnesota Press.

Schwanenflugel, P. (1991). Contextual constraint and lexical processing. In G. Simpson (Ed.), *Understanding word and sentence.* New York: North-Holland.

Schwanenflugel, P., and Shoben, E. (1985). The influence of sentence constraint on the scope of facilitation for upcoming words. *Journal of Memory and Language, 24,* 232–252.

Searle, J. (1969). *Speech acts: An essay in the philosophy of language.* London: Cambridge University Press.

Seron, X., Van der Kaa, M., Van der Linden, M., Remits, A., and Feyereisen, P. (1982). Decoding paralinguistic signals: Effect of semantic and prosodic cues on aphasics' comprehension. *Journal of Communication Disorders, 15,* 223–231.

Shadden, B. B., Burnette, R. B., Eikenberry, B. R., and Dibrezzo, R. (1990). All discourse tasks are not created equal. In T. Prescott (Ed.), *Clinical aphasiology* (Vol. 20, pp. 327–342). Austin, TX: Pro-Ed.

Sherman, J., and Schweickert, J. (1989). Syntactic and semantic contributions to sentence comprehension in agrammatism. *Brain and Language, 37,* 419–439.

Silveri, M., Carlomagno, S., Nocentini, U., Chieffi, S., and Gainotti, G. (1989). Semantic field integrity and naming ability in anomic patients. *Aphasiology, 3,* 423–434.

Simmons, N. N., Kearns, K. P., and Potechin, G. (1987). Treatment of aphasia through family member training. In R. Brookshire (Ed.), *Clinical Aphasiology Conference proceedings*. Minneapolis, MN: BRK.

Smith, R. (1988). Pragmatics and speech pathology. In M. J. Ball (Ed.), *Theoretical linguistics and disordered language*. San Diego, CA: College Hill Press.

Speedie, L. J., Coslett, H. B., and Heilman, K. M. (1984). Repetition of affective prosody in mixed transcortical aphasia. *Archives of Neurology, 41,* 268–270.

Tabossi, P. (1991). Understanding words in context. In G. Simpson (Ed.), *Understanding word and sentence*. New York: North-Holland.

Terrell, B., and Ripich, D. (1989). Discourse competence as a variable in intervention. *Seminars in Speech and Language: Aphasia and Pragmatics, 10,* 282–297.

Towey, M. P., and Pettit, J. M. (1980). Improving communication competence in global aphasia. In R. Brookshire (Ed.), *Clinical Aphasiology Conference proceedings*. Minneapolis, MN: BRK.

Tracy, K. (1984). Staying on topic: An explication of conversational relevance. *Discourse Processes, 7,* 447–464.

Ulatowska, H. K., Allard, L., and Chapman, S. B. (1990). Narrative and procedural discourse in aphasia. In Y. Joanette and H. H. Brownell (Eds.), *Discourse ability and brain and damage*. New York: Springer-Verlag.

Ulatowska, H. K., Allard, L., Reyes, B. A., Ford, J., and Chapman, S. (1992). Conversational discourse in aphasia. *Aphasiology, 6,* 325–331.

Ulatowska, H., and Bond, S. (1983). Aphasia: Discourse considerations. In K. Butler (Ed.), *Topics in language disorders* (Vol. 3). Gaithersburg, MD: Aspen Systems Corporation.

Ulatowska, H. K., and Chapman, S. B. (1989). Discourse considerations for aphasia management. *Seminars in Speech and Language, 10,* 298–314.

Ulatowska, H., Doyel, A., Stern, R., Haynes, S., and North, A. (1983a). Production of procedural discourse in aphasia. *Brain and Language, 18,* 315–341.

Ulatowska, H. K., Freedman-Stern, R., Doyel, A. W., Macaluso-Haynes, S., and North, A. J. (1983b). Production of narrative discourse in aphasia. *Brain and Language, 19,* 317–334.

Ulatowska, H., Macaluso-Haynes, S., and North, A. (1980). Production of narrative and procedural discourse in aphasia. In R. Brookshire (Ed.), *Clinical Aphasiology Conference proceedings*. Minneapolis, MN: BRK.

Ulatowska, H. K., North, A. J., and Macaluso-Haynes, S. (1981a). Production of discourse and communicative competence in aphasia. In R. Brookshire (Ed.), *Clinical Aphasiology Conference proceedings*. Minneapolis, MN: BRK.

Ulatowska, H. K., North, A. J., and Macaluso-Haynes, S. (1981b). Production of narrative and procedural discourse in aphasia. *Brain and Language, 13,* 345–371.

Van Lancker, D., and Kempler, D. (1987). Comprehension of familiar phrases by left- but not by right-hemisphere damaged patients. *Brain and Language, 32,* 265–277.

Van Lancker, D., and Nicklay, C. (1992). Comprehension of personally relevant (PERL) versus novel language in two globally aphasic patients. *Aphasiology, 6,* 37–61.

Van Petten, C., and Kutas, M. (1991). Electrophysiological evidence for the flexibility of lexical processing. In G. Simpson (Ed.), *Understanding word and sentence*. New York: North-Holland.

Waller, M., and Darley, F. (1978). The influence of context on the auditory comprehension of paragraphs by aphasic subjects. *Journal of Speech and Hearing Research, 21,* 732–745.

Wambaugh, J. L., Thompson, C. K., Doyle, P. J., and Camarata, S. (1990). Conversational discourse of aphasic and normal adults: An analysis of communicative functions. In T. Prescott (Ed.), *Clinical aphasiology* (Vol. 20, pp. 343–353). Austin, TX: Pro-Ed.

Wegner, M., Brookshire, R., and Nicholas, L. (1984). Comprehension of main ideas and details in coherent and noncoherent discourse by aphasic and nonaphasic listeners. *Brain and Language, 21,* 37–51.

Wertz, R. T., Collins, M., Weiss, D., Kurtzke, J. F. Friden, T., Brookshire, R. H., Pierce, J., Holtzapple, P., Hubbard, D., Porch, B., West, J., Davis, L., Matovitch, V., Morley, G., and Resurrecion, E. (1981). Veterans Administration cooperative study on aphasia: A comparison of individual and group treatment. *Journal of Speech and Hearing Research, 24,* 580–594.

Weylman, S. T., Brownell, H. H., Gardner, H. (1988). "It's what you mean, not what you say": Pragmatic language use in brain-damaged patients. In F. Plum (Ed.), *Language, communication and the brain*. New York: Raven Press.

Whitney, P., and Waring, D. (1991). The role of knowledge in comprehension: A cognitive control perspective. In G. Simpson (Ed.), *Understanding word and sentence*. New York: North-Holland.

Wilcox, M. J. (1983). Aphasia: Pragmatic considerations. In K. Butler (Ed.), *Topics in language disorders* (Vol. 3). Gaithersburg, MD: Aspen Systems Corporation.

Wilcox, M. J., and Davis, G. A. (1977). Speech act analysis of aphasic communication in individual and group settings. In R. Brookshire (Ed.), *Clinical Aphasiology Conference proceedings*. Minneapolis, MN: BRK.

Wilcox, M., Davis, G., and Leonard, L. (1978) Aphasics' comprehension of contextually conveyed meaning. *Brain and Language, 6,* 362–377.

Wirz, S. L., Skinner, C., and Dean, E. (1990). *Revised Edinburgh Functional Communication Profile*. Tucson, AZ: Communication Skills Builders.

Yekovich, F., Walker, C., Ogle, L., and Thompson, M. (1990). The influence of domain knowledge on inferencing in low-aptitude individuals. In A. Graesser and G. Bower (Eds.), *Inferences and text comprehension*. New York: Academic Press.

Yorkston, K., Beukelman, D., and Flowers, C. (1980). Efficiency of information exchange between aphasic speakers and their communication partners. In R. Brookshire (Ed.), *Clinical Aphasiology Conference proceedings*. Minneapolis, MN: BRK.

CHAPTER 13
Environmental Systems Approach to Adult Aphasia

ROSEMARY LUBINSKI

The concept of "functional" dominates rehabilitation in the 1990s. Rehabilitation specialists are being required by private and government health care insurers, and by consumers themselves, to demonstrate in unambiguous, realistic terms how therapeutic intervention makes a qualitative difference in the everyday life of the patient. Numerous trends in health care have spawned this focus, and the most potent of these is the rapidly escalating costs of rehabilitation, particularly to older adults. From 1984 to 1987 alone, Medicare-covered rehabilitation costs tripled from $405 million to $1.3 billion (Langenbrunner et al., 1989). Hospitals and rehabilitation departments must justify who will benefit from rehabilitation, what methods are most efficacious, and what the expected functional outcomes are. The underlying theme is "Are the outcomes of therapy worth the cost?" In the near future, we can expect to see a functional status prospective payment system for Medicare and Medicaid patients in rehabilitation programs. Such a payment plan is likely to revolutionize aphasia therapy. (See Wilkerson et al., 1992, for an in-depth discussion of functional status payment for rehabilitation.)

Speech-language pathologists have recognized for some time that functional assessment and intervention with adult aphasics must go beyond traditional approaches that focus on isolated cognitive or communicative skills (e.g., Aten, 1986; Aten et al., 1982; Davis, 1986; Davis and Wilcox, 1981; Holland 1980, 1982; Lubinski, 1981, 1988, 1991; Lyon, 1992; Wertz, 1983). ASHA (1990) recently convened an advisory committee that defined functional communication as the "ability to receive a message or to convey a message, regardless of mode, to communicate effectively and independently in a given environment." Following from this definition, functional assessment of communication involves evaluating the ability of individuals *and* their communicative environment to accommodate to the communication problem, thus achieving the highest level of quality of life possible. For aphasic individuals, accommodation entails improvement of communication skills and coping with changes in their physical and social environment. For the environment, accommodation involves learning communication strategies that facilitate interaction and ways to maintain or enhance the social role of the aphasic individual. Frattali (1992), in her discussion of functional assessment and public policy,

states that functional assessment is at odds with traditional deficit-oriented assessment and treatment. To meet individual and third-party payors' expectations of a functional communication assessment, speech-language pathologists must now reconsider the nature of their assessment protocol and the intervention that ensues from it.

One approach to aphasia assessment and intervention that appears to meet the requirements of a functional approach is that which focuses on aphasic individuals and their communicative environment as a dynamic and interdependent system. Adult aphasics and their environment create a single, inextricably interwoven unit that in turn affects the people, the events, and the relationships occurring around them. While it may be efficient to isolate the communication sequelae of the stroke from individuals and their environment, the process results in a synthetic assessment of the person. The stroke and its physical, cognitive, emotional, and communicative sequelae now serve as active agents of change for individuals, their social network, and the physical surroundings. Therefore, if communication therapy is to be comprehensive and truly tailored to the individual's needs and resources, a broader perspective on the goals of therapy, the agents of change, and the evaluation of outcomes must be offered.

This chapter aims to present a model of assessment and intervention for adult aphasics that derives from environmental and family systems theory and their application to the aphasia rehabilitation field. The philosophy discussed here is one that can be easily incorporated with other approaches presented in this text. Ideally, the environmental systems approach should complement and enhance other cognitive, linguistic, and communicative approaches while increasing their functionality for aphasic individuals in their physical and social environment.

The environmental systems approach is based on the philosophy that effective and functional therapy emanates from a comprehensive rehabilitative management model that takes into consideration the interrelatedness of individuals, their communication abilities, the effectiveness of communication partners to facilitate communication, and the physical and social environment. While therapeutic goals should rightly focus on the primary communication impairment, the goals must also facilitate and strengthen those strategies that allow aphasic individuals and their significant others to become effective communication problem solvers. If we acknowledge the principle that communication is a dyadic process, we realize that aphasia by its very nature creates problems for *both* members of that communication team. Although one individual incurs the stroke, each and every individual with whom that person communicates will face a predicament. The natural response by some communication partners is to talk for the aphasic individual; for others it is to anticipate every need; and for yet others it is to avoid communication because of potential problems. Each of these responses results in a loss of opportunity for the aphasic individual to demonstrate intact or improving communication ability. Each response may also result in fewer opportunities for the aphasic individual and partners to consider, initiate, and evaluate productive communication problem-solving strategies. The diminution of communication opportunities negatively affects the social relationships between aphasic individuals and their communication partners and reverberates to larger social systems, including family, friends, and other social groups.

The philosophy underscoring this chapter is congruent with Banja's (1990) recent definition of rehabilitation that focuses on "empowering a disabled person to achieve a personally fulfilling, socially meaningful and functionally effective interaction with the world" (p. 615). Speech-language pathologists who suspect that their aphasia therapy is incomplete, artificial, and unfulfilling to the client, to significant others, or to themselves might find this approach a starting point for answering these questions. As Lyon (1992) states, "[S]ole preoccupation with the act of communicating has failed, so far, to deliver a solution to the problem of restoring optimal function (i.e., communication use and participation in life) in natural settings" (p. 9). The approach described here helps the speech-language pathologist leave the cloister of the therapy office and enter the environment of the aphasic individual.

SYSTEM DEFINITION

A system is defined as a network of elements that has many simultaneous interactions. The interaction of any two elements produces dynamics that influence all the other elements and interactions possible within that system. In systems theory, the characteristics of the individual elements become important in how they alter the infrastructure of the whole system. Each element of subsystem affects the entire system either overtly or subtly. In the reality of human systems, individuals are part of multiple subsystems that influence each other in multidirectional ways (Brubaker, 1987). Further, the system is composed not only of human networks but also of the relationship of persons and their physical surroundings. Thus, in a comprehensive systems approach to aphasia, we might consider microsystems such as the family and macrosystems such as the cultural milieu, the physical setting, and the influence of the clinician and the rehabilitation process.

The application of systems theory to communication disorders and aphasia is not new (e.g., Andrews and Andrews, 1987; Bishop, 1982; Brocklehurst et al., 1981; Hyman, 1972; Kinsella and Duffy, 1979; Norlin, 1986; Rollin, 1987; Watzlawick and Coyne, 1980; Webster and Newhoff, 1981). What makes the present approach different is that the approach is layered rather than singularly focused on the primary system of the family.

It begins by exploring the impact of aphasia on the individual, then moves to the primary system of the family, and concludes with a discussion of extended environmental and sociocultural systems. Such a layering provides a practical model for a comprehensive approach to assessment and intervention.

The Individual

The individual is at the core of the systems approach presented in this chapter. By contributing personal characteristics to the environment, the individual becomes a member of it. Basic characteristics include age, race, sex, education, occupation, and family and socioeconomic status. To this basic framework other changing physical, psychological, and emotional characteristics are added. These characteristics have evolved through time and sociocultural experiences. Human beings enrich their environment with these distinctive features, yet must rely on other individuals and subsystems for information, support, and feedback. The individual becomes the generator of social imperatives but must also respond to social conventions.

Ideally, pressure from other individuals or subsystems will never exceed the person's ability to respond competently. This means that individuals must be sensitive to role expectations, match their characteristics to the role, self-evaluate, and modify where possible. The interplay between human beings and their environment is delicate and dynamic, creating challenges for humans' ability to adapt and survive. Lawton (1970) calls this "person-environment congruence."

Family as a Microsystem

For most of us, the family is the fundamental system within which we interact. The nucleus of the family is composed of individuals and their previous, present, and changing personal attributes. These individuals beget multiple networks, including the marital, parental, sibling, and extended family subsystems (Turnbull and Turnbull, 1991). The marital subsystem consists of the husband and wife and the stage of their family life development. McGoldrick and Carter (1982) suggest that families advance through six normative family stages, each with its particular influence on the individuals and the larger unit: (*a*) between families—the unattached young adult; (*b*) the joining of families through marriage; (*c*) the family with very young children; (*d*) the family with adolescents; (*e*) the launching of children and moving on; and (*f*) the family in later life. Jones (1989) states that this development is not a continuous process but one characterized by oscillations and vacillations. For example, one family may be in stage 4 and also in stage 5, while another family in stage 6 may have adult children return home and thus regress to stage 5.

The parental subsystem emerges in the interactions between parents and their child or children, and the sibling subsystem reflects the relationships between children of the family. As parents age and their children grow into adult roles, the relationship between parent and child evolves. Similarly, the children of the family have changing relationships as they mature and enter into new subsystems both within and outside the family.

The core family is also a part of the extended family subsystem of relatives, friends, support groups, and professionals (Turnbull and Turnbull, 1991). The family does not live in isolation but extends to many other individuals and systems. Thus, the characteristics of the family, or any of its components, will affect and be influenced by their relationships with larger social groups such as work, school, church, and leisure organizations.

Each of these subsystems is well-organized, has control mechanisms, and has energy that keeps the system going (Gray et al., 1969). Organization means that the system can be recognized by its wholeness. For example, the family is organized by its composition of members and their roles within the boundary of the family. In today's society, the organization of families can take many different forms yet conform to the definition of a family. At least 10 viable family organizations exist: (*a*) the nuclear family of husband, wife, and children; (*b*) married individuals with no children; (*c*) individuals in widowhood with or without children; (*d*) unmarried individuals with child or children; (*e*) never-married or divorced individuals; (*f*) remarried individuals with or without children; (*g*) companionate relationships; (*h*) blended nuclear family with children from one or more marriages; (*i*) any of the above with the presence of a grandparent or other family member; and (*j*) communes or collective living arrangements.

The roles that individuals have within the family emerge from tasks that need to be accomplished to keep the family in a steady state. Primary or shared roles include the financial well-being of the family, homemaking, education, caregiving, and support. The roles that individuals have are likely to change over time as the needs of the family shift and as individuals change in their ability to handle roles.

The family also has mechanisms to control itself or maintain its organization (Bonder, 1986/1987). There is potential for family disruption as the family and its individuals change over time and are influenced by the myriad systems with which they interact. Families have the self-preservation need to maintain homeostasis. Thus, the family must constantly provide feedback to its members and find ways to maintain the delicate balance of the family system. Homeostasis is generally achieved when individuals have clearly and mutually agreed on roles and an effective communication system to convey information among members. Should internal or external elements from the family cause a change in these roles, the balance of the family system is altered. Fortunately, families can be energized from within their own organization or from external systems such as professional or peer support networks. It is hoped that the resources that the individuals and the family as a system have will be strong enough to adjust family roles, to facilitate role transition with relative ease, and to minimize role strain (Maitz, 1991).

Environment as a Macrosystem

While the family has an enormous role in systems theory, an even broader concept of the environment should be considered. The environment in this chapter is defined as the aggregate of influences that impinge on individuals throughout their life cycle. These influences can be categorized into those arising from an individual's physical and social environment. The combination of these external forces with the internal characteristics of each individual forms a ''total environment'' for each person.

External Environment

The stimuli that create human beings' external environment can be grouped into two main categories: first, those generated by the physical surroundings and perceived through the senses; second, those stimuli derived from the cultural and economic climate and transmitted through the communication networks of human beings. These stimuli function in tandem, partially defining how humans will behave in any setting.

Physical Environment

The physical environment is composed of natural phenomena perceived through the senses; human contributions such as buildings and objects; and the elements of time and space. These physical stimuli create the backdrop in which human beings function and help determine where they will live, how they will live, and the rules they will develop to maintain order within that environment. The physical environment is not merely a passive stage setting for communication, but can create opportunities or barriers to people and events where communication might flourish.

Sociocultural and Economic Environment

It is through social interaction that individuals learn their roles and the expectations of others in their environment. The sociocultural milieu of an individual is a web of values, standards, and activities that define particular groups. This rule system specifies how one should behave in various roles and situations. From infancy to old age, one assumes a variety of roles. These roles are influenced by the personal characteristics of the individual and the expectations of the environment. Societies prescribe guidelines for how an individual should progress to and from various roles during the life cycle.

Formal social behavior is learned through direct, explicit communication, for example, by the rules and laws of social organizations. By contrast, mores, or traditional customs, are acquired more subtly. These are learned through informal interaction within specific subsystems such as family, work groups, and social activities (Ittelson et al., 1974). These two types of norms determine how much individual involvement, support, independence, personal growth, and expressiveness will be tolerated (Moos, 1976). Thus, each environment creates its own personality, and this unique combination of social formulae forms the social climate for the individual.

Considering that African-American, Hispanic, and Asian populations are increasing faster than the white population in the United States, aphasiologists need to be aware of the heterogeneous characteristics and expectations of numerous cultures (Friedman, 1990). Wallace and Freeman (1991) reported that in their survey of 30 university-related clinics that had a multicultural emphasis, approximately half of the neurological cases from a multicultural background were black, 28% were Hispanic, and 21% were Asians and Pacific Islanders. Most of these neurological cases were cerebral vascular accidents. Unfortunately, the majority of the individuals attended therapy for 2 months or less.

In particular, we need to understand clients' sociocultural background and how it interacts with health care systems, rehabilitation programs, and individuals from outside their usual cultural experiences. This culturally relevant sensitivity will modify our therapy goals, the agents of change, and reasonable outcomes of therapy. Cross (1988) calls this ''cultural competence.'' At a most basic level, cultural competence or multicultural sensitivity to aphasic clients necessitates that we appreciate their health care beliefs and values. Friedman (1990) states that unless health care practitioners take a transcultural perspective in working with minority clients, there will be poor communication and interpersonal tension, leading to inaccurate assessment and intervention. A clinician who does not take into consideration the sociocultural milieu of a client may find that therapy compliance and carryover to outside settings are less than expected. (See Sue and Sue, 1990, and Kavanagh and Kennedy, 1992, for discussions of communication with culturally diverse populations.)

The economic environment also influences the individual, the family, and the larger society. How health care and rehabilitation are approached may be determined to a great degree by the financial resources of the aphasic individual and his or her significant others (Ingstad, 1990). The nature and extent of one's own finances or third-party insurance to cover extensive and prolonged rehabilitation may mitigate the person's willingness to participate in therapy. While speech-language pathologists are encouraged to be culturally sensitive, they must also be "economically sensitive" to client and family concerns about the cost of therapy and the perceived cost/benefit ratio. Economic sensitivity involves understanding the cost of therapy and its impact on the everyday lives of the individuals involved. Knowing that the family cannot afford extensive therapy or that therapy costs will cut deeply into their savings may influence how therapy is done and progress is evaluated. Finally, aphasic individuals and families will appreciate a speech-language pathologist who acknowledges that financial coverage of therapy may be a burden.

RELATIONSHIP OF COMMUNICATION TO THE ENVIRONMENT

Communication is the reciprocal act of sending and receiving information. This act can assume a variety of forms. Individuals communicate through the transmission of spoken or written symbols, body language signals, vocal cues, and olfaction, as well as through manipulation of objects and space in the environment. The content of communication is limited only by the boundaries of human beings' perception of the external world and the scope of their inner world.

Communication serves human beings generously. First, it is the primary mechanism through which persons learn the rules of their environment and their social role within it. Second, communication helps humans control both their physical environment and their companions. Third, through social discourse, individuals avoid isolation and achieve a sense of belonging. Communication is a therapeutic tool when it helps individuals express their feelings and achieve psychological well-being. All individuals, especially aphasics, experience successful communication and realize its benefits when there is a physical and social environment that supports and reinforces communicative interaction, and a willingness on the part of the individual to enter into this interaction.

External Factors Related to Successful Communication

Successful communication is highly dependent on the adequate transmission and reception of the message. The environment must be structured so that communicating individuals can come within a reasonable and effective physical distance of each other. Distance is determined by one's sensory receptive

abilities and sociocultural conventions. The message must also travel between sender and receiver with a minimum of interference and distortion. Thus, the physical environment is an integral component of the communication event.

This is also true for the sociocultural environment. Simon and Agazarian (1967) explain that communicators must first establish "good maintenance." They state that communication will be successful when interactants accept each other. This is similar to Gibb's (1961) concept of a supportive communication climate. For example, an environment that places a premium on evaluation and control of its members will create defensive behavior and communication. "Defensive behavior engenders defensive listening and this in turn produces postural, facial and verbal cues which raise the defense level of the original communicator" (Gibb, 1961, p. 141).

Individual Characteristics Related to Successful Communication

For successful communication to occur, the individual must have the ability to send and receive messages. Language, speech, and hearing mechanisms must be intact and capable of sending and receiving signals. Visual acuity also contributes to effective communication, since it is through vision that one decodes many nonverbal cues. Communication will be unsuccessful when the sender transmits an unintelligible message, when he or she misperceives the availability of the receiver, and/or when the content is ambiguous, inappropriate, or irrelevant. Communication also becomes ineffectual when the individual does not comprehend the signals, receives a distorted signal, is distracted by extraneous stimuli, or loses interest.

Individuals must also contribute a sense of involvement in a situation for successful communication to occur there. They must perceive that their participation is valued by members of the group, and in turn, they must be recognized as a viable communication partner. Although physical accessibility to a variety of social occasions is important, mere presence is insufficient to stimulate interest and involvement. Social acceptance of the individual is a prerequisite for meaningful interaction.

IMPACT OF APHASIA ON SYSTEMS

When an individual suffers brain damage, the equilibrium between the person and his or her environment is disturbed. The equilibrium will be changed by many factors on immediate, short-term, and long-term bases. Few individuals or their families understand or are prepared for the numerous and complex physical, communicative, cognitive, emotional, and social changes the stroke will create. These changes have a far-reaching impact on the individual, the family, larger social groups, and the physical and social environment.

The Challenge of Being an Aphasic Individual

Brain damage and its resulting aphasia impose numerous immediate and long-term challenges for an individual: (a) the immediate health crisis; (b) long-term comorbidities; (c) communication problems; (d) the hurdles of rehabilitation; and (e) reintegration into the home and society.

Immediate Health Crisis

An individual's initial reaction to brain damage is that he or she is in an immediate life-threatening situation. There is a real possibility that the individual will die. Medical intervention and the innate forces related to recovery enable the person to cope with and relieve this initial crisis. The emergency may last for a few days or several weeks until the physical well-being of the person is stabilized. The impact of the illness is realized more fully when the health status is brought under control. The individual will survive, but now his or her physical and communicative abilities have been altered. This is the transition from the illness stage to the disability stage (Safilios-Rothchild, 1970).

Long-Term Comorbidities

Rehabilitation specialists such as speech-language pathologists, physiatrists, physical therapists, and occupational therapists may myopically view the problems of the stroke patient. In reality, physical and psychological problems following a stroke form a complex of their own that reverberates throughout the subsystems of the aphasic individual and to the rehabilitation process itself. These problems must be understood as potential influences on the effectiveness of therapy and cannot be divorced from it.

The majority of stroke patients have some physical sequelae of the stroke including physical/health problems, perceptual disabilities, and dysphagia. In addition, health problems related to the stroke, to the life-style, or to the aging process itself are likely concomitants. These may directly affect the family system, communication of the aphasic individual, and rehabilitation efforts. For example, a 75-year-old male stroke patient may also have emphysema, presbycusis, cataracts, macular degeneration, and prostate cancer. Physical and health concerns may have priority over communication rehabilitation for the individual or caregivers. For example, the elderly wife of an aphasic may perceive the major stroke-related difficulty to be her inability to assist in transfer and lifting during toileting. The nurse may be more concerned about increased dependence resulting from decrease in muscle strength, additional time in bed, and decubitus ulcers.

A second long-term comorbidity is the strong relationship between damage to the left hemisphere and psychological reactions (e.g., Starkstein and Robinson, 1988; Wahrborg, 1991). Without doubt, difficulty in expressing oneself and understanding others, physical impairments, and social changes negatively affect the individual's psychological well-being. Tanner and Gerstenberger (1988) discuss the psychological reactions to aphasia as grief arising from loss of person, loss of self, and loss of object. The stroke and its sequelae create obstacles for the maintenance of accustomed relationships with family and other social systems. Members of these social groups are usually unaware of the complex properties of stroke and have few strategies for interacting effectively with the aphasic individual. Loss of self ensues as fewer social roles are available to the aphasic individual because of active withdrawal of opportunities by the family or other social systems or because of loss of physical function to participate. Loss of external objects, such as personal items and familiar settings, can also fuel a grief response within the aphasic individual. The 80-year-old aphasic woman who finds herself institutionalized in a nursing home without her cherished possessions may have little desire to communicate or to interact socially with staff or family.

Perhaps the major psychological reaction of aphasic individuals to their predicament is depression. Thirty percent to 60%

of stroke patients exhibit depression sometimes following their insult, and this depression may be long term (e.g., Cullum and Bigler, 1991; Egelko et al., 1989; Robinson and Benson, 1981). Tearfulness and crying appear to be common long-term depressive symptoms. Such symptoms may be mistaken now as primary characteristics and lead to reduced opportunities for communication (Warhborg, 1991).

Wahrborg (1991) states that the depression following stroke can be categorized as "major poststroke depression" and "reactive poststroke depression." Major poststroke depression is that associated with the proximity of the lesion to the frontal lobe. In contrast, reactive depression is related to the ability to cope with the challenges of stroke and aphasia. Keller et al. (1989) add that depression can also emanate from a combination of the organic biochemical changes and the psychosocial challenges of aphasia. Stern and Bachman (1991) found in a recent study of depressive symptoms following stroke that dysphoria was related to site of lesion but not to the severity of aphasia. It might be added that the depression that some aphasic individuals show may be an extension of premorbid depression. Steger (1976) cautions us to remember that depression in elderly patients may be related to the complex of losses that characterize their life period as well as to the frustration involved in rehabilitation. Even without a stroke, at least 15% of the elderly are depressed, and this prevalence increases to 35% when there is a concurrent medical illness (Jenike, 1988).

The depressive symptoms that aphasic individuals may show can be multiple, ranging from pervasive sadness, dependency, and indecisiveness to physical and cognitive problems. The most extreme symptom includes suicide (Jenike, 1988). *The Diagnostic and Statistical Manual of Mental Disorders* (DSM-III-R) (American Psychiatric Association, 1987) lists major depression criteria to be related to sleep disturbance, loss of interest in activities that the person once enjoyed, feelings of guilt, loss of energy, decreased concentration, diminished appetite, psychomotor disturbance, and suicide. In general, five of these criteria persisting for at least 2 weeks may indicate clinical depression. Such depression symptomatology may be interpreted, however, by family or professionals as confusion or dementia. Comments by Jenike (1988) on "guarding against fatalistically diagnosing the cognitively impaired depressed individual as irretrievably demented and withholding a treatment as a result" (p. 128) can be applied to depressed aphasic individuals. The aphasic individual with depression is in double jeopardy because of difficulty in verbally expressing feelings. Tanner (1987) states that language is the tool for introspection and therapeutic exchange. Thus, language therapy to improve expression may be essential in addressing depressive symptoms.

Depression is not the only affective disorder exhibited among aphasic individuals. Affective changes can be any of a constellation of reactions including frustration, anger, hostility, anxiety, aggression, withdrawal, denial, regression, boasting, and catastrophic reactions (Wahrborg, 1991). Further, aphasic individuals may also incur other cognitive changes such as dementia including Alzheimer's disease, multiinfarct dementia, and dementia related to Parkinson's disease (see Chapter 29 in this text). Again, these must be differentially diagnosed from the aphasia itself and any other concomitant psychological problems such as depression.

The speech-language pathologist has an important role in identifying affective symptoms and making appropriate referral for accurate differential diagnosis and medical, psychiatric, or pharmaceutical intervention. At times, however, the speech-language pathologist, by the very nature of his or her intimate communicative experiences with the aphasic client, will need to deal directly with the psychological reactions of the aphasic individual to ensure that therapy is effective and functional. Particularly important is the speech-language pathologist's ability to use effective counseling/communicative skills with the aphasic individual. See Tanner (1987) and Tanner et al. (1989) for a more in-depth discussion of psychological reactions and their remediation in brain-damaged individuals.

Communication Difficulties

The inability to communicate successfully may be the most significant problem for aphasic persons and the greatest price they must pay for their illness. Aphasic persons are stigmatized (Goffman, 1964) by their communication problem. Each time they attempt to communicate and fail, they strengthen their negative self-perception. At a time when communication is essential for adjustment and reintegration into family and community, their skill is impaired, and opportunities to interact are often seriously reduced.

Aphasic persons face a crisis each time they cannot quickly and efficiently express or comprehend the symbols of their environment. For example, each time individuals are bombarded by communication that comes too abundantly or quickly, they must choose from among replying unintelligibly, replying inappropriately, or withholding a response. They find it difficult to fulfill their roles as an adult communicator within their family and other social groups. Similarly, a crisis occurs each time the individuals are isolated from communication contact by their voluntary withdrawal or by the retreat of significant communication partners. It may be easier to avoid communication and thereby lessen the frustration of failure.

Hurdles of Rehabilitation

Once the immediate health crisis is overcome, a new multidimensional system enters the lives of aphasic individuals and their families: the rehabilitation system. While the focus of this book is specifically on communication rehabilitation, we must remember that aphasia rehabilitation is likely to be only one of several health service programs working with the individual. Helping specialists bring unfamiliar value systems and agendas that may or may not be in concert with the aphasic individual and/or family. Rehabilitation also is influenced by the society's valuation of rehabilitation goals and outcomes. Is society willing to pay for rehabilitation and then meaningfully reintegrate the aphasic individual into the community?

The first hurdle the aphasic individual faces in the communication rehabilitation system is facing the reality that communication is impaired to some degree. Rehabilitation may be viewed as an approach-avoidance process. On one side of the scale is the potential for improvement and return to premorbid status. On the other side of the scale are numerous factors, including unknown amount of effort, fear of failure, stigmatization of being a therapy client, dependency, and imposition on others. In addition, life-long individual and societal conceptions or misconceptions of disability and rehabilitation add to the imbalance. The equation becomes more complicated when the aphasic individual is elderly and "beyond" the typical age

when rehabilitation efforts focus on return to a socially important job role (Bozarth, 1981).

The second rehabilitation hurdle the aphasic individual faces is that of being a therapy "client" or "patient." With this new and unfamiliar role comes certain expectations generated by a multilateral group of therapist, family, third-party payors, and the aphasic person. Rabinowitz and Mitsos (1964) state that at this point the client is "enrobed in a distinctive social garment" (p. 9.). Traditionally, a "good client" participates enthusiastically, carries out assignments faithfully, respects and refrains from questioning the therapist's judgment of therapy goals and methods, attends therapy promptly and regularly, is appropriately gracious and grateful, verbalizes difficulties, and so on (Rabinowitz and Mitsos, 1964). All this is seen as reflecting the good client's high motivation to improve. In fact, these very behaviors may mask confusion about therapy, indifference, and low motivation. The success of therapy rides on the shoulders of the aphasic client (Safilios-Rothschild, 1970).

According to systems theory, the "client" in actuality is the individual *and* his or her family. Rather than define a "good client," we might now consider the therapy belief system of these individuals and how this translates to positive or facilitating behaviors. For example, do they believe that therapy is more effective when client and family are actively involved? Do they believe that therapy is a problem-solving process whereby they will learn strategies to repair their communication difficulties? Do they believe that progress can be measured in multiple ways, including improvement in specific communication skills, increased willingness to enter into communication exchanges, increased ability on the part of significant others to facilitate interaction, and decreased depression or stress on the part of the client and family?

Reintegration into Home and Community

Perhaps the most difficult personal challenge for aphasic individuals is reintegration into their home and community. For some aphasic individuals, this process occurs simultaneously with outpatient therapy; for others it occurs after therapy is completed—the "ex-client" stage. Beginning with the immediate health crisis stage and afterward, the aphasic individual's accustomed family and community roles have been altered, assimilated by others, or eliminated. Carver and Rodda (1978) question whether the disabled individual is "assimilated" or "integrated" into his or her environment. With assimilation, the emphasis is on clients appropriately adapting themselves to a relatively unchanged environment. They must fit in. In contrast, in an environment that focuses on integration, there is coadaptation on the part of the physical and social environment systems. The aphasic individual and the environment now work at conforming to each other. An aphasic person who is integrated has opportunities to demonstrate accustomed, meaningful adult roles in a variety of contexts.

As a "client" or "patient," the aphasic individual is expected to passively relinquish former social roles, participate eagerly in rehabilitation, and have an ardent desire to return to normal. A dilemma arises, however, when the aphasic person declines to fulfill this model. The individual may not choose to relinquish family, vocational, or social responsibilities, nor may he or she want to participate enthusiastically in rehabilitation. Society and the individual may become adversaries during rehabilitation. For example, the aphasic person has the choice of (a) accepting the rehabilitant role that requires acceptance of disability and active participation in therapy, (b) participating impassively in therapy, or (c) refusing participation. The aphasic individual may not be able to communicate effectively his or her personal goals and consequently may resort to behaviors that society considers maladaptive or antisocial. Now, in addition to being aphasic, the individual is further stigmatized as uncooperative, unmanageable, or hostile. Consequently, fewer opportunities for reintegrating into the community materialize. Evaluation of aphasic individuals' integration into the community 5 or 10 years poststroke would provide much needed data on what the focus of therapy should be.

Microsystems Impact

Rolland (1988) states that the "family may provide the best lens through which to view other systems" (p. 17). Concurrently with understanding the impact of aphasia on the individual, we must focus on its impact on the family. "Family" is broadly defined here as the network of individuals with whom the aphasic individual is closely involved on a daily basis. This can be an immediate system of spouse and/or children, or can extend to other relatives, friends, and informal or professional caregivers. The majority of the discussion focuses on the immediate family with some discussion of more extended family systems.

Table 13.1 portrays a model for the stages through which the aphasic individual and family will evolve after the stroke. This model begins with the severe illness or crisis stage and evolves to subsequent stages of recuperation, rehabilitation, postrehabilitation, and institutionalization. While this model is presented as a sequential series of stages, in reality some stages are brief, whereas others are lengthy for individual aphasics and their families.

The family's initial concern after the stroke is coping with the sudden life-threatening illness. The family, particularly the spouse, is likely to fear that the stroke will result in death or some unknown type and degree of disability. Not only is this fear directed toward the stroke patient but there is also an amorphous fear about how their own lives will be changed by this crisis event immediately and in the long term. All sorts of feelings cloud this time: obsessive concern, anxiety, helplessness, grief, and guilt. During this time, few changes in family roles are likely to occur because the family's energy is directed toward the immediate health crisis.

Once the stroke patient's health is stabilized, the patient and the family system move into the recuperation stage. The first feeling is one of relief that the stroke patient will live. This is when the family system tries to begin the return to its precrisis state (homeostasis). In actuality, the system changes that begin to occur are likely to modify the family network forever. The changes that occur emanate from many sources, including the normative stage of the family, their historical ability to cope with problems, the immediate tasks that need to be done and the resources for accomplishing them, and other demands on the family. For example, a mature family that has clear lines of communication, a resource network of family and friends, and a history of successfully coping with problems may face a crisis differently than the family that is disengaged, interacts poorly, and has numerous conflicting demands on its members.

While stroke may occur in younger adults who are in early stages of family development, it is more likely to occur when the family is in the late life cycle. The elder spouse is likely to assume primary caregiving responsibility, although adult children play an increasingly important role in providing assistance to their parent(s). The changing demographics of our society translate into fewer middle-aged children to care for older parents (Gatz et al., 1990). Further, these children, particularly adult daughters, are likely to be employed outside the home and be caught in the "sandwich" of caring for their own children and their parents. The older family, however, has many years of experience in coping with other life problems that may assist in coping with stroke and aphasia. Rolland (1990) states that when disease occurs later in the family life cycle, the "strains are counterbalanced by a firmer relationship base" (p. 239). On the negative side, the spouse of the later-life aphasic may also exhibit health, physical, cognitive, or sensory problems that complicate the caregiving context.

During the recuperation stage, the family is likely to concentrate on activities of daily living such as walking, feeding, dressing, and toileting. These problems require direct and strenuous caregiving on the part of family members. There is a simultaneous awareness that communication is disrupted. The communication difficulties now evident between the aphasic individual and his or her family members confound provision of physical care and their social relationships. Kinsella and Duffy (1979) found that difficulty in communication results in a loss of the intimacy and support found in most marriages.

Most families with a member who has incurred a stroke do not come as units untouched by other life problems. Numerous demands concurrently have an impact on the aphasic family, including those arising from family life stage, prior family dysfunction, and financial, employment, and health problems. For example, Jones and Lubinski (b-forthcoming), in a family systems study of nine poststroke families, found that all families contended with stresses faced by maturing families such as that related to launching children, managing retirement, and coping with needs of elderly parents. Many of the families had histories of alcoholism, problems with children, unemployment, and so on. House et al. (1990) found that stroke patients as compared with controls experienced a significantly greater number of severe events in the year preceding a stroke. Evans et al. (1991a) found that poststroke patients at risk for poor-quality home care had families with caregivers who were depressed, had little knowledge about stroke care, and had prestroke family dysfunction. They concluded that "care-giver problems can have a collective effect on rehabilitation outcome" (p. 144). In another study of family characteristics related to better treatment adherence poststroke, Evans et al. (1991b) portrayed such families as having clear and direct communication exchange, effective problem-solving ability and strong emotional interest in one another. Kelly-Hayes et al. (1988) found that family and social factors were equal to medical factors in determining final outcome from stroke. Thus, these studies demonstrate that individuals and their families are vitally important in the rehabilitation process, although they bring "baggage" to the rehabilitation situation.

When medical conditions have stabilized and physical recuperation appears possible, therapies are likely to begin. These may be instigated by the medical/rehabilitation system or by the family. For many families, this will be their first encounter

Table 13.1.
Patient Stages, Possible Family Effects, and Potential Family Needs

Patient Stage	Possible Effects on Family	Potential Family Needs
Severe illness or crisis stage	Fear and shock Disequilibrium Anxiety Depression Guilt Helplessness Grief Obsessive concern	Emotional support for entire family, particularly spouse, adult child caregiver, significant other
Recuperation stage	Sense of relief from acute stage Family works toward homeostasis Members assume needed roles and jobs Search for help begins Individuals try to maintain self-image	Continued emotional support Information about family demands, resources, concerns; see ABCX model Informal education about stroke and its effects Family mobilized to work together Facilitative communication strategies modeled while communicating with aphasic adult
Rehabilitation	"Hope" that things will improve Expectation that patient will improve Solidification of new family roles Beginning of isolation from community Physical changes in home Possible logistical problems in attending therapy by patient and/or family member(s) Possible financial problems	Continued emotional support with more emphasis on self-reliance Problem-solving approach to communication difficulties Direct involvement in rehabilitation Discussion of family, individual, and clinician goals and expectations of therapy Definition of and access to community resources Peer support groups Planning for postrehabilitation stage
Postrehabilitation	Possible role-overload for primary caregiver Possible health problems for primary caregiver Long-term changes in family roles Isolation of family from extended groups Possible reduction in intimacy between aphasic and spouse or significant other Over- or underexpectations for continued improvements	Realization and support for caregiver personal needs Peer and extended group support Increase in normative features of home and aphasic person Continued emotional support—referral to community counselors
Institutionalization	Physical/psychological overload Lack of awareness of community alternatives Conflicting feelings of relief and guilt Further role changes Discomfort with setting Reduction in contact with institutionalized family member Preparation for family member deterioration or death	Help in decision making Counseling regarding alternatives Support during decision making and entry Encouragement to visit; strategies for productive visits provided Information regarding impact of institutionalization on family member Modeling of facilitative communication strategies in this setting Work with facility staff to stress importance of communication to aphasic individual Development of new roles in this setting encouraged Participation in activities with aphasic adult within and outside setting encouraged Counseling regarding deterioration and death

with a speech-language pathologist and aphasia therapy. The individual and the family are moving into the rehabilitation stage where the focus is on helping the aphasic individual improve language skills. The family system is also continuing its restructuring during this time. Role changes become more solidified so that even when aphasic individuals return to their family, the modifications are in place without their active involvement. Difficulties in communicating contribute significantly to the need for, yet impede, the aphasic's participation in family role restructuring. Unwittingly, the aphasic individual may become the marginal member of the family.

The extended family of the aphasic is also affected by the stroke and the resulting communication problems. Friends and acquaintances may feel uncomfortable during interactions with the aphasic and may withdraw from former social interaction with the entire family unit or individual members within it. The family may lose some of its opportunities for social connectedness because one member cannot communicate. This results in the disengagement of the family from the mainstream of the community.

Finally, the extended system of the aphasic individual is likely to include some new members such as professional caregivers. Nurses and nursing assistants assume a prominent role in the lives of many aphasic individuals in hospital, home, or long-term care setting. These individuals assume ''quasi-family'' roles in that they perform intimate caregiving tasks and serve as primary communication partners for the aphasic individual. Family members who are not present for therapy may look to the nursing assistant for feedback on ''how therapy is going with Dad.'' This individual may subtly influence how the aphasic individual and family perceive therapy and its progress.

Macrosystems Impact

The impact of aphasia extends beyond the immediate family to the aphasic individual's larger social and physical environments. For example, a father's aphasia has implications for resuming his coaching role on his son's soccer team and is likely to affect his ability to supervise his office staff. Most persons with whom the aphasic individual is likely to interact have had little or no experience in communicating with someone with this type of problem. Even when communication skills are greatly improved, the impression may be of someone who is less than whole. When communication problems are evident, the individual has more difficulty demonstrating his or her intelligence, social competence, and productive social role, all qualities valued by Western industrialized societies. Safilios-Rothchild (1970) says that such societies do not tolerate ''behavioral deviations [such as communication difficulties] that tend to disrupt the smooth functioning and easy flow of interpersonal relations'' (p. 127). In general, contact with an adult who has difficulty communicating arouses anxiety. The cultural norm is to mask such aversion. It therefore becomes necessary to avoid contact with the aphasic individual lest their prejudices and own inadequacies in coping with the communication difficulty become evident.

Society appears to have conflicting perceptions of someone with a disability. Rolland (1990) states that our society admires personal responsibility as the means to recovery. On the other hand, Western societies also feel a need to ''protect the less fortunate.'' Protection may lead to elimination of situations where the aphasic individual, and hence society, might face communication frustration or failure. The aphasic individual is now out of mainstream society and part of an unfamiliar minority group. Reintegration into society thus becomes more challenging.

Impact of Rehabilitation Setting and Clinician

The setting offering communication rehabilitation is itself a multifaceted system influenced by many equally complicated factors. Fundamentally, therapy is influenced by the goals of the institution and the agenda set by third-party payors. For example, restrictions set by insurers on agencies that can offer evaluation and therapy services limit patient options. Similarly,

a predetermined number of paid therapy sessions may limit scope and direction of therapy. Romano (1989) posits that many rehabilitation programs send mixed messages to the client: On the one hand, decision making is generally removed from the patient, yet on the other the patient is expected to demonstrate independence and self-motivation. The model underlying many rehabilitation programs closely resembles a biomedical model focused on the direct relationship between differential diagnosis and treatment. At present, such a medical model will not support an environmental systems approach to therapy where the emphasis is simultaneously on client, family, and environment.

The speech-language pathologist is one of the most influential factors in the aphasia therapy process. Clinician knowledge, skills, and attitudes about aphasia, aging, and rehabilitation influence who will receive therapy and how it will be delivered. Clinicians bring their own unique traits and histories that act as a ''cultural filter'' in how we communicate with, assess, and plan therapy for clients (Krefting and Krefting, 1991). In addition, clinicians contribute their professional biases that have accrued from training programs and cultural influences. Agar (1980) states that ''whether it is your personality, your rules of social interaction, your cultural bias toward significant topics, your professional training or something else, you do not go into the field as a passive recorder of objective data'' (p. 10). Clinicians are influenced by their own known and unknown biases and the expectations of the rehabilitation setting, the client, family, and society.

SYSTEM ASSESSMENT

The first step in the environmental systems rehabilitation program is to identify the impact of the stroke and the resulting aphasia on individuals, their family system, their extended social systems, and their physical and social milieu. Because of time and therapy setting constraints, we are likely to obtain the most direct information about individuals and their family and assumptions about extended social systems and the broader environment. The fact that we cannot observe aphasic individuals and their family in their home setting with their extended systems should not discourage us from developing ways to assess these components. The value added from such information contributes to a comprehensive, sensitive, and functional assessment.

A qualitative approach to assessment is presented in this chapter. What speech-language pathologists should be interested in is the quality and insight of answers given and how the questions and answers contribute to new thinking by the aphasic individual, the family members, and the speech-language pathologist. The questions presented here should be viewed as vehicles for ongoing discussion with the client and family and not just as initial assessment tools. The assessment process described here should naturally merge with communication therapy for the client and his or her family. A total picture of the client's communicative environment should develop from this layered approach to assessment of multiple systems. This information can be used in goal setting, in reassessment, and in feedback to the client, family, and third-party payors.

Individual Assessment

In addition to the traditional communicative/cognitive evaluation, we must examine (*a*) aphasic individuals' perception of

Table 13.2.
Interview Questions for Aphasic Individual Regarding Stroke and Aphasia[a]

Definition of Present Situation
1. What concerns you about your speech?
2. What problems do you have in understanding your spouse (or primary caregiver)?
3. What problems do you have in understanding other people?
4. What problems do you have in expressing yourself?
5. What problems do you have in reading? In writing?
6. How important is reading (and writing) to you?
7. In what situations do you have the most difficulty talking (or understanding)?
8. What other problems do you have besides a communication problem?
9. What is your greatest concern right now—these other problems (e.g., self-care) or communication? Why?
10. What other therapies are you receiving?

Impact of Aphasia
1. How do you feel when you have a problem communicating?
2. How do others react when you have a problem communicating?
3. Do you ever avoid a situation or a person because of your difficulty communicating? Why? Describe this.
4. How has your communication problem affected your interaction with your family?
5. How has your communication problem affected your interaction with others outside your family, such as friends or coworkers?
6. How has your communication problem affected your social life (employment)?
7. Who are the primary people you talk with every day?
8. Do you feel you have enough opportunities to talk about things that interest you? With people who are interesting to you?

Motivation to Improve Communication
1. Tell me about a typical day of yours. What do you do?
2. What would you like to improve about your communication?
3. Why is this important to you?
4. What have you done on your own that helps you communicate better?
5. Have you attended speech therapy before? If so, where? What did you work on? How successful was therapy?
6. Who in your family would you like to work with on your communication? Why this person?
7. What do you think I can do to help you in therapy?
8. What would you like to be able to do 6 months from now?
9. What concerns do you have about coming to speech therapy?
10. What motivates you to improve your speech?

[a] Note that questions should be rephrased to a simpler form or to a yes/no or gesture response format to accommodate the communication ability of the aphasic individual.

their problem(s), (*b*) the impact of these problems on everyday life, (*c*) their expectations regarding therapy and its outcomes, and (*d*) their motivation to improve their communication. The format of questions presented here should be used as a springboard to other issues that arise during interaction with the client and/or family and adapted according to the communication abilities and cultural background of the individual. Moreover, questions for the more expressively impaired aphasic individual should be phrased to elicit "yes/no" or gestural responses. Further, the questions posed here emanate from a typical "middle-class white clinician" interacting with a similar type client. These questions may need to be rephrased to sensitively meet the "self-disclosure" values of minority groups (see Sue and Sue, 1990). Further, it is important that during such discussions, the clinician convey a supportive and nonjudgmental attitude toward the client and the family.

Table 13.2 presents a series of questions under three main headings. The first area focuses on how clients define their present situation. Note that the questions target issues broader than communication per se. It is possible that the client perceives difficulties other than communication as primary burdens. Identification of such a perception helps the clinician appropriately modify therapy goals and methods, leading to greater functionality of therapy outcomes. For example, the aphasic who is more concerned about independently performing

activities of daily living so that he would not be a burden for his wife on returning home might have his communication therapy focus on vocabulary and ideas associated with these activities.

The second area of questions focuses on the clients' perception of the impact of the stroke and aphasia on their role and interaction with their family and extended systems. If clients perceive that they have a limited role within these systems and few opportunities to communicate, therapy is not likely to be productive. Identification of the complicated demands that the stroke and aphasia have placed on the aphasic leads to more functional therapy outcomes. For example, if the aphasic client perceives that his or her family avoids entering into conversations because of potential communication breakdowns, functional therapy would provide the communication partners with effective repair strategies.

The third area of questions concentrates on the client's motivation to improve. Being a "client" is a foreign role for many, if not most, aphasic adults. It is often a role associated with inadequacy, dependency, and helplessness. We need to know the client's previous experiences of being in a helping situation and what factors contributed to success or failure. The aphasic client who took his child to a speech-language pathologist for speech therapy may have a different conception about his own therapy than the client who is unsure of what a speech-language pathologist does. The final area of questions focuses on what clients would like to improve in therapy and explores their expectations for success. Answers to these questions will help the speech-language pathologist fine-tune therapy goals and make them congruent with the client's personal agenda for therapy.

Microsystems Assessment

While there are numerous models of family assessment adaptable to this environmental systems approach, one model that is especially useful is the ABCX described originally by Hill (1949) and modified by McCubbin and Patterson (1983). This model focuses on how the family deals with the stroke situation over time. Table 13.3 lists the model's components, definitions, and established formal assessment tools. Variable A is composed of the stressor event itself and the present and lingering demands faced by the family. Variable B encompasses the internal and external resources that the family may use to cope with their normative life-stage stressors, the stroke, and its sequelae. Variable C is the individual family members' definition of the problem as a source of stress. The X variable is the interaction of the above variables, resulting in the ability of the family to make productive changes to meet their challenged system. For a more complete discussion of this model, the reader is referred to Jones, 1989; Lubinski, 1991; and McCubbin and Patterson, 1983.

The ABCX model can be operationalized into an assessment tool in either of two ways. First, a number of assessment instruments are available from the family counseling literature. Jones and Lubinski (b-forthcoming) recently applied these tools to the assessment of nine poststroke mature families and found that speech-language pathologists could easily use these to assess families. Although somewhat time consuming for individual family members to complete, the instruments did provide a uniform means of assessing the ABCX factors.

Speech-language pathologists may feel more comfortable designing their own open-ended questions that reflect this model. For example, Table 13.4 offers a series of questions that probe the first three components of the ABCX model. The questions in the demand area feature the significant events prior to, during, and after the stroke that have caused hardships for individual family members and the family as a whole. Remember that in systems theory, hardships felt by one member are likely to reverberate to others. The questions are presented on a time line, beginning with prestroke hardships and proceeding to current demands. Family members may be surprised that you are interested in areas other than the aphasia, and justification for the line of questioning should be given.

The second area of questions focuses on the internal and external resources the family members bring to the current stroke situation. Through these questions, we learn more about our client's family system: their roles, family subsystems, their problem-solving style, their communication patterns, their flexibility, and their cohesion. We will also attempt to define the type, degree, and receptivity to support from extended systems such as relatives, friends, and community agencies.

The family definition of the problem constitutes the third area of questions. We must not assume that aphasia is the family's primary concern. Despite our own professional bias that communication is essential to personal well-being, we must sensitively appreciate other viewpoints. Should the family perceive other difficulties as paramount, this will lead to adjustments in therapy goals, family education, and involvement in therapy.

The analysis of the above variables helps the speech-language pathologist understand how stress develops for the aphasic person and his or her family (Variable X). Many combinations of variables are possible. Some families may have such strong resources that the demands of the stroke or aphasia result in controllable changes within the family system. Other families may have strong resources, but the immediate demands are so great that they feel out of control. Yet other families may have such weak internal or external resources that even a mild problem greatly affects their return to homeostasis.

External Environment Assessment

Two aspects of the external environment can be explored by the speech-language pathologists to further complete the

Table 13.3.
ABCX Model of Family Stress: Definitions and Tools for Assessment of Families

Variable	Definition	Self-Report Assessment Tools
A	Stressor event and its ensuing demands, negative coping strategies, lingering coexisting family problems	Questionnaire on Resources and Stress for Families with Chronically Ill or Handicapped (Holroyd, 1986)
		Family Needs Assessment Tool (Rawlins et al., 1990)
		Family Inventory of Life Events (FILE) (McCubbin et al., 1981)
		Strain Questionnaire (Lefebre and Sanford, 1985)
B	Internal and external resources to meet demands associated with stressor	Family Assessment Device (FAD) (Epstein et al., 1983)
		Family Adaptability and Cohesion Scales (FACES III) (Olson et al., 1985)
		Family Crisis Oriented Personal Evaluation Scale (F-COPES) (McCubbin et al., 1981)
C	Family definition of stressor	Family Definition Rating Scale (Jones, 1989)
X	Stress, crisis, and change exhibited by the family	Subjective analysis of interviews, observation, and above family self-report tools

total environmental systems assessments. First, careful assessment of the sociocultural and economic environment provides sensitivity to powerful but amorphous forces affecting compliance and progress in therapy. Second, assessment of the physical environment increases the aphasic client's opportunities to communicate in a setting that enhances rather than obstructs interchange.

Sociocultural and Economic Assessment

Looking at a client's surname or color of skin is no substitute for a more in-depth cultural assessment of the client and family. May (1992) further reminds us that by looking at an individual or family, we cannot assume that they fully ascribe to the dominant belief system of their culture. He states, "Cultures themselves are continually changing as they adapt to new realities" (p. 47). The speech-language pathologist should review the findings offered by other specialists, such as social workers or psychologists, for additional information on sociocultural background. It is also natural that these types of questions could be incorporated into the other areas of the interview such as in discussion of family roles.

Westby (1990) suggests that speech-language pathologists use an ethnographic interview process with multicultural clients. "Ethnographic interviews have the goal of helping the interviewer understand the social situations in which the families exist and how the families perceive, feel about and understand these situations" (p. 105). Basic to this process is the development of rapport, the use of descriptive questions, and careful wording of questions. In general, open-ended questions are most productive. These questions encourage the individuals to express their perceptions and feelings about the communication problem and its relationship to family and culture.

Table 13.5 is adapted from work on cultural assessment for nursing personnel by Friedman (1990). The initial questions elicit information regarding the cultural experiences and values of the individual and family. Again, clients from some cultural groups may be wary of such questions, and thus they should be asked with respect, judgment, and communication sensitivity.

In addition, several questions might be posed to the client or family to assess the economic impact of the stroke and therapy. Answers to these questions may be sought from other sources such as social workers and financial officers of the rehabilitation setting. It is important that the speech-language pathologist, the client, and the family understand the costs of therapy, the nature and extent of insured coverage, and the options available to supplement existing resources.

Physical Environment Assessment

Once the sociocultural milieu is better understood, we need to focus on the physical environment of our aphasic client. Particular attention should be addressed to (a) the physical accessibility to people and activities that generate communication opportunities, (b) the sensory/cognitive dimensions of the environment that contribute to adequate transmission and reception of verbal and nonverbal messages, and (c) the psychosocial environment to stimulate interaction. Specific environmental profiles to evaluate the physical environment for communication are published elsewhere (Carroll, 1978; Lubinski, 1991). In keeping with the "question format" used in this chapter, Table 13.6 presents questions that explore the nature of the

physical and social settings in which the aphasic individual resides. These questions can be adapted to hospital, nursing or rehabilitation facility, home, or other community setting.

The first series of questions explores how well the aphasic individual can access communication opportunities in his or her environment. Identification of factors that impede access to people or activities that promote conversations and cognitive stimulation is basic to carryover of therapy goals. The next two areas of questions focus on the auditory and visual environment. Answers to these questions tell us more about the sensory conditions that may facilitate or impede adequate transmission of information for the aphasic person and his or her partners. The final area tells us more about the social role available to the aphasic client. These questions help us understand the aphasic's opportunities for reintegration into family and extended social systems.

SYSTEMS INTERVENTION

Goal Planning for Environmental Systems Intervention

The line between assessment and intervention in a systems approach is less clear than in other approaches to aphasia therapy for several reasons. By the very act of interviewing and assessing, the original systems of the aphasic individual have been modified. For example, the clinician's questions regarding therapy goals force the aphasic individual and family to assess their priorities and involvement in the therapy process. Second, by asking such questions, there is an implicit assumption that the answers to these questions are meaningful to setting therapy goals. Third, during the process of assessment, the beginning of a therapeutic relationship between client, family, and clinician is being established. Interaction with the clinician during assessment sets the stage for the establishment of trust, communication, cooperation, interactive problem solving, and eventual independence.

Thus, the therapeutic goals for an environmental system approach evolve during the assessment process and therapy itself. Therapeutic objectives might be considered on both a short-term and long-term basis. Short-term environmental goals focus on that which can be accomplished during the severe illness stage, recuperation, and rehabilitation. Long-term goals concentrate on helping the individual and family cope with a communication disability and handicap, changes within the family network, and possible institutionalization. Goals are arrived at through a joint effort of the speech-language pathologist, the aphasic person, and other significant members of the aphasic individual's environment such as family members, rehabilitation specialists, and professional caregivers. An interactive approach encourages the continued reassessment and renegotiation of therapy objectives and the development of self-dependence and self-determination on the part of the client and family.

Effective and functional environmental systems goals must be operationally defined. Their effects must be measurable changes in the behaviors of the significant individuals and in the physical setting. All participants in the environmental systems management program should understand therapy goals, the importance of self-generated goals, and the relationship of goals to eventual therapy success. Goals that emanate from the aphasic individual or significant others are likely to be the most func-

Table 13.4.

Interview Questions to Explore ABCX Model of Family Coping as Applied to Adult Aphasics and Their Families[a]

A: Demands

1. What significant events were occurring in your family prior to the onset of your family member's stroke (e.g., other illnesses, death, divorce, job loss, relocation, adult child leaves home)?
2. How did these events affect your whole family when they occurred?
3. How do you think these events affect your family at this time?
4. How do you describe the impact of your family member's stroke on the family at this time?
5. How has your family member's communication difficulty affected the family?
6. Who do you think has been most affected by your family member's stroke? Why? In what way?
7. Who has primary responsibility for the care of your family member?
8. What other demands does this individual have on him/her while caring for your family member (e.g., own illness, work outside home, own family)?
9. What is involved in the care of your family member at this time?
10. How has the care of your family member affected the primary caregiver (e.g., fatigue, competing demands, illness, psychological stress)?
11. How has the care of your family member affected the social life of your family and of the primary caregiver?
12. What financial problems is your family incurring related to the stroke?
13. Do you think there will be any other major changes occurring in your family in the near future (e.g., upcoming marriage, relocation, need for home health care)?

B: Resources

1. How would you describe your family's strengths (e.g., adaptable, cohesive, good communication, opportunities for independence)?
2. How would you describe your family member's ability to cope with difficult situations in the past?
3. When your family faces a problem, what strategies do they use to solve the problem (e.g., family discussion, sharing of responsibilities, seeking outside help)?
4. How successful do you think your family is in solving difficult problems? Why?
5. How willing is your family to seek help from outside sources such as friends, medical personnel, clergy, or community counselors? Describe the circumstances in which outside help was sought previously and their effectiveness in helping the family cope.
6. Who is likely to be the leader of your family at this time? Why?
7. How are major decisions regarding the care of your family member made?
8. Who is (or will be) the primary communication partner of your family member? How willing and available is this individual to attend communication therapy?
9. What information have you received about the nature and impact of a stroke? What information have you received about communication problems following a stroke?
10. Has anyone else in your immediate family ever had a stroke? How did the family cope with this problem?
11. Has anyone else in your immediate family ever had a communication problem after a stroke? Did this person have speech-language therapy?
12. What strategies have you tried so far that facilitate communication with your family member?

C: Problem Definition

1. What do you perceive as the major problem facing your family at present?
2. Why is this problem so critical?
3. What do you think can be done about this problem?
4. If the communication problem is not mentioned, then ask the following: How does your family member's communication problem compare with the one you just mentioned?
5. What are your priorities for your family member's rehabilitation at this time?
6. How important is it to your family member to improve his or her communication at this time? Why?
7. What do you expect of communication therapy for your family member?
8. How much control do you (and other family members) feel over the present situation related to your family member's stroke and rehabilitation?

[a] The individual with aphasia is referred to as "your family member" throughout the interviews.

tional. For example, an operational goal for an aphasic client who wants and needs a greater variety of communication partners might be one of the following:

1. To encourage three individuals outside the family to talk with the aphasic person at least once daily for a period of at least 15 minutes
2. To encourage the spouse of the aphasic individual to invite one or two of her husband's friends home each week for a game of cards
3. To take the aphasic individual to a social event where he or she has the opportunity to interact with friends and acquaintances at least once weekly

Focus on the Individual

At the core of the environmental systems approach is the individual with aphasia. Rehabilitation efforts focus primarily on empowering this individual to lead as meaningful a social role as possible in his or her home and extended social groups. The most immediate need is to help the individual retain or achieve status as an active and viable communication partner. This is done by strengthening specific receptive and expressive communication skills whereby individuals can intelligibly and

Table 13.5.
Questions to Assist in Sociocultural and Economic Assessment of the Aphasic Individual and the Family[a]

Sociocultural Issues
1. Do you (or does your family) identify with a certain ethnic or racial group? If yes, which one?
2. Where were you (your family member) born?
3. If not born in the United States, when did you (your family member) come to this country?
4. Where do you live? Are there individuals from different ethnic or racial groups in the neighborhood?
5. What is the primary language spoken at home? Is there anyone in the home who does not speak English? What is the relationship between this person and you (your family member)?
6. With whom do you (your family member) socialize on a regular basis?
7. Do you (your family member) interact with individuals outside your ethnic or racial group? For what purpose (e.g., work, leisure, religious services)?
8. With whom did you (your family member) discuss the stroke or aphasia? What advice was given to you? Did you try it? How effective was it in helping you talk?
9. Do you think that your religious beliefs affect your (your family member's) participation in therapy? If so, how?

Economic Issues
1. Have you discussed financial planning for therapy with anyone? With whom?
2. Do you have insurance that will cover therapy sessions? What kind?
3. Do you understand the limitations of your insurance to cover therapy sessions?
4. Will therapy costs be a burden to your family?
5. Would you like to speak with a financial counselor in our setting to further discuss therapy costs?

[a] The individual with aphasia is referred to as "your family member" throughout the interviews.

Table 13.6.
Questions Regarding the Physical and Social Environment of the Aphasic Adult[a]

Access Within Physical Environment
1. Describe the living situation where your family member resides.
2. Does your family member spend most of his time in one area of the setting or does he have access to all areas? Where does he/she spend most of his day?
3. How well can your family member get around this setting? Independently? With help from whom?
4. Does your family member use an assistive device to get around the setting, such as a wheelchair, walker, or cane?
5. Can your family member maneuver easily within the setting? If no, why not?

Auditory Environment
1. How noisy is the situation where your family member spends most of his/her day?
2. Is this situation one where he is likely to have conversations?
3. Can noisy situations be controlled (e.g., turn off radio or TV, close door to hall)?
4. Does your family member have a hearing loss?
5. Does your family member have a hearing aid for one or both ears? An assistive listening device?
6. Does your family member wear the hearing aid (or assistive listening device) regularly?
7. Does anyone else in the immediate situation have a hearing loss (e.g., elder spouse)?

Visual Environment
1. Is there sufficient lighting to see clearly in the areas where your family member spends most of his day?
2. Is light from the windows or lamps easily available and controlled?
3. Does your family member have any visual difficulties such as cataracts, glaucoma, or macular degeneration?
4. Does your family member wear glasses regularly? Or use any type of visual assistive device such as a magnifying glass?

Psychosocial Environment
1. In what activities does your family member participate on a daily basis?
2. How personally fulfilling are these activities to your family member?
3. Is communication an important part of these activities?
4. Who is available to talk with your family member throughout the day?
5. Who would your family member enjoy talking with if he/she had the opportunity?
6. Who takes a special interest in talking with your family member?
7. What activities does your family member participate in outside his everyday setting (e.g., outside the home or nursing facility)?
8. How much does your family member participate in family decision-making activities?
9. How has your family member's social role changed since the stroke?
10. Do family members or other caregivers understand the nature of your family member's communication difficulties? Their impact on his/her quality of everyday life?
11. How well do you think your family member has been reintegrated into the family? Other favorite social groups?

[a] The individual with aphasia is referred to as "your family member" throughout the interviews.

meaningfully contribute their personal ideas and can have their physical and psychological needs appropriately met. Traditionally, this goal is achieved through individual and group speech and language therapy sessions using a variety of approaches, as offered in this text.

There are, however, other immediate goals for the individual that have long-term implications and that go beyond strengthening specific communication skills. These include helping the individual understand (*a*) what has happened to him or her (*b*) the nature of therapy, (*c*) the goal-setting process, (*d*) the mutual responsibilities of client and clinician (*e*) how progress can be measured, and (*f*) the long-term prospectus. Litman (1962), in an early study of physical rehabilitation, found that patients frequently did not know what was involved in the "disability, its limitations, implications and possibilities" (p. 569). The speech-language pathologist may need to modify how these topics are discussed with the aphasic client, depending on the client's communicative, cognitive, and emotional status.

Coping with rehabilitation and residual psychological and communication disabilities is an unfolding process for the aphasic person. The aphasic enters therapy with some degree of knowledge, however limited, regarding aphasia and rehabilitation, and this knowledge base is modified by his or her new experience as an aphasic "client" or "patient." Clients may have one set of expectations when they begin therapy and yet develop another set 6 months later. Clients who are encouraged to understand their circumstances and participate in decision making regarding them are more likely to perceive control over these circumstances and thus participate more actively in the therapeutic process. These individuals are also more likely to be perceived by significant others in their environment as more alert, more competent, and less helpless (Lubinski, 1991). Continued discussion with clients about their perceptions of aphasia and therapy should extend throughout the therapy process.

Specific topics focusing on aphasia and rehabilitation with clients might include:

1. What happened to the brain during the stroke
2. The immediate and long-term effects of the stroke on communication
3. The diagnostic process of delineating communication strengths and weaknesses
4. Tentative short- and long-term goals for therapy
5. The importance of the client's therapy goals and expected outcomes
6. How progress can be measured
7. Other effects of stroke: on social roles, on family, on extended social groups, and so on
8. Depression following stroke
9. Taking control of circumstances
10. Assets and resources to help in the rehabilitation process

The clinician must be constantly alert for signs of depression in the aphasic client. In some situations, referral to a mental health specialist is the appropriate alternative. However, several approaches to relieving symptoms of depression can be incorporated into daily aphasia rehabilitation. In fact, these approaches appear to be cornerstones of a positive approach to clients in general. Tanner et al. (1989) suggest that the speech-language pathologist incorporate frequent positive reinforcement into every session as a means of relieving depression: "Rewards permit the client to concentrate on the positive, not the negative, aspects of the disability" (p. 79). They also suggest that the

aphasic client should have opportunities to participate in private time, activities of choice, and group therapy with other aphasic clients.

Other considerations that help relieve depression include clinician willingness to temporarily put aside speech or language goals to allow aphasic patients to vent their feelings. Although some clinicians may feel uneasy when the client discusses such private feelings as inadequacy, loneliness, unhappiness, and guilt, the very act of revealing these feelings may be therapeutic. Revelation of these feelings indicates that the aphasic client has a sense of trust in the speech-language pathologist. This is the time when positive verbal and nonverbal communication skills on the part of the clinician become critical. The reader is referred to several recent resources for an in-depth discussion of communication skills during therapy and counseling (Luteman, 1991; Scheuerle, 1992; Shipley, 1992).

The speech-language pathologist also needs to consider long-term goals for the aphasic client, including strengthening coping skills to deal with residual communication difficulties, achieving independence and socially fulfilling roles in the community, returning to employment, and, for some aphasics, preparing for long-term care. Teamwork with other rehabilitation specialists provides the optimum vehicle for accomplishing these goals. Many hospitals and rehabilitation centers will have teams composed of rehabilitation counselors or psychologists, discharge planners, and vocational counselors in addition to traditional medical and rehabilitation personnel. Speech-language pathologists will need to articulate the communication needs of the aphasic patient and family to these professionals and suggest strategies for incorporating communication goals with the goals of other specialists.

Focus on the Family

Virtually every speech-language pathologist would agree that the family is important in the success of a comprehensive rehabilitation program. Two initial questions should be answered before we discuss how to involve the family: Why is the family so important? What is involvement? Answering these questions leads to defining how family involvement can be operationalized so that therapy is functional and effective for the aphasic individual and the family itself.

Importance of Family in Aphasia Rehabilitation

From the beginning of the recovery period through rehabilitation and discharge, the family performs an important role in the success of the rehabilitation program. The family has been described as "central," "critical," and "focal" to positive outcomes of rehabilitation of any kind. The literature is replete with research and clinical reports that the success of the rehabilitation process may be anchored in the family (e.g., see articles by Norlin, 1986; Power, 1989; Rau et al., 1986; Rolland, 1988; Rollin, 1987; Watson, 1989). The family is important for at least four reasons.

First, aphasic individuals' initial and continuing impressions of their communication impairment and disability will be grounded in their interactions with their family. The bewilderment, anxiety, and frustration that the family members show during interactions impress on patients the potential gravity of their communication problem. Family members' expectations of, reactions to, and ability to cope with the initial and changing social roles and communication skills may greatly influence how aphasic individuals approach communication rehabilitation. Evans et al. (1992) state that patients make conclusions about their recovery in rehabilitation based on the perceptions of family members.

Second, after hospitalization, most aphasic individuals return to their family living situation (Evans et al., 1992). Thus, the primary communication partners and sources of support for outpatient rehabilitation will be the family. The family can offer instrumental support to meet daily care needs, or expressive support, such as the feelings of caring for and being cared about (Lin, 1986). It is hoped that the family will have strong internal and external resources to meet the level of support needed for the aphasic individual. Support encompasses obtaining therapy, bringing the individual to therapy, reinforcing communication attempts, and participating in family programs. It extends to providing interesting and challenging activities that foster communication and appropriate modification of the physical environment to promote communication interchanges.

The third reason why the family is so critical in rehabilitation is that a positive, well-adapting family promotes compliance with therapy objectives (Evans et al., 1991b). Families come to the stroke rehabilitation event with preconceived beliefs regarding disability, rehabilitation, and their role in the rehabilitation process. If families are not interested in participating in communication therapy themselves, this sends a clear message to the client that the burden for improvement is his or hers alone. Further, families so enmeshed in coping with prior demands and current crises may be too overwhelmed to understand their role in therapy. Des Rosier et al. (1992), in a study of the support needs of well spouses of chronically ill individuals, found that spouses needed personal time and social support from individuals outside the home. Family members' own active participation may be dependent on first receiving physical or psychological support that will help them cope more effectively with the myriad problems facing them.

Fourth, the family serves as an important source of information to the speech-language pathologist. During initial assessment, the family is often the primary resource regarding the premorbid client and family history. Families are also excellent resources regarding goals and progress in therapy. The family is the speech-language pathologist's principal and immediate link to the everyday environment of the aphasic individual.

What is Family Involvement?

Family involvement is defined here as the inclusion of significant family members as active participants in communication assessment, goal setting, and therapy. The environmental systems approach is based on the premise that family members will be consulted, supported, and educated in each stage of recovery from the initial severe illness or crisis stage through disability and possibly institutionalization. The primary goal for the family is to become effective and independent communication problem solvers during everyday interaction. The family should feel a sense of coresponsibility for the communication life of the aphasic individual. This concept is currently defined as "empowerment" and leads to a greater sense of personal control over the course of events (Dunst et al., 1989). Family involvement must go beyond providing progress statements as the client leaves the therapy situation, sending workbooks home for practice, or mentioning the value of family support groups.

Strategies for Involving the Family

The model for working with families presented in Table 13.1 is based on the premise that the family's needs are dynamic and change over time. This is a holistic model that cannot be accomplished by the speech-language pathologist alone but should incorporate other helping professions and extended social groups. Four strategies may be used at each stage of the model: support, education, modeling, and resource referral. Support is generally provided through active, open communication between the speech-language pathologist and the family. Education involves information given about stroke, aphasia, and the therapy process. This may be done through discussion and through supplemental readings for the family. Some popular readings for family members and significant others include *Aphasia and the Family* (American Heart Association, 1986a); *An Adult Has Aphasia* (Boone, 1983); *Helping the Aphasic to Recover His Speech* (Longerich, 1986); *Pathways* (Ewing and Pfalzgraf, 1991a); *Strokes: A Guide for the Family* (American Heart Association, 1986b); *The Family's Guide to Stroke, Head Trauma, and Speech Disorders* (Tanner, 1987); and *Understanding Aphasia* (Taylor, 1958). In addition, videocassettes on aphasia for home or small-group use can supplement readings: for example, *What Is Aphasia?* (Ewing and Pfalzgraf, 1991b) and *Pathways* (Wayne State University Press, 1991). Modeling is done each time the speech-language pathologist talks to the aphasic individual in the presence of family and when family members are present during specific strategy-teaching sessions. Resource referral involves knowing hospital, community, and peer group resources that may be of benefit to the family.

Severe Illness or Crisis Stage

When the individual first has the stroke, the family is likely to be in a state of disequilibrium or crisis. Usual activities halt, and family and individual resources focus on the physical state of the stroke patient. A multitude of deep and conflicting feelings surge among family members, including shock, fear of death and disability, guilt, helplessness, sorrow, and obsessive concern. This is the time when the entire family, and in particular the spouse, needs emotional support. Emotional support involves letting the individuals know that someone in the unfamiliar and impersonal world of the hospital knows who they are and understands the trauma they have experienced. Generally, this is a time when simple introductions, active listening, and comforting nonverbal communication will be important. Such supportive counseling helps establish an atmosphere of trust whereby individual family members can eventually express their feelings and concerns to the speech-language pathologist (Ziolko, 1991). It is not a time to explain the nature of stroke or aphasia, its severity, or its impact. This initial contact alerts the family that there will be a familiar and understanding professional there during the stages of recuperation and rehabilitation.

Recuperation Stage

Once the initial life-threatening stage is completed and the patient moves into recuperation, the family is set on a new course. There is a sense of relief that the patient will survive. There is also the realization that their relative exhibits some physical and communicative difficulties. The search for help begins. Simultaneously, life outside the hospital must return to some semblance of normal; the need for family homeostasis rises. Halm (1990) states that if the family does not try to reestablish equilibrium within a few days or weeks, their efforts will eventually be redirected from "problem neutralization to anxiety reduction" (p. 62). Consequently, family members assume or are assigned new roles within the family. Family members are still highly visible and available in the hospital during their visits to the patient. This becomes an ideal time to gather information about family resources to cope with the stroke, the competing demands on them, and their general coping styles. This is also the time for our initial communication assessment and for our first formal interaction with the family. Although the initial assessment provides only baseline information, family members will be interested in knowing the nature of the communication problem and its prognosis. Common questions include "What's wrong with Dad's speech?" and "Is he going to talk normally again?" During this early contact with the family, the speech-language pathologist must help the family begin to understand their role in the communication rehabilitation process. This is the opportunity to help the family mobilize their resources and problem-solving skills to help the aphasic individual communicate.

This early stage is also the time when general communication-facilitating strategies can be modeled by the speech-language pathologist. Simple strategies include (*a*) alerting the individual that conversation is to begin, (*b*) maintaining eye contact while talking, (*c*) using well-formed short utterances, (*d*) pausing frequently and using a slow to moderate speaking rate, and (*e*) generally including the aphasic individual in conversation even if responses are limited to single words or gestures. The speech-language pathologist must also remember that the family will need continued emotional support even though the life-threatening crisis is past.

Rehabilitation

Once the stroke patient is enrolled in a therapy program, the family has a sense of "hope" that things will get better, and they "expect" the patient to invest all of his or her energies into recovery. Success of rehabilitation is partly dependent on a balance of encouragement and realistic expectations. Thus, the speech-language pathologist should discuss with the aphasic individual and the family their expectations and how these coincide with the patient's neurological status and other internal and external factors that affect the outcome of therapy. This is also the time to actively include the family in observing and participating in therapy sessions that focus on communication-facilitating strategies. The family can also be an excellent resource for sharing strategies that they have developed spontaneously to assist in interaction. To work effectively with the family during rehabilitation, we must be available to them during nontraditional therapy times. Spouses and adult children who have jobs will not be able to regularly attend therapy offered during typical daytime hours. Thus, occasional evening and weekend hours for family-centered therapy should be available.

During rehabilitation, the family continues its metamorphoses. New family roles become more solidified. There may be financial and logistical strains associated with therapy. There may be physical changes in the home and the beginning of isolation from the community. The initial support given by extended systems recedes. Spouses and adult daughters are likely to bear the burden of responsibility for managing the household, meeting the physical and rehabilitation needs of their relative, and fitting in their own personal activities. Family members may feel isolated and physically and emotionally exhausted by caregiving stresses. Throughout rehabilitation, open communication between the speech-language pathologist and the family is imperative to ensure that information regarding direct therapy is balanced with family concerns. This is an especially important time when family members should feel a sense of control about therapy decisions.

Other than the direct provision of therapy, perhaps the most important goal during rehabilitation is planning for postrehabilitation. This involves fortifying the critical family communication partners with strategies and the problem-solving mental set that normal, if not functional, communication is possible with their aphasic relative. This also involves helping the family to define their present and expected needs and helping them to access extended systems resources to meet these needs.

Postrehabilitation Stage

At some point, direct rehabilitation with a speech-language pathologist ends, and the stroke patient is likely to have some degree of residual communication disability—from imperceptible to severe. The aphasic individual and the family no longer have the cushion that rehabilitation will result in improvement. Now they must truly rely on their own internal resources and the resources provided by extended systems. The postrehabilitation stage can be less handicapping and isolating if the speech-language pathologist has helped the family plan for this period. Should this not have been a focus, the family may face many years of frustration, resentment, and anger, resulting in fewer and less fulfilling communication opportunities for the aphasic individual. The extended systems of the aphasic individual and the family become particularly important in this stage, as will be described in the next section. With careful planning and guidance, the family should be able to reintegrate the aphasic individual into the family and their extended systems in former or newly created roles.

Long-Term Care

Some aphasic individuals may need to relocate to a long-term care setting such as a nursing facility. The decision to institutionalize the aphasic individual may be made during the recuperation stage or sometime after the individual has returned to the community. This decision is difficult for families and for the aphasic person. It is likely that once the aphasic person enters a long-term care setting he or she will remain there indefinitely. The aphasic person's relationship with the family is altered by the fact that he or she is not able to participate actively in the family, and thus the individual becomes the marginal member of the family. For some families, acceptance of permanent institutionalization may instill guilt feelings; for others, institutionalization may bring a sense of relief. In either case, families continue as an important source of cognitive and social stimulation for the aphasic individual. Counseling for the family of the institutionalized individual concentrates on helping them to understand the meaning of institutionalization, their role in the communication life of the aphasic individual, and strategies for communicating with the individual in that setting. Teamwork with the social worker or nursing staff can be important in helping the family and aphasic individual adjust successfully to long-term care. Finally, families in long-term care facilities may also join family support groups or participate in institution family councils. The value of such groups will be discussed in the next section on extended systems. For more in-depth discussion of the relationship between institutionalization, communication, and aging, the reader is referred to other works by Lubinski (1988, 1991).

Focus on Extended Systems and the Sociocultural Milieu

Extended Systems

As stated previously, stroke not only affects the aphasic individual and the immediate family but reverberates to extended systems and to the larger sociocultural milieu. These social networks in turn influence how the aphasic individual and the family seek and receive help. As family structure and physical availability change in our society, extended systems assume important social support functions. These include direct instrumental assistance; psychological and emotional comfort; resource and information sharing, such as offering referrals; and attitude or value transmission (Gourash, 1978). Speech-language pathologists should never underestimate the power of nonimmediate family and friends in the success or failure of the rehabilitation process.

The questions become how to delineate the extended systems of the aphasic individual and family and how to activate these systems to become positive influences in the communication rehabilitation process and after dismissal from therapy. Network mapping can be done through interviewing of the aphasic individual and family members regarding the types and extent of assistance they need and who provides it. The Inventory of Social Support (Trivette and Dunst, 1988) is a formal caregiver self-report tool that identifies social networks and types of assistance given by network members.

During rehabilitation, a natural extended system is composed of the rehabilitation team members and other patients attending therapy simultaneously. Clinicians such as occupational and physical therapists can be catalysts for promoting the communication skills gained in speech-language therapy. They provide opportunities and reinforcement for communication. Similarly, patients who participate in the same therapy programs can become important communication partners for the aphasic individual. The speech-language pathologist might spend some time observing the interactions occurring in other therapies, provide suggestions, and model effective communication techniques for other therapists and patients who interact with the aphasic individual.

New components to the supportive extended system for the aphasic individual and the family are the ''language stimulation therapy group'' and the ''aphasia family group.'' One of the best ways to encourage reintegration of the aphasic person and his or her family into the larger sociocultural milieu is through self-help group work. A self-help group is composed of peers who share a common problem and who unite to form a collective identity. Language stimulation therapy groups may be formed as a part of formal communication therapy or as a postdirect

therapy strategy. These groups may be either a homogeneous or heterogeneous collection of aphasic individuals who meet weekly to strengthen communication skills in a more natural interactional setting. Such groups help to make direct therapy more functional, encourage a sharing of knowledge and experiences, and create a new reference group for socialization and support (Cole et al., 1979). Group work may help patients more realistically measure abilities and progress (West, 1981). Aphasic individuals assisting each other assume a helping relationship role for themselves (Glozman, 1981). These groups are usually structured by a speech-language pathologist who has the primary responsibility for the goals and activities of the sessions. Haire (1981) suggests that during such sessions, the tasks should (a) focus on communicative interaction, (b) result in communication success for the aphasic regardless of communication mode or ability, (c) be client-originated rather than clinician-directed when possible, and (d) be relevant and interesting to the clients. Luterman (1991) finds that structured experience groups effect fewer positive changes than less structured groups. See Chapter 15 in this text for more details on group therapy.

A natural adjunct to the language stimulation group is the aphasia family support or recovery group. This group can be a combination of aphasic individuals and family members or family members alone. At times, family members appreciate having their own reference group where they can exchange ideas and feelings. Mixed groups of aphasic persons and family members may be particularly good for demonstration of communication strategies and resocialization. To be effective, the group should be organized by the members, with the speech-language pathologist serving as an adjunct or informal adviser.

In some cases, the peer group may ask the speech-language pathologist to present a series of talks about aphasia and its disorders. McCormick and Williams (1976) organized a 17-week program that covered such topics as the etiology of stroke, rehabilitation services, physical and medical management, psychological/emotional changes, environmental barriers, diet, relaxation, and role changes. Pasquarello (1990) evaluated a similar type of program and found that family members specifically appreciated the opportunity to share feelings with others and find out how other families coped with a stroke. In another study of support group effectiveness, Halm (1990) found that families perceived that such groups reduced anxiety and instilled hope. Support groups may assist families in locating available services and in advocating for services where they do not exist. Thus, topics chosen for such groups should be less lecture-oriented and include more open discussion and problem solving.

Other creative extended systems might be encouraged for the aphasic individual and the family, including family-to-family programs (Williams, 1991). Bissett et al. (1978) designed a spouse advocate program in which a family member of an aphasic person assisted other aphasic individuals and their families. These individuals, by their unique kinship and empathy with the problem, can offer families special support. Such family-to-family programs are based on the premise that individuals with intimate knowledge of a problem can be excellent resources for other families while gaining positive reward from the helping experience themselves. While such programs are not intended to replace professional counseling, the families can help relieve feelings of isolation and offer practical information about logistics of obtaining funding and other assistive services. Williams (1991) states that family-to-family programs give families a "sense of control, predictability, and opportunity" (p. 305).

Family advocacy groups can take on yet another dimension. Family members may wish to affiliate and become involved with local and national family advocacy groups such as the National Stroke Foundation and the National Head Injury Foundation. These groups serve important functions such as affecting legislation on issues related to stroke and head injury and helping to change the health care and rehabilitation system. Some families assume prominent roles in such organizations.

Finally, extended systems can include other community networks such as adult day-care programs, respite programs, health care assistants in the home, and volunteers. Full-time and part-time adult day-care programs may be associated with hospitals, nursing homes, or senior citizen centers. These programs provide custodial and health care, recreation, and nutrition as well as opportunities for socialization. Respite programs may be based in a community health care setting such as a nursing home whereby the aphasic individual can reside for a limited stay while the family travels or pursues noncaregiving activities. Brief respite programs may also be available within the aphasic individual's home while a family member shops, goes to a physician, or participates in other activities. National and local volunteer programs are available through many organizations such as the Ombudsman Program offered through the American Red Cross. In this program, senior volunteers visit nursing home patients and act as patient and family advocates with nursing home administration. Bell (1990) is an excellent resource for how to build volunteer programs for patients and their families.

The speech-language pathologist should be available to the extended groups in which the aphasic individual and the family are involved. Many of these groups are open to consultation from the speech-language pathologist regarding how to facilitate communication with the aphasic individual. Most of these individuals have limited experience with aphasic individuals and are eager to learn how to communicate more effectively. The goal in working with such groups is to provide strategies for facilitating communication with the aphasic individual. Role playing and problem solving, rather than didactic information regarding the nature and etiology of aphasia, are the most effective means of instruction.

Sociocultural Milieu

What can the speech-language pathologist do to meet the cultural needs of aphasic patients and their families? While this topic could be an entire chapter unto itself, a few guidelines are suggested. The first suggestion is that more individuals from minority groups should be encouraged to become speech-language pathologists. Interaction with a variety of minority individuals and more practica experience with diverse client groups should provide white middle-class speech-language pathologists with greater cultural depth perception. Graduate training programs are encouraged by the American Speech-Language-Hearing Association to incorporate cultural issues into and across coursework and practica. In addition to understanding the communication problems of various cultural groups, coursework should also focus on understanding trans-

cultural concepts and the spectrum of health care values and beliefs outside traditional Western medicine.

Rothenburger (1990) suggests that clinicians must learn to use all senses in interacting with clients of diverse cultures. She places a special emphasis on improving verbal and nonverbal skills that increase interaction sensitivity. Most important, clinicians need to assess their own cultural history and biases and how such perceptions affect service delivery to aphasic individuals and their families. Professional speech-language pathologists could also improve their cultural awareness through increasing interaction with diverse cultural and ethnic groups, attending departmental inservices or professional meetings, and reading literature that focuses on multicultural issues. Barney (1991) suggests that professionals should have built into their quality assessment process methods for assuring that the needs of specific ethnic and racial groups have been addressed appropriately.

Focus on the Physical Environment

No matter what setting the aphasic person lives in, either family home or institution, the physical characteristics of that environment become an important backdrop for communicative interaction. The physical setting should be a source of information and stimulation for the aphasic individual. While it may be impractical to redesign the hospital or family home, some realistic modifications that facilitate communication are possible. The factors that can be manipulated in most environments include (a) lighting and visual cues, (b) acoustic treatment, (c) furniture arrangement, and (d) environmental props. For a more in-depth discussion of these topics, the reader is referred to Calkins (1988) and Lubinski (1991).

Lighting and Visual Cues

Adequate and pleasant illumination creates a visually stimulating environment for aphasic persons and their communication partners. A high proportion of aphasic individuals and their spouses will exhibit visual changes associated with aging, including glaucoma, cataracts, and macular degeneration (Carroll, 1978). These visual changes result in blindness, low or blurred vision, and changes in central or peripheral vision. Thus, rooms that are dimly lit or filled with glare will reduce the aphasic person's ability to comprehend nonverbal cues, take advantage of contextual information, and derive cognitive and social stimulation from the visual environment. When possible, the aphasic person should have visual access to windows facing outdoors or to areas where everyday activities occur, such as the kitchen and living room at home, and the nursing station and lounge areas of the nursing home. Visual access gives the aphasic person a sense of connectedness with the external environment.

The use of color in the aphasic person's environment also plays an important role. Improving visual contrasts through color enhances information and aids in visual discrimination. For example, walls painted in primary colors with contrasting colors for doors aid in identification of one's own room, as do name plates printed in large-size white letters on a contrasting dark surface. Other simple strategies that enhance visual access include eliminating slick, shiny surfaces that provide glare; adding texture to surfaces of walls, furniture, and bedding; and using warm, medium-intensity colors to facilitate orientation.

Because some aphasic individuals will be seated in wheelchairs, placement of visual information such as clocks and bulletin boards should be adjusted appropriately for a seated person.

Perhaps the simplest strategy to enhance visual access is to ensure that the aphasic individual has the best vision possible through regular referral for opthalomological or optometrical evaluations. Use of glasses or other visual assistive devices should be easily accessible to the aphasic individual. Speech-language pathologists should check the patient's chart to note if there are visual field disturbances or if glasses are used prior to evaluations and therapy. Use of large-print materials and access to magnifying glasses or magnifying sheets should be encouraged to facilitate use of pictures or printed materials. Aphasic individuals with severe visual difficulties may benefit from listening to ''talking books'' or specially adapted televisions for the visually impaired. Finally, visual access is enhanced by coming face to face with the aphasic individual or asking what positioning facilitates facial access.

Acoustic Treatment

The primary goal of enhancing the acoustic environment is to ensure that intact auditory information reaches the aphasic individual. In addition to auditory comprehension difficulties, the aphasic individual may have hearing difficulties related to the aging process or previous life experiences, such as employment in noisy environments. Again, the first step in enhancing the acoustic environment is to begin with a referral for a complete otological and audiological evaluation. Aphasic individuals with a hearing loss should be encouraged to use a hearing aid or other assistive listening device to receive auditory information more adequately. Face-to-face communication also will optimize auditory receptive abilities.

Ambient noise in the environment may reduce the aphasic person's auditory attention and comprehension skills, particularly during conversation. Ideally, areas where the aphasic person frequently communicates should be acoustically treated with sound-absorbing materials to reduce ambient noise and reverberation. Other noise control strategies include turning off the radio or television when talking with the aphasic individual, and closing a door or window to reduce noise from other areas or corridors. Each of these techniques is inexpensive.

Noise abatement, however, does not mean removing all sound from the aphasic person's environment. Everyday sounds are a source of stimulation and conversation. Stimulation from the sounds of daily life, music, radios, and television can stimulate interaction with others in the environment. Auditory stimulation gives the aphasic individual knowledge about his or her surroundings and a sense of belonging.

Furniture Arrangement

The arrangement of furniture determines where, when, and with whom the aphasic person will talk. For example, the aphasic person in a wheelchair may lack access to favorite areas and social groups. Aphasic individuals will be more likely to join a group if they feel they can enter it with a minimum of inconvenience and disruption. Furniture, when possible, should be movable to promote easy access. Circular furniture arrangement also facilitates eye contact with a variety of people. It is crucial that the aphasic person retain control over some personal space in the environment. All individuals require areas and objects that reflect their unique personalities and interests. Finally, furniture arrangement should provide opportunities for privacy and intimate talk with chosen partners.

Environmental Props

Physical props in the environment also stimulate the aphasic person's general orientation and communication. Additions such as personal items, mementos, and favorite pictures into the institutional setting give individuals consistency with their family home and their life-long identity. Other props promote comprehension and way-finding in the environment. For example, clocks, calendars, pictures, and bulletin boards serve as orientation devices. As much as possible, the physical ''stuff'' of the environment should reflect the person's history and interests while providing multisensory cuing about time and place.

THE CLINICIAN AS A SYSTEMS CATALYST

Lest we forget, the speech-language pathologist (or other rehabilitation specialist) is a new and critically important component in the environmental systems approach to aphasia. From the initial referral and reading of a client's medical chart, the speech-language pathologist has entered the environment of the aphasic and his or her family. The speech-language pathologist brings to this encounter a host of personal and professional characteristics, as well as a health care and rehabilitation value system. The setting in which the speech-language pathologist offers communication therapy and any third-party payors for such service influence the clinician and the therapy offered. While research continues to delineate aphasic characteristics, less attention has been paid to the characteristics that the clinician and the rehabilitation setting contribute to therapy delivery and effectiveness.

McNeny and Wilcox (1991) state that rehabilitation specialists have overt, distinct perspectives on rehabilitation based on their education and experiences, but they also are influenced by less conscious beliefs. McNeny and Wilcox suggest that clinicians who have insight into their underlying feelings and attitudes may understand therapy better. Dunst et al. (1989) suggest that clinician attitudes, beliefs, and behaviors associated with client empowerment can be categorized along a prehelping, helping, and posthelping continuum. During the prehelping stage, the primary characteristics needed to foster client empowerment include (a) seeing the individual and the family as having strengths and abilities rather than deficits and (b) focusing on problem solving as the goal of therapy. During the helpgiving stage, positive clinician behaviors include good listening skills, focusing on client definition of needs, and a partnership mentality. Finally, during the posthelping stage, positive clinician responses stress minimizing help seeker indebtedness, accepting of client decisions, and enhancing a sense of self-efficacy on the part of the client and the family.

Particularly in working with families, it may be difficult for the speech-language pathologist to divorce one's own family experiences from interactions with client families. Cultural differences between clinician and aphasic/family also may engender conflicts between these entities. Fatigue, frustration, and lack of positive reinforcement—which are inherent in working with long-term multiply impaired clients who evidence little progress—influence how the clinician approaches the aphasic client and family. All of these factors may lead the clinician to misinterpret or be less sensitive to the actions and beliefs of those within the aphasic environment. Maslach (1982) states that "the kind of person you are dealing with may influence what you provide, how well you do it, and even whether you will do it at all" (p. 25).

Speech-language pathologists need to become more conscious of how powerful a factor they are in the lives of clients and families. A balance must be struck between rehabilitating specific communication skills and enabling the client and family to be their own clinician. The traditional focus on remediating specific communication skills tends to be clinician-driven, while the focus on enabling stresses that the solutions to communication difficulties can be generated by client and family. The speech-language pathologist as enabler provides information, models and reinforces facilitating communication strategies, and serves as a resource and advocate for the family and the client.

FUTURE TRENDS

Each section of this chapter raises important issues for the speech-language pathologist to consider, from philosophical perspectives of aphasia rehabilitation to practical questions of effective service delivery. The first issue raised was the growing emphasis on functional assessment and rehabilitation. This will be a major challenge for speech-language pathologists and aphasiologists. A major concern is that functional assessment tools possess rigorous psychometric properties if they are to be valid and reliable components of our testing batteries. Functional assessment will mean that speech-language pathologists must include assessment of clients outside traditional therapy settings as well as rely on caregiver report. Functional assessment will need to extend to better instruments for assessment of the family's attitude toward and ability to communicate effectively with the aphasic individual. A comprehensive functional assessment may include components directed toward the individual, the family or primary caregiver, and the physical and social environment.

This chapter challenges us to specifically, rather than incidentally, target some of our treatment toward the family and other significant persons in the lives of our patients. This will mean that our preprofessional and continuing education should include more work on understanding families and the sociocultural and economic milieu of the aphasic person. Specific coursework and practica in counseling should be required. This chapter also reminds us that the physical environment can either enhance or obstruct communication opportunities for our aphasic patients.

Numerous areas of research emanate from this chapter. Although a single research study to investigate the feasibility of the environmental systems approach is impossible, more discrete components could be empirically investigated in either traditional group or single-subject studies. It is likely that to investigate the environment more carefully, we need to move toward ethnometric, descriptive field and hypothetico-deductivism studies of poststroke family interaction in their natural settings (Jones and Lubinski—a-forthcoming). Such studies would open new avenues of research opportunities for practicing clinicians and add to our much needed data on the efficacy of such therapy.

As clinicians we are faced with making many choices with and for our aphasic clients. This chapter encourages you to choose between a narrow philosophy and a broad philosophy of assessment and intervention; between clinician-directed and client/family-enabled therapy; and between progress based on quantity of speech for the aphasic and progress based on quality of communication for the aphasic and his or her partners. The communication life of the aphasic is enhanced when we choose to go beyond words to function and from function to context.

Acknowledgments

Sincere appreciation is offered to the following individuals for their invaluable assistance in the preparation of this chapter: J. B. Orange, Ph.D., University of Western Ontario, for his careful reading of the chapter; Terri Cinotti, M.A., University at Buffalo, for her help in collecting references and in preparing the bibliography; and Kathleen Jones, Ph.D., State University College at Geneso, for introducing me to the family process literature.

References

American Heart Association. (1986a). *Aphasia and the family.* Dallas, TX: American Heart Association's Communications Division.

American Heart Association. (1986b). *Strokes: A guide for the family.* Dallas, TX: American Heart Association's Communications Division.

American Psychiatric Association. (1987). *Diagnostic and statistical manual of mental disorders, III-R.* Washington, DC: APA.

American Speech-Language and Hearing Association (ASHA). (1990). *Functional Communication Scales for Adults Project: Advisory report.* Rockville, MD: ASHA.

Andrews, J., and Andrews, M. (1987). *Family based treatment in communicative disorders. Sandwich, IL: Janelle Publications.*

Agar, M. (1980). *The professional stranger: An informed introduction to ethnography.* New York: Academic Press.

Aten J. (1986). Functional communication treatment. In R. Chapey (Ed.), *Language intervention strategies in adult aphasia.* Baltimore, MD: Williams & Wilkins.

Aten, J., Caliguiri, M., and Holland, A. (1982). The efficacy of functional communication therapy for chronic aphasic patients. *Journal of Speech and Hearing Disorders, 47,* 93–96.

Banja, S. (1990). Rehabilitation and empowerment. *Archives of Physical and Medical Rehabilitation, 71,* 614–615.

Barney, K. (1991). From Ellis Island to assisted living: Meeting the needs of older adults from diverse cultures. *American Journal of Occupational Therapy, 45,* 586–593.

Bell, V. (1990). Tapping an unlimited resource: Building volunteer programs for patients and their families. In N. Mace (Ed.), *Dementia care: Patient, family and community.* Baltimore, MD: Johns Hopkins University Press.

Bishop, P. (1982). Psychological issues and behavior in stroke rehabilitation. In J. Basmajian and M. Brandstates (Eds.), *Stroke Rehabilitation.* Baltimore, MD: Williams & Wilkins.

Bissett, J., Haire, A., and Nelson, M. (1978). *Involving the aphasic's wife in the rehabilitation of other aphasics.* Poster session at the Annual Convention of the American Speech and Hearing Association, San Francisco, CA.

Bonder, B. (1986/1987). Family systems and Alzheimer's disease: An approach to treatment. *Physical and Occupational Therapy in Geriatrics, 5,* 13–24.

Boone, D. R. (1983). *An adult has aphasia.* Danville, IL: Interstate Printers and Publishers.

Bozarth, J. (1981). The rehabilitation process and older people. *Journal of Rehabilitation, 45,* 28–32.

Brocklehurst, J., Morris, P., Andrews, K., Richards, B., and Laycock, P. (1981). Social effects of stroke. *Social Science Medicine, 15,* 35–39.

Brubaker, E. (1987). *Working with the elderly: A social system approach.* Newbury Park, CA: Sage.

Calkins, M. (1988). *Design for dementia: Planning environments for the elderly and confused.* Owing Mills, MD: National Health Publishing.

Carroll, K. (1978). *Human development in aging: The nursing home environment.* Minneapolis, MN: Ebenezer Center for Aging and Human Development.

Carver, V., and Rodda, M. (1978). *Disability and the environment*. New York: Schocken Books.

Cole, S., O'Conner, S., and Bennett, L. (1979). Self-help group for clinic patients with chronic illness. *Primary Care, 6*, 325–340.

Cross, T. (1988). *Cultural competence continuum—Focal point 3 (1)*. Portland, OR: Research and Training Center to Improve Services for Seriously Emotionally Handicapped Children and Their Families.

Cullum, C. M., and Bigler, E. (1991). Short- and long-term psychological status following stroke. *Journal of Nervous and Mental Diseases, 179*, 274–278.

Davis, G. (1986). Pragmatics and treatment. In R. Chapey (Ed.), *Language intervention strategies in adult aphasia*. Baltimore, MD: Williams & Wilkins.

Davis, G., and Wilcox, M. (1981). Incorporating parameters of natural conversation in aphasia treatment. In R. Chapey (Ed.), *Language intervention strategies in adult aphasia*. Baltimore, MD: Williams & Wilkins.

Des Rosier, M., Catanzaro, M., and Piller, J. (1992). Living with chronic illness: Social support and the well spouse perspective. *Rehabilitation Nursing, 17*, 87–91.

Dunst, C., Trivette, C., Gordon, N., and Pletcher, L. (1989). Building and mobilizing informal family support networks. In G. Singer and L. Irvin (Eds.), *Support for care giving families*. Baltimore, MD: Paul Brooks.

Egelko, S., Simon, D., Riley, E., Gordon, W., Ruckdeschel-Hibbard, M., and Diller, L. (1989). First year after stroke: Tracking cognitive and affective deficits. *Archives of Physical and Medical Rehabilitation, 70*, 297–302.

Epstein, N., Baldwin, L., and Bishop, D. (1983). The McMaster family assessment device. *Journal of Marital Family Therapy, 9*, 171–180.

Evans, R., Bishop, D., and Haselkorn, J. (1991a). Factors predicting satisfactory home care after stroke. *Archives of Physical and Medical Rehabilitation, 72*, 144–147.

Evans, R., Bishop, D., Haselkorn, J., Hendricks, R., Baldwin, D., and Connis, R. (1991b). From crisis to recovery: The family's role in stroke rehabilitation. *Neurological Rehabilitation, 1*, 69–78.

Evans, R., Griffith, J., Haselkorn, J., Hendricks, R., Baldwin, D., and Bishop, D. (1992). Poststroke family function: An evaluation of the family's role in rehabilitation. *Rehabilitation Nursing, 17*, 127–132.

Ewing, S., and Pfalzgraf, B. (1991a) *Pathways: Moving beyond stroke* (video). Detroit, MI: Wayne State University Press.

Ewing, S., and Pfalzgraf, B. (1991b). *What is aphasia?* (video). Detroit, MI: Wayne State University Press.

Frattali, C. (1992). Functional assessment of communication: Merging public policy with clinical views. *Aphasiology, 6*, 63–83.

Friedman, M. (1990). Transcultural family nursing: Application to Latino and Black families *Journal of Pediatric Nursing, 5*, 214–221.

Gatz, M., Bengston, V., and Blum, M. (1990). Caregiving families. In J. Birren and K. Schari (Eds.), *Handbook of psychology of aging* (3rd ed.). San Diego, CA: Academic Press.

Gibb, J. (1961). Defensive communication. *Journal of Communication, 11*, 141–148.

Glozman, J. (1981). On increasing motivation to communication in aphasics rehabilitation. *International Journal of Rehabilitation Research, 4*, 78–81.

Goffman, E. (1964). *Stigma*. Englewood Cliffs, NJ: Prentice-Hall.

Gourash, M. (1978). Help-seeking: A review of the literature. *American Journal of Community Psychology, 6*, 499–517.

Gray, W., Dyhl, F., and Rizzo, N. (1969). *General system theory and psychiatry*. Boston, MA: Little, Brown.

Haire, A. (1981). Principles for organizing group treatment. In R. Brookshire (Ed.), *Clinical aphasiology* (pp. 146–149). Minneapolis, MN: BRK.

Halm, M. (1990). Effects of support groups on anxiety of family members during critical illness. *Heart and Lung, 19*, 62–70.

Hill, R. (1949). *Families under stress*. New York: Harper & Row.

Holland, A. (1980). *Communicative abilities of daily living*. Baltimore, MD: University Park Press.

Holland, A. (1982). Observing functional communication of aphasic adults. *Journal of Speech and Hearing Disorders, 47*, 50–56.

Holroyd, J. (1974). The questionnaire on resources and stress: An instrument to measure family response to a handicapped family member. *Journal of Community Psychology, 2*, 92–94.

House, A., Dennis, M., Mogridge, L., Hawton, K., and Warlaw, C. (1990). Life events and difficulties preceding stroke. *Journal of Neurology, Neurosurgery, and Psychiatry, 53*, 1024–1028.

Hyman, M. (1972). Social psychological determinants of patients' performance in stroke rehabilitation. *Archives of Physical and Medical Rehabilitation, 53*, 217–226.

Ingstad, B. (1990). The disabled person in the community: Social and cultural aspects. *International Journal of Rehabilitation Research, 13*, 187–194.

Ittelson, W., Proshansky, H., Rivlin, L., and Winkel, G. (1974). *An introduction to environmental psychology*. New York: Holt, Rinehart, & Winston.

Jenike, M. (1988). Depression and other psychiatric disorders. In M. Albert and M. Moss (Eds.), *Geriatric neuropsychology*. New York: Holt, Rinehart, & Winston.

Jones, K. (1989). *Impacts of cerebrovascular accidents on family systems*. Unpublished doctoral dissertation, State University of New York at Buffalo, NY.

Jones, K., and Lubinski, R. (a—forthcoming). Communication disorders research: building scientific alliances in research for clinical relevance. *Journal of Speech Language Pathology*.

Jones, K., and Lubinski, R. (b—forthcoming). Methodology for investigating impacts of strokes on family systems. *Journal of Speech Language Pathology*.

Kavanagh, K., and Kennedy, P. (1992). *Promoting cultural diversity*. Newbury Park, CA: Sage.

Keller, C., Tanner, D., Urbina, C., and Gerstengberger, D. (1989). Psychological responses in aphasia: Theoretical considerations and nursing implications. *Journal of Neuroscience Nursing, 21*, 290–294.

Kelly-Hayes, M., Warf, P., Kannel, W., Sytkowski, P., D'Agostino, R., and Gresham, G. (1988). Factors influencing survival and need for institutionalization following stroke: The Framingham study. *Archives of Physical and Medical Rehabilitation, 69*, 415–418.

Kinsella, G., and Duffy, R. (1979). Psychosocial readjustment in the spouses of aphasic patients. *Scandinavian Journal of Rehabilitation Medicine, 11*, 129–132.

Krefting, L., and Krefting, D. (1991). Cultural influences on performance. In C. Christian and C. Baum (Eds.), *Occupational therapy: Overcoming human performance deficits*. Thorofare, NJ: Slack.

Langenbrunner, J., Willis, P., Jencks, S., Dobson, A., and Lezzoni, L. (1989). Developing payment refinements and reforms under Medicare for excluded hospitals. *Health Care Financing Review, 10*, 91–107.

Lawton, M. (1970). Assessment, integration and environments for older people. *Gerontology, 10*, 38–46.

Lefebre, R., and Sanford, S. (1985). A multi-model questionnaire for stress. *Journal of Human Stress, 11*, 69–75.

Lin, N. (1986). Conceptualizing social support. In N. Lin, A. Dean, and W. Ensel (Eds.), *Social support, life events, and depression* (pp. 17–30). New York: Academic Press.

Litman, T. (1962). Self-conception and physical rehabilitation. In A. Rose (Ed.), *Human behavior and social processes*. Boston, MA: Houghton Mifflin.

Longerich, MC. (1986). *Helping the aphasic to recover his speech: A manual for the family*. Los Angeles, CA: LLU Press.

Lubinski, R. (1981). Environmental language intervention. In R. Chapey (Ed.), *Language intervention strategies in adult aphasia*. Baltimore, MD: Williams & Wilkins.

Lubinski, R. (1988). A model for intervention: Communication skills, effectiveness and opportunity. In B. Shadden (Ed.), *Behavior and aging: A sourcebook for clinicians*. Baltimore, MD: Williams & Wilkins.

Lubinski, R. (1991). Environmental considerations for elderly patients. In R. Lubinski (Ed.), *Dementia and communication* Philadelphia, PA: Decker.

Luterman, D. (1991). *Counseling the communicatively disordered and their families*. Austin, TX: Pro-Ed.

Lyon, J. (1992). Communication use and participation in life for adults with aphasia in natural settings: The scope of the problem. *American Journal of Speech-Language Pathology, 1*, 7–14.

Maitz, E. (1991). Family systems theory applied to head injury. In J. Williams and T. Kay (Eds.), *Head injury and family matters*. Baltimore, MD: Paul Brooks.

Maslach, C. (1982). *Burnout: The cost of caring*. Englewood Cliffs, NJ: Prentice-Hall.

May, J. (1992). Working with diverse families: Building culturally competent systems of health care delivery. *Journal of Rheumatology, 19*, 46–48.

McCormick, G., and Williams, P. (1976). The Midwestern Pennsylvnaia Stroke Club: Conclusions following the first year's operation of a family centered program. In R. Brookshire (Ed.), *Clinical aphasiology: Conference proceedings*. Minneapolis, MN: BRK.

McCubbin, H., Larsen, A., and Olson, D. (1981). *Family Crisis Oriented Personal Evaluation Scales (COPES)*. St. Paul, MN: University of Minnesota.

McCubbin, H., and Patterson, J. (1983). The family stress process: A double ABCX model of adjustment and adaptation. In H. McCubbin, M. Sussman, and J. Patterson (Eds.), *Advances and developments in family stress theory and research*. New York: Haworth Press.

McCubbin, H., Patterson, J., and Wilson, L. (1980). *Family Inventory of Life Events and Changes (FILE)*. St. Paul, MN: University of Minnesota.

McGoldrick, M., and Carter, E. (1982). The family life cycle. In F. Walsh (Ed.), *Normal family processes*. New York: Guilford Press.

McNeny, R., and Wilcox, P. (1991). Partners by choice: The family and the rehabilitation team. *Neurological Rehabilitation, 1,* 7–18.

Moos, R. (1976). *The human contest*. New York: John Wiley & Sons.

Norlin, P. (1986). Familiar faces, sudden strangers: Helping families cope with the crisis of aphasia. In R. Chapey (Ed.), *Language intervention strategies in adult aphasia*. Baltimore, MD: Williams & Wilkins.

Olson, D., Portner, J., and Lavee, Y. (1985). *FACES III: Family social science*. Minneapolis MN: University of Minnesota.

Pasquarello, M. (1990). Developing, implementing, and evaluating a stroke recovery group. *Rehabilitation Nursing, 15,* 26–29.

Power, P. (1989). Working with families: An intervention model for rehabilitation nurses. *Rehabilitation Nursing, 14,* 73–76.

Rabinowitz, H., and Mitsos, S. (1964). Rehabilitation as planned social change: A conceptual framework. *Journal of Health and Human Behavior, 5,* 2–14.

Rau, M. T., Schulz, R., Tompkins, C., Rhyne, C., and Golper, L. (1986). The poststroke psychosocial environment of stroke patients and their partners: Some preliminary results of a longitudinal study. In R. Brookshire (Ed.), *Clinical aphasiology*. Minneapolis, MN: BRK.

Rawlins, P., Rawlins, T., and Horner, M. (1990). Development of the family needs assessment tool. *Western Journal of Nursing Research, 12,* 201–214.

Robinson, R., and Benson, D. F. (1981). Depression in aphasia patients: Frequency, severity, and clinicopathological correlations. *Brain and Language, 14,* 282–291.

Rolland, J. (1988). A conceptual model of chronic and life-threatening illness and its impact on families. In C. Chilman, E. Nunnally, and F. Cox (Eds.), *Chronic illness and disability,* Newbury Park, CA: Sage.

Rolland, J. (1990). Anticipatory loss: A family systems developmental framework. *Family Process, 29,* 229–243.

Rollin, W. (1987). *The psychology of communication disorders in individuals and their families*. Englewood Cliffs, NJ: Prentice-Hall.

Romano, M. (1989). The therapeutic milieu in the rehabilitation processes. In D. Krueger (Ed.), *Rehabilitation psychology*. Rockville, MD: Aspen.

Rothenburger, R. (1990). Transcultural nursing overcoming obstacles to effective communication. *American Organization of Registered Nurses Journal, 51,* 1349–1363.

Safilios-Rothchild, C. (1970). *The sociology and social psychology of disability and rehabilitation*. New York: Random House.

Scheuerle, J. (1992). *Counseling in speech-language pathology and audiology*. New York: Merrill.

Shipley, K. (1992). *Interviewing and counseling in communicative disorders*. New York: Merrill.

Simon, A., and Agazarian, Y. (1967). *Sequential analysis of verbal interaction*. Philadelphia, PA: Research for Better Schools.

Starkstein, S., and Robinson, R. (1988). Aphasia and depression. *Aphasiology, 2,* 1–20.

Steger, H. (1976). Understanding the psychological factors in rehabilitation. *Geriatrics, 31,* 68–73.

Stern, R., and Bachman, D. (1991). Depressive symptoms following stroke. *American Journal of Psychiatry, 148,* 351–356.

Sue, D., and Sue D. (1990). *Counseling the culturally different: Theory and practice* (2nd ed.). New York: John Wiley & Sons.

Tanner, D. (1987). *The family's guide to stroke, head trauma, and speech disorders*. Tulsa, OK: Modern Education Corp.

Tanner, D., and Gerstenberger, R. (1988). The grief response in neuropathologies of speech and language. *Aphasiology, 2,* 79–84.

Tanner, D., Gerstenberger, D., and Keller, C. (1989). Guidelines for the treatment of chronic depression in the aphasia patient. *Rehabilitation Nursing, 14,* 77–80.

Taylor, M. (1958). *Understanding aphasia*. New York: Institute of Rehabilitation Medicine.

Trivette, C., and Dunst, C. (1988). Inventory of social support. In C. Dunst, C. Trivette, and C. Deal (Eds.), *Empowering families: Principles and guidelines for practice*. Cambridge, MA: Brookline Book.

Turnbull, A., and Turnbull, H. R. (1991). Understanding families from a systems perspective. In J. Williams and T. Kay (Eds.), *Head injury: A family matter*. Baltimore, MD: Paul Brooks.

Wahrborg, P. (1991). *Assessment and management of emotional and psychological reactions to brain damage and aphasia*. San Diego, CA: Singular Publishing Group.

Wallace, G., and Freeman, S. (1991). Adults with neurological impairment from multicultural populations. *Journal of the American Speech and Hearing Association, 33,* 58–62.

Watson, P. (1989). Indications of family capacity for participating in the rehabilitation process: Report of a preliminary investigation. *Rehabilitation Nursing, 14,* 318–322.

Watzlawick, P., and Coyne, J. (1980). Depression following strokes: Brief problem-focused family treatment. *Family Process, 19,* 13–18.

Wayne State University. (1991). *Pathways*. Detroit, MI: Wayne State University Press.

Webster, E. J., and Newhoff, M. N. (1981). Intervention with families of communicatively impaired adults. In D. L Beasley and G. A. Davis (Eds.), *Aging communication processes and disorders*. New York: Grune & Stratton.

Wertz, R. (1983). Language intervention context and setting for the aphasic adult. In J. Miller, D. Yoder, and R. Schiefelbusch (Eds.), *Contemporary issues in language intervention* (Report 12;1:116–220). Rockville, MD: ASHA.

West, J. (1981). Group treatment. In R. Brookshire (Ed.), *Proceedings of the Clinical Aphasiology Conference,* (pp. 149–152). Minneapolis, MN: BRK.

Westby, C. (1990). Ethnographic interviewing: Asking the right questions to the right people in the right ways. *Journal of Childhood Communication Disorders, 13,* 101–111.

Wilkerson, D., Batavia, A., and DeJong, G. (1992). Use of functional status measures for payment of medical rehabilitation services. *Archives of Physical and Medical Rehabilitation, 73,* 111–120.

Williams, J. (1991). Family reaction to head injury. In J. Williams and T. Kay (Eds.), *Head injury: A family matter*. Baltimore, MD: Paul Brooks.

Ziolko, M. (1991). Counseling parents of children with disabilities: A review of the literature and implications for practice. *Journal of Rehabilitation, 57,* 29–34.

CHAPTER 14
Functional Communication Treatment

JAMES L. ATEN

The purposes of this chapter are to define and describe functional communication treatment (FCT); to integrate and facilitate its inclusion into aphasia management approaches; and to discuss objectives and procedures that improve aphasic patients' communication in social contacts and everyday activities.

This topic, FCT, represents a crystallization of the concepts expressed by the other authors throughout this book. Clinical aphasiology and aphasiologists seek to improve the communicative abilities of aphasic persons. Since writing the initial version of this chapter in 1986, our medical and allied health worlds have become almost obsessed with the terms, if not the concepts, of "functional assessment" and "functional outcomes." Much else has happened very recently to enhance the status of FCT, yet much development, refinement, and documentation must be forthcoming to determine the complete role of FCT in aphasia rehabilitation.

Weniger and Sarno (1990) comment that, in terms of the future for aphasia therapy state "the pendulum appears to be swinging in the direction of a functional-holistic approach to aphasia therapy" (p. 30). As Wertz (1991) so sagely states, "certainly, aphasia treatment in 1990 has transcended only the restitution of semantics, syntax and phonology. It now involves a variety of methods designed to assist aphasic people in producing some useful, functional communication" (p. 316).

The diverse and complex nature of aphasia, both the disability and the communication impairment, presents a challenge as we attempt to define what functional communication entails. Rosenbek et al., (1989) state that "appropriate (aphasia) therapy is one that takes into account all the deficits—linguistic, cognitive, behavioral, social, familial" (p. 132). In their all-inclusive view of aphasia treatment, they have offered what this author believes is an excellent description of, and justification for, FCT.

Everyday functional communication for some patients involves little more than the capacity to convey a message to their nursing home caretakers that they want to have their wheelchair moved from the bedroom to the TV lounge. For numerous other patients, functional communicative skills might include expressing what it means to them emotionally to have experienced loss of language and their job, the limited use of

their right arm, and a diminished sense of self-esteem. The spectrum of communication needs is indeed broad for the variety of patients we treat. For example, in those very few instances where patients recover sufficiently to return to work, the functional communicative demands far exceed those of patients who spend their remaining days at home or in a board-and-care or nursing home. In actual life, "functional communication" must be individually defined for each patient and must consider the severity of the communicative disturbance, the premorbid and present self-chosen life-style of the patient, and the setting in which that person will ultimately reside.

FCT, properly defined and carefully developed according to each patient's need, should be a major focus of the aphasiologist concerned with treating the aphasic patient. Aphasia is not simply a disruption of language processes but rather involves disturbances of numerous para- and nonlinguistic processes (Katz, 1990; Lyon, 1992; McNeil et al., 1991). We need only review the recent history of aphasia treatment (Shewan, 1986) to realize that traditional treatment based on theories and principles developed by Schuell and her colleagues (1964) has been expanded from an emphasis on recovery of language functions to a position that stresses the importance of communication, as noted in the writings of Wepman (1972, 1976), Holland (1978), Martin (1978), Chapey (1981), Davis (1983), and many others. Cognizance of the limited gains from intensive application of traditional language-based treatments stimulates all but the most entrenched traditionalist to seek additional approaches to improve the amounts and levels of recovery of communication skills attained by the patients we have treated. We will consider these results in more detail later.

It has been estimated that well over 50% of communication occurs via body language. To isolate and stress auditory/oral language modalities, or semantics and syntax, or the naming function artificially limits maximization of communication processes. It is essential that we broaden our traditional views that stressed language as the major problem in aphasia.

These brief introductory comments may serve to entice the reader's continued exploration of some exciting approaches to helping the aphasic patient improve that most vital human activity—communication. Let us define our approach, see where it fits into an aphasia treatment program, and look at some ideas to help our patients get their messages across better.

FCT DEFINED

FCT is any therapeutic endeavor that seeks to improve the patient's reception, processing, and use of information germane to conducting daily activities, interacting socially, and expressing current physical and psychological needs. This formalized, operational definition emphasizes actual daily contacts and activities (functional) and information flow and exchanges (communication), in contrast to linguistically oriented, stimulus-response interactions that characterize traditional treatment interventions.

As mentioned earlier defining FCT is difficult because no sharp line of distinction exists between treatment of the language deficits in aphasia and intervention to improve daily communication. In practice, many aphasiologists engage in communicatively focused activities in treating their patients following the admonition by Schuell and colleagues (1964) "to communicate with the patient and to stimulate disrupted processes to function maximally" (p. 338). There are directional choices, however, because Schuell et al. state, "The clinician's objective is maximal recovery of language functions for each patient" (p. 342). In her wisdom she added, ". . . within the framework of the patient's needs" (p. 342). It behooves us to recognize the latter qualification. The operational model driving FCT is "whatever the patient needs."

Some aphasiologists strive to improve "processes," despite the absence of solid data to support the efficacy of such efforts. Others direct their treatments almost exclusively to remediating language deficits. The orientation of this chapter presents a break with traditionalists who stress either language or process stimulation as the sine qua non of intervention. Instead, the emphasis in FCT is on communication. Language recovery is then subsumed as an integral part but is not the sole, or even major, objective. Even contemporary writers (Holland, 1983; Wertz, 1983), in discussing the objectives of intervention and the roles of the aphasia clinician, alternate in use of the terms "language" and "communication." Semantic labels become important when they influence what we think we should do with patients.

Without clearer definitions and descriptions of the various forms of intervention, aphasiologists, particularly the less experienced, may focus on one area and fail to integrate language *and* the daily communication needs of the patient. We risk offering Band-Aids to patients who need stitches and compresses. The result is that our consumer will be treated with less than optimal efficiency, and the outcome may be a failure of treatment to maximize communication potentials in daily interactions.

CONTRASTING FUNCTIONAL COMMUNICATION APPROACHES AND TRADITIONAL REHABILITATIVE APPROACHES

Comparison of the more traditional treatment objectives and procedures with those of communication-focused treatment will clarify the role of FCT. That contrast is provided for us in Chapter 6 of this text.

Traditional treatment, as delivered by experienced aphasiologists, may often have been functionally focused. A critical

difference has been that many aphasiologists viewed language as the major deficit in the patient with aphasia. It therefore follows logically that a primary objective of traditional treatment has been to stimulate or program restoration or recovery of the patient's language functions in listening, speaking, reading, and writing. The emphasis in FCT is to recover or restore important daily communicative skills—language being only one aspect of communication, albeit an important one. For example, speaking fluently is not necessarily communicative, as patients with Wernicke's aphasia so vividly demonstrate. Conversely, the essentially mute patient, labeled mixed or Broca's type, may communicate much better (with less quantitative language) in his or her animated, head-nodding, nonlinguistic ways.

Most clinicians do not consciously reject functional approaches, however, trained as many of us were to isolate and solve problems in speech-language, we can too often stress "repairing" language deficits and discount pragmatic communicative needs. In the next section, further contrasts are presented and analyzed.

The Role of FCT in Aphasia Management

To conceptualize the role of FCT in treating aphasic patients, it is necessary to present an overview of past and contemporary forms of treatment. That overview should aid us in defining some unmet needs that FCT fulfills.

Schuell et al. (1964) stated, "We believe that the primary objective in treatment of aphasia is to increase communication" (p. 333). This same objective applies to FCT. The realization that the amount of communicative recovery will be limited necessitates emphasis on the practical or functional aspects of communication. Therefore, simply viewed, FCT and traditional aphasia therapy appear to have identical goals. Major differences do exist, however, and these differences derive from interpretations of the means for achieving the mutually desired end—communication. Despite the multiple approaches to intervention that exist today, aphasia treatment from the 1960s to present has focused primarily on Schuell's directive to achieve maximal recovery of language functions. This focus on treatment of language in aphasia and the impact on our management approaches is described next.

Traditional Focus on Language Recovery

Description of the treatment trends in aphasia over the past several years is offered by Shewan (1986) and by Wertz (1984) in his "State of the Clinical Art" discussion. Wertz classified aphasia therapies into several categories. The first he labels "traditional." It emphasizes language content and stimulus-response approaches. A second type evolved that included specific procedures for specific patient types, such as melodic intonation therapy (Sparks et al., 1974). The third type Wertz labeled "functional" treatment, and he cited Davis and Wilcox's (1981) technique, Promoting Aphasics' Communicative Effectiveness (PACE), as a solitary example. Wertz (1984) stated that PACE emphasizes language context rather than language content. Actually, this type of treatment emphasizes communication and incorporates pragmatic principles in treatment. The goals and procedures of language-based treatment can be closely integrated and fused with those of FCT rather than viewed as either separate forms of treatment or slight variations on the traditional language-based approaches.

Subsequent remarks by Wertz (1984) indicate that the concept of integrating traditional and "functional" approaches is not held by all. He observes that at the conclusion of traditional language treatment, "when improvement in language slows or stops, we consider terminating treatment or moving the patient into a maintenance group" (p. 60). Wertz recommends that at this point we should shift our attention to "caring" for the patient's function and quality of life and aid the patient in coping with the language deficits that remain. This author proposes that FCT serves a vital role in helping the patient cope initially with his or her residual language impairments. Therefore, the role of FCT should be an integrated one *with* language intervention from the *onset of treatment* and should *extend beyond* the period when language treatment, per se, is no longer effecting change.

Emphasis on Lexical Units in Isolation.   A specific example of focused language intervention is treatment aimed at improving word recall. Anomia constitutes a problem experienced by essentially all aphasic patients. Brookshire (1975) evaluated generalization that occurred when commonly employed procedures were used to reduce word-recall deficits. In a study of 10 patients, he found nonsignificant generalization to untreated words, verifying his hypothesis that drill on picture and object naming was nonefficacious. Previously, Wiegel-Crump and Keonigsknecht (1973) had found generalization to untrained words and categories, but they tested only four subjects. Brookshire's results were supported later by Seron et al. (1979), who reported that procedures to establish retrieval skills were more effective than techniques that considered word retrieval to be a loss of the lexicon.

Fodor (1983) believes that our words are organized in interconnected ways. Consequently, eliciting a word response is more likely to enrich associations and bring forth related words. We noted previously that few times in life are we asked for the specific name in isolation, yet information-bearing words are required to communicate orally. Contextual enrichment is more likely to evoke the word associations cited by Fodor.

Goodglass and Stuss (1979) noted group results may be deceptive because the type of aphasia influences how patients respond to stimulation cues. Schwartz and Whyte (1991) suggest that group research of the randomized clinical trials type does not answer efficacy questions adequately, in part because of the heterogeneity of both patients and types of treatments.

The burden on the investigator is enormous because the findings influence how we spend our clinical time. If work on naming tasks is a waste of time, it should obviously be discontinued. If, however, naming can be enhanced during FCT activities that also serve to facilitate language/communication improvement overall, precious and expensive treatment time has been used more effectively. A creative answer may be found in the investigation recently reported by Springer et al. (1991). PACE therapy alone was not efficacious unless combined with a goal-directed, structured language procedure. Further studies of this type are welcome and may show that the gap between traditional language approaches and FCT is a small one.

The role of FCT can be seen more clearly in studies that incorporate procedures such as prestimulation, description, and various other "primers." One example is a study by Podraza and Darley (1977), who looked at types of prestimulation to elicit naming responses. Direct prestimulation was relatively more effective than no stimulation and may represent one means of reducing confrontation "blockages." Waller and Darley (1978) found that paragraph-reading comprehension was enhanced by verbal descriptions that preceded the reading. Prestimulation and description are ways of putting language training into more natural or meaningful contexts, as Davis (1983) and Prutting (1982) recommend. The result is the patient is able to surmount, at least partially, the language deficits that ensue when word-comprehension or word-production tasks are demanded in isolated and artificial environments. Doyle et al. (1991) have recently shown that functional, trained responses can be generalized to unfamiliar volunteers.

Value of Redundancy.   A major reason for combining traditional language treatment and FCT principles and procedures is that it is quite likely that patients retain language content better when it is reinforced in daily contacts and use. Rosenbek et al. (1989) make a sustained plea for multiple exposures of patients to stimuli stating that once is not enough. When stimulation capitalizes on including stimuli that will be immediately heard or seen in the environment, the principle of multiple stimulation is more likely to be experienced.

The geriatric patient with severe aphasia has been repeatedly shown to comprehend and at least briefly retain information that is personally relevant. Because memory and retention play significant roles in influencing the amount and rate of aphasia recovery and learning potential or therapeutic readiness, FCT facilitates retention by providing:

1. A focus of treatment on basic language and communicative activities that are used daily;
2. An emphasis on content that is personally relevant;
3. An inclusion of principles from research on geriatric memory patterns that serve to increase retention of content. If our choice of content and materials enhances the probability that similar real-life stimulations will occur, comprehension and retention have an a priori better chance of success in generalizing to social settings.

How the Patient Views Recovery

Aphasiologists, in their predilection for repairing broken language, have been reinforced in their goal-directed language pursuits by many of the patients they treat, according to Sarno (1981). She observes that a discrepancy exists between a "patient's perception of recovery, performance on aphasia tests, and the clinical manifestations of aphasia" (p. 490). All too often, patients will not consider themselves "recovered" unless premorbid language competence is regained. We will review efficacy studies in the next section; however, the important point for now is that "a complete return to a premorbid state (of language competence) is usually the exception" (Sarno, 1981, p. 490). Indeed, as Rosenbek (1983) noted, some patients continue to insist on correcting their language errors in production, despite the clinician's insistence that "It's OK; I got your message."

In my opinion, both the aphasiologist and the patient need a therapeutic emphasis directed toward communicative focus in lieu of a language one. The goal is well stated by Rosenbek et al. (1989)—"to help them learn to live in harmony with the differences between the way they were and the way they are" (p. 131).

How the Family Views Recovery

Stroke has a cataclysmic effect on the family of the patient. They are far more likely to understand communication breakdowns in everyday interactions than they are to appreciate deficits discussed from formal language tests. Historically, Sarno's (1969) Functional Communication Profile has relied on "significant other" observation and rating. Recently, Lomas and colleagues (1989) have attempted to meet the objectives of practical assessment by developing a rating scale that is consumer oriented. Frattali (1992) points out that assessment should have social validity for the patient and family who may expect treatment on deficit skills to translate immediately into better communication between the patient and the family members.

Efficacy Studies

Objective support for Rosenbek's (1983) statement that "some patients do get better" is verified by the results of a Veterans Administration (VA) cooperative study (Wertz et al., 1986). This study was carefully designed to evaluate the efficacy of traditional, individual, language-based treatment for aphasic patients. Over 120 patients were randomly assigned to three treatment conditions. One group received approximately 100 hours of therapy offered by a trained speech pathologist immediately after enrollment and initial testing; a second group was treated by a trained volunteer for the same duration (12 weeks); a third group received the same type and amount of treatment by a Speech Pathologist as the first group, but treatment was initiated 12 weeks later. The group receiving immediate treatment by the speech pathologists made significantly more improvement than did the deferred treatment group. When the deferred group did receive treatment beginning at 12 weeks, they improved to the levels attained by the first group. The treatment effect for the group receiving immediate therapy by a speech pathologist was approximately six percentile points as measured by the Porch Index of Communicative Abilities (Porch, 1967). The result was statistically significant but not clinically robust. Traditional aphasia treatment of a carefully monitored, language-based type does improve language. Whether that language improvement is reflected in functionally significant changes in communication skills can be questioned. Overall, the functional measures employed in the VA study did not reveal significant changes. This issue will be discussed in the upcoming section on measuring treatment effects.

A previously conducted VA cooperative study (Wertz et al., 1981) was designed to compare the relative efficacy of individually administered, traditional, language-based treatment to group socialization experiences. The group treatment was designed to avoid direct treatment of language deficits and, instead, aimed to stimulate communicative skills through group discussion and social interaction. Analysis of the results indicated few differences between the groups and showed both methods of treatment to be efficacious.

The ideal, though not feasible, study would have treated a third group using combined language stimulation and social interaction procedures and would have included a fourth group that received no treatment. Nevertheless, these two well-designed studies document that language treatment helps some patients and that when group trends are analyzed, the treatment effect is statistically significant, although the gain is modest.

The group treatment result can be interpreted as support for the efficacy of communication-centered socialization treatment as well.

If FCT is to have a major role in intervention, it must be proved efficacious. Sarno (1981) cited a problem when she warned that improvement in quantitative measures of language performance of patients undergoing treatment is not always observed in functional changes in the patient's use of language. The VA cooperative study (Wertz et al., 1986) did not reveal significant change on most of the functional measures administered. Prutting (1982) comments, "At some point it will be necessary to compare clinical profiles (performance on tests, clinician-constructed tasks, and evaluation of language samples) with societal profiles (judgments of appropriateness of language use)" (p. 129).

ASSESSING FUNCTIONAL CHANGES

Aphasiologists should have assessment of functional improvement in communication as a primary objective and focus. This was noted earlier in comments by Sarno (1981, 1983) and has been recently well reviewed by Frattali (1992), who comments:

> Despite the findings that communication and language may be distinct but overlapping functions that require separate assessment, methods of integrating functional with traditional assessment approaches are seldom employed (p. 68).

As a result, the tools for assessment are few and inadequate for the task. This is true at a time when reimbursement sources are demanding functional assessment and functional treatment goals before funding treatment initiation, and functionally measured gains are required to continue funding ongoing rehabilitation.

As early as 1979, Holland directed aphasiologists' attention to recognizing communication assets in even the most severely language-impaired patient. (These are the patients who may be rejected as not suitable for language treatment and may also fail to qualify as subjects in efficacy studies because of their poor prognoses and intractability.) Holland's (1979) observation that aphasic patients "probably communicate better than they talk" (p. 173) is supported by other investigators (Wilcox, 1983). Indeed, according to Wilcox, "Aphasic persons appear to retain pragmatic abilities necessary to appropriate sociocommunicative behavior"(p. 42). Conversely, no one would seriously question the presence of specific communicative deficits requiring treatment in many aphasic patients. Therefore, we will be expected to employ the same diligence and thoroughness in diagnosing functional communication deficits as we have in assessing language prior to traditional intervention.

The need is well summarized by Blomert (1990) in saying that the primary concern of those in rehabilitation is focused on the functional performance of the patient, not simply the language deficit. He and his coworkers (Blomert et al., 1987) are developing a measure called the Amsterdam-Nijmegen Everyday Language Test. By assessing "communicative adequacy" as opposed to linguistic output, per se, the hope is to arrive at what is termed "just adequate" amounts of information that the listener can comprehend.

The testing and profiling of a patient's strengths and weaknesses in communicative acts is arduous at best because there are tools for appraisal. The Functional Communication Profile

(FCP) (Sarno, 1969) represented a beginning. The Communicative Abilities in Daily Living (CADL) (Holland, 1982) moved us farther down the functional testing path. Lomas and colleagues (1989) are refining the Communicative Effectiveness Index (CETI) to add to our scanty number of measures. Blomert's (1990) work was cited previously.

The need for assessing changes in communicative performance by other than traditional tests seems quite apparent in interpreting the results of the following study. Aten et al. (1982) found that chronic aphasic patients who had undergone extensive traditional treatment had reached a point where traditional language test scores on the Porch Index of Communicative Abilities (PICA) (Porch, 1967) were not changing over time. After these patients were enrolled in group treatment with structured, functional communication tasks and activities, their scores changed significantly on the CADL, a test purported to measure functional communication. The PICA language test scores remained static. Interestingly, Lomas and associates (1989) report that their recovering group of 11 patients revealed average changes of 11.4 on the CETI during a 6-week period but that similar changes were not evidenced on the Western Aphasia Battery (Kertesz, 1982).

Binder (1984) used an experimental form of Prutting's Pragmatic Protocol (Prutting and Kirchner, 1983) to describe spontaneous conversation in 11 aphasic patients. She documented pragmatic strengths not detectable by standard aphasia tests. A revised pragmatic profile was developed (Prutting and Kirchner, 1987) that has promise as a method for differentiating right- and left-hemisphere lesioned patients' discourse patterns.

Assessment for FCT must measure all aspects of communicative exchanges in social contexts. Horner (1984) suggests the difficulty of the task when she states, "linguistic competence and communicative competence interact in ways not completely predictable by the overall severity of the aphasia" (p. 149). This conundrum reflects the diversity of factors that directly influence communication. These factors have been well-described by Chapey (Chapter 11 in this text), Fodor (1983), Katz (1990), McNeil (1983), and others.

Byng and colleagues (1990) analyzed weaknesses in four aphasia tests currently in frequent use. They believe that the current, frequently used tests have limited value in guiding therapeutic intervention because the tests' major focus is either to classify aphasic patients into syndromes or to treat according to principles (see Chapter 8 in this text) that lack substantive or supportive data.

Lomas et al. (1989) cited above, have attempted to answer the demand for more functional measures that are consumer oriented and practical. Their 16-item rating scale was developed from a larger pool of 51 communication situations that aphasic patients and their spouses thought were important in their daily lives. The communicative areas sampled by the items are labeled *basic need* (e.g., toileting, eating, positioning); *health threat* (e.g., calling for help or exchanging information about one's medical status); *life skill* (giving or receiving information on such topics as shopping, traffic symbols, telephone); and *social need* (over dinner table, playing cards, writing a letter).

The essence of functional appraisal is to let the patient guide you. The hierarchy of losses and needs and residual strengths that are revealed become the database for intervention. This intervention is not simply an attempt to restore deficit language skills or lengthen oral responses or recover vocabulary.

Summarizing FCT Roles and Functional Testing

To summarize this section on the role of FCT in aphasia management, we have seen that traditional intervention strategies have been largely preoccupied with language improvement. Rationales have been presented to partially explain this emphasis. If language-focused or other forms of traditional treatment achieved complete recovery of language functions, the need for FCT might be debatable; however, in fact language recovery in aphasia is incomplete. Consequently, aphasic patients need improved communication in functional settings. Ultimate support for FCT will come from aphasiologists developing and administering new measures of functional communication; using FCT; and documenting a positive effect on persons with aphasia.

FCT PRINCIPLES TO GUIDE TREATMENT

FCT is structured to improve patients' reception, processing, and use of information, permitting them to interact socially, express their physical and psychological needs, and attain communication competence in a practical sense. As Wilcox (1983) stated, FCT leads to "the ability to convey and receive messages effectively and efficiently" (p. 42). Explicit principles have been proposed in the literature concerning pragmatics, cognition, and communication in the social environment. These topics will be reviewed in the next several sections.

Pragmatics

The first FCT principle is to establish communication interchanges and reinforce performances that are appropriate for that specific patient regardless of available language. Communication, not language, is primary. This principle is congruent with definitions of pragmatics such as Bates's (1976) "rules governing the use of language in context" (p. 420). Wilcox (1983) expands the definition in stating, "A pragmatic perspective focuses on *how* language is used in the communicative process. This is in direct contrast to a linguistic analysis, which focuses on *what* language is used in communication" (p. 36).

Application of pragmatics with aphasic patients (see Chapter 12), alters our traditional clinical behavior quite significantly when we elect to establish a communicative dyad rather than administering a formal language test during our initial patient contact. Prutting (1982) defined a dyad as "the minimal unit of analysis" for evaluating the communication that occurs between two people interacting in both speaker and listener roles.

Clinicians (e.g., D. R. Boone, personal communication) have recommended that the aphasiologist's first contact with a patient involve a conversational exchange as opposed to formal testing. Now, in lieu of conversation for the sake of rapport, we can converse and employ a variety of types of linguistic analyses to document the patient's communicative strengths and deficits in such areas as turn taking, intention, and topic maintenance (Prutting and Kirchner, 1987), or we analyze responses to questions and use of cohesive devices, as outlined by Wilcox (1983). This information will serve to direct our treatment focus to functions vital to communication in addition to traditional language form and content. Holland (1991) has recently addressed the issue of combining traditional language treatment with pragmatic considerations.

The dyadic type of interaction, unlike the traditional didactic one, will aid the clinician in recognizing the patient's communicative intent and attitudes beyond the grammar produced at the moment and will serve to immediately establish a better environment for FCT treatment. The range of sampling can be as brief as Helm-Estabrooks and Barresi's (1980) single-word extractions, resulting in voluntary production of involuntary expressions, to the 15-minute samples of Prutting and Kirchner (1987).

Communicative Versus Grammatical Competence

The second major FCT principle is to "stimulate and facilitate" informational exchanges. This is merely a restatement of Holland's (1978) recommendation that communication focused treatment should reinforce patients for their appropriateness in reaction to a stimulus as opposed to their linguistic accuracy. For example, incorrect yes/no answers can be evaluated as somewhat appropriate communicatively because they imply that the patient knows the interrogative condition was used by the speaker. For instance, a clinician might respond to a patient with "Good Joe! You knew that I asked a question. Now let me ask you again because I don't think you meant to say you don't want to go come tomorrow." If the objective of the session is to improve functional communication for the patient with a severe comprehension deficit, the redundancy in the natural dyadic use of language (restimulation) may accomplish the objective, and, over time, the need for repetition/clarification is reduced.

A multidimensional focus on both language used and communicative attitude/intent may help patients shift from trying so hard to produce "correct words" that they either fail or give up trying to communicate. The principle applies also to the lesser impaired, nonfluent patient who omits functors but communicates adequately with "car-wife" in response to "How did you get here today?"

Experience from clinical contacts suggests that time in treatment is better spent in giving patients multiple opportunities to use telegraphic utterances to reinforce the concept that they are communicating, in contrast to attempts to add functors and expand language. Data to support this impression are noted in Beyn and Shokhor-Trotskaya's (1966) report, which indicated that a nonpunitive, stimulating environment for Broca-type patients early in the recovery period did not evoke the typical nonfluent, agrammatical language usage frequently reported by others.

The trend away from language context to communication is exemplified by Davis and Wilcox (1981, p. 180), who presented principles for applying PACE therapy that are applicable to any communication-oriented treatment for aphasic patients. The key principles are paraphrased below:

1. An exchange of new information is promoted.
2. The aphasic patient is free—in fact is encouraged—to explore the most effective communication channel, such as gesture, writing, or speaking.
3. Both the therapist and the patient send and receive information.
4. Feedback is simply the success of communicating, the characteristic feedback of normal communication.

According to Davis (1983), "Language is but one mode by which messages are conveyed. . . . Expanding other modes of communication is helpful, also" (p. 230). He believes in train-

ing the listener to use strategies that facilitate the patient's ability to function in communication; improve the patient's use of language where the patient uses it most of the time (p. 239); and work on language content and form only to the extent that they affect message conveyance. In traditional treatment, the stimuli are clinician-selected, and interactions are contrived and unnatural. Conversely, Davis (1983) stresses developing the patient's ability to function independently from the clinician through the use of client-selected stimuli and interactions that are natural.

Cognitive Stimulation

Over the past several years, authors (Chapey, Chapter 11; Fitch-West, 1983; Hillis, Chapter 10; Lubinski and Chapey, 1978; McNeil, 1983; Myers, 1980; Wepman, 1972) have suggested that language intervention be based on stimulation of general psychological processes rather than on language. They believe that communication improvement demands greater activation of prelinguistic processes, and that language and communication treatment should indirectly follow stimulation of thoughts and images preceding the utterance, not a reverse of this order. The principle is also noted in Luria's (1970) intersystemic reorganization approaches and deblocking, defined by LaPointe (1978) as "maximizing residual skills by stimulating the channel that is most functional" (pp. 138–139). Inherent in that approach is content selection that is personally relevant to the patient's vocational or other premorbid interests.

Through use of generic stimulation and activation principles, the clinician may find that the best channel for communication is not always the best modality used by the patient in traditional language tasks or noted in test results. This clinician has always been fascinated by Global aphasic patients who are aware of time and schedules and maintain them despite the fact that they cannot correctly match the setting on a clock face when you ask them and show them how to do so.

Nonverbal Deficits

Cognitive stimulation (see Chapter 11) of an enriched, personally relevant type may help compensate for deficits in attention, memory, and informational overload that characterize some moderately or severely brain-damaged patients with aphasia. Horner (1984) cited such problems as a depressed variety of speech acts restricted language-use contexts, and noted that communication competence can be compromised by the patient's nonlinguistic abilities to use alternate channels for communicating. Chapey and colleagues (1977) noted a reduced number and variety of related ideas in aphasic patients' language.

Ulatowska et al. (1978) documented that mild aphasic patients take inordinately large amounts of time to convey or repeat a message. Such delays operate as cues for the listener to interrupt and come to the patient's aid or to simply change the topic or cease attempting to communicate. (See Lyon, 1992, for a recent, intensive treatment of these relationships in psychosocial natural settings.) In response, patients give up or struggle harder. Neither of these strategies furthers their communicative competence. Patients can also acquire attention-maintaining strategies—for example, uttering "Just a minute!" or "Hold it!" or simply extending a hand to alert others that they desire to communicate more. These patients become the more effective communicators. (See also Newhoff et al. [1982] for a discussion of some additional strategies.)

Aphasic patients show other communicative deficits that require our therapeutic attention, such as feigning understanding; failing to take turns, as commonly noted in "press of speech" patients; displaying impulsive, inappropriate response tendencies that disrupt communicative flow (e.g., answers "Fine" to "Hello" greeting); relating only to the clinician despite the presence of other communicators in the room to whom attention should be directed; and failing to initiate conversation despite retaining some communicative skills. These pragmatically inappropriate behaviors require attention that is less related to language use, per se. It is unfortunate that they may be relegated to secondary importance in traditional therapies because such behaviors are often readily modifiable and interfere with generalization and transfer of acquired language skills to the environment.

Katz (1990) and McNeil et al. (1991) alert us to the problem of extralinguistic processing and behavioral deficits that require the clinician's consideration. These problems in attending and having adequate resource cognitive energy to devote to stimuli become vital for successful, daily communication interactions. Memory is one other important factor in influencing what aphasia is and the recovery pattern (Loverso, 1986). Short-term and long-term memory deficits may help to explain one of our most common treatment problems—that is, obtaining transfer and generalization (see Chapter 31 in this text).

Confrontation Versus Spontaneity

When one observes patients in traditional language treatment reveals a sizable number for whom linguistic confrontation is detrimental. "Easing-off" and focusing less on retrieval of a specific word or phrase can result in a "freeing-up" of information flow and immediate improvement in communication. When our focus is primarily on language performance, and language is the major deficit area, we may deleteriously reinforce the "struggle for the lexicon" in patients who have other assets to use to circumvent their deficits. Martin (1981) stated, "Most processing of linguistic information is unconscious and automatic; therapy tasks that raise such processing to a conscious level may be detrimental to the therapy process" (p. 68). We can conclude from this discussion that overstressing language performance (e.g., a focus on bound morphemes) may constipate communication flow.

Summary of FCT Principles

1. Communication is stressed over linguistic accuracy (form and content).
2. Appropriate speech-act responses to stimuli are reinforced according to a particular patient's level of communication rather than his or her language impairment.
3. New and personally relevant information is preferred to arbitrary language units (e.g., random naming of objects) that exercise language processes.
4. The patient is expected to participate in receiving and sending information as opposed to acting in clinician/spouse-dictated roles.
5. Natural feedback relative to communicative efficiency is provided over reinforcement schedules restricted to efficiency of a particular modality (e.g., auditory/verbal) or language unit.
6. Communication environments are natural ones or, if contrived, stress practical exchanges of information that have immediate generalization or transfer potential to real-life situations.

7. The patient's use of the most efficient and effective communicative channel is stressed.
8. Treatment emphasizes eliminating or reducing inefficient, aberrant communicative behaviors that block or reduce the effectiveness of information flow.
9. Treatment incorporates methods for increasing the frequency of patient participation in communicative dyads and develops strategies for improving the rate of information exchange.
10. In later stages, treatment stresses the accuracy of information received and conveyed by the patient.

PROCEDURES

The procedures for FCT are only illustrative because time and length limitations prohibit an exhaustive presentation. The ultimate objective of these procedures is to enhance communicative competence.

Selecting Candidates for Treatment

Not all patients are candidates for FCT. Observation and documentation of how the patient responds to trial communication exchanges over a brief period are important in selecting patients who may benefit from FCT. There are no firm data that provide guidelines for selection, but clinical experiences suggest that patients must:

1. Be able to self-correct in some situations
2. Score higher than the 10th or 15th percentile on the PICA
3. Have sufficient auditory comprehension to respond appropriately to simple practical commands
4. Show capacity to sustain attention briefly to the clinician and tolerate at least 15 minutes of activity while sitting
5. Demonstrate ability to differentiate or match visual nonverbal stimuli and recognize some common printed words
6. Reveal during trial treatment some capacity for responding differentially to low-level stimuli with intent to communicate
7. Receive mostly one- and a few two-level scores on the CADL test

Although not validated, the above criteria are cited as clinical guidelines to stimulate aphasiologists' exploration of future prognostic indicators for selecting treatment candidates.

Trial Treatment

Eliminating Negative Communicative Behaviors

To maximize patients' ability to profit from FCT, they first need to acquire control of certain communicatively disruptive behaviors. Some of these were discussed under nonverbal deficits earlier. For impulsive patients, a clinician might ask the patient to simply "Wait a second" before giving a verbal or gestural response. (Writing usually offers its own built-in delays.) Whitney (1975) presented techniques labeled "Stop" strategies, which we find useful for the Wernicke-type of patient who has no concept of turn taking in conversational exchanges. One patient who finally acquired the strategy expressed it quite well when he said, "Oh, you want me to shut up so that I can talk, huh?" It is interesting to note that fluent patients usually require the most intensive practice and cuing before they incorporate the strategy of delayed responding combined with pauses after each phrase.

Teaching patients to delay responding serves two basic purposes. First, it allows the patient time to organize a response and, ideally, choose the most effective channel for responding. Second, it provides time to review, reauditorize, revisualize, or engage in whatever other processes that may facilitate message reception and processing. Delays should allow the patient time to think about or process more thoroughly the message as well as give more thought to the answer (Wepman, 1972, 1976). This procedure has one limitation for a minority of patients. After delaying, the patient may briefly lose some spontaneity of responding and related automatic facilitation, but increased speed in responding is relatively easy to achieve from a baseline of delay. Horner (1987) discusses some interesting clinical strategies for improving vocal output based on patients' use of pauses in their fluent/nonfluent patterns of utterance.

Patients who feign understanding, or in other ways reveal severe deficits in comprehension, benefit from the aforementioned delay/pause techniques combined with training that requires them to request repetition or clarification of the message. These patients ease their communicative burden by learning to say "What?" or "Again, please!" Rather humorous but beneficial interactions occur when the clinician purposely overloads the patient with a long grocery list, a series of left-right turns, or a telephone number, then uses the reaction to train the patient to stop the clinician much earlier during the next diatribe. Having the patient write down a phone number, asking for as many repeats as needed, has immediate transfer/generalization potential for daily functioning. Gesturing may also be effective, as documented by Feyerstein (1991).

Perseveration is one of the most commonly encountered behaviors that disrupts communication. Treating perseveration requires the use of perhaps novel, or at least less closely related, stimuli or responses demand. The patient may require a total immersion in a different conceptual framework, time-outs, or assistance in shifting attention. The fatigue that can cause perseveration in the clinic room seems less evident in natural settings. This may relate to the real world's inherent interest-maintaining qualities, or it may reflect the clinician's becoming more tyrannical in demanding quantities and qualities of responses that rapidly induce fatigue, ennui, or both.

Establishing a Communicative Set

Eliminating disruptive or noneffective emotional/behavioral reactions must be integrated with initiating successful dyadic interchanges. The severely impaired patient has had too little success in speaker exchanges and thus too few rewards since the time of insult (see Van Lancker and Nicklay, 1992). A few exchanges with the clinician wherein the patient responds appropriately and communicates at a level that represents progress should be amply and realistically rewarded. One example of a pragmatic exchange relying heavily on the traditional close procedure is presented by Cochrane and Milton (1984), with the objective of increasing output from nonverbal patients. The approach stresses "context building in the dyad of natural conversation rather than short, controlled stimulation." The clinician takes an active role to initiate conversation and uses prompts such as printed words while providing a verbal model for imitation. The latter are faded as the patient increases conversational flow. The multiple repetition of the question becomes the model for the patient.

The clinician must explore channels of response other than verbal ones. For example, a study by Katz and colleagues (1978) revealed that, despite patients' slow responding, they tend to produce an adequate number of gestures, and these gestures often add to communicative effectiveness. Our task as clinicians is not only to encourage patients to gesture but also to capture the facilitating effect of gestures on oral expression. This can be done by analyzing each patient's ability to gesture, encouraging and modeling how he or she might use gesture in concrete, simple communicative situations, and to find the "timing" wherein each patient uses gestures to best advantage.

Functional Communicative Interactions

Carlogmagno and colleagues (1991) evaluated changes in aphasia test performance and communicative abilities following PACE treatment (Davis and Wilcox, 1981). They reasoned that functional treatments that stimulated verbal and nonverbal communicative strategies would increase the information content of aphasic patients' communicative attempts. They found that patients became more accurate in choosing verbal and nonverbal strategies that were the most appropriate for the communicative context. The patients' description of the Cookie Theft picture failed to show quantitative change. They concluded that the aphasic subjects did *not* show a significant language improvement but did show more efficient communicative strategies following the PACE therapy.

Once dyadic communicative exchanges are established with the patient, the clinician's real work begins. It was stated in the principles section that FCT should be based on patient performance profiles from formal language measures and from the functional measures such as the CADL and FCP, plus whatever objective measures of spontaneous speaking can be devised. On initiating FCT, the information from diagnostic testing must be combined with observation of the patient's best channel "for getting messages across." The patient is then directed into that mode of responding on a consistent basis. The clinician must choose a relevant, personalized topic that has real-life application potential for stimulating the interaction. The clinician then must observe very closely the effectiveness and efficiency of the patient's repeated communicative modes of responding. Immediately, attention must be directed to types of feedback that are beneficial. Feedback should be allied as closely as possible to the types of reactions the real world provides. What we honestly should communicate is "I didn't get that!" when in fact, the patient has failed to communicate.

A rule to follow is that flexible and lifelike feedback will usually stimulate the patient to revise his or her communication attempt in the desired direction. Feedback that avoids overreliance on a single mode of responding is usually more efficacious. A 44-year-old aphasic/apraxic man we were seeing as an outpatient arrived for treatment after a weekend and often was unable to communicate orally other than by sterotypical utterances when initially asked about his weekend activities. Given a sheet of paper (Lyon, 1989), he drew progressively more detailed scenes that triggered verbal associations and written and spoken three- to five-word phrases.

Faber and Aten (1979) found that the stimulation/feedback phrase "I want you to tell me what you see (in this picture)" evoked as many accurate names as usually obtained with "Tell me the name of this!" while eliciting significantly more verbalization. PACE procedures (Davis and Wilcox, 1981; Hough and Pierce, Chapter 12) are potentially more effective early in treatment than the "tell me" instruction because they reinforce opportunities for multiple-channel communication.

Narrative and Discourse

In real life we seldom are asked to name things, and when we are many of us fail to retrieve the name of a particular flower or tree we just recently heard about. However, we can continue to converse about the beauty of the object and how much we like it. Fluent aphasics say "I know what it is and what you do with it" or note that they don't have one themselves, and the like. Clinician-patient interactions may often be more beneficial if they involve exchanges at discourse levels as opposed to the semantic, phrase, or even single-sentence levels. Most aphasic patients improve performance (i.e., decode and encode language better) when language is presented redundantly, as it is in natural exchanges. The type of discourse (Ulatowska and Bond, 1983) can be adjusted to the patient's severity level, as documented in formal language tests and observation of communicative strengths.

Conversational discourse may be more appropriate for the severe patient who answers yes/no questions during an informal exchange stressing turn taking. The clinician's request, in question form, is asked, then repeated, often in slightly varied, paraphrased form. (The reader should review the 1984 article by Cochrane and Milton for a more complete description of conversational prompting.) Aphasic patients, although moderately impaired, may, after several modeled questions, be encouraged to ask the clinician a question. This differs significantly from traditional treatment procedures for obtaining 80% accurate responses to singly presented, short, randomly selected questions.

The questions should be personally relevant in content and represent those most often occurring in social exchanges. By choosing questions that relate to a single theme or topic, structure is offered, redundancy is assured, and expository discourse principles are incorporated. Additionally, cognitive demands for shifting attention are reduced. Patients with milder language impairments have been shown to benefit from narrative and procedural types of discourse (Chapman and Ulatowska, 1992; Ulatowska and Chapman, 1989; Waller and Darley, 1978).

The procedure can be varied in terms of type of response, depending on whether comprehension is emphasized or verbal expression is possible and related encoding response practice is indicated. In the former instance, to assess comprehension, the clinician should allow the patient to use pictures or objects, write, or simply gesture. When verbal responses are desired, the clinician should cue and facilitate retelling at levels that accept incomplete verbal responding and grammatical inaccuracies when communication is occurring. The following questions require yes/no or short answers:

> Which branch of the service were you in? I wasn't in the service but I know you were. Which branch did you serve in? How long did you serve? That is, how long were you in the military? How many years? Did you get overseas? Did you just serve here in the States? (Repeat questions, pausing between each segment, and have props such as globes and maps.)
>
> (*Use map of the United States*)
>
> Where did you grow up? (No Answer) Show me where you grew up—I grew up in the East. Where did you live as a child?

Sample Discourse Topics

> I'll tell you how I change a tire; then you can go back over the steps with me and let me know if I left anything out.

> Here's a short article from today's newspaper. It mentions three places nearby to go to for inexpensive meals. I'll read the story then we'll discuss it.

> Here's a TV guide with sporting events for the weekend. It tells each game that will be on TV. Read aloud slowly. A variety of responses can be used from yes/no to indicating which games they'll watch, when, and who they think will win. Maps to show which cities the teams are from often facilitates communication.

Prutting and Kirchner (1987) recommend that discourse not only be considered a powerful assessment tool but also be integrated into language use management. The reader is referred to Chapter 12 in this text for more extensive application of pragmatics and diagnostic/treatment procedures.

Developing Topics and Themes

All patients benefit from being able to say their names and to exchange greetings in a socially appropriate manner. The rewards to self-esteem are obvious. We find that most patients can be trained to give either their first or last names, if only in response to close cues (i.e., Your first name is ____), after brief training. Because our early training is socially oriented, introductions and greetings are initiated as early topics in FCT. They certainly are necessary behaviors for interacting in group settings and outside the clinic. Other topics that are usually introduced early in treatment, depending on the living conditions of the patient and on the patient's severity level, include:

1. Ability to order coffee and meals in a restaurant
2. Vital information such as address and telephone number
3. Names of family members
4. Occupation and hobbies/interests
5. Jobs they have had
6. Where they have lived/grew up
7. Type of car they drive or would buy
8. Favorite foods
9. Discussion of how they like their food cooked (steak-eggs) or new foods to prevent another stroke
10. Best movie they ever saw
11. Favorite sports or TV shows or books/magazines
12. Preferred vacation spots and trips

The above listings are suggestive and must be individually profiled for the patient's background, socioeconomic and educational levels, and interests.

Materials

Many materials have appeared on the market in recent years that attempt to present materials and tasks that simulate real-life activities and demands. Personalized materials are usually preferable. Also, those materials that refer to earlier rather than more recent events in the lives of older patients may be better recalled. Famous personalities in pictorial form can serve to trigger earlier memories quite effectively. Greeting cards for birthdays and Christmas served as a stimulus for an 84-year-old woman with severe mixed aphasia who learned to write "Love, Nana" with her left hand on notes to each of 14 grandchildren and most of the 22 great-grandchildren.

Transferring Communicative Skills

Successful communication between a clinician and a patient offers no assurance that the patient will communicate effectively outside of that dyad. Abrupt confrontations in the real world may partially or totally disrupt confidence and communicative strategies that the patient demonstrates so well in the cloistered setting of the clinic. FCT offered in a group setting can provide the "halfway house" interface between the one-to-one clinical interaction and real-world demands. In Chapter 15, Kearns provides a thorough discussion of how groups may offer the opportunity to use and reinforce the tenuous communicative skills acquired in individual treatment, provide practice in a more natural setting, and simulate real-world situations such as taking turns, handling distractions, listening to a variety of speakers, and handling the stress of interruptions. The group also provides a medium for assessing the efficacy of FCT conducted in individual treatment—an issue also addressed in Chapter 15.

Holland (1982) provides numerous examples of communicative exchanges in patient's homes, on shopping trips, and in a variety of other life situations that offer opportunities for analyzing whether communication is improving. Obviously, these types of observations supply information for the clinician to revise or supplement the FCT plan of management and content. When it is not possible for the clinician or patient to travel outside the treatment environs, attempts should be made to simulate daily communicative situations within the clinic, including the creative use of videotapes and films.

Training Significant Others

A few hours of FCT per week is not sufficient to establish, transfer, and maintain functional gains. We need to include spouses and significant others in the patient's daily environment. This can begin in the acute hospital setting with medical and allied health personnel and extend to include family and friends of the patient. The family should be informed of treatment principles, objectives, and methods and be encouraged to observe successful interactions between clinician and patient. Clinicians will find Lubinski's (1981) work in nursing home settings an excellent example of using significant partners to facilitate FCT. Newhoff and colleagues (1981) provide direct training procedures for spouses. Lyon (1989) presents a complete program for incorporating significant others into the communication network of remediation for the aphasic patient. The improvement of patient-spouse communicative exchanges can serve to lengthen and intensify our clinical treatment arm.

Summarizing FCT Procedures

Communication enhancement is the goal of FCT. Guidelines have been presented for determining which approaches or models of treatment can be used appropriately with which patients. Through combining test results with trial treatments, the aphasiologist can select the channels, modalities, and processes that facilitate functional exchanges of information or better prepare the patient to try communicating in real-world settings. New advances in conversational stimulation via discourse analysis and treatment ideas have been cited. The many potential benefits from earlier exposure of the patient to group treatment were discussed. The group has value as a transfer medium and provides diagnostic information and communication-skill-building experience. Finally, it was stressed that spouses and significant others be included in the rehabilitation process as frequently and as intensively as possible.

FUTURE TRENDS

Since writing the initial version of this chapter in 1986, two events have transpired to positively alter the status of FCT with aphasic patients. First, available resources for prolonged therapeutic interventions have been rationed and show every indication of continuing to be severely limited and competitively sought. The present and future meaning for aphasiologists is that we may be forced to curtail the amount of time spent in individual therapies. Patients are discharged sooner to home/community living, which translates into fewer initial treatments delivered to inpatients. The patient is arriving in the "real world" sooner and before rehabilitation is complete or even well underway.

Second, third-party disbursers of resources require evidence of *functional* gains and objectives prior to payment for treatment. Consequently, treatment that is functionally focused is no longer simply an option in most settings; it has taken on a major and indispensable role in management of the patient with aphasia.

As Rosenbek et al. (1989) suggest, how we view aphasia and what we think it is will dictate how we treat it. This author believes that in the near future, given the reduced resources for supporting idealistic treatment of all aspects of the disorder, we will see a trend away from initial emphasis on treating the disordered language. We have learned that early treatment is not necessarily better or more complete treatment with regard to specifying language gains. The trend, already begun, will increase toward emphasis on preparing patients in the early, acute stage to live with their aphasia, to begin to communicate with each other and the rest of the world as soon as possible, and to develop a life-style that is participative with caretakers and families in real-world settings rather than individual treatment rooms.

Whatever form the treatment takes, it is mandatory that it be structured (i.e., goal focused) and that it incorporate procedures and processes that are model-driven and theory-based. Most of all, treatment should respect individual heterogeneity of the aphasic patients' potentials and their desired outcomes. Language is the single most effective method for communicating, but it is not the only way. For too many of our patients, the return of language is arduous, personally demanding, and not functionally significant. More than a decade later, Sarno's (1980) view still rings of truth:

> Measurement of spontaneous speech . . . seems to be a dimension of aphasic behavior which we have tended to neglect. . . . Until we attempt to objectify our patients' spontaneous speech behavior in everyday practice we will not have adequate, replicable means for assessing recovery . . . and designating adequate treatment programs (p. 47).

References

Aten, J., Caligiuri, M., and Holland, A. (1982). The efficacy of functional communication therapy for chronic aphasic patients. *Journal of Speech and Hearing Disorders, 47,* 93–96.

Bates, E. (1976). Pragmatics and sociolinguistics in child language. In M. Morehead and A. Morehead (Eds.), *Language deficiency in children: Selected readings.* Baltimore, MD: University Park Press.

Beyn, E. S. and Shokhor-Trotskaya, M. K. (1966). Preventive method of speech rehabilitation in aphasia. *Cortex, 2,* 96–108.

Binder, G. M. (1984). *Aphasia: A societal and clinical appraisal of pragmatic and linguistic behaviors.* Unpublished master's thesis, University of California, Santa Barbara, CA.

Blomert, L. (1990). What functional assessment can contribute to setting goals for aphasia therapy. *Aphasiology, 4* (4), 307–320.

Blomert, L., Koster, C., Van Mier, H., and Kean, M-L. (1987). *Aphasiology, 1*(6), 463–474.

Brookshire, R. (1975). Effects of prompting on spontaneous naming of pictures by aphasic subjects. *Human Communication, 5,* 63–71.

Byng, S., Kay, J., Demundson, A., and Scott, C. (1990). Aphasia tests reconsidered. *Aphasiology,* 4(1), 67–91.

Carlogmagno, S., Losanno, N., Enamuelli, S., and Casadio, P. (1991). Expressive language recovery or improved communicative skills: Effects of P.A.C.E. therapy on aphasics' referential communication and story retelling. *Aphasiology, 5,* (4 & 5), 419–424.

Chapey, R. (1981). Divergent semantic intervention. In R. Chapey (Ed.), *Language intervention strategies in adult aphasia.* Baltimore, MD: Williams & Wilkins.

Chapey, R., Rigrodsky, S., and Morrison, E. (1977). Aphasia: A divergent semantic interpretation. *Journal of Speech and Hearing Disorders, 42,* 287–295.

Chapman, S. B., and Ulatowska, H. (1992). Methodology for discourse management in the treatment of aphasia. *Clinical Communication Disorders, 2,* 64–81.

Cochrane, R., and Milton, S. (1984). Conversational prompting: A sentence building technique for severe aphasia. *Journal of Neurological Communication Disorders, 1,* 4–23.

Davis, G. (1983). *A survey of adult aphasia.* Englewood Cliffs, NJ: Prentice-Hall.

Davis, G. and Wilcox, M. (1981). Incorporating parameters of natural conversation in aphasia treatment. In R. Chapey (Ed.), *Language intervention strategies in adult aphasia.* Baltimore, MD: Williams & Wilkins.

Doyle, P., Oleyar, K., and Goldstein, H. (1991). Facilitating functional conversational skills in aphasia: An experimental analysis of a generalization training procedure. In T. Prescott (Ed.), *Clinical aphasiology.* (Chapter 22, Vol. 19, pp. 229–241). Austin, TX: Pro-Ed.

Faber, M., and Aten, J. (1979). Verbal performance in aphasic patients in response to intact and altered pictorial stimuli. In R. Brookshire (Ed.), *Clinical Aphasiology Conference proceedings.* Minneapolis, MN: BRK.

Feyerstein, P. (1991). Communicative behavior in aphasia. *Aphasiology,* 5(4 & 5), 323–334.

Fitch-West, J. (1983). Aphasia: Cognitive considerations. *Topics in Language Disorders, 3,* 49–66.

Fodor, J. (1983). *The modularity of mind.* Cambridge, MA: MIT Press.

Frattali, C. (1992). Functional assessment of communication: Merging public policy with clinical views. *Aphasiology,* 6(1), 63–83.

Goodglass, H., and Stuss, D. (1979). Naming to picture versus description in three aphasic subgroups. *Cortex, 15,* 199–211.

Helm-Estabrooks, N., and Barresi, B. (1980). Voluntary control of involuntary utterances: A treatment approach for severe aphasia. In R. Brookshire (Ed.), *Clinical Aphasiology Conference proceedings* (pp. 208–230). Minneapolis, MN: BRK.

Holland, A. (1978). Functional communication in the treatment of aphasia. In L. Bradford (Ed.), *Communication disorders: An audio journal for continuing education.* New York: Grune & Stratton.

Holland, A. (1979). Some practical consideration in aphasia rehabilitation. In M. Sullivan and M. Kommers (Eds.), *Rationale for adult aphasia therapy.* Omaha University of Nebraska Medical Center Print Shop.

Holland, A. (1980). *Communicative abilities of daily living.* Baltimore, MD: University Park Press.

Holland, A. (1982). Observing functional communication of aphasic adults. *Journal of Speech and Hearing Disorders, 47,* 50–56.

Holland, A. (1983). Language intervention in adults: What is it? In J. Miller, D. Yoder, and R. Schiefelbusch (Eds.), *Contemporary issues in language intervention* (Report 12;1:13–14). Rockville, MD: ASHA.

Holland, A. (1991). Pragmatic aspects of intervention in aphasia. 6(2), 197–211.

Horner, J. (1984). Moderate aphasia. In A. Holland (Ed.), *Language disorders in adults.* San Diego, CA: College Hill Press.

Horner, J. (1987). Pausing, planning and paraphasia in expressive language disorders. *Topics in Language Disorders,* 8(1), 24–33.

Katz, R. (1990). Intelligent computerized treatment or artificial aphasia therapy? *Aphasiology,* 4(6), 621–624.

Katz, R., LaPointe, L., and Markel, N. (1978). Coverbal behavior and aphasic speakers. In R. Brookshire (Ed.), *Clinical Aphasiology Conference proceedings.* Minneapolis, MN: BRK.

Kertesz, A. (1982). *Western aphasia battery.* New York: Grune & Stratton.

LaPointe, L. (1978). Aphasia therapy: Some principles and strategies for treatment. In R. Brookshire (Ed.), *Clinical Aphasiology Conference proceedings.* Minneapolis, MN: BRK.

Lomas, J., Pickard, L., Bester, S., Elbard, H., Finlayson, A., and Zoghaib, C. (1989). The communicative effectiveness index: Development and psychometric evaluation of a functional communication measure for adult aphasia. *Journal of Speech and Hearing Disorders, 54,* 113–124.

Loverso, P. (1986). Rehabilitation of language related memory disorders in aphasia. In R. Chapey (Ed.), *Language intervention strategies in adult aphasia* (Chapter 12, 2nd ed., pp. 239–250). Baltimore, MD: Williams & Wilkins.

Lubinski, R. (1981). Environmental language intervention. In R. Chapey (Ed.), *Language intervention strategies in adult aphasia.* Baltimore, MD: Williams & Wilkins.

Lubinski, R., and Chapey, R. (1978). Constructive recall strategies in adult aphasia. In R. Brookshire (Ed.), *Clinical Aphasiology Conference proceedings.* Minneapolis, MN: BRK.

Luria, A. (1970). The functional organization of the brain. *Scientific American, 222,* 66–78.

Lyon, J. (1989). *The challenge of generalization: The perspectives on planning, intervention, and evaluation.* Lecture presented at the Third Annual Seminar of Speech and Stroke Center, Toronto, Ontario, Canada.

Lyon, J. (1992). Communication use and participation in life for adults with aphasia in natural settings: The scope of the problem. *American Journal of Speech-Language Pathology,* 1(3), 7–14.

Martin, A. D. (1978). A proposed rationale for aphasia therapy. In R. Brookshire (Ed.), *Clinical Aphasiology Conference proceedings.* Minneapolis, MN: BRK.

Martin, A. D. (1981). The role of theory in therapy: A rationale. *Topics in Language Disorders, 1,* 63–72.

McNeil, M. (1983). Aphasia: Neurological considerations. *Topics in Language Disorders, 3,* 1–20.

McNeil, M., Odell, K., and Tseng, C. (1991). Toward integration of resource allocation into a general theory of aphasia. In T. Prescott (Ed.), *Clinical aphasiology.* (Chapter 3, Vol. 20, pp. 21–39).

Myers, P. S. (1980). Visual imagery in aphasic treatment: A new look. In R. Brookshire (Ed.), *Clinical Aphasiology Conference proceedings.* Minneapolis, MN: BRK.

Newhoff, M., Bugbee, J., and Ferreira, A. (1981). A change of PACE: Spouses as treatment targets. In R. Brookshire (Ed.), *Clinical Aphasiology Conference proceedings.* Minneapolis, MN: BRK.

Newhoff, M., Tonkovich, J., Schwartz, S., and Burgess, E. (1982). Revision strategies in aphasia. In R. Brookshire (Ed.), *Clinical Aphasiology Conference proceedings.* Minneapolis, MN: BRK.

Podraza, B. L., and Darley, F. L. (1977). Effects of auditory prestimulation on naming in aphasia. *Journal of Speech and Hearing Research. 20,* 669–683.

Porch, B. E. (1967). *Porch Index of Communicative Ability.* Palo Alto, CA: Consulting Psychologists Press.

Prutting, C. (1982). Pragmatics as social competence. *Journal of Speech and Hearing Disorders, 47,* 123–134.

Prutting, C., and Kirchner, D. (1983). Applied pragmatics. In T. Gallagher and C. Prutting (Eds.), *Pragmatic assessment and intervention issues in language.* San Diego, CA: College Hill Press.

Prutting, C., and Kirchner, D. (1987). A clinical appraisal of the pragmatic aspects of language. *Journal of Speech and Hearing Disorders, 52,* 105–119.

Rosenbek, J. (1983). Some challenges for aphasiologists. In J. Miller, D. Yoder, and R. Schiefelbusch (Eds.), *Contemporary issues in language intervention* (Report 12). Rockville, MD: ASHA.

Rosenbek, J., LaPointe, L., and Wertz, R. (1989). *Aphasia: A clinical approach.* Austin, TX: Pro-Ed.

Sarno, M. T. (1969). *The functional communication profile: Manual of direction.* New York: Institute of Rehabilitative Medicine, New York University Medical Center.

Sarno, M. T. (1980). Analyzing aphasic behavior. In M. Sarno and O. Hook (Eds.), *Aphasia: Assessment and treatment.* New York: Masson.

Sarno, M. T. (1981). Recovery and rehabilitation in aphasia. In M. Sarno (Ed.), *Acquired aphasia.* New York: Academic Press.

Sarno, M. T. (1983). The functional assessment of verbal impairment. In G. Grimby (Ed.), *Recent advances in rehabilitation medicine.* Stockholm: Almquist & Wiksell.

Schuell, H., Jenkins, J., and Jimenez-Pabon, E. (1964). *Aphasia in adults.* New York: Harper & Row.

Schwartz, M., and Whyte, J. (1991). Methodological issues in aphasia treatment research. In *Treatment of aphasia: Research and research needs.* Bethesda, MD. Proceedings of an NIDCD Workshop, June 6–7.

Seron, X., Deloche, G., Bastard, V., Chassing, G., and Hermand, N. (1979). Word-finding difficulties and learning transfer in aphasic patients. *Cortex, 15,* 149–155.

Shewan, C. (1986). The history and efficacy of aphasia treatment. In R. Chapey (Ed.), *Langauge intervention strategies in adult aphasia.* (Chapter 3, 2nd ed.). Baltimore, MD: Williams & Wilkins.

Sparks, R., Helm, N., and Albert, M. (1974). Aphasia rehabilitation resulting from melodic intonation therapy. *Cortex, 10,* 303–316.

Springer, L., Glindemann, R., Huber, W., and Willmes, K. (1991). How efficacious is PACE-therapy when "Language Systematic Training" is incorporated? *Aphasiology, 5,* (4 & 5), 391–400.

Ulatowska, H., and Bond, S. A. (1983). Aphasia: Discourse considerations. *Topics in Language Disorders, 3,* 21–34.

Ulatowska, H., and Chapman, S. (1989). Discourse considerations for aphasia management. *Seminars in Speech and Language, 10,* 293–314.

Ulatowska, H., Hildebrand, B., and Haynes, S. (1978). A comparison of written and spoken language in aphasia. Revision strategies in aphasia. In R. Brookshire (Ed.), *Clinical Aphasiology Conference proceedings.* Minneapolis, MN: BRK.

Van Lancker, D., and Nicklay, C. (1992). Comprehension of personally relevant (PERL) versus novel language in two globally aphasic patients. *Aphasiology, 6*(1), 37–61.

Waller, M. R., and Darley, F. L. (1978). The influence of context on the auditory comprehension of paragraphs by aphasic subjects. *Journal of Speech and Hearing Research, 21,* 732–745.

Weniger, D. and Sarno, M. (1990). The future of aphasia therapy: More than just new wine in old bottles? *Aphasiology, 4* (4), 301–306.

Wepman, J. (1972). Aphasia therapy: A new look. *Journal of Speech and Hearing Disorders, 37,* 203–214.

Wepman, J. (1976). Aphasia: Language without thought and thought without language. *ASHA, 18,* 131–136.

Wertz, R. (1991). Aphasiology 1990: A view from the colonies. *Aphasiology, 4* (4 & 5), 311–322.

Wertz, R. T. (1983). Language intervention context and setting for the aphasic adult: When? In J. Miller, D. Yoder, and R. Schiefelbusch (Eds.), *Contemporary issues in language intervention.* (Report 12;1:196–220), Rockville, MD: ASHA.

Wertz, R. T. (1984). Language disorders in adults: State of the clinical art. In A. Holland (Ed.), *Language disorders in adults.* San Diego, CA: College Hill Press.

Wertz, R. T., Weiss, D. G., Aten, J. L., Brookshire, R. H., Garcia-Buneul, L., Holland, A., Kurtzke, J. F., LaPointe, L. L., Milianti, F., Brannegan, R., Greenbaum, H., Marshall, R. C., Vogel, D., Carter, J., Barnes, N. S., and Goodman, R. (1986). A comparison of clinic, home, and deferred language treatment for aphasia: A Veterans Administration cooperative study. *Archives of Neurology, 43,* 653–658.

Wertz, R. T., Collins, M., Weiss, D., Kirtzke, J., Friden, T., Brookshire, R., Pierce, J., Holtzapple, P., Hubbard, D., Porch, B., West, J., Davis, L., Matovich, V., Morley, G., and Resurreccion, E. (1981). Veterans Administration cooperative study on aphasia: A comparison of individual and group treatment. *Journal of Speech and Hearing Research, 24,* 580–594.

Whitney, J. (1975). *Developing aphasic's use of compensatory strategies.* Paper presented at the Annual Convention of the American Speech-Language-Hearing Association, Washington, DC.

Wiegel-Crump, C., and Koenigsknecht, R. A. (1973). Tapping the lexical store of the adult aphasic: Analysis of the improvement made in word retrieval skills. *Cortex, 9,* 410–418.

Wilcox, M. J. (1983). Aphasia: Pragmatic considerations. *Topics in Language Disorders, 3,* 35–48.

CHAPTER 15
Group Therapy for Aphasia: Theoretical and Practical Considerations

KEVIN P. KEARNS

Group therapy for aphasia evolved in the United States as a practical response to the large influx of head-injured veterans returning from World War II. At that time, relatively few professionals were specifically trained to provide clinical services for aphasic patients, and burgeoning caseloads necessitated treating patients in groups. Group therapy has remained a common method of treating aphasia in the United States and abroad (Fawcus, 1989; Pachalska, 1991a; Tsvetkova, 1980).

Ironically, changes in reimbursement and public policy (cf Fratelli, 1992) and a renewed interest in psychosocial aspects of recovery from aphasia have stimulated a renewed interest in group treatment (Borenstein et al., 1987; Brindely et al., 1989; Pachalska, 1992; Radonjic and Rakuscek, 1991). Lyon (1992) recently argued that clinical aphasiologists should broaden their clinical perspective by incorporating psychosocial as well as functional communicative goals into therapeutic endeavors, and they should use treatment plans that facilitate or encourage "participation in life." Similarly, Fratelli (1992) has noted, "We must remember that human communication sciences and disorders is a discipline dedicated to improving the quality of life of persons with communication disorders" (p. 81).

Of course, interest in the broader aspects of recovery from aphasia are not new. Descriptive accounts of group therapy and its benefits abound in the aphasia literature (Agranowitz et al., 1954; Aronson et al., 1956; Chenven, 1953; Gordon, 1976; Holland, 1970; Inskip and Burris, 1959; Nielson et al., 1948; Schlanger and Schlanger, 1970; Wepman, 1947). Its advocates have claimed that group intervention results in widespread changes in speech and language skills and increased psychosocial adjustment to aphasia. Unfortunately, there is a paucity of objective studies to support these claims, and the efficacy of group therapy for aphasia has yet to be established. Although the results of recent investigations indicate that group therapy may be an effective form of aphasia management (Aten et al., 1982; Brindely et al., 1989; Radonjic and Rakuscek, 1991; Wertz et al., 1981) aphasiologists continue to give only meager attention to this important area of clinical investigation.

Despite these advances in our clinical science, there continues to be a dearth of information available regarding group therapy for aphasia. That is, clinical aphasiology textbooks typically contain brief descriptions of the purposes and benefits of group treatment with minimal discussion of procedures employed in therapy (Brookshire, 1992; Darley, 1982; Davis, 1992; Eisenson, 1973; Jenkins et al., 1981; Sarno, 1981), and few critical summaries of the literature are available (Fawcus, 1989; Marquardt et al., 1976). Consequently, interested clinicians must adopt techniques employed in individual treatment

to the group setting or learn group treatment approaches from experienced clinicians. In essence, the literature continues to extol the benefits of group treatment without delineating goals or procedures needed to reach rehabilitation objectives (Holland, 1975).

While recognizing the need for empirically based group treatment procedures, recent interest in broader rehabilitation goals has occurred within a conceptual and methodological framework that heretofore had been lacking. From a conceptual perspective, clinical aphasiologists have begun to appreciate the complexities associated with facilitating generalized changes in our aphasic patients (Van Harskamp and Visch-Brink, 1991). More important, an ecological perspective on intervention, which considers the complexity of environmental, personal, social, emotional, and communicative factors on treatment, is finally evolving into specific, testable treatment suggestions for both individual and group therapy for aphasia (Aten et al., 1982; Davis and Wilcox, 1981; LaPointe, 1989). Consistent with the trend toward a more ecological approach to intervention, the concomitant emphasis on methodological issues may provide a procedural framework for group therapy. For example, calls for reliable and appropriate functional (Fratelli, 1992) and psychosocial assessment tools (Lyon, 1992) as well as the development of a generalization planning approach to intervention (Kearns, 1989; Thompson, 1989) have direct relevance to group intervention for aphasia.

PURPOSE

There is a need to synthesize the group treatment literature, to describe current clinical practices, and develop specific treatment approaches that can be clinically useful and experimentally validated. Therefore, the purposes of this chapter are (a) to critically review and summarize the aphasia group therapy literature and (b) to present a perspective on group therapy for aphasia that is consistent with information in the literature on facilitating generalization. Suggestions will also be provided regarding the future role of speech-language pathologists in this area of rehabilitation.

The content and focus of group therapy for aphasia is predominantly a function of the skills and biases of the group leader (Marquardt, 1982; Marquardt et al., 1976). In general, however, most aphasia groups focus on one or more of the following parameters: psychosocial adjustment, speech-language treatment, and/or counseling (Eisenson, 1973; Fawcus, 1989). This clinical taxonomy is, of course, somewhat arbitrary, since communication and psychosocial factors are intricately related and improvement of one factor may affect the other

(Marquardt et al., 1976). Therefore, the interrelatedness and complexity of therapeutic goals in group treatment for aphasia should be kept in mind during the following discussion of group treatment approaches.

GROUP TREATMENT APPROACHES

Psychosocial Groups

Although psychotherapeutic and sociotherapeutic approaches to group management have been distinguished in the aphasia literature (Marquardt et al., 1976), these approaches share more similarities than differences. That is, despite differing descriptive labels, the purpose and procedures discussed in reports of sociotherapeutic and psychotherapeutic group therapy are often indistinguishable. Psychosocial groups provide a supportive atmosphere where aphasic individuals can ventilate feelings and learn to cope with the psychological impact of aphasia. In addition, these groups emphasize interpersonal relationships and provide social contacts with other persons "in the same boat." The primary purpose of psychosocial aphasia groups is to foster the development of emotional and psychological bonds that help group members cope with the consequences of aphasia (Inskip and Burris, 1959; Oradei and Waite, 1974; Redinger et al., 1971).

Backus and Dunn (1947, 1952) were strong advocates of psychosocial group therapy for aphasia, and they believed that the group structure provided an atmosphere of belongingness, acceptance, and security. Backus (1952) emphasized that specific behavioral procedures were less important than "creating the kind of environment in which clients become able to change" (p. 122). She viewed the interpersonal relationships as the cornerstone of therapeutic change, and a primary goal of her group was to facilitate psychosocial adjustment. Backus believed that group treatment improved her patients' observational skills and helped group members adapt to social situations outside the clinic.

Blackman (1950) and Blackman and Tureen (1948) also discussed group "psychotherapy" for aphasic clients. Their groups reportedly provided a relaxed, supportive atmosphere in which the members could socialize, ventilate feelings, and work through the psychological consequences of aphasia. Group activities included discussions, plays in which patients acted out real-life situations, and an arts and crafts exhibition. Blackman (1950) described numerous "outstanding benefits" of aphasia groups, including a decrease in feelings of isolation, reaffirmation of social acceptance, and increased self-awareness.

Godfrey and Douglass (1959) reported their experiences with a "social speech" group for aphasic patients. Occupational therapists who had minimal knowledge of aphasia or speech-language training techniques served as group leaders. Specific language treatment tasks were not employed during group sessions, but social interaction was emphasized. Godfrey and Douglass stressed that warm and natural patient-therapist relationships were instrumental in reducing the aphasic individual's levels of anxiety, defensiveness, and withdrawal. In addition, the results of subjective clinical ratings revealed that the majority of their patients improved in "psychosocial" adjustment or "language adjustment" following group therapy.

The majority of psychosocial group treatment reports have given minimal attention to subject description, procedural specification, or evaluation of treatment results. Aronson et al. (1956), however, provided a detailed description of a "social-psychotherapeutic" approach to group therapy and attempted to evaluate the effectiveness of their program. They developed a task continuum in an attempt to facilitate group discussion, provide an emotional outlet, and allow patients to develop interpersonal relationships. Tasks in the hierarchy ranged from nonverbal (e.g., music rhythm group) to solely verbal (e.g., group discussion), and they included (a) using rhythmic musical instruments, (b) participating in group singing, (c) listening to short stories read by a group leader, (d) participating in various speech games and discussion of proverbs, (e) taping and replaying speech samples, and (f) taking part in group-centered discussion. Activities from the hierarchy were introduced as needed to maintain motivation and facilitate group interaction whenever adequate group discussion could not be elicited.

The effectiveness of this approach was evaluated for 21 chronic and acute patients who attended an average of 14 hourly treatment sessions. Results of interviews and clinical ratings revealed that the patients and staff reacted quite favorably to the treatment program. The group leaders also observed a reduction in anxiety, increased intragroup support, and a heightened ability for constructive self-criticism among group members.

One additional report of psychosocial group therapy is notable for its attempt to outline specific group treatment procedures. Schlanger and Schlanger (1970) recommended the use of role playing as a method of reducing anxiety about communication and establishing spontaneous, functional discourse in the group setting. Their primary purpose was to "try to 'get something across' both inter- and intrapersonally" (p. 230) through the use of (a) gesture and pantomime, (b) role playing one's self in realistic situations, (c) role playing other individuals, and (d) psychodrama.

Gestures and pantomime were employed to enhance the communication of chronic aphasic patients who had severely limited verbal abilities. Gestural and pantomime training included the use of descriptive gestures to transmit information about pictorial referents, pantomiming daily activities such as mailing a letter, and using "universal" iconic gestures.

Following gesture and pantomime training, the patients role played themselves in nonstressful and stressful situations. Nonstressful situations included activities such as shopping or attending a picnic. Role playing in stressful situations involved having patients interact with a clinician in a "Candid Camera"-like situation. Unexpected events were blended into everyday experiences so that the patient had to problem solve and communicate in a natural situation.

In addition to role playing themselves, the aphasic patients also role played other people during simulated situations. During this activity, the patients used pantomime and verbal skills to depict people in contrived scenes from a bakery, a florist, and so on.

In the final aspect of the Schlanger and Schlanger (1970) group treatment program, psychodrama was used to act out the problems and frustrations of each group member. During this activity, patients assumed roles that allowed them to vent feelings and release hostility.

The aphasia group members gradually progressed through the four facets of training, and several benefits of the program were noted. Patients demonstrated an increased ability to cope with stressful situations, a reduction in anxiety concerning communication deficits, a feeling of accomplishment, loss of emotional inhibition, and better insight into feelings and problems. Schlanger and Schlanger (1970) concluded that role-playing activities provide an important means of adjusting to the psychosocial impact of aphasia.

Recent clinical reports have also targeted psychosocial goals within the aphasia group setting. Borenstein et al. (1987), for example, examined the psychological, linguistic, and neurological effects of a 5-day intensive residential treatment program for aphasic patients and their relatives. Eleven aphasic patients and seven family members attended the group. Sessions were conducted by a speech-language pathologist, a psychologist, and a neurologist, and formal assessments of family members' psychological adjustment and aphasic participants' language ability and neurological status were conducted. The content of the intervention program included family-centered therapy, social excursions that encouraged functional communication, and group discussions of everyday problems and adjustment strategies. Reevaluations of the participants conducted 1 year after the intensive treatment period revealed some improvements in psychological and interpersonal adjustment but not in neurological or communicative status.

Summary and Observations

There is a general consensus in the literature that psychosocial group therapy provides psychological, emotional, and social benefits for individuals with aphasia. Specific benefits that have been reported include an opportunity for increased socialization; a supportive atmosphere in which aphasic individuals can express anger, hostility, and other emotions; and the development of skills that allow patients to cope with emotional and life-style changes resulting from aphasia (Aronson et al., 1956; Backus and Dunn, 1947; Blackman, 1950; Blackman and Tureen, 1948; Eisenson, 1973; Friedman, 1961; Godfrey and Douglass, 1959; Inskip and Burris, 1959; Marquardt et al., 1976; Oradei and Waite, 1974; Redinger et al., 1971; Schlanger and Schlanger, 1970). Despite near-unanimous agreement regarding the benefits of psychosocial group treatment, it should be cautioned that the findings of reports in this area are based on subjective assessment and anecdotal observations. Data-based studies are practically nonexistent in the psychosocial group literature, and those that have been reported have not been rigorous (Aronson et al., 1956; Godfrey and Douglass, 1959; Oradei and Waite, 1974). Although the psychometric difficulties involved in measuring psychological and social parameters are substantial, there is a pressing need to begin evaluating the psychosocial impact of group treatment for aphasia.

Prerequisite to the establishment of a solid database for this approach to aphasia management is the development of specific replicable treatment procedures. Unfortunately, with few notable exceptions (Aronson et al., 1956; Schlanger and Schlanger, 1970), investigators have not delineated specific treatment principles or procedures for conducting psychosocial group therapy for aphasia. Descriptions in the literature do not provide the procedural detail necessary to translate them into clinical practice (e.g., Friedman, 1961; Oradei and Waite, 1974; Redinger et al., 1971), and psychosocial group therapy remains largely an undefined entity. Moreover, when attempts have been made to document the effectiveness of psychosocial treatment groups (e.g., Borenstein et al., 1987), failure to meet minimal psychometric standards limits the usefulness of these efforts.

Family Counseling and Support Groups

In addition to the psychosocial adjustment difficulties of aphasic individuals, the emotional, psychological, and life-style changes for family members of aphasic individuals have also been documented (Friedland and McColl, 1989; Kinsella and Duffy, 1978, 1979; Malone, 1969; Rice et al., 1987). Malone (1969), for example, interviewed spouses and family members of 20 aphasic individuals to determine the effects of aphasia on family dynamics. He found significant role changes, spouse irritability, guilt feelings, financial difficulties, job neglect, health problems, and attitudes of oversolicitousness or rejection by family members. Malone (1969) observed that "in most cases the family as a closely knit unit no longer existed" (p. 147) once a family member was stricken by aphasia. He concluded that family counseling programs are needed to help spouses and family members learn about aphasia and cope with its devastating consequences. The group setting is frequently used for counseling and educating aphasic patients and their families.

Brookshire (1992) noted that the primary objective of family support or counseling groups is to educate aphasic patients and their families about the nature of aphasia and to explore the impact of aphasia on family dynamics. Counseling groups provide a medium for discussing physical, psychological, and social consequences of brain damage. They also serve as a forum for expressing feelings and learning to adjust to newly acquired family roles and life-style changes. Brookshire observed that patient-family and spouse support groups also function as a social or recreational outlet for aphasic individuals and their families.

Friedland and McColl (1989) attempted to operationalize the definition of social support for their spouse program. Their model conceptualizes social support as having three dimensions: source of support, types of support, and how satisfied the patient is with the support received. Common sources of support may include personal, friend/family, community, and professional resources. Relatedly, the type of support received may include emotional and informational.

Numerous examples of family counseling groups are available in the aphasia literature (Bernstein, 1979; Davis, 1992; Derman and Manaster, 1967; Friedland and McColl, 1989; Gordon, 1976; Kisley, 1973; Mogil et al., 1978; Newhoff and Davis, 1978; Porter and Dabul, 1977; Puts-Zwartes, 1973; Redinger et al., 1971). Turnblom and Myers (1952) provided one of the earliest examples of group counseling for families of aphasic individuals. Following this early report, there was a virtual neglect of this area of rehabilitation for approximately 20 years. Redinger et al. (1971) subsequently described a multidisciplinary discussion group for severely impaired aphasic patients and their spouses. The purpose of the group was to facilitate emotional adjustment and help the group members work through family and social issues through problem-oriented discussions. The group consisted of several co-leaders (a speech-language pathologist, a psychiatric nurse, and a psychiatrist), six aphasic patients, and four spouses who met on a weekly basis for 1 year. Participation of the spouses was viewed as a critical element in rehabilitation, since problems discussed in the group inevitably involved adjustment difficulties that were shared by the aphasic patients and their spouses.

Redinger and his colleagues (1971) observed that the group evolved through several stages during the course of therapy. Initially, there was a period of anxiety, and group members experienced difficulty communicating with one another. During the second stage, the members expressed regrets about their condition and complained about various factors associated with rehabilitation. Finally, during the third stage of treatment, the group evolved into a friendly, understanding, and supportive unit. As the group evolved through these stages, participants gradually became better adjusted to home and social environments, and they developed a more realistic view of family problems. In addition to these benefits, the counseling group also provided a social outlet for patients and spouses.

Recent reports of spouse counseling groups highlight the importance of planning treatment to meet the specific needs of individual aphasic patients and their families. Gordon's (1976) spouse counseling group, for example, developed in response to the expressed needs of the wives of aphasic patients. The group provided an atmosphere in which spouses acquired a better understanding of aphasia, felt free to express feelings and share their reactions, and worked through problems that occurred as a result of their husband's aphasia. The ultimate goal of the group was to improve the interpersonal relationships of the aphasic individuals and their spouses.

A speech-language pathologist and a psychiatric social worker acted as co-leaders for the group. Meetings were held on a weekly basis, and attendance ranged from 4 to 10 spouses per session. The duration of individual spouse participation in the group varied from several months to 3 years. The co-leaders adopted a nondirective counseling approach in which wives increasingly assumed more responsibility for the content and direction of the group while the leaders provided information and guidance as needed. Psychosocial aspects of adjustment addressed by the social worker included feelings of resignation, guilt and loneliness, shifts in family roles, and the need to maintain interests outside of the home. The speech pathologist discussed the nature of aphasia, prognosis for recovery of language skills, and strategies for improving communication with their aphasic partners. Wives were encouraged not to demand verbal responses from their husbands, to accept nonverbal communication, and to modify their input to their aphasic partners.

Gordon (1976) concluded that wives' emotional problems hindered communication with their aphasic husbands prior to participation in the group. Relatedly, the group helped to alleviate many of the wives' emotional problems, and formal psychotherapy was seldom required. Gordon cautioned, however, that multiple repetitions were often needed before the wives comprehended group-counseling information. Some redundancy may, therefore, be necessary for spouses to receive maximum benefits from group treatment.

Bernstein (1979) also described a multidisciplinary spouse group that evolved out of concern for the emotional needs of family members. He stressed that interpersonal problems between aphasic patients and their wives may interfere with speech-language treatment attempts. More important, he believed that the family unit itself may be endangered if we ignore the emotional and psychological trauma suffered by spouses and other family members. He stressed that we cannot meet the complex emotional needs of spouses by simply providing a list of "do's and don'ts" and discussing them.

Bernstein's spouse group was conducted by a team of professionals that included speech pathologists, occupational and physical therapists, and a psychologist. The team met weekly and selected discussion topics for upcoming group meetings by reviewing the content of preceding sessions. Topics ranged from informational subjects, such as the nature of aphasic communication problems, to emotional issues, such as negative feelings toward their spouses and attitudes toward rehabilitation.

From his experience with the group, the author concluded that counseling sessions facilitated the spouses' ability to cope with their emotions and helped them acquire a better understanding of aphasia and related problems. Interestingly, Bernstein (1979) also indicated that the team leaders also benefited from the group. He stated, "We are all better clinicians for the experience" (p. 35).

Recognizing the scarcity of studies in the aphasia counseling area, Newhoff and Davis (1978) reported their attempt to objectively plan and implement a spouse-intervention program. Four spouses, two male and two female, participated in this study. Spouses were individually interviewed to determine target areas for intervention, and a questionnaire was administered before and at the termination of the study to evaluate the effectiveness of the program.

The questionnaire examined seven areas: (*a*) communication strategies, (*b*) changes in life-style and social pursuits, (*c*) spouses' feelings regarding their partner's disability, (*d*) spouses' perception of how well they understood their partner's problems, (*e*) actual level of spouse understanding, (*f*) spouse-partner independence, and (*g*) advice sought by spouses. The items in the questionnaire were all "Do you . . ." questions. For example, one item asked, "Do you talk with your spouse as you did before the accident?" (Newhoff and Davis, 1978, p. 320). The spouses circled appropriate answers on a seven-point rating scale that ranged from "very often" to "never."

The spouse intervention group met for 50-minute sessions once a week for a period of 7 weeks. A speech-language pathologist served as group leader, but the spouses provided the direction for the group. The leader served as a catalyst for discussions and provided information as needed. The purpose of the group was to accomplish the following "counseling functions": (*a*) provide information to the spouses, (*b*) receive information from spouses that might be useful during their partner's rehabilitation, (*c*) facilitate the spouses' acceptance of their own feelings and help them accept and understand their aphasic partners, and (*d*) effect change in the spouses' behavior.

After 7 weeks of group counseling, the questionnaire was readministered to evaluate the effectiveness of the intervention. A comparison of responses to pre- and poststudy questionnaires revealed considerable variability in the spouses' responding, and no discernible pattern of change was apparent.

Analysis of prestudy interviews revealed that the spouses were not well informed about factual information, and they were frustrated with their inability to communicate with their aphasic partners prior to the study. Review of actual treatment sessions, however, indicated that the spouses were better informed and demonstrated improved changes following intervention. Newhoff and Davis (1978) concluded that they had accomplished their primary counseling objectives. They also concluded that, although the measurement problems involved in evaluating group counseling are difficult, they are not insurmountable.

Rice et al. (1987) recently described their social support group for the spouses of 10 aphasic patients. The purpose of this 12-week group was to provide information and social support and enhance psychosocial adjustment. The group was also intended to facilitate communication between aphasic patients and their spouses. The authors report significant improvement on scales of psychological adjustment for those individuals who consistently attended the group. No significant differences were found in posttreatment functional communication ability of aphasic patients whose spouses regularly attended versus those whose spouses did not regularly attend. While this report is noteworthy for its attempt to evaluate the psychosocial effects of the spouse counseling group, results must be interpreted cautiously given the small number of spouses and patients included in the evaluation and the lack of a true control group.

Summary and Observations

Patient and family counseling groups have been widely advocated in the aphasia literature in recent years. The primary purpose of patient-family and spouse groups has been to provide educational information regarding aphasia and to provide emotional support for aphasic individuals and their families. Generally, speech pathologists and psychologists have acted as group co-leaders for aphasia counseling groups. Their primary function has been to lead topic-oriented discussions that center on communication and emotional adjustment issues. The emphasis in counseling groups for aphasic patients and their relatives has been on "working through" the communication, emotional, and life-style changes that affect family dynamics.

The devastating effects of aphasia on interpersonal relationships and the family unit are well documented in the literature, and the need for counseling aphasic patients and their families is unassailable. There is, however, little documentation as to the best format for accomplishing counseling objectives in the group setting. Although not specifically mentioned in most reports of group counseling, topic-oriented discussions should be accompanied by printed counseling information and/or appropriate audiovisual materials. Bevington (1985), for example, described an educational program that included the use of videotaped educational materials, lectures, and printed materials. We have adopted a similar approach to the educational component of our spouse groups. Spouses and family members of our aphasic patients receive a "counseling packet" prior to entering our spouse group. Each packet contains printed materials that explain the nature of aphasia, discuss various aspects of rehabilitation, and provide suggestions for helping family members communicate with their aphasic relatives (American Heart Association, 1981; Horwitz, 1977; National Institutes of Health, 1979). Additionally, the packets include a description of community resources such as the local "stroke club" (see Sanders et al., 1984).

Information provided in the counseling packet is supplemented by a family counseling film entitled, *A Stroke: Recovering Together* (Veterans Administration, 1983). The film reviews etiological factors, demonstrates various types of aphasia, and focuses on the life-style adjustments of several chronic patients. The film also includes comments from members of a spouse group and demonstrates their adjustment to having apha-

sic husbands. Other commercially available films found to be useful for patient and family counseling include *Pathways: Moving Beyond Stroke and Aphasia* (Adair Ewing and Pfalzgraf, 1991) and *What Is Aphasia?* (Adair Ewing and Ewing-Pfalzgraf, 1991).

Films and printed materials are shared with spouses prior to their participation in the group. Thus, they have an information base that lets them immediately interact with the other group members if they wish to do so. This approach seems to alleviate some of the anxiety that is present prior to entering the group. Discussions that are generated from the counseling materials also help the clinician determine if a spouse might benefit from individual counseling. Spouses are referred to a staff clinical psychologist for evaluation if they are not psychologically ready to share their feelings and emotions in the group setting. Similarly, spouses who discuss sensitive issues such as divorce or suicide are also referred for individual psychological counseling.

The invaluable contributions of professionals specifically trained in psychological assessment and counseling emphasize the importance of an interdisciplinary approach to family counseling for aphasia. The speech-language pathologists' expertise in communicative disorders should be augmented by the input of a clinical psychologist or counselor if maximum benefit is to be derived from the group experience. Group counseling sessions are often very emotionally laden, and speech-language pathologists are seldom specifically trained to manage the psychological and emotional impact of disability (Kearns and Simmons, 1985). Group counseling for aphasia is best conducted within a multidisciplinary approach that recognizes and treats emotional and psychological difficulties that arise from disordered communication (Friedland and McColl, 1989; Pachalska, 1991a; Radonjic and Rakuscek, 1991).

Speech-Language Treatment Groups

Speech-language treatment of aphasic patients has been conducted in group settings for nearly half a century. Yet, despite its history of longevity, group therapy for aphasia remains a controversial area. Many authors have viewed group therapy as an "adjunct" to individual therapy (Chenven, 1953; Eisenson, 1973; Marquardt et al., 1976; Makenzie, 1991; Schuell et al., 1964; Smith, 1972) or subordinate to individual therapy but not a substitute for it. Schuell et al. (1964), for example, noted that "we are unable to have confidence in group therapy as a basic method of treatment for aphasia" (p. 343), since benefits derived from group treatment are likely to be emotional or social in nature. Similarly, although he acknowledges potential speech-language benefits, Eisenson (1973) states, "The first and most important (objective) is providing psychological support for individuals within the group" (p. 188). The prevalent attitude has been that group treatment methods may not facilitate speech-language recovery in aphasia, but they are not, at least, detrimental to recovery.

In opposition to the stance that group therapy for aphasia is palliative, a number of recent authors have indicated that group intervention may be an effective means of treating speech-language deficits (Aten et al., 1981, 1982; Bloom, 1962; Fawcus, 1989; Makenzie, 1991; Wertz et al., 1981). Although the data are not yet available to conclude that individual and group therapy for aphasia are equally effective, recent data and opinions that support this conclusion are beginning to stimulate investigative interest in the group treatment approach. In the sections that follow, we will examine the speech-language treatment group literature and explore emerging trends in this area.

Advocacy Reports

For our purposes the term "advocacy reports" is used to designate articles that advocate the use of group speech-language treatment for aphasia without clearly delineating treatment procedures or presenting data to support their position. Johnston and Pennypacker (1980) originally described an advocacy research style as one in which the experimenter's prejudices interfere with his or her objectivity. That is, the experimenter "has taken the role of an advocate who defends a cause, not a scientist who searches for understanding" (p. 424).

Advocacy reports may reflect, in part, a paucity of efficacy research, strong clinical bias toward unproven techniques, and a genuine interest in sharing clinical ideas. Moreover, in related fields such as clinical psychology (Barlow et al., 1984), clinicians are often more influenced by teachers, colleagues, and non-data-based presentations than they are by clinical research. This would also appear to be the case in clinical aphasiology, where little data exist regarding the efficacy of group therapy approaches and clinicians commonly treat aphasic individuals in group settings. Unfortunately, discussions of group therapy for aphasia continue to be based primarily on clinical experience and bias. Recent descriptions of group therapy approaches have attempted to document change in psychosocial (Borenstein et al., 1987) and communication skills (Radonjic and Rakuscek, 1991) following intervention. However, failure to incorporate appropriate experimental controls, such as the use of groups of control groups and reliable measurement techniques, limits the contributions of many recent efforts and makes them comparable to earlier advocacy reports.

The current emphasis on intensive, multidisciplinary, functional, aphasia treatment groups is reminiscent of approaches that have been advocated for decades (Borenstein, et al., 1987; Pachalska, 1991a; Repo, 1991). Sheehan (1946) was among the earliest advocates of group speech-language treatment for aphasia. Her initial writings described "group speech classes" in which small groups of aphasic patients worked on everyday vocabulary. Five or six patients usually participated in the group at a given time. The specific content of "lessons" included greetings and farewells, personal identification information, money, calendar use, right-left orientation, and body part identification. As Sheehan (1946) noted, "The list is endless—a product of a little imagination and ingenuity and of observation of the things needed by the patients in their daily living" (p. 152). Sheehan (1948) was an early advocate of establishing individualized goals for each aphasic patient in treatment groups.

Wepman (1947) described a model program for inpatient rehabilitation of aphasic individuals. The program was carried out by a multidisciplinary team that included speech-language pathologists, psychologists, occupational and physical therapists, social workers, and special education teachers. Both individual and group speech therapy sessions were included in the program. The speech-language pathologist directed speech-related groups, and special educators taught writing, spelling, reading, and arithmetic in a group setting. Wepman outlined

an intensive program that included 6 to 8 hours of treatment per day, 5 days per week. He concluded that an intensive, multidisciplinary approach is necessary if aphasic patients are to make maximum gains in therapy. A similar approach for patients with "motor aphasia" was outlined by Corbin (1951).

While the earliest writers in the area emphasized the importance of functional communication therapy in the group setting, the rationale for this approach was not fully developed for several years. Bloom (1962) was the first author to clearly articulate a pragmatic philosophy of group treatment for aphasia. Her rationale for group treatment combined an awareness of contextual influences on communication and meaning with an appreciation for the power of operant training techniques.

Although several treatment groups were conducted in her setting, Bloom emphasized the feasibility of group treatment for severely impaired patients. Aphasic individuals participating in her rehabilitation program attended one session of individual treatment, one session of auditory stimulation, and an hourly group session each day. The primary goal of group treatment was to improve functional communication abilities. All treatment activities were directed toward improving performance of "activities of daily living." Unlike many of the previous reports of group treatment, this approach did not segment sessions into classroomlike activities according to separate language modalities.

Bloom (1962) emphasized a situational group approach in which language stimulation was provided in meaningful contexts. Situations that occurred in daily experience were recreated in the naturalistic group environment, while role playing and rote memorization of scripts were avoided. Verbal tasks were used to practice greetings, directions, ordering from a menu, and handling money. In addition, auditory stimulation was also provided during group sessions.

Summary and Observations. To summarize, advocacy-style treatment reports promoted the use of group therapy techniques as a primary method of intervention for aphasia. These reports described ongoing group treatment programs and presented a sampling of tasks employed in the group setting. There was consensus agreement that group speech-language treatment was efficacious, although data to support this claim were lacking.

Despite their shortcomings, advocacy reports of group treatment for aphasia were farsighted in several respects. They were, for example, ahead of their time in recommending a multidisciplinary treatment approach (Nielson et al., 1948; Sheehan, 1946; Wepman, 1947). Sheehan (1946) held regular team conferences that included speech-language pathologists, occupational therapists, and physical therapists. An effort was made to coordinate these services so that an overall plan of rehabilitation could be developed. Wepman (1947) also strongly advocated the multidisciplinary approach, and he indicated that "only by this overall cooperative approach can the maximum recovery level for the brain injured aphasic adult be achieved (p. 409). Advocacy reports laid the historical foundation for current group therapy approaches that incorporate a multidisciplinary format (Pachalska, 1991a; Radonjic and Rakuscek, 1991).

In addition to establishing a multidisciplinary approach to aphasia management, early advocates of group therapy were nearly unanimous in their call for intensive therapy regimen (Corbin, 1951; Huber, 1946; Sheehan, 1948; Wepman, 1947).

Wepman (1947) and his contemporaries suggested daily treatment, and many advocated several sessions per day. Huber (1946), for example, indicated that most aphasic patients could participate in 3 to 6 hours of therapy daily when appropriate rest periods were scheduled.

Perhaps the most impressive aspect of the early group treatment literature is the consistent emphasis on functional, real-life treatment activities (Agranowitz et al., 1954; Bloom, 1962; Corbin, 1951; Huber, 1946; Sheehan, 1946, 1948). During the embryonic stages of group therapy for aphasia, clinicians developed treatment tasks that were based on the patients' communicative needs in the living environment. Treatment approaches included a consideration of contextual factors despite the lack of a supporting theoretical basis for "pragmatic" aspects of communication.

The previous examples of advocacy reports are primarily from the post-World War II era. However, recent reports reviewed below are also advocacy in nature (Borenstein et al., 1987; Friedland and McColl, 1989; Radonjic and Rakuscek, 1991; Rice et al., 1987). These authors present data obtained from uncontrolled group treatment studies to support the effectiveness of their approaches. Whereas earlier advocacy reports presented detailed clinical information and subjective clinical impressions, more recent descriptions of group therapy have included relatively less detailed information regarding clinical techniques and quasi-experimental results.

Taken together, early and more recent advocacy reports appear to have had a subtle and perhaps significant negative impact on the cumulative growth of objective information in this area. That is, the legacy of advocacy reports has been the tacit acceptance of the effectiveness of group therapy for aphasia despite meager evidence to support this claim. Initial group therapy reports provided convincing, albeit unsubstantiated, testimonials as to the effectiveness of this method of patient management and more recent efforts have included clinical data that provide an appearance of scientific legitimacy. However, acceptance of subjective reports and uncontrolled treatment data as evidence for the efficacy of group treatment may have had the deleterious effect of retarding legitimate investigative efforts in this area. Gilbert et al. (1977) have stated that "repeated weakly controlled trials are likely to agree and build up an illusion of strong evidence because of a large count of favorable studies. Not only does this mislead us into adopting and maintaining an unproven therapy, but it may make proper studies more difficult to mount" (p. 687). It seems that advocacy reports of group therapy have seduced clinicians and researchers alike into uncritically accepting this approach, and the cumulative effect of this literature has been an "illusion of strong evidence." Recent data-based clinical efforts represent a legitimate initial effort to examine treatment effectiveness, but these efforts must be followed up with more rigorous efficacy studies that examine specific treatment approaches for clearly defined groups of aphasic patients.

In the section that follows, we will examine contributions to the group treatment literature and explore the current status of research in this area. Five types of aphasia treatment groups—direct, indirect, sociolinguistic, transition, and maintenance groups—will be considered.

Direct Language Treatment Groups

Davis (1992) has distinguished "direct" from "indirect" treatment approaches. He states that:

> Direct approaches focus the clinician-patient interaction on the exercising of specific language processes. They are referred to as stimulus-response training, in which the clinician elicits specific language responses from the patient. They are structured . . . so that the patient is using discrete functions such as auditory language comprehension or word retrieval (p. 241).

Brookshire (1992) was apparently referring to "direct" speech-language training groups when he noted that many aphasia treatment groups are didactic, relatively structured, and clinician directed. Tasks that are chosen for direct treatment groups often mimic those used in individual treatment.

Holland (1970) provided an early example of the application of "stimulus-response training" in a direct group treatment program. She applied, "shaping and reinforcement procedures to direct language work with aphasics in a group setting" (p. 385). Unlike previously discussed group treatment reports, she established specific treatment goals in an attempt to improve verbal categorization, naming, plurality, subject-verb agreement, and syntactic ordering abilities. Language tasks were arranged in hierarchies of difficulties so that patients of various severity levels could participate in the same group. Although Holland did not report objective data to support her exploratory approach, she indicated that she was able to arrange treatment so that individual patient needs were met.

Additional examples of direct language treatment groups are available from recent studies of specific training techniques. Skelly et al. (1974), for example, combined group treatment with individual treatment in their study of the effects of Amer-Ind sign on patients' verbal production. They stated that the sign group was an integral part of their gestural program. Skelly et al. did not evaluate the contributions of group training to the acquisition of Amer-Ind signs. Relatedly, Sparks et al. (1974) used "less structured" Melodic Intonation Therapy (MIT) in direct group treatment for aphasia. Although not specifically evaluated in their study, they suggested that group MIT therapy may increase patients' ability to intone basic, purposeful utterances.

More often than not, group therapy is viewed as an adjunct to individual therapy. Makenzie (1991), for example, recently examined the effectiveness of a combined regimen of direct individual and group intervention. The five subjects in this study had previously been dismissed from nonintensive speech therapy after having plateaued. All participants were at least 9 months postonset of aphasia. The primary focus of this investigation was to examine the value of an intensive period of therapy.

The stated aim of the aphasia group was "information giving." All participants were encouraged to use an available modality to communicate effectively during discussions of daily topics. In addition, each individual participated in daily individual therapy in which two verbal goals were targeted for improvement. In total, subjects received approximately 85 hours of individual and group therapy during a 1-month period. A 1-month period of no treatment followed the period of intensive therapy. A screening battery for aphasia, a test of verbal naming ability, and a test of functional communication were among the measures used to evaluate treatment gains. The results of this clinical report indicated that all five patients improved on at least one clinical measure. Some decrease in performance was found following a period of no treatment.

Indirect Language Treatment Groups

Indirect treatment approaches are unstructured and may consist of general conversation, social groups, role playing, and field trips (Davis, 1992). Many of these approaches are purported to have therapeutic merit for improving deficient language skills despite the fact that they are largely undefined. Previously presented examples of psychosocial group therapy for aphasia, which used unspecified or poorly described techniques, differ from indirect treatment approaches primarily in the orientation and general goals of the group leaders. That is, whereas the general purpose of psychosocial groups has been to facilitate emotional and psychological adjustment to aphasia, the orientation of indirect language training groups has been to stimulate language recovery.

Despite the vague nature of indirect treatment groups, there is reason to believe that loosely defined language stimulation and group discussion are commonly applied treatment methods. In a recent survey of group therapy for aphasia in a Veterans Administration Medical Center, Kearns and Simmons (1985) asked clinicians to estimate the percentage of time spent on various clinical activities during a typical aphasia group treatment session. The respondents indicated that "general, topic-oriented discussions" were the most prevalent (31%) activity engaged in during group treatment. Considerably less group treatment time was spent on "structured tasks (word retrieval, etc." (22%)).

As in all areas of group treatment for aphasia, there are little data available regarding the effectiveness of indirect language treatment groups. The poorly defined nature of these treatment approaches severely limits investigators' ability to examine the usefulness of such approaches. However, a Veterans Administration cooperative study on aphasia compared the effectiveness of individual treatment and indirect group treatment (Wertz et al., 1981). A treatment protocol was developed to help ensure uniform training within both groups. Strict selection criteria were also used in this study, and only patients having a single, left-hemisphere, cerebrovascular accident were included.

Aphasic subjects in both treatment conditions received 8 hours of therapy a week for up to 44 weeks. Subjects in the group treatment condition received 4 hours of therapy in a social setting and 4 hours of recreational activities. Group treatment activities did not include direct manipulation of speech or language abilities. That is, no specific treatment tasks were presented to improve performance in verbal, auditory, visual, or graphic language modalities. Typical group tasks included participation in discussions of current events or other interesting topics.

Subjects in the individual treatment condition received 4 hours of direct "stimulus-response" treatment of speech and language deficits. Specific tasks were presented for the various language modalities, and contingent feedback and reinforcement were provided by the clinician. In addition to individual treatment, subjects also received 4 hours per week of machine-assisted treatment.

The results of this study revealed that subjects in the individual treatment condition improved significantly more than sub-

jects in the indirect treatment group conditions on overall performance on the Porch Index of Communicative Ability (PICA) (Porch, 1967). No significant differences were apparent on other language tests. Furthermore, subjects in both the individual and group treatment conditions made significant gains in their language test scores beyond the recognized period of spontaneous recovery. The authors concluded that there were relatively few differences in the amount or type of improvement exhibited by subjects in the two treatment conditions. Wertz et al. (1981) surmised that "individual and group treatment are efficacious means for managing aphasia" (p. 593).

Sociolinguistic Treatment Groups

Sociolinguistic treatment groups have evolved as a reaction to the highly structured treatment techniques employed in direct treatment approaches. Proponents of sociolinguistic treatment approaches have pointed out that direct treatment approaches may limit the types of communicative exchanges that occur between the clinician and the patient. Wilcox and Davis (1977), for example, found that clinicians primarily produced "questions" and "requests" during direct treatment sessions, and patients responded to the clinicians with assertions. A similar pattern of restricted responding was evident in a social group setting. Clinicians and patients produced a restricted number of "speech acts" in both settings. Wilcox and Davis concluded that individual and group treatment should be less didactic and permit the exchange of a wider variety of communicative interactions including advising, arguing, and congratulating.

Davis (1992) also advocates a sociolinguistic approach to group therapy for aphasia. Rather than drilling patients on specific treatment tasks that are adapted from individual treatment, he recommended that group sessions emphasize interaction among the patients while minimizing clinician directiveness. For example, principles of Promoting Aphasic's Communicative Effectiveness (PACE) therapy (Davis and Wilcox, 1981) can be incorporated into group treatment so that patients "take turns, convey new information, practice using multiple channels, and provide each other with feedback to overcome obstacles" (p. 263).

As a participant in the panel discussion of group therapy for aphasia, conducted by Aten et al. (1981), Haire elaborated on Davis's principles of treatment. She defined the purpose of group treatment as an attempt to "maximize (the patients') communicative strengths in order to improve interpersonal communication" (Aten et al., 1981, p. 146). Her group treatment activities centered around a preplanned task or game, and PACE treatment principles were incorporated into the sessions.

Aten et al. (1982) investigated a sociolinguistic treatment approach that was described as "group functional communication therapy." Seven chronic aphasic patients participated in this study. All subjects had suffered a single, left-hemisphere, cerebrovascular accident at least 9 months prior to the initiation of treatment. The subjects participated in hourly group sessions twice weekly for a period of 12 weeks, and a total of 24 treatment sessions were administered.

The goal of treatment was to improve functional communication, and a variety of everyday communicative situations were selected for training from the Communicative Activities of Daily Living (CADL) (Holland, 1980). The "real-life" training situations included (*a*) shopping, (*b*) giving and following directions, (c) greetings, (d) giving personal information, (e) reading signs, and (f) gestural expression of ideas. Therapy activities included role playing and use of menus, grocery lists, and other materials from the patients' living environment.

The results of training were evaluated by examining pre- and poststudy performance on the PICA (Porch, 1967) and the CADL. Pre- and posttreatment PICA scores revealed nonsignificant differences, but statistically significant differences were apparent for pre- and posttreatment CADL scores. The authors concluded that group functional communication treatment is efficacious and that functional measures such as the CADL should be included in our clinical assessments.

Additional data are needed to establish the validity of sociolinguistic group treatment for aphasia. For example, evaluation of the efficacy of discourse exercises (Osiejek, 1991) and other communication-based therapies in the group setting is warranted.

Transition Groups

In addition to the direct, indirect, and sociolinguistic treatment approaches described above, several authors have described transition or maintenance group treatment for aphasia. Brookshire indicated that transition groups are conducted to help individuals make the transition between regular attendance in treatment and dismissal from treatment. Tasks employed in these groups are usually selected to help aphasic individuals adapt to communicative situations that occur in their living environment. Transition groups often meet one or more times weekly, and patients usually participate in these groups for a limited and specified period of time prior to discharge from treatment.

As a member of the group therapy panel conducted by Aten et al. (1981), West described her unique approach to transition groups. Three groups, a discharge-planning group, a community involvement group, and a stroke club group, were used to facilitate the transition between inpatient hospital services and release to the home environment. Patients in West's program participated in each of the groups in sequential order in an attempt to develop an increasing level of functional independence from the hospital staff.

The overall goals of the transition groups were (a) to help patients accept changes in physical and cognitive abilities, (b) to develop a realistic view of progress and altered ability, (c) to assist patients in finding an alternate life-style within available family and community resources, (d) to reinforce gains made in individual therapy, and (e) to help patients with community placement.

In addition to these general goals, each group had a specific purpose. For example, the main purpose of the discharge-planning group was to prepare patients for life-style changes that would occur on dismissal from the hospital. Practical difficulties encountered during home visitations were also discussed in this group.

Once patients were discharged from the hospital, they participated in the community involvement group in an attempt to facilitate emotional and psychological adjustment to their new environment. The emphasis in this group was on helping patients accept their new life-styles and assist them in developing productive alternate life-styles. The group also discussed emotional incidents that occurred in the home setting, and provided

an opportunity for emotional venting by the group members. The community involvement group attempted to "confront reality without destroying hope" (Aten et al., 1981, p. 150).

The final stage in West's transition group program was participation in a monthly "stroke club." This group provided emotional support and education, and it helped patients maintain the level of communicative ability that had been reached following individual speech-language treatment. In general, West concluded that her three-group transition process was successful because it reduced dependency on the hospital staff and integrated patients into existing family and community structures.

Maintenance Groups

In the final analysis, West's "stroke club" group appears similar in function to a "maintenance group." Brookshire notes that maintenance groups provide regular stimulation so that patients' speech-language skills do not deteriorate once they are dismissed from intensive, individual therapy. He indicates that maintenance group activities are frequently social in nature and may emphasize social interaction and communication in social contexts. Participation in maintenance groups may last from months to years, depending on the individual needs of the patient and his or her family. Brookshire observed that maintenance group meetings are seldom held more than once per week and may be held only once per month. Maintenance groups continue to be a medium for encouraging retention of therapeutic gains made during aphasia rehabilitation (Springer, 1991).

Hunt (1976) described a language maintenance group that provided support, information, and language stimulation for patients who had been dismissed from individual treatment. Eight to 12 patients participated in the groups, which met once a week for 2 hours. Family members were excluded from group participation.

The emphasis of this maintenance program was on stimulation of language in a social setting. Group activities were planned around the patients' interests and included movies, slide presentations, and guest speakers. These activities provided an opportunity for using residual language skills. Although specific language goals were not established, all attempts to communicate in the group setting were reinforced.

Hunt (1976) concluded that the social language group provided valuable language stimulation, practice of previously acquired abilities, social interaction, and entertainment. The maintenance group also acted as a source of information, support, and referral for the families of aphasic patients, and it provided a valuable training experience for student clinicians.

Kagan et al. (1990) described a unique, community-based group treatment approach that is designed to facilitate functional communication, promote independence, and maintain gains made as a result of individual therapy. An important aspect of the program is the use of community volunteers who are trained and supervised by speech-language pathologists to work on communication goals with aphasic individuals in a group setting. A comparison of the results of pre- and posttesting for chronic aphasic patients who participated in the community group versus a group of untreated community-dwelling control subjects was reported. Results revealed significant improvement in the posttreatment performance of the group participants on a test of communicative effectiveness (CETI; Lomas et al., 1989 (see Chapter 6)) but not on traditional language testing. A significant between-group difference favoring the treated patients was also found on this measure.

Efficacy of Speech-Language Treatment Groups

As in other areas of group intervention for aphasia, the efficacy of speech-language treatment groups remains largely untested (Brindely et al., 1989; Fawcus, 1989). Although several studies have explored the value of combined individual and group treatment for aphasia (Chenven, 1953; Makenzie, 1991; Smith, 1972), examination of group treatment as a primary and independent form of patient management has only recently been undertaken (Aten et al., 1982; Radonjic and Rakuscek, 1991; Wertz et al., 1981). Research evaluating the effectiveness of specific group speech-language treatment is practically nonexistent, and the scientific basis of clinical aphasiology will not be sturdy until this investigative deficiency is rectified.

Summary and Observations. Recent reports of group speech-language treatment for aphasia were reviewed, and five group therapy approaches were identified. These included (*a*) direct language treatment groups, (*b*) indirect language treatment groups, (*c*) sociolinguistic treatment groups, (*d*) transition groups, and (*e*) maintenance groups. Although each approach is unique, the common denominator among them is that their primary purpose is to facilitate recovery and/or maintenance of speech-language abilities. There is, however, considerable variability among group treatment approaches. Speech-language treatment groups range from structured, so-called "stimulus-response" approaches to essentially undefined, indirect treatment approaches. Group treatment tasks also show considerable variability and include specific techniques such as MIT (Sparks et al., 1974) as well as group discussions and recreational activities (Wertz et al., 1981). As previously noted, the variety of group treatment approaches probably reflects the training and biases of the clinicians who conduct group therapy (Marquardt et al., 1976).

There are, of course, obvious parallels between speech-language treatment group therapy and individual therapy for aphasia. Direct language treatment groups, for example, often employ the same tasks used in individual treatment and apply them in the group setting. Similarly, sociolinguistic group therapy consists of the application of recently developed treatment approaches, such as PACE therapy (Davis and Wilcox, 1981), to the group setting. Therefore, given these parallels between individual and group treatment, Holland's (1975) inquiry about the differences between these two approaches is poignant. If a group leader sequentially treats each individual in a group, and there is little interaction other than individual exchanges between the clinician and a given patient, the result may be inefficient individual treatment in a group setting. To avoid this possibility, group leaders must be aware of the strengths and communicative needs of individual group members. Ideally, tasks should be structured so that all group members can participate (Holland, 1970), but interactive aspects of communication should not be sacrificed (Davis, 1992). Moreover, the objectivity of direct approaches should be combined with the common-sense rationales for sociolinguistic group therapy. The development of data-based, pragmatic treatment approaches

will be challenging, but clinical aphasiologists have recently demonstrated the feasibility of this approach to program development (Cochrane and Milton, 1984; Davis and Wilcox, 1985; Kearns, 1986; Osiejek, 1991).

Clinicians should eschew indirect treatment approaches that have no explicit communication goals and serve as a social outlet for their aphasic patients. While socialization can be a legitimate goal of group therapy for aphasia, clinicians should be leery of letting group treatment deteriorate into totally unstructured activities that neither facilitate nor support identified communication aims. Like individual therapy for aphasia, group intervention should be based on sound clinical logic, and it should be goal directed without being overly rigid (Fawcus, 1991).

Multipurpose Groups

Taxonomies of group treatment procedures for aphasia are inherently flawed, since clinicians often identify several purposes for their groups. The results of Kearns and Simmons's (1985) survey of clinical practices indicate that 80% of the respondents listed multiple goals for their groups. As might be expected, language stimulation, often in combination with support or social goals, was the most frequent aim (84%) of aphasia groups. Following language stimulation, the next most frequently listed goals were emotional support (59%), carryover (47%), and socialization (45%). As previously indicated, attempts to classify types of aphasia group treatment approaches are generally for the sake of convenience alone, and they should not be construed as being a reflection of clinical reality. More often than not, group therapy is undertaken with several aims in mind even when a primary focus is evident.

Radonjic and Rakuscek (1991) recently described a multipurpose group that was established to decrease emotional tension; prevent social isolation; encourage the need for communication; encourage ability to search for, develop, and use communication in social situations; and develop confidence and self-respect. The group was developed by a clinical psychologist and a speech-language pathologist, and it generally ranged in size from four to seven participants with a maximum of 10 group members. Group activities included such varied activities as "learning about each other, relaxation techniques, games to strengthen psycholinguistic ability, drawing, pantomime, and therapeutic techniques involving music" (p. 451).

A five-point scale of communication was administered at the beginning and end of each patient's participation in an attempt to examine the impact of intervention. A descriptive analysis of difference scores for 108 aphasic patients revealed improvements on patients' posttreatment communication ratings as compared with pretreatment ratings. The authors concluded from their analysis that the best results were obtained for patients who participated in at least 10 treatment sessions in small groups having three to five members. Although intriguing, these clinical data must be replicated under more rigorous experimental conditions before they can be considered unassailable.

Pachalska (1991a) reviewed the group therapy literature and presented her treatment approach. Based on her review of the literature and her clinical experience, she suggests making groups as homogeneous as possible in terms of patient type and level of language involvement. Pachalska also recommends that the size of aphasia groups should not exceed four or five and that treatment sessions should last no more than an hour. A structured treatment approach is also advocated. Following her literature, Pachalska refers to a ''holistic'' method of treatment, which apparently refers to a multidisciplinary, multipurpose approach, such as her own Complex Aphasia Rehabilitation Model (CARM). Citing publications in her native language (Polish) she asserts that the holistic approach is ''the most effective approach'' (p. 547) to group treatment. CARM is described as having both individual and group treatment components, and group therapy is seen primarily as an adjunct to individual treatment. Group sessions are run by a multidisciplinary team of clinicians who provide cognitive physiotherapy, physical therapy, speech therapy, psychotherapy, and sociotherapy. Tasks are directed toward facilitating natural conversation. Pachalska (1991b) indicates that a goal on CARM is to stimulate transfer of information between the cerebral hemispheres; consequently, both linguistic and nonlinguistic stimuli are employed in treatment, and special emphasis is employed on ''language-oriented art therapy.'' Linguistic materials used in therapy include popular poems and word games. In addition to the language emphasis, other aspects of rehabilitation such as physical therapy and group discussions with family members are also included. Social activities, such as ''car rallies,'' are also considered as part of the rehabilitation process. Pachalska (1991a) makes the broad claim that ''all abilities which underwent training in the programme significantly improved, and that the disturbances in the communicative, psychological and social domains were eliminated to a considerable degree; the reintegration was more complete'' (p. 551).

The clinical forum that highlighted Pachalska's (1991a, 1991b) work included commentaries by distinguished aphasiologists (Aten, 1991: Fawcus, 1991; Loverso, 1991; Repo, 1991; Springer, 1991). Faucus (1991) emphasized that ''the whole essence of group work is its flexibility and spontaneity'' (p. 555) and cautioned against using overly structured approaches. Others agree that the mechanics of group therapy, such as group size and session length, cannot be dictated by prescription (Loverso, 1991; Springer, 1991). Our clinical experience is consistent with their suggestion that group sessions longer than 1 hour are possible and that larger groups are manageable and sometimes desirable. Larger, more heterogeneous groups may be particularly appropriate when the emphasis is not on direct communication or language training (Springer, 1991).

A final example of a multipurpose group that has recently appeared in the literature is provided by Marshall's (in press) description of problem-focused group therapy for mildly aphasic patients. The goals of this program are to provide a forum for discussing social, vocational, and recreational reintegration into society and assisting members in solving everyday communication problems. Examples of the problem-solving activities used during treatment include communicating in an emergency, meeting new people, and preparing for a physician's visit. Unique aspects of this program include the fact that it provides one of the few available descriptions of clinical management for mildly aphasic patients, and it provides a rationale for intervention that focuses on everyday problems and community reintegration.

Clinical data are presented that show the range of posttreatment improvements on standardized language test scores for the 18 patients for whom pre- and posttreatment comparisons

were available. The author recognizes the potential of functional communication assessments for evaluating progress in group therapy (Lomas et al., 1989), and he suggests that seldom used formats, such as client self report, may also provide a measure of clinical accountability. This issue is further considered in the sections that follow.

CLINICAL ACCOUNTABILITY

Measurement problems encountered in group therapy are significant but not insurmountable, and proper attention must be given to assessing speech-language treatment gains in the group setting. To date, few authors of group therapy reports have attempted to measure treatment gains, and those who have examined the success of treatment have, for the most part, relied on standardized tests of aphasia (Aten et al., 1982; Wertz et al., 1981). Although tools designed to measure functional communication ability (Holland, 1980; Lomas, et al., 1989) may be of particular value, standardized aphasia tests do not measure interactive aspects of communication, and the development and use of reliable supplemental measurement tools are sorely needed.

The importance of measurement issues in group therapy for aphasia cannot be overestimated. In a recent survey of group treatment practices within Veterans Administration Medical Centers, Kearns and Simmons (1985) reported that 73% of the respondents used periodic standardized testing to evaluate group members, and 33% employed standardized testing in combination with ''behavioral ratings of task performance.'' Surprisingly, 20% of the clinicians indicated that patient performance was *not* routinely evaluated.

A recurring problem for clinicians who run aphasia groups is the issue of clinical accountability; finding appropriate measures for assessing the effects of group therapy is problematic. As Aten (1991) points out in his commentary on Pachalska's work, treatment effectiveness will not be easily demonstrated until better assessments of psychosocial changes and conversational language are available. Similarly, Loverso (1991) addresses the need to develop and adopt tools that examine the roles of individuals within aphasia groups and the interaction of these roles during treatment. This novel suggestion is exemplified by the earlier work by Loverso et al. (1982), in which they demonstrated the reliability of a process evaluation form. Loverso et al. (1982) assessed the ''roles'' of individual group members and classified their interactions. They demonstrated that task (e.g., information giving and receiving), maintenance (e.g., encouraging following), and nonfunctional (e.g., disruptive) behaviors could be reliably rated in the small-group setting (see Chapter 6). Other novel, supplemental measures that may be employed in aphasia groups include the use of discourse analyses and interactive coding procedures (Cochrane and Milton, 1984).

Given the nature of the abilities targeted for intervention in group settings, clinicians often must devise their own clinical probes or ''minitests'' to sample skills such as turn-taking ability, initiation of interactions, and other skills, since standard assessments are not routinely available. Whatever the measurement procedure chosen, it is essential to evaluate the communicative abilities of aphasia group members routinely.

DISMISSAL CONSIDERATIONS

One final note of caution is needed regarding speech-language treatment groups that serve transition or maintenance functions. Transition groups, like previously described counseling groups, have an inherent appeal because they serve an obvious and legitimate clinical function. It is important, however, to be sure that such groups are structured so that they facilitate transition from the clinic to the home environment within a reasonable period of time. As West (in Aten et al. [1981]) has cautioned, continued group participation may foster undesirable dependence on the hospital staff, and it may actually inhibit adjustment to the posthospital environment. Patients who participated in West's program were involved in active group treatment for 4 to 6 months.

Extensive participation in maintenance groups may also not be advisable. If the purpose of maintenance groups is to help patients stabilize at their maximum performance level, then a program of periodic evaluation and occasional, brief clinical "tune-ups" may prove beneficial. However, hourly group maintenance sessions that meet monthly or even weekly may not be of sufficient intensity to truly maintain previously acquired behaviors. Therefore, when the amount of reinforcement or feedback provided in the group settings is not sufficient to help patients maintain or reacquire previously learned skills, additional, individual treatment may be needed.

The judicious use of aphasia groups as a means of maintaining treatment gains is often warranted. It is critical, however, that the specific skills to be maintained are identified prior to intervention. In addition, appropriate measurement techniques should be employed to assess performance, and a specific and reasonable period of intervention should be established and discussed with patients and their families. Surprisingly, a significant percentage (28%) of respondents in the previously noted survey of group practices indicated that *patients* decide when they should be dismissed from group treatment (Kearns and Simmons, 1985). It is apparent that more objective dismissal criteria need to be developed. Group therapy for aphasia should not be a nebulous, potentially unending process. The group setting provides an ideal atmosphere for fostering communicative independence (Pachalska, 1991a), and failure to establish clearly specified dismissal criteria may foster an unhealthy level of psychological and communicative dependency between aphasic patients and their clinicians.

GUIDING PRINCIPLES

Thus far we have considered psychosocial, family counseling and support, and speech-language treatment groups for aphasia. Among the speech-language treatment reports, we distinguished early advocacy groups from more recent speech-language treatment groups. Our review of recent speech-language treatment group reports revealed a number of distinct approaches including direct language treatment groups; indirect language treatment groups; and sociolinguistic, transition, and maintenance groups.

It should be apparent from this brief summary that no single therapeutic model can accommodate the variety of aphasia groups that have been reported in the literature. However, recent trends in the generalization literature may serve as a cornerstone for the development of eclectic, principled group treatment approaches. We will, therefore, review generalization prompt-ing tactics that may lead to testable hypotheses and generate data-based group treatment approaches. Our discussion will be limited to treatment groups that are designed primarily to facilitate improved communication abilities.

Facilitating Generalization Through Group Therapy

The ultimate goal of aphasia therapy is to develop maximum communication ability in nontraining settings and situations. In essence, generalization of target behaviors across stimuli, settings, people, behavior, and time (i.e., maintenance) is the desired end product of therapy. Treatment effects are notoriously restrictive, and generalization is the exception rather than the rule in aphasia rehabilitation and other applied fields as well. There is, however, a growing generalization literature that provides suggestions regarding specific techniques that may facilitate carryover (Baer, 1981; Horner et al., 1988; Hughes, 1985; Kearns, 1989; McReynolds and Spradlin, 1989; Spradlin and Siegel, 1982; Warren and Rogers-Warren, 1985). A philosophy of group management that is geared toward facilitating generalization may provide an opportunity to empirically test our assumptions about generalization and allow us to examine the efficacy of group therapy for aphasia.

Stokes and Baer's (1977) list of generalization-promoting techniques was generated after they reviewed over 200 published articles that had addressed questions regarding training generalization. They concluded that generalization seldom occurs spontaneously and that carryover must be actively planned for rather than anticipated. Consistent with this conclusion, reviews of the aphasia generalization literature also indicated that generalization of aphasia treatment effects is not an automatic by-product of intervention (Thompson, 1989). More often than not, clinical investigations of aphasia are what Stokes and Baer (1977) labeled "Train and Hope Studies." That is, investigators attempt to measure generalization of communicative improvements, but they seldom do anything to actively try and achieve generalized responding. Furthermore, when generalization does not occur following intervention, no additional follow-up steps are taken to obtain carryover. If the ultimate goal of aphasia therapy is to achieve maximum communicative functioning in settings and situations where patients live, work, and interact, then we have an obligation to do everything in our power to achieve functional carryover. As Horner et al. (1986) note, "[T]here is an ethical obligation, if not a responsibility, to make sure that generalization programming is incorporated into every program that endeavors to make important social and life-style changes for clients" (p. 16).

The clinical process involved in planning for generalization is described next.

Generalization Planning

Clinical practice in speech-language pathology often includes four discrete and relatively independent sequential phases involving assessment, intervention, generalization, and maintenance. As is true of other clinical specialties in speech pathology, clinical aphasiologists have attended to the assessment and intervention phases of the clinical process while placing relatively little emphasis on generalization and maintenance. In contrast to the traditional approach to treatment planning, a generalization planning approach to the clinical process is conceptualized as a means of integrating the well-known clinical phases into a continuous loop that incorporates specific procedures to maximize the possibility of promoting generalization (Baer, 1981; Horner et al., 1988; Hughes, 1985; Warren and Rogers-Warren, 1985).

Kearns (1989) notes the following differences between a generalization planning approach to intervention and the traditional discrete phase approach. First, the separation of the clinical process into discrete phases encourages the establishment of clinical goals based on performance on clinical tasks within the treatment setting. Thus, within the traditional model, an aphasia test is given during the assessment phase, and the results of testing are used to establish clinical goals. When these goals are met, clinicians may then begin to examine aspects of generalization and maintenance. By contrast, a generalization planning approach to clinical management assumes that carryover of improvements in functional communicative abilities is the primary goal of intervention, and, as a result, assessment, goal setting, and intervention are all influenced by this assumption. The desire to facilitate generalization is foremost from the initial contact with the aphasic person and his or her family. Within a generalization planning framework, carryover of functional abilities is the clinical glue that bonds all aspects of patient management into an integrated whole. Thus, all steps in the process are woven together for the express purpose of effecting change in patients' ability to communicate in nonclinical settings, and with people and in situations that they experience in daily life. Whereas generalization and maintenance are too often a clinical afterthought with the discrete phase model of clinical practice, their attainment is the driving force behind generalization planning.

The distinction between traditional treatment planning and generalization planning is far more than philosophical (Kearns, 1989). After all, most clinical aphasiologists would contend that carryover is a primary goal of group therapy. From a practical viewpoint, however, the generalization approach is procedurally more complex and sometimes more time consuming than its traditional counterpart. For example, whereas the discrete phase approach to assessment of aphasic individuals may include standard and nonstandard tests of language and functional communication, the generalization planning approach expands the evaluation process to include gathering information directly relevant to maximizing the chances of obtaining carryover of treatment effects. Expansion of the traditional assessment may include, for example, naturalistic observations in the patients' homes, interviewing significant others to determine communicative need, and recording and analyzing spontaneous interactions with familiar and unfamiliar partners. Baer (1981) suggests using every means available to make lists of all (communication) behaviors, settings, individuals, people, and actions of significant others that might affect generalization. These lists can then be narrowed down to a reasonable few and prioritized for the purposes of deciding what combination of client behaviors and environmental factors need to be altered to maximize the probability of obtaining generalization.

The primary outcome of an expanded, more ecologically valid assessment is to choose *generalization* goals. That is, based on the information gathered, the clinician attempts to determine the most critical factors that should be targeted for intervention if improved communicative ability is likely to carry over to real-life settings and conditions. On choosing these parameters of treatment, the clinician sets a criterion for evaluating whether a sufficient level of generalization occurs. The clinician is also charged with the task of determining how best to measure progress toward generalization goals. Since there are rarely specific tests available to determine if generalization of specific target behaviors improves, clinicians must develop their own means of assessing performance. For example, to measure use of self-cuing strategies to facilitate word retrieval during spontaneous interactions in the group setting, a clinician could decide to videotape PACE activities (Davis and Wilcox, 1985) and monitor the number of times patients correctly self-cue themselves during the task. These clinical probes (i.e., minitests) can be periodically given over time to evaluate progress toward generalization goals. This information can subsequently be graphed and used as a visual aid to monitor treatment effectiveness (Connell and McReynolds, 1988; Kearns, 1986a). In addition, ongoing assessment and visual-graphic data presentation also serve as a guide in making treatment decisions. For example, clinical probe data can be examined to determine if generalization occurs to targeted people, settings, and conditions, and appropriate modifications can be made to intervention strategies as needed. Since it is clear that generalization of aphasia treatment effects does not automatically occur as a result of intervention, it is imperative that progress toward generalization goals be monitored so that appropriate clinical modifications can be initiated.

Thus far we have noted that a generalization planning approach includes adopting more ecologically valid assessments, establishing criterion-based generalization goals, continuously probing performance on clinical probes, and then adjusting intervention strategies until generalization and maintenance are achieved. Another essential component of a generalization plan involves using specific treatment techniques that have been shown to facilitate generalized responding. Once an ecological assessment is completed and generalization goals and criteria are established, the clinician must decide how to shape intervention in a way that increases the likelihood of achieving generalization.

Stokes and Baer's (1977) seminal review outlined specific tactics that were found to facilitate generalized responding, and they suggested that these strategies present a list of "what to do possibilities." Elaborating on these findings, Stokes and Osnes (1986) identified three generalization programming principles that can be incorporated into a generalization plan. They are (*a*) take advantage of natural communities of reinforcers, (*b*) incorporate functional mediators, and (*c*) train diversely (loosely). A brief consideration of these principles is presented below.

Natural Maintaining Contingencies

Stokes and Osnes' (1986) first generalization prompting principle was that clinicians should take advantage of "natural maintaining contingencies" or reinforcing events in the patient's natural environment that maintain target behaviors. Communicative skills and strategies that are trained in the clinic will carry over to living settings and be maintained only if they occur with relative frequency and are sufficiently reinforced at home. Group clinicians should, therefore, train functional, frequently occurring communicative strategies that solicit reinforcement.

Baer (1981) indicates that attending to natural maintaining contingencies may be the most important generalization planning principle. The problem is that we cannot assume that we know what communication skills will be attended, reinforced, and encouraged in nonclinical environments. For example, while many adults rely on reading for information and pleasure, many others do not. In this age of mass media, a large portion of adults seldom read the newspaper, and they rely on television as their primary source of information on current events. Given these obvious facts, clinicians should not assume that improving functional reading ability is necessarily an important or useful goal for an aphasic patient. Rather, information from spouses and other sources should be used to assess the relative value of printed materials to their patients before incorporating them into therapy tasks.

Another example of common treatment goals that may be achieved in the clinic but not used or reinforced in the natural environment comes from the various forms of augmentative and alternative communication strategies. Cohelo and Duffy (1985), for example, documented the common clinical impression that even when patients learn a vocabulary of iconic signs as a means of supplementing or replacing verbal production, they often do not spontaneously use gestures for functional communication. Clinicians often lament that the same is true for augmentative communication systems. While the reasons for the poor carryover in this area are not entirely clear, it is feasible that the significant individuals with whom they attempt to use these nonverbal systems simply do not acknowledge or reinforce communicative attempts using such systems.

While it is obviously important to determine if communication goals are functional at home and in other environments, it is also worth noting that aphasic patients can be exposed to strategies that will help them enlist social attention and reinforcement from family, friends, and peers. For example, some fluent aphasic patients who have significantly impaired auditory comprehension may fail to initiate communicative exchanges because they have difficulty following a conversation. While avoidance may be a natural and rational tendency in such situations, it is not conducive to independence and reintegration into the community. As an alternative, aphasic individuals can be shown how they can control conversational opportunities, receive social reinforcement, and achieve their communicative goals by recruiting natural reinforcers. That is, fluent aphasic patients with impaired comprehension can use a "stop" strategy to cue communicative partners that they need more processing time to understand what is being said to them. They may inform a listener that they did not understand what was said to them and ask them to repeat it or rephrase it. Strategies such as these let patients solicit communicative partners as participants in exchanges that reinforce their communicative strengths.

An important corollary of the "natural maintaining contingencies" technique is that clinicians should enlist the assistance of family members or significant others when selecting individualized target behaviors. Family members' assistance can be invaluable for determining the patient's communicative needs in his or her living environment. Of equal importance, family members should be made aware of the specific target behaviors that are being practiced during group therapy so that they can attempt to prompt and reinforce the behaviors at home. In addition, any channel (e.g., verbal, gestural, writing, drawing) that can be used to communicate successfully should be accepted, reinforced, and programmed in the group setting and

at home. Too often clinicians overemphasize verbal production at the expense of other modalities only to find out that a patient communicates successfully at home with minimum reliance on verbal output. A careful examination of factors in the group members' living and social environments that encourage, reinforce, and help to develop and maintain communicative skills targeted in group therapy can be extremely useful for developing treatment strategies.

Incorporation of Functional Mediators

Another effective principle for prompting generalization described by Stokes and Osnes (1986) is to incorporate functional mediators into the generalization. The essence of this guideline is that parameters that were effective during treatment in clinic settings may be equally facilitative for fostering generalization to nonclinical settings.

Generalization can be mediated by training responses that can be used in nontraining settings to elicit appropriate responding. The systematic programming of self-cuing techniques in aphasia management can be viewed as a form of mediated generalization. Aphasic-apractic patients have, for example, been trained to use Amer-Ind gestures (Rao, 1986; Skelly et al., 1974) to facilitate verbal responding. Similarly, anomic patients have been taught to purposefully circumlocute and keep the flow of communication going when they encounter word-finding problems. Self-cuing techniques and compensatory strategies such as these allow patients to help themselves when communicative difficulties arise in nontraining settings or conditions. Functional mediators that can be controlled by the patient not only facilitate generalization but also foster communicative independence.

Aphasic individuals may reach criterion for the use of cues during structured individual tasks and be unable to rely on their cuing strategies when communication failure occurs during spontaneous interactions. When this occurs, the group setting can bridge the considerable gap between individual treatment sessions and generalization settings. Patients can practice cuing techniques during interactive communication, clinicians can identify failure to use self-cuing techniques, and remedial steps can be taken to rectify inappropriate use of cuing strategies during group sessions. Self-cuing techniques may provide an important means of mediating generalization, and group therapy for aphasia should be an integral aspect of training cuing strategies.

The probability of obtaining generalization increases when stimuli in the training situations are similar to those found in the setting in which you are trying to obtain generalization. Thus, generalization may also be facilitated when the aspects of the therapy setting resemble the natural communicative environment and vice versa. The physical setting for individual therapy is often radically different from the home environment. In fact, some treatment cubicles more closely resemble a prison cell than a living room. The group therapy environment can, however, be made to approximate a social or home setting by including appropriate furniture, decorations and accessories, or appliances. Although data are lacking to establish unequivocally that the physical setting may be critical during aphasia therapy, attempts should be made to maximize similarities between the group training setting and the natural environment.

In addition to physical setting, inclusion of peers in the training setting may facilitate generative responding. Inclusion of significant others and peers as active members of group treatment provides a means of facilitating generalization. Trained volunteers have recently been used as a means of helping aphasic patients integrate into social and communication activities (Lyon, 1992), and volunteers have been used as transitional clinicians in maintenance groups. The generalization tactics of using common physical aspects of the treatment and generalization as well as involving peers, family, and significant others into treatment may prove an effective means of planning for generalization.

Diverse Training

The second principle of generalization planning, train diversely, indicates that treatment parameters, including stimuli, responses, cues, individuals, and even settings, should be varied and diverse if treatment is to facilitate generalization. Highly structured, individualized treatment fosters situation-specific learning and inhibits generalization. Carryover may, therefore, be enhanced by exerting less control over stimuli and responses during treatment. Because of the naturalistic interaction that occurs in group, clinicians have an opportunity to vary the form of their input to patients (e.g., questions, requests), and patients receive varied feedback and social reinforcement from clinicians and other group members as well. While clinicians may be able to facilitate acquisition and carryover by exposing patients to the reduced structure of group therapy, unstructured social interaction is not an appropriate format for treatment groups. To the contrary, group sessions should be task oriented, clinician controlled and programmed to meet the individual needs of group members. Structured drill work can, however, be avoided in favor of tasks that maximize interactive communication and provide an opportunity for using target behaviors in varied, naturalistic situations. Clinicians should not lose sight of the flexibility that group settings offer (Fawcus, 1991).

To date, few treatment approaches have been developed for programming generalization. Cochrane and Milton (1984), however, have developed a conversational prompting technique that may be used to train generalization. Their sentence-building technique is intended to facilitate verbal responding during conversational exchanges. Treatment topics are selected on the basis of the patients' interests, and the clinician uses modeling and expansion to guide patient output and maintain a dialogue. In effect, the clinician orchestrates a two-way conversation concerning a relevant topic while providing appropriate cues and feedback. This approach avoids the artificiality of many highly structured tasks while maintaining therapeutic integrity. It lets the clinician elicit and reinforce novel but appropriate utterances and, in essence, program generalization (see Appendix A).

Kearns (1986a; Kearns and Scher, 1988; Kearns and Yedor, 1991) has also reported a treatment approach, Response Elaboration Training (RET), which has been adopted clinically in group settings. The thrust of this approach is to use a forward chaining technique to lengthen patient-initiated utterances and encourage response variety. Novel appropriate utterances are encouraged and reinforced. That is, any patient-initiated response that was relevant for a given stimulus item is acceptable regardless of the form or content of the response. A unique aspect of this approach is that the patient directs the content of treatment. Once treatment stimuli are selected, patients'

spontaneous utterances are used as building blocks for developing more elaborate responses. The clinician combines successive patient responses, models them for repetition by the patient, and then prompts him or her to provide additional information. Each novel elaboration is subsequently added to the chain until the patient's spontaneous responses are lengthened to preselected levels. Throughout RET an interactive, turn-taking format is maintained so that it can be readily adopted to group treatment. That is, each spontaneous conversational turn during group activities can serve as an opportunity for the clinician to prompt more elaborate verbal (and nonverbal) responses and to reinforce the use of novel but appropriate utterances (see Chapter 11).

Although the RET format has not been experimentally tested in the group setting, a series of studies has examined the efficacy and generalization of the approach for individual aphasic patients. Results to date indicate that generalized increases in verbal response length and variety have occurred following RET (Kearns, 1986; Kearns and Scher, 1989; Kearns and Yedor, 1991). In addition, this approach has also been successfully applied to facilitate improvements in nonverbal means of communication (Gaddie-Cariola et al., 1990) and communicative drawing (Kearns and Yedor, in press).

RET and other "loose training" approaches to treatment are based, in part, on the rationale that loosening and diversifying treatment parameters may facilitate generalization (Baer, 1981; Horner et al., 1988; Hughes, 1985; Stokes and Baer, 1977; Stokes and Osnes, 1986). Attempts to target generalization directly as a goal of therapy by incorporating procedures that may facilitate carryover are an integral component of a generalization planning approach to intervention for aphasia. The group setting currently provides an environment for refining this clinical process, and it also provides a rich arena for future research and development of strategies that promote generalization.

By appropriately rewarding generative responding in the group setting, we may increase the probability of obtaining carryover to the natural environment. Generalization training should, however, go beyond simply reinforcing selected responses when they occur. Task hierarchies should be developed to elicit responses under conditions that increasingly approximate the natural environment.

Summary

In summary, a generalization planning approach has been reviewed and related to group therapy for aphasia. It was suggested that group therapy for aphasia may provide a means of extending treatment beyond individual therapy by incorporating generalization prompting techniques. The group setting provides an important link between individualized treatment and the natural environment. Only future research can determine the most effective means of using group treatment to facilitate generative responding.

FUTURE DIRECTIONS

Group therapy for aphasia is at a crossroads. We can continue along our current path of investigative complacency, or we can select the more difficult but potentially rewarding path that leads to intensive research into group therapy for aphasia. Although the choice may seem obvious, the road to group therapy research will be difficult. We must begin by overcoming the unsubstantiated assumption that we already have proven group treatment methods. Group therapy for aphasia has become strongly entrenched in our clinical repertoire because of historical precedent and practical clinical exigencies. There are, however, very few experimental studies of group treatment methods to guide our clinical practice. Intensive group treatment research will not be forthcoming unless we overcome the "illusion of strong evidence" (McPeek and Mostellar, 1977) that supports current clinical practices.

The future direction of group therapy for aphasia depends on whether clinical aphasiologists can overcome this obstacle and begin to research group treatment methods aggressively. The ultimate goal of research in this area should be to identify specific, replicable, and effective group treatment procedures. Ideally, it would be desirable to be able to predict with reasonable certainty which patients would likely benefit from which types of group treatment. Thus, future research should eventually compare the relative effectiveness of group treatment methods.

In addition to investigating treatment approaches, the future direction of group therapy for aphasia will bring an increased awareness of the training needs of group clinicians. It has already been suggested that not all clinicians are appropriately trained to conduct group therapy (Eisenson, 1973; Sarno, 1981). We do not, however, have academic or training guidelines to evaluate the skill level of group leaders. Kearns and Simmons (1985) recently found that 74% of a large sample of clinicians who conduct group therapy for aphasia reported no additional training beyond their speech-language pathology coursework. Only 24% of the survey respondents indicated that they had taken coursework or training in group dynamics, counseling, or related areas. While it is not clear what type of additional training is advisable for group clinicians, this issue must be addressed in the near future. Group therapy for aphasia presents additional challenges that are not encountered in individual sessions, and investigators and academicians alike will need to consider clinical training factors relating to group intervention.

In addition to research and training, the future direction of group treatment will also be shaped by technological advances. The rapid development of computer technology will, no doubt, have an impact on group treatment methods. Individualized treatment programs that are available may be expanded to allow patients to interact with one another and jointly solve communication problems. Similarly, treatment approaches may be enhanced by the expanding video technology, and taped or simulated communicative interactions may eventually replace static picture cards as the primary stimulus material used during group sessions.

In the final analysis, the future direction of group therapy for aphasia will depend on people rather than technology. If researchers are firmly committed to this area of investigation and clinicians are willing to challenge traditional assumptions about the effectiveness of group approaches, then the potential benefits of group therapy for aphasia may eventually be realized.

References

Adair, S., and Pfalzgraf, B. (1991). *Pathways: Moving beyond stroke and aphasia.* Detroit, MI: Wayne State University Producer.

Adair Ewing, S., and Ewing-Pfalzgraf, B. (1991). *What is aphasia?* Detroit, MI: Wayne State University, Producer.

Agranowitz, A., Boone, D., Ruff, M., Seacat, G., and Terr, A. (1954). Group therapy as a method of retraining aphasics. *Quarterly Journal of Speech, 40,* 170–182.

American Heart Association. (1981). *Aphasia and the family.* Dallas, TX: Author.

Aronson, M., Shatin, L., and Cook, J. C. (1956). Sociopsycho-therapeutic approach to the treatment of aphasic patients. *Journal of Speech and Hearing Disorders, 21,* 352–364.

Aten, J. (1991). Group therapy for aphasic patients: Let's show it works. *Aphasiology, 5–6,* 559–561.

Aten, J. L., Caligiuri, M. P., and Holland, A. (1982). The efficacy of functional communication therapy for chronic aphasic patients. *Journal of Speech and Hearing Disorders, 47,* 93–96.

Aten, J., Kushner-Vogel, D., Haire, A., West, J. F., O'Connor, S., and Bennett, L. (1981). Group treatment for aphasia panel discussion. In R. H. Brookshire (Ed.), *Clinical Aphasiology Conference proceedings* (pp. 141–154). Minneapolis, MN: BRK.

Backus, O., and Dunn, H. (1947). Intensive group therapy in speech rehabilitation. *Journal of Speech and Hearing Disorders, 12,* 39–60.

Backus, O., and Dunn, H. (1952). The use of a group structure in speech therapy. *Journal of Speech and Hearing Disorders, 17,* 116–122.

Baer, D. M. (1981). *How to plan for generalization.* Austin, TX: Pro-Ed.

Barlow, D. H., Hayes, S. C., and Nelson, R. O. (1984). *The scientist practitioner: Research and accountability in clinical and educational settings.* New York: Pergamon Press.

Bernstein, J. (1979). A supportive group for spouses of stroke patients. *Aphasia Apraxia Agnosia, 1–4,* 30–35.

Bevington, L. J. (1985). The effects of a structured educational programme on relatives' knowledge of communication with stroke. *Australian Journal of Communication Disorders, 13,* 117–121.

Blackman, N. (1950). Group psychotherapy with aphasics. *Journal of Nervous Mental Disorders, 111,* 154–163.

Blackman, N., and Tureen L. (1948). Aphasia: A psychosomatic approach in rehabilitation. *Transactions of American Neurological Association, 73,* 193–196.

Bloom, L. M. (1962). A rationale for group treatment of aphasic patients. *Journal of Speech and Hearing Disorders, 27,* 11–16.

Borenstein, P., Linell, S., and Wahrborg, P. (1987). An innovative therapeutic program for aphasic patients and their relatives. *Scandinavian Journal of Rehabilitation Medicine, 19,* 51–56.

Brindely, P., Copeland, M., Demain, C., and Martyn, P. (1989). A comparison of the speech of ten chronic aphasics following intensive and no-intensive periods of therapy. *Aphasiology, 3,* 695–707.

Brookshire, R. H. (1992). *An introduction to neurogenic communication disorders* (4th ed.). Saint Louis, MO: Mosby Year Book.

Chenven, H. (1953). Effects of group therapy upon language recovery in predominantly expressive aphasic patients. Doctoral dissertation, New York University.

Cochrane, R., and Milton, S. B. (1984). Conversational prompting: A sentence building technique for severe aphasia. *Journal of Neurological Communication Disorders, 1,* 423.

Cohelo, C. A., and Duffy, R. (1985). Communicative use of signs in aphasia: Is acquisition enough? *Clinical Aphasiology, 15,* 222–228.

Connell, P., and McReynolds, L. V. (1988). A clinical science approach to treatment. In L. McReynolds, N. Lass, and D. Yoder (Eds.), *Handbook of speech-language pathology and audiology* (pp. 1058–1075). Toronto: B. C. Decker.

Corbin, M. L. (1951). Group speech therapy for motor aphasia and dysarthria. *Journal of Speech and Hearing Disorders, 16,* 21–34.

Darley, F. L. (1982). *Aphasia.* Philadelphia, PA: W. B. Saunders.

Davis, G. A. (1992). *A survey of adult aphasia.* Englewood Cliffs, NJ: Prentice-Hall.

Davis, G. A., and Wilcox, M. J. (1981). Incorporating parameters of natural conversation in aphasia treatment. In R. Chapey (Ed.), *Language intervention strategies in adult aphasia.* Baltimore, MD: Williams & Wilkins.

Derman, S., and Manaster, H. (1967). Family counseling with relatives of aphasic patients at Schwab Rehabilitation Hospital. *ASHA, 9,* 175–177.

Eisenson, J. (1973). *Adult aphasia.* New York: Appleton-Century-Crofts.

Fawcus, M. (1989). Group therapy: A learning situation. In C. Code and D. J. Muller (Eds.), *Aphasia therapy* (2nd ed.). London: Cole and Whurr.

Fawcus, M. (1991). Managing group therapy: Further considerations. *Aphasiology, 5–6,* 555–557.

Fratelli, C. M. (1992). Functional assessment of communication: Merging public policy with clinical views. *Aphasiology, 6–1,* 630–683.

Friedland, J., and McColl, M. (1989). Social support for stroke survivors: Development and evaluation of an intervention program. *Physical and Occupational Therapy in Geriatrics, 7,* 55–69.

Friedman, M. H. (1961). On the nature of regression in aphasia. *Archives of General Psychiatry, 5,* 60–64.

Gaddie, A., Kearns, K., and Yedor, K. (1989). A qualitative analysis of response elaboration training effects. *Clinical Aphasiology, 19,* 171–184.

Gaddie-Cariola, A., Kearns, K., and Defoor-Hill, L. (1990). *Response elaboration training: Treatment effects using a visual communication system.* A paper presented at the annual meeting of the American Speech-Language-Hearing Association, Seattle, WA.

Gilbert, T. P., Mcpeek, B., and Mosteller, F. (1977). Statistics and ethics in surgery and anesthesia. *Science, 198,* 684–699.

Godfrey, C. M., and Douglass, E. (1959). The recovery process in aphasia. *Canadian Medical Association Journal, 80,* 618–624.

Gordon, E. (1976). *A bi-disciplinary approach to group therapy for wives of aphasics.* Paper presented at the Annual Convention of the American Speech and Hearing Association, Houston, TX.

Holland, A. L. (1970). Case studies in aphasia rehabilitation using programmed instruction. *ASHA, 35,* 377–390.

Holland, A. L. (1975). The effectiveness of treatment in aphasia. In R. H. Brookshire (Ed.)., *Clinical Aphasiology Conference proceedings, 1972–1976* (pp. 145–159). Minneapolis, MN: BRK.

Holland, A. L. (1980). *Communicative abilities in daily living.* Baltimore, MD: University Park Press.

Horner, R. H., Dunlap, G., and Koegel, R. L. (1988). *Generalization and maintenance: Lifestyle changes in applied settings.* Baltimore, MD: Paul H. Brookes.

Horwitz, B. (1977). An open letter to the family of an adult patient with aphasia. *The National Easter Seal Society for Crippled Children and Adults, 30,* Reprint A-186.

Huber, M. (1946). Linguistic problems of brain-injured servicemen. *Journal of Speech Disorders, 11,* 143–147.

Hughes, D. L. (1985). *Language treatment and generalization: A clinician's handbook.* San Diego, CA: College Hill Press.

Hunt, M. I. (1976). *Language maintenance group for aphasics.* Paper presented at the Annual Convention of the American Speech and Hearing Association, Houston, TX.

Inskip, W. M., and Burris, G. A. (1959). Coordinated treatment program for the patient with language disability. *American Archives of Rehabilitation Therapy, 7,* 27–35.

Jenkins, J. J., Jimenez-Pabon, E., Shaw, R. E., and Sefer, J. W. (1981). *Schuell's aphasia in adults: Diagnosis, prognosis and treatment* (2nd ed.). Hagerstown, MD. Harper & Row.

Johnston, J. M., and Pennypacker, H. S. (1980). *Strategies and tactics of human behavioral research.* Hillsdale, NJ: Lawrence Erlbaum.

Kagan, A., Cambell-Taylor, I., and Gailey, G. (1990). *A unique community based programme for adults with chronic aphasia.* A paper presented at the Fourth International Aphasia Rehabilitation Congress, Edinburgh.

Kearns, K. P. (1986a). Flexibility of single-subject experimental designs II: Design selection and arrangement of experimental phases. *Journal of Speech and Hearing Disorders, 51,* 204–214.

Kearns, K. P. (1986b). Systematic programming of verbal elaboration skills in chronic Broca's aphasia. In R. C. Marshall (Ed.), *Case Studies in Aphasia Rehabilitation* (pp. 225–244). Austin, TX: Pro-Ed.

Kearns, K. P. (1989). Methodologies for studying generalization. In L. V. McReynolds and J. Spradlin (Eds.), *Generalization strategies in the treatment of communication disorders* (pp. 13–30). Toronto: B. C. Decker.

Kearns, K. P., and Scher, G. (1988). The generalization of response elaboration training effects. *Clinical Aphasiology, 18,* 223–242.

Kearns, K. P., and Simmons, N. N. (1985). Group therapy for aphasia: A survey of Veterans Administration Medical Centers. In R. H. Brookshire (Ed.), *Clinical Aphasiology Conference proceedings* (pp. 176–183). Minneapolis, MN: BRK.

Kearns, K. P., and Yedor, K. (1991). An alternating treatments comparison of loose training and a convergent treatment strategy. *Clinical Aphasiology, 20,* 223–238.

Kearns, K. P., and Yedor, K. (1992). *Artistic activation therapy: Drawing conclusions.* Paper presented at the Clinical Aphasiology Conference, Durango, CO.

Kinsella, G., and Duffy, F. D. (1978). The spouse of the aphasic patient. In Y. Lebrun and R. Hoops (Eds.), *The management of aphasia.* Amsterdam: Swets & Zeitlinger.

Kinsella, G., and Duffy, F. D. (1979). Psycho-social readjustments in the spouses of aphasic patients. *Scandinavian Journal of Rehabilitation Medicine, 11,* 129–132.

Kisley, C. A. (1973). Striking back at stroke. *Hospitals, 47,* 64–72.

LaPointe, L. L. (1989). An ecological perspective on assessment and treatment of aphasia. *Clinical Aphasiology, 18,* 1–4.

Lomas, J., Pickard, L., Bester, S., Elbard, H., Finlayson, A., and Zoghab, C. (1989). The Communicative Effectiveness Index: Development and psychometric evaluation of a functional communication measure for adult aphasia. *Journal of Speech and Hearing Disorders, 54,* 113–124.

Loverso, F. L. (1991). Aphasia group treatment, a commentary. *Aphasiology, 5–6,* 567–569.

Loverso, F. L., Young-Charles, H., and Tonkovich, J. D. (1982). The application of a process evaluation form for aphasic individuals in a small group setting. In R. H. Brookshire (Ed.), *Clinical Aphasiology Conference proceedings* (pp. 10–17). Minneapolis, MN: BRK.

Lyon, J. G. (1992). Communication use and participation in life for adults with aphasia in natural settings: The scope of the problem. *American Journal of Speech-Language Pathology, 1–3,* 7–14.

Makenzie, C. (1991). Four weeks of intensive therapy followed by four weeks of no treatment. *Aphasiology, 5* (4–5), 435–437.

Malone, R. L. (1969). Expressed attitudes of families of aphasics. *Journal of Speech and Hearing Disorders, 34,* 146–151.

Marquardt, T. P. (1982). *Acquired neurogenic disorders.* Englewood Cliffs, NJ: Prentice-Hall.

Marquardt, T. P., Tonkovich, J. D., and Devault, S. M. (1976). Group therapy and stroke club programs for aphasic adults. *Journal of the Tennessee Speech Hearing Association, 20,* 2–20.

Marshall, R. C. (in press). Problem focused group therapy for mildly aphasic clients. *American Journal of Speech-Language Pathology.*

McReynolds, L. V., and Spradlin, J. (1989). *Generalization strategies in the treatment of communication disorders.* Toronto: B. C. Decker.

Mogil, S., Bloom, D., Gray, L., and Lefkowitz, N. (1978). A unique method for the follow-up of aphasic patients. In R. H. Brookshire (Ed.), *Clinical Aphasiology Conference proceedings* (pp. 314–317). Minneapolis, MN: BRK.

National Institutes of Health. (1979). *Aphasia hope through research* (NIH Publication 80, p. 391). Bethesda, MD: Author.

Newhoff, M. N., and Davis, G. A. (1978). A spouse intervention program: Planning, implementation and problems of evaluation. In R. H. Brookshire (Ed.), *Clinical Aphasiology Conference proceedings* (pp. 318–326). Minneapolis, MN: BRK.

Nielson, J. M., Schultz, D. A., Corbin, M. A., and Crittsinger, B. A. (1948). The treatment of traumatic aphasics of World War II at Birmingham. General Veterans Administration Hospital, Van Nuys, California. *Military Surgery, 102,* 351–364.

Oradei, D. M., and Waite, J. S. (1974). Group psychotherapy with stroke patients during the immediate recovery phase. *American Journal of Orthopsychiatry, 44,* 386–395.

Osiejek, E. (1991). Discourse exercises in aphasia therapy. *Aphasiology, 5* (4–5), 443–446.

Pachalska, M. (1991a). Group therapy for aphasia. *Aphasiology, 5* (6), 541–554.

Pachalska, M. (1991b). Group therapy: A way of integrating patients with aphasia. *Aphasiology, 5* (6), 573–577.

Porch, B. (1967). *The Porch Index of Communicative Ability.* Palo Alto, CA: Consulting Psychologists Press.

Porter, J. L., and Dabul, B. (1977). The application of transactional analysis to therapy with wives of adult aphasic patients. *ASHA, 19,* 244–248.

Puts-Zwartes, R. A. (1973). Group therapy for the husbands and wives of aphasics. *Logopaed. Fomiatr., 45,* 93–97.

Radonjic V., and Rakuscek, N. (1991). Group therapy to encourage communication ability in aphasic patients. *Aphasiology, 5* (4–5), 451–455.

Rao, P. (1986). The use of Amer-Ind code with aphasic adults. In R. Chapey (Ed.), *Language intervention strategies in aphasia* (2nd ed., 360–369). Baltimore, MD: Williams & Wilkins.

Redinger, R. A., Forster, S., Dolphin, M. K., Godduhn, J., and Wersinger J. (1971). Group therapy in the rehabilitation of the severely aphasic and hemiplegic in later stages. *Scandinavian Journal of Rehabilitation Medicine, 3,* 89–91.

Repo. M. (1991). The holistic approach to rehabilitation: A commentary. *Aphasiology, 5–6*, 571–572.

Rice, B., Paul, A., and Muller, D. (1987). An evaluation of a social support group for spouses of aphasic partners. *Aphasiology, 1*, 247–256.

Sanders, S. B., Hamby, E. I., and Nelson, M. (1984). *You are not alone.* Nashville, TN: American Heart Association.

Sarno, M. T. (1981). Recovery and rehabilitation in aphasia. In M. T. Sarno (Ed.), *Acquired aphasia.* New York: Academic Press.

Schlanger, P. H., and Schlanger, B. B. (1970). Adapting role-playing activities with aphasic patients. *Journal of Speech and Hearing Disorders, 35*, 229–235.

Schuell, H., Jenkins, J. J., and Jimenez-Pabon, E. (1964). *Aphasia in adults.* New York: Harper & Row.

Sheehan, V. M. (1946). Rehabilitation of aphasics in an army hospital. *Journal of Speech and Hearing Disorders, 11*, 149–157.

Sheehan, V. M. (1948). Techniques in the management of aphasics. *Journal of Speech and Hearing Disorders, 13*, 241–246.

Skelly, M., Schinsky, L., Smith, R. W., and Fust, R. S. (1974). American Indian Sign (AMERIND) as a facilitator of verbalization for the oral verbal apraxic. *Journal of Speech and Hearing Disorders, 39*, 445–456.

Smith, A. (1972). *Diagnosis, intelligence, and rehabilitation of chronic aphasics: Final report.* Ann Arbor, MI: University of Michigan.

Sparks, R., Helm, N., and Albert, N. (1974). Aphasia rehabilitation resulting from melodic intonation therapy. *Cortex, 10*, 303–316.

Spradlin, J. E., and Siegel, G. M. (1982). Language training in natural and clinician environments. *Journal of Speech and Hearing Disorders, 47*, 2–6.

Springer, L. (1991). Facilitating group rehabilitation. *Aphasiology, 6*, 563–565.

Stokes, T. F., and Baer, D. M. (1977). An implicit technology of generalization. *Journal of Applied Behavior Analysis, 10*, 349–367.

Stokes, T., and Osnes, P. P. (1986). Programming generalization of children's social behavior. In P. S. Strain, M. Guralnick, and H. Walker (Eds.), *Chil-dren's social behavior: Development, assessment and modification* (pp. 407–443). Orlando, FL: Academic Press.

Thompson, C. K. (1989). Generalization in the treatment of aphasia. In L. V. McReynolds and J. Spradlin (Eds.), *Generalization strategies in the treatment of communication disorders* (pp. 82–115). Toronto: B. C. Decker.

Thompson, C. K. and Kearns, K. P. (in press). Analytical and technical directions in applied aphasia research: The Midas touch. *Clinical Aphasiology, 19*, 41–54.

Tsvetkova, L. S. (1980). Some ways of optimizing aphasic rehabilitation. *International Journal of Rehabilitation Research, 3*, 183–190.

Turnblom, M., and Myers, J. S. (1952). A group discussion program with the families of aphasic patients. *Journal of Speech and Hearing Disorders, 17*, 383–396.

Van Harskamp, F., and Visch-Brink, F. E. G. (1991). Goal recognition in aphasia therapy. *Aphasiology, 5–6*, 529–535.

Veterans Administration. (1983). *A stroke: Recovering together.* St. Louis V.A. Regional Learning Resources: Author.

Warren, S. F., and Rogers-Warren, A. K. (Eds.). (1985). *Teaching functional language.* Austin, TX: Pro-Ed.

Wepman, J. M. (1947). The organization of therapy for aphasia: 1. The inpatient treatment center. *Journal of Speech and Hearing Disorders, 12*, 405–409.

Wertz, R. T., Collins, M. H., Weiss, D., Kurtzke, J. F., Friden, T., Porch, B. E., West, J. A., Davis, L., Matovitch, V., Morley, G. K., and Resurreccion, E. (1981). Veterans Administration cooperative study on aphasia: A comparison of individual and group treatment. *Journal of Speech and Hearing Research, 24*, 580–594.

Wilcox, M. H., and Davis, G. (1977). Speech act analysis of aphasic communication in individual and group settings. In R. H. Brookshire (Ed.), *Clinical Aphasiology Conference proceedings* (pp. 166–174). Minneapolis, MN: BRK.

APPENDIX A[a]

Suggestions for Conversational Prompting

From Cochrane and Milton (1984)

Some general suggestions for establishing ''set,'' and promoting language retrieval during contextual support:

1. Take enough time to develop the topic or activity context (introduce appropriate vocabulary and linguistic forms, establish the affective atmosphere, etc.). Remember that patients can later draw upon this information when

---

[a]With permission from R. McCrae Cochrane and S. B. Milton (1984). Conversational prompting: A sentence building technique for severe aphasia. *Journal of Neurological Communication Disorders, 1*, 4–23.

formulating responses;

2. Introduce props or written cues on a tablet or flip chart. These can change with the topic and provide helpful cues for various points in the interchange. Thus, a patient knows he or she can glance at props or words when attempting to express ideas; and

3. Relate ongoing conversational exhange to the content of previous exchange. An individual has a higher probability of retrieving words relating to what went on 5 or 10 min ago rather than generating language on a completely new topic.

SAMPLE CONVERSATIONAL PROMPTING LEVELS

Ten conversational levels were constructed to fit the abilities and needs of a variety of patients. These are:

Concrete, Structured Context

1. Object manipulation
2. Acting out and describing sequences with props
3. Acting out and describing sequences without props
4. Picture description

5. Event description
6. Structured questions and answers

Open Context

7. Structured questions and answers—as in journalistic interview
8. Structured discussion
9. Unstructured discussion
10. Free conversation

CHAPTER 16
Computer Applications in Aphasia Treatment

RICHARD C. KATZ

Computers have gained considerable popularity over the past 15 years. The introduction of small, affordable, programmable, personal microcomputers is only the latest stage of a 40-year history that includes commercial development of hardware (e.g., integrated circuits, disk drives) and software (computer operating systems, languages, and applications). Consumers expect an imminent breakthrough that will abruptly change their lives for the better, a promise the computer industry's sales force has made since the mid-1950s, when commercial computers were first introduced. Aphasic patients and their families may be particularly vulnerable to the unsubstantiated promises made by an avid computer industry intent on increasing sales. While the world rushes forward to embrace the computer, those of us engaged in rehabilitation should step cautiously and apply accepted standards to determine the value of computer applications for each aphasic patient.

COMPUTER SYSTEMS

Clinicians considering computer use in rehabilitation should be familiar with the components of microcomputer systems. The term *microcomputer* refers to relatively small and reasonably priced ''personal'' computers currently available, for example, IBM® 386/20 and the Macintosh Classic II®. Microcomputers have numerous advantages over the larger mini- and mainframe computers used by banks and other institutions. Compared with the larger machines, microcomputers and their programs are relatively inexpensive; equipment may cost from a few hundred to a few thousand dollars, and while many programs are in the public domain and thus free, most useful programs cost about $50 to $300. Microcomputer systems automatically start running the program as soon as the disk is placed in the drive and the power is turned on; therefore, patients and students can use programs without extensive computer experience or programming skills. Many types of programs are available for popular models of microcomputers, so the computer can serve as an administrative, educational, clinical, recreational, and research tool. Clinicians in different settings can exchange files (e.g., reports, lists, tables, pictures) if the same (or a similar) model of computer is used in both settings; for example, a file from a Macintosh Classic II computer can be read by any other Macintosh Classic II. (Programs like

SoftPC® allow Macintosh computers to run programs intended for IBM computers and read from and write to disks formatted for IBM computers.) Modern microcomputers have enhanced graphic capacity that permits them to display various styles and sizes of text as well as pictures, animation (e.g., QuickTime®), and hypermedia (i.e., multimedia) material. Synthesized and digitized sounds and speech are becoming a fundamental part of new programs. Finally, many microcomputers come with built-in simple programming languages (e.g., BASIC) or authoring environments (e.g., HyperCard®), which allows nonprogrammers to create and run personalized applications that may not be available commercially.

Hardware

Hardware refers to computer equipment, both the components that are essential to the computer and the peripheral devices connected for additional or expanded functions. Five components are a part of most popular microcomputer systems.

CPU

At the heart of the computer system is the central processing unit, or CPU. The CPU is a box containing the electronic components that make up the part of the computer that does the actual work. Several parts of the CPU determine how much and the type of work the computer can do. The *microprocessor* is the ''brains'' of the computer, controlling the occurrence and timing of all computer activity. Programs contain the list of instructions that tell the microprocessor what to do and when to do it; this is how a computer can serve as many different tools. Each model of microprocessor understands a different set of instructions, which is the reason a program written for an Apple IIe computer (with a 65c02 microprocessor) cannot run on an IBM PC (with an 8088 microprocessor). *RAM* (Random Access Memory) is the working area for the microprocessor. RAM is essentially empty ''electronic'' space within memory chips. Instructions (the program read from disk) and data (values generated by the program) are both stored in RAM while the microprocessor (under the direction of the program) ''reads'' and ''writes'' values in RAM. The computer processes programs and values in RAM quickly because all activities are electrical and not mechanical. The values stored in RAM, however, exist only as long as the computer power is on; when the power is off, all information in RAM is lost. Programs usually specify the minimum amount of RAM (along with the model of computer) required to run the program. *ROM* (Read Only Memory) contains instructions and values essential to the operation of the computer. The information (called "firmware") is permanently "etched" onto the silicon ROM chip and cannot be changed, remaining in ROM even after the computer power is off. This way, routine functions that do not change (such as how to read a disk) are ready for the microprocessor each time the power is turned on.

Other components, considered "peripheral devices," connect to the CPU through slots and/or ports. Today, a *keyboard* is usually considered part of the CPU and connects to the computer through an external port. Programs usually expect special "function keys" on the keyboard to be available to the user. Also, a small pointing device, called a *mouse,* is usually included and is required for operating most new computers. The mouse is about the size of a deck of cards, with one or two buttons on the top, and contains a single rubber ball, part of which pokes through a hole in the bottom. The ball rotates as the mouse is slid over a flat surface (like the top of a desk), controlling the position on the screen of a small pointer (or *cursor*). Thus the user can point to a word or small picture (called an *icon*) and, by pressing the mouse button, activate a function associated with the word or picture. A mouse is required for operating the Macintosh®, Apple IIGs®, Amiga® and IBM computers running Windows®.

Monitor

The difference between monitors may not be evident at first glance. *Monochrome* monitors are the least expensive. They display only one foreground color and one background color (such as green letters on an otherwise black screen). Monochrome monitors are best suited for work limited to text, such as word processing or data entry. *Color* monitors come in a variety of types. *Composite* monitors are similar to commercial color televisions and are sufficient for many computer games and educational activities. They do not, however, produce clear lettering and so are unsuitable for text-based work. *RGB* (Red-Green-Blue) monitors produce sharp text and graphics in a variety of colors and are the most versatile (and expensive) monitor. Several standards exist for RGB monitors: For example, Apple® computers use analog RGB monitors, while IBM computers use digital monitors. The model of computer, job requirements, and working budget all contribute to the selection of a monitor.

Disk Drive

Programs and data are stored on disks. Computers read information from a disk into RAM in order to run the program and act on the data. Once the action is complete, the data can be saved from RAM to the disk for use later. Although disks look similar, their organization differs electronically for each type of computer. A disk from one type of computer can only be read by another type of computer under special circumstances, although this process is becoming easier and more common.

Two popular sizes of "floppy" disks exist. Large, *5.25-inch disks* store between about 135 KB (kilobytes) and 370 KB, depending on the model of computer and whether the disk is single- or double-density (referring to the concentration of magnetic particles on the disk surface) and whether the drive reads from and writes to one side (single-sided) or both sides (double-sided) of the disk. Apple II® series and IBM computers use 5.25-inch disks, but Macintosh computers do not. Newer and smaller double-density (DD) *3.5-inch disks* store between 720 KB and 800 KB and are all double-sided. "Quad" or high-density (HD) 3.5-inch disks hold about 1.44 MB (megabytes, or 1440 KB) of data. Macintosh and IBM computers can use both double- and high-density 3.5-inch disks. A drive that reads from and writes to HD disks (called, a "SuperDrive™" on Apple computers) also works with DD disks; however, HD disks do not work on DD drives.

Many computer systems also use a *hard disk drive* that consists of one to several metal disks spinning at a high speed within a sealed enclosure. Although more expensive than floppy disk drives, a hard disk provides greater storage capacity (commonly 20 MB to 100 MB) and greater speed of reading and writing data (roughly five times faster). Commonly used programs (such as the computer operating system and frequently used applications) are stored on the hard drive, significantly reducing the time needed to start up the computer system and begin running the application. Some hard drives offer removable disks (in a protected cartridge) and, although slightly slower and more expensive than nonremovable hard drives, provide discrete but unlimited storage space and added security. Many computer systems are sold with hard drives built into the CPU enclosure.

Newer, *optical disk drives* use laser technology to provide high-speed and high-storage reading and writing capacity in a small space (for example, a 128 MB cartridge is only slightly larger than a 3.5-inch disk). *CD-ROM drives* use specially produced compact discs to read information only; data cannot be written to and stored on a CD-ROM by the user. However, since a CD-ROM can hold about 550 MB of data, is virtually indestructible, and is relatively inexpensive to produce, the format has become popular as a low-cost source for large amounts of data and reference material, for example, encyclopedias, technical notes, and maps. CD-ROMs use a standard that allows data from a disc to be read by most types and models of microcomputers.

Printer

Dot matrix printers are the most popular and least expensive type of printer for computers. Letters are printed as a configuration of tiny dots on paper as pins lined up in a column on the printer head strike an ink ribbon as the head moves across the page. Printing is noisy, and the resolution of about 72 dots per inch (DPI) is adequate for drafts and informal correspondence. Some dot matrix printers provide a range of quality (e.g., draft, correspondence, near-letter) and speed of printing and can print in black or a variety of colors. *Laser printers* are quieter but more expensive and slower than dot matrix printers. Laser printers produce high-quality text and graphic images of 300 DPI (similar to, but less than, magazine print). Several other, less popular types of printers exist. Thermal printers are quick and quiet but use special paper that can fade in sunlight. Inkjet printers produce laserlike quality text, are quiet and fast, and cost less than laser printers, but do not work with some programs. Color laser printers are very expensive and still undergoing changes in technology and standards.

Modem

Modems, a component rarely seen in the past, have recently become increasingly useful. Modems are frequently packaged with communication software, the combination of which allows a computer to communicate over a telephone line with other computers of various makes and models anywhere in the office or in the world. Users can communicate directly with another single computer but often connect to a computer network or a bulletin board system (BBS). BBSs offer many services, including electronic mail (E-mail) for sending messages, software libraries (for ''downloading'' computer programs), and ''conferencing'' (where a number of users can discuss a topic ''in real time,'' while others can read the discussion and add comments later). BBSs are relatively inexpensive to set up—they require a computer, a hard disk, a BBS program, and at least one telephone line. For the cost of a telephone call, a user can connect to any one of hundreds of small BBSs throughout the world. Many large BBSs exist (e.g., CompuServe® and GEnie®) and can be accessed through a local number anywhere in the United States. BBSs offer numerous services, such as buying airline tickets, shopping for a new car, or reading the news in Prague. Special-interest BBSs are also available, such as Bitnet (popular among university faculty) and CenterNet (for discussion of case studies from the Department of Speech and Hearing Sciences, University of Arizona).

In addition to transferring files over the telephone, an increasing number of modems are sold with fax capacity, allowing transmission of documents between computers and fax machines over the telephone. A document incorporating both text and graphics (e.g., correspondence on letterhead or inclusion of a digitized photograph) can be generated and faxed to another computer, where it can be read without ever having been printed on paper.

Other Peripheral Devices

Specialized peripheral devices that can enhance the clinical usefulness of computers are available for most systems. Frequently, the device is designed by a company other than the computer manufacturer; consequently, support and compatibility with future products should not be assumed, and clinicians should make certain that the device is compatible with the software intended for its use. Peripheral devices usually connect to the computer through internal slots (using interface cards) or external ports on the CPU.

Input Devices.   A *joystick* is required for many games and allows the user to control the horizontal and vertical position of the cursor or other aspects of the program by pushing the control stick within a 360° field and pressing buttons. A *paddle* is similar to a radio volume control knob and offers more fine control than a joystick, but controls only a single dimension at a time (e.g., horizontal *or* vertical position). While a single hand is required to manipulate the stick or knob, the design requires the nondominant hand to steady the device, unless it is secured to the desk top with tape or suction cups. A *trackball* consists of a billiard ball-like object contained within a station-

ary platform that sits firmly on a desk or table, allowing the user to rotate the ball in any direction and press buttons with a single hand. Most trackballs can substitute for a joystick or mouse. Many people prefer the trackball over a mouse when desk space is limited. A *touch screen* is placed over the computer monitor display and controls placement of the cursor simply by touching that part of the screen. Some clinicians have placed touch screens over pointing boards, permitting the patient to control various actions and messages. Like trackballs, the touch screen can substitute for mouse devices and joysticks. *Graphic tablets* are rectangular, flat devices that are used primarily with a special stylus for drawing, but also can be used with a template to simulate a keyboard or pointing board. Petheram (1988) conducted the most extensive test of compatibility between aphasic subjects and computer equipment. He tested five popular input devices (mouse, joystick, trackball, touch screen, concept keyboard) with nine aphasic and three elderly-control subjects on tasks that simulated eight common exercise formats (e.g., choosing from a menu) and found the trackball best on success rate and patient preference. Petheram concluded the trackball was preferred by the subjects over the mouse and joystick because it allowed them to divide the ''point and click'' procedure into two distinct motor components: Position the cursor, then press the button.

Output Devices.   While some computers (e.g., Apple IIGS and Macintosh) have digitizers built into the CPU, other computers require that peripheral boards or devices are connected to the computer for speech and sound to be generated. Two forms of computer-controlled artificial speech are found in contemporary software. *Synthesized speech* is most often found in educational software. Two types of synthesized speech exist. *Phoneme-based* synthesized speech produces recognizable speech from a large set of ''phonemes'' and other sound combinations stored on the synthesizer card. Speech is only moderately intelligible, as many sounds are distorted. For example, the sounds for the letter ''T'' and the letter ''S'' usually differ only in duration. Also, speech is pieced together from phonemes, creating severe disruption of coarticulation, prosody, and rate, further adding to the artificial quality of the output. In *phrase-based* synthesized speech, digitized representations of entire words and phrases, rather than phonemes and sounds, are read from a disk and stored on memory chips on the synthesizer card. The prosody within words and phrases is preserved somewhat, and the quality of speech is better than with phoneme-based synthesized speech. Synthesized speech is best used when the capacity to produce unlimited novel output is required and neither the speaker nor the listener suffers from problems in hearing or auditory comprehension. This would indicate that while synthesized speech may work well to compensate for the verbal output problems of many dysarthric speakers, it would not be as appropriate for aphasic speakers, who could not understand or monitor the synthesized output. Treadwell et al. (1985) compared the two varieties of synthesized speech (using an Apple II computer and Echo II® speech synthesizer) with live speech. The nine aphasic subjects performed well on a computerized listening task when listening to phoneme-based speech; accuracy and response time were only slightly better when listening to live speech. Phoneme-based speech produced poorer performance.

Digitized speech uses an auditory digitizing device to measure the pitch (frequency) and loudness (intensity) of a sample of natural speech many thousand times each second. The frequency and intensity values of the speech sample are then stored as numbers in a file on a disk. When the sample of speech is first played back, the digitizer, controlled by special software, reads the stored frequency and intensity values from the disk and reproduces the speech sample with good clarity, prosody, and rate. Faster sampling rates result in higher speech fidelity, but require greater amounts of disk space and RAM. Computer response time can be noticeably delayed because the digitized values are read initially from a disk in a disk drive to RAM. The capacity to digitize sound provides researchers and clinicians (e.g., Conway and Niederjohn, 1988) with an excellent tool to record and study speech signals. Because digitization produces the most realistic-sounding speech, it is preferable for auditory comprehension tasks. Mills and Thomas (1983) compared intelligibility of different forms of artificial speech, specifically, synthesized speech (phoneme-based), digitized speech (4 KHz sampling rate), and analog speech (tape recorded). As a group, the six aphasic patients performed best with analog speech and worst with synthesized speech.

Because of the rapidly changing technology, little research has been reported using digitized speech to treat auditory comprehension problems in aphasic patients. Mills and Thomas (1981) and Mills (1982) used a computer to provide auditory comprehension practice for an aphasic adult. Four line drawings of common objects, presented on the screen as one-, two-, and three-part "pointing commands," were audibly presented by the computer and a speech digitizer (4 KHz sampling rate). The patient responded either by (*a*) pressing the key or keys (1–4) associated with the target picture and then pressing the return key or (*b*) by moving a joystick and pressing the joystick button. Pressing the return key alone provided the patient with a repetition of the auditory stimulus. A correct response resulted in a positive verbal message followed by presentation of the next stimulus item. An error on the first attempt resulted in feedback and a repetition of the stimulus. If a second error was produced, the auditory stimulus was again presented, the correct item was highlighted, and the next stimulus item presented. Twelve stimulus words per session were presented. Improvement over 5 months' time was observed in accuracy, response time (latency), and responsiveness (need for fewer repetitions) for one adult aphasic subject who began the computerized treatment program 2 months after suffering a left cerebral vascular accident. The influence of the program is questionable, however, because of the patient's recent time postonset.

Software

If hardware is the car, software is the driver. Software tells the microprocessor what to do to make the computer do useful work. As difficult and expensive as building a computer is, the time and costs involved in developing a body of software for a computer are even greater. Computers use several different types of software.

System Software

System software, or the operating system, is a special program (or groups of small, interrelated programs) developed for a particular type of computer and is an intimate part of how the computer works. The operating system provides instructions for the CPU to use certain internal and peripheral components

and for other programs to interact with the computer and each other. For example, to print a letter, a word processing program sends instructions to the operating system that then tells what to print and how it should look. The operating system then tells the printer how to print through a *driver,* a small program supplied by the printer manufacturer that controls the actions of the printer.

Older-style operating systems, like the Apple II's ProDOS® and MS-DOS® for the IBM, are examples of a Command Line Interface (CLI) and require the user to remember and enter coded commands and parameter values, such as "CATALOG/ HARD.DISK" or "DIR/C" to view the contents of a disk. Newer styles of operating systems, like the Macintosh System 7® and Finder®, Microsoft® DOS interface, and Windows®, are examples of a Graphic User Interface (GUI), which uses icons (pictures) to represent familiar objects and uses metaphors to activate common functions, thus operating in a more intuitive fashion. For example, the Macintosh screen looks like the top of a desk, with folders containing various applications and documents. An icon of a "trash can" in the corner of the screen is used to erase files and eject disks. When you want to write a letter, you select (point with the cursor) and open (click the button) the icon representing the word processing program; when you want to erase a letter (delete it from the disk), you select (point with the cursor) the icon of the letter and drag it (hold the button down and point with cursor) to the trash can. The GUI, first developed by Xerox in the 1960s and called Smalltalk®, is considered easier to learn and faster to use than the older CLI. Procedures for the GUI are more similar among computers than commands from the older CLI, making using and switching between different types of computers and programs easier.

A Local Access Network (LAN) is a combination of hardware and special programs that allows computers within the same office or building to be linked together and interact. LANs are commonly part of "office automation" and the "paperless office" and can even connect different types of computers (e.g., TOPS® for IBM and Macintosh). Computers on a network continue to function independently, storing programs and files on their own disks, but a LAN also enables users to share programs and files, use (E-mail), and perform other functions. Computers on a network can share expensive peripheral devices, such as laser printers, CD-ROM players, and optical disk drives. The network grows automatically as more computers are plugged into the chain.

Programming Languages and Authoring Environments

Professional programmers use a variety of computer languages to write their programs. Low-level languages, like machine language and assembly language, work quickly because they incorporate the binary code (zeros and ones) understood by the microprocessor. Although using these languages gives programmers complete control over the actions of the computer, the process of writing and testing low-level languages is a considerable investment of time and effort. Easier to learn, high-level languages were developed for special areas, enabling programmers and nonprogramming professionals to quickly write and modify certain types of programs. For example, FOR-TRAN (FORmula and TRANslation) was developed for scientists to write programs dealing with mathematics and statistical problems, and COBOL (Computer Business-Oriented Language) was developed for people writing programs dealing with common business activities, such as monitoring inventory and billing customers.

Little was available to help educators and clinicians develop software specific to the needs of their students and patients. Similar but incompatible versions of BASIC (Beginner's All-purpose Symbolic Instructional Code) were supplied on ROM with most early microcomputers. Although relatively easy to learn, BASIC was developed originally to teach students simple computer programming principles and was not used for coding complex clinical interactions. The resultant programs, although impressive, were limited in scope, depth, and speed. More flexible than small "lesson-generating" programs marketed over the years, BASIC's noble attempt met only the most rudimentary needs of aphasia clinicians seeking to shape computers into a useful therapy tool.

Programmers used sophisticated computer language, such as Pascal and C, to develop new programming languages and environments that would make developing instructional software easier. PILOT (Program Inquiry Learning Or Teaching) was developed for teachers to create educational programs and incorporated many of the elements involved in presenting educational material (e.g., graphics and color) and assessing student performance (e.g., accuracy and error responses). However, PILOT ran slowly, was expensive, and required additional hardware. The existence of several incompatible versions of the program added to the frustrations of teachers and clinicians.

In 1984, a new authoring system, HyperCard, was introduced on the Macintosh computer. Because it was supplied with every Macintosh computer sold, HyperCard quickly gained acceptance and became a standard among users and programmers (called "authors"). HyperCard allows authors to develop a series of screen displays (called "cards") that contain areas for displaying or entering text (called "fields") and other areas for controlling actions (called "buttons"). A series of cards is called a "stack" and is analogous with a program. Besides its ease of use and support directly from the computer manufacturer, HyperCard provided the user access to many of the Macintosh's special features, such as use of the mouse, menus, high-quality graphics, and digitized sound, making it a supportive environment for developing treatment activities (e.g., CLARK; Dressler, 1991) and compensatory communication systems (e.g., C-VIC; Steele et al., 1987). At the 1992 American Speech-Language-Hearing Annual Convention, a majority of the instructional labs, miniseminars, and poster sessions within the Microcomputer Applications section focused on clinical applications of HyperCard in audiology and speech pathology. Similar programs for the Apple IIGS (HyperCard IIGS® and HyperStudio®) and other computer systems are also available.

Application Software

Application software refers to programs that do the useful work for which the computer was intended. Two major divisions of application software exist. *General purpose* (or "horizontal market") programs can be applied to different professions (e.g., word processing, database, spread sheet, painting, drawing, telecommunications, and page layout). Most computer users run at least one program (usually word processing) from this list. The particular general purpose programs selected by

a computer user are determined by a number of factors, including the type of computer, price, features, prior computer experience, and compatibility with software used by others in the community.

Software also is written specifically for a particular profession or use. Examples of this vertical market include computer-assisted design (CAD) programs for engineers and architects and Individual Educational Plan (IEP) software written for public school-based speech-language clinicians. Diagnostic software for aphasia such as the *PICApad II* (© 1992 Sunset Software) program and treatment software such as *Understanding Questions II* (© 1990 Sunset Software) are examples of programs intended for a particular category of user—in this case, speech-language clinicians and their aphasic patients.

REASONS TO USE COMPUTERS IN APHASIA REHABILITATION

Speed, accuracy, reliability, and ease of use are characteristics valued wherever personal computers are used, but the power of computers in rehabilitation is not simply the result of faster microprocessors or larger storage devices. Schuell et al. (1964) stated that principles of aphasia treatment should be used through our increasing repertoire of clinical techniques. The role of computers will evolve as the technology improves. There are many areas in which computers have the potential for becoming significant tools for treating aphasia.

Supplementary Treatment

Supplementary treatment in the form of workbooks and other activities has always been an option for clinicians (e.g., Eisenson, 1973). Patients can work longer and more often on a variety of activities designed to stabilize, maintain, or generalize newly acquired skills. Contemporary commercial treatment and educational software extend controlled treatment-related language and cognitive activities beyond the confines of the treatment session if they are presented in a structured setting that incorporates important therapeutic principles and factors, such as control of both stimulus characteristics and response requirements, and recording of session performance for later review. Programs can vary along a continuum according to structure and content, ranging in complexity from simple repetitive drills to interactive tasks that not only evaluate individual responses, but also measure overall performance and adjust the type and degree of intervention provided (e.g., Katz and Wertz, 1992).

Treatment Efficacy

Measuring the effects of intervention on aphasia is an essential part of any treatment regimen. Speech-language pathologists assess the influences of various linguistic, psychological, and physical variables on communication and task performance in order to evaluate the effectiveness of a treatment approach or activity. The computer can present treatment activities in a standard manner and routinely store performance data for later descriptive and statistical analysis, thus addressing Darley's (1972) efficacy questions. Perhaps computers will help us develop a database to predict with confidence that, for example, a 55-year-old Broca's aphasic adult, who 1-year postonset is at the 50th percentile on the Porch Index of Communicative Ability (PICA) (Porch, 1981), will require between 125 and

150 trials to learn to write or print 10 functionally relevant words at the third-grade level (LaPointe, 1977). This benchmark of prognostic resolution would serve as an invaluable clinical yardstick against which the success of treatment could be measured (e.g., Matthews and LaPointe, 1981, 1983).

Generalization

Many think the value of aphasia treatment should be measured by the degree that skills acquired in treatment are observed in real-life situations. Generalization can be aided by the computer, which can administer some aspects of treatment without the familiar presence and constant conscious (and unconscious) control of the clinician. Rosenbek et al. (1989) recommended a series of clinical activities to increase the likelihood of generalization. Several of the recommendations appear well suited for the computer: (*a*) expose each patient to numerous repetitions; (*b*) train a large number of items in a given category; (*c*) extend treatment outside of the clinic; and (*d*) organize treatment to maximize independence so that patients learn to use treated responses when they want to rather than when told to by the clinician.

Independence and Emotional Factors

To foster independence and exploit availability of treatment-related activities, the patient should be able to use treatment software with minimal assistance from others. The required computer skills include selecting the treatment disk, securing the disk in the disk drive, and turning on the computer. Aphasic patients themselves can then determine when and how often they participate in supplementary language activities. This is consistent with Wertz's (1981) statement that we should allow patients to maintain as much independence as possible and that a long-term goal of aphasia treatment is to have patients become their own best therapists. The insight patients have into *their* problems and *their* strengths can be used instead of ignored, and in this way, patients can take a more active role in their treatment.

Other factors, such as motivation, dependency, and quality of life, are concerns that may become increasingly important to aphasic people and their families as recovery slows and the degree of disability and its subsequent effect on life become more apparent. Under conditions of perceived helplessness and hopelessness, people frequently become depressed (Seligman, 1975) and have greater difficulty coping with and adapting to changes and problems (Coelho et al., 1974). Bengston (1973), Langer and Rodin (1976), Schulz (1976), and others have shown that giving some options and responsibilities to persons in otherwise dependent situations (e.g., the institutionalized elderly) can have a strong positive effect on their satisfaction and physical well-being. Decision making and expression of personal preferences by each patient should be a basic part of any treatment program. Computerized activities can address this aspect of treatment by providing aphasic patients with some control over the content and frequency of treatment.

Diagnostic Activities

Testing and treatment can be a stressful experience for many patients. A good therapist can communicate empathy, honesty, and genuine concern to patients; a computer cannot. In addition, computers measure only what they have been told to measure. Using semiautonomous computers for direct patient testing is similar to using technicians or assistants who have limited experience with aphasia and patients. We can tell the assistants what to expect, but we cannot tell them everything. The inability of software to deal with unpredictable events, coupled with lack of empathy, severely limits the role of computers as a diagnostician, especially for acute patients (i.e., patients who are rapidly changing and new to the medical setting).

Computers have been shown to be useful during complex diagnostic procedures, for example, analyzing speech and voice (e.g., Conway and Niederjohn, 1988) and measuring the degree of aspiration in dysphagia (Mills, 1991). Computers are also being used routinely to help clinicians collect test data, calculate scores, print tables, draw graphs, write narrative descriptions, and finally, put all elements together to generate a diagnostic report. An appropriate diagnostic computer application, therefore, could be the routine, periodic monitoring of specific activities (e.g., attention, reading comprehension) for aphasic and cognitively impaired patients who have been involved in treatment, as these patients should already be familiar with the computer, its operation, and computer programs.

Administrative Activities

Currently, computers are assisting clinicians in the performance of administrative and clinical duties, and in all likelihood will continue to do more in the near future. However, few speech pathologists complain about having too much free time. As computers do more for clinicians, clinicians can do more for their patients and hospital administrators. As is the case for many other professions, general purpose programs have many useful applications for clinicians working with aphasic patients, for example, report and letter writing (word processing programs), organizing, recording and recalling information (database programs), and organizing, calculating, and projecting values (spread sheet programs). Recent innovations include the use of voice recognition in word processing to increase the speed of generating reports (Tonkovich et al., 1991) and the use of authoring systems to customize database data entry and retrieval (e.g., HyperCard).

Recreational Activities

Many commercial recreational programs (such as arcade and adventure games) are finding a limited but useful role in treatment (Lynch, 1983). Enderby (1987) discussed the possibility of computers providing a path toward social and intellectual stimulation for aphasic patients. While recreation therapy can be a valuable service for patients, our involvement is neither urgent nor necessary. However, computer game activities offer patients a diversion and a way of occupying their time in a novel, distracting, entertaining, and sometimes intellectually stimulating manner.

LIMITATIONS OF COMPUTERS IN APHASIA REHABILITATION

Computers cannot be all things to everyone. Four characteristics of computer programming described by Bolter (1984) emphasize the limitations of computers when applied to aphasia treatment. Computers are *discrete* (i.e., digital), making description of qualitative features difficult. Salient events must first be separated into distinct, unconnected elements before they can be acted on by a computer. Computers are *conventional;* that is, they apply predetermined rules to symbols that themselves have no effect on the rules. Regardless of the significance of the symbols or the outcome of the program, the rules never change. Computers are *finite;* their rules and symbols are limited to those defined within the program. Unforeseen problems and associations do not result in spontaneous creation of new rules and symbols. Finally, computers are *isolated;* that is, problems and solutions exist within the computer's own space, apart from the real world. Problems are stated in terms of structure so that a solution can be generated by manipulating symbols according to a specific strategy. The strategy behind the solution is called an *algorithm,* a finite series of steps described with adequate detail to guide the program to answer the questions. Computers, therefore, can consider only problems in which all the variables and rules are known ahead of time, and in which solutions can be attained in a step-by-step procedure with a finite number of steps, like a game of chess.

Aphasia treatment is very different from a game of chess. Treatment is recognized as a multilevel, interactive behavioral exchange. Not all therapeutically relevant behaviors have been identified; many that have (e.g., functionality) cannot be effectively controlled by a computer. In addition, while clinicians recognize some fundamental approaches to aphasia treatment, all the rules are not known, and those on which we agree may not be correct (Rosenbek, 1979). For example, use of linguistic rules to construct software to diagnose and treat aphasia is appealing (e.g., Guyard et al., 1990) and can ultimately teach us much about language (e.g., Fenstad, 1988) and aphasia (e.g., Wallich, 1991). However, some researchers (e.g., Katz, 1990; Kotten, 1989) believe that the pathological language behavior of aphasic people is also influenced by a variety of other factors, including cognition (e.g., attention, vigilance, memory, resource allocation); cybernetics (e.g., slow rise time, noise buildup, intermittent imperception); behavioral factors (e.g., discriminatory stimuli, chaining, extinction); pragmatics (e.g., functionality, social status); and emotion (e.g., interest, relevance, novelty, enjoyment). No one therapeutic approach currently encompasses all known intervening variables.

A program that accurately represents clinician-provided treatment will quickly exceed the capacity of modern computers. By reducing the scope of the problem to a size manageable for the computer, treatment software can be squeezed and shaped to imitate cognitive and language therapy in small, trivial, and predominantly symbolic activities. Rather than emphasize state-of-the-art aphasia treatment, the resultant computerized activity highlights the technical limitations of the computer medium. Odor (1988) referred to this problem when he wrote that computer-assisted learning defers decisions to programmers who are not physically present during the session, but must *gather* and *send* information only through the computer medium, *plan* in advance how to handle the learning interaction, and then *encode* these steps into a computer program. Consequently, the scope of treatment software is limited because computer programs are not powerful enough to represent every potentially relevant nuance of interaction during therapy. Odor (1988) concluded that computer-assisted instruction is often based on convergent rather than divergent theories of learning. Most computer treatment studies reported in the aphasia re-

search literature describe convergent activities, particularly drills, in which specific responses are learned. Dean (1987) stated that the inability to incorporate divergent strategies in computer programs severely limits their value and application to treatment of aphasic patients, particularly chronic aphasic patients, for whom such treatment appears promising (Chapey et al., 1976). Divergent treatment software is becoming commercially available (e.g., *My House: Language Activities of Daily Living,*© 1992 Laureate Learning Systems), but no data exist to support efficacy. The adaptation of divergent therapy to computer-provided treatment remains a challenge for contemporary software developers.

MODALITY CONSIDERATIONS

Face-to-face conversation (i.e., talking and listening) is our primary mode of communication. Management of auditory and verbal skills is central to the concept of aphasia rehabilitation (e.g., Schuell et al., 1964). Listening and talking are the communicative behaviors used to classify most types of aphasia (Goodglass and Kaplan, 1983; Kertesz, 1982), and are the focus of most aphasia therapy. Listening and talking, more than other language modalities, affect the likelihood of an aphasic person's successful reintegration into the community, the final demonstration of the success of therapy. For most patients, and for their families, friends, and physicians, the *perception* of recovery and treatment success is measured by improvement in listening and talking.

Contemporary treatment software seems to offer little assistance to clinicians treating the speaking and listening problems that occur for aphasic patients during conversation. The major contribution of computers to aphasia treatment appears to be in reading and writing. Computers are basically visual-motor, graphic machines. Information from the user is normally entered by typing on a keyboard; the output of the computer is displayed on the monitor screen and read by the user. This makes the computer well suited for presenting reading tasks and, through typing, writing tasks. Reading and writing skills appear to be an appropriate focus for computerized aphasia treatment for several reasons. Most aphasic patients have problems in reading (Rosenbek et al., 1989) and writing (Geschwind, 1973). Reading requires minimal response from the patient. Programs for treating reading can run on standard personal computers, without expensive modification or specialized peripheral devices. Typing on the keyboard can be used to examine many aspects central to writing (Selinger et al., 1987), with the obvious exception of the mechanics of handwriting. Also, reading and writing as communicative acts are usually done alone; having greater interpersonal distance, they are in many ways less direct and responsive than speaking and listening. As such, reading and writing are appropriate *communication* (as opposed to *therapeutic*) activities for aphasic people to practice on computers. Computerized reading and writing treatment tasks can free up valuable treatment time so that face-to-face, individual therapy can emphasize auditory comprehension and verbal output skills. While the computer can provide valuable reading and writing activities (e.g., Scott and Byng, 1989), additional noncomputerized, clinician-provided reading and writing therapy should be supplied as indicated by patient performance.

STRUCTURE OF TREATMENT ACTIVITIES

There are many elements that are common to the structure of all treatment activities regardless of the underlying principles or mode of delivery, and although some are obvious, none are trivial. An understanding of these task components is useful for describing, developing, and evaluating treatment activities for the computer.

All tasks have a *goal,* which is usually an intermediate step toward a major or long-term goal. The patient should be aware of the goal of the task, and should also be aware of the logical order or steps within the task that advance toward the goal. The clinician should provide the patient with *instructions* so that the patient knows from the beginning what is expected. The *stimuli* used and the desired *responses* should be consistent with the purpose of the task. Responses should be described and quantified using a multidimensional *scoring system* (LaPointe, 1977; Porch, 1981) whenever possible to identify and measure the occurrence of salient behaviors within the task. Care should be taken that the patient is not burdened with additional, unnecessary *response requirements* that could confound performance. Responses should be as simple as possible to reflect accurately the performance of the target behavior. *General feedback* (Stoicheff, 1960) to encourage the patient and *specific feedback* to describe the most recent response should be readily provided. The clinician should provide an *intervention* (strategy or cue) to improve performance as needed. Teaching specific responses may be the goal of some tasks; a more valuable goal commonly is to develop a task to help the patient learn an intervention (e.g., self-cue or compensatory) strategy to improve communication during actual, functional situations (e.g., Christinaz, personal communication, re. Colby et al., 1981). Criteria for *termination* of the task should be specified to provide a target against which the patient can measure progress. Responses and performance *scores should be stored* for later review and analysis. At that time, both the patient's performance and the intervention can be *evaluated* using various techniques (LaPointe, 1977; Matthews and LaPointe, 1981, 1983, McReynolds and Kearns, 1983, Prescott and McNeil, 1973).

MODELS FOR COMPUTER REHABILITATION

In contrast to the considerable attention afforded the arrival of each new treatment program, software developers have just begun to describe explicitly the treatment models influencing software evolution. As described by Wolfe (1987), early reports of computerized aphasia treatment (e.g., Katz and Nagy, 1982, 1983, 1984, 1985; Mills, 1982) provided no explicit models of rehabilitation from which the software could be evaluated. Recent studies have reversed the trend (e.g., Katz and Wertz, 1992, Loverso et al., 1985; Scott and Byng, 1989). Bracy (1986) was among the first to explicitly incorporate the work of Luria (1973, 1980) in the development of rehabilitation software. Having an explicit model facilitates the systematic development of software and provides a basis for clinicians selecting software for their patients. Three general models of rehabilitation provide clinicians with the structure to develop and evaluate software. Although they are not mutually exclusive, the models offer a basis from which the role of computers in aphasia rehabilitation can be directed and examined.

Brain-Behavior Relationships

Bracy (1986) described four theories accounting for recovery of cognitive functions, but the theory that function recovers through the retraining process (Luria, 1973) is the most closely allied to the modern concept of rehabilitation. Luria believed the return of skills involved a reorganization of brain functions so that there are new methods of performing behaviors previously executed through the structures that are now damaged. One function of computerized treatment, therefore, is to provide the patient with the direction and opportunity to retrain skills through the reorganization.

Behavior Modification

Computers in rehabilitation can serve as cues, models, or reinforcers. Computers offer extensive control over the presentation of stimuli (e.g., exposure time, visual characteristics, frequency of exposure) and reinforcement contingencies. Seron et al. (1980) used printing letters on the computer screen and verbal feedback from the clinician to reinforce correct spelling. Loverso et al. (1985) used synthesized speech presented by a microcomputer to model speech for patients in rehabilitation. The computer offers some degree of individualized presentation of materials for optimizing learning.

Educational Models

Lepper (1985) contrasted three approaches to learning with direct application to treatment software: individualized drill and practice, educational games, and simulations. Drill and practice capitalizes on the computer's advantages in providing immediate feedback, sustained attention, data analysis, and highly individualized instruction. Educational games stimulate a person's interest through gamelike activities. Educational simulations, also called, *microworlds,* involve the patient in a series of problems in an imaginary environment. The contingencies between actions and outcome should lead the patient to an understanding of basic principles relevant to real-world environments. These programs assume that active, inductive, "discovery-based" learning is better for learning general skills than direct, didactic approaches, which seem to be more effective when learning highly specified information. *My House: Language Activities of Daily Living* (© 1992 Laureate Learning Systems) is an example of computer software that is a "microworld" in which the patient is free to explore the total simulated environment rather than respond to specific stimuli.

TYPES OF COMPUTERIZED TREATMENT TASKS

Four major types of treatment activities are appropriate for presentation on the computer: stimulation, drill and practice, simulations, and tutorials. This list is not exhaustive, and types are not mutually exclusive; one treatment activity may have several purposes and demonstrate characteristics of more than one type, for example, stimulation and drill and practice (e.g., Serons et al., 1980).

Stimulation

As described by Schuell and her colleagues (1964), stimulation activities offer the patient numerous opportunities to respond quickly and usually correctly over a relatively long period of time for the purpose of maintaining and stabilizing the underlying processes or skills, rather than simply learning a new set of responses. The process, therefore, is the focus of the task. Stimuli are not selected primarily for informational content (e.g., interest and relevance), but for salient stimulus characteristics (e.g., length, number of critical elements, complexity, and presentation rate). Computer programs can easily be designed that contain a large database of stimuli and control these variables as a function of the patient's response accuracy. Overall accuracy and other salient response characteristics (e.g., latency) are usually displayed at the end of the task. An early example of a computer stimulation task is the auditory comprehension task described by Mills (1982).

Drill and Practice

The goal of drill and practice exercises is to teach specific information so that the patient is able to (or appears able to) function more independently. Stimuli are selected for a particular patient and goal, and so an authoring or editing mode is needed to modify stimuli and target responses. A limited number of stimuli are presented and are replaced when criterion is reached. Since response accuracy is the focus of the task, the program should present an intervention or cues to help shape the patient's response toward the target response. Drill and practice exercises, therefore, are convergent tasks because the accurate response must match the target response exactly. Results are displayed or stored on disk and show the effectiveness of the intervention. An example of a drill and practice exercise is the typing (writing) program described by Katz and Nagy (1984), Katz et al. (1989), and Seron et al. (1980).

Simulations

Simulations (''microworlds'') are programs that present the patient with a structured environment in which a problem or problems are presented and possible solutions are offered. Simulations may be simple, such as presenting a series of paragraphs describing stages of a problem and listing possible solutions. Complex programs more closely simulate a real-life situation by using pictures and sound. The term *virtual reality* (Rheingold, 1991) describes a totally simulated environment created through the interaction of a computer and a human along verbal and nonverbal channels. Simulations have been used in fields such as chemistry, geology, meteorology, and astrophysics to test conditions impossible to experience or to train people in situations that would otherwise be too dangerous to experience firsthand. Simulations provide the opportunity to design divergent treatment tasks that could more fully address real-life problem-solving strategies than those addressed by more traditional, convergent computer tasks, for example, by including several alternative but equally correct solutions to a problem, such as during PACE (Promoting Aphasics Communicative Effectiveness) therapy (Davis and Wilcox, 1985). The question of whether simulations can improve generalization of the new behavior to real-life settings remains to be tested.

Tutorials

Some authors (e.g., Eisenson, 1973) have suggested that aphasic patients are best served by modification of their communication environment. In that respect, tutorials offer valuable information regarding communication and quality of life to the family, friends, and others who influence the aphasic patient's world. At the most fundamental level, the computer tutorial could present information commonly found in patient information pamphlets in an interactive format, with additional modules provided when needed or requested. This type of self-paced, informational program can be appropriately realized in a hypermedia format, such as HyperCard, where a family member can navigate through text, pictures, animation, and sound describing relevant aspects of aphasia and communication. The tutorial program could incorporate features of an *expert system,* in which detailed information is provided in response to a patient/family profile, and function as a source of information for family members in the future when new problems and questions arise.

EFFICACY OF APHASIA TREATMENT SOFTWARE

According to Loverso (1987), most computer advocates focus on ''appealing'' features of computers, such as cost effectiveness and operational efficiency, while the real issue that demands attention from clinicians is treatment effectiveness; treatment activities must be effective before they can be efficient. Ineffective treatment programs would be damaging to the overall quality of treatment provided aphasic patients. If computerized treatment is to continue to develop and improve, it should undergo the same scientific scrutiny and systematic modification as do all other aspects of treatment.

Software, however, cannot reproduce every process and variable that occurs during treatment, and so computerized treatment in this sense will never be as efficacious as clinician-provided treatment. One way clinicians increase the likelihood that software is efficacious is to develop and test their own treatment programs. Mills (1988) suggested that clinicians who program with only limited programming skills tend to produce limited programs. It is important, however, that programmers have more than a limited understanding of treatment principles if treatment software is not to be limited in its effectiveness.

A range of support for the clinical application of computers exists in aphasiology. Dean (1987) wrote that existing computer treatment programs ''are not firmly grounded in a theoretical rationale for remediation'' (p. 267), thus limiting their potential. To Katz (1984, 1986), and Loverso et al. (1988), most contemporary treatment software consists of drills with no explicitly stated intervention goals; their use should be conservative and practical. Others (e.g., Bracy, 1983; Lucas, 1977; Skilbeck, 1984) have advocated the computer rather than the clinician as the primary treatment medium, and a few (e.g., Rushakoff, 1984) have described the development of clinician-independent, autonomous computerized aphasia treatment programs. Literature reviews have resulted in conflicting opinions of the efficacy of computers (e.g., Katz, 1987; Robinson, 1990). The strongest statement thus far is from Robinson (1990), who argued that research evidence is simply not available to support the use of computers for most language and cognitive problems. Robinson stated that some researchers obscured the basic issue by asking what works with whom under what conditions (see Darley, 1972), and he concluded that because computers are prematurely promoted in clinical work, their routine clinical use may be causing patients more harm than good.

There is no substitute for carefully controlled, randomized studies, the documentation of which has become the scientific foundation of aphasiology. Research reported over the last 15 years incorporated increasingly sophisticated designs and greater numbers of subjects to assess efficacy of computerized aphasia treatment, from simple A-B-A designs (Katz and Nagy, 1982, 1983, 1984, 1985; Mills, 1982) to large, randomly assigned single-subject (Loverso et al., 1992) and group studies (Katz and Wertz, 1992) incorporating several conditions. Efficacy of computerized aphasic treatment is being addressed one study at a time.

Comparison of Traditional and Computer Mediums

Comparing the effect of similar treatment activities provided by two different mediums should improve understanding of the influence of the medium and the relative effectiveness of the treatment. Many researchers are attempting to simulate currently accepted testing and treatment protocols on the computer. Some researchers think that, because of speed, reliability, and relative autonomy, computers are ideally suited to administer tests to aphasic patients, who can then work at their own pace without embarrassment or fear of humiliation (e.g., Enderby, 1987). Odell et al. (1985) developed two computerized versions of the Raven Coloured Progressive Matrices (Raven, 1975) on an IBM PC system. The program used high-resolution graphics and a touch screen input device to administer and analyze test performance quickly and accurately with minimal supervision from a clinician. The authors compared the two computerized versions of the Raven matrices with a traditional, clinician-controlled, paper booklet administration of the test. The performances of 16 aphasic subjects were essentially equivalent under all three conditions, leading the authors to conclude that the computer testing conditions did not present greater visual or cognitive demands on the subjects.

Wolfe et al. (1987) compared the real-object and computer simulation performances of non-brain-damaged and aphasic adults on another nonverbal problem-solving task, "The Towers of Hanoi" puzzle, originally administered to aphasic subjects by Prescott et al. (1984). The performance of 19 aphasic and 19 non-brain-damaged subjects was compared using two different methods of presentation: two-dimensional color computer simulation of the puzzle versus the manipulation of the actual wooden model. Non-brain-damaged subjects performed equally well under both conditions. As in the study by Odell et al. (1985), aphasic subjects demonstrated similar performance on the task under both conditions. Aphasic subjects, however, required more time to complete the puzzle in the computer condition than when manipulating the actual wooden model. The results suggest that while the computer medium did not affect the accuracy of performance for the aphasic subjects, task completion took longer and was less efficient under the computer condition.

The effectiveness of closed-circuit television, computer-controlled video laserdisk, and traditional face-to-face interaction for providing appraisal and treatment to aphasic patients in remote settings was measured by Wertz et al. (1987). Results suggested no significant differences among the three conditions in the diagnoses assigned to the subjects using standard and modified tests. In addition, subjects in all three treatment conditions demonstrated clinically significant change (between 12 and 17 percentile points on the PICA). No significant differences in improvement among the three treatment groups were

observed, indicating that aphasic patients can benefit from treatment provided in any of the three conditions. The results suggest that television and video laserdisk over the telephone could be employed to provide services for patients who live where services do not exist.

An outstanding example of the process of demonstrating efficacy in a computerized treatment program involves 14 years of published research by Loverso and his colleagues, who have documented a series of data-based reports describing the development and testing of a model-driven clinician-provided treatment approach, the "verb as core," from its origins as a "clinician-delivered therapy" (Loverso et al., 1979; Loverso et al., 1988) to its encoding and refinement as a computer/clinician-assisted program (Loverso et al., 1985; Loverso et al., 1988; Loverso et al., 1992).

Loverso et al. (1979), Loverso et al. (1988), and Selinger et al. (1987) initially developed and tested a treatment protocol for aphasic patients in which verbs were presented as starting points and paired with different *wh*-question words to provide cues to elicit sentences in an actor-action-object framework. Thirty verbs were used at each of six modules. The hierarchy was divided into two major levels, each consisting of an initial module and two submodules that provided additional cuing for subjects unable to achieve 60% or better accuracy on the initial module. Level I presented stimulus verbs and the question words "who" or "what" to elicit an actor-action sentence. Level II elicited actor-action-object sentences by presenting stimulus verbs and the question words "who" or "what" for the actor and the question words "how," "when," "where," and "why" for the object. Subjects responded verbally and graphically. Subjects were scheduled for treatment three to five times per week. During each session, 30 stimulus verbs were presented for generation of sentences. Statistically significant improvement ($p < .05$) was demonstrated on the PICA following 3.5 months of treatment for each of the two aphasic subjects.

Later, Loverso et al. (1985) compared the effects of the same treatment approach when treatment was provided by a clinician and when it was provided by a computer and speech synthesizer assisted by a clinician. The aphasic subject responded in the clinician-only condition by speaking and writing and in the clinician/computer condition by speaking and typing. Stimulus presentation and feedback in the clinician/computer condition was normally provided only by the computer. The clinician intervened only if the patient's typed response was correct but the spoken response was in error. The subject improved on the task under both conditions but took longer to reach criteria under the computer and clinician-assisted condition. Based on the subject's improvement, both on the treatment task and on "clinically meaningful" changes on successive administrations of the PICA ($p < .01$), the authors concluded that their listening, reading, and typing activities under the clinician/computer condition had a positive influence on the patient's language performance. They suggested that, although still in the early stages of development, aphasia treatment administered by computers is practical and has the capacity for success. Loverso et al. (1988) replicated the study by Loverso et al. (1985) with five fluent and five nonfluent aphasic subjects for the purpose of examining whether treatment provided under the computer/clinician condition was as effective as a clinician alone when treating various types and severities of aphasia using their cuing-verb-treatment technique. The 10 subjects required 28% more sessions (p< .05) to reach criteria under the computer/clinician condition than under the clinician-only condition. Fluent subjects required 24% more sessions and nonfluent subjects required 33% more sessions under the computer/clinician conditions than under the clinician-only condition. Of the 10 subjects, 8 showed significant improvement (p< .05) on the PICA Overall percentile measure, on the Verbal modality measure, and on the Graphic modality measure. All subjects maintained gains after a maintenance phase of 1 month posttreatment or longer. Similar results were reported following a replication of the study using 20 subjects (Loverso, et al., 1992).

Compensatory Devices

Few researchers have developed programs to compensate for aphasic verbal output problems. Colby made extensive use of computers and speech synthesizers in attempts to increase verbalization and communication in autistic and other "non-speaking" children (e.g., Colby and Kraemer, 1975; Colby and Smith, 1973). Later, Colby et al. (1981) built and programmed a small, portable microcomputer carried by a dysnomic aphasic subject on a sling and shoulder strap combination, thus allowing the use of the device in actual communicative situations. When the subject experienced word-finding problems, she pushed keys in response to prompts from the computer. On a small LCD (Liquid Crystal Display) screen, the computer printed a series of questions designed to identify the forgotten word: for example, "Do you remember the first letter of the word?" ". . . the last letter?" ". . . any other letters?" ". . . any other words that go with the forgotten word?" The subject's answers were applied according to an algorithm outlined in the program, and a list of possible words was produced and displayed across the computer screen, beginning with the most "probable" words. When the patient recognized the forgotten word, she pressed a button and the word was produced via synthesized speech. [Most dysnomic patients usually can recognize the correct word and say it after a visual or auditory model (e.g., Benson, 1975).] The subject was cued successfully by the portable computer in real-life situations that were functional and communicatively stressful. Christinaz (personal communication, 1984) indicated that the cuing algorithm subsequently generalized to noncomputer settings. Patients reported after several weeks of using the computer that they no longer required it, instead asking themselves the same series of questions previously displayed by the computer. Christinaz reasoned that the subjects had "internalized the algorithm" and now cued themselves without the need of external prompts. The frequency and success of this observation was not reported, but the implication of Christinaz's statement is certainly interesting and potentially significant. As more powerful portable computers are used as compensatory devices, acquisition and generalization of functional communication behaviors may occur if these or similar devices modeled self-cuing strategies for patients during actual communicative situations.

Dysnomic aphasic patients, such as the subject in the study by Colby et al., are usually mildly aphasic (Brown and Cullinan, 1981). Globally aphasic patients represent the other end of the severity continuum. Steele et al. (1987) and Weinrich et al. (1989) developed and tested a graphically oriented computer-based alternate communication system called the *Computer-Aided Visual Communication* system, or *C-VIC*, for chronic, global aphasic adults. C-VIC is an interactive pointing board that runs on a Macintosh computer and uses a picture-card design, or metaphor. Subjects use the mouse to select one of several pictures, called icons, each of which represents a general category. The selected icon then "opens up" to reveal pictures of the items within the selected category. After selecting the desired item, the picture is added to a sequence of other selected pictures; this "string" of pictures represents the message. The message can be read via the sequence of icons, words printed below the sequence, or, in some cases, heard through digitized speech. Much attention is given to the selection of icons. Weinrich et al. (1989) reported that concrete icons were learned and generalized faster than were abstract icons, but neither type of icon generalized well to new situations. Steele et al. (1987) noted that, although globally impaired aphasic subjects using C-VIC improve on expressive and receptive tasks, communication through more traditional modes of communication remains unchanged. A commercial version of C-VIC, called *Lingraphica*™, is currently available and incorporates animation and digitized speech on a Macintosh Powerbook© computer.

Reading Comprehension

Katz and Nagy (1982) described a program designed to test reading and also provide reading stimulation for aphasic patients. Five aphasic subjects ran the computer programs two to four times per week for 8 to 12 weeks. Although several subjects demonstrated improved accuracy, decreased response latency, and increased number of attempted items on some computer tasks, changes in pre- and posttreatment test performance were minimal. The following year, Katz and Nagy (1983) reported a drill and practice computer program for improving word recognition in chronic aphasic patients. The program was designed to accomplish a task difficult to undertake for a clinician and used the advantages of a computer. The program presented 65 words and varied the rate of exposure as a function of accuracy of response. The goal of the program was to help increase and stabilize the subject's sight vocabulary, but no changes were observed on pre- and posttreatment measures for the five chronic aphasic subjects. Later, Katz and Nagy (1985) described a self-modifying drill and practice computerized reading program for severely impaired aphasic adults. The objective of the study was to improve functional reading, and a program was developed to teach subjects to read single words without intensive clinician involvement. The program also generated, through a printer, homework (writing activities) that corresponded to the subject's performance. Four of the five subjects demonstrated pre- to posttreatment changes on the treatment items that ranged from 16% to 54%.

Scott and Byng (1989) tested the effectiveness of a computer program designed to improve comprehension of homophones (similarly sounding words) for a 24-year-old subject who suffered traumatic head injury and underwent subsequent left temporal lobe surgery. Eight months after the accident, the subject continued to demonstrate aphasic symptoms as well as surface dyslexia and surface dysgraphia. Reading was slow and labored; she was able to understand printed words by sounding them out, presenting particular problems with homophones. The computer program, based on an information-processing model, was designed to focus on this particular aspect of the subject's reading problem. The subject demonstrated steady improvement on the 136-item treatment program, which was run 29 times over a 10-week period. The subject improved in recognition and comprehension of treated ($p<$ .001) and untreated ($p<$ .002) homophones used in sentences. Improvement was also demonstrated on recognition of isolated homophones that were treated ($p<$ .05) and on defining isolated treated ($p<$ .03) and untreated homophones ($p<$ .02). Recognition of isolated untreated homophones and spelling of irregular words showed no improvement.

Writing: Typing and Spelling Words

Many reading comprehension activities are easily transferred to the computer. Writing activities, however, are less easily adapted. The most obvious problem is the inability of the common computer to evaluate handwriting and printing. The computerized writing treatment programs described in the literature substitute typing for writing during the intervention. In a comparison of writing and typing abilities of aphasic subjects, Selinger et al. (1987) examined seven subjects with left-hemisphere damage in order to assess differences between PICA graphic scores on subtests A through E using standardized PICA graphics responses, and PICA responses typed on a computer. No differences were found between scores on the PICA subtests as generated with a pencil and paper and PICA responses typed on a computer. These results suggest that the graphic language abilities of brain-damaged adults are equally represented by the two output systems.

Several investigators have incorporated complex branching algorithms in computerized writing programs to provide multilevel intervention. Seron et al. (1980) described a minicomputer/clinician combination that helped aphasic patients learn to type words to dictation. The clinician said the target word and the subject typed a response on the computer keyboard. (The clinician had to know in advance the order of the stimuli programmed in the computer.) Intervention consisted of three levels of feedback: the number of letters in the target word; whether the letter typed was in the word; and when the correct letter was typed, whether that letter was in the correct position. The five subjects completed the program in 7 to 30 sessions. Pre- and posttreatment tests required the subjects to write a generalization set of single words to dictation. A decrease ($p<$ .05) in the number of misspelled words and in the total number of errors made on the posttreatment test suggested that the computer program had improved spelling of words written by hand. Four of the five subjects maintained improved performance on a second posttreatment test administered 6 weeks later.

Katz and Nagy (1984) used complex branching steps to evaluate responses and provide patients with specific feedback in a computerized typing/handwriting confrontation/spelling task. A stimulus was randomly selected by the program, and a drawing representing the stimulus was displayed on the computer screen. The subject responded by typing on the keyboard. Feedback consisted of auditory sounds and text printed on the screen. Single and multiple cues from a hierarchy of six were selected by the program in response to the number of errors made for each of 10 stimuli. A seven-point multidimensional scoring system was used to describe performance and track the effectiveness of the various cues. Additional feedback included

repetition of the successful and most recently failed cues. At the end of the computer session, pencil-and-paper copying assignments automatically generated via the computer printer were completed by the subject. Pre- and postwriting tests revealed improved spelling of the target words for seven of the eight aphasic subjects ($p<$ .01).

Glisky et al. (1986) reported the ability of four memory-impaired, nonaphasic subjects to type words in response to definitions displayed on the computer screen. Cues included displaying the number of letters in the word and displaying the first and subsequent letters in the word, one at a time, as needed. Cues continued until either the patient typed the word correctly or the program displayed the entire word. All patients improved in the ability to type the target words without cues. Patients maintained their gains after a 6-week period of no treatment and demonstrated generalization to another typing task, although generalization to writing was not measured.

Katz et al. (1989) developed and tested a computer program designed to improve written confrontation naming of animals for nine aphasic subjects with minimal assistance from a clinician. The treatment program required subjects to type the names of 10 animals in response to pictures displayed on the computer monitor. If the name was typed correctly, feedback was provided and another picture was displayed. If an error was made, hierarchically arranged cues were presented and response requirements were modified. Five of the nine subjects reached criterion within six treatment sessions, and the performance of all nine subjects improved an average of 40% on the computer task ($p<$ .0001). In addition, improvement was measured on noncomputerized written naming tasks, such as written confrontation naming of the treatment stimuli and written word fluency for animal names ($p<$ .001). The PICA Writing modality score improved by +4.1 percentile points ($p<$ .05). Improvement did not extend to PICA Overall and Reading scores. Because the goal of the program was to teach subjects the 10 names, improvement did not, nor was it expected to, generalize to written word fluency for an unrelated category. The lack of change in these latter language activities for these 10 chronic aphasic subjects contrasts with their improved performance on treated words.

Katz and Wertz (1992) conducted a longitudinal group study to investigate the effects of computerized language activities and computer stimulation on language test scores for chronic aphasic adults. Forty-three chronic aphasic subjects who were no longer receiving speech-language therapy were randomly assigned to one of three conditions: 78 hours of Computer Reading Treatment, 78 hours of Computer Stimulation ("nonlanguage" activities), or No Treatment. The Computer Reading Treatment software consisted of 29 activities, each containing eight levels of difficulty, totaling 232 different tasks. Treatment tasks required visual-matching and reading comprehension skills, displayed only text (no pictures), and used a standard, match-to-sample format with two to five multiple choices. Treatment software automatically adjusted task difficulty in response to subject performance by incorporating traditional treatment procedures, such as hierarchically arranged tasks and measurement of performance on baseline and generalization stimulus sets, in conjunction with complex branching algorithms. Software used in the Computer Stimulation condition was a combination of cognitive rehabilitation software and computer games that used movement, shape, and/or color to focus on reaction time, attention span, memory, and other skills that did not overtly require language or other communication abilities. Subjects in the two computer conditions worked on the computer for 3 hours per week for 26 weeks. Clinician interaction during the two computer conditions was minimal. Subjects from all three conditions were tested with standardized measures (including the PICA and Western Aphasia Battery [WAB]) at baseline, 3 months, and 6 months, and revealed improved scores ($p < .05$) for the Treatment group for the PICA Overall, Reading, Writing, and Verbal modalities and for the WAB Aphasia Quotient (AQ). Additionally, the Treatment group made more improvement ($p < .05$) on the PICA Overall score than did the other two groups. No statistically significant differences in improvement were demonstrated between the Stimulation and No Treatment groups on any test measure. Results suggest that (*a*) computerized reading treatment can be administered with minimal assistance from a clinician; (*b*) improvement on the computerized treatment tasks generalizes to improvement on noncomputer language performance; (*c*) improvement results from the specific language content of the software and not simply the stimulation provided by the computer; and (*d*) chronic aphasic patients can improve performance through computerized treatment.

FUTURE TRENDS IN COMPUTER APPLICATIONS

The computer can become a very powerful clinical tool by incorporating what we know about aphasia, treatment, and computer programming. Those who are concerned that researchers are advocating computers in place of clinicians are missing the point. Aphasia clinicians selected and tested the patients, designed the treatment plans, designed and modified the treatment tasks, trained the patients to use the computers, and measured treatment efficacy in all computerized aphasia treatment studies reported. Clinicians—not the computer, software, programmer, publisher, or researcher—are responsible for treatment effectiveness. As treatment cannot be effectively "prescribed" like medicine, software should be viewed as supplementary treatment, with the clinician providing critical intervention as indicated by performance and other considerations. The role of computers and treatment software, like all tools, should extend the abilities of the clinician, allowing clinicians to intervene when skills, experience, and flexibility are required. Rather than emphasize what computers can or cannot do better than clinicians, our focus should be on an intelligent division of labor between computers and clinicians, a combination that can do more than either alone. The real danger comes from a failure to appreciate the scope and depth of clinical work. An autonomous, robotic therapist, representing the knowledge and experience of a competent aphasia clinician, is some fantasy dreamed up by people who focus too much on the *costs* of care and not enough on the *efficacy* of care. Until we can describe to others precisely how to treat specific problems in individual patients, it is unreasonable, unethical, and a misrepresentation of the complexity of aphasia therapy to assume that at this time a machine can perform the functions of a clinician.

The true value of computers in the rehabilitation of aphasia continues to be studied. Just like the question of efficacy itself in aphasia rehabilitation (Fitz-Gibbon, 1986; Howard, 1986) the effectiveness of computer use in aphasia treatment cannot be answered with a simple "yes" or "no." Much more work

is needed. Treatment software may always be an imperfect reflection of clinician-provided therapy, but by improving the software, clinicians and programmers will learn more about how and why treatment works. In the best tradition of scientific and rehabilitative efforts, aphasiologists can work together to shape this new tool of technology for the development of their professions and the benefit of all patients.

References

Bengston, V. L. (1973). Self-determination: A social psychologic perspective on helping the aged. *Geriatrics, 28*(12), 118–130.

Benson, D. F. (1975). Disorders of verbal expression. In D. F. Benson and D. Blumer (Eds.), *Psychiatric aspects of neurologic disease* (pp. 121–137). New York: Grune & Stratton.

Bolter, J. D. (1984). *Turing's man: Western culture in the computer age.* Chapel Hill: University of North Carolina Press.

Bracy, O. L. (1983). Computer based cognitive rehabilitation. *Cognitive Rehabilitation, 1*(1), 7–8, 18–19.

Bracy, O. L. (1986). Cognitive rehabilitation: A process approach. *Cognitive Rehabilitation, 4,* 10–17.

Brown, C. S., and Cullinan, W. L. (1981). Word-retrieval difficulty and dysfluent speech in adult anomic speakers. *Journal of Speech and Hearing Research. 24,* 358–365.

Chapey, R., Rigrodsky, S., and Morrison, E. (1976). Divergent semantic behavior in aphasia. *Journal of Speech and Hearing Research, 19,* 664–677.

Coelho, G. V., Hamburg, D. A., and Adams, J.E. (1974). *Coping and adaptation.* New York: Basic Books.

Colby, K. M., Christinaz, D., Parkison, R. C., Graham, S., and Karpf, C. (1981). A word-finding computer program with a dynamic lexical-semantic memory for patients with anomia using an intelligent speech prosthesis. *Brain and Language. 14,* 272–281.

Colby, K. M., and Kraemer, H. C. (1975). An objective measurement of nonspeaking children's performance with a computer-controlled program for the stimulation of language behavior. *Journal of Autism and Childhood Schizophrenia, 5*(2), 139–146.

Colby, K. M., and Smith, D. C. (1973). Computers in the treatment of nonspeaking autistic children. In J. H. Masserman (Ed.), *Current psychiatric therapies* (Vol. 11, pp. 1–17). New York: Grune & Stratton.

Conway, R. J., and Niederjohn, R. J. (1988). Generation of speech spectrograms using a general-purpose digital computer and a dot-matrix printer. *Journal of Computer Users in Speech and Hearing, 4*(1), 14–22.

Darley, F. L. (1972). The efficacy of language rehabilitation in aphasia. *Journal of Speech and Hearing Research, 37,* 3–21.

Davis, G. A. and Wilcox, M. J. (1985). *Adult aphasia rehabilitation: Applied pragmatics.* Austin, TX: Pro-Ed.

Dean, E. C. (1987). Microcomputers and aphasia. *Aphasiology, 1*(3), 267–270.

Dressler, R. A. (1991). *Beyond workbooks: The computer as a treatment supplement.* Poster session presented at the American Speech-Language-Hearing Association Annual Convention, Atlanta, GA, November 24, 1991.

Eisenson, J. (1973). *Adult aphasia.* New York: Appleton-Century-Crofts.

Enderby, P. (1987). Microcomputers in assessment, rehabilitation and recreation. *Aphasiology, 1*(2), 151–166.

Fenstad, J. E. (1988). Language and computations. In R. Herken (Ed.), *The universal Turing machine: A half-century survey* (pp. 327–348). New York: Oxford University Press.

Fitz-Gibbon, C. T. (1986). In defense of randomized controlled trials, with suggestions about the possible use of meta-analysis. *British Journal of Disorders of Communication, 21,* 117–124.

Geschwind, N. (1973). *Writing and its disorders.* Paper presented at the Second Pan-American Congress of Audition and Language, Lima, Peru.

Glisky, E. L., Schlacter, D. L., and Tulving, E. (1986). Learning and retention of computer-related vocabulary in memory-impaired patients: Method of vanishing cues. *Journal of Clinical and Experimental Neuropsychology, 8*(3), 292–312.

Goodglass, H., and Kaplan, E. (1983). *Boston diagnostic aphasia examination.* Philadelphia: Lea & Febiger.

Guyard, H., Masson, V., and Quiniou, R. (1990). Computer-based aphasia treatment meets artificial intelligence. *Aphasiology, 4*(6), 599–613.

Howard, D. (1986). Beyond randomized controlled trials: the case for effective case studies of the effects of treatment in aphasia. *British Journal of Disorders of Communication, 21,* 89–102.

Katz, R. C. (1984). Using microcomputers in the diagnosis and treatment of chronic aphasic adults. *Seminars in Speech, Language and Hearing, 5*(1), 11–22.

Katz, R. C. (1986). *Aphasia treatment and microcomputers.* New York: Taylor & Francis.

Katz, R. C. (1987). Efficacy of aphasia treatment using microcomputers. *Aphasiology, 1*(2). 141–150.

Katz, R. C. (1990). Intelligent computerized treatment or artificial aphasia therapy. *Aphasiology, 4*(6), 621–624.

Katz, R. C., and Nagy, V. T. (1982). A computerized treatment system for chronic aphasic adults. In R. H. Brookshire (Ed.), *Clinical aphasiology: 1982 conference proceedings* (pp. 153–160). Minneapolis, MN: BRK.

Katz, R. C., and Nagy, V. T. (1983). A computerized approach for improving word recognition in chronic aphasic patients. In R. H. Brookshire (Ed.), *Clinical aphasiology: 1983 conference proceedings* (pp. 65–72). Minneapolis, MN: BRK.

Katz, R. C., and Nagy, V. T. (1984). An intelligent computer-based task for chronic aphasic patients. In R. H. Brookshire (Ed.), *Clinical aphasiology: 1984 conference proceedings* (pp. 159–165). Minneapolis, MN: BRK.

Katz, R. C., and Nagy, V. T. (1985). A self-modifying computerized reading program for severely-impaired aphasic adults. In R. H. Brookshire (Ed.), *Clinical aphasiology: 1985 conference proceedings* (pp. 184–188). Minneapolis, MN: BRK.

Katz, R. C., and Wertz, R. T. (1992). Computerized hierarchical reading treatment in aphasia. *Aphasiology, 6*(2), 165–177.

Katz, R. C., Wertz, R. T., Davidoff, M., Schubitowski, Y. D., and Devitt, E. W. (1989). A computer program to improve written confrontation naming in aphasia. In T. E. Prescott (Ed.), *Clinical aphasiology: 1988 conference proceedings* (pp. 321–338), Austin, TX: Pro-Ed.

Kertesz, A. (1982). *Western aphasia battery.* New York: Grune & Stratton.

Kotten, A. (1989). Aphasia treatment: A multidimensional process. In E. Perecman (Ed.), *Integrating theory and practice in neuropsychology* (pp. 293-315). Hillsdale, NJ: Lawrence Erlbaum.

Langer, E. J. and Rodin, J. (1976). The effect of choice and enhanced personal responsibility for the aged: A field experiment in an institutional setting. *Journal of Personality and Social Psychology, 34,* 191–198.

LaPointe, L. L. (1977). Base-10 programmed stimulation: Task specification, scoring and plotting performance in aphasia therapy. *Journal of Speech and Hearing Disorders, 42,* 90–105.

Lepper, M. R. (1985). Microcomputers in education: Motivational and social issues. *American Psychologist, 40,* 1–18.

Loverso, F. L. (1987). Unfounded expectations: Computers in rehabilitation. *Aphasiology, 1*(2),157–160.

Loverso, F. L., Prescott, T. E., and Selinger, M. (1988). Cuing verbs: A treatment strategy for aphasic adults. *Journal of Rehabilitation Research and Development, 25,* 47–60.

Loverso, F. L., Prescott, T. E. and Selinger, M. (1992). Microcomputer treatment applications in aphasiology. *Aphasiology, 6*(2), 155–163.

Loverso, F. L., Prescott, T. E., Selinger, M., and Riley, L. (1988). Comparison of two modes of aphasia treatment: Clinician and computer-clinician assisted. In T. E. Prescott (Ed.), *Clinical aphasiology* (Vol. 18, pp. 297–319). Austin, TX: Pro-Ed.

Loverso, F. L., Prescott, T. E., Selinger, M., Wheeler, K. M., and Smith, R. D. (1985). The application of microcomputers for the treatment of aphasic adults. In R. H. Brookshire (Ed.), *Clinical aphasiology: 1985 conference proceedings* (pp. 189–195). Minneapolis, MN: BRK.

Loverso, F. L., Selinger, M., and Prescott, T. E. (1979). Application of verbing strategies to aphasia treatment. In R. H. Brookshire (Ed.), *Clinical aphasiology: 1979 conference proceedings* (pp. 229–238). Minneapolis, MN: BRK.

Lucas, R. W. (1977). A study of patients' attitudes to computer interrogation. *International Journal of Man-Machine Studies, 9,* 69–86.

Luria, A. R. (1973). *The working brain.* New York: Basic Books.

Luria, A. R. (1980). Higher cortical functions in man (2nd ed.). New York: Basic Books.

Lynch, W. J. (1983). Cognitive retraining using microcomputer games and commercially-available software. *Cognitive Rehabilitation, 1,* 19–22.

Matthews, B. A. J., and LaPointe, L. L. (1981). Determining rate of change and predicting performance levels in aphasia therapy. In R. H. Brookshire (Ed.), *Clinical aphasiology: 1981 conference proceedings* (pp. 17–25). Minneapolis, MN: BRK.

Matthews, B. A. J., and LaPointe, L. L. (1983). Slope and variability of performance on selected aphasia treatment tasks. In R. H. Brookshire (Ed.), *Clinical aphasiology: 1983 conference proceedings* (pp. 113–120). Minneapolis, MN: BRK.

McReynolds, L. V., and Kearns, K. P. (1983). *Single-subject experimental designs in communicative disorders.* Baltimore, MD: University Park Press.

Mills, R. H. (1982). Microcomputerized auditory comprehension training. In R. H. Brookshire (Ed.), *Clinical aphasiology: 1982 conference proceedings* (pp. 147–152). Minneapolis, MN: BRK.

Mills, R. H. (1988). Book review (*Aphasia treatment and microcomputers*). *Journal of Computer Users in Speech and Hearing, 4*(1), 40–41.

Mills, R. H. (1991). Machine vision technology: Quantification of videofluoroscopic swallowing data. *Journal of Computer Users in Speech and Hearing, 7*(1), 132–142.

Mills, R. H., and Thomas, R. P. (1981). Microcomputerized language therapy for the aphasic patient. *I.E.E.E. Proceedings of the Johns Hopkins First Search for Personal Computing Aid to the Handicapped* (pp. 45–46). Washington, DC.

Mills, R. H., and Thomas, R. P. (1983). *The Talking Apple—Comparison of three microcomputerized speech production methods.* Paper presented at the American Speech-Language-Hearing Association National Convention, Cincinnati, OH.

Odell, K., Collins, M., Dirkx, T., and Kelso, D. (1985). A computerized version of the Coloured Progressive Matrices. In R. H. Brookshire (Ed.), *Clinical aphasiology: 1985 conference proceedings* (pp. 47–56). Minneapolis, MN: BRK.

Odor, J. P. (1988). Student models in machine-mediated learning. *Journal of Mental Deficiency Research, 32,* 247–256.

Petheram, B. (1988). Enabling stroke victims to interact with a minicomputer—comparison of input devices. *International Disabilities Studies, 10*(2), 73–80.

Porch, B. E. (1981). *Porch Index of Communicative Ability, Vol. 1: Administration, scoring and interpretation* (3rd ed.). Palo Alto, CA: Consulting Psychologists Press.

Prescott, T. E., Loverso, F. L., and Selinger, M. (1984). Differences between normals and left brain damaged (aphasic) subjects on a nonverbal problem solving task. In R. H. Brookshire (Ed.), *Clinical aphasiology: 1984 conference proceedings* (pp. 235–240). Minneapolis, MN: BRK.

Prescott, T. E., and McNeil, M. R. (1973). *Measuring the effects of treatment of aphasia.* Paper presented at the Third Conference on Clinical Aphasiology, Albuquerque, NM.

Raven, J. C. (1975). *Coloured progressive matrices.* Los Angeles, CA: Western Psychologic Services.

Rheingold, H. (1991). *Virtual reality.* New York: Summit Books.

Robinson, I. (1990). Does computerized cognitive rehabilitation work? A review. *Aphasiology, 4*(4), 381–405.

Rosenbek, J. C. (1979). Wrinkled feet. In R. H. Brookshire (Ed.), *Clinical aphasiology: 1979 conference proceedings* (pp.163–176). Minneapolis, MN: BRK.

Rosenbek, J. C., LaPointe, L. L., and Wertz, R. T. (1989). *Aphasia: A clinical approach.* Austin, TX: Pro-Ed.

Rosenbek, J. C., Lemme, M. L., Ahern, M. B., Harris, E. H., and Wertz, R. T. (1973). A treatment for apraxia of speech in adults. *Journal of Speech and Hearing Disorders, 38,* 462–472.

Rushakoff, G. E. (1984). Clinical applications in communication disorders. In A. H. Schwartz (Ed.), *Handbook of microcomputer applications in communication disorders* (pp. 148–171). San Diego, CA: College Hill Press.

Schuell, H., Jenkins, J. J., and Jiménez-Pabón, E. (1964). *Aphasia in adults.* New York: Harper & Row.

Schulz, R. (1976). Effects of control and predictability on the physical well being of the institutionalized aged. *Journal of Personality and Social Psychology, 33,* 563–573.

Scott, C., and Byng, S. (1989). Computer assisted remediation of a homophone comprehension disorder in surface dyslexia. *Aphasiology, 3*(3), 301–320.

Seligman, M. (1975). *Helplessness: On depression, development and death.* San Francisco, CA: Freeman.

Selinger, M., Prescott, T. E. and Katz, R. C. (1987). Handwritten versus typed responses on PICA graphic subtests. In R. H. Brookshire (Ed.), *Clinical aphasiology: 1987 conference proceedings* (pp. 136–142). Minneapolis, MN: BRK.

Selinger, M., Prescott, T. E., Loverso, F. L., and Fuller, K. (1987). Below the 50th percentile: Application of the verb as core model. In R. H. Brookshire (Ed.), *Clinical aphasiology: 1987 conference proceedings* (pp. 55–63). Minneapolis, MN: BRK.

Seron, X., Deloche, G., Moulard, G., and Rouselle, M. (1980). A computer-based therapy for the treatment of aphasic subjects with writing disorders. *Journal of Speech and Hearing Disorders, 45,* 45–58.

Skilbeck, C. (1984). Computer assistance in the management of memory and cognitive impairment. In B. A. Wilson and N. Moffat (Ed.), *Clinical management of memory problems.* Rockville, MD: Aspen Publications.

Steele, R. D., Weinrich, M., Kleczewska, M. K., Wertz, R. T., and Carlson, G. S. (1987). Evaluating performance of severely aphasic patients on a computer-aided visual communication system. In R. H. Brookshire (Ed.), *Clinical aphasiology: 1987 conference proceedings* (pp. 46–54). Minneapolis, MN: BRK.

Stoicheff, M. L. (1960). Motivating instructions and language performance of dysphasic subjects. *Journal of Speech and Hearing Research, 3,* 75–85.

Tonkovich, J. D., Horowitz, D. M., Kawahigashi, J. N., Krainen, G. H., and Kronick, D. (1991). *An application of voice recognition technology for clinical documentation.* Computer poster session presented at the 1991 American Speech-Language-Hearing Association Annual Convention, Atlanta, GA.

Treadwell, J. E., Warren, L. R., and Wilson, M. S. (1985). The influence of three types of speech production upon auditory comprehension in aphasia.

In R. H. Brookshire (Ed.), *Clinical aphasiology: 1985 conference proceedings* (pp. 280–286). Minneapolis, MN: BRK.

Wallich, P. (1991, October). Digital dyslexia: Neural network mimics the effects of stroke. *Scientific American,* p. 36.

Weinrich, M., Steele, R. D., Kleczewska, M., Carlson, G. S., Baker, E., and Wertz, R. T. (1989). Representation of ''verbs'' in a computerized visual communication system. *Aphasiology, 3*(6), 501–512.

Wertz, R. T. (1981). Aphasia management: The speech pathologist's role. *Seminars in Speech, Language and Hearing, 2,* 315–331.

Wertz, R. T., Dronkers, N. F., Knight, R. T., Shenaut, G. K., and Deal, J. L. (1987). Rehabilitation of neurogenic communication disorders in remote settings. *Journal of Rehabilitative Research and Development, 25*(1), 432–433.

Wolfe, G. R. (1987). Microcomputers and treatment of aphasia. *Aphasiology, 1*(2), 165–170.

Wolfe, G. R., Davidoff, M., and Katz, R. C. (1987). Nonverbal problem-solving in aphasic and non-aphasic subjects with computer presented and actual stimuli. In R. H. Brookshire (Ed.), *Clinical aphasiology: 1987 conference proceedings* (pp. 243-248). Minneapolis, MN: BRK.

APPENDIX

Sources for Treatment Software

BrainTrain
727 Twin Ridge Lane
Richmond, VA 23235
(804) 320-0105

Clinical Solutions, Inc.
1800 Meidinger Tower
Louisville, KY 40202
(502) 589-3100

Developmental Learning Materials
One DLM Park
Allen, TX 75002

Edu-Ware Services, Inc.
22222 Sherman Way
Canoga Park, CA 91303

Hartley Courseware
P.O. Box 431
Dimondale, MI 48821

HyperStudio Network
Box 103
Blawenburg, NJ 08504
(609) 466-3196

Interactive Learning Materials
150 Croton Lake Road
P.O. Box S
Katonah, NY 10536
(914) 232-4682

Laureate Learning Systems, Inc.
110 East Spring Street
Winooski, VT 05404
(800) 562-6801

Madenta Communications Inc.
Box 25
Advanced Technology Centre
Edmonton, Alberta
Canada T6N 1G1
(800) 661-8406

Mayer-Johnson Co.
P.O. Box 1579
Solana Beach, CA 92075-1579
(619) 481-2489

MECC
2520 Broadway Drive
St. Paul, MN 55113

Medical Software Products
591 W. Hamilton Avenue
Suite 205
Campbell, CA 95008
(800) 444-4570

Micro Video
P.O. Box 7357
Ann Arbor, MI 48107
(800) 537-2182

Parrot Software
190 Sandy Ridge Road
State College, PA 16803
(800) PARROT-1

Prentke Romich Company
1022 Heyl Road
Wooster, OH 44691
(800) 262-1984

Pro-Ed
8700 Shoal Creek
Austin, TX 78758-6897
(512) 451-3246

Psychological Corp.
Harcourt Brace Jovanovich, Inc.
555 Academic Court
San Antonio, TX 78204-2498
(800) 228-0752

Roger Wagner Publishing
1050 Pioneer Way, Suite P
El Cajon, CA 92020
(800) 421-6526

Software Excitement
6475 Crater Lake Highway
Central Point, OR 97502
(800) 444-5457

Spinnaker Software Corp.
215 First Street
Cambridge, MA 02142

StatSoft
2325 E. 13th Street
Tulsa, OK 74104
(918) 583-4149

Sunburst Communications, Inc.
39 Washington Avenue
Pleasantville, NY 10570

Sunset Software
9277 East Corrine Drive
Scottsdale, AZ 85260
(602) 451-0753

Systat, Inc.
1800 Sherman Avenue
Evanston, IL 60201-3793
(800) 428-STAT

Tiger Communication System, Inc.
155 East Broad Street, S-325
Rochester, NY 14604
(716) 454-5134

Tolfa Corporation
1860 Embarcadero Road
Palo Alto, CA 94303
(800) 332-4913

APPENDIX

Trademarks

Amiga is a registered trademark of Commodore, Inc.
Apple, Apple II, Apple IIGS, Finder, HyperCard, HyperCard IIGS, Macintosh, Macintosh Classic II, ProDOS, QuickTime, and System 7 are registered trademarks of Apple Computer, Inc. SuperDrive is a trademark of Apple Computer, Inc.
CompuServe is a registered trademark of CompuServe, Inc.
Echo II is a registered trademark of Street Electronics, Inc.
GEnie is a trademark of General Electric Company.
HyperStudio is a registered trademark of Roger Wagner Publishing, Inc.

IBM is a registered trademark of International Business Machines Corporation.
Lingraphica is a trademark of Tolfa Corporation.
Microsoft and MS-DOS are registered trademarks of Microsoft Corporation.
Windows is a trademark of Microsoft Corporation.
Smalltalk is a registered trademark of Xerox Corporation.
SoftPC is a registered trademark of Insignia Solutions, Inc.
TOPS is a registered trademark of Sun Microsystems, Inc.

CHAPTER 17
Augmentative and Alternative Communication for Persons with Aphasia

KAREN HUX, DAVID R. BEUKELMAN, AND KATHRYN L. GARRETT

Many adults with aphasia have temporary or permanent difficulty meeting their daily communication needs through natural speech. Despite this, aphasia is one of the few severe communication disorders that augmentative and alternative communication (AAC) professionals have minimally addressed. The reasons for this lack of attention are not well understood but probably stem, at least in part, from the intricacy of the language-processing deficits typical of aphasia and the difficulty of applying interventions designed primarily for motor-impaired individuals to persons with language and cognitive limitations.

Although aphasiologists are far from agreeing unanimously about fundamental aphasia treatment issues, they have progressed considerably toward acknowledging that aphasia has long-term effects on an individual's life-style. For a long time, practitioners focused remediation efforts on specific modalities of communication (e.g., reading, speaking, listening). More recently, there has been increased recognition that aphasia disrupts the integrity of the whole person. Aphasiologists now acknowledge that most persons with aphasia do not recover "normal" communication skills. As a result, speech-language pathologists are currently redefining successful communication as it pertains to aphasia and are establishing more realistic expectations for language therapy outcomes (Marshall, 1987). There is a potential for many of these revised definitions and expectations to incorporate AAC strategies and technology.

The philosophical foundations of AAC and aphasiology, once understood more clearly, can provide complementary support to theorists and practitioners of both fields. This chapter provides information about these two related, yet unique, areas. First, a definition of AAC and a brief historical perspective of AAC approaches relative to aphasia are presented. Second, candidacy for AAC services is discussed with respect to the philosophy and knowledge base of clinicians and the capabilities and needs of stroke survivors. Third, the assessment of persons with unmet communication needs is outlined in a section describing the authors' framework for AAC process analysis for adults with aphasia. This section includes a discussion of factors that influence the communication needs of persons with aphasia, and, because most persons with aphasia are over 65 years of age, special attention is given to the communication

patterns of elderly persons. The interaction patterns of persons with severe communication disorders are also reviewed. Finally, five case reviews illustrating AAC interventions are presented to demonstrate the application of AAC strategies to adults with aphasia and the impact such strategies have on communicative interaction.

DEFINING AAC

A committee of the American Speech-Language-Hearing Association provided a commonly used definition of AAC.

> Augmentative and alternative communication is an area of clinical practice that attempts to compensate (either temporarily or permanently) for the impairment and disability patterns of individuals with severe expressive communication disorders (i.e., the severely speech-language and writing impaired) (ASHA, 1989, p. 107).

The primary goal of AAC intervention is the facilitation of an individual's participation in various communicative contexts. Depending on the individual's circumstances and extent of disability these communicative contexts will vary. For example, the communication needs of persons who live at home differ from those of persons who live in extended care facilities; communication needs of persons attending school differ from those who are working or are retired; and communication needs of persons who interact only with familiar persons differ from those who also converse with strangers. These variations in contexts necessitate different AAC strategies.

An AAC system should consist of "an integrated group of components, including symbols, strategies, and techniques used by individuals to enhance their communication" (ASHA, 1991, p. 10). AAC systems can no longer be conceptualized as technology alone. Instead, successful AAC systems often combine high-technology, low-technology, and communication interaction strategies.

HISTORICAL PERSPECTIVE OF AAC APPROACHES

For centuries, physical, cognitive, and language impairments have prevented some people from speaking well enough to meet their daily communication needs. Only during the past 20 to 30 years, however, has society made a systematic effort to provide assistance to these communication-impaired individuals using AAC strategies and devices.

Early AAC Interventions

Much of the early effort in augmentative communication focused on persons who could not communicate because of physical impairments but who were literate and able to spell their messages—that is, persons with impairments such as cerebral palsy or spinal cord injuries. Early augmentative communication systems usually involved modifications of electric typewriters using devices such as key guards, head sticks, enlarged key pads, and light-activated devices. Although these systems served the writing needs of some individuals, the approaches were not particularly supportive of conversational interactions. Furthermore, persons who were illiterate could not use these early augmentative communication systems.

In time, alternative symbol systems emerged to support the communication efforts of preliterate children. Actual objects, miniature objects, and photographs were used to represent messages. Eventually, communication professionals developed specialized systems of line drawings—such as Blissymbolics (Kates and McNaughton, 1975), Picture Communication Symbols (Johnson, 1981, 1985), and Picsyms (Carlson, 1985)—to substitute for earlier, concrete symbol systems. The number of symbol sets and systems has grown substantially over the years, and a large number are now in widespread use.

In an effort to provide technology that was accessible to persons with physical impairments and that accommodated symbol-based communication, AAC professionals introduced a number of technological advances. For example, some AAC devices can be activated with finger or head sticks or have scanning or headlight pointing options. Typically, these systems require considerable training and expertise to operate and are relatively expensive. Their complexity makes them ineffective options for individuals with cognitive limitations.

In the mid-1980s, the augmentative communication field began to consider seriously the communication needs of persons with cognitive, as well as physical, limitations. The result was development of simplified symbol systems, easy to operate electronics with high-quality speech synthesis, and a large number of communication strategies. A consequence of these efforts has been that many persons with cognitive impairments have learned to communicate using augmentative options. Unfortunately, individuals with language disorders acquired during adulthood (i.e., aphasia) have continued to receive little consistent attention from the augmentative communication field.

AAC Interventions for Adults with Aphasia

Speech-language professionals have been considerably less effective in designing AAC interventions for adults with aphasia than they have been for literate and nonliterate persons with physical limitations and, more recently, for persons with cognitive impairments. Despite this, AAC includes many strategies for people who cannot meet all of their communication needs through natural speech, including aphasic persons (Garrett and Beukelman, 1992). Some of these strategies are "unaided" in that they require no external equipment. Others are "aided" AAC strategies that require either high- or low-technology materials or equipment.

Unaided AAC Strategies

Unaided AAC strategies include gestures, pantomime, and facial expressions. Sometimes, such strategies are formalized into codes that are understood only by groups of people trained specifically in their use. Skelly's (1979) code of hand gestures is one such example. At other times, unaided AAC strategies occur naturally within a culture and are easily interpreted by members of that culture without special training. For example, most people readily interpret an upturned hand to mean "I don't know," a head nod to mean "yes," or an extended palm to indicate that an activity should stop. Other unaided AAC strategies are idiosyncratic to an individual. For example, individuals with severe aphasic impairments often develop and use idiosyncratic gestures—sometimes routinely and sometimes sporadically—to compensate for their limitations in verbal communication.

Aided AAC Strategies

Aided AAC strategies include a wide assortment of devices and materials that function to increase the efficiency and effectiveness of an individual's communication. A complete review of specific AAC options is beyond the mission of this text. Also, the rapid development of AAC technology discourages the discussion of specific technology in a textbook. For information on specific technology, interested readers can refer to the following, regularly updated sources:

1. *Trace ResourceBook: Assistive Technologies for Communication, Control, and Assess,* Madison, WI: Trace Research and Development Center.

2. Hyper-ABLEDATA (Compact Disk) Madison, WI: Trace Research and Development Center.

The simplest of aided AAC techniques use materials such as paper and pencil for drawing (Lyon and Helm-Estabrooks, 1987), picture and word books for identifying referents (Garrett et al., 1989), photograph albums for specifying individuals (Beukelman et al., 1985), and maps for locating places. A number of companies publish extensive symbol sets for use in augmentative devices (see Appendix 17.1). Some of these products are available in multiple formats, including line-drawings, computer graphics, and graphic stickers.

More technically sophisticated materials include a range of electronic devices, some of which may be helpful to persons with aphasia. For example, because nearly all persons with aphasia retain physical control of at least one hand, they can use "direct selection" devices that allow selection of choices from a screen, keyboard, or touch-sensitive surface. A variety of these direct selection devices have been designed to meet the communication needs of persons with differing language and cognitive capabilities. However, as was mentioned earlier in this chapter, many selection devices serve to augment the communication only of persons with functional literacy skills because messages must be spontaneously spelled, selected from a menu of printed words or phrases, or retrieved through abbreviated codes (e.g., OD = open the door). Because of the language limitations of many persons with aphasia, such literacy-based systems are difficult, if not impossible, for aphasic individuals to operate.

A second group of direct selection AAC devices allows users to choose preprogrammed or prestored messages by selecting printed or graphic symbols associated with specific messages. Usually, selection and activation of a symbol triggers the speaking or printing of a corresponding message. When a unique symbol corresponds with each message, the size and complexity of the symbol display dictate the number of messages possible. For young children or individuals with cognitive impairments, the resulting limitation of messages may not be of initial concern. However, persons with aphasia may have extensive numbers of messages they wish to communicate. When this is the case, the "one symbol = one message" strategy may be unsatisfactory.

To overcome these message limitations, AAC professionals have designed devices that allow users to select symbols in different combinations and sequences (called iconic encoding) (Baker, 1982, 1986). Each combination of symbols corresponds with a different message. For example, an *apple* symbol may represent "eat"; an *apple* and a *building* may represent "restaurant"; an *apple* and a *?* may represent "When do we eat?" Iconic encoding is available, with variations, in a number of aided communication products, including Minspeak (Intro-Talker, TouchTalker, LightTalker, and Liberator by Prentke-Romich Company), symbol sequencing (DAC by Adaptive Communication Systems, Dynovox by Sentient Systems, and Talking Screen by Words +, Inc.) and keylinking (Macaw by Zygo Industries). (See Appendix 17.1 for addresses of AAC manufacturers.)

The ability of persons with severe aphasia to learn multiple symbol sequences has received little research or clinical study. To reduce the learning involved in symbol sequencing, AAC products with dynamic screen display capabilities have recently been introduced (Dynovox by Sentient Systems; Talking Screen by Words +, Inc.; Talking Symbols by Mayer-Johnson, Inc.; Lingraphica by Tolfa Corporation). With these devices, a user selects an option from a screen of general category symbols (e.g., people, food, activities, calendars), and the screen changes dynamically to present numerous options within the selected category. By selecting a symbol from this new page, the user can identify a specific item. Although dynamic display devices hold some promise of compensating for the language limitations of aphasic persons, research and clinical studies testing this hypothesis have not yet been performed.

Many of the problems associated with applying existing AAC technology to persons with aphasia relate to system-specific limitations such as inappropriate or limited vocabulary, poor physical design, limited relevance to adult topics of conversation, and complexity in constructing multiword messages. Other problems relate directly to disturbances of language processing such as decreased comprehension of syntactic structures or poor retrieval of specific words. The challenge for speech and language professionals is to match the available AAC strategies and technologies with the particular needs and capabilities of aphasia individuals. A first step to meeting this challenge is appropriate identification of those adults with aphasia who can benefit from AAC intervention. This identification has been a persistent problem in both AAC and aphasiology fields.

CANDIDACY FOR AAC INTERVENTION

The goal of AAC—to improve the effectiveness and ease with which a person communicates—is in accordance with the needs of the majority of persons with aphasia. Although AAC strategies will not benefit all aphasic individuals and, even when beneficial, will not eliminate all communication difficulties, a substantial number of persons with aphasia can use AAC strategies effectively to meet a portion of their communication needs.

Unfortunately, persons with aphasia currently represent a neglected subgroup of AAC candidates. Only a small number of those aphasic individuals who are AAC candidates are fortunate enough to receive AAC services. Many persons with aphasia are not exposed to AAC options and, consequently, are unaware of the possible benefits such strategies and devices can provide.

The discrepancy between the number of persons with aphasia who are AAC candidates and the number who are AAC recipients exists for several reasons. First, the field of aphasiology has poorly described the possible benefits of applying augmentative communication strategies. In other words, the role that AAC strategies can play in the treatment of persons with aphasia remains largely undefined. This absence of role definition is evident in the varying philosophies clinicians have about the appropriateness of introducing AAC strategies to aphasic individuals. For example, some clinicians do not introduce augmentative approaches unless it is clear that recovery of natural speech will be insufficient to meet an individuals' daily communication needs. Other clinicians limit the introduction of augmentative strategies to stroke survivors whose language skills are relatively intact but who have significant difficulty with motor speech control. Still other clinicians introduce augmentative strategies when an aphasic individual needs temporary communication facilitation before regaining natural speech.

A second reason for the discrepancy between the number of AAC candidates and recipients is that aphasiologists have restricted views of what AAC is. For many, augmentative communication implies complex technology. At the other extreme, some clinicians associate AAC only with picture/photograph books or communication boards. Both views reflect limited awareness of the range of AAC possibilities currently available and reduce the number of aphasic individuals who receive AAC intervention.

A third reason for the candidacy-recipient discrepancy is that clinical aphasiologists vary greatly in their exposure to the AAC field. Because AAC is relatively new, many persons in clinical practice have had limited opportunities for in-depth learning about AAC options. As is true of all clinical practice, clinicians' limitations have a direct negative impact on treatment outcomes. In the case of AAC, the impact is evident in the small number of persons with aphasia who historically have received treatment incorporating AAC strategies.

Fourth, the discrepancy between the number of AAC candidates and recipients exists because clinicians differ in their views of the purpose of aphasia intervention. Some aphasiologists perceive the purpose of intervention to be the improvement of natural speech. These clinicians have minimal use for AAC strategies. In contrast, clinicians who have a broader goal of preparing stroke survivors for "a lifetime of aphasia" (Rosenbek et al., 1989, p. 132) and who recognize survivors' needs to compensate for residual communication deficits (Rosenbek et al., 1989) typically encourage multimodal communication. Multimodal approaches include AAC strategies as well as natural speech.

A final reason for the discrepancy between the number of aphasic AAC candidates and recipients reflects the diversity of capabilities and needs displayed by adults with aphasia. These differences stem from several factors. First, differing premorbid communicative competencies and needs lead adults with aphasia to vary in their needs and expectations for poststroke communication interactions. Second, variations in health, emotional status, and social supports affect how adults with aphasia cope with the medical, physical, psychosocial, and cognitive problems that accompany stroke. Third, differences in the cause, severity, location, and extent of brain damage from strokes affect outcomes and recovery patterns. Fourth, although groups of aphasic adults may share similar clusters of communication behaviors, every individual responds uniquely to brain damage and displays a distinctive pattern of intact and deficient language processes. In combination, these factors lead to vast differences in the communication characteristics of adults with aphasia—characteristics that professionals must match with AAC strategies and techniques.

As aphasiologists gain awareness of the range and potential applications of AAC options, it is probably that the number of stroke survivors receiving AAC services will increase substantially. AAC strategies are already gaining recognition as important parts of aphasia assessment and intervention programs. Despite this growth, aphasiologists provide AAC-based intervention to only a small portion of the many AAC candidates within the population of aphasic adults.

ASSESSMENT

AAC assessment of adults with aphasia has five phases: (*a*) identification of AAC candidates, (*b*) identification of communication patterns and needs, (*c*) assessment of communication capabilities, (*d*) analysis of current communication interactions, and (*e*) documentation of communication constraints (Beukelman and Mirenda, 1992; Beukelman et al., 1985). Information gathered during the assessment allows selection and personalization of AAC strategies.

Identifying Aphasic AAC Candidates

Two types of aphasic adults are AAC candidates: (*a*) those persons who do not regain sufficient natural speech for communicating daily needs and (*b*) those persons who rely on natural speech to meet many of their communication needs but find it inadequate or inefficient in certain instances. Individuals of the first type usually display severe and persistent expressive communication difficulties, sometimes with accompanying receptive language impairments. Individuals of the second type often have less severe expressive disabilities but find that specific speech and language deficiencies interfere significantly with their communication. For example, some persons with aphasia have difficulty establishing new topics of conversation, although they can communicate successfully once their listeners know the topic. AAC techniques can assist these individuals to introduce topics. Other persons with aphasia have naming difficulties that interfere with the recall of specific words. These individuals can improve the efficiency of their communication by using augmentative techniques to cue word retrieval. Still other individuals have impaired comprehension of verbal language and can benefit from AAC strategies that present information through multiple modalities. Finally, some persons with aphasia communicate effectively until a communication failure forces repair or revision of an utterance. The attempt to repair a miscommunication may tax fragile speech and language skills to the point that further breakdown occurs. For these individuals, AAC strategies are useful in resolving communication breakdowns.

Identifying Communication Patterns and Purposes

Communication Patterns

As reported by Rosenbek et al. (1989), most strokes occur in elderly persons; 80% occur in people over 65 years of age. In contrast, most professionals who assist persons with aphasia are young or middle-aged adults. This age difference can lead to conflicting expectations about forms and functions of communication. Young professionals must guard against superimposing their communication expectations on elderly clients and should be aware of the communication patterns typical of elderly adults.

Unique Communication Patterns of Elderly Adults. Elderly adults have several unique communication patterns. An example of one of these is the manner in which they relate information. Requests for information often prompt elderly adults to present material in storylike modes in which the speaker assumes the role of transmitter of "cultural lore" (Mergler and Goldstein, 1983). As a storyteller, the elderly person can use narratives in a variety of ways. In some instances a narrative may serve to relate historical information; in other instances, a similar narrative may relate to an ongoing activity. For example, Stuart (1991) found that conversations about the Gulf War of 1991 prompted many elderly individuals to recount personal experiences from World War II. At times, the purpose of such conversation was to provide an account of historical events; at other times, it was to relate current and past events, perhaps as a means of facilitating the elderly adult's participation in the conversation.

Another unique communication pattern of elderly speakers reflects a shift from focusing conversations on family members to talking primarily about friends and acquaintances (Stuart, 1991). This shift is quite common as people age and probably relates to several factors. One factor is that siblings and spouses become less available topics of conversation as they die or become disabled. Another contributing factor is that children of an elderly person often establish families of their own and are no longer in geographic proximity to their parents; hence, there is decreased contact and involvement in children's lives.

A third distinction between the conversation of different aged adults results from a tendency for elderly persons to engage in extensive amounts of game playing (Stuart, 1991). Elderly adults use board games and card games much more frequently to establish social contact than do young adults. The effect is a striking difference between elderly and young adults in what topics of conversation typically arise.

Implications for AAC Systems. Unique communication patterns of elderly persons lead to differences in the communication needs of elderly and young adults. AAC systems should reflect these differences. In particular, AAC systems for elderly persons should contain materials and strategies that foster storytelling modes of communication. Also, AAC selection sets should include lexical items that allow users to greet people, inquire about their current situations and backgrounds, reveal biographical and personal information, and engage in activities typical of elderly adults.

Observations about the communication patterns of elderly adults are from investigations of persons without disabilities. Information is not yet available about the impact of physical, cognitive, or linguistic disability on communication forms and functions. Despite this absence of information, it seems logical to assume that physical and cognitive impairments would substantially affect styles, topics, and patterns of communication. Information that is available about the communicative purposes prominent in the interactions of people who use AAC systems can serve as a basis for speculation about the communication needs of persons with aphasia.

Communication Purposes

Light (1988) outlined four communicative purposes prominent in the interactions of people who use AAC systems. These purposes include the use of communication to express wants and needs, to share information, to foster social closeness, and to comply with rules of social etiquette. These communicative functions are not unique to AAC users; instead, they are common to virtually all persons with or without communication impairments. Differences exist, however, in the extent to which individuals with differing abilities need assistance with each of the purposes.

Expressing Wants and Needs. One obvious function of communication is the expression of wants and needs. It is easy to imagine that persons with aphasia would require assistance with this type of communication, especially because their experience with stroke may have dramatically changed their ability to perform daily activities independently. However, on closer examination, aphasic persons' need to communicate wants and needs may not be nearly as prevalent as one might expect.

A person with aphasia may have less need to communicate basic desires than other individuals. This reduction is due, in part, to the structured environment of most hospitals and rehabilitation centers. During acute care hospitalization, the routine of the hospital generally determines how a patient's wants and needs are met: Meals occur at routine times, toileting programs are established, visiting hours are regulated, and physicians' visits occur at preset times. During inpatient rehabilitation, the structure is equally tight: Therapies occur on a schedule, food appears at certain times, and family members and friends are told when they can visit. This high degree of structure—along with the familiarity of the hospital staff in interacting with and caring for stroke survivors—greatly reduces the amount that the person with aphasia must communicate about his or her basic wants and needs.

After returning home, the physical capabilities of the person with aphasia and the involvement of caretakers affect the need to communicate wants and needs. For those individuals able to walk or use a wheelchair effectively, there is a certain pride taken in self-sufficiency. Many persons with aphasia have struggled to regain independence following their strokes and have little desire to ask for assistance in performing daily activities. Consequently, they may remain less likely than other individuals—disabled or nondisabled—to engage in communication about basic wants and needs.

Even persons with aphasia who engage in minimal communication about wants and needs must have some means of expressing these desires. As such, it is important to ensure that the individual can communicate certain wants and needs either through natural speech or through use of an augmentative strategy. Clinical aphasiologists, however, must take care not to over-stress this type of communication or over-represent it within an AAC system.

Information Sharing. The sharing of novel information is an important communicative purpose for most individuals. Desire for this type of interaction does not change with the occurrence of stroke and, consequently, AAC strategies must provide a means for persons with aphasia to participate in communication acts directed at sharing information.

The need to share information is especially prominent during the early stages of a stroke survivor's recovery. During acute stages of illness, hospital staff may ask a person with aphasia for information that will permit evaluation of cognitive, language, or physical status. At the same time, family members and business associates may need information from the patient regarding such things as legal papers, business operations, and financial obligations. Augmentative communication strategies can facilitate transfer of these types of information.

During later stages of recovery, the need to communicate new information may lessen, but an intermittent communication need usually remains. Persons with aphasia who return to their communities, retirement centers, or nursing facilities may find that their greatest need to share information is when meeting new people.

Social Closeness. Social closeness is an important communication goal for individuals of any age. With increasing age, a substantial proportion of interactions revolve around the establishment and maintenance of social relationships. In fact, communicative interaction involving social closeness is a predominant communication activity of elderly persons (Stuart et al., 1993). Because of this, inclusion of communication that supports social closeness is important in augmentative communication systems.

The need to express social closeness is evident throughout the recovery process from stroke. During acute hospitalization, stroke survivors need communication to maintain social closeness with their family members and friends. This communication serves as an important source of support while struggling with changes brought on by sudden illness. During rehabilitation, the opportunities for social closeness expand as relationships with additional friends are reestablished and new relationships are formed. Following discharge, some stroke survivors return to environments where they can easily become isolated. To prevent this, it is important that persons with aphasia have a method of communicating for social interaction that allows resumption of activities typical of elderly adults.

Social Etiquette. Social etiquette is another communicative function that tends to increase in importance with advancing age. The desire to use communication for social etiquette does not change with the occurrence of illness. In contrary, the increase in the number of caregivers that accompanies a serious illness makes the need for communicating social etiquette information even greater for a stroke survivor than it would be for an elderly adult living independently. As such, inclusion of social etiquette phrases in AAC systems is important. Personalizing these messages to match those that the individual used prior to his or her stroke may be an especially important consideration for persons with aphasia. However, it should also be noted that many persons with aphasia retain the ability to communicate social information through natural gestures and automatic phrases. When this is the case, it is unlikely that they will opt to use external augmentative strategies to meet social etiquette needs and, hence, inclusion of such phrases in an AAC system is not advantageous.

Assessing AAC Capabilities

A capabilities assessment provides a profile of an aphasic individual's strengths and weaknesses. Because traditional aphasia assessment batteries focus on identifying and measuring communication deficits—and often do so in decontextualized settings—AAC professionals must identify the communication strengths that persist following a stroke through additional, nonstandardized assessments. Garrett and Beukelman (1992) identified several areas of residual skills important to the application of AAC strategies with adults with aphasia. These areas include perceptual, communication, motor, visual, and pragmatic skills, as well as the individual's experiential base.

Perceptual Skills

Individuals with aphasia often understand many of the visual symbols found in maps, logos, and signs. They may retain the ability to recognize photographs and line drawings related to familiar people and places and may have knowledge of shape, size, goodness, and importance relations. Some are able to draw and can communicate aspects of intended messages through this modality (Garrett and Beukelman, 1992). During a capabilities assessment, an AAC professional evaluates a range of perceptual skills to determine the role that such skills can play in an AAC system.

Communication Skills

Limitations in linguistic functioning are the hallmark of aphasic performances. However, many adults with aphasia demonstrate relatively functional communication capabilities when linguistic information is presented to them within a communication context. Because many standard aphasia tests assess language rather than communication skills and do so primarily in decontextualized ways, additional contextually based assessments may be informative. Such assessments emphasize the aphasic person's comprehension and expression of information given maximum contextual assistance. For example, a conversation partner may provide pragmatic, environmental, social, and nonverbal cues in addition to linguistic information to facilitate comprehension of a message by the person with aphasia. Likewise, the communication partner may accept any successful transmittal of information by the individual with aphasia, even if it relies on nonlinguistic modalities.

Motor Skills

Most aphasic individuals retain sufficient motor skills to use AAC strategies and devices. Of fundamental importance is the individual's ability to select items directly from a language board or an electronic device. Occasionally, a stroke survivor may have a limb apraxia that interferes with this ability. Thus, AAC professionals perform brief screening tests to confirm that individuals with aphasia have sufficient residual motor skills to control various AAC devices.

Visual Skills

Often, strokes do not affect the visual system. However, visual field cuts sometimes occur, usually on the right side when the left hemisphere sustains damage. If a right-field cut is present, the individual will not see images positioned in the right visual field. During assessment, the AAC professional confirms the integrity of the visual fields through performance of informal tasks. Also, because AAC techniques rely heavily on visual skills, it is helpful to confirm that glasses are of the appropriate strength to correct visual acuity.

Pragmatic Skills

Most persons with aphasia have extensive prestroke experience with communicating through speech and writing. Hence, they understand how communication works and are aware of the importance of pragmatic aspects of communication such as turn taking, speaker-listener roles, and topic coordination. Occasionally, if an aphasic individual has been an unsuccessful communicator for a sustained time period, he or she may need encouragement to resume appropriate interaction roles. The AAC professional must determine the status of the stroke survivor's pragmatic skills in various types of communication settings.

Experiential Base

Most persons with aphasia have lived many years and have experienced relatively normal life-styles. Therefore, their knowledge bases are extensive. An AAC assessment will need to solicit from them, their families, and their friends the content of this knowledge base so that it can be incorporated into their AAC system. Asking families to write a brief biography of the aphasic individual is an efficient way of obtaining this information.

Assessing AAC Constraints

When considering an AAC system for an adult with aphasia, it is necessary to determine if there are professional, psychosocial, and/or financial factors that will constrain the effectiveness of intervention.

Professional Support

The knowledge and skill of the speech-language pathologist serving an individual with aphasia often influences the effectiveness of an AAC intervention. If a professional not directly involved with the AAC team is to manage the intervention, it is necessary to ensure that he or she agrees about the need for an AAC system and has sufficient background to provide the appropriate services. However, the crucial factor is not always the amount of actual AAC experience the clinician has had. Instead, his or her willingness to explore and learn new strategies, techniques, and technologies is more important.

Family and Communication Partner Skill and Support

Family and social support for AAC interventions is necessary if an aphasic individual is to achieve effective and efficient use of an augmentative system. The screening form displayed in Figure 17.1 can be helpful in determining the skill and

Partner Skill Screening Form

Patient _____ Date _____

Partner _____

Directions: For sections 1–3, check the appropriate box or fill in the answer while interviewing the partner. For section 4, observe the partner with the patient. Readminister this section after training.

Basic Skills

Hearing	Poor _____	Good _____	Corrected? _____
Vision	Poor _____	Good _____	Corrected? _____
Reading _____	Nonreading _____		Reads news, magazines _____
Writing Legibility	Poor _____	Good _____	
Spelling	Poor _____	Good _____	

Knowledge of Patient

How many years have you known _____? _____ years

What is your relationship to the patient? _____

_____

What activities have you done together? _____

_____

_____

_____

Knowledge of Deficits

What have you been told about _____'s stroke?

_____

_____

_____

Describe some of the things that are different.

_____

_____

_____

Would you like to learn more?   Yes _____   No _____

Partner Skill Screening Form (*continued*)

Interactional Skills

Does partner have good eye contact with patient?	Yes_____	No _____
Does partner provide alerting cues if necessary?	Yes_____	No _____
Does partner choose topics of interest to discuss?	Yes_____	No _____
Does partner ask questions using appropriate language complexity?	Yes_____	No _____
Does partner pause long enough for patient to respond?	Yes_____	No _____
Does partner respond immediately to patient's efforts to gain attention?	Yes_____	No _____
Does partner revise messages if patient does not understand?	Yes_____	No _____
Does partner supplement spoken communication with written words when necessary?	Yes_____	No _____
Does partner avoid asking open-ended questions when patient has no means of answering?	Yes_____	No _____
Does partner provide appropriate written choices when necessary?	Yes_____	No _____
Does partner move materials into patient's visual field?	Yes_____	No _____
Does partner encourage patient to use alternative modes of communication when the primary mode is unsuccessful?	Yes_____	No _____
Does partner interpret alternative modes of communication successfully?	Yes_____	No _____
Does partner respond to patient's use of control phases?	Yes_____	No _____
Is partner able to maintain consecutive turns in the course of an augmented conversation?	Yes_____	No _____
Does partner persevere until patient has communicated the message?	Yes_____	No _____
Does partner enjoy interacting with patient?	Yes_____	No _____

Figure 17.1. Partners skills screening form.

knowledge base of potential communication partners (Garrett and Beukelman, 1992).

Financial Support

Professional services and AAC equipment are often quite expensive. Although AAC interventions may be potentially effective for an individual with aphasia, there may be insufficient financial support to provide the needed services. Assurance that an individual has adequate finances to cover costs should be established prior to introducing an expensive AAC system or one that will require substantial training to master. Otherwise, the person with aphasia may be left with an AAC system that he or she cannot use and, hence, will continue to experience frequent communication breakdowns.

AAC Process Analysis Framework for Aphasia

As stated earlier, it is essential to match the capabilities, needs, and constraints of persons with aphasia with effective AAC strategies. One method of achieving this match is for AAC professionals to perform analyses of communication interactions between persons with aphasia and representative communication partners. Such a system of analysis is represented in the flowchart depicted in Figure 17.2. Each node of the flowchart represents a point where communication breakdowns can occur. AAC support at these breakdown points may facilitate progress toward achieving successful communication exchanges. Shaded boxes on the flowchart indicate that the person with aphasia has adequately performed given steps in the communication process. Each of these steps is explained in the following sections.

Contextual Awareness

Contextual awareness refers to an individual's environmental awareness, interaction, comprehension, and interpretation. It is a cognitive skill fundamental to all forms of communication and is susceptible to damage from stroke.

Stroke survivors are distinguishable on the basis of their level of contextual awareness. Their behavior can be categorized into four awareness levels—profound impairment, severe impairment, moderate to mild impairment, and intact contextual awareness.

Profound Impairment. The profound level of impaired contextual awareness is evident in comatose individuals. Persons in a coma display little or no awareness of the environment, demonstrate no purposeful behaviors, and fail to interact communicatively with others (Miller et al., 1990). Although extended periods of coma are not typical of stroke survivors, when

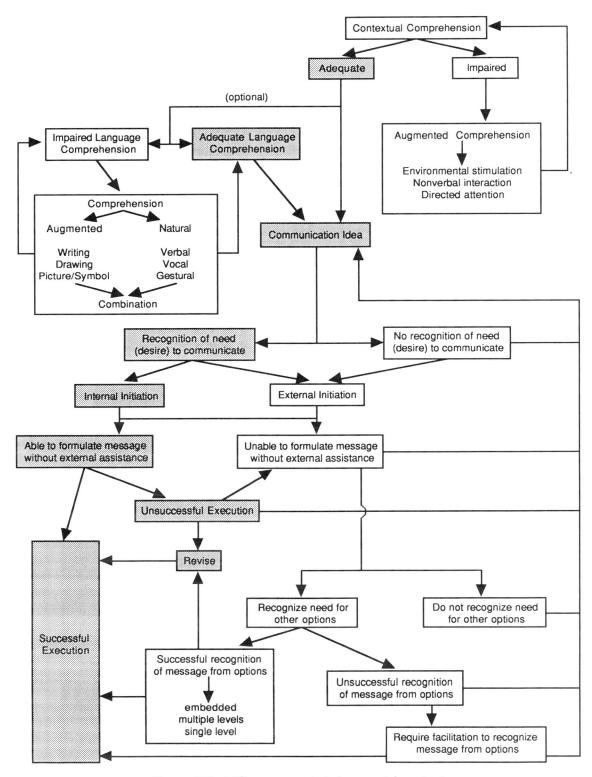

Figure 17.2. AAC process analysis framework for aphasia.

they do occur, multimodal sensory stimulation may facilitate improvement in the level of consciousness (Ansell, 1991).

Severe Impairment. Severe impairment of contextual awareness implies a failure to comprehend environmental and contextual information. It differs from profound impairment primarily in the survivor's level of arousal and alertness. Stroke survivors with severely impaired contextual awareness may engage in motor activities given constant physical assistance and guidance but do not follow verbal directions, appropriately interpret nonverbal information, initiate or complete meaningful tasks independently, or attempt communication with others.

Moderate to Mild Impairment. Stroke survivors with moderate to mild impairments of awareness are inconsistent in their interpretation of contextual information. Although they actively interact with the environment and other individuals, they are prone to occasional errors in interpreting contextual information. For example, adults with moderate contextual impairment may misinterpret nonverbal cues, especially ones inconsistent with verbal content; or, what appears as a loss of social tactfulness may, in fact, be a reflection of moderate to mild impairment in contextual awareness.

Intact Contextual Awareness. Intact contextual awareness indicates no apparent deficiency in a stroke survivor's interpretation of contextual information. Many adults with aphasia display this level of awareness as evidenced in the consistency with which they correctly interpret nonverbal and contextual cues. Cognitive problems experienced by these survivors appear to center around speech and language functions.

Language Comprehension

Language comprehension is fundamental to communicating with others on a linguistic level but is not a prerequisite to the information of communication ideas; individuals can conceptualize ideas solely through experiencing and interacting with their surroundings. However, when speakers desire conversational interactions with others, they must have at least rudimentary comprehension of linguistic input.

Both natural and augmentative communication strategies provide means to compensate for impaired language comprehension. Natural communication supplements include message repetitions and revisions and the addition of simple gestures. Augmented supplements include such strategies as writing salient words, drawing pictures or diagrams to illustrate messages, and displaying related pictures or symbols to communicate portions of messages.

Communication Ideas

A communication idea is simply a thought, feeling, or concept that an individual wishes to express to others. Many adults with aphasia independently generate communication ideas; others, however, appear unable to generate communication ideas from internal needs or external events. Communication ideas may or may not relate to preceding contextual events or linguistic information. The communication idea must be transformed into a communication act for transmittal to another person.

Recognition of Communicative Desire and Need

Comprehension of a linguistic or contextual message and identification of an internal communication idea does not ensure recognition of the need or desire to communicate. A lack of communicative desire can stem from a variety of sources. For example, an individual with a pragmatic deficit may not realize that a speaker expects a response; a severely fatigued, inattentive, or depressed individual may not wish to communicate; an individual who believes he or she is faced with a demeaning or difficult communicative task may choose not to interact linguistically.

One step in analyzing communication breakdowns is determining whether a person with aphasia recognizes communicative needs and has a desire to communicate. If the individual does not consistently recognize communicative needs, initiation of communication acts may have to be external. For example, the communication partner may have to initiate communication acts repeatedly and provide clear encouragement for the stroke survivor to respond. If the adult with aphasia recognizes communicative needs but shows little or no interest in communicating, the speech-language pathologist and caregivers must determine what factors are discouraging communication attempts and work to minimize those factors. Only after a person with aphasia recognizes a communicative need and wants to interact communicatively with others will he or she be ready to initiate the formulation of messages.

Initiation

The initiation of messages can be either internal or external. Internal initiations originate with the speaker; external initiations originate with someone other than the speaker—typically a communication partner. External initiation often takes the form of providing key words to the adult with aphasia or repeatedly prompting the initiation of responses with semantic or phonological cues.

Message Formulation

Formulation refers to an individual's attempt to symbolize an intended message. Some adults with aphasia can formulate messages with natural speech, gestures, and vocalizations. Others need augmentative strategies to formulate messages but can implement these strategies independently. Still others can only formulate messages given external assistance in the form of aided AAC strategies or another person.

Whether message formulation is performed independently or with assistance, it is successful only when the listener comprehends the speaker's intended meaning (Arwood, 1983). This means that the message must be accurate, complete, and presented in a comprehensible form (Grice, 1975; Searle, 1969). If it is not, some form of message revision will have to precede successful communication.

Message Revision. Many persons with aphasia attempt to revise messages that they have not executed successfully. Speakers can perform revisions by repeating messages, altering semantic and/or syntactic forms, or adding additional modalities for conveying information (e.g., supplementing speech with gestures, pictures, or written words). Some adults with aphasia successfully and independently revise the majority of their messages; others experience intermittent success in revising messages; still others are rarely successful and require assistance to initiate and perform meaningful revisions.

Externally Assisted Message Formulation. When persons with aphasia cannot independently formulate messages, they may benefit from external assistance. This assistance can be from other people or from augmentative devices or materials such as partner-generated written choices or picture books. In either case, the first step is recognition of the need for external assistance. As with other steps in the communication process, some persons with aphasia fail to recognize or act on this need and, hence, experience communication breakdowns. The reason for these breakdowns is not always clear but may relate to (a) limited awareness of the potential benefit of seeking assistance in particular communication situations; (b) limited technical competence in using AAC technology; (c) perceived negative attitudes of listeners, family members, and friends about the need for assistance with communication; or (d) limited self-confidence in operating AAC devices.

Recognition of Messages from Options.   Once the person with aphasia recognizes and acts on the need for external assistance, successful exchange of a communication idea is dependent on the individual's skill at identifying the appropriate message from available options. This is sometimes a relatively simple task requiring only identification of a target word or picture from a limited choice group. At other times, the task is considerably more complex, such as when the individual must recall a message's location in a multilevel AAC system. Although some adults with aphasia can access messages or symbols stored in multilevel systems and simultaneously keep pace with the time demands of ongoing conversation, many more experience difficulty recognizing and selecting appropriate communication messages. This difficulty may reflect a problem locating the AAC device itself, selecting the appropriate category or level, or identifying the target message. When such difficulties are encountered, partner support in the form of cues to locate a specific message area or to generate choices that are relevant to the immediate situation may be beneficial.

A listener's comprehension of a message marks the end of a communication act. At that point, the speaker and listener have the choice of ceasing their interaction or continuing with a new communication idea.

Styles of Social Interaction

In addition to the assessment information outlined above, the selection of an appropriate AAC intervention is dependent on an understanding of the person's anticipated level of interaction with others and participation in the community. Some individuals may have participated minimally in family and community interactions prior to their aphasia. It is unrealistic to expect that aphasia will encourage them to become more active participants. On the other hand, other individuals may have played active roles in family and community communications and may want to resume much of this interaction. For these individuals, the anticipated level of participation interaction with others may be quite high. AAC strategies and devices should appropriately complement an individual's level and style of social interaction.

AAC INTERVENTION: ENHANCING SOCIAL PARTICIPATION

Once the preliminary assessment of an aphasic individual's communication needs, capabilities, and constraints has been performed, AAC intervention can be initiated. The basic goal of this intervention is to enhance the individual's participation in social interactions.

Each person with aphasia has unique communication needs, capabilities, and constraints. As a consequence, a personalized approach to AAC intervention is necessary, with modifications made as needs and capabilities change. To illustrate intervention processes, five case reviews are presented in the following section. The reviews describe AAC approaches developed for persons with widely differing communication needs and capabilities. Included are examples of (a) augmented message initiation and formulation, (b) augmented language comprehension, (c) independent augmented communication, (d) augmented verbal revisions, and (e) augmented contextual comprehension. Each review provides general background information, a brief summary of speech and language assessment findings, an analysis of AAC processes following the framework outlined earlier, and a description of the AAC strategies and techniques used to maximize the individual's communicative effectiveness.

Case Review One: Augmented Message Initiation and Formulation

Background

Warren was a 63-year-old teacher who sustained a massive left cerebrovascular accident (CVA). He remained in an acute care hospital for 1 month. Warren was slow to regain general alertness because of the severity of his stroke and complications related to blood sugar fluctuations. He was most alert when family members were present but did not speak and made infrequent attempts to nod his head when asked yes/no questions.

Warren's awareness of his surroundings improved steadily during the second week of his hospitalization. The nursing staff determined that he knew basic hospital routines and schedules because he consistently looked at a clock just prior to the arrival of his medication or meal tray. His communication attempts continued to be limited to basic gestures. After 4 weeks, Warren was transferred to a rehabilitation hospital for intensive therapy. By then, his blood sugar levels were relatively stable and his overall endurance had improved significantly.

Assessment of Capabilities and Communication Needs

Capabilities.   On initial evaluation, Warren's rehabilitation team rated his prognosis for functional recovery as fair. His physical therapist focused on wheelchair mobility and prevention of chronic spasticity in his right extremities. His occupational therapist worked on increasing functional movements in his right arm and improving living skills necessary for his return home. Warren's speech-language pathologist focused intervention efforts on regaining basic receptive and expressive communication skills.

Warren received an aphasia quotient of 4.6 on the Western Aphasia Battery (Kertesz, 1982), placing him in the category of global aphasia. Warren's clinician observed extreme difficulty in his processing of decontextualized auditory information but relatively good environmental awareness. For example, Warren would anticipate his clinician's arrival and would clear his lap tray of extraneous materials in preparation for therapy sessions. However, he could not initiate or repeat any verbalizations, relied solely on gesturing to communicate basic needs, and became easily frustrated when asked anything other than routine social questions (e.g., "How are you?").

Communication Needs. Warren had been working as a teacher/administrator until his stroke. He participated extensively in community organizations and was an extremely social individual with many close friends and colleagues. His children no longer lived in the immediate area, but he called them frequently and visited with them several times a year.

Warren's communication needs assessment (Beukelman et al., 1985) indicated wide-ranging needs. Most basic was his inability to communicate physical needs to the nursing staff. Also, because Warren could not relate specific information and was inconsistent in matching communication ideas to externally provided messages, he needed guidance in comprehending the verbal choices presented by others.

Another of Warren's communication needs was to reestablish social interactions. Warren could not answer questions posed by others and could not communicate important information about himself or the events of his day. Hence, his speech and language difficulties severely limited his use of communication to interact socially. Despite this, Warren was still capable of communicating social etiquette information by greeting and thanking visitors with a warm handshake or nod of his head.

Assessment of Communication Partner Capabilities. Warren was clearly dependent on others to support his communication efforts. To determine the capabilities and needs of his primary communication partner, Warren's wife completed a partner skill screening form (see Fig. 17.1). From her responses, it was evident that she needed to learn to pause after her husband's communication efforts, to alert him before she spoke, to reduce the complexity of her questions, and to use alternative means of facilitating Warren's communication.

Analysis of Warren's Communicative Interactions

The speech-language pathologist analyzed Warren's interactions using the AAC process analysis framework (see Fig. 17.2). The analysis revealed that:

1. Warren's strength was contextual comprehension. He demonstrated recognition of others, appreciation of his grandchildren's antics, readiness for therapy sessions, and interest in local newspapers and family photographs.
2. Warren had many communication ideas and had a strong desire to communicate. He frequently pointed and gestured to indicate immediate physical needs. He attempted to participate in social conversations but did not persevere when communication breakdowns occurred.
3. Because of receptive aphasia, Warren sometimes needed external initiation to respond to questions.
4. The severity of Warren's expressive aphasia was such that he needed encouragement to attempt message formulations. His difficulty mapping language onto ideas interfered with his ability to formulate messages without external assistance. He could not retrieve or encode symbolic units and was dependent on externally available symbols to communicate information. Furthermore, Warren could not locate external symbols without direct assistance from others.

Components of Warren's AAC System

Conversational Written Choices. Warren's speech-language pathologist selected social communication as the initial focus of intervention. Because Warren had extreme difficulty

Instructions

1. Start a conversation by writing a topic at the top of the page. Use your knowledge of the person to come up with an interesting topic. For example, if the person has an obvious physical or medical need, write the word "need" or "pain" on the top of the page. Interesting conversational topics include hobbies, current events, politics, sports teams, advice, pets, and family.
   Hint: Write in large, clear block letters.
2. Ask a starter question. Anticipate possible answers and write them in the form of word choices or rating scales (see example).
   Hint: Write choices vertically with a dot in front of each.
   Read the choices aloud while you write them.
3. Encourage the person to point to his or her answer.
   Hint: Sometimes you have to provide physical assistance to help the person initiate pointing.
4. Circle his or her answer. Then add your own thoughts or comments.
5. Follow up with another question.
6. Continue until you have exhausted the topic.

Example

Friend:	Can you give me advice on what to make for the school bake sale tomorrow?
Aphasic:	[nods yes]
Friend:	Should I take an angel food cake, brownies, or cookies? [writes choices vertically in notebook] * ANGEL FOOD CAKE * BROWNIES * COOKIES
Aphasic:	[points to brownies]
Friend:	Yes, those always sell fast! [circles brownies] Should I make them from scratch or get a box mix? [writes choices] * SCRATCH * BOX MIX
Aphasic:	[laughs and points to box mix]
Friend:	[laughs and circles box mix] Yeah, it's more work to make them from scratch! [pause] What do you think about the kids' elementary school? Do you think they're getting a good education or a so-so one? [writes rating scale]

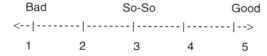

Aphasic:	[hesitates, points to 4]
Friend:	[circles 4] Yeah, we're pretty happy with the school district. Too bad the classes are so big, though!
Aphasic:	[nods yes]

Figure 17.3. Written choice explanation.

processing decontextualized information, treatment materials were restricted to personally relevant information in hopes of facilitating his language comprehension. Warren's clinician employed the technique of Written Choice Conversation (Garrett and Beukelman, 1992) to ask questions about a topic of interest to Warren (see Fig. 17.3). After asking each question, the clinician wrote possible answers in large capital letters. She read the answers aloud as she wrote them and encouraged Warren to point to his response selection. Warren initially needed assistance scanning the written options and pointing to his answer. Gradually, however, he improved and could participate in conversations requiring answers to a series of questions, each with three to five response options presented.

Warren's therapist realized that he would not continue interacting with others unless his communication partners learned the written choice technique. She encouraged Warren's wife and sons to attend therapy sessions to learn the technique. After mastering written choice communication, family members were able to ask Warren for his opinions about school and home events. The family also used the written choice strategy to resolve communication breakdowns when Warren initiated messages.

Stored Information System.   Warren's wife constructed a photo album depicting his life and accomplishments. Warren often used the album to share information with others. As Warren gained competence in using the album to facilitate communication, other materials were added, such as a map of his home state, a list of his fellow teachers, and his children's phone numbers. This prestored information allowed Warren to communicate some specific information without being dependent on a partner to offer appropriate choices. However, Warren could not initiate a complete communication sequence with these materials, seldom thought to open the album himself, and typically needed assistance to locate target pages.

Gestures.   Warren slowly developed a repertoire of self-initiated gestures to express basic needs such as drinking, opening a window, and going to the bathroom.

Case Review Two: Augmented Language Comprehension

Background

Dennis was a 52-year-old construction worker who sustained a CVA without warning in late July. During his brief hospitalization, a computed tomography (CT) scan revealed a small to moderate infarct in the third temporal gyrus of the left hemisphere. Within a week, Dennis regained his ability to walk and use his right hand for gross motor and fine motor activities. The slower recovery of his communication skills prompted Dennis's participation in outpatient speech and language therapy.

Assessment of Capabilities and Communication Needs

Capabilities.   Dennis's ability to manage independently at home was his speech-language pathologist's primary concern. Dennis displayed moderate to severe anomia and semantic paraphasias coupled with auditory comprehension breakdowns for linguistic material beyond the level of social speech and simple commands. He could not recognize errors in his language production.

Communication Needs.   Dennis's speech-language pathologist performed an analysis of his communicative interactions and met with his wife and son to discuss their concerns about his speech and language. The family initially focused on difficulties related to word retrieval and word substitutions. With time, however, family members improved at interpreting Dennis's messages, and their primary concern shifted to Dennis's comprehension difficulties. These were most evident with presentation of complex or specific information. Dennis's family was also concerned about the difficulty he had changing topics; Dennis would often continue commenting about one subject long after his communication partner(s) had switched to a new topic.

Dennis demonstrated needs in all communication domains: expressing wants and needs, sharing information, and using language for social closeness and social etiquette purposes. However, unlike some other expressively impaired communicators, Dennis's needs originated primarily from his difficulties understanding others.

Assessment of Communication Partner Capabilities. Dennis's wife completed the Partner Skill Screening Form (see Fig. 17.1). Although she was effective in facilitating some aspects of communicative interactions with Dennis, she was not effective with others. Specifically, she did not alert him before beginning a message and did not supplement her messages with written words or gestures.

Analysis of Dennis's Communicative Interactions

Dennis's pattern of communication interactions was analyzed with the AAC process analysis framework (see Fig. 17.2). His strengths and deficits included the following:

1. Good contextual awareness
2. Intact communication ideas, recognition of need to communicate, and adequate formulation of messages without external assistance
3. Moderate impairment of language comprehension

Components of Dennis's AAC System

Written Key Words.   Dennis's clinican devised a relatively simple intervention technique to support the comprehension of auditory information. She noticed that writing key words as they were spoken greatly facilitated Dennis's understanding. He could appropriately answer questions and add information to conversations given this supplemental written information. Dennis quickly began to rely on written words to augment his comprehension, and the technique was easily taught to his wife and son. Dennis was given a card (see Fig. 17.4) describing his disability and instructing unfamiliar communication partners to write key words as they conversed. Dennis taped the card to the cover of a notepad that he carried with him at all times.

Supplemental Gestures.   The clinician also observed that Dennis comprehended more of her conversation when she provided simultaneous gestures. For instance, when asking about his physical therapy sessions, Dennis's clinician pointed in the direction of the gym and pantomimed riding an exercise bicycle. Dennis responded to supplemented questions quickly and accurately. This strategy was also taught to Dennis's wife and son.

Ultimately, Dennis's clinician, wife, and son learned to supplement all auditory messages with a combination of writing, drawing, and gesturing. Dennis learned to wait for this supplemental input and, at times, requested it if unclear about the meaning of a message. By late August, Dennis still had moderate auditory comprehension problems that prevented his return to work. However, he was successfully using augmented comprehension strategies with friends and community members, thereby minimizing communication breakdowns.

```
I HAVE HAD A STROKE. SOMETIMES IT IS DIFFICULT
FOR ME TO UNDERSTAND WHAT YOU SAY.

IF I LOOK PUZZLED, DON'T TALK LOUDER.
DO USE THIS NOTEBOOK TO:

   1. WRITE DOWN IMPORTANT WORDS YOU SAY
   2. WRITE DOWN WHAT YOU THINK I SAID—THAT
      WAY I CAN CHANGE IT IF IT'S WRONG
   3. WRITE DOWN THE NAME OF THE TOPIC
      (ESPECIALLY IF YOU CHANGE IT FAST)

SEEING OUR CONVERSATION IN PRINT REALLY
HELPS. THANKS FOR TAKING THE TIME.

_____

   NAME:
   ADDRESS:

   PHONE:
```

Figure 17.4. Disability description and AAC instruction card.

Case Review Three:* Independent Augmented Formulation

Background

Mike was 74 years of age and had sustained two left-hemisphere CVAs during a 4-year period. Both strokes affected Mike's speech and language functioning and prompted his participation in rehabilitation programs. Three years of individual and group therapy at a university speech and hearing clinic followed Mike's inpatient rehabilitation for severe aphasia resulting from the second stroke. Even with this extended period of treatment, Mike's natural speaking abilities were insufficient to meet his communication needs.

Assessment of Capabilities and Communication Needs

Capabilities. A review of Mike's speech and language intervention records revealed that he had a mild receptive language deficit compounded by a moderate, bilateral sensorineural hearing loss for high frequencies. Expressively, Mike experienced much greater difficulty than he did receptively. He successfully expressed his communicative intent only about 20% of the time using natural speech, thus experiencing extensive communication failure. Even with familiar partners, communication interactions were lengthy and inefficient. With unfamiliar partners, who had no knowledge of his communication strategies or personal background, communication breakdowns were virtually constant.

Mike's performance on the Western Aphasia Battery gave him an aphasia quotient of 34.6. Table 17.1 summarizes his performance results.

An analysis of Mike's communication strengths revealed that he was aware of his environment and the principles of interpersonal communication. He demonstrated a strong desire to communicate and used some compensatory strategies to resolve communication failure. His compensatory strategies included using a number of supplementary, nonformalized gestures; attempting to spell words that he could not say; and identifying locations on simple maps. He did not spontaneously draw to clarify messages, although he could replicate simple line drawings.

Communication Needs. Mike was retired and lived with his wife, daughter, and granddaughter. Despite his age and medical problems, Mike had a relatively active life-style and participated in activities such as visiting friends and going to restaurants and the racetrack. He traveled alone much of the time, using buses and taxis.

Mike's communication needs assessment (Beukelman et al., 1985) revealed a complex set of communication needs. He interacted with many different communication partners and in multiple contexts. He needed to communicate a wide variety of messages depending on the partner and the context.

Analysis of Mike's Communicative Interactions

Conversations between Mike and his daughter, Mike and his wife, and Mike and an unfamiliar student clinician were videotaped. These interactions were analyzed using the AAC process analysis framework (see Fig. 17.2). The analysis revealed that:

1. Mike was contextually aware.
2. Mike comprehended the spoken and gestured messages of familiar and unfamiliar partners with only occasional requests for repetition. He never required augmented comprehension strategies to understand his partners.
3. Mike expressed many communication ideas and displayed a strong, almost irrepressible, desire to communicate. The tapes revealed both internally and externally initiated communication interactions.
4. Mike demonstrated a number of different message formulation patterns. At times, he successfully formulated and expressed messages on the first attempt. Often, however, he was unsuccessful either in formulating a complete message or in expressing it so that his partner understood. Occasionally, he successfully revised a message, but frequently he experienced communication failure after several revision attempts. He waved his hand to signal that he was abandoning a message and moving on to a new communication idea.
5. Mike spontaneously attempted to resolve communication breakdowns by using alternative modes of communication. His most frequent supplement to natural speech was to gesture or pantomime a message or an element of a message. Although some of his gestures were well executed, Mike tended to use single gestures for a variety of different messages, thus confusing his communication partners. In addition, some gestures were contextually confusing to listeners. For example, Mike tried to indicate that his wife had made an emergency phone call by lifting his hand to his ear and moving it in a rotary motion. To the young adult who was his communication partner at the time, the gesture was incomprehensible because she had grown up with push button rather than "crank" phones.

   When Mike could locate an alternative representation of a message, he willingly used augmentative communication strategies. For example, he often "unloaded" his billfold to search for a small calendar or a Nebraska football schedule to clarify a date. One time he selected a five dollar bill from his billfold to indicate the number "5." Mike actively scanned his environment for people, objects, and characteristics (size, color, category, etc.) that he could use to clarify a message. He had no difficulty selecting specific items from large groups of objects and did not require a facilitator to select and present objects for him.

---

*Portions of this case study were previously reported by Garrett et al., 1989.

Table 17.1.
Test Data from the Western Aphasia Battery

Subtest	Results
I. Spontaneous speech	
Content	6 (Correct response to 4 of 6 items)
Fluency	4 (Halting, telegraphic speech)
II. Auditory verbal comprehension	60/60
Auditory word recognition	53/60
Sequential commands	51/60
III. Repetition	26/100
IV. Naming	31/60
Word fluency	8/20
Sentence completion	5/10
Responsive speech	6/10
Aphasia quotient: 34.6/100	

From Garrett, K., Beukelman, D. R., and Low-Morrow, D. (1989). A comprehensive augmentative communication system for an adult with Broca's aphasia. *Augmentative and Alternative Communication, 5,* 56. Copyright 1989 by Williams & Wilkins. Reprinted by permission.

6. Occasionally, the identification of an object or item would cue Mike to name the item; however, he usually communicated by simply pointing to the item.

Reviewing Mike's interaction skills assisted his speech-language pathologist in developing an AAC system to supplement his natural speech and gestures. Because Mike's communication needs were extensive and varied, the AAC system contained a number of components.

Components of Mike's AAC System

Word Dictionary. Because Mike could accurately identify single words and short phrases, because he could sometimes cue his verbalization of single words by reading printed words, and because he could receptively identify single words and phrases, a word dictionary served as a valuable augmentative communication device for him. Over several months, Mike, his family, and his clinican identified an extensive number of words to include in the dictionary. Words were classified into eight categories: family, food and restaurants, sports, personal history, places, personal care items, phone numbers, and time references (month, o'clock, etc.) Mike's relatively intact semantic organization system prompted organization of the words by category. Additional structure resulted from alphabetizing the words within each category. Some words were also organized according to narratives that Mike was particularly fond of relating. This supplemental organizational strategy allowed rapid selection of words and issues related to specific topics.

Alphabet Card. Mike was limited in his ability to spell words. However, he was sometimes successful in identifying the first letter of a word or spelling common abbreviations. To facilitate letter identification and spelling, the 25 alphabet letters were displayed on a card for him. Although his accuracy was inconsistent, Mike's identification of a word's initial letter sometimes facilitated his listener's comprehension. In addition, Mike frequently was able to produce a word after identifying its first letter.

New Information Pocket. The new information pocket allowed Mike to carry remnants about current events. His favorites were clippings from the newspaper and mementos from the race track—items that sometimes became tattered from

	CLUES
IT'S A:	PERSON
	PLACE
	EVENT
	THING
	TIME
I'LL DESCRIBE IT:	COLOR
	SIZE
	WHAT IT'S MADE OF
	WHAT IT DOES
	SOMETHING ELSE

Figure 17.5. Clue phrases in communication notebook.

their repeated use. These remnants allowed Mike to transfer information from one context to another and to introduce new conversation topics. He selected items for the new information pocket by himself and decided when to discard each item.

Breakdown Resolution Clues. A card containing communication breakdown resolution clues was developed so that Mike could guide his communication partners in efforts to rectify communication breakdowns (see Fig. 17.5). This card contained clues guiding a communication partner through a structured form of "20 questions" to arrive at the desired information. For example, Mike could use the breakdown resolution card to encourage his partner to confine guesses to a person, place, thing, event, or time.

Conversational Control Strategies. Although Mike appeared to be quite competent in conversational pragmatics, he had some difficulty "managing" conversations to ensure effective interactions. This problem most often occurred during efforts to resolve communication breakdowns. A card listing conversational control strategies (see Fig. 17.6) was included at the end of Mike's communication notebook. He used these strategies most frequently when interacting with new communication partners. With familiar partners, he only needed to signal topic changes and terminations.

DIRECTIONS

GUESS THE WORD
ASK ME QUESTIONS
I'M CHANGING TOPIC
WE WILL STOP

Figure 17.6. Control phrases in communication notebook.

Natural Communication Modalities

Mike used his AAC system to supplement his speech and natural gestures. He continued to rely extensively on natural communication modalities and, consequently, was encouraged to systematize his use of informal gestures. Prior to intervention on gesture usage. Mike tried to communicate multiple messages with single gestures. The result, of course, was confusion on the part of his listeners.

Mike's clinician also encouraged him to write and draw as augmentative communication strategies. Although quite willing to attempt writing, Mike was initially reluctant to draw pictures. He viewed himself as having little artistic ability. However, given time and encouragement, drawing eventually became an option for Mike—although always one that he chose reluctantly.

Before development of his communication system, Mike wrote on whatever scraps of paper he could find. This led to problems when Mike wanted to refer to something written earlier. To eliminate this problem, Mike learned to insert blank pages in his communication notebook to write abbreviations or initial letters of words or to sketch diagrams or drawings.

System Consolidation

To consolidate the elements of Mike's communication system, a 5- by 8-inch communication notebook was constructed. Each component was identified with a tab. Within some components, especially the word sections, subtabs further organized information.

Although Mike had demonstrated use of the various components of his AAC system when they were presented separately, he initially had difficulty choosing the most efficient mode of communication when presented with the entire system. This was especially true during conversations in which a communication breakdown occurred. At these times, Mike sometimes repeated a communication attempt seven or eight times before shifting to an alternative strategy. To combat this problem, Mike's clinician divided the various components of his AAC system into three different levels or tiers (see Fig. 17.7). During intervention, Mike was to attempt communication through natural speech first. If that was unsuccessful, he was to use a Level 1 strategy followed, if necessary, by a Level 2 strategy and then a Level 3 strategy. All strategies were represented with color codes and labels on a large chart, which was in full view during intervention sessions. After several months of practice, Mike had fully mastered his AAC system and used it effectively to supplement his speech.

A final aspect of Mike's AAC system was a list of instructions to his communication partners. Because Mike frequently conversed with unfamiliar partners, instructions on the front cover of his communication book (see Fig. 17.8) served to introduce people to Mike's communication system. When Mike

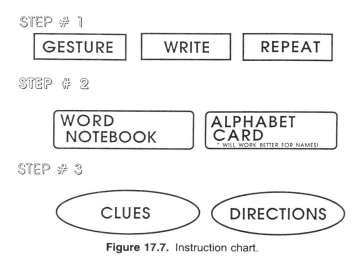

STEP # 1

| GESTURE | WRITE | REPEAT |

STEP # 2

| WORD NOTEBOOK | ALPHABET CARD *WILL WORK BETTER FOR NAMES! |

STEP # 3

| CLUES | DIRECTIONS |

Figure 17.7. Instruction chart.

MIKE J.
STREET ADDRESS
LINCOLN, NE ZIP
(PHONE)

HELLO.
MY NAME IS MIKE J.
I HAVE HAD A STROKE.
THIS IS NOT A WALLET.
IT HELPS ME COMMUNICATE.
I WILL SHOW YOU WHAT I NEED OR WOULD LIKE
TO SAY BY POINTING TO THE WORDS IN THE BOOK.

IF THE WORD I WANT IS NOT IN THE BOOK, I WILL TRY
TO POINT TO THE FIRST LETTER OF THE WORD.

I WILL ALSO POINT TO SOME DEFINITIONS IF WE NEED
EXTRA HELP.

THANK YOU FOR HELPING ME.

Figure 17.8. Communication book instructions.

initiated a conversation with a new partner, he would first present the list of instructions to the individual. Then, this energetic, elderly man could interact with and entertain anyone who was willing to cooperate with his augmented communication system.

Case Review Four: Augmented Verbal Revisions

Introduction

Although persons with relatively mild aphasia often experience communication deficits that interfere with their life-styles, professionals seldom consider AAC approaches when attempting to facilitate their communication interactions. The following case study documents one man's use of AAC techniques to compensate for mild anomia.

Background

Don was 37 years old when he fell down a flight of stairs and struck his head. He was unconscious when he was found.

An initial neurological examination revealed a large hematoma covering much of the parietal lobe of his left hemisphere. Don was transported by air ambulance to a regional medical center where surgeons evacuated the hematoma and removed damaged brain tissue. Following this surgery, Don had great difficulty communicating simple messages. He was confused and demonstrated extensive word-finding problems. Over the next few months, he recovered rapidly but continued to display a persistent anomia.

Assessment of Capabilities and Communication Needs

Capabilities. While Don was in rehabilitation, he spoke fluently despite severe anomia. His ability to say specific words was not enhanced by phonemic cuing or verbal imitation; however, seeing a word in print often cued his production of it. Although Don experienced extreme difficulty in verbal naming, he could spontaneously write the words that he could not verbalize.

Don's auditory comprehension skills were much less impaired than his verbal naming. He correctly identified common objects, pictures, and printed words in response to verbal stimuli. Don could also follow verbal commands with good accuracy.

Communication Needs. Prior to his accident, Don had completed a masters degree and taught in a community college. He lived alone and enjoyed a wide variety of outdoor activities. Six months after the accident, Don returned to independent living. Although he no longer taught, Don worked at the community college in a maintenance/landscaping position.

Don reported significant improvement in his communication during inpatient rehabilitation. Although he thought that his communication had continued to improve following discharge from the rehabilitation unit, Don's persistent word-finding problems prevented his return to a postsecondary teaching position.

During the communication needs assessment (Beukelman et al., 1985), Don reported that spoken and written anomia interfered with his ability to express precise information such as names, locations, and events. Aside from his word-finding problems, he experienced no difficulties interacting with a wide range of individuals. Don believed that his communication problems resulted from his failure to relate sufficient content and were minimally affected by listener or contextual changes.

Analysis of Don's Communicative Interactions

Conversations between Don and a speech-language pathology intern and between Don and a medical resident were videotaped. With the intern, Don discussed his communication needs; with the medical resident, he discussed the status of his seizure disorder. The videotaped interactions were analyzed using the AAC process analysis framework (see Fig. 17.2) and yielded the following observations:

1. Don was contextually aware.
2. Don comprehended spoken and gestured messages adequately.
3. Don initiated communication ideas promptly and appropriately.
4. Don demonstrated an eagerness to communicate that was appropriate for the context.
5. Don engaged in both internally and externally initiated interactions.
6. Don successfully formulated and expressed most messages; however, he was often unsuccessful when relating specific content. At

times, he experienced communication failure. At other times, his communication partner resolved breakdowns by providing a correct target word.
7. When shown the written form of a target word, Don could usually say the word accurately.

To assist Don's compensation for anomia, his clinican developed an AAC system for him. Don needed very little training to use the system and, within a month, had taken responsibility for selecting items for inclusion in the system.

Components of Don's AAC System

The purpose of Don's AAC intervention was development of a communication notebook to supplement his natural speech. Within a few weeks, Don decided that he preferred several small notebooks to the single large one that his clinician had suggested. Don's final AAC system consisted of three notebooks, each 3 by 5 inches in size.

For the most part, Don refers to the notebooks to remind himself of a target word and say it. He then continues with his conversation. Occasionally, when he cannot say a target word or message, he turns the notebook around so that his communication partner can read the target word or message. The contents of the three notebooks are organized according to (*a*) general conversation; (*b*) medical, financial, and legal information; and (*c*) current events and experiences.

General Conversation. Don uses one of his AAC notebooks to support general conversation. The first several pages list the complete names, addresses, and phone numbers of many different people. Additional information, such as occupations, hobbies, and family relationships, is included after some of the names. The names are organized by contexts (e.g., work, friends, church, family), and there is a location subheading under each. For example, Don organizes the names of people from his church according to the town or region where they live. As Don meets new people, he has them add their names under the appropriate headings.

Don has a large number of names listed in his AAC notebook. He has reported that remembering people's names is one of his most difficult tasks. He has also indicated that, because he lives alone, knowing the last names of people and their phone numbers is important to him.

Don's general conversation book also contains a list of places, towns, business, and buildings. Where appropriate, phone numbers and names of key people are listed as well. In addition, Don has a small paperback atlas of national and state maps included in his general conversation notebook. At the back of the atlas, he has glued a fold-out map of his county. Don refers to these maps when he recounts stories of his vacations and the experiences of his extended family.

Medical, Financial, and Legal Information. Don's second AAC notebook contains medical, financial, and legal information. Included are several sections for the names of people, companies, facilities, and places associated with Don's medical, financial, and legal affairs. The notebook contains detailed information about Don's insurance policies, agents, and companies. In addition, there is a section containing words associated specifically with insurance, such as *liability, comprehensive, term, permanent,* and *maturity.*

The medical section of Don's AAC notebook contains brief notes—probably entered by physicians and nurses—regarding his ongoing medical treatment. Apparently, Don requests that someone jot down a few sentences each time he has a medical visit. Pharmaceutical information is also listed with the date of each prescription and the person who authorized it.

In addition, the medical section contains a narrative about Don's medical history since his accident. The medical history information is surprisingly detailed. In addition to general information about his injury, treatment, recovery, and continuing problems, Don included the names of the professionals with whom he has worked and described their involvement in his recovery process. When asked about the detail of the narrative, Don smiles and says, "Doctors like that."

Current Events and Experiences. Don's third AAC notebook consists of several small manila envelopes. The envelopes contain remnants about recent episodes in Don's personal and community life. These include such items as newspaper articles, ads for fishing equipment and clothing, recent church bulletins, and a list of "things to do this month" from a local newspaper. Don uses these items to supplement his narratives and cue his production of detailed information. For example, while visiting with a group of people, Don used a newspaper article describing his nephew's high school basketball team to supplement his conversational interactions.

Maintenance of Don's AAC System

Don's anomia persists. He continues to use his AAC system and has assumed responsibility for keeping it current. Occasionally, a friend types handwritten pages that Don has added to his notebooks, but, other than this, Don is independent in using and maintaining his communication system.

Case Review Five: Augmented Contextual Comprehension

Background

Verna was an 82-year-old woman with a history of cardiac problems. She sustained a left CVA of embolic origin along with a heart attack and a brief period of anoxia. Verna had difficulty regaining consciousness and did not respond to any stimulation for 2 weeks. During the third week, she occasionally opened her eyes for brief periods.

Verna was seen for initial speech-language and occupational therapy consultations at the beginning of the fourth week of hospitalization. The medical team and the rehabilitation therapists decided that the most appropriate placement for Verna would be a subacute rehabilitation unit until her stamina and responsiveness improved.

Assessment of Capabilities and Communication Needs

Capabilities. A speech-language pathologist saw Verna twice daily for 15-minute sessions. When Verna was seated in a wheelchair, she maintained alertness during most treatment sessions; however, she quickly fell asleep during bedside sessions. Verna opened her eyes in response to her name approximately 75% of the time.

Verna had severe communication and cognitive limitations. She displayed a right-sided neglect and probable right visual field cut. She did not follow any simple commands or imitate sounds, words, or oral postures. When asked to point to pictures of family members, Verna occasionally picked up pictures to examine but did not point to any. She did not respond when asked her about personal care needs or comfort and communicated protest, discomfort, and pleasure solely through body postures and movements.

One of the few positive signs of Verna's cognitive status was her ability to track visually the movement of people in her room. Despite this, she appeared minimally aware of routine events and activities around her. Her sole interaction with the environment was to pick up a deck of cards placed on her night stand and randomly shuffle it.

Communication Needs. Because of Verna's extensive language and cognitive impairments, her treatment team doubted that she would regain social interaction skills or the ability to communicate specific information. The immediate need was to assist Verna in communicating basic wants about her care. The burden of initiating and interpreting communication attempts fell on Verna's communication partners.

Analysis of Verna's Communicative Interaction

Verna demonstrated extremely severe deficits that interfered with all levels of communication processing. She had a profound impairment in contextual comprehension that prevented her participation in communicative interactions. Until the contextual comprehension deficits diminished, concerns about Verna's language comprehension, generation of communication ideas, recognition of the need to communicate, and formulation and revision of messages were irrelevant.

AAC Treatment Strategies

Treatment focused on improving Verna's environmental awareness and participation in functional routines. Her clinician targeted two prelinguistic treatment goals: (*a*) enhancing visual attention to the environment and (*b*) encouraging functional choice selection on a nonlinguistic level.

To address the treatment goals, the clinician capitalized on natural opportunities to direct Verna's attention to events in the environment and to make choices about personal care routines. For instance, the clinician observed that Verna sometimes looked in the mirror and touched and primped her hair. This prompted him to begin each treatment session with a discussion about Verna's hairdo. He held out a small mirror and said, "How does your hair look?" Initially, Verna required assistance to reach out and grasp the mirror but soon began reaching for it herself. Then, Verna's clinician asked if she liked her hair and verbally interpreted her facial expression. If her expression was of puzzlement or dislike, Verna's clinican would offer her a choice of styling aids such as a brush, curlers, bobby pins, or hairspray. He offered her only two items at a time, presenting each slowly and pantomiming its function. He then placed her hands on both items and gave her the one she held for the longest. By interpreting Verna's facial expressions and physical actions, her clinician encouraged her to associate behaviors with events.

By the end of the second week of treatment, Verna was making one or two choices per session about her personal care. With continued practice, her visual attention to people and target objects gradually increased. Although she still could convey her desires only in highly contextualized situations, Verna was able to indicate preferences about her personal care.

Follow-Up

Verna was dismissed from speech and language therapy at the end of 1 month because of lack of funding. Her family continued to use highly contextualized, choice-making activities to determine her personal care preferences. She was given the opportunity to make personally relevant choices (e.g., selecting an outfit) whenever possible. Verna eventually learned to answer some questions when presented with written choices but died before progressing to more advanced levels of communication.

FUTURE TRENDS IN AAC FOR PERSONS WITH APHASIA

Continuing advances in AAC intervention are likely to have substantial effects on the treatment of persons with aphasia. One probable effect will be the increased use of AAC strategies and techniques to enhance the early and long-term communication effectiveness of aphasic adults. A second likely effect will be the development of assessment materials and training programs to further the application, transfer, and acceptance of AAC systems in hospital, rehabilitation, and community settings. In particular, clinicians will need tools to determine the status of the residual communication skills necessary for the use of AAC strategies and will need materials to teach partners to interact with AAC users. The third area likely to be affected by growth in the field of AAC concerns the efforts of researchers to document effective communication intervention for aphasia. Studies will focus on how AAC interventions affect natural speech recovery for some individuals with aphasia, as well as how AAC affects the communicative effectiveness of those who have more limited residual speech and language skills. In addition, investigations will serve to identify the skill and knowledge levels necessary for adults with aphasia to achieve communicative competence using various AAC strategies and devices.

References

American Speech-Language-Hearing Association. (1989). Competencies for speech-language pathologists providing services in augmentative communication. *ASHA, 31,* 107–110.

American Speech-Language-Hearing Association. (1991). Report: Augmentative and alternative communication. *ASHA, 33* (Suppl. 5), 9–12.

Ansell, B. J. (1991). Slow-to-recover brain-injured patients: Rationale for treatment. *Journal of Speech and Hearing Research, 34,* 1017–1022.

Arwood, E. (1983). *Pragmaticism: Theory and Application.* Rockville, MD: Aspen Systems Corp.

Baker, B. (1982). Minspeak: A semantic compaction system that makes self-expression easier for communicatively disabled individuals. *Byte,* pp. 186–202.

Baker, B. (1986). Using images to generate speech. *Byte,* pp. 160–168.

Beukelman, D. R., and Mirenda, P. (1992). *Augmentative and alternative communication: Management of severe communication disorders of children and adults.* Baltimore, MD: Paul H. Brookes.

Beukelman, D. R., Yorkston, K., and Dowden, P. (1985). *Communication augmentation: A casebook of clinical management.* Austin, TX: Pro-Ed.

Carlson, F. (1985). *Picsyms categorical dictionary.* Lawrence, KS: Baggeboda Press.

Garrett, K., and Beukelman, D. R. (1992). Augmentative communication approaches for persons with severe aphasia. In K. Yorkston (Ed.), *Augmentative communication in the medical setting.* Tucson, AZ: Communication Skill Builders.

Garrett, K., Beukelman, D. R., and Low-Morrow, D. (1989). A comprehensive augmentative communication system for an adult with Broca's aphasia. *Augmentative and Alternative Communication, 5,* 55–61.

Grice, H. (1975). Logic in conversation. In P. Cole and J. Morgan (Eds.), *Syntax and semantics: Speech acts.* New York: Academic Press.

Hyper-ABLEDATA (Compact Disk). Madison, WI: Trace Research and Development Center.

Johnson, R. (1981). *The picture communication symbols* (Book 1). Solana Beach, CA: Mayer-Johnson Co.

Johnson, R. (1985). *The picture communication symbols* (Book 2). Solana Beach, CA: Mayer-Johnson Co.

Kates, B., and McNaughton, S. (1975). *The first application of Blissymbolics as a communication medium for nonspeaking children: History and development, 1971–74.* Don Mills, Ontario: Easter Seals Communication Institute.

Kertesz, A. (1982). *Western Aphasia Battery.* New York: Grune & Stratton.

Light, J. (1988). Interaction involving individuals using augmentative and alternative communication systems: State of the art and future directions. *Augmentative and Alternative Communication, 4,* 66–82.

Lyon, J., and Helm-Estabrooks, N. (1987). Drawing: Its communicative significance for expressively restricted aphasic adults. *Topics in Language Disorders, 8,* 61–71.

Marshall, R. (1987). Reapportioning time for aphasia rehabilitation: A point of view. *Aphasiology, 1,* 59–73.

Mergler, N., and Goldstein, M. (1983). Who are these old people? *Human Development, 26,* 72–90.

Miller, J. D., Pentland, B., and Berrol, S. (1990). Early evaluation and management. In M. Rosenthal, E. R. Griffith, M. R. Bond, and J. D. Miller (Eds.), *Rehabilitation of the adult and child with traumatic brain injury* (2nd ed., pp. 21–51). Philadelphia, PA: F. A. Davis.

Rosenbek, J., LaPointe, L., and Wertz, R. (1989). *Aphasia: A clinical approach.* Austin, TX: Pro-Ed.

Searle, J. (1969). *Speech acts.* London: Cambridge University Press.

Skelly, M. (1979). *Amer-Ind gestural code based on universal American Indian hand talk.* New York: Elsevier-North Holland.

Stuart, S. (1991). Topic and vocabulary use patterns of elderly men and women of two age cohorts. Unpublished doctoral dissertation, University of Nebraska–Lincoln, NB.

Stuart, S., Vanderhoof, D., and Beukelman, D. R. (1993). Topic and vocabulary use patterns of elderly women. *Augmentative and Alternative Communication.*

Trace resourcebook: Assistive technologies for communication, control, and assessment. Madison, WI: Trace Research and Development Center.

Appendix 17.1

AAC Symbol Sets Cited in the Chapter

Blissymbolics, Blissymbolics Communication International, 250 Ferrand Dr., Suite 200, Don Mills, Ontario M3C 3P2, Canada.

Brady-Dobson Alternative Communication Symbols, Ginny Brady-Dobson, 89623 Demming Rd. Elmira, OR 97437.

Oakland Schools Picture Dictionary, Oakland Schools Communication Enhancement Center, Waterford, MI 48328.

Pictogram IdeoGrama Communication Symbols, George Reed Foundation for the Handicapped, 1919 Scarth St., P.O. Box 1547, Regina, Saskatchewan, S4S 1V5, Canada.

Picsyms, Baggeboda Press, 1128 Rhode Island Ave., Lawrence, KS 66044.

Pick 'N Stick, Imaginart Communication Products, 307 Arizona St., Bisbee, AZ 85603.

Picture Communication Symbols, Mayer-Johnson Company, P.O. Box AD, Solana Beach, CA 92075-0838.

Rebus Symbols, American Guidance Services, Circle Pines, NM 55014.

Self Talk, Communication Skill Builders, 3830 E. Bellevue, P.O. Box 42050, Tucson, AZ 85733.

Sigsymbols, Don Johnston Developmental Equipment Company, P.O. Box 639, Wauconda, IL 60084.

Talking Pictures, Crestwood Company, 6625 Sidney Pl., Milwaukee, WI 53209.

Trace Research and Development Center, S-151 Waisman Center, 1500 Highland Ave., Madison, WI 53705.

Prentke-Romich Company, 1022 Heyl Rd., Wooster, OF 44691.

Adaptive Communication Systems, Inc., 354 Hookstown Grade Rd., Clinton, PA 15206.

Zygo Industries, Inc., P.O. Box 1008, Portland, OR 97207.

Sentient Systems Technology, Inc., 5001 Baum Blvd., Pittsburgh, PA 15123.

Words +, Inc., P.O. Box 1229, Lancaster, CA 93535.

Tolfa Corporation, 1860 Embarcadero Rd., Palo Alto, CA 94303.

CHAPTER 18
Use of Amer-Ind Code by Persons with Aphasia

PAUL R. RAO

OVERVIEW OF APHASIA AS A HANDICAPPING CONDITION

Aphasia has been defined as "an acquired impairment of language processes underlying receptive and expressive modalities and caused by damage to areas of the brain which are primarily responsible for the language function" (Davis, 1983). Persons with severe aphasia are among the most likely candidates for a nonverbal approach to functional communication. Collins (1990) provides an operational definition of the most severe variety of aphasia as a "severe, acquired impairment of communicative ability, which crosses all language modalities, usually with no single communicative modality substantially better than any other. In addition, visual, non-verbal problem solving abilities, as well as other cognitive skills, are often severely depressed and are usually compatible with language performances" (p. 113). This chapter will concentrate on persons with severe aphasia for whom traditional approaches of aphasia treatment may not have been beneficial or productive.

Another way of operationalizing the "functional issues" with severe communication impairment is to place this discussion with the framework of the World Health Organization's (1980) Model of Consequences of Pathology: "Impairment (dysfunction at the organ level), disability (functional consequences of impairment that affect performance of daily tasks), and handicap (social disadvantage resulting from an impairment or a disability)." Hence, in this context, severe aphasia would be an impairment that results in a functional communication disability that may often pose some degree of communication handicap.

A simple definition of handicap is that it is a "limitation of choice." It is precisely in this area of "choice" that the rehabilitation professional must attempt to minimize the handicap in severe aphasia by maximizing communication options. The following three macro approaches to aphasia rehabilitation may be employed to meet this challenge:

- *Enhance functional capacity* by assisting the person with severe aphasia to change behavior through functional communication treatment. (See Aten's Chapter 14 for an elaboration of the myriad of methods for getting a message across.)
- *Reduce demands of the environment* by removing noise in the system (e.g., turning off the TV) and optimizing transmission of signals (e.g., having action pictures in a communication book available). (See Lubinski's Chapter 13 for amplification on the environmental approach to rehabilitation.)
- *Provide assistive devices and/or alternative methods* by determining the menu of core needs and abilities, then training the person with severe aphasia in the use of alternative communication options to convey wants and needs (the use of Amer-Ind Code is an example of this approach). (See Beukelman's Chapter 17 for an extensive review of the augmentative communication issues.)

NATURE OF LANGUAGE AND COMMUNICATION

Although the terms "language" and "communication" are frequently employed interchangeably, for the purposes of this chapter it is essential to distinguish them. Language and communication are not synonymous. Indeed, according to Holland (1975), adults with aphasia are better communicators than they are language users. She adds that "every aphasia therapist has experienced moments of superb communication with patients whose language was either minimal or unintelligible" (p. 4). Oral or manual language is a code with structured properties characterized by a set of rules for producing and comprehending spoken or signed messages. Functional communication, as defined by the ASHA Advisory Panel (ASHA, 1990), is "the ability to receive a message or to convey a message, regardless of the mode, to communicate effectively and independently in a given environment." While spoken language usually serves as the primary means for communication, the communication process also makes use of a variety of other tools such as intonation, facial expression, eye movements, and body gestures, including motions of the hand and the head. When language is used to communicate, language and communication may be said to overlap. However, when the language-impaired adult attempts to communicate, the differences between language and communication become clearly evident. This dissociation between language and communication is noted by Holland (1975): "It is usually suprasegmental, gestural, and contextual cues that are most heavily relied upon by the aphasics we have observed" (p. 4). This chapter will focus on Amer-Ind Code, a form of gestural communication that has been used as a functional communication tool to meet needs when language no longer works.

AMER-IND CODE: A NONLANGUAGE GESTURAL SYSTEM

Amer-Ind Code is based on Native American Hand Talk. According to Skelly-Hakanson et al. (1982), Hand Talk was developed thousands of years ago to provide communication among Native American tribes with widely different linguistic systems. In establishing the Amer-Ind Code adaptation, Skelly (1979) has deleted the more culturally specific of the historical signs as well as those deemed inappropriate for clinical use. Novel signals were created (e.g., drive) and several historical signals were modified before the system was standardized by Skelly (1981a) over the past decade. Amer-Ind Code is primarily a demonstrable, expressive system that was designed to meet the functional daily needs of adult surgical patients such as those with normal cognitive abilities who have had a laryngectomy (Skelly et al., 1975).

Since signals represent concepts rather than words, Amer-Ind Code signals are discussed in terms of a repertoire instead of a vocabulary. Each concept may stand for several English words, since Amer-Ind Code does not follow a signal-for-word translation. Hence the current, clinically tested signal repertoire of 236 labels has an English vocabulary equivalent of nearly 2,500 words. Of the 236 concept labels, 131 are normally executed by one hand and the remaining 105 signals are normally produced with two hands. The latter signals were adapted for one-hand execution for use with individuals who do not have both hands available for signaling, such as hemiplegic stroke patients.

The advantages of Amer-Ind Code are that it is concrete, pictographic, highly transparent, easily learned, and telegraphic, and it does not make use of functors or grammar (Rao and Horner, 1980). Amer-Ind Code is recognized cross-culturally, since its iconic basis provides a concrete representation of the referent object. The Amer-Ind Code repertoire is said to be universally recognizable, similar to the international road signs. Hence, when a signaler indicates thumbs down with a frown, the viewer recognizes the message as "bad." This "guessability" factor has been referred to as the signal's transparency.

The transparency of Amer-Ind Code is an important research and clinical issue. Skelly (1979) and her colleagues completed several projects to document signal transmission, with the resultant claim that the corpus of Amer-Ind Code signals is between 80% and 88% "guessable" to naive viewers. More recent evidence suggests that Amer-Ind Code may be more accurately described as approximately 50% transparent to naive viewers (Daniloff et al., 1983; Kirschner et al., 1979). Although this transparency factor is much less than Skelly reports, it remains significantly more transparent than the 10% to 30% reported for American Sign Language (ASL) signs (Griffith et al., 1981). This latter form of gestural communication is often confused with Amer-Ind Code. ASL is the manual language of the deaf and is distinct from nonlanguage gestural systems such as Amer-Ind Code. One who does not know ASL would require each ASL symbol to be translated into his or her own language in order to understand what the message is. Griffith et al. (1981) reported that normal viewers found ASL to be only 20% transparent. However, one who has never encountered Amer-Ind Code before would not require the Code to be translated, because of the aforementioned iconicity and transparency (Daniloff et al., 1983). Kirschner et al. (1979) have demonstrated

that Amer-Ind Code is easier to learn in a brief period of time and is retained more easily than ASL signs. Even within ASL signs, the role of iconicity in sign language learning has been found to be a crucial factor in sign recognition and retention. Lieberth and Gamble (1991) found that "iconicity may play an important role in the selection of an initial lexicon for the non-verbal client. Iconic signs may be learned more easily and quickly and retained longer than non-iconic signs" (p. 90). (See also Lloyd et al. [1985] for a comprehensive discussion of iconicity in sign acquisition.)

Amer-Ind Code's superior gestural transparency and retention, in conjunction with its relative ease of production, has prompted several investigators to suggest that iconic, simple signals are the easiest ones to teach individuals with a severe communication impairment (Coelho, 1990, 1991; Duncan and Silverman, 1978; Fristoe and Lloyd, 1980; Lloyd and Daniloff, 1983; Rao and Horner, 1980; Skelly 1979). If this intuitive clinical hypothesis is accurate, Amer-Ind Code would indeed be an appropriate gestural system to facilitate functional communication in brain-injured adults.

Amer-Ind Code Populations

Amer-Ind Code has been used successfully with the following four populations (Skelly, 1979):

1. Linguistically intact, for example, after glossectomy or patients on voice rest
2. Linguistically delayed, for example, developmentally delayed
3. Linguistically disordered, for example, persons with aphasia
4. Linguistically intact with a phonological or motor speech disorder, for example, persons with verbal apraxia or anarthria.

Amer-Ind Code Validation Studies

The ability for adults with aphasia to recognize Amer-Ind Code signals was first studied by Daniloff et al. (1982). This study examined the relationship between the impairment of Amer-Ind Code recognition and the severity of aphasia and primary language skills. Administration of an Amer-Ind Recognition Test to 15 subjects with aphasia resulted in all subjects performing equally well, regardless of their aphasia severity classification. These data contrast markedly with the school that studied pantomime rather than Amer-Ind Code. Duffy and Duffy (1981), who studied pantomime rather than Amer-Ind Code, concluded that there is a clear and significant association between gesture recognition and production and language under the umbrella term "asymbolia." According to these authors, "Aphasia is best understood as a general impairment of symbolic communication that includes nonverbal as well as verbal deficits." This line of research was further investigated by Coelho and Duffy (1987) when they studied the relationship between successful acquisition of manual signs ($N = 37$, 23 of which were Amer-Ind Code signals) and degree of aphasia severity in 12 subjects with chronic, varying degrees of severe aphasia. This study demonstrated a clear and significant relationship between aphasia severity and success in the acquisition and generalization of manual signs. Results also suggest that there may be a threshold of aphasia severity below which acquisition of manual signs is negligible (e.g., a PICA below the 35th percentile). The apparent discrepancy between intact (Daniloff et al., 1982) and impaired gestural recognition (Duffy and Duffy, 1981) was investigated by Rao (1985), who found no differences between normal persons and brain-injured subjects on the Amer-Ind Recognition Test (N = 50 Amer-Ind Code signals), but a significant difference on Amer-Ind imitation (subject imitating examiner's 50 signals) and production tasks (subject demonstrating object usage of 10 pictured items).

Beyond the transparency issues between Amer-Ind Code and ASL that were discussed earlier, several studies also examined other contrasting issues between these two distinct gestural systems. Daniloff et al. (1986) examined Amer-Ind Code versus ASL recognition and imitation in aphasia and found that Amer-Ind Code signals were consistently easier to recognize and imitate than matched ASL signs. In another study, Guilford et al. (1982) explored the acquisition and use of Amer-Ind Code versus ASL. Their eight adult subjects with aphasia received 2 hours of instruction for 4 weeks on 20 signs from each system. Results indicated that there was no difference in the subjects' ease of acquisition between the sign systems. However, this study defined "acquisition and use" as the ability to produce a sign on command. It must be cautioned that this ability does not ensure that the patient will be able to *use* these signs spontaneously to meet activities of daily living (ADL) needs. Finally, Daniloff and Vegara (1984) studied the motoric constraints for Amer-Ind Code formation versus ASL. They compared the 236 Amer-Ind Code signals and their ASL counterparts. It was found that ASL signs were indeed more complex than Amer-Ind Code signals, since ASL requires the use of two hands rather than one, involves a greater variety of hand shapes, requires more overall movement, and necessitates a greater number of changes in hand orientation during production. In sum, Amer-Ind Code has generally been found to be superior to ASL in terms of the recognition, imitation, and production of the two systems by adults with aphasia.

Amer-Ind Code Selection Considerations

Prior to selection of Amer-Ind Code for use with a communicatively impaired individual, the clinician must decide if the patient's skills are appropriate for such a system and if the system has the potential for meeting the patient's functional communication needs. Yorkston and Dowden (1984) concluded that appropriate selection of a gestural system is dependent on the clinician's understanding of the characteristics of each system, "specifically the symbolic load, motoric complexity, and communicative function of the system." Musselwhite and St. Louis (1988) list many other factors that must be considered in matching an unaided signal or symbol system to an individual with a severe communication impairment. These other factors include cognitive abilities, size of vocabulary, grammatical structure of system, and ease of learning (transparency, availability of communication partners, and availability of support methods and training). Analyzing these potent factors and considering the above validation studies, it may be concluded that, at least for severely impaired adults with aphasia, Amer-Ind Code is superior to ASL in achieving functional communications.

USES OF AMER-IND CODE BY PERSONS WITH APHASIA

Amer-Ind Code has three potential applications for the person with aphasia: (*a*) as an alternative means of communication, (*b*) as a facilitator of verbalization, and (*c*) as a deblocker of

other language modalities. In 1979, Skelly reported on six earlier projects summarizing the use of Amer-Ind Code by 161 adults with aphasia. The results of these projects, although fairly positive, were often flawed by poor subject controls, no therapy control, and haphazard designs. Christopoulou and Bonvillian (1985) provide a comprehensive literature review regarding the use of sign language, pantomime, and gestural processing in persons with aphasia. They conclude that many individuals with aphasia who fail to regain spoken language skills may retain the ability to acquire aspects of a manual communication system. "Overall, the aphasia subjects appeared to be less impaired in their visuomotor processing than in their auditory-vocal processing. The results, however, are not definitive enough to resolve the long standing debate as to whether or not a central deficit is present aphasia" (Christopoulou and Bonvillian, 1985). Several case studies are presented below to highlight the various uses of Amer-Ind Code with adults with aphasia.

Alternative Means of Communication

Heilman et al. (1979) reported on a patient with global aphasia following a left cerebrovascular accident (CVA). The patient was trained to communicate effectively with Amer-Ind Code. He learned 100 signals and was able to sequence them in a series of three or more. This study supports the impression that Amer-Ind Code can be used successfully with severe, even global, aphasics for meeting their daily needs. Rao et al. (1980) reported on the use of Amer-Ind code by four adults with severe aphasia who had no functional expressive language skills. Two subjects who had plateaued in traditional treatment were enrolled in an Amer-Ind Code program. The remaining two subjects were enrolled in both traditional and code programs concurrently on the commencement of their rehabilitation program. All subjects made progress as reported by the patient's significant other and supported by the clinician's impression, though pre- and postaphasia test results did not reflect significant change. It was suggested that pre- and postmeasures that tap linguistic skills do not appear to be the best indicators of a patient's communication progress using Amer-Ind Code. As Skelly (1977) pointed out in an early Amer-Ind workshop, "Just as we do not measure apples with a ruler, so we should not measure use of the *code* with a language measure."

J.C., who presented with severe Broca's aphasia following a left CVA, was enrolled in a 6-month Amer-Ind Code treatment program. His admission Aphasia Quotient (AQ) on the Western Aphasia Battery (WAB) (Kertesz, 1980) was 17.4, and his discharge AQ was 27.10. However, perhaps more reflective of J.C.'s excellent attainment of functional communication skills was his discharge score of 129/136 on the Communication Abilities of Daily Living (CADL) (Holland, 1980). In addition, he demonstrated a 94% acquisition level of the Amer-Ind Code core repertoire on command and on written word stimulation. The patient served as a nonverbal volunteer at a VA Medical Center for 5 years after the conclusion of treatment, as a superior patient escort, demonstrating the merits of Amer-Ind Code on a daily basis.

Finally, R.J., a 72-year-old male with jargon aphasia, demonstrated the efficacy of aphasia treatment in general and a combined graphic and gestural approach specifically. R.J. presented with global aphasia as a result of a CVA in 1985. He had a

2-year history of aphasia treatment without notable results, followed by a 3-year hiatus from any form of therapy. At the request of the patient's daughter, a speech-language pathology (SLP) reevaluation was conducted nearly 5 years postonset and more than 3 years after the termination of any form of communication intervention. R.J. served as his own control in a single-subject experimental design examining the efficacy of a novel, intensive, treatment regimen commenced 5 years postonset. Treatment effects and/or spontaneous recovery were clearly absent as extraneous variables. Initially, R.J.'s aphasia was so severe and his language so perseverative that no formal testing could be administered. Following 10 weeks of aphasia treatment that focused on gesture and drawing as expressive modalities, R.J. was discharged home. The patient's initial and final functional communication status was rated using the ASHA Functional Communication Measures (Larkins, 1987), in which 0 = totally dependent and 7 = totally independent. The results were as follows:

Functional Communication Measures	Admission Status	Goal	Discharge Status
Comprehension of Spoken Language	3	5	4
Comprehension of Written Language	2	5	4
Comprehension of Nonspoken Language	4	6	6
Production of Spoken Language	2	4	3
Production of Written Language	2	4	3
Production of Nonspoken Language	4	6	5

Results of Treatment: At discharge, R.J. had demonstrated:
1. Functional repertoire of 30 Amer-Ind Code signals
2. 90% accuracy on WAB (Kertesz, 1980) Word Reading subtest
3. 90% accuracy on WAB (Kertesz, 1980) Yes/No Questions subtest
4. The ability to draw ADL needs with a high degree of transparency

Customer Satisfaction: R.J.'s daughter corresponded 3 months postdischarge with the following testimonial:

This is to keep you abreast of how dad has sustained his progress since working with you. He has initiated "letters" to his son in California who writes to him every week. He also has written to me several times and enclosed a bird's-eye view drawing of his neighborhood with the streets labeled correctly and the route of his daily walk marked in red. His salutation and signature are correct, but the words in the text of the letter are copied randomly from books. Nevertheless, they are extremely heartwarming to receive and make us feel more connected to him. He is able to negotiate his medication with housekeepers and relatives now. As you know, most of his medication was withdrawn, and so now he sometimes feels pain from his arthritis. Previously he would have panic attacks if he noticed any change of medication routine. Now he is able to trust that he is communicating, both sending and receiving accurately enough to adjust his own pain medication. At his son's wedding in Chicago, his brothers and sisters-in-law noted that he seemed more relaxed, happy, and healthy. *He indeed gestured and drew pictures for them and clearly indicated that he was happy with the results of his hospitalization.* I game him a VCR when he left here. He now indicates to his housekeeper through drawing that he wants a National Geographic, opera, or drama video rented for him. He also communicated with a drawing to my aunt that he needed a new razor. I can't tell you how full of gratitude my heart is toward you and everyone who worked with us at the hospital. Bless you and thank you. Sincerely, K.J.

Conclusion: Results of R.J.'s 6-week SLP treatment regimen highlight significant receptive and expressive gains that were documented by formal tests, functional outcome measures, a consumer satisfaction measure, and periodic patient and family correspondence. Efficacy issues as well as significant implications for using unconventional treatment approaches with persons exhibiting chronic, severe aphasia, were outlined in this case study. It is worth noting that the entire inpatient and outpatient stay was preauthorized, paid, and well documented. Can one put a dollar value on a 72-year-old individual, 5 years post left CVA, who finally began to live life more fully as a result of rehabilitation? The customers (the patient, the daughter, and the payor) appeared to be quite satisfied with the outcome.

Facilitator of Verbalization

Skelly et al. (1974) reported on the effects of Amer-Ind Code as a facilitator of verbalization for apraxic patients without aphasia. She noted that all six patients had mastered 50 signals within the first 6 months and were able to interpret over 200 signals. In addition, Skelly reported an increase in verbal output when speech was accompanied by gesture. This increase of verbal output was confirmed by an increase in verbal scores on the Porch Index of Communicative Ability (PICA) (Porch, 1967). Skelly concluded that Amer-Ind Code was an effective facilitator of verbalization in nonlanguage-impaired patients with verbal apraxia. (See Rosenbek et al. [1989] for a detailed description of an Amer-Ind Code training program that was designed to facilitate verbalization. The three-step program consists of sign selection, training, and combining gesture with speech.)

Dowden et al. (1982) attempted to answer the question, "Does Amer-Ind Code facilitate aphasic-apraxic verbal communication?" Using only two severely aphasic/apraxic subjects, they attempted to replicate the earlier study by Skelly et al. (1974). Unfortunately, their results fail to replicate the earlier Skelly study, since they found no measurable change from baseline on the PICA overall or on the verbal percentile following either training or maintenance. What they did find, however, was that one of their two subjects demonstrated a sharp decrease in the proportion of verbal responses and a marked increase in the proportion of nonverbal and combined responses on the CADL (Holland, 1980) following completion of the Amer-Ind Code treatment regimen.

Deblocker of Other Language Modalities

Snead and Solomon (1977) found that some global aphasics comprehended more when Amer-Ind Code was employed. They therefore suggested that Amer-Ind Code should be incorporated in diagnostic and treatment strategies to increase the likelihood of "gaining entry into each global aphasic." Gesture has been included as part of a cuing hierarchy in testing (Porch, 1967) and as a language facilitator in treatment (Rao and Horner, 1978). (See section on "Efficacy and Prognosis" in this chapter for a fuller description of the latter case.)

AMER-IND CODE TREATMENT

Core Lexicon

The selection of an initial Amer-Ind Code signal repertoire for adults with severe aphasia (Rao et al., 1980) was based on:

1. Ease of production
2. ADL relevance to a veteran population
3. High transparency

The Amer-Ind Code limited repertoire consisted of five sets of 10 signals that met the above selection criteria. It is suggested that clinicians consider each patient's unique ADL needs and motoric constraints and also consult the transparency data by Daniloff et al. (1983) and the Amer-Ind recognition data by Rao (1985) before arriving at a decision regarding a core Amer-Ind Code repertoire (consult also Lloyd and Daniloff [1983]). Sample contrasting needs that were included in the core lexicon were hot and cold, eat and drink, shave and comb, and yes and no. Rao (1985) found near-perfect performance of the left CVA patients with aphasia ($N = 12$ patients) on the Amer-Ind Recognition Test ($N = 50$ signals).

The fact that subjects with aphasia (Rao, 1985) were able to recognize Amer-Ind Code signals—even with difficult foils (motor, semantic, and semantic/motor)—as well as were normals underlines the obvious dissociation between language and signal processing. The following eight Amer-Ind Code signals were recognized by all normals, left CVAs, and right CVAs on the Amer-Ind Recognition Test: drink, glasses, fight, telephone, sleep, time, cold, and dive (Rao, 1985). Hence an initial core of treatment signals should include ADL-type needs such as drink, sleep, cold, and time. Amer-Ind Code is an iconic signal system that appears to be well suited for use with adults with aphasia whose sign system is disordered, but whose signal system is intact. (See Appendix 18.1 for a partial listing of Amer-Ind Code signals and corresponding transparency levels.)

Treatment Suggestions

Skelly (1981b) has highlighted six procedures that enhance Amer-Ind Code signal transmission and comprehension:

1. *Slow down.* According to Skelly, 70% of problems of transmission are due to speed of signaling.
2. *Additive signal(s).* Generally, the fewer the signals, the better, though on occasion, more signals may be called for to convey a message.
3. *Alternative signal(s).* Patient and clinician should be able to signal a message in at least two different ways.
4. *Negative contrast.* Employ the negative to rephrase a message (e.g., Mad Not = Happy).
5. *Questions.* In the event of a confused message, the receiver should clarify the message by signaling who, what, where, etc.
6. *Reality testing.* Set up a "mock" interaction with a patient and a trained Amer-Ind Code receiver to work out what the patient's real ADL needs are, such as buying medicine or getting a haircut.

Amer-Ind Code Treatment Hierarchy

Once the clinician has selected Amer-Ind Code as a treatment modality, the clinician then must determine where to begin. Periodically, one may see a person with global aphasia who not only is nonverbal but also is nonstimulable for using hand gestures. This nonstimulable, nonverbal patient would not yet be a good Amer-Ind Code candidate. Helm-Estabrooks et al. (1982) developed a treatment program to get just such a patient ready for a gestural treatment program. Their visual action therapy (VAT) is a method designed to train persons with global aphasia to produce symbolic hand gestures for hidden items. VAT employs a hierarchically structured, trilevel program that ranges from tracing eight objects with the hand, such as a hammer and a razor, to producing pantomimed gestures for absent objects. According to Helm-Estabrooks et al. (1982), VAT is a means to an end, and not an end unto itself. Once the patient has demonstrated the ability to produce simple hand gestures, VAT may be discontinued and the Amer-Ind Code treatment hierarchy initiated.

Rao et al. (1980) developed a treatment hierarchy for training persons with aphasia in the use of Amer-Ind Code. The hierarchy moves along the following task continuum:

1. *Demonstration.* The clinician demonstrates the use of gestures in functional communication situations before and after the treatment session in order to validate the code's communication value as well as its acceptability.
2. *Recognition.* The concept that "recognition precedes production" is probably valid in a gestural training program as well as in a verbal one. Can the patient point to an object from an array, once the function of a given object is demonstrated?
3. *Imitation.* The patient imitates selected gestures under various stimulus conditions.
4. *Replication.* Remember, practice makes permanent. The patient gestures a signal without a model in response to either a spoken or written command.
5. *Consolidation.* Review and refine recognition, imitation, and replication of signals. Begin use of signals with the patient in a natural communication environment outside of the clinic, stressing the use of the patient's core repertoire.
6. *Retrieval.* The patient is required to demonstrate/use the core repertoire in context and without a model.
7. *Initiation.* The patient initiates basic messages during gestural communication with the clinician or a significant other.

A potentially useful training paradigm at the consolidation stage is a matrix approach introduced by Tonkovich and Loverso (1982). They trained four adults with chronic aphasia using various pairs of signals in a 4×8 matrix (four verbs and eight nouns), and found that each subject was able to acquire novel gestures in a relatively short period of time and to maintain these gestures over time. This last stage, generalization, is indeed the most difficult to achieve and the most critical one for independent functional communication. The crux of the training complaints with severely aphasic patients is that clinicians may establish gestural recognition and imitation and some use in therapy, but there is little or no carryover to functional communication situations. Coelho (1990) did find that moderately to severely aphasic subjects can acquire single manual signs and a variety of basic combinations. The key was severity—that is, those subjects who acquired the most signs were the least impaired. Generalization was attainable, but subjects required additional "extraclinical" training to become proficient in the use of signs to convey a message. This finding is consistent with that of Coelho (1991), who concluded that propositional use of manual signs by aphasic subjects rarely follows a routine of simple acquisition and generalization of signs to untrained settings. This crucial step *does not* occur without additional training in natural communication situations.

The case of R.J. presented previously illustrates the following training strategies that proved invaluable in fostering generalization.

- *Address other nonverbals:* Prior to addressing a gesture for a given stimulus, facial expression, tone of voice, and other nonverbals were prompted. On presentation of a picture of ice cream, a smile and "mmm" sound preceded the gesture for eat or hungry.

Table 18.1.
Amer-Ind Scale of Progress[a]

Level	Label	Description	Use
X	Transfer	Verbal more than 50%	
IX	Facilitation	Verbal less than 50%	Facilitation of verbalization
VIII	Propositional	Equivalence	
VII	Conversational	At least three interchanges	Alternative means of communication
VI	Initiation	One interchange	
V	Transition	Wavers between IV and VI	
IV	Retrieval		
III	Replication	Long-term memory—no model	
II	Imitation	Short-term memory	
		Model present	
I	Recognition	Appropriate behavioral response to clinician's signal	Deblocker of other language modalities

[a] Adapted from Skelly, M. (1979). *Amer-Ind Gestural Code based on Universal American Indian Hand Talk.* New York: Elsevier.

- *Involve consumer in signal selection:* The original repertoire of 50 was "cut down" to 30 by the patient, who wished to delete gestural signals he did not need and signals for referents that he could either point to or draw just as easily or did not need.
- *Build in environmental support:* R.J.'s primary communication partners were oriented to Amer-Ind Code and were instructed to encourage R.J.'s use of gesture. Staff who were so oriented were housekeeping, nursing, dietary, the unit manager, and the receptionist for each therapy area.
- *Encourage risk taking:* Much preparatory time was spent fostering more and varied responses to a given stimulus. The patient was constantly advised that the absence of *any* response or initiative guarantees the absence of communication.

Amer-Ind Code Scale of Progress

The Amer-Ind Scale of Progress (Table 18.1) describes 10 levels of increasing competence in the use of Amer-Ind Code signals (Skelly, 1979). Skelly recommends that the scale be followed in training patients to use the signals, because it is believed that signal recognition, execution, and retrieval lead to self-initiation and propositional use. The highest levels include gestural facilitation of verbalization and, finally, verbalization with some gestural support. Hence the scale of progress is a task continuum, the goal of which is achievement of any of the three potential uses of the code with adults with aphasia.

The Amer-Ind Scale of Progress should be regarded as a treatment barometer that can be used to document progress in the use of Amer-Ind Code over time. It can also be used to determine which use of the Code is most appropriate for the patient, and which level is ultimately attainable.

EFFICACY AND PROGNOSIS

The crucial question in discussing a novel approach to aphasia treatment is, "Does it work?" Aphasiologists are concerned not only about whether aphasia therapy is efficacious but also about whether specific approaches are efficacious. The following case (Rao and Horner, 1978) supports the impression that not only does aphasia therapy work, but Amer-Ind Code in particular works. In this case, gesture was used to deblock

Table 18.2.
Deblocking via Gesture[a]

Auditory vs. Gesture Recognition		
Listen (object name)	—Point	60%
Watch gesture	—Point	100%
Point vs. Gesture Response		
Listen	—Point	60%
Listen	—Gesture	100%
Deblocking via Gesture		
Listen—then—gesture—then	—Point	90%

[a] From Rao, P., and Horner, J. (1978). Gesture as a deblocking modality in a severe aphasic patient. In R. Brookshire (Ed.), *Clinical Aphasiology Conference proceedings.* Minneapolis, MN: BRK.

listening, reading, and speech through a systematic pairing procedure (Table 18.2).

P.J. is a right-handed 38-year-old male with a B.S. degree who was self-employed. He presented with aphasia following left-hemisphere surgery for aneurysm repair. The patient awakened from surgery "with a profound right hemiplegia and was mute. He was initially evaluated at 6 months postonset (*with no history of speech treatment*), at which time he was described as profoundly aphasic, receptively and expressively. There was a paucity of speech overall; speech was spontaneously neologistic with poor imitation. Before Amer-Ind Code Treatment, the most striking residual ability was in the *gestural modality*. He recognized gestures, and he spontaneously produced gestures. P.J. was provided an intense Amer-Ind Code treatment program, and within 8 months learned 80 Amer-Ind Code signals.

During training and stabilization of Amer-Ind Code, a deblocking program was conducted. That is, gesture by the clinician and by the patient was systematically paired on "both" receptive tasks of listening and reading and expressive tasks of imitation and naming.

To summarize this case (see Table 18.3), prior to the Amer-Ind plus Traditional treatment course, *gesture was relatively spared* both *receptively* and *expressively*. Treatment involved systematic pairing of gesture with auditory stimuli and gesture with printed

Table 18.3.
Receptive-Expressive Language Deblocking via Gesture[a]

PRETREATMENT			POSTTREATMENT	
Input	Output		Input	Output
GST	GST		AUD	GST
			VIS	VBL

TREATMENT	
Input	Output
GST	GST
+	+
AUD	VBL
+	
(VIS)	

[a] From Rao, P., and Horner, J. (1978). Gesture as a deblocking modality in a severe aphasic patient. In R. Brookshire (Ed.), *Clinical Aphasiology Conference proceedings.* Minneapolis, MN: BRK.
GST = gesture, AUD = auditory, VIS = visual, VBL = verbal.

words (on the input side) and systematic pairing of gesture with verbal imitation and naming performances (on the output side).

Posttreatment status found input and output modalities to be significantly improved. It was thought that this was due to the increased automaticity of transcoding processes effected through gestural deblocking procedures. Using Amer-Ind Code signals, alone or in combination with speech, P.J. was a functional communicator at 18 months postonset. Specifically, this means that P.J. could get his message across by using gesture expressively in three ways: gesture alone, a contemporaneous gesture-verbal combination, or a sequence of gestures followed by verbals.

Possible Prognostic Indicators for Amer-Ind Code Treatment

A tentative list of prognostic variables includes the following: residual language ability, visual recognition and reasoning ability, learning ability, modality preference (Is this patient willing to use gesture in place of, or accompanying, speech?), limb praxis, motivation, and acceptance. Pretreatment abilities specifically pertinent to Amer-Ind Code, and perhaps the most salient prognostic indicators, include gesture recognition and gesture production, including object use, imitation, and spontaneous use.

Horner (1980) summarized the Amer-Ind Code prognostic issue by noting that a patient is a good Amer-Ind Code treatment candidate if:

1. A preference for the verbal modality can be shifted to a preference for gestures.
2. Gestural recognition is preserved.
3. Manual/limb praxis is preserved in the presence of severe oral-verbal apraxia.
4. Manifest limb apraxia is predominantly ideomotor rather than ideational.

Table 18.4.
Patient G.G.: Biographical and Medical Data

Biographical	Medical
Age: 56	Date of onset: 10-24-76
Sex: Male	Type of CVA: Left cerebral thrombosis
Education: High school	Sequelae: Aphasia and right hemiplegia
Marital status: Married, 8 children	Perception: Moderate high-frequency sensorineural
Handedness: Dextral	hearing loss bilaterally;
Environment: Home	wears corrective lenses
Occupation: Retired lumber inspector	Earlier medical history: Myocardial infarction (1972)

Table 18.5.
Patient G.G.: Initial Speech and Language Findings (September, 1979)[a]

ALPS (max 10):	Listening = 5.5; Talking = 1 Reading = 4.5; Writing = 5.5		
BDAE (auditory):	Word Discrimination = 64.5/72 Body Part Identification = 18/20 Commands = 14/15 Complex Ideational = 2/12		
PPVT (max = 50):	89		
Ceiling:	115		
TACL (max = 101):	82		
YES/NO (max = 20):	19		
Boston Naming Test (max = 85):	7		
		Oral	Limb
Apraxia Battery	Imitation	2.3	3.6
(max = 4):	Command	0.7	2.3
Initial Diagnosis: Moderate to severe Broca's aphasia and severe oral apraxia			

[a] ALPS = Aphasia Language Performance Scales; BDAE = Boston Diagnostic Aphasia Examination; PPVT = Peabody Picture Vocabulary Test; TACL = Test of Auditory Comprehension of Language.

5. Manifest limb apraxia is mild or moderate rather than severe in degree, and perseveration is minimal or absent.
6. Dependence on real object and/or imitative cues for gestural production can be resolved rather quickly.
7. Transient cues are as effective as static cues in eliciting gestures.
8. Gestures can be stimulated with a broad range of stimulus types and methods rather than idiosyncratic cues.
9. Impulsivity can be controlled.
10. Most important, the patient demonstrates an ability to learn elicited or responsive gestures after trial therapy, and evidence for generalization across setting, however rudimentary, is observed.

APPLICATIONS OF AMER-IND CODE TO PACE THERAPY

G.G. is one of three subjects reported on by Rao and Koller (1982). He was 35 months postonset before he was referred for a speech and language evaluation. As Table 18.4 reveals, the patient's biomedical background was fairly unremarkable, except for the fact that he had no prior history of speech treatment. Table 18.5 presents pertinent speech and language data that corroborate the initial diagnosis of moderate to sever Broca's aphasia and severe oral apraxia. Initially, Amer-Ind Code was employed with G.G. However, since G.G. rejected Amer-Ind Code as a sole means of communication, an attempt was made to incorporate the principles of Promoting Aphasic's Communicative Effectiveness (PACE) (Wilcox and Davis, 1981) into the treatment program. In general, PACE's multimodality approach incorporates the natural rules of communication. Figure 18.1 indicates the greater flexibility in the patient's responsorium as a result of treatment incorporating the principles of PACE. Specifically, at treatment Session 1, the patient described pictures employing graphic or written responses 100% of the time. By Session 5, roughly half of the responses were graphic, one-third were gestural, and one-tenth were verbal. By Session 10, approximately 20% of the responses were graphic (writing a key word or drawing an action picture), 50% were gestural (Amer-Ind Code), and 30% were verbal (telegraphic but intelligible spoken descriptors). Hence, although overall communication accuracy may not have changed, G.G. did achieve greater communicative flexibility and success. (His spouse and 11 children verified that G.G. was a more effective communicator with more means to communicate.) His handicap was minimized by increasing his options.

Although both Amer-Ind Code and PACE have essentially an expressive communication bent, Table 18.6 reveals a significant pre- and posttreatment change on the Boston Diagnostic Aphasia Examination's (Goodglass and Kaplan, 1972) complex ideational subtest (from 2/12 to 9/12). Also worthy of note on follow-up were the results of the Aphasia Language Performance Scales (Keenan and Brassell, 1975), wherein a nearly equal performance on each scale was obtained following an aggressive, multimodal therapy regimen. The discharge diagnosis of moderate Broca's aphasia was consistent with the clinician and family report that G.G. had improved considerably in this overall functional communication skills.

In G.G.'s case, Amer-Ind Code played a definite, although ancillary, role in PACE therapy. Rather than resorting to simple pantomime as part of PACE therapy, Amer-Ind Code was used because of its well-documented high transparency (Daniloff et al., 1983) and ease of production (Daniloff and Vegara, 1984). Within the context of PACE therapy, it became obvious that the standardized corpus of Amer-Ind Code enhanced the efficiency and transparency of messages sent and received by the patient.

FUTURE DIRECTIONS

Amer-Ind Code has a bright future in aphasiology. The study of the code with this population is really just in its youth. This chapter has reviewed the various uses of the Code with persons with aphasia and concluded that the Amer-Ind Code approach appears to be singularly beneficial with persons with severe

Table 18.6.
Patient G.G.: Pre-, Post-, Follow-Up Data[a]

	Pre	Post	Follow-Up
ALPS (max = 10)			
Listening	5.5	8.5	6
Talking	1	2.5	6
Reading	4.5	7	6
Writing	5.5	6	4.5
TACL (max = 101)	82	91	97
YES/NO Battery (max = 10)			
PPVT (max = 150)	89	103	95
Ceiling	115	114	127
BDAE Complex Ideational (max = 12)	2	9	9
Apraxia Battery (max = 4)			
Oral: Imitation	2.3	3.0	DNT
Command	.7	2.7	DNT
Limb: Imitation	3.6	4.0	DNT
Command	2.3	3.0	DNT

Final Diagnosis: Moderate Broca's aphasia and mild oral apraxia

[a] ALPS = Aphasia Language Performance Scales; BDAE = Boston Diagnostic Aphasia Examination; PPVT = Peabody Picture Vocabulary Test; TACL = Test of Auditory Comprehension of Language.

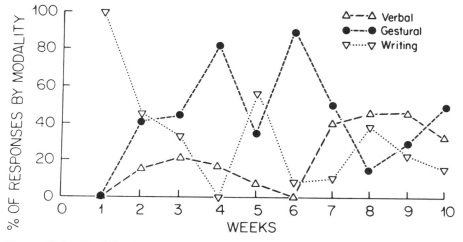

Figure 18.1. Flexibility in patient response as a result of treatment incorporating the principles of PACE.

aphasia. Future study should focus on clarifying the candidacy issue even further. Are persons with Broca's aphasia better candidates than those with Wernicke's aphasia for the various uses of the Code? Is there a certain PICA or CADL profile that suggests that Amer-Ind Code might be warranted? What level of the Skelly (1979) Scale of Progress predicts ultimate attainment and use of the Code? These questions must be answered if clinicians are to make an informed decision on when and why to use the Amer-Ind Code.

Once the candidacy issue has been resolved, several treatment issues must be clarified. The first treatment priority is to involve the significant other in Amer-Ind Code treatment. Future case studies should include reports on the family's recognition and use of the code in concert with the patient. If the patient and the family are trained to "think action," then the family and the patient will be more efficient in their "interactions." Once the patient and family are gesturally oriented, should the clinician avoid the use of language in treatment? There is controversy on this issue even among long-time Amer-Ind Code users. Skelly (1981b) strongly encourages a nonvocal approach with severe and global aphasics, while Rao et al. (1980) have noted improved auditory comprehension when employing a "talk and hand talk" approach to Amer-Ind Code. Tomorrow's clinicians deserve to know the optimal mode of signal presentation.

The future will also see discussion of the following issues:

- Refined lexicon prioritized in terms of easiest to hardest to teach
- Group versus individual treatment
- Amer-Ind Code plus Talking Pictures
- Action Amer-Ind Code Pictures versus Amer-Ind Code itself

These, as well as many other issues, will require much time and effort to resolve. However, based on its efficacy and popularity in many nations, it is not unreasonable to expect that Amer-Ind Code will become the International Code of aphasiologists.

Acknowledgments

Dr. Rao wishes to acknowledge the two hospitals where this work was conducted (the Ft. Howard VA Medical Center and the National Rehabilitation Hospital) and the patients who were studied, particularly G.G., J.C., P.J., and R.J. Finally, Dr. Rao wishes to thank Dr. Madge Skelly for her significant contributions to the communicatively impaired and Ms. Therese Goldsmith for her editorial contributions to this manuscript.

References

American Speech-Language-Hearing Association. (1990). Functional Communication Scales for Adults Project: Advisory Report. Rockville, MD: ASHA.

Christopoulou, C., and Bonvillian, J. D. (1985). Sign language, pantomime, and gestural processing in aphasic persons. *Journal of Communication Disorders, 18,* 1–20.

Coelho, C. A. (1990). Acquisition and generalization of simple manual sign grammars by aphasic subjects. *Journal of Communication disorders, 23,* 383–400.

Coelho, C. A. (1991). Manual sign acquisition and use in two aphasic subjects. In T. Prescott (Ed.), *Clinical aphasiology* (Vol. 19). Austin, TX: Pro-Ed.

Coelho, C. A., and Duffy, R. J. (1987). The relationship of the acquisition of manual signs to severity of aphasia: A training study. *Brain and Language, 31,* 328–345.

Collins, M. J. (1990). Global aphasia. In L. L. LaPointe (Ed.), *Aphasia and related neurogenic language disorders.* New York: Thieme Medical Publishers.

Daniloff, J., Frittelli, G., Hoffman, P. R., and Daniloff, R. G. (1986). Amer-Ind versus ASL: Recognition and imitation in aphasic subjects. *Brain and Language, 28,* 95–113.

Daniloff, J., Lloyd, L., and Fristoe, M. (1983). Amer-Ind transparency. *Journal of Speech and Hearing Disorders, 48,* 103–110.

Daniloff, J., Noll, J. D., Fristoe, M., and Lloyd, L. (1982). Gesture, recognition in patients with aphasia. *Journal of Speech and Hearing Disorders, 47,* 43–49.

Daniloff, J., and Vegara, D. (1984). Comparison between the motoric constraint for Amer-Ind and ASL sign formation. *Journal of Speech and Hearing Research, 27,* 76–88.

Davis, G. A. (1983). *A survey of adult aphasia.* Englewood Cliffs, NJ: Prentice-Hall.

Dowden, P. A., Marshall, R. C., and Tomkins, C. A. (1982). Amer-Ind as a communicative facilitator of aphasic and apraxic patients. In R. Brookshire (Ed.), *Clinical Aphasiology Conference proceedings.* Minneapolis, MN: BRK.

Duffy, R. J., and Duffy, J. R. (1981). Three studies of deficits in pantomimic recognition in aphasia. *Journal of Speech and Hearing Research, 46,* 70–84.

Duncan, J. L., and Silverman, F. H. (1978). Impact of learning Amer-Ind sign language on mentally retarded children. In J. R. Andrews and M. S. Burns (Eds.), *Remediation of language disorders.* Evanston, IL: Institute for Continuing Professional Education.

Fristoe, M., and Lloyd, L. (1980). Planning an initial lexicon for persons with severe communication impairment. *Journal of Speech and Hearing Disorders, 45,* 170–180.

Goodglass, H., and Kaplan, E. (1972). *Assessment of aphasia and related disorders.* Philadelphia, PA: Lea & Febiger.

Griffith, P. L., Robinson, J. H., and Panagos, J. M. (1981). Perception of iconicity in ASL by hearing and deaf subjects. *Journal of Speech and Hearing Disorders, 46,* 405–412.

Guilford, A. M., Scheuerle, J., and Shirek, P. G. (1982). Manual communication skills in aphasia. *Archives of Physical Medicine and Rehabilitation, 63,* 601–604.

Heilman, K. M., Rothi, L., Campanella, D., and Wolfson, S. (1979). Wernicke's and global aphasia without alexia. *Archives of Neurology, 36,* 129–133.

Helm-Estabrooks, N., Fitzpatrick, P., and Barresi, B. (1982). Visual action therapy for global aphasia. *Journal of Speech and Hearing Disorders, 47,* 385–389.

Holland, A. (1975). *Aphasics as communicators: A Model and its implications.* Paper presented at the Annual Convention of the American Speech-Language-Hearing Association, Washington, DC.

Holland, A. (1980). *Communicative abilities of daily living.* Baltimore, MD: University Park Press.

Horner, J. (1980). *Amer-Ind candidacy.* Paper presented at a George Washington University Medical Center Neuropathology Symposium, Washington, DC.

Keenan, J. S., and Brassell, E. G. (1975). *Aphasia Language Performance Scales.* Murfreesboro, TN: Pinnacle Press.

Kertesz, A. (1980). *Western Aphasia Battery.* London, Ontario: University of Western Ontario.

Kirschner, A., Algozzine, B., and Abbott, T. B. (1979). Manual communication systems: A comparison and its implications. *Education and Training in the Mentally Retarded, 14,* 5–10.

Larkins, P. (1987). Program evaluation system. Rockville, MD: American Speech-Language-Hearing Association.

Lieberth, A. K., and Gamble, M. E. (1991). The role of iconicity in sign language learning by hearing adults. *Journal of Communication Disorders, 24,* 89–99.

Lloyd, L. L., and Daniloff, J. (1983). Issues in using Amer-Ind Code with retarded persons. In T. M. Gallagher and C. A. Prutting (Eds.), *Pragmatic assessment and intervention issues in language.* San Diego, CA: College Hill Press.

Lloyd, L. L., Loeding, B., and Doherty, J. E. (1985). Role of iconicity in sign acquisition: A response to Orlansky and Bonvillian (1984). *Journal of Speech and Hearing Disorders, 50,* 299–301.

Musselwhite, C. R., and St. Louis, K. W. (1988). *Communication programming for persons with severe handicaps* (3rd ed.). Boston: College Hill Press.

Porch, B. (1967). *Porch Index of Communicative Ability.* Palo Alto, CA: Consulting Psychologists Press.

Rao, P. (1985). *An investigation into the neuropsychological basis of gesture.* Ph.D. dissertation, College Park, MD, University of Maryland.

Rao, P., Basil, A. G., Koller, J. M., Fullerton, B., Diener, S., and Burton, P. (1980). The use of Amer-Ind Code by severe aphasic adults. In M. Burns and J. Andrews (Eds.), *Neuropathologies of speech and language diagnosis and treatment: Selected papers.* Evanston, IL: Institute for Continuing Professional Education.

Rao, P., and Horner, J. (1978). Gesture as a deblocking modality in a severe aphasic patient. In R. Brookshire (Ed.), *Clinical Aphasiology Conference proceedings.* Minneapolis, MN: BRK.

Rao, P., and Horner, J. (1980). Non-verbal strategies for functional communication by aphasic adults. In M. Burns and J. Andrews (Eds.), *Neuropathologies of speech and language diagnosis and treatment: Selected papers.* Evanston, IL: Institute for Continuing Professional Education.

Rao, P., and Koller, J. (1982). *A total communication approach to aphasia treatment in three chronic aphasic adults.* Paper presented at the Semi-Annual Conference of the International Neuropsychological Society, Pittsburgh, PA.

Rosenbek, J., LaPointe, L. L., Wertz, R. T. (1989). *Aphasia: A clinical approach.* Austin, TX: Pro-Ed.

Skelly, M. (1977). Amer-Ind Code Basic Workshop, sponsored by the Washington Hospital Center, Washington, DC.

Skelly, M. (1979). *Amer-Ind Gestural Code based on Universal American Indian Hand Talk.* New York: Elsevier.

Skelly, M. (1981a). *Amer-Ind Code repertoire* (videocassette). St. Louis, MO: Auditec.

Skelly, M. (1981b). Amer-Ind Code Presentors Workshop, sponsored by the St. Louis Speech and Hearing Center, St. Louis, MO.

Skelly, M., Schinsky, L., Smith, R., Donaldson, R., and Griffin, J. (1974). American Indian sign (Amerind) as a facilitator of verbalization for the oral-verbal apraxic. *Journal of Speech and Hearing Disorders, 39,* 445-456.

Skelly, M., Schinsky, L., Smith, R., Donaldson, R., and Griffin, P. (1975). American Indian sign: Gestural communication for the speechless. *Archives of Physical Medicine and Rehabilitation, 56,* 156–160.

Skelly-Hakanson, M., Wollner, B., Bornhemer, K., Drollinger, K. (1982). Questions and answers about the code. *AMICIL Newsletter, 1.* Wales, WI: Somed.

Snead, N. S., and Solomon, S. J. (1977). *The effects of various stimulus modalities on global aphasics' phrase reception.* Paper presented at the Annual Convention of the American Speech-Language-Hearing Association, Chicago, IL.

Tonkovich, J., and Loverso, F. (1982). A training matrix approach for gestural acquisition by the agrammatic patient. In R. Brookshire (Ed.), *Clinical Aphasiology Conference proceedings.* Minneapolis, MN: BRK.

World Health Organization. (1980). *International classification of impairments, disabilities, and handicaps.* Geneva Switzerland: World Health Organization.

Wilcox, M. J., and Davis, A. J. (1981). Incorporating parameters of natural conversation in aphasia treatment. In R. Chapey (Ed.), *Language intervention strategies in adult aphasia.* Baltimore, MD: Williams & Wilkins.

Yorkston, K., and Dowden, P. A. (1984). Non-speech language and communication systems. In A. Holland (Ed.), *Language disorders in adults.* San Diego, CA: College Hill Press.

APPENDIX 18.1

Amer-Ind Code Signals (*N* = 38) with 90% or Better Transparency Using Either Liberal or Conservative Scoring[a,b]

100%	97.5%–90% (*N* = 23)
Bird	Automobile
Cold	Break
Cry	Telephone
Drink	Yes
No	Glasses
Pour	Pen
Quiet	Stir
Scissors	Dive
Swim	Nailfile
Toothbrush	Dig
Come	Pain
Fight	Comb
Ball	Grab
Sleep	Wash
Book	Stop
	Time
	Write
	Ring
	Good-bye
	Mirror
	Look
	Laugh
	Think

[a] Listed in rank order from 100% to 90%.
[b] From Daniloff, J., Lloyd, L., and Fristoe, M. (1983). Amer-Ind transparency. *Journal of Speech and Hearing Disorders, 48,* 103–110.

CHAPTER 19
Melodic Intonation Therapy

ROBERT W. SPARKS AND JOHN W. DECK

Numerous studies have indicated that an unimpaired right cerebral hemisphere is dominant for music in right-handed persons. This explains why aphasic persons can sing the melody of a familiar song. However, their accurate emission of the words of the song is of greater interest because of its contrast with their inability to communicate the most basic needs. This preserved skill also includes recitation of prayers, some social gesture phrases, and premorbid use of profanity. Jackson (1931) classified such utterances as nonpropositional language because they do not involve encoding of a message that contains specific information. He theorized that such utterances are processed in an undamaged so-called nondominant hemisphere of an aphasic. Today we can produce no better word to describe such language, although we no longer label the right hemisphere as being a nondominant one. Indeed, research indicates that the right hemisphere is involved in processing the prosody of propositional language.

Sparks et al. (1974) reviewed some of the literature on right-hemisphere processing of the prosodic elements of speech. Their analysis suggests that in normal right-handed persons and many left-handed persons the right hemisphere functions in a tandem relationship with the left hemisphere for both encoding and emission of propositional language. However, the final integrative process takes place in the temporal lobe of the left hemisphere. Reorganization of this interhemispheric process with increased participation of the right hemisphere probably occurs only when recovery is slow and incomplete. Of equal importance in this reorganization are preserved interhemisphere pathways for language. Indeed, Gordon (1972) states that a long period may be involved in increasing the function of the right hemisphere. The reader is referred to Code's discussion of the role of the right hemisphere in the treatment of aphasia (see Chapter 20 in this text). The probability that this is increased by melodic intonation therapy (MIT) is even more likely when we consider the right hemisphere's dominance for music. Studies of adult aphasia that have described language performance from a phonological model have included Blumstein (1973), Martin and Rigrodsky (1979), and Whitaker (1970).

The intentions of the authors of this chapter are to instruct the clinician in the technique of melodic intonation, describe the verbal behavior of both good candidates and poor candidates for MIT, discuss the administration of the MIT hierarchy, offer suggestions for involving the families of the aphasics who are selected for exposure to this language intervention strategy, and suggest future trends in further development of MIT.

Melodic Intonation Therapy involves singing. The specific techniques we call intonation is described in some detail later in the chapter. This type of singing is an ancient form dating back at least to the Judeo-Christian period. It is distinct from other forms of singing in that each intoned utterance is based on the *melody pattern*, the *rhythm*, and the *points of stress* in the spoken model. Use of an intoned utterance that resembles a familiar song may produce disastrous results, therapeutically speaking. The familiar melody will stimulate recall of the nonpropositional words of that song.

PRINCIPLES OF LANGUAGE THERAPY AFFECTING MIT

Objectives of MIT

The original intention for developing MIT for severely nonfluent aphasics was to achieve at least a basic recovery of ability to use some language accurately. Good candidates demonstrate extreme paucity of speech and show concern about such an incapacity. Reasonable priorities of therapeutic purpose for such patients would relegate the quality of articulation and syntax to secondary consideration. Emphasis on the linguistic or semantic aspects of verbal utterances for these aphasics is the primary goal of MIT. However, some clinicians are using the technique as a more phonological intervention for verbal apraxia. A review of our physiological model implies that the right hemisphere controls prosody. This, then, justifies the use of MIT for the phonological defects of such patients.

Speech Pathology Principles Applied to MIT

The Examination

A preference as to standardized aphasia examinations that are used to evaluate a potential candidate for MIT is not an issue. Sparks (1978) has presented guidelines for supplementary parastandardized examination of aphasics that make it possible to investigate more specific language skills in addition to those sampled in standardized examination batteries. In any event,

MIT depends on evidence from the examination that the aphasic candidate has a distinct potential for some recovery of language.

Eight Principles of Language Therapy Involved in MIT

The first principle is concerned with gradual progression of the length and difficulty of the tasks in the therapeutic hierarchy. Such progression involves the type of linguistic material used, a gradual withdrawal of participation by the clinician in the purely repetition tasks, and reduction of reliance on melodic intonation in the last level of the MIT hierarchy.

The second principle, one endorsed by Schuell et al. (1964), maintains that direct attempts to correct the aphasic's verbal errors fail because he cannot recall the specific nature of his errors. Attempts to correct errors accomplish little and may do some harm if they detract from the smooth progression of the hierarchy. The severely handicapped aphasic who is considered to be a candidate seldom can effectively correct his verbal errors by retrial. Such retrials often result in a perseverated repetition of the error, which thus reinforces it. MIT attempts to achieve correct responses by means of a second trial that involves the technique of "backup." Specifically, when the aphasic fails a step, he is immediately guided through a repetition of the previous step and then a second attempt of the step that he failed. He may or may not be aware of the purpose of this procedure, but it is not drawn to his attention. A second backup retrial is never attempted if failure occurs again.

The third principle maintains that repetition is a highly effective therapeutic device. It serves as the core of MIT. Actually, repetition involves a rather complex process. The fact that normal persons can repeat familiar or simple sentences more efficiently than more difficult sentences suggests that a process of decoding the stimulus and then reencoding it for emission is involved. Accurate repetition deteriorates in longer units. However, the paraphrased repetition of the longer sentence does not alter the meaning. The stimulus has been accurately received and decoded, but some word substitutions have been used for the restatement. Perhaps the most difficult repetition task involves unknown words of another language or nonsense syllables. In this task, the usual decode-encode process is less efficient. As stated previously, the use of repetition in MIT gradually decreases as the level of difficulty of tasks increases.

The fourth principle is concerned with latencies of response. One such control is use of latency between completion of stimulus presentation by the clinician and permission for response by the aphasic so that the complete stimulus is received and decoded. Another use of latency is between the completion of one sentence-item progression in the hierarchy and the beginning of the next.

The fifth principle is avoidance of practice effect by using the same material or carrier phrases repeatedly. This is often tedious and not therapeutically effective. A well-constructed program of intervention will include many useful high-probability utterances that trigger recall of premorbid language skills. Language that is alien to the aphasic should not be used. Therefore, enough variety of meaningful material is encouraged for MIT so that no utterance is used more often than every 9th or 10th session of therapy.

The sixth principle maintains that the clinician should pay scrupulous attention to the purpose and semantic value of each of his or her verbal utterances. For example, exuberant reinforcements within a sequence of steps are disruptive. A smile of encouragement will serve just as well or better. This is not an indictment of a warm, holistic approach to therapeutic intervention in general. However, clinicians should practice restraint during MIT.

The seventh principle maintains that written or pictorial materials should not be used as added stimuli. We believe that the presumption that such material is supportive to the auditory stimulus is very suspect. Our premise is that these materials actually distract rather than support the MIT therapeutic process. This is particularly true for good candidates for MIT who have auditory comprehension that permits them to understand and retain spoken stimuli in a variety of contexts. Aphasics with severe auditory deficits may respond better to auditory stimuli when they are accompanied by pictures. However, such patients are not candidates for MIT.

The eighth principle pertains to the frequency of therapy sessions. Treatment sessions twice daily are essential for the aphasic with severe impairment of language. Where restrictions of time, resources, or transportation are involved, the training of family members to function as assistants in the MIT program may be very effective.

CANDIDACY FOR MIT

Assessment of the efficacy of MIT has proved that no single language intervention strategy for aphasia is a panacea. Indeed, MIT is effective for only a portion of the aphasic population. This then implies a need for careful evaluation of each aphasic who is being considered for exposure to this method.

Chapter 3 of this text describes computed tomography (CT) scan findings of cortical and subcortical lesions as predictions of candidacy for MIT. Such studies contribute much. Language profiles of both good and poor candidates are presented here as guides for selection. Emphasis is placed on auditory comprehension, several aspects of verbal expression, and nonlanguage behavior.

The Good Candidate

Auditory Comprehension

Examination of auditory comprehension indicates that the good candidate's understanding and retention of spoken language is essentially normal in a variety of contexts.

It is simplistic to presume that the process of monitoring one's own verbal utterances is solely through auditory feedback. Actually, kinesthetic feedback probably alerts us to phonological or semantic errors immediately before the auditory feedback has commenced. In any event, evidence of preserved self-criticism in the good candidate is important.

Verbal Language

The clinical impression of the good candidate is that of an aphasic with a marked paucity of any kind of verbal output. In other words, he or she is a nonfluent aphasic. This is accompanied by demonstration of frustration and despondency concerning his or her language impairment. A curious and enigmatic perseveration of a neologistic utterance has been observed in some aphasics who have subsequently responded well to MIT. It is enigmatic because it is similar to the stereotypical jargon utterances of some global aphasics. However, there are two points of difference. Good candidates will modify the prosody of the utterance so that it reflects their intention to make a declarative, interrogative, or forceful imperative statement. Second, they will be annoyed by the meaningless morphology of the utterance. With the exception of such stereotyped jargon utterances, little speech is initiated except for an occasional single substantive word that is always an appropriate communication.

Phonological performance by the good candidate who has no language impairment other than speech production includes effortful but indistinct speech that is interrupted by pauses for attempted initiation of each utterance and attempts to correct himself or herself. Speech is phonologically distorted. When the articulation is analyzed, a systematic reorganization of sound patterns may seem to occur.

A summary of results of the examination of verbal expression produces a profile of the good candidate as follows:

1. Almost no responses occur in confrontation naming, responsive naming, word and phrase repetition, or sentence completion. However, an occasional response will be poorly articulated but accurate enough to indicate correct encoding of the target word.
2. Effort at self-correction is often vigorous. This is to be expected in aphasics who are acutely aware of making errors in their verbal output. Unfortunately, the product is usually not improved by this effort.

Nonverbal Behavior

Good candidates are often reasonably depressed, but they are almost always emotionally stable with a mature response to counseling by the clinician. They manifest a strong desire to enter into intensive efforts to rehabilitate their speech, and they accept MIT.

Concurrent Abnormalities

The good candidate usually demonstrates a significant buccofacial apraxia and has a hemiplegia that is more severe in the arm than in the leg.

Language Profile After MIT

A diagnosis of "classical" this or "classical" that is usually careless, but it is tempting to describe the verbal output of the post-MIT aphasic as having evolved into that of a classical Broca's aphasic. Some of the aphasic's utterances continue to be poorly articulated and agrammatical but telegraphically appropriate. An example is, "home—weekend—Saturday an' Sunday. Hospital—you—Monday." Considering the graduate's almost total inability to communicate prior to the therapy, this telegram is a triumph.

Further Improvement After MIT

The question as to whether achieved language improvement will be retained by the aphasic following successful MIT produces some concern for clinicians. Fortunately, follow-up examinations of MIT graduates have shown that not only do they maintain their new competency but they continue to improve in their own home environment. Syntactic substance begins to appear in their verbal output. MIT graduates and their families should be advised that a review of the final steps of the hierarchy will be beneficial in the continuing improvement. The clinician should discuss the extent of the family's participation and be available as a continuing consultant.

The Poor Candidate

Three aphasic syndromes are not responsive to the present form of MIT. These three types of aphasia are *Wernicke's*, *Transcortical*, and *Global*. The labels are not as important as brief reviews of the verbal behavior involved in each of the three types. They all are clearly distinct from the profile of the good candidate that has been presented.

Wernicke's Aphasia

Achieving therapeutic success with Wernicke's aphasics is a very difficult and challenging task. Concerted effort by some speech pathologists to produce more effective language therapy for persons with this type of aphasia is essential. The following characteristics of the Wernicke's aphasic are in marked contrast to those of the good candidate:

1. Auditory comprehension is poor and variable. Wernicke's aphasics show no evidence of being aware that they fail to be understood. As a matter of fact, they usually reject language therapy, and their reaction to MIT is either explosive or one of amused condescension.
2. Verbal utterances are overly fluent, syntactically normal, and clearly articulated. However, they include abundant paraphasic errors for the substantive words, and the end result is bizarre and meaningless.
3. The Wernicke's aphasic is often emotionally unstable, often hostile, but sometimes extremely cordial.

The application of MIT techniques to patients with Wernicke's aphasia has produced poor results. Wernicke's aphasics accurately duplicate intonation patterns, including the melody, rhythm, and points of stress. This is in contrast to their replacement of the words in the stimulus model with their own paraphasic jargon.

Transcortical Aphasia

The aphasic demonstrating this profile may be similar in some ways to the good candidate and in other ways to the person with Wernicke's aphasia. The important feature of this form of aphasia is an isolated skill at accurately repeating long phrases and sentences, seemingly without the normal decoding process mentioned earlier. The aphasic performs perfectly in MIT, but there is no carryover to improved functional language. Investigation of repetition skill as a candidacy factor would suggest that ability to repeat even single words may be a negative prognostic factor for MIT candidacy.

Global Aphasia

The history of language therapy for persons with global aphasia indicates that such therapy has been unsuccessful in improving their functional verbal language. This was pointed out by Albert and Helm-Estabrook (1988), by Sarno et al. (1970), and by Schuell et al. (1964). MIT is no more effective than other language therapy in reestablishing any useful verbal communication.

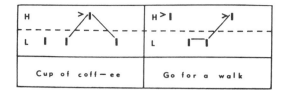

Figure 19.1. Prosodic patterns of speech. H indicates higher pitch. L indicates lower pitch. A single-syllable word is indicated by a single vertical bar. Vertical bars that are connected represent multisyllabic words or clusters of words. An arrow preceding a vertical bar indicates stress on that word or syllable.

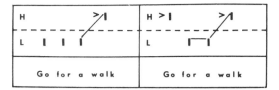

Figure 19.2. Two equally acceptable spoken prosody patterns using the same figure legend as Figure 19.1.

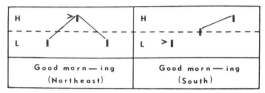

Figure 19.3. Regional differences in patterns of spoken prosody for one sentence.

MELODIC INTONATION

Sparks and Holland (1976) briefly describe the difference between songs and melodic intonation. Specifically, songs have distinct melodies. In contrast, melodic intonation is based solely on the spoken prosody of verbal utterances. The latter uses a vocal range that is limited to three or four whole notes. This is all that is necessary to achieve an adequate variety of melodic patterns. The range is about the same as that of the melodic line of speech.

This limited range of sung notes is comfortable for the untrained voice of adults. It is important to point out the necessity of avoiding melodic intonation patterns that are similar to those of long-lasting popular songs.

The Form of Melodic Intonation

Melodic intonation is based on three elements of spoken prosody: the melodic line or variation of pitch in the spoken phrase or sentence, the tempo and rhythm of the utterance, and the points of stress for emphasis. Certainty as to the appropriateness of the intonation pattern is essential in MIT. The need for this appropriateness becomes essential in the final level of the hierarchy when intoned utterances are gradually transposed back to spoken prosody.

Some exaggeration of the three elements of a spoken prosody model occurs when that utterance is intoned. First, the tempo is lengthened to a more lyrical utterance. Second, the varying pitch of speech is reduced and stylized into a melodic pattern involving the constant pitch of intoned notes. Third, the rhythm and stress are exaggerated for purposes of emphasis. This usually involves increased loudness and elevation of intoned notes. These three modifications of spoken prosody serve as a means of emphasizing the prosodic structure of the utterance.

Acceptable Variety of Melodic Patterns and Regional Differences

There are several alternative prosody patterns for any verbal utterance. The clinician must exercise his or her own judgment as to which one will be used for a phrase or sentence in any one session of language therapy. Using a different intonation pattern in a subsequent session is a means of achieving variety of stimulation. Two such variations are illustrated in Figure 19.1 and will be discussed.

Regional differences of speech prosody are sometimes quite pronounced. This is not a matter of concern if the clinician and the aphasic come from and are in the same region. However, the emigration of a clinician from one prosodically distinct area

to another implies that he or she must make an adjustment when MIT is involved. Samples of regional differences are presented in Figure 19.2 and will be discussed.

Plotting Spoken Prosody Patterns

Two illustrations of the method of graphically plotting verbal utterances along with an explanation of the plotting technique are presented in Figure 19.1. This method, an adaptation of the one developed at the Kodaly Musical Training Institute and presented by Knighton (1973), will be used in all subsequent illustrations.

In the first phrase, "cup of coffee," the utterance starts on a lower pitch for "cup," but the substantive importance of the word places it alone. This is followed by the cluster of words, "_____ of coffee." Emphasis stress is on the first syllable of "coffee" along with the higher pitch that such stress produces. The last syllable of this declarative phrase has the customary drop in pitch. In the second illustration, "Go for a walk," there is stress on "go" with accompanying higher pitch, then a drop in pitch for the two functor words in the cluster, then a return to the higher pitch along with stress for the substantive word, "walk."

Figure 19.2 plots the difference of two variations for the phrase "Go for a walk." The first is as illustrated in Figure 19.1. The second illustrates a model where the word "for" is detached from the rest of the cluster that follows. This may be desirable as the aphasic improves and the clinician thinks that therapy should begin to attack absence of functor or relational words in the patient's speech.

In Figure 19.3, a comparison of prosody for the social gesture utterance "good morning," shows a rise-fall melody pattern of the northeastern parts of the United States and a gradually rising inflectional pattern of at least some parts of the South.

Transposing Speech to Intonation

Illustrations of the transposition of plotted speech prosody models into melodic intonation are presented in Figure 19.4, using those phrases illustrated in Figure 19.1. The placing of the notes on a musical staff in these illustrations does not imply

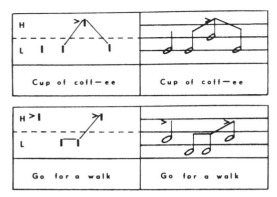

Figure 19.4. Transposition of spoken prosody models to melodic intonation. Key of C in treble cleff is used for illustration. No attempt is made to present accurate musical tempo.

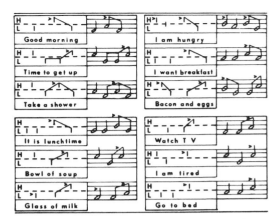

Figure 19.5. Four thematic three-item illustrations of melodic intonation material using the same figure legend presented in Figure 19.1.

that ability to read music is a prerequisite to administering MIT, although such skill is an advantage. The primary purpose here is to duplicate graphically the pattern of spoken prosody that has served as the model. Considerable musical license has been taken, and musicians are requested not to take issue. For those who are interested, however, the key of C is used in the illustrations so that variations of sung note combinations may be demonstrated.

Sprechgesang

The fading of melodic intonation and a return to spoken prosody occurs in the fourth level of the MIT hierarchy. It is a technique that lies halfway between speech and singing. It is used in choral reading but more lyrically by Schoenberg in his *Ode to Napoleon* and *Pierrot Luraire*. Schoenberg defined the technique as *sprechgesang*, or "spoken song."

The exaggerated tempo, rhythm, and points of stress in *sprechgesang* are the same as in the intoned model. However, the more variable pitch of speech replaces the more constant pitch of intoned notes. The utterance is lyrical but spoken rather than sung.

The senior author lays claim to the use of this art form as a bridging technique in the MIT hierarchy after having heard a performance of *Ode to Napoleon* by the Boston Symphony Orchestra in 1973. He will furnish a cassette sample of *sprechgesang* on request provided the request is accompanied by phrases to be illustrated and a cassette.

LINGUISTIC CONTENT

The importance of a linguistically sophisticated control of the grammatical structure of phrases and sentences used in MIT depends largely on the severity of the individual aphasic's inability to communicate and the usefulness of the verbal material. The selection of phrases and short sentences should be high-priority communication. This involves investigation of basic aspects of the aphasic's premorbid milieu that may be used, and then some creativity on the part of the clinician to produce stimulating material. In other words, all material should be egocentric for the individual aphasic. This should be the case in all therapy for the traumatized aphasic, but it is of particular importance as a counterbalance in MIT, where the technique is so atypical of normal verbal behavior. Information

about such things as basic family routines, family relationships and customs, personal needs, and personal likes and dislikes will suggest an abundance of material of both universal and individual appeal. Clusters of sentences that have a spherical relationship add an even greater significance. This is illustrated in Figure 19.5, which presents four three-item themes as an illustration of thematic relationship of therapy material along with further illustration of melodic intonation plotting. Additional illustration of the thematic arrangement of material presented by Sparks and Holland (1976) is included here with the permission of the senior author of that article:

Sample Material for Level II

1. twelve o'clock
2. time for lunch
3. bowl of soup
4. salt and pepper
5. ham sandwich
6. apple pie
7. glass of milk
8. I am sleepy
9. take a nap

Sample Material for Levels III and IV

1. Sit down in a chair.
2. Read the newspaper.
3. Look at the sports page
4. Turn on the TV.
5. Go for a walk.
6. I am very tired.
7. It is getting late.
8. Time to go to bed.
9. It is ten o'clock.

Meaningful stimulus items for the aphemic candidate who has no impairment other than phonological errors should, in addition to being meaningful for the individual patient, focus on facilitating more intelligible speech. The creative clinician will meet with the candidate and family and explain the importance of gaining information about specific linguistic preferences the patient used in his or her premorbid speech. Therapeutic concern for consistent phonological errors makes it more difficult to select meaningful material. Table 19.1 illustrates the use of phonological patterns in selecting stimulus materials.

MELODIC INTONATION HIERARCHY

The hierarchy of MIT is highly structured for gradual progression of difficulty. Therefore, it is presented in explicit detail because attention to every specification has contributed to its success. We are sympathetic with those clinicians who prefer less structured language intervention strategies, and we assure them that their reservations about using hierarchies is understood. Sparks and Holland (1976) referred to the dilemma of presenting a hierarchy in a way that is too detailed and seemingly dogmatic for some clinicians and perhaps not explicit enough for others. The presentation here will include a description of the technique of intoning, a detailed and illustrated discussion of the four levels of the hierarchy, and a suggested method of scoring each MIT session.

Specific Aspects of the Technique

Discussion of the hierarchy will be made more explicit by first describing the several techniques that are involved.

Use of Verbal Cuing

Phonemic cues, along with their important visual components, are used in the second level of the program and to a lesser extent in the subsequent levels. The use of such cues is limited to assisting aphasics in initiation of their responses when it is apparent that they are having difficulty. It is *never* used as a means of repeating the task for purposes of correcting errors in the aphasic's responses.

Backups and Patient's Failures

A means of attempting indirect correction of errors, called "backups," is used in the third and fourth levels of the program. If the aphasic's response in any step is considered not to be adequate, the clinician has the aphasic repeat the preceding step and then attempt the failed step again. This second trial is often effective in producing the correct response without distracting the patient or making him or her directly aware of the error. As illustrated, if the third step of a level is failed, the second is repeated and the third is then attempted again. If the fourth is failed, the third is repeated as a backup, and so forth. If the aphasic again repeats the error or produces a different one after a backup sequence, the clinician terminates any further effort with that sentence-item and proceeds to the first step of the level with a new sentence. This is consistent with the concept that overt attempts to correct errors are not useful with the type of aphasic who is a candidate for MIT.

Hand Tapping and Control by Hand Signals

It is recommended that the clinician seat himself across the table from the aphasic so that his participation is visible to the aphasic and the aphasic's performance is clearly visible to him. The clinician grasps the patient's left hand so that he can engage it in tapping out the rhythm of the stimulus as it is presented, and then the rhythm of the responses. Many subjects begin to exercise some control of the hand tapping. This should be encouraged provided it is accurate. The clinician's participation may then be faded to that of monitoring the accuracy while continuing to hold the aphasic's hand. Hand tapping has proved to be an important and effective supportive stimulus. It has a cuing value that often seems as effective as the verbal component it accompanies.

The clinician's use of his or her left hand as a means of controlling onset of the aphasic's responses is recommended as a nonverbal and nondistracting means of exercising such control. Held up, the left hand advises the aphasic to remain silent and listen. Dropped with a finger pointed at the aphasic, it signals him to respond. This method is useful in enforcing latency if it is used consistently. The clinician may feel like a traffic officer and may wish he or she could develop a means of also using his or her feet.

Unison Repetition and Fading Participation by the Clinician

An early step in all the levels of the hierarchy involves clinician-aphasic unison repetition of the stimulus that the clinician has just presented. The clinician fades her participation, first the audible and then the visible component, so that the aphasic is repeating the sentence "solo." It is often necessary for the clinician to rejoin the aphasic when it is evident that he is not quite ready to proceed in the repetition on his own.

Adapting to the Aphasic's Modification of Melody Patterns

The clinician should be prepared to change the key of the melody to that of the aphasic's inadvertent modification. Attempts to correct such modifications is an unnecessary distraction. Rather, accurate repetition of the verbal material is the primary goal. Modification of the rhythm or number of intoned

Table 19.1.
Sample Phonological Patterns for MIT Stimuli

	Facilitation of Velar Production	
cup of coffee	corn on the cob	piece of cake
calico cat	good cookie	call a cab
make music	big lake	can of coke
	Facilitation of Cluster Production	
ask the man	pass the salt	small price
stamp please	go back home	last street
deep snow fall	spare room	sports coat
	Facilitation of Syllable Sequencing	
build a snowman	light the Christmas trees	more ice cubes
it's a democracy	open the refrigerator	fix the machine
read it in the paper	time for breakfast	play the music box

syllables, however, cannot be permitted because of their effect on the substance of the sentence.

MIT Session Scoring

The best way of judging the effectiveness of any highly structured form of language therapy for aphasia is to use or develop an objective system of scoring each therapy session. This principle is recommended for MIT as a means of measuring the efficiency of the method for producing steady improvement by any one aphasic. The method suggested here involves a two-point score for an accurate response that has not required a phonemic cue to initiate a response or a backup, a one-point score for an accurate response achieved with cuing or after a backup, and a reduction of the maximum possible score for any sentence-item if steps have not been completed.

The Hierarchy of MIT

The discussion of each of the four levels of the MIT hierarchy will include a fully detailed description, and Tables 19.5 to 19.7 provide a quick reference. A second table for each level presents a sample therapy session that includes management of errors and scoring, and a review of the types of errors most frequently encountered.

Level I

The first level is a one-step preliminary means of establishing a set for holding hands and, as far as the aphasic may see it, singing odd little nothings. The melodies are those that are used for intoning phrases and sentences. They should increase in length and complexity of melody and stress points as the aphasic adapts to the technique. Our good candidate can usually be introduced to the idea by a simple description of the process and its purpose. The clinician hums a melody twice while hand tapping the rhythm-tempo-stress pattern with the aphasic. Humming is suggested rather than a vowel of ''la-la'' because of its less distinct phonemic quality. Melody patterns similar to those illustrated in Figure 19.5 should be used. Second, the clinician signals the aphasic to join her in unison humming of the melody along with the hand tapping. The patient may use a more phonemic verbal utterance when he joins in with the clinician. This is acceptable in this first nonverbal level. When the clinician thinks, the aphasic is ready for a solo effort, she fades her vocal participation but continues hand tapping with the aphasic. When the aphasic has completed his unaccompanied repetition, the clinician reinforces the performance by saying ''good'' and proceeding to the next melody pattern. No scoring takes place in Level I. The time required to complete this first level varies from 15 minutes for some aphasics to two therapy sessions for others. In any event, moving to the second level occurs as soon as the aphasic is comfortable in the set of intoning, hand tapping, and complying with the hand-signal controls of the clinician.

Level II

At Level II, linguistic material is added to the type of intonation patterns introduced in the first level. Each of the four steps in the level is presented in detail below. The model presented by Sparks and Holland (1976) had five steps. The present model

has combined the first two steps of that model. The use of phonemic cuing is indicated when applicable. Scoring involves two points for a response from the aphasic that does not require a cue to initiate it, and one point if the response is acceptable when initiated by a cue from the clinician. Hand tapping by the clinician and the aphasic occurs in all stimuli and responses.

Step 1.   The clinician hums the melody-tempo-stress intonation pattern that is to be used with the sentence while hand tapping it with the aphasic, then repeats it with the sentence added. He pauses briefly and then repeats it. Then he signals the aphasic to join him in unison repetition of the intoned sentence. If the aphasic's performance is acceptable, the clinician proceeds to Step 2. If the aphasic's performance is not acceptable, the clinician pauses for several seconds to produce decay of the strength of the stimulus and then proceeds to the next sentence. The maximum score for an acceptable performance by the aphasic is one point.

Step 2.   After a brief pause, the clinician and the aphasic begin a unison intoning of the same sentence along with hand tapping. The clinician then fades his verbal participation in the manner described earlier but continues to hand tap the rhythm stress pattern with the aphasic. An acceptable performance implies progression in the third step, and the maximum score is again one point. An unacceptable performance terminates further progression; the clinician pauses for several seconds and then proceeds to the next sentence to be attempted.

Step 3.   The aphasic is signaled to listen. Then the clinician presents the same intoned sentence. This is accompanied by the hand tapping. Then the aphasic is signaled to repeat it, unaccompanied by the clinician except for his participation in the hand tapping. If the aphasic has difficulty initiating the repetition, the clinician gives a phonemic cue for the first phoneme of the sentence. Again, this is accompanied by the hand tapping and, it is hoped, the aphasic will respond to the cue accurately. If this third step is completed without cuing, the score is two points. If it is unacceptable only after cuing for initiation, the score is one point. Failure to initiate the utterance after one cuing effort or failure to produce it accurately enough to be acceptable terminates progression to the fourth step. After a suitable pause, the clinician proceeds to the next sentence.

Step 4.   In the final step of the second level, the clinician, without hand tapping, intones the question, ''What did you say?'' immediately after successful completion of the third step. He then signals the aphasic to repeat the intoned sentence. Cuing along with the hand tapping is offered once if the aphasic is having difficulty initiating the repetition. Occasionally, the aphasic may modify the sentence slightly by omitting a functor word or by a slight paraphrase of the sentence. This may be acceptable to the clinician. We maintain that any appropriate near-target response is evidence of progress. Scoring is the same as that of the third step. Two points are given for an acceptable uncued response; only one point is given when a cue was necessary for initiation. The aphasic is reinforced if he successfully completes the four steps for the sentence.

Level II Accomplishment.   The aphasic who succeeds in Level II has acquired the skill of repeating intoned sentences immediately after hearing the model, and then in response to a question. The latter is more difficult because the question not only acts as a masking intrusion but also initiates the process of reencoding the stimulus for responsive speech. Attention to this becomes progressively more active in the subsequent levels.

Table 19.2.
Sample MIT Level II Session with Step and Summation Scores

Aphasic's Performance	Scores			
	Step 1	Step 2	Step 3	Step 4
First sentence: Aphasic succeeds in all steps. Maximum scores attained.	1	1	2	2
Second sentence: Succeeds in all steps but requires a cue to initiate response in Steps 3 and 4.	1	1	1	1
Third sentence: Succeeds in Steps 1 and 2, requires a cue to initiate response in Step 3, and fails Step 4 because of an unacceptable response after backup.	1	1	1	0
Fourth sentence: Succeeds in Steps 1 and 2, requires a cue to initiate response in Step 3, and requires a backup to initiate Step 4.	1	1	1	1
Fifth sentence: Succeeds in Step 1, fails in Step 2. Progression stopped and no scores given for Steps 3 and 4.	1	0	–	–
Scores Total:	5/5 18/24 (75%)	4/5	5/8	4/6

The Most Common Errors Occurring in Level II. First, the aphasic may be so surprised by his solo repetition when the clinician fades her participation that he will falter. The clinician should be generous in reentering the unison repetition as much as she considers it useful in producing improvement of the aphasic's performance. Second, increasing repetition skill may disclose significant evidence of poor articulation, and this will continue throughout the MIT program for that aphasic. As stated previously, we give greater priority to increasing linguistic skill.

Sample MIT Session and Scoring for Level II. A brief five-item therapy session and its scoring is presented in Table 19.2 to illustrate management of errors in the aphasic's performance.

Level III

The third level is actually a liaison between the aphasic's recovery of ability to repeat during participation in Level II and the return to speech prosody and responsive speech in the fourth level. Latency of permitted responses and less specific questions in the last step begin to put more stress on the encoding of responsive speech. In this level, phonemic cuing by the clinician is replaced by the backup system already discussed. In addition to their use as an aid for initiation of responses, backups are also used as an indirect means of correcting an error in a response. As in cuing, only one backup and retrial of a failed step is permitted if the hierarchy is followed without modification. Again, the Sparks and Holland (1976) hierarchy has been modified by combining their first and second steps into one. The detailed description of this third level follows.

Step 1. The clinician presents the intoned sentence with the usual hand tapping once, then signals the aphasic to join in unison intoning and hand tapping the sentence. As the aphasic shows evidence that he can continue, the clinician fades her verbal participation, returning briefly if necessary and then fading again until the aphasic can continue alone. The maximum score is one point for acceptable performance, and the clinician proceeds to Step 2. It would be unusual for the aphasic to fail this step, but if he does the progression for that sentence is discontinued.

Step 2. The clinician intones the same sentence once with the usual patient-clinician hand tapping. The aphasic's response

will be intoned repetition, but delay in his response of 1 or 2 seconds is imposed by a hand signal from the clinician; then she signals him to repeat the intoned sentence. Failure involves an immediate backup to Step 1, unison intoning with clinician fading, and then retrial of the second step. If the step is completed without a backup, the score is two points. One point is given for an adequate response following a backup if it is necessary. Failure after one retrial terminates progression to the third step for that sentence.

Step 3. There is no hand tapping in this step. The clinician intones a question asking for a substantive response concerning some element of information in the sentence that has been presented. For instance, if the sentence used in the preceding steps was, "I want some pie," the question for Step 3 could be, "What kind of pie?" Perhaps the encouraging early indications of language recovery during MIT are the occasional appropriate but nondirected responses to the question. Such responses seem to be ahead of any other evidence of recovery in the aphasic's functional language. They please and surprise the aphasic and reward the clinician. These responses are usually uttered in normal speech prosody, and they certainly should be accepted. Failure to respond appropriately to the question implies an immediate backup to Step 2, delayed repetition, and then a retrial of Step 3. The clinician should not solicit some response of her own choosing. Scores are the same as for Step 2: two points without a backup and one point after a backup.

Level III Accomplishment. Satisfactory completion of this third level of MIT has begun the modification of the aphasic's responses from simpler repetition that is well supported by the clinician's participation to more difficult responses involving some retrieval and a beginning of attempts at encoded responses to specific questions.

The Most Common "Errors" Occurring in Level III. - Although not a verbal error, the aphasic's burgeoning confidence and enthusiasm may prompt him to respond before the clinician has signaled him to do so, particularly when delayed response is required. Because of the increasing difficulty of the tasks, the clinician must insist on compliance with her controls. Second, the aphasic may omit an occasional functor word. Perhaps this is an error of omission, but we believe that any improvement should be free of criticism and should not be inhibited by too much attention to syntax at this point in the progression of the hierarchy. Third, the variety of appropriate but unanticipated responses to the question in Step 3 should be praised even though they may not be what was expected. They are not errors, particularly if the questions are open-ended enough to make it possible for a variety of responses to occur.

Sample MIT Session and Scoring of Level III. As in Level II, a brief five-item therapy session and its scoring are presented in Table 19.3 to illustrate management of errors.

Level IV

In this last level, the return to normal speech prosody by way of the *sprechgesang* technique described earlier occurs for each sentence used, longer delays are imposed by the clinician before he permits the aphasic to respond, and more spontaneous and appropriate verbal intrusions by the aphasic may be expected.

Step 1. The clinician signals the aphasic to listen, then intones the sentence. He then pauses briefly and presents the sentence twice in *sprechgesang* accompanied by hand tapping with the aphasic. He invites the aphasic to join him in unison *sprechgesang* repetition of the sentence with continued hand tapping. Failure of the aphasic to respond appropriately calls for a backup to the clinician's solo presentation accompanied by hand tapping, then a second trial of the unison repetition. A second failure terminates further effort with that sentence. If the step is completed without a backup, the score is two points; the score is one point if a backup is necessary.

Step 2. The clinician again signals the aphasic to listen. Then he presents the same sentence in *sprechgesang* with hand tapping, delays permission for the aphasic to respond for 2 or 3 seconds, and then signals him to repeat it in *sprechgesang* with hand tapping. Failure involves an immediate backup to the first step, unison repetition in *sprechgesang* with hand tapping and fading participation by the clinician, and then a retrial of Step 2. If the step is completed without a backup, the score is two points; the score is one point if a backup is necessary to get an acceptable response. Failure to respond appropriately after one backup terminates progression to the third step for that sentence.

Step 3. Hand tapping is now discontinued for the remainder of Level IV for each sentence. The clinician signals the aphasic to listen, then presents the same sentence twice but now in normal speech prosody. After delaying permission to respond for 1 or 2 seconds, the clinician signals the aphasic to repeat the sentence as presented in normal speech prosody. The length of the delay may be lengthened as the aphasic develops proficiency. Failure involves a backup to the second step; delayed repetition in *sprechgesang*, with hand tapping; then a retrial of Step 3. Scoring is the same: two points without a backup, one point after a backup produces an acceptable response. Failure after a backup terminates progression to the fourth step for that sentence.

Step 4. As in the last step of the third level, the clinician asks questions concerning substantive information contained in the same sentence immediately after successful completion of Step 3, but the number of such questions may be increased. Then the clinician asks questions that are more associative in nature. As illustration, the following example is given:

> Sentence: I want to watch TV.
>
> Sequence of questions: (a) What do you want to watch? (b) Who wants to? (c) When do you like to do that? (d) What programs do you enjoy most?

The guidelines for decisions as to what may be considered acceptable responses and when a backup should be used are less specific as this last step in the hierarchy becomes less rigidly structured. One suggested solution is to demand accurate responses to the specific questions based on material in the sentence and reward the aphasic with extra credit for appropriate responses to the less specific questions. Backups should be used only for failures to initiate responses to the specific questions or when such responses are inferior to the aphasic's current ability. Principles of suggested scoring are modified to conform to the above guidelines for acceptability of responses. If a backup is used, it will be Step 3, delayed repetition of the sentence in normal speech prosody, and then a retrial of this fourth step. Backups should be restricted to use with the first specific questions, as responses to the less specific ones are bonus items. Response to the specific questions yields two points for each one, but only one point if a backup was necessary. Response to one or more of the less specific questions would yield a single score of three points, an added bonus that is a nice reinforcement the aphasic will enjoy.

This last level of the MIT hierarchy is more permissive than the first three and demands significantly more from the aphasic because he has recovered enough speech to reach it. The somewhat less stringent form lends itself to transition to any other language therapies that the clinician may want to employ after completion of MIT.

Level IV Accomplishments and Post-MIT Therapy. The aphasic who has completed the MIT program has

Table 19.3.
Sample MIT Level 3 Session with Step and Summation Scores

Aphasic's Performance	Scores		
	Step 1	Step 2	Step 3
First sentence: Aphasic succeeds in all steps. Maximum scores attained.	1	2	2
Second sentence: Succeeds in all steps but requires backups for Steps 2 and 3.	1	1	1
Third sentence: Succeeds in Step 1, requires a backup to initiate Step 2, succeeds in Step 3.	1	1	2
Fourth sentence: Succeeds in Step 1, requires a backup for Step 2 because of inaccurate response, fails to initiate response in Step 3 after a backup.	1	1	0
Fifth sentence: Succeeds in Step 1, fails to repeat accurately in Step 2, and fails again after a backup. Progression stopped and no score may be given for Step 3.	1	0	—
Scores Total:	5/5	5/10	5/8
	15/23 (65%)		

Table 19.4.
Sample MIT Level IV Session with Step and Summation Scores

Aphasic's Performance	Scores			
	Step 1	Step 2	Step 3	Step 4
First sentence: Aphasic succeeds in Steps 1 and 2, requires a backup to initiate normal prosody in Step 3. Succeeds in Step 4 but no bonus because of failure on last associative question.	2	2	1	2
Second sentence: Succeeds in Step 1, requires backups for Steps 2 and 3. Succeeds with bonus in Step 4.	2	1	1	3
Third sentence: Aphasic requires a backup to succeed in Step 1 and then succeed in subsequent steps.	1	2	2	3
Fourth sentence: Succeeds in Steps 1, 2, and 3, requires a backup for Step 4, fails to answer any associative question.	2	2	2	1
Fifth sentence: Succeeds in Steps 1, 2, and 3, requires a backup for one specific question in Step 4, but answers all associative questions.	2	2	2	2
Scores	9/10	9/10	8/10	11/15
Total:	37/45 (82%)			

Table 19.5.
Quick Reference Hierarchy Guide MIT Levels I and II

LEVEL I

Single Step
  C (HT) Hums melody twice.
  C and **A** (U) Hum melody twice. **C** fades.
  Score and progression: No score. Proceed to next melody.

LEVEL II

Step 1
  C (HT) hums melody → intones sentence.
  C signals **A**.
  C and **A** (HT) (U) intonation of sentence.
  Score and progression:
    Acceptable—1 point. Proceed to Step 2, same sentence.
    Unacceptable—Discontinue progress for sentence.

Step 2
  C (HT) hums melody → intones same sentence.
  C signals **A**.
  C and **A** (HT) (U) intone of sentence. **C** fades.
  Score and progression:
    Acceptable—1 point. Proceed to Step 3, same sentence.
    Unacceptable—Discontinue progression for sentence.

Step 3
  C (HT) intones same sentence → **C** signal **A**.
  C and **A** as **A** intones sentence. **C** intones sentence. **C** intones cue if necessary.
  Score and progression:
    Acceptable without cue—2 points. Proceed to Step 4, same sentence.
    Acceptable with cue—1 point. Proceed to Step 4, same sentence.
    Unacceptable—Discontinue progression for sentence.

Step 4
  C intones "What did you say?" → **C** signals **A**.
  A repeats intoned sentence. **C** intones cue if necessary.
  Score and progression:
    Acceptable without cue—2 points.
    Acceptable with cue—1 point.
    Proceed to Step 1 for next sentence.

Symbols: **A**, aphasic; **C**, clinician; **(HT)** handtapping by clinician with aphasic; **(U)** unison.

Table 19.6.
Quick Reference Hierarchy Guide MIT Level III

Step 1
  C (HT) intones sentence → **C** signals **A**.
  C and **A** (HT) (U) intonation of sentence. **C** fades.
  Score and progression:
    Acceptable—1 point. Proceed to Step 2, same sentence.
    Unacceptable—Discontinue progression for sentence.

Step 2
  C intones same sentence → **C** signals **A** to wait.
  C signals **A** after 1 or 2 seconds.
  A (HT) repeats intoned sentence.
  (B) to Step 1 if **A** fails → retrial of Step 2.
  Score and progression:
    Acceptable without (B)—2 points. Proceed to Step 3, same sentence.
    Acceptable after (B)—1 point. Proceed to Step 3, same sentence.
    Unacceptable after (B)—Discontinue progression for sentence.

Step 3
  C intones a question → **C** signals **A**.
  A gives an appropriate answer, intoned or spoken.
  (B) to Step 2 if **A** fails → retrial of Step 3.
  Score and progression:
    Acceptable without (B)—2 points.
    Acceptable after (B)—1 point.
    Proceed to Step 1 for next sentence.

Symbols: **A**, aphasic; **C** clinician; (HT) handtapping by clinician with aphasic; (B) backup to previous step; (U) unison.

maintained the skills he acquired earlier in the program and has carried them over to normal speech prosody along with an ongoing recovery of ability to encode and emit at least basic verbal communication. Perhaps this recovery now exceeds or will exceed the limits of what MIT is currently designed to offer. Some clinicians may think that the goals should be expanded to help the less severely impaired aphasic whose language profile is essentially that of the good candidate but with less acute impairment. This would place the method alongside other tech-

Table 19.7.
Quick Reference Hierarchy Guide MIT Level IV

Step 1
C (HT) intones sentence → C signals A to wait.
C (HT) presents sentence twice in *sprechgesang*.
C signals A.
C and A (HT) (U) *sprechgesang* of sentence.
(B) to C (HT) presentation in *sprechgesang* if aphasic fails.
Retrial of C and A (HT) (U) *sprechgesang*.
Score and Progression:
   Acceptable *sprechgesang*—2 points. Proceed to Step 2, same sentence.
   Acceptable after (B)—1 point. Proceed to Step 2, same sentence.
   Unacceptable—Discontinue progression for sentence.

Step 2
C (HT) presents same sentence in *sprechgesang* → C signals A to wait.
C signals A after 2 or 3 seconds.
A (HT) repeats sentence in *sprechgesang*.
(B) to Step 1 if A fails → retrial of Step 2.
Score and Progression:
   Acceptable without (B)—2 points. Proceed to Step 3, same sentence.
   Unacceptable—Discontinue progression for sentence.

Step 3
No handtapping.
C presents same sentence twice in normal speech prosody.
C signals A to wait 2 or 3 seconds → then signals to repeat.
A repeats sentence in normal speech prosody.
(B) to C presentation in normal speech prosody if A fails.
Retrial of A repetition.
Score and Progression:
   Acceptable without (B)—2 points. Proceed to Step 4, same sentence.
   Acceptable after (B)—1 point. Proceed to Step 4, same sentence.
   Unacceptable—Discontinue progression for sentence.

Step 4
C Question about substantive content, same sentence.
A Any appropriate response.
(B) to Step 3 if response if unacceptable → retrial of Step 4.
C Questions about associative information.
A Any appropriate responses.
Score and Progression:
   2 points without (B), substantive content, 1 point after (B).
   3 bonus points, one or more responses to associative questions.
   Proceed to next sentence.

Symbols: **A**, aphasic; **C**, clinician; (HT) handtapping by clinician with aphasic; (B) backup; (U) unison.

niques that are concerned with improving syntax, articulation, and efficiency of retrieval. MIT might be used concurrently with these techniques in post-MIT language therapy. Many of us have modified the hierarchy for limited use after completion of the four levels. The issue could be raised as to how long language therapy should continue when the improving aphasic person reaches a point where he can experience some continuing recovery in his own milieu. However, that discussion does not belong here.

A fifth, less structured postgraduate step has been used to retire melodic intonation. Its design includes only *sprechgesang* and normal speech prosody repetition along with an increased emphasis on answering questions such as those used in Step 4 of the last level. It is useful to encourage the aphasic to use *sprechgesang* as an auto-therapy when he is experiencing difficulty with word finding and the phonemic structure of words. Most MIT graduates find it difficult to use the technique unless some prompting takes place before final discharge from the realm of MIT.

Sample MIT Session and Scoring for Level IV.   A five-item therapy session with scoring for the fourth level is presented in Table 19.4.

Quick Reference Guide for the Hierarchy

The four levels of the MIT hierarchy are presented in Tables 19.5 to 19.7 for the convenience of the clinician during administration of the therapy.

Concurrent Language Therapies

Because MIT involves a marked departure from normal speech, and because of its carefully planned program of progression, we recommend that no other therapy that is directed specifically to improved verbal output should be used concurrently. The aphasic may easily be confused if one form demands intoning all verbal output and another uses a procedure involving normal speech prosody. The gradual transition in MIT to therapy that involves normal prosody makes it possible to transfer to other language intervention strategies easily after completion of the hierarchy. This has been discussed earlier.

Progression from One Level to the Next One

Progression from Level II to Level III or from Level III to Level IV, or from Level IV to post-MIT therapy should occur after sufficient evidence that the aphasic has developed a stable proficiency. Our hypothesis that increased participation of the right hemisphere occurs in MIT implies that a somewhat prolonged process is involved. Whether the clinician who uses MIT agrees with our hypothesis is less essential than that he or she progresses slowly to ensure maintained improvement from this method. Actually, the rate or progress made by the good candidate will be slow.

Suggested Means of Controlling Rate of Progression

We recommend that moving from one level to the next higher one should occur only after a mean score of 90% or better for 10 consecutive therapy sessions has been achieved. This may often involve some approach-retreat before the 90% mean is achieved when we consider the usual fluctuation of aphasic performance from day to day.

Participation of the Aphasic's Family During and After Clinical MIT

Much emphasis is placed on members of the aphasic's family participating in the process of attempted rehabilitation of his language. However, participation of the family in the early period when the focus is entirely on intonation and accuracy of intonation patterns is viewed with reservations unless supervision is provided by the clinician. The family of the aphasic should be encouraged to assist in selection of useful phrases used frequently by themselves and the aphasic premorbidly. It is important that these lists be extensive to provide great variety of word orders. Experience with this selective process makes it possible for the aphasic and his family to offer information and vocabulary based on observations and experience in their daily activities.

The role of the family to encourage *sprechgesang* as a means of word-retrieval efficiency for the aphasic in the home and among selected friends is strongly recommended for words and phrases that have a high frequency of use in the household.

SUMMARY

In summary, six major elements of MIT are covered. They are as follows: certain principles of language therapy for aphasia and associated phonological disorders that have influenced the design of the MIT strategy; a discussion of the candidacy that contrasts the language profiles of good and poor candidates for this type of language intervention; a description of the technique of intoning and plotting intonation patterns; a detailed instruction of administration of the MIT hierarchy; a discussion of post-MIT strategies; and participation of members of the aphasic's family during clinical intervention and after its completion.

FUTURE TRENDS

The family of the aphasic who is receiving or has received MIT should be systematically involved as a support team. Future development of Melodic Intonation Therapy should include the development of published guidelines that the family may use. Their support is particularly essential when the aphasic is receiving less than one therapy session each day with the clinician.

Further collection of data on candidacy is essential as a means of further evidence of the efficacy of melodic intonation therapy. The contributions of careful language examination and scientific studies are of equal importance.

REFERENCES

Albert, M. L., and Helm-Estabrook, N. (1988). Diagnosis and treatment of aphasia, Part II. *Journal of American Medical Association, 259,* 1208–1209.

Blumstein, S. E. (1973). *A phonological investigation of aphasic speech.* The Hague: Mouton.

Gordon, H. W. (1972). *Verbal and non-verbal cerebral processing in man for audition.* Doctoral thesis, California Institute of Technology.

Jackson, H. (1931). *Selected writings of John Hughlings Jackson.* London: Hodder & Stoughton.

Knighton, K. (1973). Beginning teaching techniques. *Teaching music at beginning levels.* Wellesley: Kodaly Musical Training Institute.

Martin, A. D. and Rigrodsky (1979). An investigation of phonological impairment in aphasia, Part I. *Cortex, 10,* 318–328.

Sarno, M., Silverman, M. and Sands, E. (1970). Speech therapy and language recovery in severe aphasia. *Journal of Speech and Hearing Research, 13,* 607–623.

Schuell, H., Jenkins, H. and Jimenez-Pabon, E. (1964). *Aphasia in adults.* New York: Harper & Row.

Sparks, R. (1978). Parastandardized examination guidelines for adult aphasia. *British Journal Disorders of Communication, 41,* 135–146.

Sparks, R., Helm, N., and Albert, M. (1974). Aphasia rehabilitation resulting from melodic intonation therapy. *Cortex, 10,* 303–316.

Sparks, R., and Holland, A. (1976). Method: Melodic intonation therapy. *Journal of Speech and Hearing Disorders, 41,* 287–297.

Whitaker, H. A. (1970). A model for neurolinguistics. *Occasional Papers.*

CHAPTER 20

Role of the Right Hemisphere in the Treatment of Aphasia

CHRIS CODE

In this chapter we will examine the idea that the right cerebral hemisphere can have a special role in the treatment of aphasia. We will examine this claim with reference to two fundamental assumptions that underlie much therapy for aphasia: (*a*), that the right hemisphere processes certain kinds of cognitive material in a relatively superior way, and that for aphasic individuals with damage limited to the left hemisphere, the right hemisphere can be used to *compensate* for lost language functions; (*b*), that, following damage to the left, the right hemisphere can be encouraged to *restore* lost functions.

We will consider the variety of approaches that have been advocated and tried that claim at some level to engage cognitive processing in the right hemisphere. Some have simply employed techniques and methods that make use of the right hemiphere's compensatory functions, whereas others have sought to examine the claim that we can influence right-hemisphere processing directly using lateralization techniques.

LANGUAGE PROCESSING IN THE RIGHT HEMISPHERE

The right hemisphere appears to be a sophisticated visuospatial processor, and damage often results in impairments of functions that appear to require intact visuospatial processing. Patients may present with a range of perceptual problems including facial and object agnosia, unilateral neglect, tactile and visual recognition of complex geometric patterns, spatial disorientation, and constructional apraxia (Perecman, 1983; Young and Ratcliff, 1983), as well as disturbances in emotional expression and reception (Ley and Bryden, 1981). From the perspective of aphasia treatment, as we will see later, intact perceptual processing has been used in developing approaches to treatment that use the right hemisphere.

It is no longer a secret that the right hemisphere has significant language abilities, and it will not be our mission in this chapter to review these in detail. (See the reviews by Chiarello, 1988; Code, 1987; and Joanette et al., 1990.) What is still a mystery, however, is the nature and extent of the right hemisphere's involvement in language in the normal brain. The major barriers to demystification result to a large extent from the population and methodological differences between studies. Studies have looked at a large range of subject types including normal subjects, stroke patients, head-injured patients, and individuals who have undergone radical and major brain surgery—hemispherectomies and commissurotomies. Methodologies have included examination of lesion sites, cerebral blood flow and metabolism, electrical activity, and the effects of anesthetizing the hemispheres. Behavioral methods that are thought to measure "lateral preference" for a wide range of language material have proliferated over the years. These methods have been used to assess the contribution of the left and right hemispheres to language processing by examining and measuring laterality effects in the auditory, visual, and tactile modalities; eye and eyebrow movements; finger tapping; and degree of lateral mouth opening during speech. The data from these studies too are mainly inconclusive. While this has produced a rich and varied database for neuropsychology, it has resulted in incompatibility and lack of agreement between studies and a poor replication record. A general belief now is that there are significant individual differences in cognitive style and response to experimental tasks (Segalowitz and Bryden, 1983), brain organization and representation of language (Ojemann, 1979), and cerebral circulation (Hart et al., 1991).

Bearing in mind the cautions outlined in the previous paragraph, what does the research tells us about the right hemisphere's role in language processing in the normal brain? It may be best to deal with this complex question with reference to a standard linguistic framework.

The study of aphasic symptomatology over the last 100 years or so confirms that the left hemisphere's role in language is in terms of those aspects that can be characterized through a formal unit-and-rule generative linguistic model. Aphasic individuals have problems at the strict linguistic levels of phonology, morphology, syntax, and lexical semantics (Code, 1991a). In contrast, an essential characteristic of the right hemisphere's involvement is in aspects of language processing not covered by straight linguistic processes. In this way, underlying the syntactic, morphological, and phonological processing associated with the left hemisphere is a serial, analytical, segmental processing mode. In comparison, some have suggested that the right hemisphere's fundamental processing mode is holistic and parallel. Thus, left-hemisphere damage produces problems in context-free linguistic processes (e.g., syntax, phonology), whereas right-hemisphere damage effects context-dependent complex linguistic entities like verbal jokes, metaphors, narratives, and indirect speech acts, as well as semantic discrimination and intonation (for reviews see Chiarello, 1988; Code, 1987; Joanette et al., 1990).

Not everyone is happy with dichotomizing the contributions of the right and left hemispheres to mental activity in this way (see Bradshaw and Nettleton, 1981, and accompanying commentaries), although the fact remains that much of the research in the area is concerned with testing the predictions of the analytical-holistic characterization.

Actually, although rudimentary, the right hemisphere does appear to have some straight linguistic competence. It cannot process active versus passive, distinguish singular from plural, or process future tenses, but it appears to be able to differentiate affirmatives and negatives and comprehend concrete nouns, adjectival phrases, and object definitional phrases. Assessment of the right hemisphere of split-brain individuals on standardized tests has indicated that it has a vocabulary roughly equivalent to a 13-year-old child, but its syntactic competence is around the 5-year-old level. Although it may have this auditory comprehension ability, the right hemisphere appears to possess little or no facility for processing phonological and phonetic information (Code, 1987; Searleman, 1977).

The right hemisphere has some abilities to process lexical-semantic information. Right-hemisphere-damaged patients have impairments in comprehending the meaning of individual words (Gainotti et al., 1983); have deficits in the understanding of connotative but not denotative meaning (Brownell et al., 1984; Gardner and Denes, 1973), and do not appear to be able to make judgments of semantic relatedness involving picture-word matching (Hart et al., 1991).

As indicated earlier, there is more to language than that which can be handled by a strictly linguistic model. Wapner et al. (1981) have summarized the findings from a series of studies of right-hemisphere-damaged subjects. The left hemisphere deals with the context-free, componential domains of syntax, phonology, and so on, whereas the right hemisphere handles noncomponential, context=bound, nonliteral, complex features of language, such as understanding stories, jokes, and metaphors; integrating complex linguistic information; appreciating indirect speech acts; and using contextually bound discourse (Bryan, 1989; Code, 1987; Wapner et al., 1981).

Finally, there is now a large body of research that shows that the right hemisphere is engaged in the processing of various suprasegmental features of prosody (Ross, 1983) as well as emotional prosody and emotional language (Ley and Bryden, 1981). There are close relationships between the processing of music and prosody, and the right hemisphere is engaged in the processing of both.

The Right Hemisphere Language Battery (Bryan, 1989) is a battery of standardized procedures tested for reliability for patients with right-hemisphere damage. It includes tests of lexical semantics, verbal and written metaphor, verbal humor, stress, and discourse.

RECOVERY AND THE RIGHT HEMISPHERE

We should start with one assumption: The right hemisphere is very clearly involved in normal mental activity. Following left-hemisphere damage, we should expect the right hemisphere to be involved.

The notion that following left-hemisphere damage the right hemisphere is involved in the spontaneous recovery of aphasia takes more than one form. One form of the idea is that all or some of the symptoms that characterize aphasia—agrammatism, paraphasia, speech automatisms, dyslexia, and so on—are produced not by a damaged left hemisphere but by an intact right hemisphere. The evidence for this view is sparse and mainly inferential. Right-hemisphere hypotheses have been developed for some kinds of speech automatisms (Code, 1987, 1991b) and for some of the features of acquired dyslexia (Coltheart, 1980; Landis and Regard 1988; Weniger et al., 1988). The strongest claim, what we can identify after Code (1987) as *the lateral shift hypothesis*, is based on the conventional dominance model, which sees the left hemisphere as dominant over the right in the normal brain. Following damage to the left hemisphere, perhaps to some control mechanism, the right hemisphere is released from the inhibition of the dominant left, and there is a shift in control from left to right. Related to this is the notion that linguistic abilities that have been latent can emerge from the right hemisphere following damage to the left (Moscovitch, 1973). The weakest claim is that the right hemisphere's contribution following left-hemisphere damage is a straight and simple compensatory one in which, for instance, visuospatial processing is used by the patient to compensate for lost linguistic skills. These two last broad notions have relevance for ideas on how to employ the right hemisphere in treating aphasia, as we will see later.

Little is certain in this area, but there are strong indications from a range of studies that the involvement of the right hemisphere in aphasic individuals varies as a function of severity and time since onset: The more severe the aphasia and the more time has elapsed since the damage, then the more involved the right hemisphere appears to be (Cappa and Vallar, 1992; Code, 1987; Gainotti, in press; Weniger et al., 1988).

Now that we have some basic background on the issues in the area, and some understanding of the nature of the right hemisphere's contribution to mental activity and its contribution to recovery from aphasia, we can ask some questions about the role of the undamaged right hemisphere in the treatment of aphasia following left-hemisphere damage.

ROLE OF THE RIGHT HEMISPHERE IN THE TREATMENT OF APHASIA

In the remainder of this chapter, we will examine attempts to cause improvement in communication for aphasic individuals by influencing processing in the right hemisphere. We can divide up these various approaches in a number of ways. We can use the established notions of *restitution* and *compensation*, as outlined earlier, to guide us. Some approaches are unquestionably experimental, insofar as they are not designed to be employed in everyday rehabilitation.

Using the Right Hemisphere to Compensate for Aphasia

The most obviously compensatory approaches are those that use intact, traditionally termed "nonverbal" processing associated with the right hemisphere.

Glass et al. (1973) and Gardner and his associates (Baker et al., 1975; Gardner et al., 1976) developed artificial languages that they taught to groups of globally aphasic patients. Glass et al. (1973) used the system developed by Premack (1971) to test the abilities of chimpanzees to acquire and use a symbolic system. The system employs left-to-right sequencing of arbitrary shapes, which are functionally equivalent to words. Seven severely aphasic but alert patients with good nonverbal skills and high motivation, but no apparent syntactic competence with natural language, were able to achieve a level of skill far beyond their abilities with natural language. Training entailed teaching a vocabulary of nouns and verbs and symbols for interrogation and negation. "Sentences" were gradually built up until patients could ask questions like "Anthea (therapist's name) give John (patient's name) water" (Glass et al., 1973, p. 98).

VIC (visual communication) was the name of the system developed by Baker et al. (1975) and Gardner et al., (1976). Like the Premack system, VIC employs some arbitrary geometric shapes, but also ideographic-representational symbols. Some were actually schematic object pictures. The symbols were on small cards and were used in a left-to-right syntax. A small group of globally aphasic patients of more than 6 months post-onset who were able to match objects to pictures were trained to carry out commands, answer questions, and describe events. Some patients went on to a further level that explored the ability to express needs, feelings, and desires using VIC. Patients' comprehension of VIC symbols was 94% compared with 50% comprehension of spoken commands. Naming using VIC was 89%, with natural naming at 14%.

Both studies report significant success. The globally aphasic patients could learn the systems and use them in a propositional fashion at a level far superior to their abilities with natural language. With these systems, globally aphasic patients were able to create novel sentences by arranging and rearranging the symbols, not simply match shapes to pictures.

More recently, the VIC system has been developed for the Apple Macintosh computer and has become C-VIC. Using the mouse, the patient is able to select the "cards" from a range of domains, for example, nouns and verbs. By using the mouse, these can be arranged into a simple left-to-right syntax. The most up-to-date version (which is known as Lingraphica) runs on the highly portable Mac Powerbook and has been much augmented. The vocabulary of icons has been increased, with verb icons becoming animated for ease of recognition, editing, and composition. Also sound and text displays have been added. Careful single-case treatment studies are verifying that it can be learned and used by severely aphasic individuals such that they can communicate with it better than with natural language (Steele et al., 1989; Steele et al., 1992; Weinrich et al., 1989).

The patients trained on VIC and C-VIC, like those trained on the Premack system, are using a syntactic code, demonstrating a retained linguistic competence. What appears to be happening is that the patient is using a nonlinguistic syntactic analysis, some kind of implicit functional syntactic mechanism employed in decoding a meaningful visual array (Gazzaniga, 1974).

Carrier and Peak (1974) have developed the Non-Slip (Non Speech Language Initiation Program) based on the VIC research and the research by Glass et al. (1973). It includes various sizes of arbitrary geometric colored shapes with the words the shapes represent printed on them and the stimulus.

RESTORATION VIA COMPENSATION OF FUNCTION USING THE RIGHT HEMISPHERE

There is a class of therapeutic methods that probably use right-hemisphere processing to restore lost functions. Melodic intonation therapy (MIT) (Sparks, 1981; Sparks, et al., 1974) is consciously based on the findings that the right hemisphere has particular involvement in the processing of some features of music and prosody. It is well recognized that Broca's-type patients and global patients, particularly, often retain remarkable abilities to sing and use intonation. There is an ability to articulate the words of songs with a level of skill far in excess of their ability to pronounce the same words in a nonmusical context (Yamadori et al., 1977). We will not go into MIT in detail here, as the method is well known and highly accessible elsewhere (Sparks, 1981). The method entails a strict behavioral training program involving several levels and stages within levels. First, the patient is trained to use a slightly exaggerated intonation (like the sort of "speechsong" operatic characters use to communicate in between the main songs of the opera) for short utterances with the help of the therapist, who gradually fades out his or her assistance. As the program and the patient progress, utterances become longer, therapist help fades out, and the patient reduces reliance on the exaggerated intonation. While certain features of musical processing seem to be processed by the left hemisphere, depending on a complex interaction of individual levels of musical expertise and degree of familiarity with the material (Gordon, 1978), the evidence from aphasia and hemispherectomy cases confirms that the right hemisphere for these patients can articulate when an utterance is carried with the coupling of a musical contour (Yamadori et al., 1977).

Words can be contrasted on an imageable (concrete)–nonimageable (abstract) dimension (Paivio, 1971; Richardson, 1975). Paivio's dual-coding theory proposes that information can be processed using an abstract verbal system or a concrete imagery system. The former is a left-hemisphere system for most people and the latter is associated with visuoperceptual processing in the right hemisphere (Bakan, 1980). Studies show that normal subjects perform better on a variety of cognitive tasks with words high in imagery and concreteness than on words low in imagery and concreteness. West (1983) proposes a form of therapy based on the observation that this holds for aphasic individuals also who have good retained abilities in imagery. Using Paivio's (1971) model as a basis, West suggests that an intact visual imagery system may have the capacity to arouse the verbal system for some patients. Myers (1980) also advocates that stimulus materials used with aphasic patients should aim to encourage imagery, not simply with pictures of concrete objects but through use of highly imageable actions, entailing complex relationships and interactions with the ability to invoke rich associations.

There have been some intriguing indications that there may be a role for the hypnotized right hemisphere in the treatment of aphasia. There is evidence that the right hemisphere is markedly more affected by hypnosis than the left. Gur and Gur (1974) found significant interactions between lateral eye movements during verbal and spatial tasks in 60 subjects under hypnosis and Frumkin et al. (1978) found significantly more right-hemisphere involvement in dichotic presentation of CVC (consonant-vowel-consonant) syllables during hypnosis than before and following hypnosis. McKeever et al. (1981) provide some support for the idea that there might be a role for hypnosis in aphasia therapy from their study, which examined the effects of hypnosis on the right hemisphere of a commissurotomized patient. The 28-year-old female patient was tested for left-hand tactile anomia before, during, and following hypnosis. Because of the disconnection between the left-hand tactile input and the left hemisphere caused by the sectioning of the corpus callosum, such patients are unable to name objects palpated with the left hand. Before hypnosis, the patient successfully named 2 out of 20 objects palpated with the left hand; but during hypnotic regression, 7 days later, she was able to name 7 of 21 objects. Her speech was slow and effortful. When tested following hypnosis, she could name only one item. During further sessions of hypnosis with and without regression, the subject was able to name between 3, 5, 11, and 12 objects from 21. The remarkably improved performance under hypnosis is unlikely to be due simply to the relaxing effect of hypnosis. The authors conjecture that it may be due to suppression of guessing by the left hemisphere, which they suggest may be responsible for poor guessing without hypnosis. The labored speech may have been due to control of the left-hemisphere speech production mechanism by the right via her intact anterior commissure.

Hypnosis and imagery have been applied to aphasic patients in an attempt to improve naming. Thompson et al. (1986) trained three Broca's patients on a single-subject design to use imagery and visualization. Items were split so that five were retained for testing only and five were used for treatment. Therapy sessions ranged between 15 and 17 sessions over 8 to 17 weeks. Results showed that combined imagery and hypnosis training was effective for two of the subjects. For one subject, improvement appeared to generalize to items not used in treatment, and for the other, improvement was limited to items used in treatment. While these were interesting results and encourage further research, the authors acknowledge that the patients may not have been fully hypnotized, as there are no valid measures of hypnotic susceptibility for aphasic patients. They may not have been using imagery, as the only way to assess this is via self-report—by asking people if they are imaging items.

RESTORATION OF FUNCTION IN THE RIGHT HEMISPHERE VIA DIRECT LATERALIZATION RETRAINING

The approaches discussed thus far use the apparent natural abilities of the right hemisphere to compensate or substitute for lost functions. Finally, in this chapter we will examine some exploratory approaches into reestablishing language skills via hemispheric retraining and/or stimulation.

The final kind of approach that aims to use the intact right hemisphere attempts to influence recovery via a direct access to the right hemisphere using such techniques as dichotic listening and hemifield viewing. This can involve the reestablishment of lost functions via some kind of hemispheric specialization retraining. We will consider the few single case studies that have been completed.

Buffery and Burton (1982) describe the treatment of a male Wernicke's-type patient through the visual, auditory, and tactile modalities, first separately and then progressing to a cross-trimodal semantic discrimination stimulation task. A typical task entailed presentation of the word "lad" to the left visual field

via a tachistoscope, "boy" to the left hand, and "toy" to the left ear. The patient's task was to identify "toy" as the odd one out. At the separate visual stage, single letters progressed to words presented to the left visual field. For training in the auditory condition, verbal material was presented to the left ear while white noise was presented to the right ear, and haptic (tactile) training involved presentation of raised letters and words to the left hand while the right hand felt a sponge.

The patient was treated for 2 years and 6 months with this kind of semantic stimulation, with tasks progressing from simple to more complex, making semantic odd-one-out decisions. As the material was presented to the left of body and space, the assumption was that it was ending up in the right hemisphere for processing. The patient made gradual and significant improvement in Wechsler Adult Intelligence Scale (WAIS) verbal IQ to a near average level. There was also an increase in left lateral responses (i.e., left ear, left visual field, and left-hand scores) over the treatment period.

Buffery and Burton's (1982) approach essentially entailed semantic stimulation, or "bombardment" as they called it, based on the assumption that the right hemisphere has some semantic discrimination abilities to build on, as indeed the literature reviewed earlier appears to suggest.

A similar study (Code, 1983, 1989) was underway at the same time as Buffery and Burton's. The patient, J.W., was 37 years old and 2 years, 9 months postonset when the study began. He had suffered a unilateral posterior left-hemisphere lesion. He had been well educated and worked as a civil servant prior to his stroke. Following the stroke, he worked as a gardener for the city. Detailed pretreatment assessment revealed a partially recovered patient classified as Wernicke's. Under normal, everyday conditions he was fluent and made occasional paraphasic errors but could conduct a normal conversation provided the other participant was prepared to interrupt occasionally for clarification; J.W. himself had to request repetitions at times. Auditory verbal comprehension was clearly J.W.'s main problem, with particular difficulties on nonredundant tests. On DeRenzi and Faglioni's (1978) Shortened Token Test he scored 11, which places him in the Severe category (there are five categories from Normal to Very Severe).

J.W. was also tested on the Digit Span Test described by Albert and Bear (1974). Albert and Bear showed that the temporal aspects of speech perception are clearly implicated in comprehension loss, such that patients require more time to understand. When the rate of presentation of sets of digits is reduced, many aphasic patients are able to retain significantly more digits. For J.W., recorded sets of three digits were presented at three different rates: with a 5-second pause, with a 3-second pause, and with a 0.5-second pause between digits. From 10 presentations of 3-digit trigrams, J.W. reported back 11 at the 0.5 second condition (36.6%) but managed no complete trigrams; 20 digits (66.6%) in the 3-second condition with two complete trigrams; and 25 digits (83.3%) with six complete trigrams in the 5-second condition. This would indicate, first, that J.W. had severe auditory verbal retention problems at relatively normal rates (0.5 seconds) and, second, that J.W. benefited considerably from additional time to process the incoming information.

J.W. underwent additional exhaustive pretreatment testing, including tests of lateral preference for visual, auditory, and haptically presented verbal material. On three dichotic, two tachistoscopic, and two haptic verbal tests he showed a preference for material presented to his left ear, visual field, and left hand, respectively. This suggests that J.W. was already using his right hemisphere more than his left for language.

We took about 19 months to work through a three-part program aimed at improving his comprehension using specially prepared dichotic tapes (Part 1) and hemifield viewing (Part 2) only, first separately and then in a combined cross-modal program (Part 3). Each of the three parts took approximately 6.5 months. J.W. was seen twice weekly with sessions lasting about 40 minutes. The specific aim of Part 1 was to improve his right hemisphere's ability to discriminate between phonemes and to improve its auditory verbal retention capabilities. Therefore, so during Part 1, he was asked to use his left ear, in competition with his right, in the discrimination of dichotically presented syllables and the auditory retention of strings of digits and syllables.

For the visual program (Part 2), the tachistoscopic hemifield viewing technique was used to present visual-verbal material to J.W.'s right hemisphere via his left visual field (LVF). A range of tasks involved letter, digit, and CVC word identification and semantic discrimination of words using a three-word odd-one-out task (e.g., car, bus, hat). In addition, there was a phonological two-word task where two words that could be phonologically fused were presented in the left field for processing. Two words such as sun-pun (spun) and sin-kin (skin) were presented, and J.W. was expected to report both words and to deduce the fused word.

Part 3 of the program concentrated on the cross-modal capabilities of dichotic listening and hemifield viewing. Material was presented simultaneously to the right hemisphere via the auditory and visual modalities. A same-different paradigm was employed in which verbal auditory retention and phonemic discrimination were combined. In one cross-modal treatment task, two pairs of digits were presented dichotically via tape (two to each ear), with a pause of 1.5 seconds between each pair. Simultaneous with presentation of the second digit pair, two digits appeared in the subject's left visual field via the tachistoscope. Either both the auditory and visual digits were either identical (a same response) or both visually presented digits were different to the dichotically presented digits. The tasks making up the program increased in difficulty as J.W. progressed: The number of digits increased to three digits at the left ear and in the left visual field; one of the three visually presented digits was the same as one of the three dichotically presented digits for a different response; and two of the three visual digits were the same as the dichotic digits for a different response. A further cross-modal subprogram in Part 3 of the treatment program combined phonemic discrimination with verbal auditory retention by presenting pairs of minimally paired words simultaneously with words in J.W.'s left visual field for a same/different response.

Both Buffery and Burton (1982) and Code (1989) report statistically significant improvements in their patients on standardized tests and changes in laterality scores. Buffery and Burton used the WAIS (Wechsler, 1955) for pre- and posttreatment measurement, and Code (1989) used a range of standard tests including the PICA (Porch Index of Communication Ability) (Porch, 1967, 1971), the Shortened Token Test (DeRenzi and Faglioni, 1978), and the Reporter's Test (DeRenzi and

Ferrari, 1978), as well as ongoing monitoring of J.W.'s performance using the Base-10 methodology (LaPointe, 1977).

Despite the apparent positive effects of the treatment in both these cases, there are many problems with the laterality methods used and the assumptions made, some of which reflect a fairly naive appreciation of the power of the methodology. In fact, it is simply impossible to determine whether the improvements were really due to direct stimulation of the right hemisphere or to other uncontrolled factors.

First, we now have a better understanding of the limitations and unreliability of the behavioral "laterality" techniques, especially with brain-damaged individuals. It is clear that it is simply not possible to measure hemispheric processing in many brain-damaged patients using behavioral laterality methods (see Code, 1987, for a critical review of the main techniques). Additionally, lateralization techniques actually used in treatment, as in both of these case studies, cannot be considered as reliable and uncontaminated measures of hemispheric processing. The only control for this factor used in the studies under discussion was the tactile (haptic) test used in Code's (1989) study. Here measures were taken before treatment and after each part of the treatment with verbal haptic tests involving the presentation of verbal material to the hands and fingers of the subject. While both left dichotic and visual hemifield advantages increased (usually interpreted within the paradigm as indicating increased right-hemisphere activity), haptic scores did not. However, this statement is also subject to the same proviso concerning the reliability of haptic processing. So the indications are that either there was no real change in hemispheric processing as a result of the treatment or the methods used were not reliable enough to answer the question.

In neither study was there any guarantee that the treatment material was being processed by the right hemisphere. There was no real evidence to exclude the possibility that the material was not passing over to the left hemisphere for processing, even if the material was actually reaching the right hemisphere initially in the intended order.

Recently, Burton et al. (1987) have attempted to apply a tighter experimental design in a single-case study that employed a modified dichotic listening task to examine the effects of semantic "priming" of the right hemisphere on picture-naming performance. The subject was a 55-year-old aphasic man some 2 years postonset. The aim of the study was to assess short-term effects over six treatment sessions. The design entailed treating (priming) and testing on four sets of pictures in a pre- and posttest and a priming condition.

Forty object pictures were split into four sets of 10 each (A1, A2, A3, A4) in which the patient had to say whether the dichotically presented name at the attended ear matched the picture presented in free vision. All that was required from the patient was a "Yes" or "No" response. Set A1 was used in all tasks (pretest, priming treatment, and posttest); set A2 was used for pre- and posttest only; set A3 was used for priming and posttest only; and set A4 was used just for posttest. With this design, the authors hoped to determine the effects of priming in the separate conditions and of generalization.

In two sessions, material was presented in dichotic competition where the patient had to attend to his left ear; in two other sessions, material was presented for attention by the right ear; and in the final two sessions, material was presented binaurally, first for the attention of the left ear and then for the attention of the right ear.

The patient's performance in naming following the right and left dichotic sessions was contrasted with the binaural sessions. At posttest, the patient was assessed on all four sets of pictures, and little support was found for the view that the right hemisphere can be selectively primed to increase its contribution to language processing, at least in the short term. There was also little evidence for any difference in the effects of left or right dichotic versus binaural presentation from this study. The patient's speed of naming *decreased* significantly after left ear and binaural priming, but latencies showed improvement following repeated presentation of pictures for naming. On the control set of pictures (A4) not used during treatment, there was no evidence of improved naming. Overall, the results seem to suggest that semantic priming using dichotic or binaural presentation fails to produce improvement in naming, at least for this individual patient and in the short term.

USING THE RIGHT HEMISPHERE IN THE TREATMENT OF APHASIA: FUTURE TRENDS

Although it is probable that the right hemisphere is involved during much of the treatment we do with aphasic people, the research thus far has not been able to demonstrate beyond doubt that it is possible to directly influence the rate or amount of right-hemisphere involvement in recovery.

What does the future hold? First, it seems reasonable to conclude that the right hemisphere is involved in the recovery of aphasia, although its involvement may vary depending on, at least, severity and time since onset and individual differences. Second, while there is little hard evidence to support specific effects in individual patients, it would appear reasonable to conclude that the by now well-known functions of the right hemisphere can play a role in therapy in the kinds of approaches we have discussed above, such as melody and imagery. When it comes to evaluating the possibilities of a more direct role for the right hemisphere in treatment, an obvious conclusion must be that there is no solid experimental evidence to support an approach to treatment involving direct stimulation of the right hemisphere.

Perhaps a future approach to using the right hemisphere to the full in the treatment of aphasia will look something like that advocated by Horner and Fedor (1983). These authors bring together a whole range of traditional and contemporary ideas and research findings to provide the framework for an approach to aphasia treatment with its foundation in the idea of hemispheric reorganization. The approach of these authors aims to access impaired left-hemisphere functions through intact homologous areas in the right hemisphere and their connecting neural pathways. The therapy tasks essentially entail deblocking and facilitation. Horner and Fedor (1983) detail treatment for a range of impairments. The treatment for agrammatism centers on prosody, phonology, and syntax. At each level of treatment an intact function, assumed to be under the control of the right hemisphere, is paired with an impaired function. The initial aim at the level of prosody is to restore control of phonation, which may be achieved by pairing intact emotional facial expression (prosodic-affective deblockers) and whole-body movements (spatial-holistic deblockers) with vocalization.

There is no shortage of ideas in our search for successful treatment for aphasia. What there is still a shortage of, however, are clear indications that the treatments we devise are really helping the people who depend on us. We will end this chapter in the traditional manner, with a plea for more, and better, research. We need a series of tightly designed single cases that aim to control for the factors mentioned earlier in this chapter: Is the patient improving? If so, is the patient improving as a direct result of the treatment? If so, is directing the treatment to the right hemisphere a necessary feature of the effectiveness of the treatment?

References

Albert, M. L., and Bear, D. (1974). Time to understand: a case study in word deafness with reference to the role of time in auditory comprehension. *Brain, 97*, 373–384.

Bakan, P. (1980). Imagery, raw and cooked: A hemispheric recipe. In J. E. Shorr, G. E. Sobel, P. Robin, and J. A. Connella (Eds.), *Imagery: Its many dimensions and applications.* New York: Plenum Press.

Baker, E., Berry T., Gardner, H., Zurif, E., Davis, L., and Veroff, A. (1975). Can linguistic competence be dissociated from natural language functions? *Nature, 254*, 509–510.

Bradshaw, J. L., and Nettleton, N. C. (1981). The nature of hemispheric specialization in man. *Behavioral and Brain Sciences, 4*, 51–91.

Brownell, H.H., Potter, H.H., and Michelow, D. (1984). Sensitivity to lexical denotation and connotation in brain-damaged patients: A double dissociation? *Brain and Language, 22*, 253–265.

Bryan, K. (1989). *The Right Hemisphere Language Battery.* London: Whurr Publishers.

Buffery, A., and Burton, A. (1982). Information processing and redevelopment: Towards a science of cognitive rehabilitation. In A. Burton (ed.), *The pathology and psychology of cognition.* London: Methuen.

Burton, A., Kemp, R., and Burton, E. (1987). Hemispheric priming and picture naming in an aphasic patient. *Aphasiology, 1*, 41–51.

Cappa, S. F., and Vallar, G. (1992). The role of the left and right hemispheres in recovery from aphasia. *Aphasiology, 6*, 359–372.

Carrier, J., and Peak, T. (1974). Non Speech Language Initiation Program. Lawrence, KS: H & H Enterprises.

Chiarello, C. (Ed.). (1988). *Right hemisphere contributions to lexical semantics.* Berlin: Springer-Verlag.

Code, C. (1983). Hemispheric specialization retraining in aphasia: Possibilities and problems. In C. Code and D. J. Muller (Eds.), *Aphasia therapy.* London: Edward Arnold.

Code, C. (1987). *Language, aphasia, and the right hemisphere.* Chichester: Wiley.

Code, C. (1989). Hemispheric specialization retraining in aphasia: possibilities and problems. In C. Code and D. J. Muller (Eds.), *Aphasia therapy,* (2nd ed.). London: Whurr Publishers.

Code, C. (1991a). Symptoms, syndromes, models: the nature of aphasia. In C. Code (Ed.), *The characteristics of aphasia.* Hove: Lawrence Erlbaum.

Code, C. (1991b). Speech automatisms and recurring utterances. In C. Code (Ed.), *The characteristics of aphasia.* Hove: Lawrence Erlbaum.

Coltheart, M. (1980). Deep dyslexia: A right hemisphere hypothesis. In M. Coltheart, K. Patterson, J. Marshall (Eds.), *Deep dyslexia.* London: Routledge and Kegan Paul.

DeRenzi, E., and Faglioni, P. (1978). Normative data and screening power of a shortened version of the Token Test. *Cortex, 14*, 41–49.

DeRenzi, E., and Ferrari, C. (1978). The Reporter's Test: A sensitive test to detect expressive disturbances in aphasics. *Cortex, 14*, 279–293.

Frumkin, L. R., Ripley, H. S., and Cox, G. B. (1978). Changes in cerebral hemispheric lateralization with hypnosis. *Biological Psychiatry, 13*, 741–750.

Gainotti, G. (in press). The riddle of the right hemisphere's contribution to the recovery of language. *European Journal of Communication Disorders.*

Gainotti, G., Caltagirone, C., and Miceli, G., Selective impairment of semantic-lexical discrimination in right-brain-damaged patients. In E. Perecman (Ed.), *Cognitive processing in the right hemisphere.* London: Academic Press.

Gardner, H., and Denes, G. Connotative judgements by aphasic patients on a pictorial adaptation of the semantic differential. *Cortex, 9*, 183–196.

Gardner, H., Zurif, E. B., Berry, T., and Baker, E. (1976). Visual communication in aphasia. *Neuropsychologia, 14,* 275–292.

Gazzaniga, M. S. (1974). Cerebral dominance viewed as a decision making system. In S. J. Dimond and J. G. Beaumont (Eds.), *Hemispheric function in the human brain.* London: Elek Science.

Glass, A. V., Gazzaniga, M. S., and Premack, D. (1973). Artificial language training in global aphasics. *Neuropsychologia, 11,* 95–103.

Gordon, H. W. (1978). Hemispheric asymmetry for dichotically presented chords in musicians and non-musicians, males and females. *Acta Psychologia, 42,* 383–395.

Gur, R., and Gur, R. E. (1974). Handedness, sex, and eyedness as moderating variables in the relation between hypnotic susceptibility and functional brain asymmetry. *Journal of Abnormal Psychology, 83,* 635.

Hart, J., Lesser, R. P., Fisher, R. S., Schwerdt, P., Bryan, R. N., and Gordon, B. (1991). Dominant-side intracarotid amobarbital spares comprehension of word meaning. *Archives of Neurology. 48,* 55–58.

Horner, J. and Fedor, K. (1983) Minor hemisphere mediation in aphasia treatment. In H. Winitz (Ed.), *Treating language disorders: For clinicians by clinicians.* Baltimore, MD: University Park Press.

Joanette, Y., Goulet, P., and Hannequin, D. (1990). *Right hemisphere and verbal communication.* New York: Springer-Verlag.

Landis, T., and Regard, M. (1988). The right hemisphere's access to lexical meaning: A function of its release from left-hemisphere control? In C. Chiarello (Ed.), *Right hemisphere contributions to lexical semantics.* New York: Springer-Verlag.

LaPointe, L. L. (1977). Base 10 programmed stimulation: Test specification, scoring and plotting performance in aphasia therapy. *Journal of Speech and Hearing Disorders, 42,* 90–105.

Ley, R. G., and Bryden, M. P. (1981). Consciousness, emotion, and the right hemisphere. In G. Underwood and R. Stevens (Eds.), *Aspects of consciousness. Vol. II: Structural issues.* London: Academic Press.

McKeever, W. F., Larrabee, G. J., Sullivan, K. F., Johnson, H. J., Ferguson, S., and Rayport, M. (1981). Unimanual tactile anomia subsequent to corpus callosotomy: Reduction of anomic defect under hypnosis. *Neuropsychologia, 19,* 179–190.

Moscovitch, M. (1973). Language and the cerebral hemispheres: Reaction-time studies and their implications for models of cerebral dominance. In P. Pliner, L. Krames, and T. Alloway (Eds.), *Communication and affect: Language and thought.* New York: Academic Press.

Myers, P. (1980). Visual imagery in aphasia treatment: A new look. In R. H. Brookshire (Ed.), *Clinical Aphasiology Conference proceedings.* Minneapolis, MN: BRK.

Ojemann, G. A. (1979). Individual variability in cortical localization of language. *Journal of Neurosurgery. 50,* 164–169.

Paivio, A. (1971). *Imagery and verbal processing.* New York: Holt.

Perecman, E. (Ed.) (1983). *Cognitive processing in the right hemisphere.* New York: Academic Press.

Porch, B. (1967). *The Porch Index of Communicative Ability. Vol. I: Theory and development.* Palo Alto, CA: Consulting Psychologists Press.

Porch, B. (1971). *The Porch Index of Communicative Ability. Vol. II: Administration and scoring.* Palo Alto, CA: Consulting Psychologists Press.

Premack, D. (1971). Language in chimpanzee? *Science, 172,* 808–822.

Richardson, J. T. E. (1975). Further evidence of the effect of word imageability in dyslexia. *Quarterly Journal of Experimental Psychology, 27,* 445–449.

Ross, E. D. (1983). Right hemisphere lesions in disorders of affective language. In A. Kertesz (Ed.), *Localization in neuropsychology.* London: Academic Press.

Searleman, A. (1977). A review of right hemisphere linguistic capabilities. *Psychological Bulletin, 84,* 503–528.

Segalowitz, S. J., and Bryden, M. P. (1983). Individual differences in hemispheric representation of language. In S. J. Segalowitz (Ed.), *Language functions and brain organization.* London: Academic Press.

Sparks, R. (1981). Melodic intonation therapy. In R. Chapey (Ed.), *Language intervention strategies in adult aphasia.* Baltimore, MD: Williams & Wilkins.

Sparks, R., Helm, N., and Albert, M. (1974). Aphasia rehabilitation resulting from melodic intonation therapy. *Cortex, 10,* 303–316.

Steele, R. D., Weinrich, M., Wertz, R. T., Kleczewska, M. K., and Carlson, G. S. (1989). Computer-based visual communication in aphasia. *Neuropsychologia, 27,* 409–426.

Steele, R. D., Kleczewska, K. K., Carlson, G. S., and Weinrich, M., Computers in the rehabilitation of chronic, severe aphasia: C-VIC 2.0 cross-modal studies. *Aphasiology, 6,* 185–194.

Thompson, C. K., Hall, H. R., and Sison, C. E. (1986). Effects of hypnosis and imagery on naming behavior in aphasia. *Brain and Language, 28,* 141–153.

Wapner, W., Hamby, S., and Gardner, H. (1981). The role of the right hemisphere in the apprehension of complex linguistic materials. *Brain and Language, 14,* 15–33.

Wechsler, D. (1955). *Wechsler Adult Intelligence Scale.* New York: The Psychological Corporation.

Weinrich, M., Steele, R. D., Kleczewska, M. K., Carlson, G. S., Baker, E., and Wertz, R. T. (1989). Representation of ''verbs'' in a computerized visual communication system. *Aphasiology, 3,* 501–512.

West, J. F. (1983). Heightening visual imagery: A new approach to aphasia therapy. In E. Perecman (Ed.), *Cognitive processing in the right hemisphere.* New York: Academic Press.

Weniger, D., Kitteringham, V., and Eglin, M. (1983). The variability of right-hemisphere reading capacities in global aphasia. In C. Chiarello (Ed.), *Right hemisphere contributions to lexical semantics.* New York: Springer-Verlag.

Yamadori, A., Osumi, Y., Masuhara, S., and Okubo, M. (1977). Preservation of singing in Broca's aphasia. *Journal of Neurology, Neurosurgery and Psychiatry, 40,* 221–224.

Young, A. W., and Ratcliff, G. (1983). Visuospatial abilities of the right hemisphere. In A. W. Young (Ed.), *Functions of the right cerebral hemisphere.* London: Academic Press.

SECTION THREE
LANGUAGE STRATEGIES FOR SPECIFIC IMPAIRMENTS

CHAPTER 21
Management of Fluent Aphasic Clients

ROBERT C. MARSHALL

Mr. Wells was my first fluent aphasic patient. He entered my office and said, "Is this where I'm supposed to be?" I asked, "Are you Mr. Wells?" He replied, "That would be the little one without a gridle-bridle or anything else." I thought he might be lost or in the wrong clinic, and I said, "Psychiatry is next door." He replied, "I don't know why you want to know all that crap; I always do that up there." Embarrassed, I noted that his ID bracelet said G. Wells. In a very "professional manner," I told him that his doctor wanted me to see him because he was having communication problems, and I would do some testing. He looked at me seriously and asked, "Tell me, am I getting better or will I always be a doctor?"

Seeking safety, I grabbed the Minnesota Test for Differential Diagnosis of Aphasia (Schuell, 1965) and gave instructions for subtest A-1, pointing to pictures. When asked to point to "the cup," "the pencil," and "the spoon," he said, "There's one," "That's another one," and "Whiddie," respectively. He didn't point to anything, except a picture of Lyndon B. Johnson, about which he commented, "Isn't he a crackerjack?" I switched to a repetition task. I said, "Say pie," and he replied enthusiastically, "Pie, I love it." My spirits soared, but this was his last relevant response, except for "screw." Here, he brought his thumb and index finger of his left hand together and formed a circle. Next, he inserted the index finger of his right hand in the circle. He then looked at me incredulously, made a back-and-forth motion, and said, "You mean like this?"

In 30 minutes, I had no information about Mr. Wells, so I listened. He was angry because he wanted to tell me something important, and I did not understand. With a lot of trial and error, we connected. He was worried because his dog was at home and there was no one to feed him. I volunteered to check with a neighbor, and he clasped his hands prayerfully and said, "Thank the Lord."

Patients like Mr. Wells challenge clinical aphasiologists. They seem incompetent when speaking or responding to questions, yet they display surprising abilities in other areas. They arouse feelings of discomfort because they (*a*) talk rather than listen, (*b*) fail to recognize errors (*c*) are difficult to assess formally, and (*d*) may not appreciate or acknowledge the need for treatment. These behaviors frustrate clinicians accustomed to being "in charge." With clients like Mr. Wells it seems the client is in charge.

This chapter (*a*) provides guidelines for addressing the communicative needs of fluent aphasic persons in the early postonset or "pretherapeutic" period, and (*b*) presents strategies for management of auditory comprehension and verbal production deficits for fluent aphasias during the long-term postonset when the use of more structured treatment becomes possible.

ABOUT THIS CHAPTER

Language Intervention Strategies in Adult Aphasia is an advanced textbook. Readers should be familiar with (*a*) the anatomical organization of language in the brain, (*b*) the speech and language characteristics, and (*c*) the loci of causative lesions in the fluent aphasias (Wernicke's, conduction, anomic, and transcortical sensory aphasia). For an overview see Goodglass and Kaplan (1983) or Kertesz (1979).

This chapter approaches management of fluent aphasias by focusing on clients as individuals instead of members of taxonomic groupings. Disruptions in cognitive/language abilities due to brain injury differ for each client. It has been suggested that further exploration of the classical aphasic taxonomies will not enhance our knowledge about the systems and subsystems that support language processing, nor will it guide practitioners in the management of persons with language processing deficits (Caramazza, 1984; Margolin, 1991; Schwartz, 1984).

Other data also support a case-by-case approach. Only 40% to 50% of aphasic patients can be classified reliably as members of one taxonomic group or another (Goodglass, 1981). It is widely accepted that aphasic symptoms change during the patient's poststroke improvement course (Creary and Kertesz, 1988; Kertesz and McCabe, 1977; Pashek and Holland, 1988; Whitaker, 1984). Thus, treatment plans and procedures will continuously need to be adjusted to meet the individual's needs, because a patient may move from one classification to another during the course of treatment.

This chapter emphasizes treatment of impaired auditory and speaking components in the fluent aphasias. Limited attention is given to reading and writing because the chapters on treatment of aphasic reading (Chapter 24) and writing (Chapter 25) cover this material in depth.

The author has provided examples of fluent aphasic clients' communications. These are, in most cases, events that actually occurred with real patients. Every effort has been made to preserve patient anonymity. Finally, the author is indebted to all of those fluent aphasic individuals who supplied the examples and gave inspiration to this work.

MANAGEMENT IN THE PRETHERAPEUTIC PERIOD

The pretherapeutic period encompasses the first month following onset of aphasia. The patient may be in the acute care hospital, in an extended care facility (ECF), or starting outpatient treatment. During this time, the clinician provides support and guidance. Van Harskamp and Visch-Brink (1991) and others (Marshall, 1987; Wepman, 1972) indicate that aphasia treatment studies make no distinction among support and guidance and the later "structured therapy" that addresses permanent residuals of stroke. They point out that all aphasic clients do not improve sufficiently to qualify for "structured treatment" but that early support and guidance is needed by all patients.

The Case for Early Intervention

In the fluent aphasias, the affected areas of the brain are those served by the posterior branches of the left middle cerebral artery: the primary auditory cortex (Areas 41 and 42), Wernicke's area (Area 22), and portions of the second temporal gyrus and angular gyrus, with possible white-matter extension (Bachman and Albert, 1990). These areas are integral to the interpretation of "meaningful sound patterns" and speech and language activities containing an auditory component (Goodglass and Kaplan, 1983). Immediately after stroke, cerebral edema will cause many patients to have severe comprehension problems. The client's world may be chaotic and confusing. Some patients feel as if they are listening to a foreign language. Suspiciousness, mistrust, and paranoia are not uncommon reactions (Edwards, 1987; Marshall, 1982).

Timely referral to the communication specialist is problematic because lesions causing fluent aphasias spare the primary motor and sensory areas. Fluent aphasic clients have few obvious physical rehabilitation needs (e.g., physical therapy, occupational therapy, kinesiotherapy). Early discharge from the primary care center may prevent the patient from seeing the communication specialist.

The importance of early referral to the communication specialist is seen with the following cases. VL was hospitalized after a left-hemisphere hemorrhagic stroke. He tried to tell his caregivers that his wife had a "drinking problem" and that without supervision she would squander their meager savings. He became so agitated when they could not understand him that he was restrained, sedated, and sent to an ECF. BC fared less well because his aphasia was mistaken for something else. His stroke occurred in a tavern. Police and paramedics interpreted his fluent, paraphasic speech and his inappropriate responses as "a psychiatric disturbance." He spent a month in a state mental hospital before anyone learned that he had suffered a stroke.

Patient Needs and Clinician Roles

Clinicians treating fluent aphasic patients in the pretherapeutic period fill a "special role." Many clients miscomprehend; in turn, their utterances are incomprehensible. Caregivers don't know what the patient is thinking, because thoughts are usually expressed verbally and/or in response to questions. The patient needs an advocate with the time to "listen" and provide consistent structure. Determining that Mr. Wells was worried about his dog was time well spent. It prevented later frustration for other caregivers who may not have taken the time to work through the problem.

Early management is not an exact science. Treatment should be flexible, eclectic, and positive (Edwards, 1987; Kennedy, 1983; Marshall, 1983). Flexibility indicates a willingness to switch, to deviate from a plan, and to make on-line decisions to enhance communication. Eclecticism entails experimentation, use of different strategies and combinations of strategies to improve message understanding, and message exchange. "Positive" clinicians tolerate and adjust to clients' day-to-day fluctuations in language processing. Clinicians can be "upbeat" and honest and can add a touch of humor when the patient may not yet grasp the purpose of treatment.

Communicate About Something Important

Given the severity of the communicative deficits presented by most clients after a stroke, early treatment should deal with issues of importance to the patient. The cases of Mr. Wells, VL, and BC suggest that the client often wishes to communicate something important but has difficulty doing so. An example of how something important to the patient was used in early treatment follows.

MA was an 88-year-old woman seen in a nursing home for assessment and treatment of a severe fluent aphasia. She had no physical impairments. MA communicated one thought clearly: She wanted to go home. The physician thought that her aphasic deficits would prevent her from living independently. Early intervention focused on what MA did at home: fixing meals, shopping, paying bills, and other activities. It became clear that everything she did occurred in her neighborhood. MA did not drive. Her weekly outing was going to church with a friend. She convinced the clinician, and the clinician convinced the physician, that her needs were few. A neighbor agreed to provide emergency assistance, and MA went home and functioned without difficulty.

Breaking the Garbage In–Garbage Out Cycle

In the pretherapeutic period, clients have problems comprehending what is said. These problems affect recognition and correction of speech errors (Albert et al., 1981; Marshall and Tomkins, 1982). Speech output contains paraphasic errors and lacks content (Goodglass, 1981; Marshall et al., 1985; Martin, 1981). Some clients cannot inhibit their speech output (Benson, 1979). The feeding back of defective output into an impaired auditory system creates a garbage in–garbage out cycle that needs to be interrupted.

Stop Strategy

One obvious strategy for breaking the cycle is to have the patients become better listeners and monitor their errors. Whitney's (1975) "stop strategy" proposes this. The client is directed to listen to himself and to stop when he hears an error. If necessary, the clinician signals occurrence of an error, but the ultimate goal is to have the client identify and correct his errors, first in therapy, then outside the clinic. In the pretherapeutic period, however, this may be difficult because comprehension and self-monitoring skills are too impaired.

Interpreting

Martin (1981) offers an alternative to the "stop strategy" for clients who do not comprehend well enough to monitor their speech errors. This method is very useful in breaking the cycle of events that impedes early communication. Martin suggests that the clinician become a better interpreter and not "correct the patient's speech." By being a translator of the client's defective utterances, the clinician breaks the cycle and improves message exchange. An example of Martin's approach follows:

> *PR*: (Waving an issue of *American Kennel Club Magazine*) "Here's the one smasher, master boy, oh nuts! It's there, where is it? My caster, the ones out there where I live. I know it. What's wrong with me? (Pause) Smas, M-A-T-T-E-R. Matteree. Oh God!"
> *Clinician*: "I understand you are a dog breeder. What types of dogs do you raise?"
> *PR*: (Opening the magazine) "Well they're not in here but they are big and mean." (Opens the page to show bulldogs) "Almost like this but bigger. Smashbees, masters, mastees, oh nuts. Why can't I say it?" (Now frustrated)
> *Clinician*: "Do you mean Bull Mastiffs? They are big fellows."
> *PR*: "Bull Mastiffs, Bull Mastiffs, that's it. You got it. Those are my boys." (Now enthusiastic)
> *Clinician*: "Mean animals."
> *PR*: "Yeah, they'll bite your head right off, and once they get a hold, they don't let go."

The clinician knew that PR raised Bull Mastiffs, and he interpreted his utterances to mean that PR was talking about dogs. He interrupted PR with a statement that the client was likely to understand. PR's response indicated an interest, and he paused long enough for the clinician to model "Bull Mastiffs." This prevented the PR's defective productions from feeding back into his system. It broke the cycle without stopping communication.

Staying on Familiar Ground

In the pretherapeutic period it helps to communicate about something that the client has gone over before. This may prevent the garbage in–garbage out cycle from starting. For example, MA (see prior example) began each treatment session with the question "When am I going home?" or "Have you talked to my doctor about me going home yet?" It was useful to allow her to pursue this. Another client, CH, told and retold a "favorite story" of carrying two 100-lb sacks of grain 2 miles to win a bet. Personally relevant conversations are comforting because they occur in a context. The client produces or tries to produce words and phrases that have been used before, and she listens to statements that have been made earlier.

Humor

Humor, emotion, and descriptive language also interrupt the cycle. HN was seen 4 days postonset laughing at a group of painters putting up a scaffold. He tried to explain what was so funny, but his response was not intelligible. The clinician, knowing that HN was a house painter, joked, "You just can't get good work with cheap labor?" HN smiled and produced his business card, saying, "You gotta go to the right place." He tried to convince the clinician to have his house painted. Cochrane (1983) writes of the "language and the atmosphere of delight." She suggests that much spontaneous language is not consciously generated but is generated in response to emotional events. The clinician's quip about "cheap labor" was a catalyst for a successful communicative interchange.

Cycle breaking can be accomplished with use of expressions ("Here's mud in your eye"), expletives ("Oh, shit!"), and colloquialisms (a bird nest on the ground) that are familiar to the client. Humor and emotion get the patient's attention. The following shows how using a World War II slang term promoted a successful communicative exchange with a client, TL, during the pretherapeutic period.

> *Clinician*: (Seeing TL eating in his room) "What's that shit on a shingle?"
> *TL*: (Brightly) "You ain't just a whistling Dixie. Would you please get me a hammer and nails?"
> *Clinician*: (Pause) "I'll bet you would rather have a hamburger."
> *TL*: "Oh, lovely. With lots uf ughburns, uggums, oh you know they make you cry."
> *Clinician*: "You want onions on your hamburger. I'll ask your wife to get you one when she comes to visit."

Maximizing Input

Shortly after a stroke, most fluent aphasic clients are not ready for direct work on auditory comprehension. They respond poorly to single words and short phrases, and in general they have problems with anything out of a meaningful context. This does not mean, however, that efforts to help them understand verbal messages should be abandoned. The time the client spends with the clinical aphasiologist is minimal compared with that spent with the family, the rehabilitation staff, and other caregivers. In the pretherapeutic period, we want to maximize input in all situations. We need help, and we need to guide patients in helping themselves.

Getting Some Help from Others

Caregivers need to know how to maximize input when speaking to fluent aphasic clients. This increases clients' communication opportunities, and the more of these, the better. Hospital staff usually welcome the chance to be of assistance, but family members do not always acknowledge the patient's comprehension deficits. Czvik (1977) found that family members did not agree with the speech pathologist's test results documenting the patient's auditory comprehension deficits. They even disputed this diagnosis following a demonstration of the patient's problems, blaming fatigue, depression, stubbornness, or the ridiculousness of the comprehension task.

Czvik's (1977) report and the trend for most individuals to see aphasia only as "an expressive problem" suggest that demonstrations of how poorly the patient comprehends may be counterproductive. A positive approach demonstrating the benefits of getting the patient's attention, slowing down, talking about something meaningful, and various "cycle-breaking" techniques may yield better results. If the patient miscomprehends, the clinician can "take the blame" (e.g., I spoke too fast).

Being fallible is humbling, but it gains caregiver cooperation. In short, caregivers want to know what they can do to help, not that George did poorly on the Token Test.

Visual Supplements

Spoken messages can be visually supplemented. Some fluent aphasic clients do better reading than listening to single words and short phrases. Written words can aid comprehension. Gesturing is another form of visual supplementation. For example, the question, ''Did you shave today?'' can be accompanied by a shaving gesture. Alternatively, the same question can be asked while holding a can of shaving cream. When the spouse wants dinner at ''Dominick's,'' the aphasic client may miss the restaurant's name. Showing him the menu, a matchbook cover, or yellow page listing helps. Other useful visual aids for all clients during the pretherapeutic period are a Road Atlas, city map, and telephone directory.

Paralinguistic Information

Prosodic features such as rate, phrase length, stress, and pitch (Albert et al., 1981) convey specific linguistic information. Aphasic persons use these cues to extract auditory information (Blumstein and Goodglass, 1972; Green and Boller, 1974). Pitch elevation at the end of an utterance signals a question; falling pitch contours signal an information-carrying statement. One's ''tone of voice'' can reflect anger, disappointment, joy, boredom, fatigue, sickness, disgust, and other emotions. Facial expressions convey similar information. In combination, prosodic cues, tone of voice, and facial expression are a powerful team. They are useful in supplementing spoken messages and maximizing input to the fluent aphasic patient.

Category-Specific Deficits

Some clients have category specific auditory comprehension deficits (Goodglass et al., 1978). If this affects day-to-day function, a category-specific visual aid can be developed. For example, a picture of a human body, with an accompanying label for each part, may help the patient respond to questions about pain, sensation, or motor functioning. When numbers are problematic, a sheet with Arabic numbers (1, 2, . . . 100) and their written equivalents (one, two, . . . one hundred) may help understanding of prices, bill totals, and other financial issues.

Caregivers as Assistants

Not all caregivers are adept at maximizing input for fluent aphasic clients. Deciding who can help is difficult. Clinician instruction is necessary, but how well these instructions will be carried out depends on two factors: (a) caregiver communicative skills (e.g., listening) and (b) caregiver attitudes toward the aphasic person. The clinician gets this information by observing caregiver-client communications and by obtaining an understanding of the ''quality'' of the relationship. Sometimes, caregivers do naturally what aphasia clinicians would like them to do when talking to the client. We can learn from these persons and avoid embarrassing ourselves. Some caregivers, however, talk too rapidly, don't talk at all, don't listen, and change topics abruptly. They may be unable to think about maximizing input because they are too overwhelmed with the impact of stroke and aphasia on the family. They need guidance.

The importance of the quality of the patient-caregiver relationship and its effect on education is reflected in the following examples. Mrs. B wanted to help her husband. Before his stroke she took little interest in policy decisions (e.g., finances, insurance, driving). His aphasic deficits required her to assume these responsibilities, but Mrs. B feared making a mistake. Therefore, she welcomed suggestions that would help Mr. B ''understand'' the problems so that he could give input and help her make major decisions. Mrs. R, on the other hand, came to a support group and described her husband's severe fluent aphasia and the problems of a ''difficult'' marriage of 25 years. When the group members empathized, she stated, ''I'm doing fine. He's treated me terribly all of my life, and now I've got him just where I want him.'' Education was not called for.

Develop the Client's Concern for Comprehension

In the pretherapeutic period, we want patients to help themselves. Comprehensional concern is reflected by active listening, asking for repetitions, and verifying message understanding (Marshall, 1983). If the client is unsure of the message's meaning, the clinician can help him or her show this by using nonverbal (looking quizzical, puzzled, etc.) or nonvocal (Huh?) queries. The clinician can model the appropriate queries for the patient. When the patient does something that represents increased comprehensional concern, the clinician provides informational feedback (e.g., ''I'm glad you asked me to say that again; it's important that you understand me'').

Interpersonal Monitoring

Interpersonal monitoring limitations merit attention during the pretherapeutic period. Poor interpersonal monitors fail to heed signals to switch roles, be quiet, listen, or respect a social convention (e.g., speak softly). One client, ME, a master teacher before his stroke, talked nonstop to a fellow passenger on a long flight. This embarrassed his wife, who thought the passenger wanted to read but didn't know how to stop ME from talking. ME missed the passenger's obvious ''clues'' (e.g., opening his book, turning away) that he wanted to read.

Patients with interpersonal monitoring deficits put family members in awkward situations socially. While the caregiver may be apprehensive about offending the client, a direct approach is best. The clinician may take the role of ''bad guy'' and show or tell the client what is expected of him or her. For example, CW would not stop interrupting as the clinician was talking to his wife. The clinician looked at CW and signaled (hand gesture) him to ''stop.'' This was followed by a ''be quiet'' gesture. The sequence was repeated with each interruption. After three sequences, CW understood that the conversation did not concern him and stopped interrupting. Family members may want to prepare for important social events that include the client with an interpersonal monitoring problem (e.g., Thanksgiving dinner). Guests can be warned that ''George will probably talk your leg off'' and that it is permissible to excuse themselves or ask George to be quiet.

Maintaining Communication Flow

Many fluent aphasic clients are actually more fluent immediately postictus. As they become aware of their speech errors and recognize how others respond to them, they start to struggle.

Table 21.1.
Examples of Fluent Aphasic Struggle Behavior to Produce Specific Words During the Pretherapeutic Period. Target Word is Shown in Brackets

Example 1 [cigarette]

Patient PJ: "You smoke a cig, a sigg, oh what is it? I want one now. Smittering, ciggerthing, almost, what's it called. You put in in your mouth and smuch it. Smucher, smuch, smukker, chitter. No." (Patient spent about three minutes in this endeavor).

Example 2 [Alaska]

Patient HB: "I always wanted to go to Alasta, where its cold. Alasta, Alaskan, Alasker (pause)

Clinician: (Signals HB to go on)

HB: "Alaska."

Example 3 [coffee]

Patient BB: "Well since my heart went bad, my Dr. said no more cokkee, I mean cottee. It is not good for my blood pressure."

Example 4 [cigarette]

Patient SA: Approaches nurses station. "Hey, Miss, yoo hoo." (Gesture that he is smoking) "Please, OK."

Nurse: "Say cigarette!"

Example 5 [hospital]

Patient RG: "They took me right to the hottle, hopil, hosital, for the sick people, lots of doctors, you know, hostitle, hosital, where you work of course. I just can't get today. Maybe I'll get it tomorrow."

While productive self-correction is desirable, the success with which aphasic patients can correct their speech production errors is variable (Marshall and Tompkins, 1981, 1982). Some patients react maladaptively to these disruptions in speech fluency. At times, prolonged struggle to produce a word interferes with communication. Table 21.1 shows some examples of how clients struggle when "stuck" on a particular word.

Fill In. In example 1, a woman who became aphasic following removal of a left temporal lobe tumor tries to say "cigarette." She worked at this for 3 minutes. Her efforts suggest that she is not going to produce the desired word. The best decision is to move on. The clinician stops the patient by saying or writing the missing word.

Keep Trying. In the second example (Table 21.1), a patient tells about a trip to Alaska. The response suggests the word is on the "tip of his tongue." It's appropriate to say "Tell me more" or provide a gesture that suggests "Try a bit harder." This decision is based on the clinician's intuition and the patient's past performance.

Let It Go. In example 3, the client reports that he doesn't drink coffee because of a heart condition that caused his stroke. The essence of the communication, his medical condition, is fulfilled. Spending time with the word "coffee" when the message has been conveyed interrupts the communication unnecessarily. The best decision is to acknowledge understanding of the message (e.g., "I drink too much coffee myself") and move on.

Take What the Patient Gives. It's desirable for the patient to initiate communication. When he does this, and it is clear what he wants, form is often unimportant. SA's gesture (example 4) is unambiguous. The nurse's response "Say cigarette" is not appropriate at this early stage. She might have said, "I'll get you a cigarette right away" or "This is a nonsmoking hospital."

Reward Persistence. When the patient tries to work through a communication snag, acknowledge the effort regardless of its success. This can minimize the effects of failure. Some comments that might do this for the patient's response shown in example 5 are the following: "I like the way you stuck with that," "You really tried to say that word," or "That word 'hospital' is a toughie today."

Variability. LC called his wife "Mildred" on one day and "Bernice" (his ex-wife's name) the next. This upset LC, and he usually hit his head and said, "Mildred, Mildred, Mildred—damn it, why can't I say it?" Many clients don't attribute day-to-day fluctuations to their strokes and berate themselves unnecessarily. It's helpful to counsel them that this variability is expected, that they are not stupid or crazy but have disrupted language circuitry because of a stroke. Using a visual aid to explain what a stroke is and how it disrupts language may help the patient understand variability and make him less critical of himself or herself.

STRUCTURED TREATMENT

Structured treatment begins about 4 to 8 weeks postictus when the client is comprehending more, is aware of his deficits, and can be assessed thoroughly. Intervention now addresses the permanent speech and language deficits of the stroke. Candidates should be motivated to respond, to attend therapy, and to understand the treatment's intent. Patient and caregiver understanding that the period of rapid change (e.g., spontaneous recovery) is slowing and that improvement will require hard work and practice is also important. The long-term goal of structured treatment is to help the patient become the "best possible communicator" within the limits of his neurological insult, in accordance with his personal wishes and his life situation. The frequency, duration, goals, and outcomes of treatment will depend greatly on the extent to which the patient's language-processing system has been compromised by brain injury and on other factors.

Managing Auditory Comprehension Deficits

Models of Auditory Comprehension

"Bottom-up" models suggest that comprehension begins with analysis of the physical characteristics of the message and works its way up to assignment of meaning. Multiple processes (reception of the acoustic speech signal, phonemic perception, discrimination, lexical/semantic comprehension, syntactic comprehension) are involved in understanding spoken messages (Bachman and Albert, 1990). "Top-down" models stress listeners' general knowledge of the world and expectations about what will be said. Participants sharing common knowledge anticipate that messages will make sense (be cohesive) in light of what has been said earlier. Cohesive ties permit the listener to compute backward and establish a linkage with what was said earlier, when a specific element is not understood

(Brownell, 1988). Comprehension of spoken messages by normal and aphasic listeners involves both bottom-up and top-down processing (Brookshire, 1992).

Auditory comprehension and auditory memory are interdependent and cannot be separated (Brookshire, 1986). Most memory models postulate a three-stage process through which spoken messages pass. The first is the sensory register, which stores acoustic signals briefly. In the second stage, short-term (STM) or working memory, the listener performs acoustic, semantic, and some syntactic analysis. STM, however, has a limited capacity, and the verbatim structure of a sentence can be retained only with rehearsal; it will also be replaced with new information. If the information in STM is important and can be maintained in STM for a sufficient length of time to be decoded, it may be transferred to long-term (LTM) or secondary memory, which has a relatively large capacity and within which information decays slowly (Brookshire, 1986). With fluent aphasic clients, the best overall strategy is to do whatever is needed to get the message into long-term memory. This involves manipulating message components, using context, and compensating for specific deficits.

Manipulating Message Components

Linguistic, timing, and contextual variables influence aphasic persons' auditory comprehension (Shewan and Canter, 1971). These have been reviewed extensively elsewhere (Bachman and Albert, 1990; Boller et al., 1977; Darley, 1976; Marshall, 1986) and an in-depth presentation will not be made. Most of what is known about aphasic persons' comprehension comes from investigations of aphasic subjects' performances on "bottom-up" processing tasks, for example, distinguishing acoustic differences and showing comprehension of single words and isolated sentences.

Generally, the more syntactically complex the message, the greater the likelihood of miscomprehension (Brookshire and Nicholas, 1980; Caramazza et al., 1978; Goodglass et al., 1979; Parisi and Pizzamiglio, 1970; Shewan and Canter, 1971). Clients understand semantically reversible sentences (e.g., John is looking at Mary) less well than nonreversible sentence (e.g., John is eating cake) (Deloche and Seron, 1981; Kudo, 1984; Pierce and Beekman, 1985). Passive sentences (e.g., John ate lunch) are more difficult than active sentences (e.g., John is eating lunch) (Pierce 1981, 1982). Negative sentences are harder than affirmative sentences (Just et al., 1977; West et al., 1976). Comparatives (Bill is taller than Kathy) are tougher than noncomparatives (Bill is tall and Kathy is short) (Berndt and Caramazza, 1980). Infrequently occurring words such as "gnu" are harder to understand than frequently occurring words (e.g., bear) (Goodglass et al., 1970). Longer sentences pose more problems than shorter ones (Boller and Dennis, 1979; Goodglass et al., 1979).

From this body of research some important suggestions emerge that are helpful in treating auditory comprehension deficits of the fluent aphasias.

Stimulus Saliency

Goodglass (1973) defines saliency as "the psychological resultant of the stress, the informational significance, the phonological prominence, and the affective value of a word." Darley (1976) translates this as giving the patient a "word he can hold

on to." Select salient words and incorporate these words into treatment. For example, PS was an avid student of biblical studies. Words such as "Genesis," "Proverbs," and "Samuel" were salient for him. Asking him to find "Genesis, chapter 4, verse 3" was a good way to work on auditory comprehension. Saliency may also be increased by using direct wording (e.g., "Tell me your address!") rather than indirect wording ("Tell me your address so that I can fill out this form") (Boller and Green, 1974; Darley, 1976) and by placing the information-bearing elements in a prominent position (beginning or end) of the sentence (Darley, 1976).

Redundancy

Message redundancy is increased with "props" of the communicative situation. For example, the client knows what is coming when he sees the physician's white coat, stethoscope, and tongue blade. Comprehension improves if the questions match the communicative situation and its props. For example, McKenzie Buck (1968) complained that he thought it inappropriate for his therapist to ask him questions about toileting as he was eating. Message redundancy further includes supportive information within the utterance (Clark and Flowers, 1987; Gardner et al., 1975; Gravel and LaPointe, 1983). The client is more likely to respond to "delicious, juicy, T-bone steak" than to "steak." Repetitions and revisions (e.g., "I like your hat. Do you always wear a hat?") provide yet another mechanism for increasing redundancy and heightening comprehension.

Attention

Attentional deficits cause clients to miss the beginning of a message or to miss short messages entirely (Brookshire, 1974; Loverso and Prescott, 1981; Marshall and Thistlethwaite, 1977). Signaling that a message is on the way with alerters such as "Listen to me" or "I'd like to say something now" may help. Frequently, however, the inattentive patient gets lost because of a topic change. Client CH was talking about cold weather. He stated that the thermometer dropped to "39 degrees" and he turned up the electric blanket. The clinician, however, wanted to ask CH about his recent birthday and said, "You had a birthday Tuesday. How old are you?" CH replied, "You want to know about the cold—the cold—cold—C-O-L-D." CH may have confused "old" with "cold," but this snag might have been averted by preparing CH for the topic switch by writing "happy birthday," providing a gesture, or saying, "Let's change the subject."

Using Context

Treatment of comprehension deficits in aphasia has stressed the use of "bottom-up" comprehension tasks. Schuell's intensive auditory stimulation (Schuell et al., 1964) stresses "bombarding" the patient with 20 or more repetitions of the same stimulus. Typically, treatment begins with single words and phrases; length and complexity of stimuli are increased as the patient improves (Darley, 1982; Marshall, 1978; Pierce, 1983). There are several reasons, however, why this didactic approach using "bottom-up" and off-line tasks may not be appropriate for treatment of aphasic comprehension deficits.

Recently, several studies have shown that aphasic persons' comprehension of words and unrelated sentences does not predict comprehension of discourse (Pashek and Brookshire, 1982; Stachowiak et al., 1977; Waller and Darley, 1978; Wegner et al., 1984; Wilcox et al., 1978).

There is no solid evidence that treatment of comprehension deficits using forced-choice picture-pointing tasks improves comprehension of spoken discourse (Brookshire, 1992). With these types of activities, understanding of the stimuli (pictures and words) and the patient's ability to "translate" between verbal and pictorial representations are assumed, not known (Tyler, 1992).

Conventional procedures for both assessment and treatment of comprehension disorders in aphasia involve "off-line" tasks that are quite different from what occurs in normal comprehension (Marslen-Wilson and Tyler, 1980). That is, these procedures assess only the end point of comprehension. The entire message needs to be put in before the patient responds, and the patient's response must be organized and executed before the examiner sees any evidence of comprehension success or failure.

Comprehension in most communicative situations involves listening to spoken discourse. Discourse is processed "on-line." On-line studies of aphasic persons' miscomprehension are rare, with the exception of a recent work from Tyler (1992). The fact that fluent aphasic patients' spoken discourse is "on-line," but often faulty, coupled with the fact that these individuals do poorly on off-line tasks (e.g., picture-pointing), suggests that comprehension deficits in the fluent aphasias might be better addressed within a meaningful context. HB is a fluent aphasic man who demonstrates this point quite adequately.

HB is a 69-year-old man who became aphasic as a result of a left cerebral hemorrhage. His score on the 62-item Token Test (DeRenzi and Vignolo, 1962) is 38; his percentile scores on the word-discrimination subtest (53 of 72 correct) and on complex ideational material (6 of 12 correct) from the Boston Diagnostic Aphasia Examination (Goodglass and Kaplan, 1983) are 50% and 60%, respectively. HB, however, operates successfully, and without assistance, a multi-million-dollar company. How can he do this?

Several factors account for HB's success. Aphasic patients respond better to personally relevant material (Busch and Brookshire, 1982; Gray et al., 1977; Van Lancker and Nicklay, 1992; Wallace and Canter, 1985). Focusing treatment on HB's business provides a familiar script. Brookshire (1992) suggests that comprehension is enhanced if messages follow the patient's life script. A script or schema is a mental device by which the individual organizes his or her knowledge of a situation. HB's script is his 40-year business. When treatment employs the vocabulary of "the business," HB has expectations about what events are likely and when and in what order they will occur. With clients like HB, single-word "point-to" tasks, isolated sentences, unrelated questions, and following of commands are a disservice.

Treatment of Specific Auditory Comprehension Deficits

Many clients improve enough in auditory comprehension to understand a conversation. For these patients, comprehension deficits may be addressed in conjunction with other problems

(e.g., word retrieval). There are, however, specific areas that may require direct clinical intervention.

Retention Problems

Aphasic persons have short-term or working memory deficits (Brookshire, 1986). These are seen on span tasks, for example, remembering digits forward and backward, remembering words, and following sequential commands (Goodglass et al., 1970; Marshall and Brown, 1974). Deficits are also seen in the verbatim recall of sentence- and paragraph-length material (Caramazza et al., 1978; Flowers and Danforth, 1979; Wegner et al., 1984). Span deficits are more evident than sentence retention difficulties because patients frequently retain the "gist" of the sentence, and meaning may not be affected (Hanson, 1976; Marshall et al., 1991; Wegner et al., 1984).

The client may pretend to understand because he fears forgetting the message and "looking stupid." He may panic and fail to listen carefully or selectively. Treatment of retention deficits should relate to life demands. For example, improving retention span from four to five digits forward is good, but if it doesn't help in remembering phone numbers or addresses, does it make a difference? The goal is to lessen the patient's panic and allay fears that forgetting the message is the end of the world. The patient needs encouragement to remain calm under pressure. The following strategies are offered to assist retention of the message that Mr. Edwards from Sears has called and asked the patient to call him at 284-6541 about a new dishwasher.

Asking for Help. The patient can request assistance, for example, "I didn't get all of that. Would you please say it again?" He can restate the gist of the message to verify that he understood: for example, "Excuse me, did you say your name was Edwards? Tell me that number to call on the dishwasher again." The patient can assist himself. He will probably remember that the call came from Sears and can consult the Yellow Pages for the phone number.

Chunking. The patient might ask the caller to repeat the number in smaller segments, for example, 284-65-41. Different methods of presenting the phone number in "chunks" can be practiced in treatment to determine the best way to remember the phone number.

The Message Machine. Some clients don't answer phone calls. They record the message on a machine, play it back several times, and return the call after they are sure they have comprehended the message.

Write It Down or Make a List. It helps to write things down. "Post-its" come in all colors and sizes. When the patient needs to take his medicine at 3:00 P.M., his wife can post a note on the refrigerator. If the patient goes to the market for "milk, eggs, and bread," she can give him a list rather than asking him to remember the three items.

Comprehension of Specific Syntactic Constructions

In sentence verification tasks, the patient sees a picture. A spoken message is presented (e.g., John is giving a present to Mary), and the patient decides if the message is or is not a true representation of the picture. In another form of sentence verification, a sentence is presented alone (e.g., Elephants are larger than dogs), and the aphasic person makes a decision about the truthfulness of the sentence based on his or her general knowledge. In each case, the clinician can measure the number

Table 21.2.
Stages in the Word-Retrieval Process. Adapted From Lesser (1987)

Stage	Disorder
Semantic lexicon	Category loss or degradation
	Generalized degradation
	Access problems
Phonological lexicon	Impaired word-form representations
	Plus a disorder of phonological control
Phonological assembly	Impaired phoneme selection and seriation
Phonetic planning	Impaired mapping from phonemic to phonetic realization
Articulation	Neuromotor damage

of accurate responses and the time it takes the patient to arrive at the decision. Sentence verification provides a convenient means of working on auditory comprehension of specific constructions.

Discourse Comprehension

Brain-injured aphasic patients are limited in terms of the "neural resources" they can devote to a language-processing task (McNeil et al., 1991). Patients complain, "I can't do two things at once," "Driving is difficult with the radio on," "It's impossible to understand at a party," and "It's hard to concentrate when the television is playing." Background noise (Basili et al., 1980), distractions (DeRenzi et al., 1978), and competing tasks (LaPointe and Erickson, 1991) affect comprehension. Treatment seeks to help the patient identify life situations where comprehension breaks down and to devise strategies to prevent this and to optimize his or her comprehension performance.

Withdraw.   Patients may recover by seeking a moment of quiet. They remove themselves from the competitive listening situation. This is called "taking a break." Some patients communicate better if they have a nap before the significant other gets home from work. Others need counseling that it is not necessary to be "macho." When a rest helps, the patient should be encouraged to get it.

Previews and Summaries.   When clients know what to listen for, they usually comprehend better. They can be "prestimulated" for a film, a play, or a television show by reading or listening to a synopsis of the program before viewing it. This alerts patients to the "unexpected." Similarly, patients and their significant others (or the clinician) can discuss the program immediately afterward. This practice is ideal when shared in treatment (group or individual) and serves as a vehicle to work on other deficits (e.g., organization, word retrieval, syntax).

Word Retrieval

Word-retrieval problems interfere with communication, but not all aphasic word-retrieval problems are the same (Benson, 1979). Table 21.2 depicts stages in retrieval of an object's name, as described by Lesser (1987). The first three stages—the cognitive/semantic system, the phonological output lexicon, and phonological assembly—are pertinent to management of fluent aphasias. The later stages, phonetic planning and articula-

tion, represent the mapping of a phonemic pattern onto phonetic realization and include the articulatory process itself. Problems at these stages occur in the motor speech disorders apraxia of speech and dysarthria and are not within the domain of this chapter.

Semantic/Cognitive System

The semantic system is organized (Buckingham, 1979; Lesser, 1987; Rinnert and Whitaker, 1973). Semantic fields are hierarchically (superordinate) arranged (e.g., fruit to apple to Washington delicious). Buckingham (1979) hypothesizes that the semantic system is organized in lexical sets such as like objects (e.g., hoe, shovel, rake), synonyms (e.g., building, structure, edifice), or antonyms (e.g., big-little, fast-slow).

Table 21.3 provides some examples of responses of fluent aphasic patients with semantic-level impairments for the word "blanket." Investigators have sought to determine whether these types of responses represent degradation of the semantic system (loss of word knowledge) or impaired access to it (Goodglass and Baker, 1976; Grober et al., 1980; Grossman, 1981; Whitehouse et al., 1978; Zurif et al., 1974). Information with regard to consistency, comprehension, priming effects, and categorization skills helps make this determination.

Consistency of the Retrieval Deficit.   One clue to the nature of semantic problems is the consistency with which the patient evokes specific target words or category members (e.g., fruits, body parts, numbers). This is assessed by repeated testing with the same items the patient has failed to name on confrontation, under other conditions (e.g., naming to description, naming in a pictorial sequence, oral word reading). Fluctuation and variation should occur when the problem is one of access. With a degraded semantic lexicon, clients should be consistent in their failure to retrieve specific words or words within categories (Benson, 1979).

Comprehension of the Target Word.   Benson (1979) suggests that clients with true semantic deficits may not always recognize the object's spoken or written name. Marshall (1983) notes that some fluent aphasic clients lack awareness of the content words in their speech. Gainotti (1976, 1987) and his colleagues (Gainotti et al., 1981; Gainotti et al., 1986; Silveri et al., 1989) identified a group of patients with word-retrieval deficits who also had lexical comprehension difficulties. They suggested that these patients' word-retrieval difficulties result from impairments in accessing semantic representations or loss of information at the level of representations associated with some lexical items. It is reasonable to suspect that these are patients who began as Wernicke's aphasics (primary deficit is a severe comprehension deficit) and evolved to end-stage anomic aphasia (primary deficit is word retrieval), as suggested in several studies (Creary and Kertesz, 1988; Pashek and Holland, 1988). Their comprehension deficits are now manifested subtly, such as in taking more time to recognize a semantic target or an associated word (Goodglass and Baker, 1976), or in other ways. Conversely, the patient with accessing problems recognizes the target name immediately.

Sensitivity to Semantic Priming.   Priming studies involve lexical decision tasks where the patient judges if a stimulus presented is a word or a nonword. Preceding the stimulus with a prime affects the speed of this judgment. Milberg and Blumstein (1981) illustrated that Wernicke's aphasic patients respond

Table 21.3.
Examples of Fluent Aphasic Persons' Word-Retrieval Behaviors at Different Stages of the Lexical Retrieval Process. Target Word is Shown in Brackets

	Semantic Lexicon	
[blanket]	"Just blank."	Degradation/access
	"Pillow."	Degradation/access
	"Bed thing."	Degradation/access
	Phonological Lexicon	
[ballet]	"The kind of dancing where they are up on their toes."	Access
[taxi]	"Black and white' Gestures that he is driving.	Access
[chair]	"This thing right here." Touches the arms of the chair.	Access
[tea]	Pantomimes steps in brewing tea.	Access
[jury]	"The 12 people who tell the judge if he did it or not."	Access
	Phonological Assembly	
[blanket]	"baksets"	Phoneme selection/sequencing
[matches]	"patches, batches, hatches, close but not quite."	Phoneme selection
[elephant]	"efalunt, elfant, elafant, elephant OK."	Phoneme selection/sequencing
[snakes]	"godes and goat wheels."	Phoneme selection/Access

faster to real-word targets (e.g., dog) when they are preceded by a related prime (e.g., cat) than when they are preceded by an unrelated prime (e.g., land) or a nonword (e.g., spado). Their findings indicate that patients with severe language problems retain semantic information that can be activated by priming and that access may be the primary problem in aphasic word retrieval.

Category Sorting Tasks. Category-specific naming deficits occur in aphasia (Hart et al., 1985; Yamaduri and Albert, 1973). Deficits have been reported for colors (Geschwind and Fusillo, 1966), body parts (Gentilini et al., 1988), and animate and inanimate objects (Hecaen and Ajuriaguerra, 1956) for individual cases. Posteriorly lesioned aphasic subjects have been shown to be more impaired than anteriorly damaged subjects in semantic categorization skills (Grober et al., 1980) and "lexical creativity" (making up words by combining morphemes in a novel way, e.g., map ball = globe) (Liederman et al., 1983). Poor category sorting would be anticipated for patients with degraded systems or category-specific problems, whereas clients with an access problem should be more proficient on these types of tasks.

Phonological Lexicon

The phonological (having to do with sounds) lexicon (having to do with words) includes the entire pool of words in one's vocabulary (Margolin, 1991). Lesser (1987) and others (Hillis, 1991; Kempen and Huijbers, 1983) suggest that this stage in word retrieval involves mapping of items from the semantic lexicon onto their phonological shapes in the phonological lexicon. Problems result from impaired word-form representations or selection difficulties in going from one lexicon to another (Gainotti, 1987; Lesser, 1987). Benson (1979) refers to this problem as word selection (word dictionary) anomia. While these patients often fail to name an item on confrontation, they inform us in other ways (e.g., definition, pantomime, description, showing) of their semantic knowledge of it (see Table 21.3). They always recognize the target when it is provided for them.

Phonological Assembly

After an item has been retrieved from the phonological lexicon, the phonemic pattern needed for its outputting needs to be selected and ordered. Patients with phonological assembly problems have the target in mind but cannot always select and order its phonemes correctly. The final examples of Table 21.3 represent those of clients with problems selecting and assembling phonemic sequences for outputting. These responses are usually associated with the syndrome of conduction aphasia (Green and Howes, 1977), but phonological assembly problems are also seen in other fluent aphasias. With such clients, we hear an abundance of literal paraphasias (e.g., eflalent for elephant); frequent, excessive, but usually unsuccessful self-corrections (Marshall and Tompkins, 1982); and successive approximation (Joanette et al., 1980).

Treatment of Word-Retrieval Deficits in Fluent Aphasia

Management requires recognizing how impairments at different stages of word retrieval are manifested behaviorally, understanding their impact on communication, and deciding what can be done to compensate for them. It is important to distinguish *behaviors* (what the patient does in reaction to failure to retrieve a desired word) from word-retrieval *strategies* (what the patient does purposefully or what the clinician teaches the patient to do in order to compensate for the missing word). Behaviors tell the clinician what to target for treatment. Getting the client to develop and use strategies is the treatment. Strategies may be developed from some behaviors, but many behaviors are counterproductive (e.g., excessive struggle) and need to be unlearned or replaced.

Other Considerations

Stage Identification. It would be convenient to confirm the stage at which the patient is having word-retrieval problems and then to develop a treatment plan to reactivate or reorganize functions at that stage. Unfortunately, patients don't always cooperate. They have problems at multiple stages. Difficulties within one stage may exacerbate those of other stages. Combinations of problems at more than one stage create unique deficits. For example, the patient with problems at the phonological lexicon and with phonological assembly produces neologistic jargon (Lesser, 1987).

Task. Clinical aphasiology has more treatment programs for confrontation naming than for anything else. The reason for this is that it is easier to treat word-retrieval problems using confrontation naming because the target is known and documentation is simplified. This procedure, however, may not be the most effective treatment approach. Rarely is the aphasic client approached in the grocery store with a banana and asked, "What is this?" There is also some compelling evidence that fluent aphasic clients do better at retrieving words in speaking tasks that allow more freedom (e.g., picture description) than on confrontation naming tasks (Joanette et al., 1980; Williams and Canter, 1982). This, as well as the fact that spontaneous speech makes up most communicative interactions, suggests it might be better to focus on word-retrieval deficits occurring at the discourse level.

Discourse, however, poses a different set of problems. When the patient has freedom to compose and the listener doesn't know the target word, the client may revise, substitute, or talk around the word. This may lead the client astray from his or her original thoughts (Wepman, 1972). German (1992) has developed an assessment procedure for the assessment of word-finding difficulties in the connected speech of language-impaired adults and children. Marshall and Blake (1992) have used this tool successfully with fluent aphasic adults. In the final analysis, the clinician will need to do what is best for the individual patient.

Adjusting to the Client's "Shutter Openings"

Wepman (1972) suggests that the mind functions similarly to a camera shutter. It is amenable to stimulation when it is open; it does not respond during its closed phase. Clinicians should present treatment stimuli in accordance with the rhythm of the patient's "shutter openings." Response delays, self-corrections, and related errors may reflect that the client's "shutter is about to close" and more time for internalizing of the stimulus and integration by association is needed. According to Wepman (1972), presentation of additional stimuli at this time (while the shutter is closed) can lead to perseverative responses or errors. Regardless of the stage of the word-retrieval process targeted for treatment, it is important to take the time to strengthen, enrich, and consolidate "weak" responses rather than add something new. An example follows:

> *Patient*: "It's a cakker-cacsus-cactus-yeah—Whew."
> *Clinician*: "OK, say it again—cactus."
> *Patient*: "Catter, no (pause) cactus, cactus, yeah."
> *Clinician*: "A cactus grows where?"
> *Patient*: "In the desert of course."
> *Clinician*: "When you sit on a cactus, what happens?"
> *Patient*: "Pain, it has sharp things—thorns."
> *Clinician*: "Try that word again."
> *Patient*: "OK, cactus, cactus."

Here the clinician "strengthened" the response with semantic information and gave the patient time to practice the re-sponse. It took more of the clinician's time, but in the long run it may be worth it.

Treatment of Semantic Deficits

Patients with word-retrieval problems rooted in semantic lexicon are slow to recognize target words and have problems distinguishing category boundaries. They are less sensitive to primes and cues. Treatment aims (a) to strengthen semantic associative fields and (b) to activate semantic representations.

Enriching Semantic Fields

In Von Stockert's (1978) program, the clinician presents a picture (e.g., milk) surrounded by five related (coffee, tea, soda, cow, baby) and five unrelated pictures (house, cactus, pencil, chair, boat). The client orders the related pictures under the target and puts the unrelated items aside. Errors are acknowledged, and the patient is helped to correct them. Next, the clinician names the target and then the five related words, pointing to each one. Step two uses written names of the pictures. The clinician takes a written name, reads it aloud, and matches it with its target picture. Then the patient does the same thing with the remaining cards. Training is supplemented with reading of the word cards and pointing to the appropriate picture by the clinician. The program does not require the patient to speak, nor does it curtail spontaneous responses to name the item.

A feature analysis program described by Massaro and Tompkins (1992) provides another means for shoring up semantic networks. The clinician gives a concept word (e.g., cat), and the client is asked to provide information about certain semantic features. These include group membership (animals), actions (meowing, hunting), use (pet), location (inside or outside), properties (furry, four-legged), and associations (makes me think of dog, Calico, etc.).

SORRT stands for Semantic, Oppositional, and Rhyming Retrieval Training (Logue and Dixon, 1979). First, the client listens to word pairs consisting of rhymes (dog-hog), synonyms (dog-canine), or antonyms (dog-cat) and designates the nature of the relationship. Then the target (e.g., dog), rhyme (hog), synonym (canine), and antonym (cat) are presented on cards, and the patient selects the appropriate item. Next, the patient is asked to produce the same antonyms, synonyms, and rhymes previously supplied by the clinician. Finally, the patient produces additional rhymes, synonyms, and antonyms.

Hillis (1991) suggests that patients who make semantic errors do not always distinguish among category members. Her treatment of an aphasic client highlighted differences among category members following error responses. For example, if the patient said "cherry" for "lemon," the clinician might ask him to draw a lemon and point out the differences among the two constituents (e.g., sour/sweet, red/yellow, hard/soft, rough skin/smooth skin).

Activating Semantic Representations

Word retrieval is facilitated by treating a modality in which the patient can produce responses to items he or she cannot name. For the client who cannot name "bridge," auditory word and picture-matching practice, in which the clinician says a

Table 21.4.
Examples of Facilitation Tasks That Have Potential for Activating Semantic Representations to Aid Later Word Retrieval

	Self-cue	
Target word	Clinician	Client
[palamino]	What can you think of to help you remember this type of horse?	"Horse, Roy Rogers rode one."
	Semantic judgment	
[brick]	Is this item heavy?	"Yes."
[clouds]	Tell me two things about these.	"They are fluffy." "In the sky."

word (e.g., bridge) and the patient points to "bridge" within an array of items, may aid later naming of the item.

Several lines of evidence suggest that facilitators that do the best job at aiding later word retrieval are those that activate semantic representations (Howard et al., 1985a, 1985b; Marshall et al., 1992a; Marshall et al., 1992; Marshall et al., 1990; Patterson et al., 1983; Pring et al., 1990). In contrast, facilitators who supply only phonological information about the target to be named fare less well than those activating semantic representations (Howard et al., 1985a; Marshall et al., 1991a, 1991b, 1992; Patterson et al., 1983).

Table 21.4 describes some facilitation tasks that activate semantic representations related to the target word. In example 1, the client creates a self-cue to aid later recall. Here, the clinician presents the item and asks the client to use the self-cue to aid in its naming. In the next example, the client has to make a semantic judgment about the target. In example 3, the client provides two characteristics about the item. Craik and Lockhart (1972) suggest that activation of semantic processes causes the stimulus to be processed at a "deeper level." They indicate that persistence of a memory trace is a positive function of the "depth" of stimulus processing (depth refers to degree of semantic involvement). It should also be noted that activation of semantic representations takes more time. It is possible that this time allows the patient to internalize the stimulus and to integrate it by association (Wepman, 1953). Treatment tasks that activate semantic mechanisms are only limited by clinician imagination and willingness to give the patient time to respond.

Treatment at the Phonological Lexicon Level

Word-retrieval deficits involving the phonological lexicon require a different approach. Examples in Table 21.3 reflect that the target has been retrieved from the semantic lexicon but that accessing phonological representations and moving from the semantic to phonological lexicon is a problem. These clients usually say, "I know it but I can't say it." They compose another group identified by Gainotti et al. (1986), who differ from the one discussed earlier in that they do not have lexical comprehension deficits.

Clinician Decisions

Before targeting treatment, the clinician needs to answer more questions. Are the patient's word-retrieval behaviors reac-

tions to a problem, or are they intentionally derived? Does the patient become "upset" with failure to come up with the specific target word? Does the behavior seen (e.g., pantomime, description, oral spelling) lead to production of the target word or promote self-correction? Does the information supplied in the patient's word-retrieval behaviors permit the listener to "guess" the target word without the patient saying it?

An example of how these decisions are made is seen with patients HB and RP. HB referred to Alaska as "the biggest state," Africa as "lion country," and salespersons as "peddlers." When his listeners learned to fill in the missing words, HB's descriptive behaviors became a strategy. Patient RP tried to spell words that he had problems retrieving; he usually spelled them incorrectly. He recognized his misspelling and tried again and again. Frustration followed and communication suffered. His wife was "trained" to do a lot of guessing, and usually she was wrong. This created more frustration for both parties.

With HB, the clinician could choose to fill in the blanks and keep the communicative exchange moving forward. Alternatively, it might be helpful to encourage HB to rephrase his descriptions such as "the biggest state" and see if this would assist him in producing the target word "Alaska." What to do is determined by success and by the patient's reaction to the intervention. Conversely, RP's oral-spelling tactic is not productive. The clinician needs to help RP replace it with something more productive.

Does the Behavior Lead to Production of the Target?

Marshall (1976) examined word-retrieval behaviors in the conversational speech of an unselected sample of adult aphasics with respect to their frequency of use and the success with which they led to production of a target word. They included delay (taking more time), semantic association, phonetic association, description, and use of general proforms (e.g., "thing," or "it"). Delayed responses, in the form of requesting more time, and unfilled and filled pauses occurred infrequently, but delays led to production of the target word more frequently than any other behavior. The optimum time for word retrieval is not known, but the best evidence, from aphasic picture naming, is 3 to 5 seconds; the client also may dictate the pace (Brookshire, 1971). Possibly, more time in combination with having the patient "review" his or her behavior (e.g., description, associated words, approximations) would make a delay strategy even more effective. Since most aphasic persons complain of listener time pressure, getting the patient to use a delay strategy will require some education of conversational partners.

Communication Without Saying the Words

Informative behaviors help the listener "guess" the target word without the patient saying it. Some patients supply one or two letters of the word or write in the air. Others demonstrate with pantomime and gesture. Descriptions may be so complete that the target word is easily guessed. Tompkins and Marshall (1982) examined these phenomena experimentally. They determined listeners' ability to determine target-word information in subjects' self-cues by presenting videotape samples of word-retrieval behaviors for which target words were deleted. Listeners, in many cases, could determine the target word on the basis of the behavior (e.g., gesture, pantomime, description), and there was little relationship among behavior type and eventual production of the target utterance.

Some fluent aphasic clients communicate well with few specific words, but unfortunately they do not know this, and continuously berate themselves. Marshall (1983) described them as "unknowing compensators." He noted that these clients became upset with failure to produce specific target words and did not participate in social activities because they felt "foolish." With such patients, the aims of treatment should be communication and information exchange, not lexical specificity. These individuals need positive experiences and counseling to understand just how well they do "in life" without specifics.

Oral Reading of Familiar Material

PS, a 77-year-old teacher, manifested severe deficits at both the phonological lexicon and the phonological assembly stages. This combination resulted in speech consisting of neologistic jargon (Lesser, 1987). His productions were much more likely to be successful during oral reading, when he could sound out words (phonics) and determine their meaning. In the beginning, it helped for the clinician to read with PS and to fill in words the client faltered on. Ultimately, however, the clinician "faded out," and PS continued on his own. Patients who rely on phoneme-to-grapheme conversion for reading success may have problems with irregularly spelled words such as "pneumonia" (Margolin, 1991); PS was no exception. Here, the clinician followed a suggestion by Hillis (1991) and used phonetic spellings (e.g., numonia). Reading material used in treatment was previewed. Irregularly spelled words were highlighted, and their phonetic spellings were written above the words. This helped PS to continue reading without a break, and, eventually, the pairings were learned. PS improved markedly in oral reading, and these improvements generalized to spontaneous speech and conversations with his family.

Treating Phonological Assembly Problems

Clients with problems assembling the phonemes of words and phrases for outputting have high self-correction effort (Kohn, 1989; Marshall and Tompkins, 1982), and low self-correction success (Marshall and Tompkins, 1982; Marshall et al., 1980).

Overcorrection

Clients' repeated attempts to produce a target word may be random (Alajouanine et al., 1939; Lecours and Lhermitte, 1969) or regular (Joanette et al., 1980). The former do not seem to approximate the target utterance; the latter do (Joanette et al., 1980). Successful treatment requires that the clinician be aware of the behavior and make appropriate decisions about what aids or hinders communication.

Marshall (1983) used the term "monitor" to describe the fluent aphasic client who does not stop correcting and revising his or her speech errors, no matter how slight. Monitors do not accept approximations but rather want "perfection." Sometimes, these excessive efforts interfere with communication, and the client ends up worse off than if he had "left well enough alone." When the patient is "almost right," informational feedback (e.g., That's close enough) from the clinician may be useful in signaling the patient to move on. If this doesn't

work and the patient continues to try and produce the target word correctly, the clinician can "model" with a spoken or written word. When a client becomes upset with unsuccessful self-correction attempts, the clinician needs to be more forceful. The patient needs to be supplied with the target word, and told in no uncertain terms that it is time to move on and that tomorrow is another day.

Repetition

The nature of the speech task has some relationship to successful phonological assembly. Joanette et al. (1980) and others (Valdois et al., 1989) studied sequences of phonemic approximations of aphasic patients for known target words in oral reading, spontaneous speech, automatic speech, and repetition of real and nonsense words. They found that series of phonemic approximations more closely approached targets for spontaneous speech, oral reading, and automatized sequences than repetition tasks.

At face value, the results of Joanette et al. (1980) make a case for avoiding repetition tasks in the management of phonological assembly problems. The argument has a practical side because in real life, one seldom needs to repeat speech. A counterargument can also be made. This is that in many communicative interactions, phonological assembly problems at the word, phrase, or sentence level "turn into" a repetition task as the patient focuses on production. In the following example, client EH is commenting about the regulations on keeping Pit Bulldogs on private property.

> *Clinician*: They (Pit Bulldogs) are dangerous.
> *EH*: I just don't think they should allow "piffles, I mean pit pulls, Bulldogs, no not Bulldogs, pibbles. What's happening? You know what I mean. Pit (pause) Bulls, that's it, Pit Bulls. What was I saying now? Oh, I don't think they should allow (pause), here I go again. Anyway, they should not be allowed on private property."

When EH has problems assembling the phonemes for "Pit Bulldogs," he recognizes and tries to correct the error. Saying "Pit Bulldogs" becomes a repetition task. It is hoped that EH will learn to deal with these problems more productively so that communication will not be disrupted. Specific work on repetition may help him do this.

Two basic explanations for repetition errors of fluent aphasic clients exist. One involves a deficit in the sequential selection and combination of target phonemes (Strub and Gardner, 1974; Tzortzis and Albert, 1974). The other implicates a short-term auditory-retention memory deficit as the responsible factor (Caramazza et al., 1981; Shallice and Warrington, 1977). Patients in the former category make phonemic errors; those in the latter category do not. Repetition work may be helpful to both types of patients.

Oral Reading Tasks. Sullivan et al. (1986) suggested that an intact visual-verbal system can facilitate performance of an impaired auditory-verbal system. They used oral-reading tasks (sentences and questions) to treat the repetition deficit of a single conduction aphasic patient. Stimuli involved a vocabulary "personalized" for the client. The patient improved in repetition of questions and sentences, as evidenced by fewer paraphasic errors and more accurate responses. Generalization to untreated stimuli was minimal, however Beard and Prescott (1991), who replicated the study by Sullivan et al. (1986) obtained similar results with another conduction aphasic patient. Boyle (1989) used an oral reading program consisting of overlapping words (chair), phrases (big chair), and sentences (The big chair is red) to reduce instances of phonemic paraphasia in a conduction aphasic subject. She assessed the impact of this treatment on the patient's production of trained items, as well as its impact on connected speech. Oral-reading treatment resulted in fewer phonemic paraphasias and a slower rate of speech. The patient's connected speech also improved as a consequence of treatment.

Unblocking.   The author has found that some fluent aphasic clients are more successful at repetition if they try to produce the target word or phrase (name or read) before being asked to ''repeat.'' Rarely is the attempt to name or read aloud successful, but for some reason it facilitates repetition. Joanette et al. (1980) suggested that phonemic approximations to the target may indeed be related to the initial strength and permanence of the internal representation of the target. Thus, it is possible that an attempt to name ''unblocks'' the repetition response by strengthening the internal representation of the target.

Beyond the Word Level

Several writers have suggested that treatment of fluent aphasias should take place in a context and that the convergent tasks of traditional stimulation should be avoided (Edwards, 1987; Marshal, 1982; Martin, 1981; Wepman, 1972). Most communications take place in a context requiring interchange of speaker and listener roles. The speaker tries to make the listener's task as easy as possible by providing the necessary information, without giving unnecessary information or misleading the listener (Grice, 1975). Aphasic subjects give a better representation of their communicative abilities in contextual situations than in artificial situations (Holland, 1977; Holland, 1983; Pierce, 1988; Pierce and Beekman, 1985; Schienberg and Holland, 1980). They respond better to personally relevant, plausible statements (Busch and Brookshire, 1982; Deloche and Seron, 1981; Gray et al., 1977). Finally, aphasic subjects' performance on didactic tasks does not predict how well they will perform in a context (Wilcox et al., 1978).

Establishing Contexts

Establishing a context requires background information, observation of the patient in situations outside the speech clinic (Holland, 1982, 1983), and consideration of client communication needs and interests. Green (1984) suggests obtaining information about preaphasia communications in several areas.

Style.   Was the client talkative, quiet, argumentative, or responsive to chit chat? Was she a good or poor listener? Did the individual dominate the conversation, correct others, and in general enjoy talking to people?

Activities.   Did the client initiate communication freely or speak when spoken to? Did the client speak in public, at club meetings, on the telephone, or to strangers?

Partners.   Who does the client talk to most often: family members, friends, colleagues? With whom would the client be most likely to share something emotional?

Situations.   What types of communication situations does the client talk in: public-private, quiet-noisy, one to one, home-work?

Topics.   What does the client like to talk about: news, TV, sports, religion, politics, family, children?

Guiding Principles

The existing aphasia literature provides helpful information to aid clinicians in developing contextually rich, communicatively based treatment for the fluent aphasias.

Stress Everyday Contexts

The difference between contextual communication and performance on convergent treatment tasks (e.g., naming, repetition, and oral reading) is astounding for many fluent aphasic clients (Marshall, 1983, 1982; Wepman, 1972). Treatment should stress the vocabulary and demands associated with the places the patient goes, the persons he or she communicates with, and other daily living activities.

Make Effective Communication a Priority

All communication is not done with words. Reward the patient for initiating communication and for using novel efforts to get his or her point across. NP, a very severe fluent aphasic, wanted a submarine sandwich. He knew he could not come up with the words. He ''pretended'' to be deaf; he copied the words ''roast beef and turkey combination'' on a paper and presented them to the clerk. The clerk produced a checklist, and NP indicated what he wanted on his sandwich. NP got his sandwich without speaking. He communicated effectively.

Put Some PACE in Treatment

The Promoting Aphasic Communicative Effectiveness (PACE) program of Davis and Wilcox (1985; Davis, 1980) was developed to make treatment situations more like natural communicative interactions. PACE stresses the use of new information, equal participation for both speaker and listener, freedom of communication channel selection (patient can communicate by writing, gesturing, drawing, or speaking), and use of natural feedback based on communicative adequacy, not production accuracy. PACE has been efficacious in the treatment of aphasic persons (Carlomagno et al., 1991; Davis, 1980; Davis and Wilcox, 1985; Li et al., 1988; Pulvermuller and Roth, 1991; Rau, 1986). Its principles are applicable in the management of fluent aphasias.

Pulvermuller and Roth (1991) present PACE modifications well suited to work on conversation in a context. These involve a series of communicative treatment settings similar to everyday conversations called language games. The requesting (for severe patients) and bargaining (for mild aphasic clients) games require the client to use sequential actions and strategies that parallel those of actual communicative situation, much like a role-playing situation.

Another PACE modification reported by Springer et al. (1991) involved presenting the patient with an array of 22 pictures, a subset of which the patient had to sort out as specific semantic classes (e.g., tools). The superordinate category was written on a card, and the card and pictures were given to the patient and the therapist, who were separated by a screen. The patient and the therapist took turns conveying class membership of each picture. The investigators compared results of this modi-

Table 21.5.
Response Elaboration Training (RET) With a Fluent Aphasic Patient (Kearns, 1986)

Step 1
Verbal Instruction and Stimulus Presentation

Clinician: Tell me about this picture, as completely as you can.
Patient: "He took it right to that sucker. To the hole, to the hole."

Step 2
Elaboration, Model, Reinforce

Clinician: "Bill Walton dunks the ball over Kareem - Good."
Patient: No response

Step 3
"Wh Cue"

Clinician: "What is going on here?"
Patient: "Playing in the Western Conference finals. Wowie. Gonna beat the Lakers four straight. Wait and see.

Step 4
Combine Patient Responses, Model, Reinforce

Clinician: "Bill Walton dunks the ball over Kareem in the Western Conference finals against the Lakers - Great."
Patient: No response

Step 5
Request Repetition and Model

Clinician: "You try and say the whole thing. Bill Walton dunks the ball over Kareem in the Western Conference finals against
              the Lakers.
Patient: "Walton dunks on Kareem in the finals with the Lakers."

Step 6
Reinforce, Model

Clinician: "Good work. Bill Walton dunks the ball over Kareem in the Western Conference against the Lakers."

---

fied approach with the traditional PACE approach and found that the modified approach had a more effective impact on verbal naming and general communication.

Train Loosely

Loose training permits clients to communicate in a flexible, creative manner (Kearns, 1986; Kearns and Scher, 1989; Kearns and Yedor, 1991). Emphasis is on divergent tasks that demand variety, quantity, relevance, and production of logical alternatives (Chapey, 1986) instead of the traditional convergent tasks (e.g., sentence completion, repetition) used to facilitate language improvement. Loose training is particularly well suited for the fluent aphasic patient who has difficulty with specific words but can communicate in a context.

Response Elaboration Training (RET).   Kearns's RET is a "loose training" method for increasing the verbal elaboration skills of aphasic patients (Kearns, 1986; Kearns and Scher, 1989; Kearns and Yedor, 1991). It stresses shaping and chaining *patient-initiated* rather than *clinician-selected* responses. The rational for RET is that didactic training inhibits creative, flexible language use and generalization. The end goal of RET is to facilitate generalized improvement in aphasic patients' ability to elaborate on conversational topics and share the communicative burden. To this point, reports of RET have been limited to results obtained with nonfluent clients; however, the author has found the procedure to be very useful with the fluent aphasias as well. The example in Table 21.5 came from a RET

session with client LB. The stimulus was a *Sports Illustrated* cover picture of a local professional basketball player (Bill Walton) making a "slam dunk" over an even more famous basketball player (Kareem Abdul Jabbar) in a 1977 playoff game.

Context-Centered Therapy

Wepman's (1972) context-centered therapy is one of few approaches that has a direct impact on the aphasic patient's functioning in real-life situations. This is an indirect method focusing on the "thoughts" underlying verbal messages rather than on specific words. Treatment materials include topics of prestroke interest (e.g., vocations, hobbies, family, activities). These are introduced, and the patient is encouraged to respond verbally. Clinician-patient exchanges are used to formulate, perceive, and revise messages until consensus about meaning is reached (Martin, 1981a). The clinician does not correct the patient's verbal efforts but keeps the conversation "on track" by reflecting back the client's intended thoughts and paraphrasing when word-retrieval difficulties interfere. In the short term, this method seeks to maintain continuity of content; in the long term, it endeavors to increase the exploration of nuances and embellishment of ideas about a topic (Wepman, 1972).

The following vignette came from a context-centered treatment session with client HB. The purposes of the clinician's comments are in brackets.

Clinician: "Let's talk about the time you were in college." [Introduction of topic]

HB: "The good old days, at the University of (pause) not Corvallis, the other one (pause) I was a duck."

Clinician: "You did *not*[Stress negative] go to Oregon State. You went to the University of. . ." [Gestures for patient to continue]

HB: "Oregon, in Eugene. I started there in 1965, and I got out in (pause) 66, 67, 68, 69. That's it, 1969."

Clinician: "You graduated from the University of Oregon in 1969." [Paraphrase]

HB: "Right. And then I lost my student (pause) whatchimacallit (pause) referral, not that, enlistment (pause), that's not it either, anyway things got bad."

Clinician: "You had a student deferment [fills in] and lost it after graduation from Oregon. What happened then?" [Lets client know consensus achieved on "deferment" and gets client back on the topic]

HB: "I got drafted of course and got sent to (pause) VC, V something, the war. It wasn't any fun and here I am now."

Clinician: "Vietnam was a tough situation. [Fills in the missing word without correcting the client] What branch of the service were you in?" [Gets conversation back on track with a highly redundant, related question]

HB: "The army."

Context-centered therapy has been stressed for the fluent aphasias throughout much of this chapter. Wepman (1972) reported that this approach was successful with clients who had failed with traditional approaches. He described these patients as pragmatic aphasics, or "the talking aphasics." His comments appear to fit the patient population dealt with in this chapter. This communicatively based treatment places words in a subservient position to thoughts and not vise versa. It allows clinicians to emphasize the social needs of the patient and the family, as well as the patient's linguistic deficits.

FUTURE TRENDS IN MANAGEMENT OF THE FLUENT APHASIAS

The fluent aphasias have been studied extensively, but efforts have largely focused on "symptoms" (e.g., repetition, single-word reading, naming) rather than treatments to ameliorate symptoms and improve communication. For example, Howard and Franklin (1988) devote an entire book to the study of single-word processing of one aphasic subject. There are several specific treatment programs for nonfluent and nonspeaking aphasic clients, but few procedures have been derived from research findings for fluent patients. It is hoped that one trend of the future will be to correct this imbalance.

Margolin (1991) points out that behavioral analyses of aphasic deficits "lag" behind technology. Advances in neuroimaging procedures such as PET (positron emission tomography), CAT scan (computerized axial tomography), MRI (magnetic resonance imaging), and other methods have advanced knowledge of the role of the brain in language. Clinicians now ask to see the CAT scan before testing reasonable hypotheses about which disrupted neural circuits are affecting disordered communication and how they are doing this. Another trend of the future will be that of behavioral analyses "catching up" with technology (Margolin, 1991).

There are signs that times are changing. Researchers (Byng et al., 1990; Caramazza, 1984; Schwartz, 1984) are conducting the painstaking case studies that teach us so much about the effects of brain injury on language. These studies show that brain damage can selectively impair one or more components of the cognitive-linguistic system (Caramazza, 1984). From this work, procedures have been developed to conduct the necessary analyses to develop model-driven assessment and treatment procedures applicable not only to the fluent aphasias but to all who suffer from this devastating problem (Byng et al., 1990; Weniger and Sarno, 1990; Weniger et al., 1987). Largely, treatment applications derived from process-oriented case-by-case approaches have focused on reading (Andreewsky et al., 1991; Friedman and Robinson, 1991) and writing (Carlomagno et al., 1991; Hillis and Caramazza, 1987). It is hoped that a future trend will be to give equal attention to speaking and listening, abilities that are far more important to day-to-day functioning for the aphasic person.

What fluent aphasic persons do best is to talk, but not perfectly. Any clinician that has tried to transcribe a speech sample of one of these clients understands how difficult it is to determine (*a*) if the patient is getting better or worse, (*b*) if he or she is communicating more effectively, and (*c*) if he or she is coming up with more specific words. Discourse analyses are time consuming, and valid, reliable measures are lacking. Recent efforts have been made to develop measures of connected speech analysis that are valid and reliable (Nicholas and Brookshire, 1992). These will be of immense help to clinicians working with the fluent aphasias.

References

Alajouanine, Th., Ombredane, A., and Durand, M. (1939). *Le syndrome de desintegration phonetique dans l'aphasia.* Paris: Masson.

Andreewsky, E., Desi, M., and Parisse, C. (1991). Deep dyslexia: theoretical implications for reading and rehabilitation. *Aphasiology, 5,* 335–340.

Bachman, D. L., and Albert, M. L. (1990). Auditory comprehension in aphasia. In H. Goodglass (Ed.), *Handbook of neuropsychology* (pp. 281–306). New York: Elsevier.

Basili, A. G., Diggs, C. C., and Rao, P. R. (1980). Auditory processing of brain–damaged adults under competitive listening conditions. *Brain and Language, 9,* 362–371.

Beard, L. C., and Prescott, T. E. (1991). Replication of a treatment protocol for repetition deficit in conduction aphasia. *Clinical Aphasiology, 19,* 197–208.

Benson, D. F. (1979). Neurologic correlates of anomia. In H. Whitaker and H. A. Whitaker (Eds.), *Studies in neurolinguistics* (Vol. 4, pp. 293–328). New York: Academic Press.

Berndt, R. S., and Caramazza, A. (1980). Semantic operations deficit in sentence comprehension. *Psychological Research, 41*(2–3), 169–176.

Blumstein, S. E., and Goodglass, H. (1972). The perception of stress as a semantic cue in aphasia. *Journal of Speech and Hearing Research, 15,* 800–806.

Boller, F., and Dennis, M. (Eds.). (1979). *Auditory comprehension: Clinical and experimental studies with the Token Test.* New York: Academic Press.

Boller, F., and Green E. (1972). Comprehension in severe aphasics. *Cortex, 8,* 382–394.

Boller, F., Kim, Y., and Mack, J. L. (1977). Auditory comprehension in aphasia. In H. Whitaker and H. A. Whitaker (Eds.), *Studies in neurolinguistics* (Vol. 3, pp. 1–63). New York: Academic Press.

Boyle, M. (1989). Reducing phonemic paraphasias in the connected speech of a conduction aphasic subject. *Clinical Aphasiology, 18,* 379–393.

Brookshire, R. H. (1971). Effects of trial time and inter–trial interval on naming by aphasic subjects. *Journal of Communication Disorders, 3,* 289–301.

Brookshire, R. H. (1974). Differences in responding to auditory verbal materials among aphasic patients. *Acta Symbolica 1,* 1–18.

Brookshire, R. H. (1986). *An introduction to aphasia* (3rd ed.). Minneapolis, MN: BRK.

Brookshire, R. H. (1992). *An introduction to neurogenic communication disorders* (4th ed.). St. Louis, MO: Mosby Yearbook.

Brookshire, R. H., and Nicholas, L. E. (1980). Sentence verification and language comprehension of aphasic persons. In R. H. Brookshire (Ed.), *Clinical Aphasiology Conference proceedings* (pp. 53–63). Minneapolis, MN: BRK.

Brownell, H. H. (1988). The neuropsychology of narrative comprehension. *Aphasiology, 3/4,* 247–250.

Buck, M. (1968). *Dysphasia: Professional guidance for family and patient.* Englewood Cliffs, NJ: Prentice–Hall.

Buckingham, H. W. (1979). Linguistic aspects of lexical retrieval disturbances in the posterior aphasias. In H. Whitaker and H. A. Whitaker (Eds.), *Studies in neurolinguistics* (Vol. 4, pp. 269–291). New York: Academic Press.

Busch, C., and Brookshire, R. H. (1982). Aphasic adults' auditory comprehension of yes–no questions (unpublished manuscript).

Byng, S., Kay, J., Edmundson, A., and Scott, C. (1990). Aphasia tests reconsidered. *Aphasiology, 4,* 67–92.

Caramazza, A. (1984). The logic of neuropsychological research and the problem of patient classification in aphasia. *Brain and Language, 21,* 9–20.

Caramazza, A., Basili, A., Koller, and Berndt, R. S. (1981). An investigation of repetition and language processing in a case of conduction aphasia. *Brain and Language, 14,* 235–271.

Caramazza, A., Zurif, E., and Gardner, H. (1978). Sentence memory in aphasia. *Neuropsychologia, 16,* 661–669.

Carlomagno, S., Colombo, A., Casadio, P., Emanuelli, S., and Razzano, C. (1991). Cognitive approaches to writing rehabilitation in aphasics: Evaluation of two treatment strategies. *Aphasiology, 5,* 355–360.

Carlomagno, S., Losanno, N., Emanuelli, S., and Casadio, P. (1991). Expressive language recovery or improved communicative skills: Effects of P. A. C. E. therapy on aphasics' referential communication and story retelling. *Aphasiology, 5,* 419–424.

Chapey, R. (1986). Cognitive intervention: Stimulation of cognition, memory, convergent thinking, divergent thinking, and evaluative thinking. In R. Chapey (Ed.), *Language intervention strategies in adult aphasia* (2nd ed., pp. 215–238). Baltimore, MD: Williams & Wilkins.

Clark, A. E., and Flowers, C. R. (1987). The effect of semantic redundancy on auditory comprehension in aphasia. In R. H. Brookshire (Ed.), *Clinical aphasiology* (pp. 174–179). Minneapolis, MN: BRK.

Cochrane, R. M. (1983). Language and the atmosphere of delight. In H. Winitz (Ed.), *Treating language disorders: For clinicians by clinicians* (pp. 143–162). Baltimore, MD: University Park Press.

Craik, F. L., and Lockhart, R. S. (1972). Levels of processing: A framework for memory research. *Journal of Verbal Learning and Verbal Behavior, 11,* 671–684.

Creary, M. A., and Kertesz, A. (1988). Evolving error profiles during aphasia syndrome remission. *Aphasiology, 2,* 67–78.

Czvik, P. (1977). Assessment of family attitudes towards aphasic patients with severe auditory processing disorders. In R. H. Brookshire (Ed.), *Clinical Aphasiology Conference proceedings* (pp. 160–164). Minneapolis, MN: BRK.

Darley, F. L. (1976). Maximizing input to the aphasic patient. In R. H. Brookshire (Ed.), *Clinical Aphasiology Conference proceedings* (pp. 1–21). Minneapolis, MN: BRK.

Darley, F. L. (1982). *Aphasia.* Philadelphia, PA: W. B. Saunders.

Davis, G. A. (1980). A critical look at PACE therapy. In R. H. Brookshire (Ed.), *Clinical Aphasiology Conference proceedings* (pp. 248–257). Minneapolis, MN: BRK.

Davis, G. A., and Wilcox, M. J. (1985). *Adult aphasia: Applied pragmatics.* San Diego, CA: College Hill Press.

Deloche, G., and Seron, X. (1981). Sentence understanding and knowledge of the world: Evidence from sentence–picture matching task performance by aphasic patients. *Brain and Language, 14,* 57–69.

DeRenzi, E., Faglioni, P., and Prevedi, G. (1978). Increased susceptibility of aphasics to a distractor task in the recall of verbal commands. *Brain and Language, 14,* 14–21.

DeRenzi, E., and Vignolo, L. (1962). The Token Test: A sensitive test to detect receptive disturbances in aphasia. *Brain, 85,* 665–678.

Edwards, S. (1987). Assessment and therapeutic intervention in a case of Wernicke's aphasia. *Aphasiology, 1,* 271–276.

Flowers, C. R., and Danforth, L. C. (1979). A step–wise auditory comprehension improvement program administered to aphasic patients by family members. In R. H. Brookshire (Ed.), *Clinical Aphasiology Conference proceedings* (pp. 196–202). Minneapolis, MN: BRK.

Friedman, R., and Robinson, S. (1991). Whole–word training therapy in a stable surface alexic patient: It works. *Aphasiology, 5,* 521–528.

Gainotti, G. (1976). The relationship between semantic impairment in comprehension and naming in aphasic patients. *British Journal of Disorders of Communication, 11,* 57–61.

Gainotti, G. (1987). The status of the semantic–lexical structures in anomia. *Aphasiology, 1,* 449–462.

Gainotti, G., Miceli, G., Caltagirone, C., Silveri, M. C., and Masullo, C. (1981). The relationship between type of naming error and semantic–lexical discrimination in aphasic patients. *Cortex, 3,* 401–410.

Gainotti, G., Silveri, M. C., Villa, G., and Miceli, G. (1986). Anomia with and without lexical comprehension disorders. *Brain and Language, 29,* 18–33.

Gardner, H., Albert, M. L., and Weintraub, S. (1975). Comprehending a word: The influence of speed and redundancy on auditory comprehension in aphasia. *Cortex, 11,* 155–162.

Gentilini, M., Faglioni, P., and DeRenzi, E. (1988). Are body part names selectively disrupted by aphasia? *Aphasiology, 2,* 567–576.

German, D. J. (1992). *Test for word finding in discourse.* Allen, TX: DLM.

Geschwind, N., and Fusillo, M. (1966). Color naming defects in association with alexia. *Archives of Neurology, 15,* 137–146.

Goodglass, H. (1976). Studies on the grammar of aphasics. In H. Whitaker, and H. Whitaker (Eds.), *Studies in neurolinguistics* (Vol. 1, pp. 237–259). New York: Academic Press.

Goodglass, H. (1981). The syndromes of aphasia: Similarities and differences in neurolinguistic features. *Topics in Language Disorders, 1,* 1–15.

Goodglass, H., and Baker, E. (1976). Semantic field naming and auditory comprehension in aphasia. *Brain and Language, 3,* 359–374.

Goodglass, H., Barton, M., and Kaplan, E. (1978). Sensory modality and object naming in aphasia. *Journal of Speech and Hearing Research, 11,* 488–496.

Goodglass, H., and Blumstein, S. (Eds.). (1973) *Psycholinguistics and aphasia* (pp. 183–215). Baltimore, MD: Johns Hopkins University Press.

Goodglass, H., Blumstein, S. E., Gleason, J. B., Hyde, M., Green, E., and Statlender, S. (1979). The effect of syntactic encoding on sentence comprehension in aphasia. *Brain and Language, 7,* 201–209.

Goodglass, H., Gleason, J. B., and Hyde, M. (1970). Some dimensions of auditory comprehension in aphasia. *Journal of Speech and Hearing Research, 13,* 595–606.

Goodglass, H., and Kaplan, E. (1983). *The assessment of aphasia and related disorders* (2nd ed.). Philadelphia, PA: Lea & Febiger.

Gravel, J., and LaPointe, L. L. (1983). Length and redundancy in health care providers' speech during interactions with aphasic and non–aphasic individuals. In R. H. Brookshire (Ed.), *Clinical Aphasiology Conference proceedings* (pp. 208–211). Minneapolis, MN: BRK.

Gray, L., Hoyt, P., Mogil, S., and Lefkowitz, N. (1977). A comparison of clinical tests of yes/no questions in aphasia. In R. H. Brookshire (Ed.), *Clinical Aphasiology Conference proceedings* (pp. 265–268). Minneapolis, MN: BRK.

Green, E., and Boller, F. (1974). Features of auditory comprehension in severely impaired aphasics. *Cortex, 10,* 133–145.

Green, E., and Howes, D. (1977). The nature of conduction aphasia: A study of anatomic and clinical features and of underlying mechanisms. In H. Whitaker and H. A. Whitaker (Eds.), *Studies in neurolinguistics* (Vol. 3, pp. 123–156). New York: Academic Press.

Green, J. (1984). Communication in aphasia therapy: Some of the procedures and issues involved. *British Journal of Disorders of Communication, 19,* 35–46.

Grice, H. P. (1975). Logic and conversation. In P. Cole and J. L. Morgan (Eds.), *Syntax and semantics, Vol. 3. Speech acts.* New York: Academic Press.

Grober, E., Perecman, E., Kellar, L., and Brown, J. (1980). Lexical knowledge in anterior and posterior aphasics. *Brain and Language, 10,* 318–330.

Grossman, M. (1981). A bird is a bird is a bird: Making reference within and without superordinate categories. *Brain and Language, 12,* 313–331.

Hanson, B. R. (1976). Recall of sentence meaning in aphasic and nonaphasic adults. *Journal of Communication Disorders, 9,* 235–246.

Hart, S., Berndt, R. S., and Caramazza, A. (1985). Category-specific naming deficit following cerebral infarction. *Nature, 316,* 439–440.

Hecaen, H., and Ajuriaguerra, J. de (1956). Visual agnosia for inanimate objects due to left occipital disease. *Revue Neurologique, 94,* 222–233.

Hillis, A. G. (1991). Effects of separate treatments for distinct impairments within the naming process. *Clinical Aphasiology, 19,* 255–266.

Hillis, A. G., and Caramazza, A. (1987). Model–driven treatment of dysgraphia. In R. H. Brookshire (Ed.), *Clinical Aphasiology Conference proceedings* (pp. 84–105). Minneapolis, MN: BRK.

Holland, A. L. (1977). Some practical considerations in aphasia rehabilitation. In M. Sullivan and M. S. Kommers (Eds.), *Rationale for adult aphasia therapy* (pp. 167–180). Lincoln, NB: University of Nebraska.

Holland, A. L. (1982). Observing functional communication in aphasic adults. *Journal of Speech and Hearing Disorders, 47*, 50–56.

Holland, A. L. (1983). Remarks on observing aphasic people. In R. H. Brookshire (Ed.), *Clinical aphasiology conference proceedings* (pp. 345–349). Minneapolis, MN: BRK.

Howard, D., and Franklin, S. (1988). *Missing the meaning* (a cognitive neuropsychological study of processing of words by an aphasic patient). Cambridge, MA: MIT Press.

Howard, D., Patterson, K., Franklin, S., Orchard-Lisle, V., and Morton, J. (1985a). The facilitation of picture naming in aphasia. *Cognitive Neuropsychology, 2*, 49–80.

Howard, D., Patterson, K., Franklin, S., Orchard–Lisle, V., and Morton, J. (1985b). Treatment of word retrieval deficits in aphasia. *Brain, 108*, 817–829.

Joanette, Y., Keller, E., and Lecours, A. R. (1980). Sequences of phonemic approximations in aphasia. *Brain and Language, 11*, 30–44.

Just, M. A., Davis, G. A., and Carpenter, P. A. (1977). A comparison of aphasic and normal adults in a sentence-verification task. *Cortex, 13*, 402–423.

Kearns, K. P. (1986). Systematic programming of verbal elaboration skills in chronic Broca's aphasia. In R. C. Marshall (Ed.), *Case studies in aphasia rehabilitation* (pp. 225–244). Austin, TX: Pro-Ed.

Kearns, K. P., and Scher, G. P. (1989). The generalization of response elaboration training effects. *Clinical Aphasiology, 18*, 223–242.

Kearns, K. P., and Yedor, K. (1991). An alternating treatments comparison of loose training and a convergent treatment strategy. *Clinical Aphasiology, 20*, 223–238.

Kempen, G., and Huijbers, P. (1983). The lexicalization process in sentence production and naming: Indirect election of words. *Cognition, 14*, 185–209.

Kennedy, J. L. (1983). Treatment of Wernicke's aphasia. In W. H. Perkins (Ed.), *Language handicaps in adults* (pp. 15–24). New York: Thieme-Stratton.

Kertesz, A. (1979). *Aphasia and associated disorders*. New York: Grune & Stratton.

Kertesz, A., and McCabe, P. (1977). Recovery patterns and recovery in aphasia. *Brain, 100*, 1–18.

Kohn, S. E. (1989). The nature of the phonemic string deficit in conduction aphasia. *Aphasiology, 3*, 209–240.

Kudo, T. (1984). The effect of semantic plausibility on sentence comprehension in aphasia. *Brain and Language, 21*, 208–218.

LaPointe, L. L., and Erickson, R. J. (1991). Auditory vigilance during divided task attention in aphasic individuals. *Aphasiology, 5*, 511–520.

Lecours, A. R., and Lhermitte, F. (1969). Phonemic paraphasias: Linguistic structures and tentative hypotheses. *Cortex, 5*, 193–228.

Lesser, R. (1987). Cognitive neuropsychological influences on aphasia therapy. *Aphasiology, 1*, 189–200.

Li, E., Kitselman, K., Dusatko, D., and Spinelli, C. (1988). The efficacy of PACE in the remediation of naming deficits. *Journal of Communication Disorders, 21*, 491–503.

Liederman, J., Kohn S., Wolf, M., and Goodglass, H. (1983). Lexical creativity during instances of word–finding difficulty: Broca's vs. Wernicke's aphasia. *Brain and Language, 20*, 21–32.

Logue, R. D., and Dixon, M. M. (1979). Word association and the anomic response: Analysis and treatment. In R. H. Brookshire (Ed.). *Clinical Aphasiology Conference proceedings* (pp. 248–260). Minneapolis, MN: BRK.

Loverso, F. L., and Prescott, T. E. (1981). The effect of alerting signals on left brain damaged (aphasic) and normal subjects' accuracy and response time to visual stimuli. In R. H. Brookshire (Ed.), *Clinical Aphasiology Conference proceedings* (pp. 55–67). Minneapolis, MN: BRK.

Margolin, D. I. (1991). Cognitive neuropsychology: Resolving enigmas about Wernicke's aphasia and other higher cortical disorders. *Archives of Neurology, 48*, 751–762.

Marshall, J., Pound, C., White-Thomson M., and Pring, D. (1990). The use of picture/word matching tasks to assist word retrieval in aphasic patients. *Aphasiology, 4*, 167–184.

Marshall, R. C. (1976). Word retrieval behavior of aphasic adults. *Journal of Speech and Hearing Disorders, 41*, 444–451.

Marshall, R. C. (1978). Clinician controlled auditory stimulation for aphasic adults. Tigard, OR: C. C. Publications.

Marshall, R. C. (1982). Treatment of Wernicke's aphasia. *AAO Exchange, 2*, 3–7.

Marshall, R. C. (1983). Communication styles of fluent aphasic clients. In H. Winitz (Ed.), *Treating language disorders: For clinicians by clinicians* (pp. 163–180). Baltimore, MD: University Park Press.

Marshall, R. C. (1986). Treatment of auditory comprehension deficits. In R. Chapey (Ed.), *Language intervention strategies in adult aphasia* (2nd ed., pp. 370–393). Baltimore, MD: Williams & Wilkins.

Marshall, R. C. (1987). Reapportioning time for aphasia rehabilitation: A point of view. *Aphasiology, 1*, 59–76.

Marshall, R. C., and Blake, P. (1992). Word finding difficulties of fluent aphasic adults in conversational speech (unpublished manuscript).

Marshall, R. C., and Brown, L. J. (1974). Effects of semantic relatedness upon the verbal retention of aphasic adults. In B. Porch (Ed.), *Clinical Aphasiology Conference proceedings* (pp. 3–13). New Orleans: B. Porch Publisher.

Marshall, R. C., Freed, D., and Phillips, D. (in press). Labeling of novel stimuli by aphasic subjects: Effects of phonological and self–cueing procedures. *Clinical Aphasiology*.

Marshall, R. C., Neuburger, S. I., and Phillips, D. S. (1991a). Sentence comprehension and repetition in conduction aphasia: Results of parallel testing. *Clinical Aphasiology, 19*, 151–162.

Marshall, R. C., Neuburger, S. I., and Phillips, D. S. (1991b). An experimental analysis of aphasia treatment tasks. *Clinical Aphasiology, 19*, 77–90.

Marshall, R. C., Neuburger, S. I., and Phillips, D. S. (1992). Effects of facilitation and cueing on labelling of "novel" stimuli by aphasic subjects. *Aphasiology, 6*, 567–583.

Marshall, R. C., Neuburger, S. I., and Starch, S. A. (1985). Aphasic confrontation naming elaboration. In R. H. Brookshire (Ed.), *Clinical Aphasiology Conference proceedings* (pp. 295–300). Minneapolis, MN: BRK.

Marshall, R. C., and Thistlethwaite, N. (1977). Verbal and nonverbal alerters: Effects on auditory comprehension of aphasic subjects (unpublished manuscript).

Marshall, R. C., and Tompkins, C. A. (1981). Identifying behavior associated with verbal self–corrections of aphasic clients. *Journal of Speech and Hearing Disorders, 6*, 168–173.

Marshall, R. C., and Tompkins, C. A. (1982). Verbal self-corrections of fluent and nonfluent aphasic subjects. *Brain and Language, 15*, 292–306.

Marshall, R. C., Tompkins, C., Rau, M., Phillips, D., Golper, L., and Lambrecht, K. (1980). Verbal self–correction behavior of aphasic subjects for single word tasks. In R. H. Brookshire (Ed.), *Clinical Aphasiology Conference proceedings* (pp. 39–46). Minneapolis, MN: BRK.

Marslen-Wilson, W., and Tyler, L. K. (1980). The temporal structure of spoken language understanding. *Cognition, 8*, 1–71.

Martin, A. D. (1981a). Therapy with the jargonaphasic. In J. Brown (Ed.), *Jargonaphasia* (pp. 305–326). New York: Academic Press.

Martin, A. D. (1981b). An examination of Wepman's thought centered therapy. In R. Chapey (Ed.), *Language intervention strategies in adult aphasia* (pp. 141–154). Baltimore, MD: Williams & Wilkins.

Massaro M., and Tompkins, C. A. (1992). *Feature analysis for treatment of head–injured patients: An efficacy study*. Paper presented at the Clinical Aphasiology Conference, Durengo, CO.

McNeil, M. R., Odell, K., and Tseng, C. (1991). Toward the integration of resource allocation into a general theory of aphasia. *Clinical Aphasiology, 20*, 21–40.

Milberg, W., and Blumstein, S. (1981). Lexical decision and aphasia: Evidence for semantic processing. *Brain and Language, 14*, 371–385.

Nicholas, L. E., and Brookshire, R. H. (1993). A system for quantifying the informativeness and efficiency of the connected speech of adults with aphasia. *Journal of Speech and Hearing Research, 36*, 338–350.

Parisi, D., and Pizzamiglio, L. (1970). Syntactic comprehension in aphasia. *Cortex, 6*, 204–215.

Pashek, G. V., and Brookshire, R. H. (1982). Effects of rate of speech and linguistic stress on auditory paragraph comprehension of aphasic individuals. *Journal of Speech and Hearing Research, 25*, 377–383.

Pashek, G. V., and Holland, A. L. (1988). Evolution of aphasia in the first year post-onset. *Cortex, 24*, 411–423.

Patterson, K., Purell, C., and Morton, J. (1983). Facilitation of word retrieval in aphasia. In C. Code and D. Muller (Eds.), *Aphasia therapy* (Studies in Language Disability and Remediation, 6) (pp. 76–87). London: Edward Arnold.

Pierce, R. S. (1981). Facilitating the comprehension of tense related sentences in aphasia. *Journal of Speech and Hearing Research, 24*, 364–368.

Pierce, R. S. (1982). Facilitating the comprehension of syntax in aphasia. *Journal of Speech and Hearing Research, 25*, 408–413.

Pierce, R. S. (1983). *Aphasia treatment manual: A research-directed guide*. Kent, OH: Blaca Enterprises.

Pierce, R. S. (1988). Influence of prior and subsequent context on comprehension in aphasia. *Aphasiology, 2,* 577–582.

Pierce, R. S., and Beekman, L. A. (1985). Effects of linguistic and extralinguistic context on semantic and syntactic processing in aphasia. *Journal of Speech and Hearing Research, 28,* 250–254.

Pring, T., White–Thomson, M., Pound, C., Marshall, J., and Davis, G. (1990). Picture/word picture matching tasks and word retrieval: Some follow-up data and second thoughts. *Aphasiology, 4,* 479–484.

Pulvermuller, F., and Roth, V. M. (1991). Communicative aphasia treatment as a further development of PACE therapy. *Aphasiology, 5,* 39–50.

Rau, M. T. (1986). Beyond our usual treatment goals. Treatment of a high level aphasic person. In R. C. Marshall (Ed.), *Case studies in aphasia rehabilitation* (pp. 31–44). Austin, TX: Pro-Ed.

Rinnert, C., and Whitaker, H. A. (1973). Semantic confusions by aphasic patients. *Cortex, 9,* 56–81.

Schienberg, S., and Holland, A. L. (1980). Conversational turn-taking in Wernicke's aphasia. In R. H. Brookshire (Ed.), *Clinical Aphasiology Conference proceedings* (pp. 106–110). Minneapolis, MN: BRK.

Schuell, H. (1965). *Minnesota Test for Differential Diagnosis of Aphasia.* Minneapolis, MN: University of Minnesota Press.

Schuell, H., Jenkins, J., and Jiminez-Pabon, E. (1964). *Aphasia in adults.* New York: Harper & Row.

Schwartz, M. F. (1984). What the classical aphasia categories can't do for us, and why. *Brain and Language, 21,* 3–8.

Shallice, T., and Warrington, E. K. (1977). Auditory-verbal short-term memory impairment and conduction aphasia. *Brain and Language, 4,* 479–491.

Shewan, C. M., and Canter, G. J. (1971). Effects of vocabulary, syntax, and sentence length on auditory comprehension in aphasic patients. *Cortex, 7,* 209–226.

Silveri, M. C., Carlomagno, S., Nocentini, U., Chieffi, S., and Gainottti, G. (1989). Semantic field integrity and naming ability in anomic patients. *Aphasiology, 3,* 423–434.

Sparks, R. (1978). Parastandardized examination guidelines for adult aphasia. *British Journal of Disorders of Communication, 13,* 135–146.

Springer, L., Glindemann, R., Huber, W., and Willmes, K. (1991). How efficacious is PACE–therapy when ''Language Systematic Training'' is incorporated? *Aphasiology, 5,* 391–400.

Stachowiak, F. J., Huber, W., Poeck, K., and Kerchensteiner, W. (1977). Text comprehension in aphasia. *Brain and Language, 4,* 177–195.

Strub, R. L., and Gardner, H. (1974). The repetition deficit in conduction aphasia: Mnestic or linguistic? *Brain and Language, 1,* 241–255.

Sullivan, M. P., Fisher, B., and Marshall, R. C. (1986). Treating the repetition deficit in conduction aphasia. In R. H. Brookshire (Ed.), *Clinical aphasiology conference proceedings* (pp. 172–180). Minneapolis, MN: BRK.

Tompkins, C. A., and Marshall, R. C. (1982). Communicative value of self–cues in aphasia. In R. H. Brookshire (Ed.), *Clinical Aphasiology Conference proceedings* (pp. 75–82). Minneapolis, MN: BRK.

Tyler, L. K. (1992). *Spoken language comprehension: An experimental approach to disordered and normal processing.* Cambridge, MA: MIT Press.

Tzortzis, D., and Albert, M. L. (1974). Impairment of memory for sequences in conduction aphasia. *Neuropsychologia, 12,* 355–366.

Valdois, S., Joanette, Y., and Nespoulous, J. (1989). Intrinsic organization of sequences of phonemic approximations: A preliminary study. *Aphasiology, 3,* 41–54.

Van Harskamp, F., and Visch-Brink, E. G. (1991). Goal recognition in aphasia therapy. *Aphasiology, 5,* 529–540.

Van Lancker, D., and Nicklay, C. K. (1992). Comprehension of personally relevant (PERL) versus novel language in two globally aphasic patients. *Aphasiology, 6,* 37–62.

Von Stockert, T. R. (1978). A standardized program for aphasia therapy. In V. Lebrun and R. Hoops (Eds.), *The management of aphasia* (pp. 97–107). Amsterdam: Swets & Zeitlinger B. V.

Wallace, G., and Canter, G. J. (1985). Effects of personally relevant language materials on the performance of severely aphasic individuals. *Journal of Speech and Hearing Disorders, 50,* 385–390.

Waller, M. R., and Darley, F. L. (1978). The influence of context on the auditory comprehension of paragraphs in aphasic subjects. *Journal of Speech and Hearing Research, 21,* 732–745.

Wegner, M. L., Brookshire, R. H., and Nicholas, L. E. (1984). Comprehension of main ideas and details in coherent and noncoherent discourse by aphasic and nonaphasic listeners. *Brain and Language, 21,* 37–51.

Weniger, D., and Sarno, M. T. (1990). The future of aphasia therapy: More than just new wine in old bottles? *Aphasiology, 4,* 301–306.

Weniger, D., Springer, L., and Poeck, K. (1987). The efficacy of deficit–specific therapy materials. *Aphasiology, 1,* 215–222.

Wepman, J. M. (1953). A conceptual model for the processes involved in recovery from aphasia. *Journal of Speech and Hearing Disorders, 18,* 4–13.

Wepman, J. M. (1972). Aphasia therapy: A new look. *Journal of Speech and Hearing Disorders, 37,* 203–214.

West, J. A., Gelfer, C. E., and Rosen, J. S. (1976). Processing of true and false affirmative sentences by aphasic subjects. In R. H. Brookshire (Ed.), *Clinical aphasiology conference proceedings* (pp. 248–254). Minneapolis, MN: BRK.

Whitaker, H. A. (1984). Two views on aphasia classification. *Brain and Language, 21,* 1–2.

Whitehouse, P., Caramazza, A., and Zurif, E. (1978). Naming in aphasia: Interacting effects of form and function. *Brain and Language, 6,* 63–74.

Whitney, J. (1975). *Developing aphasics' use of compensatory strategies.* Paper read at the convention of the American Speech and Hearing Association, Washington, D.C.

Wilcox, M. J., Davis, A. G., and Leonard, L. B. (1978). Aphasics' comprehension of contextually conveyed meaning. *Brain and Language, 3,* 362–377.

Williams, S. E., and Canter, G. J. (1982). The influence of situational context on naming performance in aphasic syndromes. *Brain and Language, 17,* 92–106.

Yamadori, A., and Albert, M. L. (1973). Word category aphasia. *Cortex, 9,* 112–125.

Zurif, E., Caramazza, A., Myerson, R., and Galvin, J. (1974). Semantic feature representations for normal and aphasic language. *Brain and Language, 1,* 167–187.

CHAPTER 22
Treatment of Nonfluent Broca's Aphasia

CYNTHIA K. THOMPSON

Broca's aphasia is one of the nonfluent aphasias often associated with lesions of the left frontal lobe in left-hemisphere language-dominant individuals. The lesion itself may occupy the fontal operculum (Brodmann's areas 44 and 45), the adjacent premotor and motor regions, the underlying white matter and basal ganglia, and the insula (H. Damasio, 1991; H. Damasio and Damasio, 1989). The general pattern of language breakdown associated with the diagnostic classification of Broca's aphasia is a reduction in language production in the presence of relatively spared auditory comprehension. The disorder, as described by Goodglass and Kaplan (1983), has the following characteristics: Broca's aphasic individuals produce halting, effortful speech that frequently results in incomplete, fragmented sentences in which syntactic complexity is reduced from normal levels, and content words (especially nouns) are produced much more frequently than are grammatical words (articles, pronouns, auxiliary verbs, and some prepositions). Bound grammatical elements (especially verb inflections) are frequently omitted, and auditory comprehension is relatively spared.

Consider the following excerpts of two patients diagnosed with nonfluent Broca's aphasia resulting from a left frontal lesion, telling the story of *Cinderella*.

Patient 1: Male, 41 years old
''The girl was washing . . . UH . . . washing the dishes and all this. And the . . . UH . . . girls were . . . UH . . . cleaning up her. The girls are . . . UH . . . fixing . . . UH . . . the girls are fixing . . . UH . . . UH . . . UH . . . proper attire you know. And UH then she's . . . UH . . . out . . . UH . . . she's brushing clothes or iron . . . UH . . . washing dishes you know. And then going up outside you know. She's talking to the . . . UH . . . UH . . . farm an animals you know. She thinks about . . . UH . . . the . . . UH . . . nice . . . UH . . . UH . . . dress. And the girls tearing . . . UH . . . off . . . UH . . . off the . . . UH . . . dress. And UH . . . UH maiden . . . UH . . . a fair maiden. The girl outa the west or something . . . UH . . . UH . . . says why go and . . . UH . . . go and go out and . . . UH . . . UH . . . the . . . UH wedding started and all this. And . . . UH . . . she's . . . UH . . . says oh maiden appear. And wop she . . . UH . . . great . . . UH . . . gown. And she's . . . UH . . . go out and to a wedding. Not a wedding . . . UH . . . the ball, the ball. And UH . . . UH . . . UH . . . the man . . UH . . . oh the . . . UH . . . guests hosts I guess. I guess so. And the girl she dances with him. And . . . UH . . . clock started to tick. And the . . . UH . . . going down stairs . . . UH . . . a foot

slip. And she's . . . UH . . . UH . . . she's . . . UH . . . UH. And she says well . . . UH . . . men are going around . . . UH . . . checking on the . . . UH . . . the girls . . . . UH . . . UH . . . foots. And UH . . . girls says no wrong know big and little and everything else. And she . . . UH . . . says well. The . . . UH . . . the woman says well maybe . . . UH . . . UH. UH well no forget it . . . UH . . . she's the maid. And . . . and . . . UH . . . she's . . . UH . . . the girl fits. UH . . . and the guy is oh my God it fits you know. And the . . . UH . . . carriage . . whatever. And . . . UH . . . she looks at the princess and married you know.''
Patient 2: Male, 56 years old
''I don't know. Cinderella want . . . . . . I don't know. Well . . . she lost her . . . UH . . . shoe. And . . . UH . . . I . . . they . . . she . . . she had two big sister. They want the shoe. I think she was go to . . . fit the shoe. There it was. It all started. I think the shoe is . . . the one thing. Tie in with . . . marrying the . . . UH . . . prince . . . prince. The shoe didn't fit . . . no . . . no. Oh shit. The was going the marry the prince . . . except the shoe weren't fit her except one. What is the name . . . I don't know. What people . . . no . . . no. I think she marry the prince. I think the prince and her . . . real well. Get it to the prince and her . . . yeh. I think the . . . to the prince . . . and her because . . . I think they do.''

Indeed, these patients present with many of the characteristics described by Goodglass and Kaplan (1983). Production patterns are halting, effortful, and incomplete, and fragmented sentences are frequently produced in which syntactic complexity is reduced. Content words are produced much more frequently than are grammatical words, however, both patients appear to have the most difficulty with verb production, and both produce articles and pronouns and even some auxiliary verbs and prepositions. Further, bound grammatical elements (especially verb inflections, plural forms) are sometimes omitted or produced incorrectly; however patient 1 appears to have retained the ability to produce at least some of these elements as well. Clearly, although these patients belong to the same diagnostic category, they present with different patterns of productive language disruption.

A close inspection of the complete language profiles of these patients—based on administration of the Western Aphasia Battery (WAB [Kertesz, 1982]) and other language tests—indicates that in addition to the apparent expressive language disruption, they also evince some difficulty with auditory comprehension, especially for lengthy and grammatically complex material. Additionally, they have difficulty in confrontation naming tasks and they have both reading and writing difficulty.

Such clinical observations, as well as research demonstrating dissociations among the various symptoms that have been taken to be the hallmark of Broca's aphasia, have spurred debate in the clinical aphasiology literature concerning the homogeneity of patients diagnosed with Broca's aphasia. Specifically, dissociations have been found in individual patients (a) between grammatical morpheme omission and other sentence structural abnormalities (Berndt, 1987; Kolk and Van Grunsven, 1985; Miceli et al., 1983; Saffran et al., 1980); (b) between bound and free-standing grammatical morphemes (Miceli and Mazzucchi, 1990; Saffran et al., 1989) and (c) among specific elements within the class of free-standing and bound grammatical morphemes (Miceli et al., 1989). Clearly, not all patients diagnosed with nonfluent Broca's aphasia present with the same patterns of language disruption. Production patterns may differ and, further, the extent to which auditory comprehension is "spared" may vary considerably from patient to patient (Caramazza and Hillis, 1989; Caramazza and Zurif, 1976; Miceli et al., 1983; Nespoulous et al., 1988). Additionally, reading and writing are often disrupted in the nonfluent Broca's aphasic patient, with qualitative differences noted in these domains as well (Morton and Patterson, 1980; Patterson et al., 1985).

Although the debate is yet to be resolved, patients fitting into the general classification of nonfluent Broca's aphasia require treatment. The purpose of this chapter is to address these treatment needs. Because of the heterogeneity among so labeled nonfluent Broca's patients, a thorough assessment of language behavior is essential prior to application of treatment such that the specific patterns of deficit may be delineated. In addition to standardized testing, in-depth assessment of lexical semantic processing, grammatical and syntactic processing, and pragmatic abilities is necessary (Byng et al., 1990). The remainder of this chapter will address treatment of these types of deficits. Following a brief philosophical discussion of intervention, approaches to treatment of disrupted lexical processes will be discussed. Treatment of grammatical deficits then is addressed, and, finally, functional/pragmatic approaches to training will be presented.

A PHILOSOPHY OF INTERVENTION

Treatment for aphasia is not an exact science. Until recently, controlled research investigating the effects of treatment provided to aphasic patients was virtually nonexistent. Early attempts to document the efficacy of treatment were undertaken with groups of aphasic patients—often with no control group being studied—who presented with a wide variety of language impairments. Nonspecific treatment—for example, "traditional, individual stimulus-response type treatment of speech and language deficits in all communicative modalities" (Wertz et al., 1981, p. 583)—then was applied, and language changes noted on administration of standardized tests were documented. In light of the above discussion, the shortcomings of this approach to documentation of treatment effects are obvious. Aphasic patients are not all the same—even those diagnosed as having a particular aphasic syndrome. Therefore, it follows that all aphasic patients will not respond optimally to the same

treatment. That is, documenting the effects of generic treatment may not provide the best information regarding the effects of specific treatments for specific language impairments. Further, standardized tests do not capture specific changes within the language-processing system. Indeed, improvements in language have been documented in patients who have *not* demonstrated improvement on standardized tests (Thompson, 1989).

The importance of studying language breakdown in individual patients with aphasia has recently gained popularity, precisely because of the heterogeneity evident among aphasic individuals. For example, in the cognitive neuropsychological literature, the case study approach has been widely used to delineate specific deficit patterns within and across language domains in aphasic patients (Caramazza, 1986). While clearly this approach has been subject to criticism (Bates et al., 1991), it has heightened awareness of the individual patterns of language disruption that may occur in aphasic individuals, and it has provided information for formulating models of language processing that will later need to be experimentally examined and verified.

In the treatment domain, individual aphasic patients also have come into focus. However, the individual subjects approach to studying treatment effects has taken a more scientific line than the individual approach in the cognitive neuropsychological literature. That is, recent examinations of treatment effects have used single-subject experimental paradigms that closely examine treatment effects in individual subjects while demonstrating experimental control. These designs also require replication of treatment effects across subjects presenting with similar language disruption patterns (Kearns, 1986; Kearns and Thompson, 1991; McReynolds and Thompson, 1986; Thompson and Kearns, 1981). In this sense, single-subject experimental research is not synonymous with studying single subjects. This approach to treatment research in aphasia has brought us closer to understanding the effects of certain treatments for certain language deficits.

Unfortunately, research of this sort is in an embryonic state, and much additional research of this nature is needed. Because we have only just begun to gather scientific data concerning the effects of treatment for the language problems seen in nonfluent aphasic individuals, the clinician is charged with a difficult task in prescription and delivery of treatment. In doing so, it is important to consider carefully the exact language problems of the individual patient and to design treatments to focus on each of these problems. Perhaps most important, the treatment design must consider *generalization* of treatment effects or the extent to which treatment has influenced not only the responses focused on in treatment but also other untrained responses. Further, the extent to which these trained and untrained responses are used across language contexts must be considered.

Generalization is an important and often overlooked aspect of aphasia treatment. Although aphasiologists have historically assumed that generalization is a natural and expected outcome of treatment (e.g., Schuell et al., 1964), this has turned out to be an erroneous assumption. Indeed, well-controlled treatment research has indicated that most often generalization *does not* occur naturally. Clearly, if generalization to untrained responses does not occur as a result of treatment, then, "in theory we must endeavor to train all responses that the aphasic patient will ever use . . . . and if generalization across contexts does not occur ... our treatment may be deemed unsatisfactory, because it is this carry-over of responding from the clinic to natural contexts that is the ultimate goal of treatment'' (Thompson, 1989, p. 83). Therefore, in the design of treatment for the nonfluent aphasic patient (as well as for all other aphasias)—whether treating lexical semantic deficits, morphosyntactic deficits, or pragmatic deficits—assessment of generalization should be systematically undertaken throughout treatment. This can be easily accomplished by extending the principles of single-subject experimental research design into the design of treatment. This entails selecting and measuring a variety of responses in a variety of language contexts in the baseline or pretreatment phase, applying treatment to only a few of these responses in one or more contexts, and periodically measuring generalization (*a*) to the untrained responses and (*b*) in the untrained language contexts. If generalization does not occur as a natural outcome of treatment, then steps must be taken to facilitate generalization (see Thompson, 1989, for review of these methods).

LEXICAL DEFICIT IN NONFLUENT APHASIA

Lexical deficits, defined simply as deficits in processing of words resulting from impairment to one or more of the mechanisms thought to be involved in the processing of words, are pervasive in all types of aphasia. However, the specific aspect of the lexical system that is impaired differs across aphasic syndromes and across patients carrying the same diagnostic classification. Depending on which aspects of lexical processing are disrupted in a particular patient, difficulties with naming of pictures or objects in either written or spoken form or in matching either spoken or written words to pictures or objects may be exhibited. For example, some nonfluent aphasic patients may have word-retrieval difficulty or anomia in the absence of a single-word auditory comprehension deficit. Others may have both single-word anomia and comprehension difficulty for at least some types of words, for example, low-frequency words (Warrington and Shallice, 1984) or categories of words (Hart et al., 1985; Warrington, 1981).

Models of lexical processing may assist in understanding the complexity of lexical deficits. For example, Ellis and Young (1988), Rapp and Caramazza (1991), and others have discussed models of the functional architecture of the lexical system, delineating the basic components of the system and how these components are interrelated. Such models include a central semantic system that is interconnected with both input and output modules, as is shown in Figure 22.1. Input modules consist of a written word recognition component or the orthographic input lexicon, a spoken word recognition component or phonological input lexicon, and a visual object recognition component. These input modules feed into the lexical semantic system or repository of the meanings of words (Jackendoff, 1983; Miller and Johnson-Laird, 1976). Prior to gaining access to these input lexicons, perceptual mechanisms process the stimulus, visual or phonological as the case may be, in order to represent information regarding the letters or phonemes in the stimulus. The output modules consist of written and spoken forms of words, the orthographic output lexicon, and the phonological output lexicon, respectively. Using such a model, which appreciates the complexities of lexical processing, the locus of a particular lexical deficit for a particular patient may be

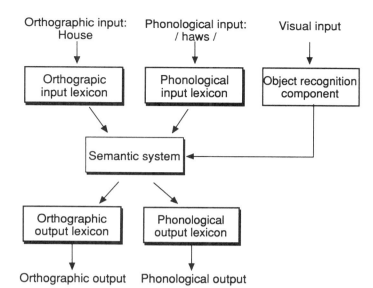

Figure 22.1. Model of the lexical processing system.

estimated. For example, a patient with a deficit in the semantic system would evince difficulty with tasks designed to test both input and output components. The patient would be unable to match written or spoken words to pictures or objects; would be unable to match pictures by semantic category or by other features; and would be unable to perform confrontation written or verbal naming of objects or pictures.

Clearly, other components or combinations of components of the lexical system may be involved. Nonfluent aphasic individuals most often evince primary difficulty with output. That is, in the presence of often (but not always) relatively spared single-word written and auditory comprehension and spared ability to match pictures or objects according to certain semantic variables, they have difficulty with written and/or spoken naming of words and pictures. This deficit pattern has most often been considered an *access* problem that delimits the ability to retrieve the phonological form of desired words either from the phonological word store or from the semantic system itself. This deficit pattern also is sometimes considered a *degradation* problem in which case patients may experience more difficulty with abstract words as compared with concrete words; they may experience greater difficulty in naming low-frequency words as compared with high-frequency words; they may fail to appreciate characteristic attributes of items within word categories (e.g., they may not select ''legs'' as being a feature of all animals); and their naming errors will be consistent (i.e., they will consistently have difficulty naming certain items). For example, Hart et al. (1985) described a patient with a category-specific naming deficit who had difficulty naming fruits and vegetables but no difficulty naming a large range of other pictures and objects. As well, the patient retained ability to sort written words by category and point to pictures when named. Patients experiencing access problems may not show category-specific effects, and their naming errors will be inconsistent. It is postulated that these patients have uncompromised semantic representations but that they have difficulty in accessing the semantic system and/or the phonological form of the desired word.

The specific locus of impairment(s) in the lexical system underlying the naming deficit patterns in nonfluent aphasic individuals is yet unclear. However, by careful testing of both input processes (i.e., pointing to pictures or objects of written or spoken words) and output processes (i.e., written and oral naming) using both low- and high-frequency words, words from various semantic and grammatical categories, and so on, as well as assessing the semantic system (e.g., appreciation of word meaning, category sorting), the deficit pattern in an individual patient may be estimated. Model-based assessment of lexical-semantic deficits has been described in detail in several sources. The reader is referred to these for further clarity of assessment practices along these lines (Byng et al., 1990; Rothi et al., 1991). Treatment may then be applied in accordance with the deficit pattern noted. This principled approach to treatment is the focus of the following discussion.

Approaches to Treating Lexical Deficits

Treating the Access Problem

Treatment approaches for access problems are more abundant in the literature than those for degradation problems. Indeed, the earliest writings concerned with treatment of aphasia were based on the premise that aphasia is characterized by reduced efficiency in accessing language—that it is a restriction of language availability and not an actual loss of language (Schuell et al., 1964). Based on this premise, a number of so-called "stimulation" treatments or access treatments were developed. For treatment of word-level deficits, such treatments emphasize the adequacy of the clinician's stimulus for facilitation of a response—with the idea being that if the various dimensions of the stimulus (e.g., volume, rate of presentation, frequency of presentation, modality of presentation, clinical cues) are made adequate, then a naming response is facilitated. The assumption is that with this practiced facilitation, access to the lexicon is improved. It is interesting to note here that with this approach, generalization to untrained responses is an assumed natural outcome of treatment. That is, if treatment improves access to the lexicon, then improvement in numbers of lexical responses should improve simultaneously. As will be subsequently discussed, this is not always the case.

Approaches to training access to the lexicon have been posed by several researchers. These approaches have used various forms of cuing and cuing hierarchies, or what I will refer to as intermodal facilitation methods (i.e., use of relatively spared language or nonlanguage processes as facilitators of impaired processes).

Cuing and Cuing Hierarchies. One of the first studies to focus on word retrieval in which cuing was used as a primary treatment method was that reported by Wiegel-Crump and Koenigsknecht (1973). Lexical items from several word categories (e.g., living things, clothes, household items, action verbs) were selected. From these categories, certain words were chosen for treatment, and following a treatment period untrained words from trained categories and words from an untrained category (foods) were tested for naming. Using both auditory and visual stimulation, target words were presented repeatedly as single words and in sentences, and a host of auditory-verbal cues including gestures, associated words, synonyms, carrier phrases, and initial phonemes or syllables of the desired response were used to facilitate naming responses. Results indi-

Table 22.I.
Cuing Hierarchies Used for Treatment of Lexical Retrieval

Thompson & Kearns (1981)
    Picture
    Picture + Sentence completion ("You fly in
      a _____")
    Picture + Sentence completion + Initial phoneme ("You
      fly in a /p/")
    Picture + Sentence completion + verbal model
Linebaugh (1990)
    Picture
    Picture + "Tell me what you do with it."
    Picture + "Show me what you do with it."
    Picture + Descriptive statement
    Picture + Sentence completion
    Picture + Sentence completion + Initial phoneme
    Picture + "Say _____."
    Picture + "Show me what you do with it."
    Picture + Functional gesture
    Picture + Sentence completion + Printed target word and
      two foils
    Picture + Sentence completion + Printed target word
    Picture + Sentence completion + target word + initial
      phoneme
    Picture + "Say _____."
Thompson, Raymer & leGrand (1991)
    Picture + "Tell me the name of this."
    Picture + Rhymed word
    Picture + Initial phoneme
    Picture + Auditory model
    Picture + "Tell me the name of this."

cated that all four of the aphasic patients receiving treatment improved; naming improved for both trained and untrained words within trained categories and generalization to the untrained category was noted as well. The authors concluded that the naming deficit evinced by their patients was indicative of an access problem or an "underlying loss of efficiency in retrieving words from the lexical store" (p. 410).

Other treatment studies using cuing have resulted in mixed findings (Linebaugh and Lehner, 1977; Seron et al., 1979; Thompson and Kearns, 1981). For example, Thompson and Kearns (1981) presented an in-depth treatment study of a woman with a 4-year history of anomic aphasia. Four lists of words were selected, with items on the first list being semantically paired with items on the third list and items on the second list being semantically paired with items on the fourth list. For example, the word "plane" appeared on the first list, and the word "train" appeared on the third list. Using a single-subject multiple-baseline design across behaviors, one word list was trained at a time while generalized naming of untrained words on the untrained lists was assessed. Treatment used a cuing hierarchy, as is indicated in Table 22.1. Results indicated limited generalization effects of treatment. That is, the aphasic woman began to name items successfully as they were trained; however, no generalization to untrained naming responses—even to semantically related responses—was noted.

The discrepant findings noted in these studies regarding the efficacy of this type of treatment are not surprising. Most treatment research concerned with establishing the efficacy of these treatments has not specified the locus of impairment within the lexical processing system of the patients under study.

Therefore, it may be that patients who present with differing patterns of breakdown across naming tasks may respond to naming treatment in different ways. Indeed, based on our current knowledge, it is highly possible that the patients studied in early treatment reports of naming intervention did not present with homogeneous naming problems. Further, many studies were not experimentally controlled. That is, they did not include control groups or within-subject controls such that the effects of variables other than treatment on the derived results could be discerned. Further, in some studies spontaneous recovery was not controlled and, therefore, the naming improvement noted may have been due, at least in part, to natural recovery processes.

In recent years, several researchers including Hillis (1989, 1991), Howard et al. (1985), Marshall et al. (1990), Pring et al. (1990), Raymer et al. (in press), Thompson et al. (1991), and others have begun to delineate certain treatments for certain types of naming deficits in aphasia. For example, Howard et al. (1985), recognizing that the functional basis for anomia can relate to semantic or to phonological mechanisms, examined separate semantic and phonological treatments sequentially in a group of 12 patients with varied aphasia classifications. Their semantically based treatment consisted of tasks that tap into the semantic nature of words, including (a) pointing to pictures named out of a set of four semantically related pictures, (b) matching written words to one of four semantically related pictures, and (c) answering yes/no questions pertaining to the superordinate category of a pictured item. Conversely, phonological treatment consisted of tasks concerned more with the phonological form of words: (a) repetition of target words, (b) provision of a phonemic cue to aid in production, and (c) presentation of rhyming and nonrhyming word pairs for the patient to recognize as rhyming or not rhyming. Findings from the study did not show clear distinctions between the two treatments in that both forms of treatment were effective in improving naming performance for trained items, with some advantage of semantic over phonological treatment and a small amount of generalization to untrained control words. However, by 6 weeks posttreatment, improvement in naming performance had diminished substantially. From the perspective that naming deficits are heterogeneous, the findings derived by Howard et al. (1985) are not surprising. That is, it is possible—and rather likely—that the patients under study presented with varying patterns of impairment to the lexical processing system. It is suggested that perhaps greater and more lasting treatment effects might have resulted if the types of treatment applied were matched with the types of deficit patterns displayed by the aphasic patients.

The work of Hillis (1989), Raymer et al. (in press), Thompson et al. (1991), and others has more clearly delineated the deficit patterns of their aphasic patients and then designed treatment directly focused on these deficits. For example, Thompson et al. (1991) developed a phonological treatment based on the work of Patterson et al. (1985) and treated two nonfluent aphasic individuals using this treatment. Prior to administration of treatment, it was determined, through a battery of seven lexical tasks, that both subjects evinced a primary locus of verbal impairment at the level of the phonological output lexicon. The lexical tasks included oral picture naming, oral word reading, repetition, written picture naming, auditory word/picture verification, and written word/picture verification.

As well, it was determined that one of the subjects had some lexical-semantic impairment. Two lists of words were sequentially trained using picture stimuli. During each training trial, the subject was instructed to name a picture such as "bat," and when naming was unsuccessful, a rhyming cue was presented (i.e., in this example, the clinician said, "It rhymes with cat"). When this did not assist with correct naming, a phonemic cue coinciding with the target word was provided. Finally, if necessary, the target word was modeled (see Table 22.1). Throughout treatment, naming of target items as well as rhymed and semantically related words was assessed. In addition, testing of oral reading and written naming of both trained and untrained words was undertaken. Results of the study indicated improved naming of trained items for both subjects and some evidence of generalization to untrained items. Interestingly, improvement in oral reading also was noted for one subject, coinciding with his improvement in oral naming. In consideration of the model of lexical processing presented in Figure 22.1, it is interesting to note that both oral naming and oral reading rely on the phonological output lexicon. Therefore, this generalization could have been predicted. In a study extending the previous work, Raymer et al. (1993) demonstrated similar findings in additional subjects.

Intermodal Facilitation Methods. Another general method for improving naming in aphasic patients exploits relatively intact language or nonlanguage modalities in the naming treatment process. For example, the graphic modality may be used to facilitate naming. When written naming is relatively unimpaired as compared with oral naming, pairing written naming with oral naming may strengthen oral naming. Indeed, in some discussions of lexical processing, a link between these two output lexicons is postulated. Gestures or object pantomimes also have been used to facilitate access to naming responses, and more recently, drawing has been used along these lines (Lyon and Helm-Estabrooks, 1987). The idea underlying these types of treatments is that this intervention might strengthen the likelihood of correct oral verbal naming and that it might also provide the patient with a self-cuing strategy that may be used for facilitating naming during naming failures. Additionally, this treatment provides patients with an alternative method of responding in the event that an oral response is not forthcoming even with the self-cued response.

Research along these lines, in which gestural responses are used, is the most abundant, although only a few studies have been reported. Usually, iconic gestures (those that visually resemble the target response) are selected and paired with oral naming in treatment. Skelly et al. (1974) was perhaps the first to publish a report of the effects of gestural treatment on verbal responding. However, a close inspection of Skelly's work indicates that the patients provided with this treatment received not only gestural training, but also practice with oral verbal responding.

Questioning the direct effect of gestural responses on verbal output, Kearns et al. (1982) trained two nonfluent aphasic patients to produce selected gestural responses one at a time, taking special care *not* to provide opportunity for verbal practice of the target words. To measure the effects of this gestural treatment on verbal responding, they repeatedly tested both gestural and verbal production of target words throughout the gestural training period. Results indicated that gestural training alone had no effect on verbal production. Only later when the trained gestural responses were paired with verbal production practice was verbal production improved. These data suggested that verbal plus gestural training is superior to gestural training alone for facilitating verbal naming responses. However, the authors did not address the effects of verbal training alone in their study. Therefore, the role of the gestural training was not completely clear. That is, it is possible that verbal training alone might have resulted in naming at the same levels as the verbal plus gestural training.

Hoodin and Thompson (1983) addressed this issue. Using an alternating treatments design, they investigated the effects of three treatment methods on oral verbal naming of familiar nouns. The three treatments included (a) gestural treatment alone, (b) verbal treatment alone, and (c) gestural plus verbal treatment. Picturable nouns matched for frequency of occurrence were selected and randomly divided into three sets. Two nonfluent aphasic patients then received the three treatments simultaneously with each set of words paired with a particular treatment in a counterbalanced manner. Gestures only were trained for the first set of nouns, verbal labels only were trained for the second set of nouns, and both gestural and verbal labels were trained for the third set. To assess the effects of each treatment on verbal naming, verbal production of all sets of nouns was tested throughout treatment by presenting all pictures and asking the subjects to name them. The results were interesting and supported the previous findings of Kearns et al. (1982). Gestural training alone had no effect on naming; verbal training alone had some effect; however, gestural plus verbal treatment was by far the most effective for all patients studied. It is important to note that we have repeated this experiment in our lab with four additional nonfluent aphasic patients. All have responded similarly, with gestural plus verbal treatment always being superior.

Treating the Degradation Problem

Approaches to treatment of degradation problems are not common. Indeed, inspection of the treatment literature indicates limited research concerned with treating such problems. Perhaps the rarity of treatments for degradation problems reflects the rarity of these reported problems in the literature. Hillis (1991) reported the results of treatment for a 22-year-old woman with a history of cerebral contusions. Results of administration of an extensive lexical evaluation indicated that the patient's naming failure resulted from two levels of impairment: (a) the semantic system and (b) the phonological output lexicon. The initial treatment was applied to teach semantic distinctions for items whose names were then written. Improvement subsequently was noted in written naming, oral picture naming, writing to dictation, repetition, and matching pictures to spoken words. Because phonological deficits persisted, a subsequent phonemic treatment for oral reading was administered in which phonetic spellings of words were pronounced. As a result, oral reading of trained words improved and generalization was noted for the pronunciation of the same words in oral naming and repetition tasks.

Jacobs and Thompson (1992) developed a treatment for a presumably pervasive semantic system deficit in a globally aphasic patient. The treatment used five semantic categories with seven common objects per category. Items from four of these semantic categories (foods, clothing, eating utensils, and

body parts) were selected for training, while some items from each of these categories as well as all items from an untrained category (furniture) were used for generalization testing. For treatment purposes, general (superordinate category) and specific (object function) semantic cues were developed to (a) improve comprehension of words first with unrelated picture distractors and then with semantically related distractors and (b) improve category sorting. Throughout treatment, auditory word recognition, written word recognition, written and oral naming, and category sorting were assessed. Although the effects of treatment for this globally impaired patient were minimal—only slight improvement in auditory comprehension and category sorting was noted—such an approach for training category-specific deficits in Broca's aphasic patients may be beneficial. At least a trial period of such treatment that includes assessment of both input and output components of lexical processing throughout treatment would be appropriate.

SENTENCE-LEVEL DEFICITS IN NONFLUENT APHASIA

Sentence-level deficits are perhaps the most salient diagnostic indicator of nonfluent Broca's aphasic individuals. Indeed, these deficits comprise a diagnostic label—albeit a controversial one—of their own. That is, this aspect of the disorder is sometimes referred to as *agrammatism*—a complex disorder characterized, in the case of production, by the omission/substitution of grammatical morphemes, the omission/nominalization of main verbs, and the misordering of sentence constituents or arguments. In the case of comprehension, agrammatism is characterized by asyntactic comprehension co-occurring with surprisingly spared ability to judge grammatical well-formedness of sentences (Berndt, 1987; Caplan and Hilebrandt, 1988; Linebarger, 1990; Saffran and Schwartz, 1988; Schwartz et al., 1985; Schwartz et al., 1987). As discussed previously, some of these patients may present with more or less difficulty with bound versus free-standing morphemes and with grammatical morphemes versus ordering of sentence constituents. Further, they may present with more or less difficulty with comprehension versus production of grammatical morphemes and sentence strings. Thus, the diagnostic category of agrammatism has been challenged for the same reasons as the diagnostic classification of Broca's aphasia (Badecker and Caramazza, 1985; Miceli et al., 1989). It cannot be questioned that patients presenting with language behaviors indicative of agrammatism represent a heterogeneous patient group.

Treatment of these grammatical impairments is not an easy task, and little treatment research focused on these problems is available. Part of the reason for this is the fact that grammatical deficits as seen in nonfluent aphasic patients are not well understood and there is not agreement in the literature regarding the nature of the disorder. Further, most studies of agrammatism have been based on comprehension patterns as opposed to careful analysis of production patterns. Only recently have researchers begun to collect systematic data concerned with aspects of sentence production. Indeed, there are a number of theoretical explanations for the various aspects of agrammatism including, but not limited to (a) difficulty with thematic role assignment (Saffran et al., 1980), (b) difficulty ''mapping'' thematic role information onto grammatical categories (noun phrases) in sentences (Saffran and Schwartz, 1988; Schwartz et al., 1987), (c) a deficit in phonological working memory (Baddeley, 1986; Kolk and Van Grunsven, 1985); (d) deletion or misselection of terminal nonlexical elements (e.g., inflections, agreement, and complementizers) in the phrasal geometry of a sentence (Grodzinsky, 1990); and (e) patient adaptation to performance limitations (Kolk and Van Grunsven, 1985; Kolk et al., 1985). These and other theoretical positions are reviewed elsewhere (see, for example, Berndt, 1991) and, therefore, they will not be discussed here. The point here is that we are only beginning to understand the nature of the agrammatic symptom complex and, therefore, it is not surprising that treatment for grammatic aspects of nonfluent aphasia also is in an embryonic state.

Assessment of Sentence-Level Deficits

Assessment of grammatical aspects of nonfluent aphasia presents a challenge. Clearly, given the various aspects of sentence production that may be aberrant in these patients, an in-depth assessment of the impairment is imperative, including testing of both comprehension and production of grammatical morphemes as well as various sentence types. Unfortunately, at present, published assessment tools are not available for accomplishing this completely, and aphasia test batteries do not provide adequate testing of salient grammatical and syntactic language variables. Available tests for comprehension such as the Revised Token Test (McNeil and Prescott, 1978) and the Auditory Comprehension Test for Sentences (Shewan, 1981) do not address all types of sentence-level problems that need to be tested with this patient population, and virtually no published tests for sentence production are available.

Goodglass et al. (1972) developed a story completion technique for testing production of 14 different English sentence structures rarely heard in the free speech of agrammatic patients. Using this method with agrammatic aphasic subjects, they reported a hierarchy of sentence difficulty (Gleason et al., 1975; Goodglass et al., 1972). This story completion method, known as the Story Completion Test, is presented in Table 22.2. In our early work with treatment of agrammatism, we often used this method. However, because we found that it did not always elicit the desired sentence types, and because not all relevant sentence types are included on the test, we no longer recommend using it as the primary test of sentence production. It is recommended instead that clinicians develop stimuli of their own to test various types of sentences as well as free-standing and bound morphemes both for comprehension and production until comprehensive, well-standardized tests in this area are available.

Saffran and colleagues have developed and have begun standardization procedures on a test for sentence comprehension—the Philadelphia Comprehension Battery for Aphasia (Saffran et al., unpublished). To date, the test has been used primarily for research, but it may be available for clinical use in the future once standardization has been completed. This test addresses important aspects of sentence comprehension, providing sections for contrasting lexical comprehension versus comprehension of sentences of several types, including reversible active (e.g., *The man serves the woman*), passive (e.g., *The woman was served by the man*), object-relative clause (e.g., *The dog that the boy washed was dirty*), and subject-relative clause sentences (e.g., *The policeman that shot the robber was lucky*).

Each of these and other sentence types are tested using a picture-pointing task. Another test that may be available soon is that being developed by Caplan (1988 -- **get ASHA magazine presentation**). This linguistically based test purportedly tests both comprehension and production and includes sections concerned with lexical, morphological, and sentence-level processing.

Additionally, during the course of assessment, it is important to analyze spontaneous language. Saffran et al. (1989) have developed a method for undertaking this analysis, although revisions of their analysis system are currently underway (Thompson et al., 1992; Thompson et al., in press). Saffran et al. (1989) recommend using a story retelling task to collect the language sample. Specifically, they use the story of *Cinderella*. After collection of the story sample, it is transcribed; segmented into utterances according to syntactic, prosodic, and semantic criteria; and coded. Utterances are coded for utterance type (e.g., complete sentence, embedded utterance); words are coded according to lexical class (e.g., nouns, verbs); verb inflections are coded; and other bound and free-standing grammatical morphemes are coded. As well, sentence constituents (e.g., noun phrases, verb phrases) are coded. From these data, both lexical and sentence structural analyses are undertaken to derive information such as noun:verb ratio, open class:closed class ratio, noun:pronoun ratio, number of words produced in sentences, mean length of sentences, and the proportion of utterances with complete sentences. Although this coding system is quite complex, it is worthwhile for clinicians to become familiar with analyses of this type because changes in these language variables may become the focus of treatment. However, the system by Saffran et al. (1989) does not address types of sentences produced or aspects of verb-argument structure as does the research presently underway by Thompson and colleagues.

Approaches to Training Sentence Comprehension

To the author's knowledge, no treatment studies or treatment approaches for training comprehension of grammatical morphemes have been published. Therefore, this section focuses on approaches to training sentence-level comprehension deficits.

Mapping Therapy

As is well known, nonfluent Broca's aphasic individuals with agrammatism have sometimes marked comprehension difficulty at the sentence level. This deficit is reliably revealed by tests that require patients to interpret semantically reversible sentences that allow for role-reversal errors (Caramazza and Zurif, 1976; Jones, 1984; Schwartz et al., 1980). For example, patients with so-called agrammatic comprehension deficits have difficulty performing sentence-picture matching tests using sentences such as *The boy is chased by the dog* when the target picture is presented with a reversed-role distractor (i.e., a picture of a boy chasing a dog). In spite of this recognized difficulty, these patients often retain aspects of grammatical processing. For example, aphasic patients appear to perform normally on grammaticality judgment tasks (Linebarger et al., 1983). These findings led Schwartz and colleagues (1980) to conclude that the core problem in agrammatic comprehension is not failure to perform syntactic analysis (i.e., to parse sentences for their syntactic function) so much as it is a difficulty in assigning

Table 22.2.
The Story Completion Test **format. Sample sentences from Goodglass, Gleason, Bernholtz, and Hyde (1972).**

1. IMPERATIVE INTRANSITIVE
   My friend comes in. I want him to sit down. So I say to him: What? (Sit down!)
2. IMPERATIVE TRANSITIVE
   The grass needs to be cut. I give my son the lawn mower, and I tell him: What? (Cut the grass!)
3. DECLARATIVE INTRANSITIVE
   The baby smiles. I want the baby to laugh. I tickle the baby. What happens? (The baby laughs).
4. DECLARATIVE TRANSITIVE
   Mr. Jones wants to hear the news. The radio is off. What happens? (He turns the radio on.)
5. DIRECT + INDIRECT OBJECT
   My dog is hungry. I get a bone to give the dog. What next? (I give the dog the bone.)
6. YES-NO QUESTION
   John is in his room. He thinks he hears his mother call. Se he goes downstairs to see if she called him, and he asks. . . what? (Did you call me?)
7. WH QUESTIONS
   Jane can't find her shoes. Her mother has just cleaned the room. She knows her mother put them somewhere. So she asks . . .what? (Where did you put my shoes?)
8. FUTURE
   Father smokes his pipe every evening after supper. Supper is just over now. What will happen now? (He will smoke his pipe.)
9. EMBEDDED SENTENCE
   The soldier's gun was dirty. The sergeant was annoyed. So he called the soldier over and told him he wanted . . . what? (He wanted him to clean the gun.)
10. PASSIVE
    A man was walking on the railroad tracks. A train came along. The man didn't hear it. What happen to him? The man . . . what? (The man was killed by the train.)
11. COMPARATIVE
    Mrs. Jones tried to open the jar. She wasn't strong enough. So she called her husband and he did it the first try. How come? (He was stronger.)
12. CARDINAL NUMBER + NOUN
    There are some cups on the table. There are twelve of them. What is on the table? (Twelve cups.)
13. ADJECTIVE + NOUN
    He told a story. It was funny. He told a . . . what? (A funny story.)
14. ADJECTIVE + ADJECTIVE + NOUN
    I sold her a small car. The car was red. In other words, I sold her . . . what? (A small red car.)

the correct interpretation to the parsed constituents, that is, **mapping** syntax-to-semantics.

A treatment method for overcoming this mapping deficit is known as *mapping therapy* (Byng, 1988; Jones, 1986; LeDorze et al., 1991; Schwartz et al., 1992). Jones (1986) reported an initial case study examining the effects of this approach in a patient presenting with long-standing language patterns considered indicative of a mapping deficit. In essence, the patient was taught the meaning relations existing around the verbs in sentences using a series of comprehension tasks. Results indicated improved sentence comprehension for this patient. However, experimental control was not demonstrated; therefore, it is not possible to attribute this patient's improvement directly to the treatment provided.

In a similar study, LeDorze et al. (1991) partially replicated the work of Jones. LeDorze et al. trained one chronic agrammatic aphasic patient who presumably presented with a mapping deficit to identify the verb, actor, patient, and locative arguments in subject-verb, subject-verb-object (S-V-O), and subject-verb-prepositional phrase sentences. This training improved the patient's verb and noun-verb comprehension and production using both training stimuli and untrained stimuli of the type trained. However, the extent of improvement on untrained sentence types was not addressed. Further, experimental control was not maintained throughout the course of

the study; therefore, it is not certain that the results reported were a direct result treatment.

Byng (1988) reported two additional case studies using this approach—one with an agrammatic patient (B.R.B.) who received treatment on reversible locatives and the other with a more severely involved patient (J.G.) who received treatment on reversible passive constructions because he was unable to learn reversible locatives. Improvements were noted over the course of treatment for both patients. However, experimental control again was not demonstrated; neither control subjects nor control phases were incorporated into the treatment design. Further, close inspection of the data indicated that generalization beyond the structure trained was noted for only one of the subjects (B.R.B.). For this subject, generalization occurred to additional semantically reversible sentences (i.e., from reversible locative to reversible passive constructions).

Saffran et al. (1993) provided mapping therapy for eight nonfluent Broca's aphasic subjects presenting with varying deficit patterns and severity. Again using input tasks concerning the thematic role carried by a verb's arguments, subjects were first trained on canonical (S-V-O) sentences with action verbs and various ''padding'' (additions of modifying words and phrases to the subject and/or object noun phrase). Next, subjects were trained on the same sentence types, this time using verbs referring not to actions but to so-called ''states of mind'' (e.g., *knowing, seeing*). Finally, noncanonical sentences including passives, object relative sentences, and subject relative sentences were trained. The main point of mapping therapy is to train patients to pick out the logical subject and logical object of these sentences. During treatment, the patient is presented with a typed sentence that the examiner reads aloud after the patient first attempts to read it. This is followed by the examiner asking three probe questions. The first probe results in the subject identifying the verb by underlining it. Then using *wh*-questions such as, "Which one is doing the V-ing?" and "What is she/he V-ing?" to query the logical subject and logical object, respectively, the subject underlines the appropriate sentence constituent. Although the percentage of errors was low prior to treatment, results indicated that when the first sentence type was trained, improved comprehension of both sets of canonical sentences occurred. However, this training resulted in little improvement in comprehension of the more complex, noncanonical sentences. The treatment also did not seem to markedly improve comprehension of these sentences for all subjects even when treatment was extended to them. It is interesting to note, however, that some improvement in productive language resulted for some patients receiving mapping therapy. For example, increases in the percentage of words used in sentences was noted following treatment on *Cinderella* narratives.

At present, mapping therapy continues to be researched to refine its methodology and to examine its effectiveness in greater numbers of aphasic patients. It is anticipated that this work will provide an important method for training sentence comprehension difficulties in some patients and that concomitant improvement in sentence production also may occur.

Approaches to Training Production of Sentences

Improving Production of Grammatical Morphemes

There are few treatment studies concerned with production of grammatical morphemes in the aphasia treatment literature. Here, a few sample studies will be reviewed primarily to provide a basis for clinicians to organize their treatment program. Clearly, treatment of grammatical morphology should be principled; that is, it should be guided by what is known about inflectional morphology, the relation between and among freestanding grammatical morphemes, and theories of insertion of grammatical morphemes into sentence frames (see, for example, Garrett, 1980, for discussion of representational levels of grammatical elements in sentence production).

Cannito and Vogel (1987) undertook a simple demonstration study concerned with teaching production of regular plural forms to a 66-year-old woman with moderately severe nonfluent aphasia. The purpose of the study was twofold. First, the investigators queried whether their patient could be trained to produce plural morphemes correctly; second, they examined the carryover of this training both to untrained irregular plural forms and to a discourse task. The training procedure used pictured objects as singletons and in pairs and a sentence closure task. The clinician pointed to the single-object pictures, for example, and said "one car" and then pointed to the pictured objects in pairs and said, "two _____." Results indicated that after approximately 12 training sessions, the production of regular plurals was established in the patient and, as would be predicted, this training had no effect on irregular plural forms. Interestingly, this patient did not overregularize the irregular plurals

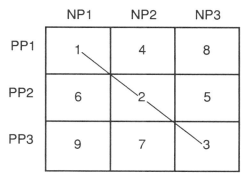

Figure 22.2. Matrix utilized for training production of locative prepositions in simple declarative sentences.

as is often the case in children's language. It was reported that the patient seemed to avoid irregular plurals; instead of producing *childs* for *children*, for example, the subject produced "one boy and one girl," indicating that the subject retained knowledge that irregular plurals do not take the regular plural form. Reportedly, the subject did demonstrate correct use of the plural form in the discourse task following treatment, although the data documenting this generalization were not presented. It would be interesting to note the effect of this training on sentence production. That is, the extent to which this type of treatment influenced verb usage and/or noun-verb agreement in sentences would be of interest.

Another treatment study concerned with production of grammatical morphemes—namely locative prepositions—was reported by Thompson et al. (1982). In this study, two nonfluent, agrammatic aphasic subjects were trained to produced locative prepositions in simple declarative sentences of the form noun phrase (NP)-verb (V)-prepositional phrase (PP). The locatives *behind* and *beside* were selected for treatment because both patients evinced difficulty with both comprehension (discrimination) and production of these spatially related locatives. The treatment design used a matrix-training approach (Foss, 1968; Goldstein, 1985) in which NPs and PPs used in the study were arranged in a 3 x 3 matrix as is shown in Figure 22.2. Treatment, using a modeling and forward-chaining procedure, then was applied to train combined NP-V-PP responses located on the diagonal of the matrix (i.e., cells 1, 2, and 3 in Figure 22.2). In this manner, generalized production of untrained NP-V-PP combinations could be assessed to the untrained cells (i.e., cells 4, 8, 6, 5, 9, and 7 in Figure 22.2). The matrix-training approach is an excellent way to arrange stimuli during treatment to systematically assess generalized use of trained forms in untrained contexts. Results of the study indicated rapid acquisition and generalized production of trained locatives in untrained sentence contexts, but no effect on production of the untrained locative in its sentence contexts was seen.

A final study fitting into this discussion of treatment for production of grammatical morphology is one undertaken by Kearns and Salmon (1984). Two chronic nonfluent aphasic patients considered to be agrammatic based on the Boston Diagnostic Aphasia Examination (BDAE [Goodglass and Kaplan, 1983]) spontaneous speech samples participated in the treatment study. Both patients produced primarily nouns and verbs in the absence of the copula, auxiliary verbs, and verb inflections. Therefore, subjects were taught to produce the third-person singular auxiliary *is* in sentence contexts, as in, for example, *boy is drinking*, using action pictures and verbal modeling of target sentences. Throughout treatment, generalized production of the auxiliary *is* and the copula *is* in untrained sentence contexts was tested. Results indicated improved production of the trained auxiliary in both trained and untrained sentence contexts. As well, concomitant improvement was noted in some, but not all, copula *is* sentence contexts. That is, strong generalization was noted to copula *is* + predicate adjective (e.g., *man is tall*) contexts, but not to copula *is* + predicate nominative (e.g., *man is a sailor*) or predicative locative (e.g., *ball is on table*) contexts.

The generalization contexts set up by Kearns and Salmon (1984) are perhaps the most important for clinicians to consider in developing their treatment protocols for patients presenting with difficulty with verb morphology. That is, despite the unexpected relation between auxiliary *is* forms and copula *is* (i.e., the copula *is* functions as a main verb, whereas *is. . .ing* serves to refine another required main verb), this generalization did occur. It would have been more likely for generalization to occur from auxiliary *is* to auxiliary *are* because both forms require identical sentence frames for production, and according to some theories of inflectional morphology, the *aux . . . ing* operate as a unit and are thus inserted into sentence-planning frames together (Garrett, 1980, 1982; Lapointe, 1983, 1985). On the other hand, the lack of generalization to copula + predicate locative contexts could have been predicted because locatives are unrelated to the copula *is* by most theoretical accounts of language. The spread of effect resulting from treatment, however, is sometimes unpredictable; therefore, both plausible and implausible contexts for measuring generalization should be undertaken as part of treatment.

Strategies for Improving Production of Specific Sentence Types

Several researchers have undertaken studies concerned with treatment of sentence production deficits in agrammatic patients. The majority of this work has approached treatment along traditional lines, focusing intervention on aberrant sentence structures by means of presenting repeated opportunities for production of grammatically correct sentences. Until recently, treatment studies concerned with improving sentence production have not considered underlying representational or processing deficits that might have resulted in the abnormal structural forms noted. The following discussion focuses first on the more traditional approaches to treating sentence production deficits. Namely, the syntax stimulation approach developed by Helm-Estabrooks and colleagues (Helm-Estabrooks et al., 1981; Helm-Estabrooks and Ramsberger, 1986) and a direct production training approach studied by Thompson and colleagues (Thompson and McReynolds, 1986; Wambaugh and Thompson, 1989) will be addressed. Following presentation of these training approaches, neurolinguistic treatment paradigms will be discussed together with other recently reported theoretically based treatment strategies.

Syntax Stimulation.   Based on the early work of Goodglass and colleagues (Gleason et al., 1975; Goodglass et al., 1972), in which a hierarchy of syntactic difficulty for agram-

matic aphasic patients was described, Helm-Estabrooks et al. (1981) developed an approach to sentence production training. The Helm Elicited Language Program for Syntax Stimulation (HELPSS [Helm-Estabrooks, 1981]) uses the story completion format by Goodglass et al. (1972) to train production of the sentence types shown in Table 22.3. Multiple exemplars of each of the sentence types are trained at two levels of difficulty using published picture stimuli. At the first level, the clinician provides a story completion stimulus together with the target sentence response, and the patient is required to produce the target response after a delay. At the second level, the target sentence is not modeled by the clinician. Instead, the patient is required to produce the target response immediately after the story completion stimulus.

Mixed findings have been reported by researchers attempting to establish the effects of this training procedure on sentence production in agrammatic aphasic patients. Helm-Estabrooks et al. (1981) and Helm-Estabrooks and Ramsberger (1986) reported positive effects for seven chronic agrammatic aphasic patients. That is, improved performance on the expressive portion of the Northwestern Syntax Screening Test (NSST [Lee, 1969]) and on the BDAE (Goodglass and Kaplan, 1983) Cookie Theft Picture description task was noted for all subjects. Conversely, Doyle et al. (1987) found this treatment approach to be less successful with their four Broca's aphasic patients. Using a well controlled single-subject experimental research paradigm, Doyle et al. (1987) trained patients to produce 5 of the 11 HELPSS sentence types, one sentence type at a time, using the HELPSS training procedure. Results indicated that, although all subjects learned to produce each sentence type as it was trained, little generalization to untrained sentence types was noted, and no change in spontaneous speech scores derived from administration of the Western Aphasia Battery (WAB [Kertesz, 1982]) was seen. Further, only one of the subjects showed any change in performance on the NSST. Improvement in production of some sentence types was noted, however, for all subjects using a stimulus generalization probe procedure designed to elicit each sentence type in a nontraining language context. For example, to elicit imperative intransitives, the clinician instructed the patient to "Tell me to do something." Then the clinician banged a pen on the table, stood on a chair, and so on in order to elicit sentences such as *Stop it*, and *Get down*.

Direct-Production Training.   A training approach similar to the HELPSS is a direct-training approach used by Thompson and colleagues for training *wh*-interrogative productions (Thompson and McReynolds, 1986; Wambaugh and Thompson, 1989). For example, Wambaugh and Thompson (1989) used a story completion format (see Table 22.4) paired with a modeling and forward-chaining treatment paradigm for training *what* and *where* questions in *wh* + copula (is) + NP sentence contexts (e.g., *What is the price? Where is the pen?*) in agrammatic aphasic adults. To train these sentences, the examiner verbally presented a story completion stimulus. If the story was not successful in eliciting production of the desired sentences, the correct response was modeled using a forward-chaining procedure. The examiner modeled the first two words of the target response and then the remaining two, instructing the subject to repeat each portion as it was modeled.

Table 22.3.
Sentence Types Utilized in the *Helm Elicited Language Program for Syntax Stimulation* **(Helm-Estabrooks, 1981 [HELPSS])**

Sentence	Sentence Type	Example
1.	Imperative Intransitive	Wake up.
2.	Imperative Transitive	Lock the door.
3.	Wh-Interrogative	What are you eating?
4.	Declarative Transitive	He paints houses.
5.	Declarative Intransitive	He sings.
6.	Comparative	He is taller.
7.	Passive	The car was towed.
8.	Yes-No Questions	Did you buy the paper?
9.	Direct-Indirect Object	He gives his son a toy.
10.	Embedded Sentences	He wanted him to be rich.
11.	Future	He will travel.

Table 22.4.
Example Story Completion Probe Items Used by Wambaugh and Thompson (1989) for Elicitation of Wh-Interrogative Sentence Productions

Where + V copula (is) + NP

1. Mary is going to a party. She wants to know where her dress is. So, Mary asks Mother . . . (Where is my dress?).
2. Jim wants to feed the dog. He wants to know where the dog is. So Jim asks Dad . . . (Where is the dog?).
3. Mary wants to go bike riding. She wants to know where her bike is. So, Mary asks Jim . . . (Where is my bike?).
4. Dad wants to wear Jim's coat. He wants to know where the coat is. So, Dad asks Jim . . . (Where is the/your coat?).
5. Mom wants to butter her toast. She wants to know where the butter is. So, she asks Dad . . . (Where is the butter?).

What + V copula (is) + NP

1. The children are having math class. The teacher wants to know what the answer is. So, she asks Jim . . . (What is the answer?).
2. There is a new girl at school. Jim wants to know what the new girl's name is. So, he asks Mary . . . (What is her name?).
3. Dad sees something strange. He wants to know what it is. So he asks Mom . . . (What is that?).
4. Jim is going to visit John. He wants to know what John's address is. So, he asks Mary . . . (What is John's/his/the address?).
5. Jim has a problem. Mom wants to know what the problem is. So, she asks Jim . . . (What is the/your problem?).

Where + VP (present progressive)

1. Jim went fishing. Dad wants to know where Jim is fishing. Dad asks Mary . . . (Where is Jim fishing?).
2. Mom went shopping somewhere. Mary wants to know where Mom is shopping. So, Mary asks Dad . . . (Where is Mom shopping?).
3. Dad is hunting somewhere. Jim wants to know where Dad is hunting. so she asks Mom . . . (Where is Dad hunting?).
4. Mary is hiding. Jim wants to know where Mary is hiding. So, Jim asks Mom . . . (Where is Mary hiding?)
5. Mom and Dad see Mary going somewhere. Dad wants to know where Mary is going. So, Dad asks Mom . . . (Where is she going?).

What + VP (present progressive)

1. Mom and Dad are watching Jim eat something. Dad wants to know what Jim is eating. So, he asks Mom . . . (What is he/Jim eating?).
2. Jim and Mary smell Mom cooking something. Mary wonders what Mom is cooking. So, she asks Jim . . . (What is she/Mom cooking?).
3. Mom and Mary see Dad building something. Mary wants to know what Dad is building. So, she asks Mom . . . (What is he/Dad building?).
4. Mom and Dad see Mary drinking something. Mom wants to know what Mary is drinking. So she asks Dad . . .(What is she/Mary drinking?).
5. Dad and Jim see Mom sewing. Jim wants to know what Mom is sewing. So, he asks Dad . . . (What is she/Mom sewing?).

Throughout training, generalization was tested from *what* sentences to *where* sentences and from *where* sentences to *what* sentences in untrained sentence contexts—in both *wh* + copula (is) + NP sentence contexts and in sentences using present progressive verbs (e.g., *What is he eating? Where is he sleeping?*). Results were similar to those obtained by Doyle et al.

(1987) using the HELPSS program. All subjects (a total of eight agrammatic patients across two separate treatment studies received direct-production treatment) acquired the ability to produce the trained *wh*-question forms on training probes. However, no generalization to untrained question forms—even those in which the same *wh*-interrogative was required—was noted.

That is, no generalization was seen from sentences such as *What is the price?* to sentences such as *What is he eating?* or to sentences such as *Where is the money?*

Neurolinguistic Approaches. In search for an understanding of the limited generalization that has resulted from traditional sentence production treatment, researchers recently have begun to consider formal linguistic theory. It has been reasoned, for example, that generalization has not occurred across sentence types because linguistic processes have not been considered either in selecting sentences for training or for analysis of generalization. That is, targeted sentences are most often selected based on patients' presenting sentence production deficits. Practice in producing surface structural forms then ensues without regard to the linguistic rules and principles underlying production of these sentence forms.

Treatments in which linguistic theory has been considered have recently been developed. Specifically, two treatment approaches—one that considers Chomsky's Government Binding (GB) (Chomsky, 1981, 1982, 1986; Lasnik, 1988) theory and one that considers Case grammar (Fillmore, 1968)—have been developed and studied.

Linguistic-Specific Treatment. To develop their linguistic-specific approach to sentence production treatment, Thompson and colleagues examined the findings derived by Wambaugh and Thompson (1989) in their *wh*-interrogative training (see Thompson, 1992, for a complete discussion). Aspects of GB theory, which is concerned with the underlying psychological competences of grammar, were considered. Additionally, findings from the neuropsychological and neurolinguistic literature concerned with sentence processing were considered (Clifton et al., 1991; Friederici and Frazier, 1992; Shapiro and Levine, 1989; Shapiro et al., 1992; Zurif et al., in press).

The lexical properties of verbs are at the heart of linguistic-specific treatment. There is considerable evidence that some aphasic patients demonstrate a strong dissociation between the relative accessibility of nouns versus verbs (Kohn et al., 1989; Zingeser and Berndt, 1988). That is, agrammatic patients appear to have more difficulty retrieving verbs than they do nouns. Therefore, it is possible that the sentence production problems seen in agrammatism are related to this difficulty with verbs. Verbs are represented in the mental lexicon, or dictionary, with set phrases and thematic roles that each verb idiosyncratically selects. For example, the verb *hit* requires a direct object NP, as in *Zack hit the ball*; the verb *put*, if followed by a direct object NP, also requires a PP, as in *Zack put the book on the table*; and the verb *sleep* does not require a direct object NP, as in the sentence *Zack sleeps*. This phrasal (and clausal) information, known formally as **strict subcategorization**, also carries **semantic/thematic** information that is determined by the verb (e.g., agent, theme, goal). This thematic information when considered in syntax is termed *argument structure* (Jackendoff, 1990). For example, the two NPs required by the verb *hit* take the thematic roles of Agent and Theme, each occupying an **argument position** in the sentence:

1. [Zack_Agent] hit [the ball _Theme];

The verb *put* requires three arguments, with the final argument having the role of Goal:

2. [Zack _Agent] put [the ball _Theme] on [the table _Goal]

and the verb *sleep* requires only one argument, the subject:

3. [Zack _Experiencer] sleeps.

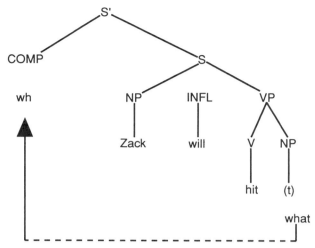

Figure 22.3. Diagram illustrating the movement rule "Move-alpha" for formation of a *wh*-interrogative sentence from the d-structure representation to s-structure.

Another important aspect of verbs is the manner in which the lexical properties of verbs interact with the syntax. According to the **projection principle**, lexical properties are observed at all levels of syntax. That is, the argument positions of a particular verb must be represented in a sentence using that verb or the sentence will be ungrammatical. For example, the verb *put* requires Agent-Theme-Goal as shown in (2); therefore sentences such as those in (4) and (5) are ungrammatical.

4. Zack put.
5. Zack put the ball.

Wh-interrogatives also must consider the lexical properties of verbs in their formation. According to GB theory, the s-structure representation (referred to as surface structure in Chomsky's early work) of *wh*-interrogatives are derived from d-structures (formerly referred to as deep structure) by application of a general movement rule—"move-alpha." The *wh*-word originates in d-structure where thematic role assignment occurs, and it is moved to sentence-initial position by a **transformation**. An example of this transformation is shown in Figure 22.3, which illustrates formation of a *wh*-interrogative sentence from d- to s-structure. Note that the underlying structure allows for representation of all of the arguments required by the verb used: *hit*. The role of Agent is assigned to the subject NP, and Theme is assigned to the direct object NP position. To form a *wh*-interrogative, the object NP is replaced by a *wh*-morpheme and moved to the sentence-initial position—COMP (for **complementizer**), the "landing site" for *wh*-morphemes. When the direct object NP is moved it leaves behind a trace (t) of its movement, which is coindexed with its antecedent—the *wh*-word.

When the underlying representations of the *wh*-interrogative sentences trained by Wambaugh and Thompson (1989) were considered, we discovered that indeed *what* and *where* are different. That is, while the surface realizations of sentences used in treatment such as *What is he cooking?* and *Where is he hunting?* are identical, their d-structure representations are not. *Cook* and *hunt* have different lexical properties (*cook* is a **transitive** verb taking a direct object NP, and *hunt* is an **intran-**

sitive verb that does not allow a direct object NP), as is shown in (6) and (7) below:

6. [$_{NP}$ He] [$_{VP}$ [$_V$ is cooking] [$_{NP}$ a steak]]

7. [$_{NP}$ He] [$_{VP}$ [$_V$ is hunting]] [$_{PP}$ in the woods]

In verbs like *cook*, then, the object NP is within the domain of the verb phrase—*cooking a steak*; whereas in verbs like *hunt*, the locative falls outside the domain of the verb phrase—*in the woods*. Indeed, the focus of the *wh*-question with verbs such as *hunt* is a locative **adjunct** specifying where the action is taking place.

When deriving *wh*-interrogatives from (6) and (7), *a steak* is replaced by *what*, and *in the woods* is replaced by *where*, as shown in (8) and (9).

8. [$_{S'}$ [COMP] [$_S$ [$_{NP}$ He] [$_{VP}$ is cooking [$_{THEME}$ what]]]]

9. [$_S$ [COMP] [$_S$ [$_{NP}$ He] [$_{VP}$ is hunting] [$_{LOC}$ where]]]

The thematic role of Theme is assigned to the direct object position occupied by *what*, but a Location role is assigned by the preposition to the position occupied by *where*. Such is the underlying distinction between verbs that subcategorize for a direct object NP, like *cook*, and intransitive verbs, like *hunt*, that do not.

Recent psycholinguistic and neurolinguistic work has shown that virtually all of these theoretical constructs have processing implications. For example, it has been shown that a verb's lexical properties directly affect sentence processing (Shapiro et al., 1987). That is, as the verb becomes more complex in terms of the number of different argument structure arrangements that are possible for a given verb, processing load increases in the immediate temporal vicinity of the verb. Additionally, it appears that adjuncts may be computationally more expensive than arguments of the verb (Shapiro et al., 1993); that is, processing load increases in the temporal vicinity of a preposition heading an adjunct PP (as in, for example, "The old man sent the toy *in the box*") relative to a preposition heading a PP that contains an argument (as in "The old man sent the toy *to the girl*"). Because an adjunct is not coded by the verb, adjuncts are always optional. Therefore, in processing sentences no information concerning the adjunct can be derived when the verb is processed—thus adjuncts are processed more slowly than arguments.

Agrammatic Broca's aphasic patients also normally activate a verb's multiple argument structure possibilities (Shapiro and Levine, 1989), suggesting that verb properties need to be controlled in treatment research. However, such patients appear to have difficulty with "complex" sentences—those in which arguments have been moved out of their canonical (S-V-O) positions such as *wh*-interrogatives, passive sentences, and relative clause constructions (Grodzinsky, 1990; Schwartz et al., 1987).

The sentence production treatment developed by Thompson et al., is based on these facts (Shapiro and Thompson, in press; Thompson, 1992; Thompson and Shapiro, in press; Thompson et al., 1993). For example, fully specified lexical entries seem to be available at d-structure for some, if not all, Broca's aphasic patients. The problem for some of these patients lies either in the derivation of the s-structure representations (e.g., traces, see Grodzinsky, 1990) or in the sentence-processing routines computing these representations (see, for example, Prather et al., 1991; Schwartz et al., 1987; Zurif et al., in press). Inasmuch as surface realizations of sentences result from their underlying linguistic representation, this treatment approach focuses on the underlying form with the idea being that generalization across sentence structures sharing similar linguistic properties may result. That is, this treatment addresses linguistic or grammatical rules, processes, and representations that are used for more than single-sentence types.

Treatment strategies have been developed for training *wh*-interrogative and object cleft sentences (e.g., *It was the girl that the boy hit*). Wh-interrogative treatment focuses on *what* and *who* questions—both of which take transitive verbs requiring a direct object NP to which the role of Theme can be assigned in the d-structure. When *wh*-movement is applied to the sentences, *wh*-interrogatives with similar s-structure also result, as in, for example, "She is fixing *the car*" yields "What is she fixing?" and "She is hitting *the boy*" yields "Who is she hitting?"

This treatment uses a set of sentences made up of the underlying linguistic representation of target *wh*-interrogatives with the word/phrase constituents of sentences depicted on individual 3 x 5 cards. Subjects are trained to recognize the verb, its argument structures, and their thematic role assignments. Then instructions concerned with replacement of the direct object NP with a *wh*-morpheme are given, and movement of the d-structure sentence constituents to derive target surface forms is demonstrated. Steps for *wh*-interrogative training are depicted in Table 22.5. Thompson et al. have shown positive effects of this treatment in their preliminary work. That is, for some subjects, generalization across *wh*-sentence types was noted (i.e., from *who* to *what* sentences)—generalization that has not been forthcoming in other syntax-training work.

Object cleft sentence training also has been developed and studied with regard to its effect on *wh*-interrogative sentence production and vice versa. Leaving important details aside, these two sentence types rely on the same "move alpha" rule for their derivation (*wh*-movement), even though the surface realizations of these sentences are very different. In this training, again the d-structure representations of the desired surface forms are used and sentence constituents are printed on cards. For example, sentences such as *The boy hit the girl* are used. Treatment is again focused on the verb, its argument structures, and their thematic role assignments. Instructions are given concerned with movement of d-structure sentence constituents to surface form position (e.g., *It was the girl who the boy hit*). The treatment protocol for object cleft training is shown in Table 22.6. Using this treatment, generalization as predicted from object cleft sentences to *wh*-questions, and from *wh*-questions to object cleft sentences, has been noted in some agrammatic aphasic patients (Thompson and Shapiro, in press).

Cuing Verb Treatment. Another neurolinguistic approach to treatment of sentence production deficits for aphasic individuals was developed by Loverso et al. (1986, 1992). This treatment approach uses Case grammar (Fillmore, 1986)—which considers the verb as the "motor" of the sentence's propositional structure—as a basis for training production of **simple** sentences. The treatment begins with verb training and then, in a series of graduated steps, expands the verb to include its subject and, depending on the type of verb, either its object or a location, adverbial of time, and so on. The sentence expansion is produced by using *wh*-words. For example, after the verb *run* has been trained, an index card with *who run*? written

Table 22.5.
Protocol for Training Wh-Interrogative Sentences: Thompson and Shapiro's Linguistic Approach

Step 1. E presents d-structure sentence constituents printed in upper and lower case letters on 3' x 5' cards. WHAT, WHO, and ? cards also are presented (e.g., *The man is sending flowers WHAT WHO?*). E says: "You want to know *the thing* the man is sending so you ask . . . " A 5-second response interval is provided.

Step 2. E identifies the verb, the subject NP, and the object NP of the sentence and (a) explains that the object NP is either "the thing" (for *what* questions) or "the person (for *who* questions) receiving the action of the verb, and (b) that it is re-placed by WHAT or by WHO, respectively. E replaces the object NP with the appropriate *wh*-morpheme, by selecting either the WHAT or WHO card, and places the ? card at the end, forming an echo question (e.g., *The man is sending WHAT?*). The echo question is read/repeated by S.

Step 3. E demonstrates subject/auxiliary verb inversion by physically moving the subject NP cards and the auxiliary verb card (e.g., *is the man sending WHAT?*).

Step 4. E demonstrates movement of the wh-morpheme to the sentence initial position. The correct question is read/repeated by S (e.g., *WHAT is the man sending?*).

Step 5. Sentence constituent cards are rearranged in their d-structure order. WHAT, WHO, and ? cards are presented. Steps 2, 3, and 4 are repeated with the S replacing/selecting/moving cards. E provides assistance at each step if needed. Once formed, the correct question is read/repeated by S.

Note. E = examiner; S = subject; NP = noun phrase.

Table 22.6.
Protocol for Training Object Cleft Sentences: Thompson and Shapiro's Linguistic Approach

Step 1. E presents d-structure sentence constituents printed in upper and lower case letters on 3' x 5' cards together with two pictures: one depicting the target sentence and one depicting the reversed action (e.g., *The girl hit the boy/The boy hit the girl*). IT, WAS, and WHO cards also are presented. E says, pointing the foil picture: "In this picture the boy hit the girl, but in this picture (pointing to the target picture) . . ." A 5-second response interval is provided.

Step 2. E identifies the verb, subject NP, and object NP in the sentence and (a) explains that the object NP is the object of the verb (e.g., "This is the person who the girl hit") and that (b) the WHO card is placed next to the person who was hit (e.g., *The girl hit the boy WHO*).

Step 3. E explains that "to make the new sentence, the object NP and WHO cards are moved to the beginning of the sentence" (e.g., *The boy WHO the girl hit*). E demonstrates movement and reads the newly formed utterance.

Step 4. E instructs that to make the sentence grammatically correct, the elements IT WAS are added to the sentence initial position. The correct sentence is read/repeated by S (e.g., *IT WAS the boy WHO the girl hit*).

Step 5. Sentence element cards are rearranged in their d-structure order. IT WAS WHO cards are presented. Steps 2, 3, and 4 are repeated with S replacing/selecting/moving cards. E provides assistance at each step if needed. Once formed, the correct question is read/repeated by S.

Note. E = examiner; S = subject; NP = noun phrase.

on it is presented, and the patient is expected to produce "I run." Then *who run when* is presented to yield "I run yesterday," and so on.

Increases in the Porch Index of Communicative Abilities (PICA) subtest scores have been noted in patients receiving this treatment; however, it is unknown whether generalization to untrained verb and verb-argument combinations resulted. Because the verbs used in treatment are not controlled for the number and types of arguments that they entail, generalization may be limited. For example, intransitive verbs that do not allow a direct object NP, like *run* and *look*, "psychological" verbs like *think*, *feel*, and *like* are used; and transitive verbs like *hit* and *read* are used in training. Because the lexical properties of verbs have direct consequences in sentence comprehension and production, it may be that using this approach with verbs of a particular type might result in maximal generalization.

Other Model-Based Approaches

Other current approaches to treatment of sentence production deficits in aphasia espouse the use of Garrett's (1980, 1982)

model of sentence production for guiding interventions (Mitchum, 1992; Mitchum and Berndt, 1988). The model, based on the relative frequency of speech errors made by normal speakers, has provided a useful—albeit nonspecific—framework for interpretation of sentence production impairments in aphasia (Garrett, 1982; Kohn et al., 1989; Pate et al., 1987; Schwartz, 1987).

Five levels of representation in the sentence production process are described by Garrett, as shown in Figure 22.4. The five levels of representation include the (*a*) message level, (*b*) functional level, (*c*) positional level, (*d*) phonetic level, and (*e*) articulatory level. The claims made by the model are simply that these levels of representation must be established at some point during construction of a sentence and that the levels of representation are roughly serial and unidirectional. A major distinction made in the model concerns differences between sentence-planning processes, involved in selection of content words, and processes involved in determining the choice and location of function words and inflectional morphemes in the sentence. The message level is a conceptual one where the speaker conceptualizes what he or she intends to say, presum-

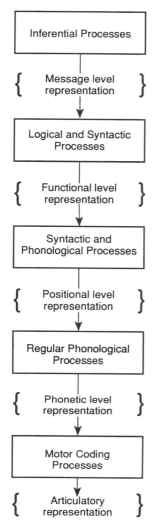

Figure 22.4. A model of sentence production formulated by Garrett (1975, 1980).

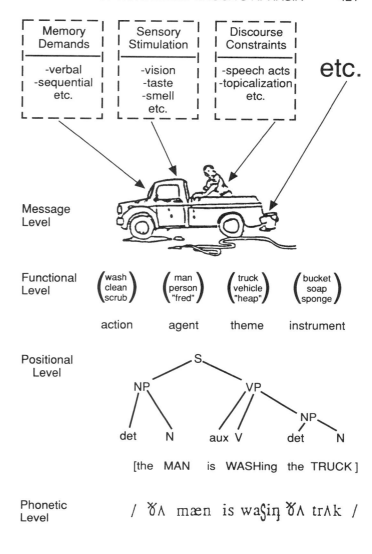

Figure 22.5. Schematic representation of sentence production training using Garrett's model of sentence production (Mitchum and Berndt, 1992).

ably stimulated by a variety of inferential processes or sensory experiences. At the functional level, the speaker accesses abstract lexical semantic representations for those concepts (i.e., people, places, things, actions, and attributes), and the logical relations among these lexical entities are established. That is, information about aspects of meaning that are related to the sentence such as thematic roles (i.e., argument structures of verbs) is specified. It is at the positional level that the phonological representation of words and the syntactic form of a sentence are designated. That is, the phonological forms of words from major lexical categories are inserted into their appropriate position in the syntactic structure of the sentence. At this level, grammatical elements, including function words and inflectional morphemes for both nouns and verbs, also are inserted into the sentence frame. Thus, at the positional level is a phonologically specified, syntactically ordered, and morphologically complete sentence that expresses the original message. Finally, the phonetic form of words and morphemes in the sentence frame is specified at the phonetic level, and at the articulatory level, motor aspects are performed for production of the sentence.

Mitchum and Berndt (1988) use this framework for treatment of aphasic individuals with sentence production deficits, arguing that reference to some model of normal processing is crucial in understanding the surface structure deficits that characterize aphasic sentence production. They suggest that linking observed production deficits, however loosely, to models of normal production is beneficial for treatment planning. For example, deficits appearing to arise from later levels of sentence production (e.g., phonetic/articulatory) may be treated best by focusing training here. Conversely, if disrupted sentence production appears to result from earlier levels in the case, for example, in which semantic paraphasias are produced for major lexical items, then treatment might focus on improving retrieval of appropriate lexical items (see Fig. 22.5).

This approach to intervention also has been studied primarily with respect to the observed verb retrieval deficits in agrammatic aphasic patients (Saffran et al., 1980). Mitchum and Berndt (1988) described a 54-year-old, right-handed patient (M.L.) presenting with sentence production deficits characterized by poor verb retrieval, impaired verb inflection, underuse of auxiliary verbs, and disrupted ordering of nouns around the verb. Although this patient was described as fluent, these sentence production deficits are consistent with some aspects of agrammatism. Treatment for this patient first began by focusing on verb retrieval using a small set of verbs—an exercise presumably tapping into several levels of the sentence production process. That is, naming of the verb engages message-level extraction, establishes some sort of functional representation of the action, and requires phonological specification at the positional level. Results of treatment indicated that the patient improved in verb retrieval; however, no change in his sentence production patterns was noted. Given this patient's poor use of grammatical elements that support the verb, this result was not surprising.

Subsequently, the patient was subjected to additional treatment, this time focusing on tasks that would presumably strengthen phonological and syntactic verb representation at the positional level (Mitchum, 1992). That is, treatment focused on constructing sentence elements contained in the grammatical frame. Specifically, using 14 sets of sequential action pictures representing the future, present, and past tenses, the patient was trained to produce sentences such as, *The man will wash the car*, *The man is washing the car*, and *The man has washed the car*. The patient was instructed to describe each ordered sequential frame using the auxiliary verb and the appropriate inflection of the main verb to denote if the action was "about to happen," "happening right now," or "already done." These cues were provided as needed during sentence production attempts by the patient. Results of treatment indicated improved sentence production on both trained and untrained sets of temporally sequenced pictures. Additionally, pre- to posttreatment changes were noted in sentence formulation both on sentence production probe tasks and in narrative conversation.

The results reported for this patient are encouraging; however, this approach to intervention requires caution. First, as is pointed out by Mitchum (1992), Garrett's model can only loosely be used to describe aphasic errors. Although it may be possible to infer that certain errors result from disruption of certain level(s) of the production process, it is not possible to make causal inferences. That is, the reasons for the noted disruptions cannot be known because the actual processes occurring at each level of production are unspecified by Garrett. For example, according to the model, verb specification and thematic role assignment occur at the functional level of representation; however, the processes required for accomplishing this are not delineated. In this regard, linguistic theory that more clearly describes rules and processes involved—for example, in verb-argument structure and the interrelation between lexical properties of verbs and syntax (as described above)—may also need to be considered. Further, there is nothing inherent in Garrett's model that explicitly addresses the treatment methods that might be used to improve certain levels of impairment. Therefore, if this approach is taken, the clinician will need to select his or her own treatment methods that will **intuitively** ameliorate a particular problem. Certainly, more work needs to be accomplished with a greater number of patients before clinicians may come to rely on this approach to treatment.

However, this theoretically informed approach holds promise for advancing our data base for treatment of sentence production deficits. As with other more recently developed treatments, the complete extent of its effectiveness awaits further research.

FUNCTIONAL APPROACHES TO TREATMENT

Functional approaches to treatment of nonfluent Broca's aphasia, defined here as those that address the patient's disrupted **use** of language for communication, have been advanced for several reasons. As pointed out earlier, some functional training approaches have arisen from the noted lack of success with other approaches to treatment. For example, early studies of syntax training indicated limited treatment effects. And even the more recently studied approaches to training sentence production have not completely addressed the extent to which improved sentence production results in improved ability to use language in functional contexts. Therefore, to advance the patient's ability to express his or her thoughts, wants, needs, and so on, in spite of his or her impaired language system, these important functionally based treatments have been developed.

Functional treatments need not replace, but instead may be viewed as an extension of, lexical and/or syntactic treatments. That is, patients may benefit most from a trial of treatment aimed toward maximal improvement of lexical and syntactic aspects of the language system. Concurrently, language **use** should be tested in various functional contexts. When generalized use of language is not evident in these extralinguistic contexts, treatment should be instituted to facilitate this carryover. Any of the following techniques for promoting functional language may prove beneficial in this regard.

To varying degrees, a number of functional or pragmatic approaches to treatment have been emphasized in this volume (see, for example, Chapter 12). Several of these treatments attempt to simulate naturalistic speaking contexts to some extent through the use of role play (Aten et al., 1982) or through turn-taking activities. Using a naturalistic intervention setting serves as the basis for the intervention protocol developed by Wilcox and Davis (1977)—Promoting Aphasics' Communicative Effectiveness (PACE). This method, discussed in more detail below, attempts to replicate the structure of natural conversation. In a similar vein, Kearns (1985, 1990) developed a treatment approach designed to expose the client to numerous and varied parameters that occur in naturalistic conversational settings. A discussion of this "loose training" approach, referred to as Response Elaboration Training (RET [Kearns, 1985, 1990]), also is presented below. Finally, in this section conversational training approaches will be discussed in which (*a*) the conversational behavior of the aphasic patient is directly altered during the course of conversation, and (*b*) the behavior of the conversational partner serves as a basis for intervention.

PACE

PACE was developed out of recognition that traditional intervention techniques do not replicate the structure of natural conversation. In this approach, the following four principles apply:

1. The clinician and client participate equally as senders and receivers of messages.
2. There is an exchange of new information between the clinician and the client.

3. The speaker has free choice as to which modality is used to convey a message.
4. Feedback to the listener focuses on the adequacy of the message.

Essentially, PACE intervention involves the clinician and the client taking turns describing pictures presumably unknown to each other. A stack of pictures is placed face down on a table, and the clinician and client alternate choosing a card and describing it. The primary goal of this treatment is for the speaker to adequately convey the intended message to the listener; when the clinician takes his or her turn, desired response styles are modeled for the client to later emulate. Task variety is possible by varying the type of pictures used. For example, action pictures depicting certain types of verbs, sets of locative prepositions, or noun sets arranged by category or by some other dimension could be used. Similarly, if a patient has difficulty providing information in a logically ordered sequence, a series of pictures representing an event or story also could be used. Pulvermuller and Roth (1991) have recently presented creative ideas for extending the PACE format to elicit a range of speech acts.

Barrier activities (Muma, 1978) are a variation of PACE, described by Newhoff and Apel (1990). As the name implies, this technique involves the use of an opaque barrier that is placed on the table between the client and the clinician. Also placed on each side of the barrier are duplicate "board" tasks that the client and the clinician must identically complete. For example, both participants may be given a set of objects and a 3 x 3 grid. Through conversational dialogue between the two participants, decisions as to where to place the items on the grid are made. The task requires each conversational partner to take a turn describing a potential "move" in the materials, requesting information about the move, and/or directing the other partner to move the materials. Wambaugh and Thompson (1989) used this technique with 10 Broca's aphasic individuals, transcribed the language samples obtained, and coded them for speech acts. Interestingly, this method resulted in the subjects producing many statements; however, they used few requests in completion of the task.

Response Elaboration Training (RET)

Response Elaboration Training (RET [Kearns, 1985, 1990]) was developed as a method for increasing the length and information content of verbal responses produced by nonfluent aphasic patients. RET is based on "loose training" procedures advanced by Stokes and Baer (1977). Loose training procedures operate on the premise that generalization may occur when the treatment environment approximates stimulus conditions and response variations found in the natural environment. Not to be confused with unstructured training, treatments of this nature are designed to avoid restricted stimulus control by introducing a rich and varied set of stimuli and conditions that sample relevant dimensions of the subject's natural environment and by allowing for variation in response topography.

To this end, RET loosens the response parameters. Rather than restricting responding to a narrow range of clinician-selected responses, as is the case in many production training paradigms, client-initiated responses are used as the primary content of treatment. Picture stimuli depicting actions using transitive and intransitive verbs are used, and the client is encouraged to elaborate on "whatever he or she is reminded of."

The simplicity of the picture stimuli is an important aspect of this treatment. That is, patients are discouraged from simply describing the action; instead, they are encouraged to talk about their personal history and world knowledge in response to the pictures. Specifically, Kearns (1990) delineates the following steps for elaborating client-initiated utterances:

1. An initial response is elicited to a picture stimulus.
2. This response is modeled and reinforced by the clinician.
3. "Wh" cues are provided to prompt clients to elaborate on their initial responses.
4. The subsequent client-attempted response is reinforced, and then sentences that combine the initial and all subsequent responses to a given stimulus picture are modeled.
5. A second model of sentences that combine previous responses are modeled, and then the client is instructed to repeat the sentence
6. Repetitions of combined sentences are reinforced, and a final model of the sentence is provided.

Kearns and colleagues have shown that this treatment results in an increase in the number of content units produced to trained and untrained picture stimuli. In addition, a moderate degree of generalization has been reported across stimuli, people, and settings following this treatment (Kearns, 1985; Kearns and Potechin, 1988). It is interesting to note that this treatment protocol also has been used to train nonverbal aphasic patients to elaborate on their drawing responses (Kearns, 1989).

Conversational Training

It is well known that aphasic patients evince difficulty in communicative situations requiring informational exchange between communicative partners and that they often rely heavily on the conversational partner for successful communication (Kagen and Gailey, in press; Linebaugh and Young-Charles, 1981; Lyon, in press). Clearly, conversation is a basic and unique form of communication that, as pointed out by Kagen and Gailey (in press), is essential for maintaining psychosocial well-being. From this perspective, the consequences of reduced ability and/or opportunity to engage in conversation are viewed as a distinct handicap for the aphasic individual. A few treatment approaches that directly focus on improving conversational skills have been advanced. Two of these will be discussed here. One approach focuses intervention on the aphasic patient, providing him or her with practice in production of appropriate, comprehensible, and meaningful utterances in conversational contexts. The other approach focuses on the conversational partner, providing him or her with appropriate strategies for improving the informational exchange in conversational dyads and in groups.

Conversational Skills Training (CST)

Doyle and colleagues developed a rather elaborate protocol for training aphasic patients to produce requests and statements in conversational contexts (Doyle et al., 1989; Doyle et al., 1991). Again using principles derived from loose training, this treatment loosens the stimuli used in treatment, the responses expected from the client, and the feedback provided. The stimuli are loosened by using several clinicians with the idea being that generalization across speaking partners will be enhanced if during treatment the client has practice in conversing with more than one person. The responses trained are loosened by

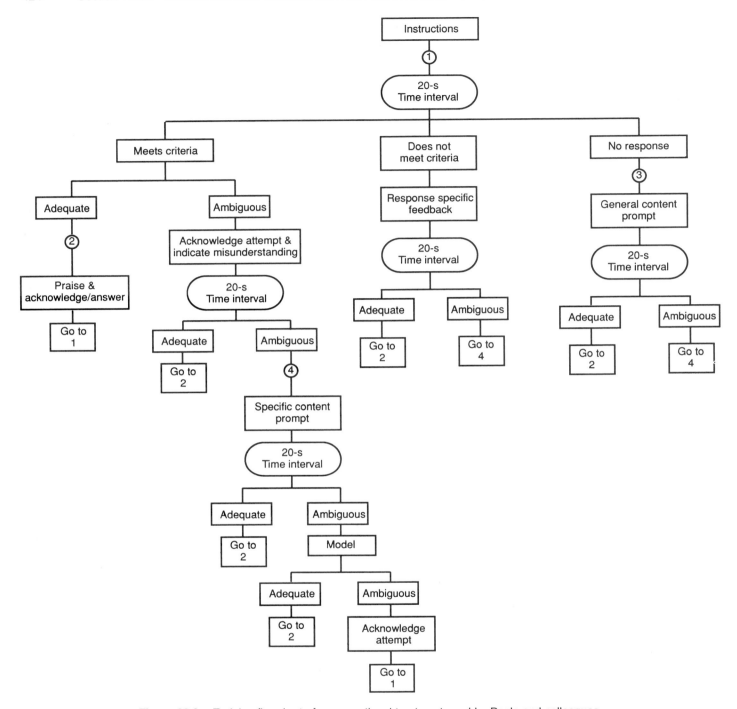

Figure 22.6.   Training flowchart of conversational treatment used by Doyle and colleagues.

allowing production of several types of questions and statements with response requirements being only that they are intelligible, that they contain at least one content word, and in the case of requests, that they either contain a question morpheme or are produced with rising inflection. Finally, to loosen the feedback dimension of treatment, naturalistic feedback is provided.

The treatment itself uses a flowchart as shown in Figure 22.6. The subject first is instructed to ask questions or to make

statements about a particular topic. Usually these topics are provided for the subject; for example, the client may be instructed to ask questions about personal information. In more recent uses of this treatment, the client and the clinician together view a short TV news segment, and afterward the clinician instructs the client to either ask questions or make statements about what was viewed (Doyle and Thompson, in progress). Adequate responses are reinforced either by the clinician answering the client-posed questions or by the clinician providing a follow-up, salient statement. When inadequate responses are produced, a modeling procedure is implemented whereby the client-initiated response is modeled either in question form or in statement form for the subject to repeat. In instances in which no response is produced even after additional instruction, a question or statement relevant to the topic under discussion is modeled for the subject to repeat. Each time an adequate response is produced by the client, the clinician responds in a conversational manner, again, by answering the client-posed question or by providing a follow-up statement. Periodically throughout this intervention, conversational probes are administered with the client conversing with either a familiar partner (e.g., family member or friend) or an unfamiliar partner. Results have shown increases in the use of both statements and requests in these conversational contexts following treatment.

Presently, work is underway to refine this conversational training approach as well as the methods for measuring its effectiveness. It has been noted, for example, that some conversational contexts are more conducive to asking questions than others. Doyle et al. (in press) found that open conversations as opposed to conversations about videotaped news segments resulted in aphasic subjects producing more questions. Conversely, a richer variety of statements were made by aphasic patients when conversing about videotaped news segments. Therefore, revisions are being made along these lines.

Conversational Partner Training

Simmons et al. (1987) presented an interesting and somewhat atypical approach to conversational treatment. During observations of a chronic, nonfluent Broca's aphasic patient conversing with his spouse, it was noted that the spouse frequently used conversational behaviors that were deemed to impede the aphasic patient's use of available language. For example, she frequently interrupted the patient's sentences before they were complete and asked direct questions that required only a yes or no response. Both of these spouse behaviors appeared to frustrate the aphasic patient even more than his struggle to express his thoughts. Therefore, Simmons et al. (1987) undertook a training program with the **spouse**. Using videotaped conversational samples between the spouse and the aphasic patient, the spouse was trained to recognize and then to modify her interruptive behavior. When this was accomplished, she was then trained to replace her closed-ended question-asking behavior with a convergent question-asking strategy.

Throughout training, videotaped conversations between the spouse and her aphasic partner were collected in open discussion, in conversation about TV sports shows, and in conversation about TV talk shows. Results showed a decrease in spouse interruptions and an increased use of convergent questions during these conversations. Unfortunately, the effect of this training on the aphasic patient's conversational speech was not directly measured, although it reportedly improved his language as well (Simmons, personal communication).

Another approach to treatment that has recently been described is a novel one that uses volunteers as conversational facilitators with groups of chronic aphasic individuals (Kagen and Gailey, in press). This conversational approach was developed by the spouse of an aphasic patient who became "desperate for posttherapy service" for her aphasic partner. With the assistance of other spouses of aphasic individuals as well as a group of dedicated volunteers, the Aphasia Center in North York, Ontario, Canada was developed. Small groups of aphasic individuals meet several times weekly together with a volunteer in discussion groups. Volunteers, ranging from university students to senior citizens, participate in organized volunteer training that emphasizes methods for facilitating natural and spontaneous conversational exchange.

Volunteers are provided with training for facilitating conversation using a simple framework that stresses:

1. That the message gets in (to the aphasic adult);
2. That the aphasic adult has a mechanism for getting the message out;
3. That the flow of conversation be maintained.

Specifically, volunteers are trained to use resource material (i.e., calendars, photographs, and personal information about the aphasic individuals, maps, newspapers, and so on) for facilitating both understanding and expression of ideas. Additionally, they receive instruction in the use of question-asking strategies (e.g., closed-ended versus open-ended); the use of nonverbal stimuli such as gesture and pantomime, writing, and drawing; and the use of topic-changing devices. Additionally, volunteers are given instruction as well as opportunity to practice methods for maximizing understanding (e.g., using of repetition, slowing down, providing adequate processing time) and for facilitating maximal output through the use of modeling and expansion techniques. To maintain the flow of conversation, volunteers are encouraged to use humor and verbal confirmation and to verbally link the ideas of the group members together. In the groups, discussions are centered on broad and sometimes complex topics including, for example, discussions on aphasia, current political crises or other events, or personal problems.

This approach to conversational training departs significantly from others that are typically described. First, as is apparent, trained volunteers instead of professional staff engage in the treatment. This aspect of the treatment is particularly compelling. By virtue of being volunteers, they may choose to discontinue participation at any time. Therefore, it is assumed that the volunteers *want to* communicate with these aphasic individuals. Second, all conversations are accomplished in groups to foster group membership and friendships; and third, the aphasic individuals are encouraged to *talk to* each other rather than direct their responding to a therapist.

Although this approach to treatment has not been scientifically tested, it represents a novel and important dimension to the treatment process. Indeed, over 100 chronic aphasic individuals are presently receiving treatment at the Aphasia Center, and some will remain "members" for the remainder of their lives. Aphasia is a lifelong communication deficit and, therefore, opportunities for improving communication should be provided for these individuals into the chronic phases of the disorder.

FUTURE TRENDS IN TREATMENT OF NONFLUENT, BROCA'S APHASIA

This chapter has highlighted current trends and practices for treatment of nonfluent Broca's aphasia. Emphasizing the heterogeneity of so-labeled aphasic individuals, methods for improving lexical processing, sentence production deficits, and functional communication have been discussed. In consideration of the information presented here, it should be apparent that we have yet to discover which of these treatments, if any, are the most beneficial. Clearly, continued research is needed in all areas of treatment addressed.

There presently is a move away from diagnostic classifications such as Broca's aphasia, Wernicke's aphasia and the like as researchers and clinicians have noted that these terms are not helpful either for treatment or for research. Instead, these labels are being replaced by terms that more explicitly delineate the language and communication deficits seen in aphasic individuals. This change, however, cannot be completely accomplished until such time as we obtain a better understanding of aphasic language deficits and develop methods for testing them. Once this is accomplished, treatments for these deficits also will become more precise.

Acknowledgment

The author wishes to acknowledge Sandra Schneider for her assistance with researching portions of this chapter.

References

Aten, J., Caliguri, M., and Holland, A. (1982). The efficacy of functional communication therapy for chronic aphasic patients. *Journal of Speech and Hearing Disorders, 47,* 93–96.

Baddeley, A. D. (1986). *Working memory.* Oxford: Oxford University Press.

Badecker, W., and Caramazza, A. (1985). On consideration of method and theory governing the use of clinical categories in neurolinguistics and cognitive neuropsychology: The case against agrammatism. *Cognition, 20,* 97–126.

Bates, E., Appelbaum, M., and Allard, L. (1991). Statistical contraints on the usage of single cases in neuropsychological research. *Brain and Language, 40,* 295–329.

Berndt, R. S. (1987). Symptom co–occurrence and dissociation in the interpretation of agrammatism. In M. Coltheart, G. Sartori, and R. Job (Eds.), *The cognitive neuropsychology of language.* Hillsdale, NJ: Lawrence Erlbaum.

Berndt, R. S. (1991). Sentence processing in aphasia. In M. T. Sarno (Ed.), *Acquired aphasia* (2nd ed.) pp. 223–270. New York: Academic Press.

Byng, S. (1988). Sentence processing deficits: Theory and therapy. *Cognitive Neuropsychology, 5,* 629–676.

Byng, S., Kay, J., Edmundson, A., and Scott, C. (1990). Aphasia tests reconsidered. *Aphasiology, 4,* 67–91.

Cannito, M. P., and Vogel, D. (1987). Treatment can facilitate reacquisition of a morphological rule. In R. H. Brookshire (Ed.). *Clinical aphasiology* (Vol. 17, pp. 23–28). Minneapolis, MN: BRK.

Caplan, D. (1990). *Psycholinguistic assessment of language disorders.* Paper presented at the American Speech–Language–Hearing Association Annual Convention.

Caramazza, A. (1986). On drawing inferences about the structure of normal cognitive systems from the analysis of patterns of impaired performance: The case for single patient studies. *Brain and Cognition, 5,* 41–66.

Caramazza, A., and Hillis, A. E. (1989). The disruption of sentence production: Some dissociations. *Brain and Language, 36,* 625–650.

Caramazza, A., and Zurif, E. (1976). Dissociation of algorithmic and heuristic processes in language comprehension: Evidence from aphasia. *Brain and Language, 3,* 572–582.

Chomsky, N. (1981). *Lectures on government and binding.* Dordrecht: Foris.

Chomsky, N. (1982). *Some concepts and consequences of government and binding.* Cambridge, MA: MIT Press.

Chomsky, N. (1986). *Knowledge of language: Its nature, origin, and use.* New York: Praeger.

Clifton, C., Speer, S., and Abney, S. (1991). Parsing arguments: Phrase structure and argument structure as determinants of initial parsing decisions. *Journal of Memory and Language, 30,* 251–271.

Damasio, H. (1991). Neuroanatomical correlates of the aphasias. In M. T. Sarno (Ed.), *Acquired aphasia* (2nd ed.). New York: Academic Press.

Damasio, H., and Damasio, A. R. (1989). *Lesion analysis in neuropsychology.* New York: Oxford University Press.

Doyle, P. J., Goldstein, H., and Bourgeois, M. (1987). Experimental analysis of syntax training in Broca's aphasia: A generalization and social validation study. *Journal of Speech and Hearing Disorders, 52,* 143–155.

Doyle, P. J., Goldstein, H., Bourgeois, M. S., and Nakles, K. O. (1989). Facilitating generalized requesting behavior in Broca's aphasia: An experimental analysis of a generalization training procedure. *Journal of Applied Behavior Analysis, 22,* 157–170.

Doyle, P. J., Oleyar, K. S., and Goldstein, H. (1991). Facilitating functional conversational skills in aphasia: An experimental analysis of a generalization training procedure. In T. Prescott (Ed.), *Clinical aphasiology* (Vol. 19, pp. 229–241). Austin, TX: Pro–Ed.

Doyle, P. J., Thompson, C. K., Oleyar, K., Wambaugh, J. L., and Jackson, A. (in press). The effects of setting variables on conversational discourse in normal and aphasic adults. *Clinical aphasiology* (Vol. 21).

Ellis, A. W., and Young, A. W. (1988). *Human cognitive neuropsychology.* Hillsdale, NJ: Lawrence Erlbaum.

Fillmore, C. J. (1986). The case for case. In E. Bach and T. Harms (Eds.), *Universals in linguistic theory.* New York: Holt, Rinehart, and Winston.

Foss, D. (1968). Learning and discovery in the acquisition of structured material: Effects of number of items and their sequence. *Journal of Experimental Psychology, 77,* 341–344.

Friederici, A., and Frazier, L. (1992). Thematic analysis in agrammatic comprehension: Syntactic structure and task demands. *Brain and Language, 42,* 1–29.

Garrett, M. F. (1980). Levels of processing in sentence production. In B. Butterworth (Ed.), *Language production* (Vol. 1). New York: Academic Press.

Garrett, M. F. (1982). The organization of processing structure for language production: Applications to aphasic speech. In D. Caplan, A. R. Lecours, and A. Smith (Eds.), *Biological perspectives on language.* Cambridge, MA: MIT Press.

Gleason, J. B., Goodglass, H., Green, E., Ackerman, N., and Hyde, M. K. (1975). The retrieval of syntax in Broca's aphasia. *Brain and Language, 24,* 451–471.

Goldstein, H. (1985). Matrix and stimulus equivalence training. In S. Warren and A. Rogers-Warren (Eds.), *Teaching functional language.* Baltimore, MD: University Park Press.

Goodglass, H., Gleason, J. B., Bernholtz, N. D., and Hyde, M. K. (1972). Some linguistic structures in the speech of a Broca's aphasic. *Cortex, 8,* 191–212.

Goodglass, H., and Kaplan, E. (1983). *The assessment of aphasia and related disorders* (2nd ed). Philadelphia, PA: Lea and Febiger.

Grodzinsky, Y. (1990). *Theoretical perspectives on language deficits.* Cambridge, MA: MIT Press.

Hart, J., Berndt, R., and Caramazza, A. (1985). Category-specific naming deficit following cerebral infarction. *Nature, 316,* 439–440.

Helm-Estabrooks, N. (1981). *Helm elicited language program for syntax stimulation.* Austin, TX: Exceptional Resources, Inc.

Helm-Estabrooks, N., Fitzpatrick, P., and Barresi, B. (1981). Response of an agrammatic patient to a syntax stimulation program for aphasia. *Journal of Speech and Hearing Disorders, 46,* 422–427.

Helm-Estabrooks, N., and Ramsberger, G. (1986). Treatment of agrammatism in long–term Broca's aphasia. *British Journal of Disorders of Communication, 21,* 39–45.

Hillis, A. E. (1989). Efficacy and generalization of treatment for aphasic naming errors. *Archives of Physical Medicine and Rehabilitation, 70,* 632–636.

Hillis, A. E. (1991). Effects of separate treatment for distinct impairments within the naming process. *Clinical Aphasiology, 19,* 255–265.

Hoodin, R., and Thompson, C. K. (1983). Facilitation of verbal labeling in adult aphasia by gestural, verbal or verbal plus gestural training. In R. H. Brookshire (Ed.), *Clinical Aphasiology Conference Proceedings* (pp. 62–64). Minneapolis, MN: BRK.

Howard, D., Patterson, K., Franklin, S., Orchard-Lisle, V., and Morton, J. (1985). Treatment of word retrieval deficits in aphasia. A comparison of two therapy methods. *Brain, 108,* 817–829.

Jackendoff, R. (1983). *Semantics and cognition.* Cambridge, MA: MIT Press.

Jackendoff, R. (1990). *Argument structure.* Cambridge, MA: MIT Press.

Jacobs, B., and Thompson, C. K. (1992). *Effects of semantically based training on lexical processing in severe aphasia.* Paper presented at the American Speech-Language-Hearing Association Annual Convention. San Antonio, TX.

Jones, E. V. (1984). Word order processing in aphasia: Effect of verb semantics. In F. C. Rose (Ed.), *Advances in neurology. Vol. 42. Progress in aphasiology.* New York: Raven.

Jones, E. V. (1986). Building the foundations for sentence production in a non-fluent aphasic. *British Journal of Disorders of Communication, 21,* 63–82.

Kagen, A., and Gailey, G. F. (in press). Functional is not enough: Training conversation partners for aphasic adults. In: A. Holland (ed.).

Kearns, K. P. (1985). Response elaboration training for patient initiated utterances. In R. H. Brookshire (Ed.), *Clinical Aphasiology Conference Proceedings* (pp. 196–204). Minneapolis, MN: BRK.

Kearns, K. P. (1986). Flexibility of single-subject experimental designs. Part II. Design selection and arrangement of experimental phases. *Journal of Speech and Hearing Disorders, 51,* 204–214.

Kearns, K. P. (1989). Methodologies for studying generalization. In L. McReynolds and J. Spradlin (Eds.). *Generalization strategies in the treatment of communication disorders* (pp. 13–30). Toronto: BC Decker.

Kearns, K. P. (1990). Broca's aphasia. In L. L. Lapointe (Ed.), *Aphasia and related neurogenic language disorders.* New York: Thieme Medical Publishers, Inc.

Kearns, K. P., and Potechin, G. (1988). The generalization of response elaboration training effects. In T. Prescott (Ed.), *Clinical aphasiology* (pp. 223–246). Boston, MA: College Hill Press.

Kearns, K. P., and Salmon, S. (1984). An experimental analysis of auxiliary and copula verb generalization in aphasia. *Journal of Speech and Hearing Disorders, 49,* 152–163.

Kearns, K. P., Simmons, N. N., and Sisterhen, C. (1982). Gestural sign (Amer-Ind) as a facilitator of verbalization in patients with aphasia. In R. H. Brookshire (Ed.), *Clinical Aphasiology Conference proceedings* (pp. 183–190). Minneapolis, MN: BRK.

Kearns, K. P., and Thompson, C. K. (1991). Technical drift and conceptual myopia: The Merlin Effect. In T.E. Prescott (Ed.), *Clinical aphasiology* (Vol. 19). Austin, TX: Pro-Ed.

Kertesz, A. (1982). *The Western Aphasia Battery.* New York: Grune and Stratton.

Kohn, S. E., Lorch, M. P., and Pearson, D. M. (1989). Verb finding in aphasia. *Cortex, 25,* 57–69.

Kolk, H. H., and Van Grunsven, M. (1985). Agrammatism as a variable phenomenon. *Cognitive Neuropsychology, 2,* 347–384.

Kolk, H. H., Van Grunsven, M., and Keyser, A. (1985). On parallelism between production and comprehension in agrammatism. In M. L. Kean (Ed.), *Agrammatism.* (pp. 165–206). Orlando, FL: Academic Press.

Lapointe, S. G. (1983). Some issues in the linguistic description of agrammatism. *Cognition, 14,* 1–39.

Lapointe, S. G. (1985). A theory of verb form use in the speech of agrammatic aphasics. *Brain and Language, 28,* 196–234.

Lasnik, H. (1988). *A course in BG syntax: Lectures on binding and empty categories.* Cambridge, MA: MIT Press.

LeDorze, G., Jacobs, A., and Corderre, C. (1991). Aphasia rehabilitation with a case of agrammatism: A partial replication. *Aphasiology, 5,* 63–85.

Lee, L. (1969). *Northwestern Syntax Screening Test.* Evanston, IL: Northwestern University Press.

Lineberger, M. C. (1990). Neuropsychology of sentence parsing. In A. Caramazza (Ed.), *Cognitive neuropsychology and neurolinguistics: Advances in models of cognitive function and impairment* (pp. 55–122). Hillsdale, NJ: Lawrence Erlbaum.

Linebarger, M. C., Schwartz, M. F., and Saffran, E. M. (1983). Sensitivity to grammatical structure in so–called agrammatic aphasics. *Cognition, 13,* 361–394.

Linebaugh, C. W., and Lehner, L. H. (1977). Cueing hierarchies and word retrieval: A therapy program. In R. H. Brookshire (Ed.), *Clinical Aphasiology Conference Proceedings.* Minneapolis, MN: BRK.

Linebaugh, C. W., and Young-Charles, H. Y. (1981). Confidence in ratings of aphasic patients' functional communication: Spouses and speech–language pathologists. In R. H. Brookshire (Ed.), *Clinical Aphasiology Conference proceedings* (pp. 226–233). Minneapolis, MN: BRK.

Loverso, F. L., Prescott, T. E., and Selinger, M. (1986). Cueing verbs: A treatment strategy for aphasic adults. *Journal of Rehabilitation Research, 25,* 47–60.

Loverso, F. L., Prescott, T. E., and Selinger, M. (1992). *Aphasiology, 6,* 155–163.

Lyon, J. G. (in press). Optimizing communication and participation in life for aphasic adults and their prime caregivers in natural settings: A use model for treatment. In G. Wallace (Ed.), *Adult aphasia: Clinical management for the practicing clinician.* Baltimore, MD: Andover Medical Publishing Co.

Lyon, J. G., and Helm-Estabrooks, N. (1987). Drawing: Its communicative significance for expressively restricted aphasic adults. *Topics in Language Disorders, 8,* 61–71.

Marshall, J., Pound, C., White-Thomson, M., and Pring, T. (1990). The use of a picture/word matching tasks to assist word retrieval in aphasic patients. *Aphasiology, 4,* 167–184.

McNeil, M. R., and Prescott, T. E. (1978). *Revised Token Test.* Baltimore, MD: University Park Press.

McReynolds, L. V., and Thompson, C. K. (1986). Flexibility of single-subject experimental designs. Part I. Review of the basics of single-subject design. *Journal of Speech and Hearing Disorders, 51,* 194–203.

Miceli, G., and Mazzucchi, A. (1990). The nature of speech production deficits in so-called agrammatic aphasia: Evidence from two Italian patients. In L. Menn and L. K. Obler (Eds.), *Agrammatic aphasia: Cross-language narrative source book.* Baltimore, MD: Johns Benjamina.

Miceli, G., Mazzucchi, A., Menn, L., and Goodglass, H. (1983). Contrasting cases of Italian agrammatic aphasia without comprehension disorder. *Brain and Language, 19,* 65–97.

Miceli, G., Silveri, M. C., Romani, C., and Caramazza, A. (1989). Variation in the pattern of omissions and substitutions of grammatical morphemes in the spontaneous speech of so-called agrammatic patients. *Brain and Language, 36,* 447–492.

Miller, G. A., and Johnson-Laird, P. N. (1976). *Language and perception.* Cambridge, MA: Harvard University Press.

Mitchum, C. C. (1992). Treatment generalization and the application of cognitive neuropsychological models in aphasia therapy. In *Aphasia treatment: Current approaches and research opportunities.* NIDCD Monograph (pp. 99–116). Bethesda, MD: The National Institute of Deafness and Other Communication Disorders.

Mitchum, C. C., and Berndt, R. S. (1988). Aphasia rehabilitation: An approach to diagnosis and treatment of disorders of language production. In M. G. Eisenberg (Ed.), *Advances in clinical rehabilitation. II.* New York: Springer.

Morton, J., and Patterson, K. (1980). A new attempt at an interpretation, or, an attempt at a new interpretation. In M. Coltheart, K. Patterson, and J. Marshall (Eds.), *Deep dyslexia.* London: Routledge and Kegan Paul.

Muma, J. R. (1978). *Language handbook: Concepts, assessment and intervention.* Englewood Cliffs, NJ: Prentice-Hall.

Nespoulous, J. L., Dordain, M., Perron, C., Ska, B., Bub, D., Caplan, D., Mehler, J., and Lecours, A. R. (1988). Agrammatism in sentence production without comprehension deficits: Reduced availability of syntactic structures and/or grammatical morphemes? A case study. *Brain and Language, 33,* 273–295.

Newhoff, M., and Apel, K. (1990). Impairments in pragmatics. In L. L. Lapointe (Ed.), *Aphasia and related neurogenic language disorders* (pp. 221–233) New York: Thieme Medical Publishers, Inc.

Pate, D. S., Saffran, E. M., and Martin, N. (1987). Specifying the nature of the production impairment in a conduction aphasic: A case study. *Language and Cognitive Processes, 2,* 43–84.

Patterson, K. E., Marshall, J. C., and Coltheart, M. (Eds.). (1985). *Surface dyslexia.* London: Lawrence Erlbaum.

Prather, P., Shapiro, L. P., Zurif, E. B., and Swinney, D. (1991). Real time examination of lexical processing in aphasia. *Journal of Psycholinguistic Research, 23,* 271–281.

Pring, T., White-Thomson, M., Pound, C., Marshall, J., and Davis, A. (1990). Picture/word matching tasks and word retrieval: Some follow–up data and second thoughts. *Aphasiology, 4,* 479–483.

Pulvermuller, F., and Roth, V. R. (1991). Communicative aphasia treatment as a further development of PACE therapy. *Aphasiology, 5,* 39–50.

Rapp, B., and Caramazza, A. (1991). Lexical deficits. In M. Sarno (Ed.), *Acquired aphasia.* New York: Academic Press.

Raymer, A. M., Thompson, C. K., Jacobs, B., and le Grand, H. (1993). Phonological treatment of naming deficits in aphasia: Model–based generalization analysis. *Aphasiology, 7,* 27–53

Rothi, L. G., Raymer, A. M., Maher, L., Greenwald, M., and Morris, M. (1991). Assessment of naming failures in neurological communication disorders. *Clinics in Communication Disorders, 1,* 7–20.

Saffran, E. M., Berndt, R. S., and Schwartz, M. F. (1989). The quantitative analysis of agrammatic production: Procedure and data. *Brain and Language, 37,* 440–479.

Saffran, E. M. and Schwartz, M. F. (1988). "Agrammatic" comprehension it's not: Alternatives and implications. *Aphasiology, 2,* 389–394.

Schwartz, M. F., Saffran, E. M., Fink, R. B., Myers, J. L., and Martin, N. (1992). Mapping therapy: An approach to remediating agrammatic sentence comprehension and production. In *Aphasia treatment: Current approaches and research opportunities.* NIDCD Monograph (pp. 77–90). Bethesda, MD: The National Institute of Deafness and Other Communication Disorders.

Saffran, E. M., Schwartz, M. F., and Marin, O. (1980). The word order problem in agrammatism: production. *Brain and Language, 10,* 263–280.

Saffran, E. M., Schwartz, M. F., Linebarger, M., Martin, N., and Bochetto, P. (1991). *The Philadelphia Comprehension Battery for Aphasia.* Unpublished test.

Schuell, H., Jenkins, J. J., and Jimenez-Pabon, E. (1964). *Aphasia in adults: Diagnosis, prognosis and treatment.* New York: Harper and Row.

Schwartz, M. F. (1987). Patterns of speech production deficit within and across aphasia syndromes: Application of a psycholinguistic mode. In M. Coltheart, G. Sartori, and R. Job (Eds.), *The cognitive neuropsychology of language.* Hillsdale, NJ: Lawrence Erlbaum.

Schwartz, M. F., Linebarger, M. C., and Saffran, E. M. (1985). The status of the syntactic deficit theory of agrammatism. In M. L. Kean (Ed.), *Agrammatism* (pp. 83–104). New York: Academic Press.

Schwartz, M. F., Linebarger, M. C., Saffran, E. M., and Pate, D. S. (1987). Syntactic transparency and sentence interpretation in aphasia. *Language and Cognitive Processes, 2,* 85–113.

Schwartz, M. F., Saffran, E. M., and Marin, O. (1980). The word order problem in agrammatism. 1. Comprehension. *Brain and Language, 10,* 249–262.

Seron, X., Deloche, G., Bastard, V., Chassen, G., and Hermand, N. (1979). Word finding difficulties and learning transfer in aphasic patients. *Cortex, 15,* 149–155.

Shapiro, L. P., and Levine, B. A. (1989). Verb processing during sentence comprehension in aphasia. *Brain and Language, 38,* 21–47.

Shapiro, L. P., McNamara, P., Zurif, E., Lanzoni, S., and Cermak, L. (1992). Processing complexity and sentence memory: Evidence from amnesia. *Brain and Language, 42,* 431–453.

Shapiro, L. P., Nagel, H. N., and Levine, B. A. (1993). Preferences for a verb's complements and their use in sentence processing. *Journal of Memory and Language, 32,* 96–114.

Shapiro, L. P., and Thompson, C. K. (In press). The use of linguistic theory as a framework for treatment studies in aphasia. In P. Lemme (Ed.), *Clinical aphasiology* (Vol. 21).

Shapiro, L. P., Zurif, E., and Grimshaw, J. (1987). Sentence processing and the mental representation of verbs. *Cognition, 27,* 219–246.

Shewan, C. M. (1981). *Auditory Comprehension Test for Sentences.* Chicago, IL: Biolinguistics Clinical Institutes.

Simmons, N. N., Kearns, K. P., and Potechin, G. (1987). Treatment of aphasia through family member training. In R. H. Brookshire (Ed.), *Clinical aphasiology* (Vol. 17, pp. 106–116). Minneapolis, MN: BRK.

Skelly, M., Schinsky, L., Smith, R. W., and Fust, R. S. (1974). American Indian sign (Amerind) as a facilitator of verbalization for the oral verbal apraxic. *Journal of Speech and Hearing Disorders, 39,* 445–456.

Stokes, T., and Baer, D. M. (1977). An implicit technology of generalization. *Journal of Applied Behavior Analysis, 10,* 349–367.

Thompson, C. K. (1989). Generalization in the treatment of aphasia. In L. V. McReynolds and J. E. Spradlin (Eds.), *Generalization strategies in the treatment of communication disorders.* Philadelphia, PA: B.C. Decker, Inc.

Thompson, C. K. (1992). A neurolinguistic approach to sentence production treatment and generalization research in aphasia. In *Aphasia treatment: Current approaches and research opportunities.* NIDCD Monograph. Bethesda, MD: The National Institute of Deafness and Other Communication Disorders.

Thompson, C. K., Doyle, P. J., and Jacobs, B. (1992). *Toward a technology of generalization assessment in aphasia: Effects of setting variables on sentence structure in conversational discourse.* Paper presented at the Clinical Aphasiology Conference.

Thompson, C. K., and Kearns, K. P. (1981). An experimental analysis of acquisition, generalization, and maintenance of naming behavior in a patient with anomia. In R. H. Brookshire (Ed.), *Clinical Aphasiology Conference proceedings* (pp. 35–45). Minneapolis, MN: BRK.

Thompson, C. K., and Kearns, K. P. (1989). Analytical and technical directions in applied aphasia analysis: The Midas touch. In T. Prescott (Ed.), *Clinical aphasiology* (Vol. 19, pp. 31–40). Austin, TX: Pro-Ed.

Thompson, C. K., Raymer, A. M., and Le Grand, H. (1991). Treatment of phonological naming deficits in aphasia: A model-based approach. In T. Prescott (Ed.), *Clinical aphasiology* (Vol. 20, pp 239–261).

Thompson, C. K., and McReynolds, L. V. (1986). *Wh*-interrogative production in agrammatic aphasia: An experimental analysis of auditory-visual stimulation and direct-production treatment. *Journal of Speech and Hearing Research, 29,* 193–206.

Thompson, C. K., McReynolds, L. V., and Vance, C. (1982). Generative use of locatives in multiword utterances in agrammatism: A matrix training approach. In R. H. Brookshire (Ed.), *Clinical Aphasiology Conference proceedings.* Minneapolis, MN: BRK.

Thompson, C. K., and Shapiro, L. P. (in press). A linguistic-specific approach to treatment of sentence production deficits in aphasia. In P. Lemme (Ed.), *Clinical Aphasiology* (Vol. 21).

Thompson, C. K., Shapiro, L. P., and Roberts, M. M. (1993). Treatment of sentence production deficits in aphasia: A linguistic-specific approach to wh-interrogative training and generalization. *Aphasiology, 7,* 111–133.

Thompson, C. K., Shapiro, L. P., Li, L., and Schendel, L. (in press). Analysis of verbs and verb argument structure: A method for quantification of aphasic language production. *Clinical Aphasiology* (Vol. 23).

Wambaugh, J. L., and Thompson, C. K. (1989). Training and generalization of agrammatic aphasic adults' wh-interrogative productions. *Journal of Speech and Hearing Disorders, 54,* 509–525.

Wambaugh, J. L., and Thompson, C. K. (1989). *Speech act analysis using conversational barriers.* Unpublished manuscript.

Warrington, E. (1981). Concrete word dyslexia. *British Journal of Psychology, 72,* 175–196.

Warrington, E., and Shallice, T. (1984). Category specific impairments. *Brain, 197,* 829–854.

Wertz, R. T., Collins, M. J., Weiss, D., Kurtzke, J. F., Friden, T., Brookshire, R. H., Pierce, J., Holtzapple, P., Hubbard, D. J., Porch, B. E., West, J. A., Davis, L., Matovitch, V., Morley, G. K., and Ressureccion, E. (1981). Veterans Administration cooperative study on aphasia: A comparison of individual and group treatment. *Journal of Speech and Hearing Research, 24,* 580–594.

Wiegel-Crump, C., and Koenigsknecht, R. A. (1973). Tapping the lexical store of the adult aphasic: Analysis of the improvement made in word retrieval skills. *Cortex, 9,* 411–418.

Wilcox, M. J., and Davis, G. A. (1977). Speech act analysis of aphasic communication in individual and group settings. In R. H. Brookshire (Ed.), *Clinical Aphasiology Conference proceedings.* Minneapolis, MN: BRK.

Zingeser, L., and Berndt, R. S. (1988). Grammatical class and context effects in a case of pure anomia: Implications for models of language production. *Cognitive Neuropsychology, 5,* 473–516.

Zurif, E., Swinney, D., Prather, P., Solomon, J., and Bushell, C. (in press). An on-line analysis of syntactic processing in Broca's and Wernicke's aphasia.

CHAPTER 23
Treatment of Global Aphasia

RICHARD K. PEACH AND SCOTT S. RUBIN

Global aphasic patients constitute a significant proportion of the acute stroke population (Brust et al., 1976). Though myths exist as to the reversibility of this syndrome (Schuell et al., 1964), the largest percentage of aphasic patients referred for speech-language pathology is composed, nonetheless, of those presenting with global aphasia (Sarno and Levita, 1981). This incongruous finding is likely due, at least in part, to the overwhelming devastation of global aphasia for patients, families, and friends relative to other types of aphasia.

Despite the limited success reported previously regarding language rehabilitation for these individuals, the clinical management of global aphasia has received renewed emphasis recently. The evidence to support this claim can be found in (a) the development of new assessment measures designed to be particularly sensitive to the preserved abilities of patients with global aphasia (e.g., The Boston Assessment of Severe Aphasia [BASA], Helm-Estabrooks et al., 1989b); (b) technological advances using computed tomography (CT) scans to assist in clinical decision making regarding verbal versus nonverbal treatment approaches for severe aphasia (e.g., see Naeser et al., 1989); (c) the development of computer-based programs for the treatment of global aphasia (e.g., Computer-aided Visual Communication [C-ViC], Steele et al., 1989); and (d) the redirection in the clinical management of these patients to methods that emphasize their functional communicative capabilities.

In this context, we provide an overview of the clinical management of global aphasia. We provide a philosophy for intervention and review current methods for rehabilitation with these patients. These topics are introduced by a discussion of the features of global aphasia, its etiology, the patterns of evolution and outcome in global aphasia, and some factors that are related to recovery from this syndrome.

FEATURES

Incidence

Global aphasia may be one of the most frequently occurring types of aphasia. Previously, incidence rates between 10% and 40.6% have been reported for global aphasia (Basso et al., 1987; Brust et al., 1976; Collins, 1986; De Renzi et al., 1980; Eslinger and Damasio, 1981; Kertesz, 1979; Kertesz and Sheppard, 1981). Some recent reports, however, suggest that the incidence rate during the acute stage may be even higher. Scarpa

et al. (1987) reported an incidence of 55.1% in an acute sample. All of the 108 aphasic patients included in the study by Scarpa et al. (1987) were assessed between 15 and 30 days postonset and were right-handed, with a single left-hemisphere lesion. When these data are combined, they provide evidence indicating that global aphasic patients are prominent among aphasic patients as a whole. As a result, they constitute a significant demand on the resources of clinical aphasiologists from the acute stages of illness through the time of maximal recovery.

Characteristics

Age and Sex

There appears to be no observable difference in the distribution of global aphasia when patients are compared by either age or sex (Habib et al., 1987; Scarpa et al., 1987; Sorgato et al., 1990). In relation to sex, Davis (1983) suggested that there is a general bias toward males in the data generated among Veterans Affairs Medical Centers because of the nature of the population seen at these hospitals. Further studies including more representative patient distributions may be necessary for reliable data regarding the influence of sex on global aphasia. Regarding age, Sorgato et al. (1990) reported no effect of age on aphasia types, including global aphasia. The older patients in their sample, however, did tend to show atypical aphasias including global aphasia from brain damage that was restricted to either anterior or posterior areas. Nonetheless, age and sex may not be considered to have a differential effect on the incidence of global aphasia.

Site of Lesion

Cerebrovascular lesions producing global aphasia have been described as involving Broca's (posterior frontal) and Wernicke's (superior temporal) areas (Kertesz, 1979) or, alternatively, both the prerolandic and postrolandic speech zones (Goodglass and Kaplan, 1983). The global aphasic subjects described by Murdoch et al. (1986) exhibited large lesions extending from the cortical surface inferiorly to subcortical areas including the basal ganglia, internal capsule, and thalamus. The previously described lesions producing a global aphasia were extensive, dominating the left hemisphere. However, numerous exceptions have been reported in the literature, suggesting that such an extensive lesion may not be necessary to produce a global aphasia.

Mazzocchi and Vignolo (1979) found global aphasia in 3 of 11 cases following lesions that were confined to anterior regions. In four additional cases, the lesions were deep and confined to the insula, the lenticular nucleus, and the internal capsule. Varying lesion effects were also described by Cappa and Vignolo (1983). Basso et al. (1985) observed global aphasia following discrete lesions confined to anterior (sparing of postrolandic centers) or posterior sites. Further, Basso et al. (1985) reported other forms of aphasia following lesions that would have been suggestive of global aphasia. Alexander et al. (1987) found global aphasia in association with one lesion or a series of primarily subcortical lesions that collectively damaged the striatum-anterior limb of the internal capsule; the anterior, superior, anterior-superior, and extraanterior periventricular white matter; and the temporal isthmus. Yang et al. (1989) also identified global aphasia in patients with lesions involving the internal capsule, basal ganglia, thalamus, and anterior-posterior paraventricular (sic) white matter. Lüders et al. (1991) produced global aphasia during electrical stimulation of the basal temporal region. This region has its white matter in contact with the white matter deep to Wernicke's area, thereby favoring close interaction between these two areas.

Ferro (1992) investigated the influence of lesion site on recovery from global aphasia. Fifty-four subjects were initially seen during either the first month (34 subjects), third month (7 subjects), or after 6 months postonset (13 subjects). They were followed at 3, 6, and 12 months and yearly thereafter when possible. The lesions in this group of global aphasic subjects were grouped into five types with differing outcomes. Type 1 included patients with large pre- and postrolandic middle cerebral artery infarcts. These patients had a very poor prognosis. The remaining four groups were classified as follows: type 2, prerolandic; type 3, subcortical; type 4, parietal; and type 5, double frontal and parietal lesion. Patients in these latter groups demonstrated variable outcomes, improving generally to Broca or transcortical aphasia. Complete recovery was observed in some cases with type 2 and type 3 infarcts.

Language

The hallmark of global aphasia is a loss of language comprehension with concomitant deficits in expressive abilities (Damasio, 1991; Davis, 1993; Kertesz, 1979). Wallace and Stapleton (1991) suggested that the linguistic deficit in global aphasia has been traditionally interpreted as a loss of language competency (i.e., the knowledge for linguistic rules and operations). According to these authors and others (Rosenbek et al., 1989), the recent clinical evidence demonstrating preserved areas of language functioning in global aphasia suggests that the loss for these patients may be viewed more appropriately as a variable mix of competence and performance deficits.

Comprehension. A number of isolated areas of comprehension following global aphasia have been identified in the literature. These include recognition of specific word categories (McKenna and Warrington, 1978; Wapner and Gardner, 1979), familiar environmental sounds (Spinnler and Vignolo, 1966), and famous names (Van Lancker and Klein, 1990) and rela-

tively better comprehension of personally relevant information (Van Lancker and Nicklay, 1992; Wallace and Canter, 1985).

Wallace and Stapleton (1991) analyzed the responses of global aphasic subjects on the auditory comprehension portion of the Boston Diagnostic Aphasia Examination (BDAE) (Goodglass and Kaplan, 1983) to identify patterns of preserved and impaired performance. Although their results generally supported previous claims that distinct patterns of preserved components are absent in global aphasia, two or three of their subjects did evidence differential performance within and across tasks. Interestingly, the scores for each of these subjects were collected during the acute stage of their recovery. The authors speculate that differential auditory comprehension performance during acute aphasia may be a useful prognostic indicator.

Expression. It has been suggested that globally aphasic patients may be most severely impaired in their expressive abilities. This may be due to the greater contributions of the right hemisphere for comprehension than for expressive behaviors (Collins, 1986). The verbal output of many global aphasic patients consists primarily of stereotypical recurring utterances or speech automatisms (Kertesz, 1979). Stereotypes have been described as being either nondictionary verbal forms (unrecognizable) or dictionary forms (word or sentence) (Alajouanine, 1956).

Blanken et al. (1990) examined 26 patients demonstrating the nondictionary forms of speech automatisms. Of these cases, 24 were classified as being globally aphasic. The other patients demonstrated signs more closely associated with Broca's and Wernicke's aphasia. Although speech automatisms were frequently associated with comprehension disturbances, the observed variability in language comprehension among these patients suggests that speech automatisms cannot be used to infer the presence of severe comprehension deficits. Blanken et al. (1990) proposed that speech automatisms relate only to speech output and do not necessarily indicate the presence of severe comprehension deficits.

Cognition

The cognitive abilities of brain-damaged patients are often assessed by administration of Raven's Coloured Progressive Matrices (RCPM) (Raven, 1965). Conflicting results have been reported regarding aphasic subjects' performances relative to performances of nonaphasic left brain-damaged patients. Some studies have found that aphasic subjects perform at lower levels (Basso et al., 1981; Basso et al., 1973; Colonna and Faglioni, 1966), while others have failed to show any significant difference between these two groups (Arrigoni and De Renzi, 1964; Piercy and Smith, 1962). Collins (1986) has reported significant positive correlations between the language ability of global aphasic subjects and their performance on the RCPM. The subjects in the Collins study were in the early stages of recovery, and eventually these subjects achieved RCPM scores similar to less severe aphasics.

Using a new version of the RCPM, modified to minimize the potential effect of unilateral spatial neglect, Gainotti et al. (1986) compared acute and chronic subjects with varying types of aphasia to normal controls, right-hemisphere damaged subjects, and nonaphasic left-hemisphere damaged subjects. In the study by Gainotti et al. (1986), the aphasic subjects performed worse than the other groups. Further, the global aphasic and Wernicke's aphasic patients scored the poorest in comparison to the other aphasic groups (anomic, Broca's, and conduction). These results were similar to those obtained by Kertesz and McCabe (1975). Gainotti et al. (1986) did not obtain differences relative to severity of aphasia but did link poor performance on the RCPM to the presence of receptive semantic-lexical disturbances. Gainotti et al. (1986) conclude that "a specific relationship exists in aphasia between cognitive nonverbal impairment and breakdown of the semantic-lexical level of integration of language" (p. 48).

Communication

The presence of recurring utterances among individuals with global aphasia was addressed previously. There are those who exhibit only recurring consonant-vowel (CV) syllables (for example, do-do-do or ma-ma-ma). As described by Collins (1986), these global aphasic patients often give the impression of somewhat preserved communicative abilities in that they may make use of the suprasegmental aspects of speech. The use of suprasegmentals, in a conversational turn-taking exchange, may appear to indicate that the aphasic patient is producing utterances with some communicative intent. deBlesser and Poeck (1984) studied a group of global aphasic patients and found that they did not exhibit prosodic variability to the extent necessary for conveying communicative intent. The utterances used for analysis, however, were limited to those elicited during formal testing and may not have reflected the spontaneous use of inflection to convey intent (Collins, 1986). deBlesser and Poeck (1985) subsequently analyzed the spontaneous utterances of a group of global aphasic subjects with output limited to CV recurrences. Utterances were sampled during interviews in which the examiner asked a series of open-ended questions. The length of the utterances and their pitch contours were analyzed for variability. The authors concluded that both length and pitch appeared to be stereotypical and that the prosody of these patients did not seem to reflect communicative intent. The appropriateness of these CV recurring utterances with regard to turn taking remains questionable. These findings highlight the marked discrepancy that exists between research outcomes and clinical reports. deBlesser and Poeck (1985) suggest that the contributions to conversation for which these patients are credited may be, in fact, the result of the communicative partner's need for informative communication rather than the patient's use of prosodic elements to convey intent.

In a study by Herrmann et al. (1989), a group of chronic and severe nonfluent aphasic subjects were described in terms of their communication strategies and communicative efficiency. The patients presented with either severe Broca's or global aphasia (50%). The results showed that the efficiency of the patients' communication was dependent on the type of question to which they were asked to respond. As might be expected, superior performance was observed for responses to yes/no questions ("Did your illness occur suddenly?") when compared to interrogative pronoun questions ("How long have you had language problems now?") and narrative requests ("Tell me what happened to you after you took ill"). Herrmann et al. (1989) reported that the patients used mostly gesture in their responses to the yes/no questions. The other types of ques-

tioning required increased verbal output and thus created the need for more complex communicative responses from the patients.

In examining the communication strategies used, Herrmann et al. (1989) found that patients rarely took initiative or expanded on topics. The most frequent strategies reported by these authors were those enabling the patients to secure comprehension (e.g., indicating comprehension problems, requesting support for establishing comprehension). Herrmann et al. (1989) concluded that this population relies most heavily on nonverbal communication.

Affect

Depression following cerebrovascular accidents and aphasia has been well established (Fromm et al., 1984; Robinson and Price, 1982; Robinson et al., 1984). It may be that the depression evident in some patients is the result of a grief reaction and is common to many catastrophic illnesses (Horenstein, 1970). Davis (1983) recommends that patients' depression be addressed early in treatment so that a chronic depressed state does not emerge.

Signer et al. (1989) reviewed and analyzed the charts of 61 aphasic patients who had been hospitalized because of behavioral disturbances. The subjects were divided into three groups: (a) anteriorly lesioned, (b) posteriorly lesioned, and (c) nonlocalizing syndrome. For the purposes of this study, the nonlocalizing syndrome group was composed of global, anomic, and mixed transcortical aphasic subjects. Of the 61 patients included in this study, 48% had been hospitalized for the presence of delusions (primarily persecutory). The largest number of delusional patients was found in the posterior lesion group (58% of this group exhibited delusions). Twenty-seven percent of the nonlocalizing syndrome group was delusional.

Depression was the most common mood disorder, occurring in 31% of the patients studied. The majority of the patients with depression were from the anteriorly lesioned group. Depression was present in 33% of the nonlocalizing group. Of the nonlocalizing patients with delusions, 75% also suffered from depression. Elation was present in 11 subjects in the posterior group. One of the patients in the nonlocalizing group and none in the anterior group exhibited elation.

Results of the study by Signer et al. (1989) are applicable to aphasic patients who require hospitalization for delusional or mood disorders. The findings refer to this population only and are not indicative of aphasic patients in general. The reported differences in affective states varying in relation to anterior or posterior lesions are consistent with previous findings (Robinson and Benson, 1981). Additional research specifically focusing on the global aphasic patient is needed to delineate the presence and nature of affective disorders in this population.

ETIOLOGY

As described, the majority of lesions producing global aphasia are extensive and involve both prerolandic and postrolandic areas. The blood supply for these areas is via the middle cerebral artery. The middle cerebral artery is the largest branch of the internal carotid artery, branching at the point of the Sylvian fissure. Because of the extent of the lesion, global aphasia most commonly results from a cerebrovascular event, the locus of which is in the middle cerebral artery at a level inferior to the point of branching. Further, the event causing global aphasia is more commonly thrombotic than embolic (Collins, 1986).

Not all occurrences of global aphasia are due to a cerebrovascular event in the middle cerebral artery. Interestingly, Wells et al. (1992) reported a temporary case of global aphasia due to simple partial status epilepticus. The aphasia lasted during a period in which there were periodic lateralized epileptiform discharges. Wells et al. (1992) reported that the patient's language returned to near normal during the 24 hours following the seizures.

RECOVERY

The recovery from the global aphasic symptoms seen in the patient of Wells et al. (1992) (i.e., language recovery over a 24-hour period) is not typical. The common course of recovery is bleaker for these patients. Kertesz and McCabe (1977) reported that the group of global aphasic subjects in their study generally demonstrated limited language recovery, a pattern similar to that reported by Wapner and Gardner (1979). When assessing the language recovery that does occur, better improvement is demonstrated in comprehension than in expression (Lomas and Kertesz, 1978; Prins et al., 1978). With regard to recovery of nonverbal cognitive abilities, Kertesz and McCabe (1975) found a precipitous and parallel rate of improvement for RCPM and language performance during the first 3 months postonset. During the next 3 months, RCPM performance continued to increase substantially, surpassing language performance that was only mildly improved from levels attained at the end of the first 3 months. Patients appeared to reach a plateau in both RCPM and language performance during the period between 6 and 12 months postonset. Overall, RCPM performance in the global aphasic patients did not exceed approximately 50% of the maximum attainable score.

In relation to the recovery observed in other aphasia types, Kertesz and McCabe (1977) described global aphasia as having the lowest recovery rate. With regard to the temporal aspects of recovery in global aphasia, differences have been reported depending on whether the subjects were receiving speech and language treatment. For global aphasic patients not receiving treatment, improvement appears to be greatest during the first months postonset (Kertesz and McCabe, 1977; Pashek and Holland, 1988). Siirtola and Siirtola (1984) observed the greatest improvement in their untreated subjects during the first 6 months postonset. Global aphasic patients receiving treatment, however, demonstrated substantial improvements during the first 3 months but also continued improvement during the period between 6 and 12 months or more postonset (Kertesz and McCabe, 1977; Sarno and Levita, 1979, 1981). In the study of Kertesz and McCabe (1977), significantly greater improvement was noted in treated versus untreated global aphasics during this period, although the authors attributed this gain at least partially to subject heterogeneity. In the studies of Sarno and Levita (1979, 1981), improvement was most accelerated between 6 and 12 months poststroke.

Evolution

During the recovery process, the symptoms of global aphasia may evolve to warrant reclassification to other aphasia syndromes. These changes have been documented in at least four reports, each of which used the Western Aphasia Battery

(WAB) (Kertesz, 1982) to assess language performance during the acute period of recovery and at regular intervals up to 1 year (or more) postonset. Kertesz and McCabe (1977) tested 93 aphasic subjects between 0 and 6 weeks postonset and found that 5 of their 22 global aphasic subjects progressed to other syndromes, including Broca's, transcortical motor, conduction, and anomic aphasia after 1 year or more. Siirtola and Siirtola (1984) classified aphasic subjects within the first 2 weeks after hospitalization. At 1 year postonset, 6 global aphasic subjects from among 14 had evolved to other syndromes including Broca's, conduction, anomic, and Wernicke's aphasia or, in the case of one subject, had recovered completely. Holland et al. (1985) followed 15 patients for 1 year who had been classified as globally aphasic immediately after stroke. In this study, classifications were based on results obtained from the WAB as well as from clinical impressions. A variety of patterns were observed at the end of the first year: two patients (in their 30s) returned to normal language functioning; two (in their 40s) evolved to Broca's aphasia; two (59 and 61 years of age) evolved to anomic aphasia; two (in their 70s) evolved to Wernicke's aphasia; and two (in their 80s) remained globally aphasic. The five remaining subjects died during the course of the study. Finally, Pashek and Holland (1988) described the evolution of 11 global aphasic subjects from among a larger group of 32 subjects who were followed for at least 6 months. While language performance was assessed by repeated administration of the WAB, these aphasic subjects were classified on the basis of descriptive criteria rather than WAB typology. All subjects were evaluated within the first 5 days after stroke. Four of these patients evolved to less severe syndromes including Broca's, Wernicke's, and anomic aphasia. Two patients evolved to a less severe but unclassifiable aphasic syndrome. One subject recovered normal language, and two subjects demonstrated symptoms of dementia.

Holland et al. (1985) and Pashek and Holland (1988) also found that patients who progressed to some other form of aphasia demonstrated change early in the sequence of recovery (i.e., within the first months postonset). In some cases, the global aphasia may not begin to evolve until after the first month has passed. Recovery from global aphasia was also investigated by Sarno and Levita (1979) using standard language measures including selected subtests of the Neurosensory Center Comprehensive Examination for Aphasia (NCCEA) (Spreen and Benton, 1977) and the Functional Communication Profile (Sarno, 1969). Classification of aphasia was based on clinical impressions as well as language test scores. In this study, however, the earliest language observations were collected at 4 weeks postonset with a variation of no greater than plus or minus 1 week. Repeated testing was continued until 1 year after the stroke. In contrast to the above studies, none of these 14 global aphasic subjects evolved to another type of aphasia by the end of the year. Similar results were observed in a follow-up study of seven global aphasic subjects (Sarno and Levita, 1981). One apparent explanation for these discrepancies might be a greater stability of language scores and, therefore, aphasia classifications obtained after the first month postonset versus those obtained during the first 4 weeks after stroke. However, Reinvang and Engvik (1980) assessed their aphasic subjects initially between 2 and 5 months after their injuries (mean = 3 months) and found that 4 of the 7 global aphasic subjects had evolved to a less severe Broca's, conduction, or unclassifiable syndrome at retesting. The retesting was completed no sooner than 1 month after initial testing, with a mean time of 7.5 months after injury and a range of 3 to 30 months. Based on these findings, the discrepancies in recovery from global aphasia reported in these studies do not appear to be simply the result of the time at which the initial language observations were recorded. Apparently, evolution from global aphasia is the result of a complex interaction among a number of heretofore incompletely understood factors.

Prognostic Factors

Age

Following global aphasia, a patient's age appears to have an impact on recovery: The younger the patient, the better the prognosis (Holland et al., 1985; Pashek and Holland, 1988). Age may also relate to the type of aphasia at 1 year poststroke. For example, in the study reported by Holland et al. (1985), younger global aphasic patients evolved to a nonfluent Broca's aphasia, while older patients evolved to increasingly severe fluent aphasias with advancing age. Their oldest patients remained globally aphasic (see above).

Whether age can be considered a prognostic indicator has yielded differing conclusions. Advanced age has been found to have a negative influence on recovery (Holland and Bartlett, 1985; Holland et al., 1989; Marshall and Phillips, 1971; Sasanuma, 1988) and to be an insignificant predictor of recovery (Hartman, 1981; Kertesz and McCabe, 1977; Sarno, 1981; Sarno and Levita, 1971). Pashek and Holland (1988) noted specifically that age appeared to predict a poor prognosis for change in global aphasia, but they also identified a number of exceptions to this rule. Thus, age cannot be considered an absolute predictor. The variability in evolution patterns and age effects identified by these authors is intriguing and suggests the need for further large-scale research studies in this area.

Hemiplegia

The occurrence of global aphasia without hemiparesis has previously been described in the literature (Bogousslavsky, 1988; Ferro, 1983; Van Horn and Hawes, 1982). Such preservation of motor abilities may result from dual discrete lesions occurring in both frontal and temporoparietal regions, a single frontotemporoparietal lesion, or a single temporoparietal lesion. The lack of hemiparesis, in the presence of global aphasia, is a positive indicator for recovery (Legatt et al., 1987; Tranel et al., 1987). Tranel et al. (1987) described global aphasic patients with dual discrete lesions (anterior and posterior cerebral) that spared the primary motor area. These patients' global aphasia improved significantly within the first 10 months postonset. Deleval et al. (1989) reported two cases of global aphasia without hemiparesis following discrete prerolandic lesions. Though both of these patients exhibited mild right arm weakness initially, this motor disturbance cleared within 48 hours of onset. The patients of Deleval et al. (1989) showed rapid recovery, yet they continued to exhibit what the authors referred to as a residual motor aphasia.

Mouth Asymmetry

The right hemisphere has been thought to be responsible for increases in propositional speech following severe left-hemisphere lesions (Papanicolaou et al., 1988). One potential indicator of the hemispheric contribution to propositional speech is mouth asymmetry. Graves and Landis (1985) studied the mouth asymmetry of a group of aphasic patients during both propositional and automatic speech acts. Greater right-sided mouth opening during speech acts was considered to represent left-hemisphere control. Conversely, greater left-sided mouth opening is assumed to signify right-hemisphere control. Differences were apparent in the aphasic subjects studied by Graves and Landis (1985). As suspected, propositional speech acts produced greater mouth opening on the right, while automatic speech acts revealed greater mouth opening on the left. As Graves and Landis (1985) have suggested, these techniques may be applied to global aphasia to investigate the reacquisition of propositional speech in these patients. That is, degree of mouth-opening shift may prove useful in predicting the amount of speech that may reemerge.

Handedness

Another factor that has been associated with aphasia recovery is handedness. It has been suggested that left-handers may recover better than right-handers from aphasia (Luria, 1970; Subirana, 1969). The premise underlying this proposal is that left-handers may have language more bilaterally represented. Thus, if there is a lesion in the left hemisphere, the right hemisphere is better able to accept the increased language load. In a study involving left-handed and right-handed aphasic subjects, Basso et al. (1990) obtained conflicting results. Basso et al. (1990) found that their left-handed subjects displayed the same type of aphasia as the right-handed subjects. They concluded that language may not be more bilaterally represented in left-handed patients. Given these findings, handedness does not appear to be a reliable prognostic indicator for recovery following global aphasia.

Radiological Findings

CT scans may provide one of the strongest prognostic tools. In a two-part study, Pieniadz et al. (1983) investigated the relationship between hemispheric asymmetries and recovery from aphasia. The first part of the study involved the analysis of hemispheric asymmetry in a large group of aphasic subjects and in a group of nonaphasic control subjects. The results demonstrated significant similarity and consistency in hemispheric asymmetry for both groups. The most frequent asymmetry involved greater left than right occipital width. Frontal width was greater in the right hemisphere than in the left hemisphere. Length was also greater in the left occipital region. For frontal length, the hemispheres were typically equal.

In the second part of the study by Pieniadz et al. (1983), recovery patterns were examined in a group of global aphasic subjects. These researchers found larger right occipital widths and lengths on CT scans for subjects demonstrating superior recovery of single-word comprehension, repetition, and naming. Pieniadz et al. (1983) suggested that these atypical asymmetries may indicate a right-hemisphere dominance for language. Evaluation of hemispheric asymmetries may be used, therefore, to predict recovery of single-word functions, with atypical patterns suggesting superior long-term gains.

Naeser et al. (1990) used CT scans to compare lesion location and language recovery in a group of global aphasic subjects.

The primary foci in the study by Naeser et al. (1990) were recovery of comprehension abilities and differentiation between temporal lobe lesions involving Wernicke's area and those restricted to the subcortical temporal isthmus. The subjects in this study had either frontal, parietal, and temporal lobe lesions or lesions involving the frontal and parietal lobes with temporal lobe lesions restricted to the subcortical temporal isthmus. The results of Naeser et al. (1990) showed significantly better recovery of auditory comprehension for the group without damage to Wernicke's area (lesions limited to the subcortical temporal isthmus). Over the course of 1 to 2 years, the majority of these subjects reportedly obtained auditory comprehension scores on the BDAE (Goodglass and Kaplan, 1983) that were consistent with only mild to moderate comprehension deficits (Naeser et al., 1990). None of the subjects in this study made significant gains in speech output.

A particularly severe group of global aphasic subjects, with extreme loss of both verbal and nonverbal communication (including comprehension), was studied by De Renzi et al. (1991). De Renzi et al. (1991) found a variety of lesion patterns, only 35% of which involved the entire language area. Attempts to correlate specific types of lesions with some recovery of language abilities were unsuccessful. For the patients who showed some comprehension improvement, there was no common lesion pattern.

Language Scores

Performance on the Porch Index of Communicative Ability (PICA) (Porch, 1981) may be used to predict recovery. According to Collins (1986), global aphasic patients will invariably obtain scores below the 25th percentile. However, high intra- and intersubtest variability suggests at least the potential for recovery. Variability in this instance is defined as the difference between the mean score for a PICA subtest and the highest score within that subtest. A total variability score is derived by adding the variability scores for all PICA subtests. Variability scores above 400 suggest excellent potential for recovery, while scores below 200 suggest poor potential for recovery.

Using medical and PICA data, Collins (1986) suggests that global aphasic patients demonstrating some variability within subtests and variability scores around 100, but relatively flat scores across all modalities, have a poor prognosis for recovery. Imitation, copying, and matching may be better than other test behaviors. Patients showing additional variability, such that their variability scores are well above 100 and there is greater divergence among modality scores, have a fair prognosis for recovery. Performance is generally characterized by mostly correct object matching, good copying skills, the ability to name one or two of the objects, and production of some differentiated responses on the verbal subtests. Significant increases in overall variability relative to the previous two categories and occasionally higher scores (7 or above) on auditory comprehension, reading, and naming subtests are consistent with a good prognosis for recovery. One patient described by Collins (1986) achieved a variability score over 400 while still performing at the 9th percentile.

Collins's recommendations should be tempered by recent work. Wertz et al. (1993) tested the influence of PICA intrasubtest variability on prognosis for improvement in aphasia. Negative and nonsignificant correlations were obtained between vari-

ability scores at 1 month postonset and improvement in PICA Overall performance at 6 and 12 months postonset. In addition, no significant differences in improvement were found at 6 and 12 months postonset between two groups with high variability (over 350) and low variability (under 300) at 1 month postonset. Wertz et al. (in press) concluded that intrasubtest variability has no influence on prognosis.

For other aphasia measures, it generally appears that a lack of variability between auditory comprehension scores and other language scores may be viewed as a negative indicator. The more performance differs among tasks, the more the prognostic outlook improves. Further, a higher percentile rank is consistent with a better prognosis.

INTERVENTION

Before we discuss clinical intervention for global aphasia, a few introductory remarks are in order to provide a philosophy for the management strategies that follow. Included among the issues addressed here are (a) some influences regarding the timing of intervention for global aphasia, (b) the nature of the language assessment, and (c) the behavioral targets for treatment.

Influences Regarding the Timing of Intervention

Recovery Patterns

As described previously, the prognosis for recovery from global aphasia is generally poor (Kertesz and McCabe, 1977). Nonetheless, approximately one-fourth to three-fourths or more of these global aphasic patients will recover to a less severe aphasic or normal condition by the end of the first year after their stroke. Whether this figure is more or less appears to be somewhat related to the time of initial classification. The closer to the aphasia-producing episode that the initial language assessment is completed, the greater will be the proportion of global aphasic patients who evolve to a less severe syndrome (see Table 23.1). While such a trend appears to be evident, these data should be interpreted with caution, especially given the results reported by Reinvang and Engvik (1980).

Do these findings argue against early intervention for global aphasia? Collins (1986) describes the position of some practitioners who would withhold assessment and treatment for these patients until a stable language profile is achieved. We, like Collins, would disagree with such an approach for a number of reasons.

Prognostic Limitations

Primary among the reasons for advocating early intervention is the current clinical inability to identify accurately those global aphasic patients who will evolve to less severe syndromes and those who will not. Even if it could be established that withholding early treatment from patients who have a high or low probability for good recovery is an acceptable clinical practice, current methodologies prevent clinicians from accurately identifying the recovery potential for these patients. Global aphasia cannot be reliably discriminated in the early stage (Wallesch et al., 1992). Conflicting findings with regard to many of the factors identified above continue to present problems for estimating clinical prognosis.

Table 23.1.
Proportion of Global Aphasic Subjects Evolving to Less Severe Aphasia Syndromes or Normal Language With Time of Initial Testing After Cerebral Injury

Study	N	Initial Testing	% Evolved[a]
Holland, Swindell, & Forbes (1985)	10	Immediately	80
Pashek & Holland (1988)	11	0–5 days	64
Siirtola & Siirtola (1984)	14	0–2 weeks	43
Kertesz & McCabe (1977)	22	0–6 weeks	23
Sarno & Levita (1979)	11	4 weeks	0
Sarno & Levita (1981)	7	4 weeks	0
Reinvang & Engvik (1980)	7	2–5 months	57

[a] End-stage assessments were completed between 6 to 12 months postinjury in all studies except Kertesz and McCabe (1977) and Reinvang and Engvik (1980). Only 10 of the global aphasic subjects studied by Kertesz and McCabe (1977) were assessed at 1 year or more postonset. Specific data for the global aphasic subjects of Reinvang and Engvik (1980) were not reported; the mean time postonset for the end-stage observations of all aphasic subjects in their study was 7.5 months with a minimum time of 3 months postonset.

New developments in technology may soon remedy this problem. The potential for recovery of auditory comprehension following global aphasia can be estimated by examining the CT scan lesion site patterns for these patients. As described earlier, better recovery can be expected at 1 to 2 years postonset in patients whose temporal lesions spare Wernicke's area and involve only the subcortical temporal isthmus. Patients having temporal lesions that include more than half of Wernicke's cortical area, however, will likely continue to demonstrate moderate to severe comprehension deficits at 1 to 2 years after their injuries (Naeser et al., 1990). Naeser et al. (1989) also have identified two neuroanatomical areas—the medial subcallosal fasciculus (initiation of spontaneous speech) and the middle one-third periventricular white matter (motor/sensory aspects of spontaneous speech)—that can be examined to assess potential for recovery of spontaneous speech in severely nonfluent stroke patients with infarction in the branches of the left middle cerebral artery (MCA). For patients with lesions outside the left MCA, these authors suggest examination of other specific structures as well (e.g., supplementary motor area, cingulate gyrus).

While these findings provide a promising approach to prognosis for global aphasia, their application appears to warrant discretion on several accounts when making decisions regarding early intervention for global aphasia. For example, the findings of Naeser et al. (1989) are limited in the current context because many of the patients in their most severe subject groups were not globally aphasic. In addition, these authors recognized that exceptions to expected patterns of recovery exist even in patients who meet their suggested neuroanatomical profile. Fi-

nally, the lack of any clear CT scan patterns that could be associated with recovery from global aphasia in other studies (DeRenzi et al., 1991) suggests that these approaches are in need of further data before they can be applied rigorously.

Besides CT scan analysis, patients' levels of alertness or attention at the outset of global aphasia might also be assessed to predict superior recovery. Patients who are initially more alert or have better attention appear to show greater recovery from their global aphasia (Kertesz and McCabe 1977; Sarno and Levita, 1981). However, since the evidence for these latter findings is primarily anecdotal, their application as a clinical guideline might also be considered tenuous until additional information becomes available. These observations, along with differing profiles in the evolution of global aphasia, underscore the fact that global aphasic patients are a heterogeneous group. It is evident that research is needed to identify the particular factors and the way that they interact. Clinicians might then more accurately identify the subgroups of globally aphasic patients who will demonstrate substantial language recovery and those who will not. This information can then be applied in management decisions regarding treatment (Ferro, 1992; Sarno et al., 1970).

In the absence of accurate techniques for predicting recovery from global aphasia, the most powerful reason for providing early treatment is the latent recovery observed in those patients who receive acute speech and language treatment. As described previously, global aphasic patients receiving early treatment, as a group, show continued language improvement during the period between 6 and 12 months postonset (Kertesz and McCabe, 1977; Sarno and Levita, 1979, 1981); this improvement is not observed in untreated patients (Pashek and Holland, 1988; Siirtola and Siirtola, 1984). Until more is known about the individual global aphasic patient, these data suggest that clinicians should continue to intervene at the earliest opportunity to assist these patients at a time when such treatments may be most crucial to long-term recovery.

Treatment Objectives

A second reason for early intervention in global aphasia concerns the purpose of treatment. In deliberating this issue, consider a scenario where the clinical limitations described above no longer applied in predicting recovery from global aphasia. With full awareness of whether a patient will experience a good versus a minimal recovery, which outcome would suggest the need for early treatment? For patients who are expected to evolve to a less severe aphasia, would treatment be deferred necessarily to obtain the more stable language profile that might subserve a more effective long-term management plan? Or might treatment be initiated immediately to accelerate the patient's anticipated recovery? And, for patients who are not expected to demonstrate substantial recovery, would treatment be withheld because of the poor prognosis, thus allowing clinical and financial resources to be allocated more effectively? Or would these patients become primary candidates for treatment to develop a functional communication system from the outset of their aphasia that will provide them the primary means through which they will communicate subsequently? When considering the purpose of treatment in either case, the arguments for early intervention with global aphasic patients, no matter their outcome, are more compelling than otherwise. The recovery patterns per se following global aphasia, therefore, do not provide an adequate rationale for postponing aphasia treatment for these patients.

Global aphasia will be greatest during the acute phase of recovery. Often, as alluded to above, treatment during this phase focuses on the remediation of language deficits via stimulation of disrupted cognitive processes. However, depending on the degree to which the condition renders the patient unable to communicate even the most basic of needs, the first goals of treatment also focus on establishing some means of communication, no matter how simple. Some methods to accomplish this would include establishing reliable yes/no responding or a basic vocabulary of functional items through oral or gestural means such as head nodding, eye blinking, and pointing to pictures or specific icons. Interestingly, the activities associated with establishing these communication systems may, in and of themselves, be considered stimulatory for language. During this phase, clinicians also provide information to family, friends, and health care staff regarding the patient's particular language profile, that is, preserved versus deficient areas, his or her prognosis, and suitable ways to improve communication with the patient. Early intervention in global aphasia, therefore, has the multiple purposes of language stimulation directed toward cerebral reorganization and recovery, identification of successful communicative strategies, and patient, family, and staff counseling. None of these activities can or should be deferred until a stable language profile is achieved.

Goal Revisions

Global aphasic patients do demonstrate varying improvements in linguistic, extralinguistic, and nonverbal communicative functioning (Kenin and Swisher, 1972; Mohr et al., 1973; Prins et al., 1978; Sarno and Levita, 1979, 1981; Wapner and Gardner, 1979). As discussed, these improvements may result in recovery to a less severe form of aphasia in some cases, while in others, the changes may be insufficient at as much as 1 year postonset to suggest reclassification to another form of aphasia (Sarno and Levita, 1979, 1981). For this latter group, improvement can be anticipated in at least one of these categories, especially that of functional communication.

Most, if not all, clinical aphasiologists recognize the dynamic nature of aphasia. Early testing, therefore, is viewed only as a measure of the patient's language functioning at one point in time that will be used to establish a baseline for intervention during the acute period. Because of recovery, frequent probes for improvement in treated and untreated behaviors during this early period, as well as reevaluation using formal instruments, are not only encouraged but expected.

Those who would advocate withholding early treatment until more stable language profiles have been obtained for treatment planning fail to acknowledge that establishment and revision of short-term treatment goals are inherent principles of aphasia rehabilitation. Whether treatment is provided before or after the first month postonset, this process will be repeated regularly throughout the term of the patient's rehabilitation, regardless of the type of aphasia. There is little sense, therefore, in accepting that this process is less valid in global aphasia when treatment is initiated before the first month after injury.

As described above, clinicians have much to offer global aphasic patients and their families during the acute period of recovery. When patients improve, the treatment objectives reflect this change; when patients fail to change, concerted rehabilitative efforts continue in the areas of the patients' greatest functional communicative needs. After weighing these issues, we strongly consider early intervention in global aphasia to be the accepted practice for these patients.

The Nature of the Assessment

Assessment of aphasic individuals encompasses more than simple diagnosis. Ideally, assessment provides a profile not only of the patient's areas of weakness but also of their strengths. Reasonable treatment plans require both types of data. Formal tests provide one method for gathering such data and, in addition, facilitate discussion of patient findings among colleagues. To that end, Collins (1986, p. 62) provides a summary of the severity ratings for a number of these tests that are suggestive of global aphasia. But formal tests may sometimes be inadequate for treatment planning (Rosenbek et al., 1989), especially in the case of severely impaired patients such as those with global aphasia. Little can be gained about patients' preserved areas of communicative functioning from test scores that are consistently near the floor for a given test. For these patients, information regarding their residual communicative capacities may be more readily available from a variety of informal (i.e., nonstandardized) measures. Such measures consist of patient observation to determine functional communication and the diverse methods for cuing behaviors that, when logically varied, allow a practical test of approaches that result in the most favorable responses. Methods that are successful in eliciting target behaviors are incorporated into treatment and provide an initial approach for developing subsequent behaviors.

Our approach includes both formal and informal measures of assessment to establish a communication profile for the global aphasic patient. From a practical point of view, our initial contact with the patient is preceded by a review of medical records and interviews with knowledgeable others to glean information about the patient's communicative status. To the degree possible, we complete a formal language assessment using a standardized aphasia battery, sampling behaviors across tasks at least minimally in each language domain (i.e., speaking, listening, reading, writing), and describing the patient's responses to each item. Given this baseline, our assessment continues through what might be viewed as diagnostic treatment to identify the conditions that further promote successful language performance. Included here would be an analysis of patient responses during interviews focusing on familiar topics or in selected situations and the evaluation of hierarchical cues within language tasks.

In this "qualitative" approach, as described by Helm-Estabrooks (1986), neither type of language assessment (formal or informal) is seen as simply augmenting the other. For the global aphasic patient, both types are deemed mandatory to describe communication functioning adequately. A host of procedures are available to accomplish these objectives. These will be reviewed in the following sections.

Behavioral Targets for Treatment

Perhaps because the impairment in aphasia is, first and foremost, a linguistic one, the primary target for aphasia treatment traditionally has been language performance. As a result, the success of this intervention has been most often evaluated by the extent of changes occurring exclusively in the aphasic patient's grammatical and lexical behaviors. In such an approach, of course, the potential for these changes is diminished with increases in the initial severity of the language impairment. Too often, this approach has resulted in an underestimation of what has been accomplished regarding recovery of communication skills.

Nowhere might this problem be more prevalent than in the case of the global aphasic patient. Since the report of Sarno et al. (1970) suggesting that severe aphasic stroke patients do not benefit from speech and language treatment, rehabilitative attempts for this group of patients have been viewed by many as senseless. However, the conclusions in this study, as well as others like it, were based solely on statistical comparisons of pre- and posttreatment language scores and failed to account for positive changes that may have occurred in other communication behaviors. In a subsequent study involving global aphasic patients, Sarno and Levita (1981) examined the changes occurring not only in language scores but also in communication performance as assessed by the Functional Communication Profile. These authors observed clinically significant improvements in the patients' language scores that were nonetheless insufficient to warrant reclassification to another aphasia syndrome. However, inspection of nonverbal communication abilities revealed recovery of alternate skills (e.g., gesture, pantomime, and other extralinguistic behaviors) that exceeded the reported language changes. According to Sarno and Levita (1981), these improvements resulted in limited but effective communication by the end of the first year after stroke.

These findings suggest that a fundamental revision in the treatment approach to global aphasia is in order. Propositional speech may no longer be an appropriate goal for global aphasic patients during or after the acute period of recovery. Instead, increased emphasis might be placed on those areas of language performance where some signs of residual capacity exist (Wapner and Gardner, 1979) or on other functional abilities that improve not only communication but also the patient's quality of life. Such an emphasis is apparent in many of the more recent treatment methods that have been developed for global aphasic patients.

ASSESSMENT

Assessment of communication functioning in patients with global aphasia is best achieved using both formal and informal measures. These measures are summarized in Table 23.2.

Formal Test Measures

General Language

The language features of global aphasia are described in a previous section. Some standardized aphasia test batteries that specifically address global aphasia in their classification schemes include the Language Modalities Test for Aphasia (Wepman and Jones, 1961); the Minnesota Test for Differential Diagnosis of Aphasia (irreversible aphasia syndrome) (Schuell, 1974); the Boston Diagnostic Aphasia Examination (Goodglass and Kaplan, 1983); the Sklar Aphasia Scale (Sklar, 1973); and the Western Aphasia Battery (Kertesz, 1982). Additional batteries that comprehensively assess language performance to

Table 23.2.
Formal and Informal Measures for Assessment of Global Aphasia

Formal Assessment
  General Language
    Aphasia Language Performance Scales
    Boston Assessment of Severe Aphasia
    Boston Diagnostic Aphasia Examination
    Examining for Aphasia
    Language Modalities Test for Aphasia
    Minnesota Test for Differential Diagnosis of Aphasia
    Neurosensory Center Comprehensive Examination for Aphasia
    Porch Index of Communicative Ability
    Sklar Aphasia Scale
    Western Aphasia Battery

  Modality-Specific
    Auditory Comprehension Test for Sentences
    Boston Naming Test
    Functional Auditory Comprehension Test
    Nelson Reading Test
    Reading Comprehension Battery for Aphasia
    Token Test

  Functional Communication
    Functional Communication Profile
    Communicative Abilities in Daily Living

Informal Measures
  General Language
    Behavioral Assessment (Salvatore and Thompson, 1986)
    Auditory Comprehension Assessment (Edelman, 1984)

  Functional Communication
    Natural Communication (Holland, 1982)
    Communicative Effectiveness Index (Lomas et al., 1989)
    Functional Rating Scale (Collins, 1986)

provide the clinical data for a diagnosis of global aphasia include Examining for Aphasia (Eisenson, 1954); the Porch Index of Communicative Abilities (Porch, 1981); the Neurosensory Center Comprehensive Examination for Aphasia (Spreen and Benton, 1977); and the Aphasia Language Performance Scales (Keenan and Brassell, 1975). The performance pattern for global aphasic patients on any of the tests identified above is generally one of severe impairment in all language abilities.

Information derived from a number of modality-specific assessment instruments can also be combined to arrive at a diagnosis of global aphasia. These tests include the following:

> *Auditory Comprehension*
> Token Test (De Renzi and Vignolo, 1962)
> Auditory Comprehension Test for Sentences (Shewan, 1979; Shewan and Canter, 1971)
> Revised Token Test (McNeil and Prescott, 1978)
>
> Functional Auditory Comprehension Task (LaPointe and Horner, 1978; LaPointe et al., 1985)
> *Reading Comprehension*
> Reading Comprehension Battery for Aphasia (LaPointe and Horner, 1979)
> Nelson Reading Test (Nelson, 1962; Nicholas et al., 1985);
> *Naming*
> Boston Naming Test (Goodglass and Kaplan, 1983)

Unlike the foregoing instruments, the Boston Assessment of Severe Aphasia (BASA) (Helm-Estabrooks et al., 1989b) was developed "for the specific purpose of identifying and quantifying preserved abilities that might form the beginning steps of rehabilitation programs for severely aphasic patients" (p. 1). The BASA assesses performance on 61 items in 15 areas: social greetings and simple conversation; personally relevant yes/no question pairs; orientation to time and place; buccofacial praxis; sustained phonation and singing; repetition; limb praxis; comprehension of number symbols; object naming; action picture items; comprehension of coin names; famous faces; emotional words; phrases; and symbols; visuospatial items; and signature. Responses are scored for response modality (verbal, gestural, or both); communicative quality (fully communicative, partially communicative, noncommunicative, unintelligible, irrelevant, incorrect, or unreliable, or task refused or rejected); affective quality; and perseveration. Raw scores are summed according to seven clusters of items: auditory comprehension, praxis, oral-gestural expression, reading comprehension, gesture recognition, writing, and visuospatial tasks. Norms are provided to convert the total raw score and item cluster raw scores to standard scores and percentile ranks. "Because an important goal of the BASA is to help determine whether a severe case of aphasia may be classified as global" (p. 42), two separate sets of norms are provided, one for cases of severe aphasia and one for global aphasia.

Functional Communication

Two measures for the formal assessment of functional communication include the Functional Communication Profile (FCP) (Sarno, 1969) and Communicative Abilities in Daily Living (CADL) (Holland, 1980). The FCP assesses 45 communication behaviors in a conversational situation that are considered to be common functions of everyday life. Behaviors are rated as normal, good, fair, or poor and transformed to raw scores within five dimensions: movement, speaking, understanding, reading, and other behaviors. The raw scores are converted to a percentage and a weighted score representing the patient's performance relative to normal behavior for that dimension. An overall score is obtained by summing the weighted scores to represent the patient's percentage of normal communication.

The CADL includes 68 items that assess communication skills in structured, simulated daily life activities. Responses can be communicated by a variety of verbal and nonverbal means and are scored as either correct, adequate, or wrong. Norms are provided to determine whether the functional communication of patients varying in age, sex, and institutionalization is normal or aphasic.

Informal Measures

General Language

As described previously, informal measures of language assessment are conducted following formal assessment with a standardized battery to identify the conditions that further promote successful language performance. Such measures aim to identify isolated areas of preserved performance such as those found above under features of comprehension. Hierarchical cues are used to evaluate such residual areas within language tasks.

Salvatore and Thompson (1986) provide an example of informal assessment procedures designed to assess verbal and nonverbal communication systems in global aphasic patients. The model used in their approach uses one stimulus to evoke a variety of responses. When stimuli are presented to evoke all levels of responding, stimulus-response relations that are preserved and those that are impaired are identifiable. For example, patients may be asked to provide several responses to a pictured stimulus including matching it to an identical picture and both writing and saying its name. Responses are analyzed in different modes including gesturing, drawing, reading, writing, and verbalizing. A matrix is developed to categorize the various relations that are tested. The results of the assessment supply important information that provides a basis for treatment.

Edelman (1984) provides an outline for the assessment of comprehension in global aphasia that specifically takes into account research findings identifying areas of residual function in global aphasia and factors that facilitate understanding. The suggested framework permits a systematic evaluation of understanding both contextually and acontextually while manipulating variables found to be facilitative. Performance is assessed using commands and questions at simple linguistic levels. Commands are divided into two sections. Those relating to self involve whole-body movements, limb movements, and orofacial movements. Those relating to objects in the environment are divided into object recognition and object manipulation. These tasks are assessed respectively in a natural verbal context ("Have you any water?" "Can you pass the tissues?") and acontextually ("Show me the comb"; "Pick up the comb"). Questions require affirmation or negation only and include those relating to self and those of less personal saliency. Responses are accepted when communicated either verbally or nonverbally. In addition, hierarchical cuing is incorporated, consisting of repetition, utterance expansion, and gestural accompaniment, and responses are scored using a modified PICA system.

Functional Communication

A number of informal procedures that can be used to evaluate the functional communication of global aphasic patients systematically have also appeared in the literature. Holland (1982) developed a procedure to score observations of natural communication in normal family interactions. The categories of behaviors included verbal and nonverbal output, reading, writing, and math, as well as other communicative behaviors such as talking on the phone and singing. The verbal behaviors were further subcategorized to capture the form, style, conversational dominance, correctional strategies, and metalinguistics of the production. Holland's (1982) procedure is "primarily concerned with the frequency and form of successful and failed verbal and nonverbal communicative acts" (p. 52).

Lomas et al. (1989) constructed the Communicative Effectiveness Index (CETI) using communicative situations provided by aphasic patients and their families that were thought to be important in day-to-day life. The CETI quantitatively assesses aphasic persons' performance over time in 16 situations using judgments provided by spouses or significant others. Performance is rated relative to the aphasic persons, premorbid abilities using a visual analogue scale. The situations range from getting

Table 23.3.
Treatment Approaches for Global Aphasia

Stimulation Approaches
  Auditory Comprehension
    Matching pictures
    Eliciting appropriate responses
    Playing cards
  Verbal Expression
    Associating meaning with speech movements
    Conversational prompting
    Voluntary Control of Involuntary Utterances
Compensatory Approaches
  Gestural Programs
    Amer-Ind Code
    Visual Action Therapy
    Pantomime
    Limited manual sign systems
  Gestural-Assisted Programs
    Communication Boards
    Blissymbols
    Drawing
    Computer-aided Visual Communication

somebody's attention to describing or discussing something in depth. The index was found to be internally consistent, to have acceptable test-retest and interrater reliability, and to be a valid measure of functional communication when compared with other measures. The authors conclude that the CETI is an instrument that is capable of measuring the functional changes occurring during the aphasic patient's recovery that have been difficult to measure previously.

Finally, a less systematic but often effective assessment of functional communication can be derived from patient interviews or questionnaires completed by individuals who are familiar with the global aphasic patient. Collins (1986) reviews several of these questionnaires and provides one such example, an adaptation of the FCP called the Functional Rating Scale.

TREATMENT

Given the poor outcome in chronic global aphasia (Kertesz and McCabe, 1977; Sarno and Levita, 1981) and the negative results that have been reported for treatment programs aimed specifically at remediating verbal skills (Sarno et al., 1970), treatment for these patients largely emphasizes compensatory rather than stimulatory approaches to language rehabilitation (Peach, 1993). Compensatory approaches include those techniques that exploit the patient's residual linguistic and nonlinguistic cognitive skills to increase successful communication, while stimulatory approaches use structured methods that are carefully controlled for levels of difficulty to provide a context that will facilitate successful language responses and shape succeeding language behaviors of increasing complexity. Both approaches, however, may be used appropriately in treatment during the course of recovery from global aphasia. Table 23.3 provides a summary of these approaches.

Stimulation Approaches

Auditory Comprehension

Collins (1986, 1990) suggests that a realistic goal for treatment with the global aphasic patient consists of improving auditory comprehension, supplemented with contextual cues, to permit consistent comprehension of one-step commands in well-controlled situations. For the most severe comprehension deficits, picture matching, accompanied by the clinician's production of the name of the items to be matched, may provide the most basic level of auditory stimulation. Even in those cases where the patient has no understanding of the auditory stimulus accompanying the pictures, it is assumed that the response elicited by the matching task evokes auditory representations of the visual stimuli that may underlie subsequent association of meaning with the name of the pictures (Peach, 1993). Complexity may be increased within this task by (*a*) increasing the size of the response field; (*b*) moving from pairing real objects to realistic pictures of objects to line drawings of the objects; (*c*) matching objects to pictures and pictures to objects, a technique that is incorporated in Visual Action Therapy (Helm-Estabrooks et al., 1982); and (*d*) using sets of pictures that represent nouns with decreasing frequency of occurrence in language usage. As performance improves, these tasks may be followed by word recognition for objects, pictures, or body parts and responses to simple questions.

Marshall (1986) provides an approach to treating auditory comprehension in global aphasic patients that is presented in four phases: (*a*) eliciting responses, (*b*) eliciting differentiated responses, (*c*) eliciting appropriate responses, and (*d*) eliciting accurate responses. In the first phase, clinicians focus on attending, pointing, and yes/no responding; at a minimum, the clinician should help the patient to express himself or herself through head nods, smiles, or frowns. Patients who cannot respond to spoken messages may engage in visual matching or orientation tasks. They may also be provided spoken messages accompanied by gestures. Questions and statements about personally relevant topics may constitute one of the best ways to elicit responses during this phase. In the second phase, the materials and techniques to elicit responses are not unlike those used in the first phase. At this time, however, the clinician accepts and reinforces any response that is different from the previous response given for those stimuli (e.g., varied facial expressions, head nods, gestures, and stereotypical utterances). To do this, the clinician records the patient's responses to a standard set of simple questions, looking for a variety of responses between stimuli and from session to session. With progress, the patient will move into the third phase, demonstrating appropriate responses with occasional accurate responses such as pointing to a calendar when asked to show the date, saying "yes" instead of "no," and shrugging the shoulders when asked how he or she is feeling. Other appropriate responses consist of performing one command for another or producing jargon in response to a question or a request for information. Marshall (1986) suggests that for some patients, appropriate responses may represent their best performance and should therefore be encouraged by clinicians and others in the patient's environment. Finally, in the fourth phase, clinicians seek accurate responses to such tasks as object and picture identification, following commands, and responding to yes/no and *wh-* questions. Nonverbal responses may be facilitated with accompanying props, including pages with words and numbers written on them; a clock with movable hands; a calendar; a road atlas; lists of families; relatives, and friends; and a communication notebook.

Collins (1986, 1990) has designed a program to treat auditory comprehension using playing cards. The approach is based on the observation that global aphasic patients can often recognize names that contain two salient features (e.g., "queen of hearts"), differentiate cards by suit, and place cards in a sequence when they are unable to perform similarly with other stimuli. Although not all patients achieve the highest levels of performance, Collins suggests that portions of the program are useful at some stage for most patients.

Verbal Expression

Despite conclusions that traditional treatment focused on verbal communication skills may be ineffective for global aphasia (Salvatore and Thompson, 1986; Sarno and Levita, 1981), short-term attempts to establish or expand verbal expression with global aphasic patients may be a legitimate therapeutic activity during both the acute and chronic phases of recovery (Rosenbek et al., 1989). Rosenbek et al. (1989) do this by first attempting to associate meaning with speech movements. To do this, patients use available methods (e.g., showing fingers, pointing, gesturing, writing, matching, selecting objects) to confirm the meaning of any successfully elicited verbalizations. Included among these may be serial productions, imitated words and phrases, or automatic, meaningful responses to conversations relating to a variety of topics. As described previously, conversational topics that are personally relevant will improve performance (Van Lancker and Klein, 1990; Van Lancker and Nicklay, 1992; Wallace and Canter, 1985). Patients who succeed in these tasks are taught to produce at least a small repertoire of useful spoken or spoken plus gestured responses. They suggest that these items include at least one greeting, the words "yes" and "no", a few proper names, single words that express important needs, and perhaps one or more phrases, especially if they appear in the patient's spontaneous verbal productions. Imitation, either alone or supplemented by gesture and reading, is used to establish these responses (see also Collins, 1986, 1990 for a detailed approach to establishing an unequivocal yes/no response). Imitated responses are then practiced in more functional contexts using questions or practical situations to facilitate response generalization.

Conversational prompting, a method reported by Cochran and Milton (1984), uses modeling, expansion, and feedback to develop the verbal responses of severe aphasic patients in conversational contexts. Props and written cues are provided to facilitate verbal expression. Ten conversational levels are identified ranging from concrete, structured contexts (e.g., manipulating objects, acting out and describing sequences) to more open contexts (e.g., structured interview, structured discussion). A cuing hierarchy is described to promote language retrieval. With its emphasis on conversational interaction, this technique may be particularly useful in developing contextually appropriate communication for global aphasic patients. It may also provide a suitable means for overcoming some of the problems traditionally associated with the generalization of trained responses to conversational contexts.

As described above, the verbal output of many global aphasic patients consists primarily of stereotypical recurring utterances or speech automatisms. For many of these patients, productive usage of single words or phrases may not be a realistic goal. The treatment program Voluntary Control of Involuntary Utterances (VCIU) (Helm and Barresi, 1980; Helm-Estabrooks and Albert, 1991) can be used with these patients to bring these stereotypes into more productive usage. In this program, words that are involuntarily and inappropriately produced in the contexts of testing and treatment are identified and used as later targets in treatment. The words are trained in a sequence including oral reading, confrontation naming, and finally, conversational usage until a vocabulary of between 200 and 300 words is established.

Compensatory Approaches

Gestural Programs

Amer-Ind Code. Probably the best known of the gestural programs is Amer-Ind Code (Rao, 1986; Skelly, 1979). Amer-Ind Code is adapted from Native American sign, a gestural system based on the concepts underlying words rather than on the word themselves (Skelly et al., 1975). According to Rao and Horner (1980), Amer-Ind is concrete, pictographic, highly transmissible, easily learned, agrammatical, and generative. The system can be applied in aphasia rehabilitation as an alternative means of communication, as a facilitator of verbalization, and as a deblocker of other language modalities (Rao, 1986). While a few reports exist demonstrating the usefulness of Amer-Ind Code as an alternative means of communication (Rao et al., 1980; Tonkovich and Loverso, 1982), the greatest utility of the technique appears to be as a facilitator of verbalization although reports of its effectiveness vary (Hanlon et al., 1990; Hoodin and Thompson, 1983; Kearns et al., 1982; Rao and Horner, 1978; Raymer and Thompson, 1991; Skelly et al., 1974). Rosenbek et al. (1989) describe a treatment program for gestural reorganization that uses Amer-Ind Code as the primary system of gestures and has as its end goal verbalization without gestural accompaniment.

Visual Action Therapy (VAT). VAT (Helm-Estabrooks and Albert, 1991; Helm-Estabrooks et al., 1982; Helm-Estabrooks et al., 1989a; Ramsberger and Helm-Estabrooks, 1989) uses gestures to reduce apraxia and improve the patient's verbal expression or ability to use symbolic gestures as a means of communication. Three programs constitute the approach, including proximal limb, distal limb, and buccofacial VAT. A hierarchical procedure is used in each program to "move the patient along a performance continuum from the basic task of matching pictures and objects to the communicative task of representing hidden items with self-initiated gestures" (Helm-Estabrooks and Albert, 1991, p. 178). The authors suggest that the method produces improvements not only in the area of pantomime, as indicated by formal assessments, but also in the areas of auditory and reading comprehension, verbal repetition, and graphic copying.

Conlon and McNeil (1991) proposed that the efficacy of VAT has not been established because of experimental limitations in the original work of Helm-Estabrooks et al. (1982). Therefore, they investigated the effects of VAT on the communication abilities of two global aphasic patients. Using a modified program for experimental purposes, positive treatment effects were observed on most steps of the program for their first subject and on about half the steps for their second subject. While these results were generally consistent with those of Helm-Estabrooks et al. (1982), generalization of these effects to untreated items was not observed. This lack of generalization suggested that the learned behaviors did not influence performance on untreated but similar behaviors. Conlon and McNeil (1991) determined that VAT is not effective in achieving the program's stated purpose of establishing "symbolic representation" as defined by Helm-Estabrooks et al. (1982). These authors concluded that further research is needed before VAT can be confidently recommended for the treatment of global aphasic patients.

Some other gestural programs include pantomime; limited manual sign systems for hospitals and nursing homes such as manual shorthand, manual self-care signals, or a hand-talking chart; gestures for yes and no; eye-blink encoding; and pointing (Silverman, 1989). Silverman (1989) offers a number of suggestions for the selective use of each of these approaches. For example, pantomime may be appropriate for the aphasic patient who cannot use Amer-Ind Code. Limited manual sign systems may be used initially on an interim basis until other communication systems can be developed but may ultimately provide the only means of communication for the most severely impaired patients (for example, see Coelho, 1990, 1991). Pointing is desirable for the patient who is going to use a communication board.

Gestural-Assisted Programs

Silverman (1989) also describes gestural communication strategies assisted by nonelectronic or electronic means. Strategies using nonelectronic assistance include transmission of messages by communication boards, manipulation of symbol sequences, and drawing. One of the most prominent gestural-assisted strategies in the rehabilitation of global aphasic patients using electronic means is computer-aided visual communication (C-ViC) (Weinrich et al., 1989a).

Alexander and Loverso (1993) developed a specific treatment program for global aphasia that supports the capacity to make categorical and associational semantic discriminations but that is sufficiently easy to allow an understanding of the nature and purpose of the tasks. They contend that treatment of this sort establishes a necessary precondition for subsequent treatment with gestural-assisted programs using iconic/substitutional language (e.g., communication boards, C-ViC). Twenty-four common everyday objects, realistic pictures of those objects, and realistic pictures of the locations in which those objects would be found were used as treatment stimuli. The stimuli were described as being representationally similar to those adopted for communication boards or C-ViC. Eight hierarchically arranged treatment levels were identified, beginning with object-to-object matching in a field of one and increasing to picture sorting into locatively related groups. Two of five global aphasic patients studied reached the proposed goal of treatment—demonstration of semantic capacity across categorical and associational boundaries. The remaining global aphasic patients were unable to recognize the nature of the response required at more complex levels. The authors concluded that, even if only 40% of the cases respond successfully to the program, these patients constitute the appropriate group for substituted language systems.

Communication Boards. Communication boards vary in type and complexity. For severely impaired patients, a typical board will contain personally relevant words and pictures, num-

bers, and the alphabet. Specific treatment is required for effective use of the board. Collins (1986, 1990) suggests a training procedure where target items are identified in isolation, then after an imposed delay, and finally from among increasing numbers of foils until a temporary ceiling is obtained for the number of items contained on one board. Alternative boards containing pictures within only one domain (e.g., family, familiar objects) may be used to increase the number of items available to the patient.

Bellaire et al. (1991) investigated the acquisition, generalization, and maintenance effects of picture communication board training. Although their two subjects were not globally aphasic, their findings have potential application to the treatment of this population.

Treatment and acquisition probes were administered in a traditional treatment room, while generalization probes and training occurred during a coffee hour in a nursing home care unit. Pictures were divided into three sets for communicating social responses, requests for food and other items, and personal information. Stimulus presentations were followed by a 5-second response interval. If an accurate response was not observed, cues consisting of a verbal cue, a model, and a physical assist were provided. Subjects received response-contingent verbal feedback. Generalization training was conducted using a role-playing procedure in the treatment room using a script employed during the coffee-hour probes or within the coffee-hour setting. Maintenance data were collected for up to 6 months.

Following treatment, requesting and personal information responses were acquired but not social responses. No response generalization to untrained responses was observed, nor was there generalization of board use during the coffee hour. Of the two procedures for training generalization, only training within the actual coffee-hour setting resulted in generalized use of all responses except for social responses. Based on these results, the authors recommended that (*a*) communication boards include primarily pictures that communicate specific content items and (*b*) treatment for the use of picture communication boards take place in the natural environments where the board is to be used.

Blissymbols. Johannsen-Horbach et al. (1985) assessed the benefits of treating four global aphasic patients with Blissymbols, a visual symbol system of pictograms and ideograms. All patients had previously received at least 6 months of traditional aphasia therapy without significant improvement in expressive language. For the procedures using Blissymbols, patients received individual treatment twice per week for a period of at least 2 months. Treatment was designed to (*a*) provide a basic lexicon of nouns, verbs, adverbs and function words; (*b*) teach the production and comprehension of simple sentences in the symbol language; and (*c*) acquaint relatives with the symbol system to use in communicating with the patients. Symbols were introduced verbally along with simultaneous presentation of pictures or objects or the pantomime of the therapist. Training consisted of associating symbols and pictures for nouns, verbs, and function words in multiple-choice arrays and subsequently incorporating these items into Blissymbol sentences.

All patients acquired a symbol lexicon; three patients produced Blissyntactically correct sentences in response to pictures. Two of the patients successfully used the symbols in their communication with their relatives. In an important related finding, three patients evidenced the ability to articulate the correct words while pointing to the corresponding symbols, and one patient articulated grammatical sentences. Variable outcomes with regard to continued use of the symbols with these four patients were reported.

Drawing. Drawing has received considerable attention both as a communicative medium and as a means to deblock verbal and written communication. Morgan and Helm-Estabrooks (1987; see also Helm-Estabrooks and Albert, 1991) designed a program entitled Back to the Drawing Board (BDB) to teach patients to communicate messages through sequential drawings. Patients are trained to draw cartoons from memory using verbal instruction, demonstration, and practice through copying. The cartoons range from one panel up to three panels. Criterion performance consists of reproducing a recognizable drawing that contains the critical details relevant to the humorous aspects of the cartoon. Treatment outcome is evaluated by increased accuracy in the patients' drawings of nine "accidents of living." Morgan and Helm-Estabrooks (1987) provide an operational definition of accuracy to facilitate comparison and interpretation of the drawings. Their posttreatment results for two patients indicated an improved ability to convey information through the use of drawing alone.

Lyon and Sims (1989) undertook a study to determine the degree to which severely aphasic patients can communicate through drawing and to evaluate the effectiveness of a treatment program emphasizing drawing-aided communication. Eight aphasic patients and eight comparable normal adults participated in the study. The eight aphasic subjects were enrolled in a treatment program focused on refining primary drawing skills (form, visual organization, detail, and perspective) within defined communicative contexts. Verbal and graphic cuing and requests for enlargement of distorted parts were used to improve the recognizability of the drawings. The drawings were then placed in a communicative interaction between the patient and a trained interactant who used specific strategies to optimize communicative effectiveness.

Communicative effectiveness was assessed using a 40-item drawing outcome measure to evaluate pre- and posttreatment performance with and without the use of drawings. A scale of communicative effectiveness was designed to rate performance on the outcome measure. A second scale was designed to rate the recognition of drawings. Pre- and posttreatment performance on the PICA was also used to measure communicative effectiveness.

Substantial pretreatment gains in aphasic subjects' communicative effectiveness were observed through the introduction of drawing. Performance further improved following treatment to 88% of the communicative effectiveness score attained by the normal adults. The aphasic subjects also improved in the recognizability of their drawings following treatment, achieving 65% of the normal adults' scaled value. Based on these data, the authors concluded that drawing serves as an important facilitator of communication by providing aphasic patients a fixed representation of a concept that is readily available for subsequent modification. However, specific programming may be needed to establish the spontaneous use of drawing for communicative purposes (Kearns and Yedor, 1992).

Computer-aided Visual Communication (C-ViC). C-ViC (Steele et al., 1987; Steele et al., 1989; Weinrich et al., 1989b) provides one of the most promising approaches to estab-

lishing alternative communication in severely impaired patients. Using procedures similar to those of visual communication (ViC) (Gardner et al., 1976) but in a microcomputer environment, C-ViC is an iconographic system in which patients construct communications by selecting symbols from six "card decks" and arranging them according to certain syntactic conventions. The card decks contain interjections, animate nouns, verbs, prepositions, modifiers, and common nouns. Using C-ViC, global aphasic patients are able to develop a formal visual syntax in the absence of natural language that may be used successfully in a visual communication system (Weinrich et al., 1989a). Formal procedures have been developed that extend training from introductory phases that teach the patient to follow simple commands to later phases designed to transfer C-ViC communication skills to use in a home setting (Baker and Nicholas, 1992).

Similar to that reported with other gestural strategies, we have also noted verbal facilitation in patients using C-ViC that results in successful naming not seen in these same patients in other communicative contexts (e.g., conversation, formal testing). While the ultimate goal of C-ViC is not verbalization without computer assistance (as might be the case with some of the foregoing gestural strategies), these observations suggest that C-ViC is a powerful verbal reorganizer that enhances language production in patients using the system. Further investigation of this point is needed to fully understand its long-term effects for language recovery. Nonetheless, for the severely impaired aphasic patient, a patient for whom successful treatment approaches are too often lacking, C-ViC offers an important tool for communication.

The last approach that will be considered here is Promoting Aphasics' Communicative Effectiveness or PACE treatment (Davis, 1980, 1986; Davis and Wilcox, 1981, 1985; Wilcox and Davis, 1978). Because PACE procedures allow patients to freely choose the channel(s) through which they will communicate, the technique provides opportunities for patients to use a verbal strategy or any of the gestural or gestural-assisted strategies described above, with or without verbal accompaniment, to convey messages. In this way, the approach emulates natural conversation by allowing participants to exchange information through multiple modalities. In addition to free selection, some of the other characteristics of natural conversation that provide guiding principles for PACE treatment include the following: (*a*) Clinician and patient participate equally as senders and receivers of messages, (*b*) the interaction incorporates the exchange of new information between clinician and patient, and (*c*) the clinician's feedback is based on the patient's success in communicating a message (Davis and Wilcox, 1985). PACE treatment uses a multidimensional scoring system to better capture the full range of behaviors that may be observed in this interactive approach. Generalization of language gains observed following PACE treatment has been demonstrated on formal language assessment instruments. Given its emphasis on the pragmatic aspects of language, PACE is well suited as a means to incorporate compensatory strategies into communication treatment. An additional strength of the approach, however, lies in its use as a framework for incorporating traditional language stimulation techniques into a communicatively dynamic context.

FUTURE TRENDS IN TREATING GLOBAL APHASIA

It is clear that future clinical research must better identify the conditions under which treatment for global aphasia is maximally effective. To do so, several issues must receive further exploration. One of these concerns outcome in global aphasia and includes (a) identifying the factors that differentially account for evolution in some global aphasic patients to less severe aphasia syndromes, (b) establishing or refining prognostic indicators or profiles that can reliably predict outcome in global aphasia, (c) specifying the relationships between site and extent of lesion for outcome in global aphasia, and (d) defining the role of attention as an early indicator of outcome. A second issue concerns how this outcome information can be better applied to management decisions for global aphasic patients. Naeser (1991) provides one example of the use of outcome information obtained during the acute phase of recovery for these purposes. This approach must be further developed to improve specificity and accuracy. Finally, clinicians must continue to identify specific assessment and treatment approaches that are sensitive to the capabilities of global aphasic patients and produce reasonable outcomes in functional communication relative to the time and effort expended during the rehabilitation process.

References

Alajouanine, M. S. (1956). Verbal realization in aphasia. *Brain, 79,* 1–28.

Alexander, M. P., and Loverso, F. L. (1993). A specific treatment for global aphasia. *Clinical Aphasiology, 21,* 277–289.

Alexander, M. P., Naeser, M. A., amd Palumbo, C. L. (1987). Correlations of subcortical CT lesion sites and aphasia profiles. *Brain, 110,* 961–991.

Arrigoni, G., and De Renzi, E. (1964). Constructional apraxia and hemispheric locus of lesion. *Cortex, 1,* 170–197.

Baker, E., and Nicholas, M. (1992). *C-ViC training manual.* Unpublished manuscript.

Basso, A., Capitani, E., Luzzati, C., and Spinnler, H. (1981). Intelligence and left hemisphere disease: The role of aphasia, apraxia and size of lesion. *Brain, 104,* 721–734.

Basso, A., Della Sala, S., and Farabola, M. (1987). Aphasia arising from purely deep lesions. *Cortex, 23,* 29–44.

Basso, A., De Renzi, E., Faglioni, P., Scotti, G., and Spinnler, H. (1973). Neuropsychological evidence for the existence of cerebral areas critical to the performance of intelligence tasks. *Brain, 96,* 715–728.

Basso, A., Farabola, M., Grassi, M. P., Laiacona, M., and Zanobio, M. E. (1990). Aphasia in left-handers: Comparison of aphasia profiles and language recovery in non-right-handed and matched right-handed patients. *Brain and Language, 38,* 233–252.

Basso, A., Lecours, A. R., Moraschini, S., and Vanier, M. (1985). Anatomoclinical correlations of the aphasias as defined through computerized tomography: Exceptions. *Brain and Language, 26,* 201–229.

Bellaire, K. J., Georges, J. B., and Thompson, C. K. (1991). Establishing functional communication board use for nonverbal aphasic subjects. *Clinical Aphasiology, 19,* 219–227.

Blanken, G., Wallesch, C. W., and Papagno, C. (1990). Dissociations of language functions in aphasics with speech automatisms (recurring utterances). *Cortex, 26,* 41–63.

Bogousslavsky, J. (1988). Global aphasia without other lateralizing signs. *Archives of Neurology, 45,* 143.

Brust, J. C., Shafer, S. Q., Richter, R. W., and Bruun, B. (1976). Aphasia in acute stroke. *Stroke, 7,* 167–174.

Cappa, S. F., and Vignolo, L. A. (1983). CT scan studies of aphasia. *Human Neurobiology, 2,* 129–134.

Cochran, R. M., and Milton, S. B. (1984). Conversational prompting: A sentence building technique for severe aphasia. *Journal of Neurological Communication Disorders, 1,* 4–23.

Coelho, C. A. (1990). Acquisition and generalization of simple manual sign grammars by aphasic subjects. *Journal of Communication Disorders, 23,* 383–400.

Coelho, C. A. (1991). Manual sign acquisition and use in two aphasic subjects. *Clinical Aphasiology, 19,* 209–218.

Collins, M. (1986). *Diagnosis and treatment of global aphasia.* San Diego, CA: College Hill Press.

Collins, M. J. (1990). Global aphasia. In L. L. LaPointe (Ed.), *Aphasia and related neurogenic language disorders* (pp. 113–129). New York: Thieme.

Colonna, A., and Faglioni, P. (1966). The performance of hemisphere-damaged patients on spatial intelligence tests. *Cortex, 2,* 293–307.

Conlon, C. P., and McNeil, M. R. (1991). The efficacy of treatment for two globally aphasic adults using Visual Action Therapy. *Clinical Aphasiology, 19,* 185–195.

Damasio, A. (1991). Signs of aphasia. In M. T. Sarno (Ed.), *Acquired aphasia* (2nd ed., pp. 27–43). San Diego, CA: Academic Press.

Davis, G. A. (1980). A critical look at PACE therapy. *Clinical Aphasiology, 10,* 248–257.

Davis, G. A. (1983). *A survey of adult aphasia.* Englewood Cliffs, NJ: Prentice-Hall.

Davis, G. A. (1986). Pragmatics and treatment. In R. Chapey (Ed.), *Language intervention strategies in adult aphasia* (2nd ed., pp. 251–265). Baltimore, MD: Williams & Wilkins.

Davis, G. A. (1993). *A survey of adult aphasia and related language disorders* (2nd ed.). Englewood Cliffs, NJ: Prentice-Hall.

Davis, G. A., and Wilcox, J. (1981). Incorporating parameters of natural conversation in aphasia. In R. Chapey (Ed.), *Language intervention strategies in adult aphasia* (pp. 169–194). Baltimore, MD: Williams & Wilkins.

Davis, G. A., and Wilcox, M. J. (1985). *Adult aphasia rehabilitation: Applied pragmatics.* San Diego, CA: College Hill Press.

deBlesser, R., and Poeck, K. (1984). Aphasia with exclusively consonant-vowel recurring utterances: Tan-Tan revisited. In F.C. Rose (Ed.), *Advances in neurology: Vol. 42. Progress in aphasiology* (pp. 51–57). New York: Raven Press.

deBlesser, R., and Poeck, K. (1985). Analysis of prosody in the spontaneous speech of patients with CV-recurring utterances. *Cortex, 21,* 405–416.

Deleval, J., Leonard, A., Mavroudakis, N., and Rodesch, G. (1989). Global aphasia without hemiparesis following prerolandic infarction. *Neurology, 39,* 1532–1535.

De Renzi, E., Colombo, A., and Scarpa, M. (1991). The aphasic isolate: A clinical-CT scan study of a particularly severe subgroup of global aphasics. *Brain, 114,* 1719–1730.

De Renzi, E., Faglioni, P., and Ferrari, P. (1980). The influence of sex and age on the incidence and type of aphasia. *Cortex, 16,* 627–630.

De Renzi, E., and Vignolo, L. A. (1962). The token test: A sensitive test to detect receptive disturbances in aphasics. *Brain, 85,* 665–678.

Edelman, G. M. (1984). Assessment of understanding in global aphasia. In F. C. Rose (Ed.), *Advances in neurology: Vol. 42. Progress in aphasiology* (pp. 277–289). New York: Raven Press.

Eisenson, J. (1954). *Examining for aphasia* (rev. ed.). New York: The Psychological Corporation.

Eslinger, P. J., and Damasio, A. R. (1981). Age and type of aphasia in patients with stroke. *Journal of Neurology, Neurosurgery, and Psychiatry, 44,* 377–381.

Ferro, J. M. (1983). Global aphasia without hemiparesis. *Neurology, 33,* 1106.

Ferro, J. M. (1992). The influence of infarct location on recovery from global aphasia. *Aphasiology, 6,* 415–430.

Fromm, D., Holland, A. L., and Swindell, C. S. (1984). Depression following left hemisphere stroke (Abstract). *Clinical Aphasiology, 14,* 268–270.

Gainotti, G., D'Erme, P., Villa, G., and Caltagirone, C. (1986). Focal brain lesions and intelligence: A study with a new version of Raven's colored matrices. *Journal of Clinical and Experimental Neuropsychology, 8,* 37–50.

Gardner, H., Zurif, E. B., Berry, T., and Baker, E. (1976). Visual communication in aphasia. *Neuropsychologia, 14,* 275–292.

Goodglass, H., and Kaplan, E. (1983). *The assessment of aphasia and related disorders* (2nd ed.). Philadelphia, PA: Lea & Febiger.

Graves, R., and Landis, T. (1985). Hemispheric control of speech expression in aphasia: A mouth asymmetry study. *Archives of Neurology, 42,* 249–251.

Habib, M., Ali-Cherif, A., Poncet, M., and Salamon, G. (1987). Age-related changes in aphasia type and stroke localization. *Brain and Language, 31,* 245–251.

Hanlon, R. E., Brown, J. W., and Gerstman, L. J. (1990). Enhancement of naming in nonfluent aphasia through gesture. *Brain and Language, 38,* 298–314.

Hartman, J. (1981). Measurement of early spontaneous recovery from aphasia with stroke. *Annals of Neurology, 9,* 89–91.

Helm, N. A., and Barresi, B. (1980). Voluntary control of involuntary utterances: A treatment approach for severe aphasia. *Clinical Aphasiology, 10,* 308–315.

Helm-Estabrooks, N. (1986). Severe aphasia. In J. M. Costello and A. L. Holland (Eds.), *Handbook of speech and language disorders* (pp. 917–934). San Diego, CA: College Hill Press.

Helm-Estabrooks, N., and Albert, M. L. (1991). *Manual of aphasia therapy.* Austin, TX: Pro-Ed.

Helm-Estabrooks, N., Fitzpatrick, P. M., and Barresi, B. (1982). Visual action therapy for global aphasia. *Journal of Speech and Hearing Disorders, 47,* 385–389.

Helm-Estabrooks, N., Ramsberger, G., Brownell, H., and Albert, M. (1989a). Distal versus proximal movement in limb apraxia. *Journal of Clinical and Experimental Neuropsychology, 7,* 608.

Helm-Estabrooks, N., Ramsberger, G., Morgan, A. R., and Nicholas, M. (1989b). *Boston assessment of severe aphasia.* Chicago, IL: Riverside Press.

Herrmann, M., Koch, U., Johannsen-Horbach, H., and Wallesch, C. W. (1989). Communicative skills in chronic and severe nonfluent aphasia. *Brain and Language, 37,* 339–352.

Holland, A. L. (1980). *Communicative abilities in daily living.* Baltimore, MD: University Park Press.

Holland, A. L. (1982). Observing functional communication of aphasic adults. *Journal of Speech and Hearing Disorders, 47,* 50–56.

Holland, A. L., and Bartlett, C. L. (1985). Some differential effects of age on stroke-produced aphasia. In H. K. Ulatowska (Ed.), *The aging brain: Communication in the elderly* (pp. 141–155). San Diego, CA: College Hill Press.

Holland, A. L., Greenhouse, J. B., Fromm, D., and Swindell, C. S. (1989). Predictors of language restitution following stroke: A multivariate analysis. *Journal of Speech and Hearing Research, 32,* 232–238.

Holland, A. L., Swindell, C. S., and Forbes, M. M. (1985). The evolution of initial global aphasia: Implications for prognosis. *Clinical Aphasiology, 15,* 169–175.

Hoodin, R. B., and Thompson, C. K. (1983). Facilitation of verbal labeling in adult aphasia by gestural, verbal or verbal plus gestural training. *Clinical Aphasiology, 13,* 62–64.

Horenstein, S. (1970). Effects of cerebrovascular disease on personality and emotionality: Presentation 17. In A. L. Benton (Ed.), *Behavioral change in cerebrovascular disease* (pp. 171–194). New York: Harper & Row.

Johannsen-Horbach, H., Cegla, B., Mager, U., Schempp, B., and Wallesch, C. W. (1985). Treatment of global aphasia with a nonverbal communication system. *Brain and Language, 24,* 74–82.

Kearns, K., Simmons, N. N., and Sisterhen, C. (1982). Gestural sign (Amer-Ind) as a facilitator of verbalization in patients with aphasia. *Clinical Aphasiology, 12,* 183–191.

Kearns, K. P., and Yedor, K. (1992, June). *Artistic activation therapy: Drawing conclusions.* Paper presented at the Clinical Aphasiology Conference, Durango, CO.

Keenan, J. S., and Brassell, E. G. (1975). *Aphasia language performance scales.* Murphreesboro, TN: Pinnacle Press.

Kenin, M., and Swisher, L. P. (1972). A study of patterns of recovery in aphasia. *Cortex, 8,* 56–68.

Kertesz, A. (1979). *Aphasia and associated disorders: Taxonomy, localization, and recovery.* Orlando, FL: Grune & Stratton.

Kertesz, A. (1982). *Western aphasia battery.* New York: Grune & Stratton.

Kertesz, A., and McCabe, P. (1975). Intelligence and aphasia: Performance of aphasics on Raven's Coloured Progressive Matrices (RCPM). *Brain and Language, 2,* 387–395.

Kertesz, A., and McCabe, P. (1977). Recovery patterns and prognosis in aphasia. *Brain, 100,* 1–18.

Kertesz, A., and Sheppard, A. (1981). The epidemiology of aphasia and cognitive impairment in stroke. *Brain, 104,* 117–128.

LaPointe, L. L., Holtzapple, P., and Graham, L. F. (1985). The relationships among two measures of auditory comprehension and daily living communicative skills. *Clinical Aphasiology, 15,* 38–46.

LaPointe, L. L., and Horner, J. (1978, Spring). The functional auditory comprehension task (FACT): Protocol and test format. *FLASHA Journal,* pp. 27–33.

LaPointe, L. L., and Horner, J. (1979). *Reading comprehension battery for aphasia.* Tigard, OR: C. C. Publications.

Legatt, A. D., Rubin, M. J., Kaplan, L. R., Healton, E. B., and Brust, J. C. M. (1987). Global aphasia without hemiparesis: Multiple etiologies. *Neurology, 37,* 201–205.

Lomas, J., and Kertesz, A. (1978). Patterns of spontaneous recovery in aphasic groups: A study of adult stroke patients. *Brain and Language, 6,* 388–401.

Lomas, J., Pickard, L., Bester, S., Elbard, H., Finlayson, A., and Zoghaib, C. (1989). The communicative effectiveness index: Development and psychometric evaluation of a functional communication measure for adult aphasia. *Journal of Speech and Hearing Disorders, 54,* 113–124.

Lüders, H., Lesser, R. P., Hahn, J., Dinner, D. S., Morris, H. H., Wyllie, E., and Godoy, J. (1991). Basal temporal language area. *Brain, 114,* 743–754.

Luria, A. R. (1970). *Traumatic aphasia.* The Hague: Mouton.

Lyon, J. G., and Sims, E. (1989). Drawing: Its use as a communicative aid with aphasic and normal adults. *Clinical Aphasiology, 18,* 339–355.

Marshall, R. C. (1986). Treatment of auditory comprehensive deficits. In R. Chapey (Ed.), *Language intervention strategies in adult aphasia* (2nd ed., pp. 370–393). Baltimore, MD: Williams & Wilkins.

Marshall, R. C., and Phillips, D. S. (1971). Prognosis for improved verbal communication in aphasic stroke patients. *Archives of Physical Medicine and Rehabilitation, 64,* 597–600.

Mazzocchi, F., and Vignolo, L. A. (1979). Localization of lesions in aphasia: Clinical CT scan correlations in stroke patients. *Cortex, 15,* 627–654.

McKenna, P., and Warrington, E. K. (1978). Category-specific naming preservation: A single case study. *Journal of Neurology, Neurosurgery, and Psychiatry, 41,* 571–574.

McNeil, M. R., and Prescott, T.E. (1978). *Revised Token Test.* Baltimore, MD: University Park Press.

Mohr, J. P., Sidman, M., Stoddard, L. T., Leicester, J., and Rosenberger, P. B. (1973). Evolution of the deficit in total aphasia. *Neurology, 23,* 1302–1312.

Morgan, A. L. R., and Helm-Estabrooks, N. (1987). Back to the Drawing Board: A treatment program for nonverbal aphasic patients. *Clinical Aphasiology, 17,* 64–72.

Murdoch, B. E., Afford, R. J., Ling, A. R., and Ganguley, B. (1986). Acute computerized tomographic scans: Their value in the localization of lesions and as prognostic indicators in aphasia. *Journal of Communication Disorders, 19,* 311–345.

Naeser, M. A. (1991, November). *How to analyze CT scans to predict potential for recovery and good response to specific verbal and nonverbal treatment programs in aphasia.* Symposium conducted at the annual scientific meeting of the Academy of Neurologic Communication Disorders and Sciences, Atlanta, GA.

Naeser, M. A., Gaddie, A., Palumbo, C. L., and Stiassny-Eder, D. (1990). Late recovery of auditory comprehension in global aphasia: Improved recovery observed with subcortical temporal isthmus lesion vs. Wernicke's cortical area lesion. *Archives of Neurology, 47,* 425–432.

Naeser, M. A., Palumbo, C. L., Helm-Estabrooks, N., Stiassny-Eder, D., and Albert, M. L. (1989). Severe non-fluency in aphasia: Role of the medial subcallosal fasciculus plus other white matter pathways in recovery of spontaneous speech. *Brain, 112,* 1–38.

Nelson, M. J. (1962). *The Nelson Reading Test.* Boston, MA: Houghton-Mifflin.

Nicholas, L. E., MacLennan, D. L., and Brookshire, R. H. (1985). Validity of multi-sentence reading comprehension subtests in aphasia tests. *Clinical Aphasiology, 15,* 29–37.

Pashek, G. V., and Holland, A. L. (1988). Evolution of aphasia in the first year post-onset. *Cortex, 24,* 411–423.

Papanicolaou, A. C., Moore, B. D., Deutsch, G., Levin, H. S., and Eisenberg, H. M. (1988). Evidence for right-hemisphere involvement in recovery from aphasia. *Archives of Neurology, 45,* 1025–1029.

Peach, R. K. (1993). Clinical intervention for aphasia in the Unites States of America. In A. L. Holland and M. M. Forbes (Eds.), *Aphasia treatment: World perspectives* (pp. 335–369). San Diego, CA: Singular Publishing Group.

Pieniadz, J. M., Naeser, M. A., Koff, E., and Levine, H. L. (1983). CT scan cerebral hemispheric asymmetry measurements in stroke cases with global aphasia: Atypical asymmetries associated with improved recovery. *Cortex, 19,* 371–391.

Piercy, M., and Smith, V. O. G. (1962). Right hemisphere dominance for certain non-verbal intellectual skills. *Brain, 85,* 775–790.

Porch, B. E. (1981). *Porch Index of Communicative Ability* (3rd ed.). Palo Alto, CA: Consulting Psychologists Press.

Prins, R. S., Snow, E., and Wagenaar, E. (1978). Recovery from aphasia: Spontaneous speech versus language comprehension. *Brain and Language, 6,* 192–211.

Ramsberger, G., and Helm-Estabrooks, N. (1989). Visual Action Therapy for bucco-facial apraxia. *Clinical Aphasiology, 18,* 395–406.

Rao, P. R. (1986). The use of Amer-Ind code with aphasic adults. In R. Chapey (Ed.), *Language intervention strategies in adult aphasia* (2nd ed., pp. 360–367). Baltimore, MD: Williams & Wilkins.

Rao, P. R., Basili, A. G., Koller, J., Fullerton, B., Diener, S., and Burton, P. (1980). The use of Amer-Ind code by severe aphasic adults. In M. S. Burns and J. R. Andrews (Eds.), *Neuropathologies of speech and language: Diagnosis and treatment* (pp. 18–35). Evanston, IL: Institute for Continuing Professional Education.

Rao, P. R., and Horner, J. (1978). Gesture as a deblocking modality in a severe aphasic patient. *Clinical Aphasiology, 8,* 180–187.

Rao, P. R., and Horner, J. (1980). Nonverbal strategies for functional communication in aphasic persons. In M. S. Burns and J. R. Andrews (Eds.), *Neuropathologies of speech and language: Diagnosis and treatment* (pp. 108–133). Evanston, IL: Institute for Continuing Professional Education.

Raven, J. C. (1965). *Guide to using the Coloured Progressive Matrices.* London: H. K. Lewis.

Raymer, A. M., and Thompson, C. K. (1991). Effects of verbal plus gestural treatment in a patient with aphasia and severe apraxia of speech. *Clinical Aphasiology, 20,* 285–295.

Reinvang, I., and Engvik, H. (1980). Language recovery in aphasia from 3 to 6 months after stroke. In M. T. Sarno and O. Hook (Eds.), *Aphasia: Assessment and treatment* (pp. 79–88). New York: Masson.

Robinson, R. G., and Benson, D. F. (1981). Depression in aphasic patients: Frequency, severity, and clinical-pathological correlations. *Brain and Language, 14,* 282–291.

Robinson, R. G., and Price, T. R. (1982). Poststroke depressive disorders: A follow-up study of 103 stroke outpatients. *Stroke, 13,* 635–641.

Robinson, R. G., Starr, L. B., and Price, T. R. (1984). A two-year longitudinal study of post-stroke mood disorders: Prevalence and duration at six-month follow-up. *British Journal of Psychiatry, 144,* 256–262.

Rosenbek, J. C., LaPointe, L. L., and Wertz, R. T. (1989). *Aphasia: A clinical approach.* Austin, TX: Pro-Ed.

Salvatore, A. P., and Thompson, C. K. (1986). Intervention for global aphasia. In R. Chapey (Ed.), *Language intervention strategies in adult aphasia* (2nd ed., pp. 403–418). Baltimore, MD: Williams & Wilkins.

Sarno, M. T. (1969). *The Functional Communication Profile: Manual of directions* (Rehabilitation Monograph 42). New York: New York University Medical Center, Institute of Rehabilitation Medicine.

Sarno, M. T. (1981). Recovery and rehabilitation in aphasia. In M. R. Sarno (Ed.), *Acquired aphasia* (pp. 485–529). New York: Academic Press.

Sarno, M. R., and Levita, E. (1971). Natural course of recovery in severe aphasia. *Archives of Physical Medicine and Rehabilitation, 52,* 175–178.

Sarno, M. R., and Levita, E. (1979). Recovery in treated aphasia during the first year post-stroke. *Stroke, 10,* 663–670.

Sarno, M. T., and Levita, E. (1981). Some observations on the nature of recovery in global aphasia after stroke. *Brain and Language, 13,* 1–12.

Sarno, M. T., Silverman, M. G., and Sands, E. S. (1970). Speech therapy and language recovery in severe aphasia. *Journal of Speech and Hearing Research, 13,* 607–623

Sasanuma, S. (1988). Studies in dementia: In search of the linguistic/cognitive interaction underlying communication. *Aphasiology, 2,* 191–193.

Scarpa, M., Colombo, A., Sorgato, P., and De Renzi, E. (1987). The incidence of aphasia and global aphasia in left brain-damaged patients. *Cortex, 23,* 331–336.

Schuell, H. M. (1974). *The Minnesota Test for Differential Diagnosis of Aphasia* (rev. ed.). Minneapolis, MN: University of Minnesota Press.

Schuell, H. M., Jenkins, J. J., and Jimenez-Pabon, E. (1964). *Aphasia in adults: Diagnosis, prognosis, and treatment.* New York: Harper & Row.

Shewan, C. M. (1979). *Auditory Comprehension Test for Sentences.* Chicago, IL: Biolinguistics Clinical Institutes.

Shewan, C. M., and Canter, G. J. (1971). Effects of vocabulary, syntax, and sentence length on auditory comprehension in aphasic patients. *Cortex, 7,* 209–226.

Signer, S., Cummings, J. L., and Benson, D. F. (1989). Delusion and mood disorders in patients with chronic aphasia. *Journal of Neuropsychiatry, 1,* 40–45.

Siirtola, T., and Siirtola, M. (1984). Evolution of aphasia. *Acta Neurologica Scandinavica, 69* (Suppl. 98), 403–404.

Silverman, F. H. (1989). *Communication for the speechless* (2nd ed.). Englewood Cliffs, NJ: Prentice-Hall.

Skelly, M. (1979). *Amer-Ind gestural code based on universal American Indian hand talk.* New York: Elsevier.

Skelly, M., Schinsky, L., Smith, R., Donaldson, R., and Griffin, P. (1974). American Indian Sign (Amerind) as a facilitator of verbalization for the oral-verbal apraxic. *Journal of Speech and Hearing Disorders, 39,* 445–456.

Skelly, M., Schinsky, L., Smith, R., Donaldson, R., and Griffin, P. (1975). American Indian Sign: Gestural communication for the speechless. *Archives of Physical Medicine and Rehabilitation, 56,* 156–160.

Sklar, M. (1973). *Sklar Aphasia Scale* (rev. ed.). Los Angeles, CA: Western Psychological Services.

Sorgato, P., Colombo, A., Scarpa, M., and Faglioni, P. (1990). Age, sex, and lesion site in aphasic stroke patients with single focal damage. *Neuropsychology, 4,* 165–173.

Spinnler, H., and Vignolo, L. (1966). Impaired recognition of meaningful sounds in aphasia. *Cortex, 2,* 337–348.

Spreen, O., and Benton, A. L. (1977). *Neurosensory Center Comprehensive Examination for Aphasia* (rev. ed.). Victoria, B.C.: University of Victoria.

Steele, R. D., Weinrich, M., Kleczewska, M. K., Carlson, G. S., and Wertz, R. T. (1987). Evaluating performance of severely aphasic patients on a computer-aided visual communication system. *Clinical Aphasiology, 17,* 46–54.

Steele, R. D., Weinrich, M., Wertz, R. T., Kleczewska, M. K., and Carlson, G. S. (1989). Computer-based visual communication in aphasia. *Neuropsychologia, 27,* 409–426.

Subirana, A. (1969). Handedness and cerebral dominance. In P. J. Vinken and G. W. Bruyn (Eds.), *Handbook of clinical neurology: Vol. 4. Disorders of speech, perception, and symbolic behavior* (pp. 248–272). Amsterdam: North-Holland.

Tonkovich, J. D., and Loverso, F. L. (1982). A training matrix approach for gestural acquisition by the agrammatic patient. *Clinical Aphasiology, 12,* 283–288.

Tranel, D., Biller, J., Damasio, H., Adams, H. P., and Cornell, S. H. (1987). Global aphasia without hemiparesis. *Archives of Neurology, 44,* 304–308.

Van Horn, G., and Hawes, A. (1982). Global aphasia without hemiparesis: A sign of embolic encephalopathy. *Neurology, 32,* 403–406.

Van Lancker, D., and Klein, K. (1990). Preserved recognition of familiar personal names in global aphasia. *Brain and Language, 39,* 511–529.

Van Lancker, D., and Nicklay, C. K. H. (1992). Comprehension of personally relevant (PERL) versus novel language in two globally aphasic patients. *Aphasiology, 6,* 37–61.

Wallace, G. L., and Canter, G. J. (1985). Effects of personally relevant language materials on the performance of severely aphasic individuals. *Journal of Speech and Hearing Disorders, 50,* 385–390.

Wallace, G. L., and Stapleton, J. H. (1991). Analysis of auditory comprehension performance in individuals with severe aphasia. *Archives of Physical Medicine and Rehabilitation, 72,* 674–678.

Wallesch, C. W., Bak, T., and Schulte-Monting, J. (1992). Acute aphasia—patterns and prognosis. *Aphasiology, 6,* 373–385.

Wapner, W., and Gardner, H. (1979). A note on patterns of comprehension and recovery in global aphasia. *Journal of Speech and Hearing Research, 29,* 765–772.

Weinrich, M., Steele, R., Carlson, G. S., Kleczewska, M., Wertz, R. T., and Baker, E. H. (1989a). Processing of visual syntax in a globally aphasic patient. *Brain and Language, 36,* 391–405.

Weinrich, M., Steele, R., Kleczewska, M., Carlson, G. S., Baker, E. H., and Wertz, R. T. (1989b). Representation of "verbs" in a computerized visual communication system. *Aphasiology, 3,* 501–512.

Wells, C. R., Labar, D. R., and Solomon, G. E. (1992). Aphasia as the sole manifestation of simple partial status epilepticus. *Epilepsia, 33,* 84–87.

Wepman, J. M., and Jones, L. V. (1961). *The Language Modalities Test for Aphasia.* Chicago, IL: Education-Industry Service.

Wertz, R. T., Dronkers, N. F., and Hume, J. L. (1993). PICA intrasubtest variability and prognosis for improvement in aphasia. *Clinical Aphasiology, 21,* 207–211.

Wilcox, M. J., and Davis, G. A. (1978, November). *Procedures for promoting communicative effectiveness in an aphasic adult.* Symposium conducted at the annual meeting of the American Speech and Hearing Association, San Francisco, CA.

Yang, B. J., Yang, T. C., Pan, H. C., Lai, S. J., and Yang, F. (1989). Three variant forms of subcortical aphasia in Chinese stroke patients. *Brain and Language, 37,* 145–162.

CHAPTER 24
Treatment of Acquired Reading Disorders

WANDA G. WEBB AND RUSSELL J. LOVE

HISTORICAL PERSPECTIVES

The first clearly defined case report of a reading disorder accompanying aphasia is credited to Dejerine in 1891 (Benson and Geschwind, 1969). Since then there have been numerous studies or case reports concerning different types of acquired reading disorders. Depending on the type, the disorders are known as both *alexias* and *dyslexias*. Notable among the descriptions or studies are those by Benson (1977), Coltheart (1980), and Deloche et al. (1982) Hecaen and Kremin (1976), Newcombe et al. (1975). Reports such as these have helped us specify and describe the features of the disorders as well as understand the recovery patterns. Leading clinicians such as Davis (1983), LaPointe and Kraemer (1983), and Schuell et al. (1964) have offered treatment suggestions as well. The literature describes several different types of acquired reading disorders.

TYPES OF READING DISORDERS

Traditional Classifications

The reading problems associated with aphasia were traditionally classified by their association with other symptoms of language disorder and/or the location of the damage thought to cause the reading disorder. The severity of the disorder was based on the results of the assessment of reading comprehension, but reading aloud was not a standard component of the testing and classification. The traditional classifications follow (Benson, 1979).

Alexia Without Agraphia

The patient with alexia without agraphia, or "pure" alexia, shows greatly compromised reading comprehension, with oral language normal or nearly normal. The ability to copy is usually impaired and may tend to worsen over time. Written acalculia and color anomia are often present. A right homonymous hemianopsia is almost always present, but a right hemiparesis is rare. A visual agnosia for objects and/or colors occasionally accompanies the syndrome.

The patient with alexia without agraphia often is noted to read in a "letter-by-letter" fashion. Each letter of the word is named, often aloud, before the word is identified. Comprehension of words spelled aloud is usually good.

Alexia with Agraphia

Alexia with agraphia is the second traditional classification but can be subdivided into aphasic alexia and agraphic alexia (Friedman and Albert, 1985). Aphasic alexia refers to the disorder that is a part of the aphasia. The two most frequently cited reading disturbances are those accompanying Wernicke's aphasia and those accompanying Broca's aphasia. The reading problems tend to parallel the overall language disorder. In Wernicke's aphasia, part of speech is not an important predictor, although the patient may read function words somewhat better than contentives. Paralexic errors are frequent, like the paraphasic errors of oral language. The degree of reading disturbance usually parallels auditory comprehension deficit, although case studies have shown that there may be a strong modality bias in Wernicke's patients (Hier and Mohr, 1977; Kirshner and Webb, 1982).

Frontal Alexia

Broca's aphasia shows reading disturbance similar to that referred to as the "third alexia," anterior alexia or frontal alexia (Benson, 1977). As in the speech of the Broca's patient, word class and frequency show an important effect, with concrete nouns being read more accurately than abstract nouns or function words. The Broca's patient may comprehend more than would be expected because comprehension of the contentives may be good. Sentences in which the meaning is derived from syntax may be very difficult. These patients tend to read with a whole-word or "gestalt" attack rather than a letter-by-letter or syllable approach. Comprehension of words spelled aloud is impaired.

Aphasic Alexia

Aphasic alexia is implicated when reading and writing are impaired in the absence of a significant aphasia. This has also been referred to as a parietotemporal alexia (Benson, 1979). There is difficulty with identification of letters and words as well as a significant impairment of writing in all aspects of written tasks. Often, but not always, these patients will show elements of the Gerstmann syndrome; agraphia, acalculia, impairment of finger identification, and right-left disorientation. Hemianopsia is sometimes present, and apraxia is often found to accompany it.

Psycholinguistic Classification

In the 1970s researchers, primarily in Britain, began to describe classifications of acquired reading disorders based on errors made in reading aloud (Beauvois and Derousne, 1979; Coltheart, 1978; Marshall and Newcombe, 1973; Saffran and Marin, 1977; Shallice and Warrington, 1975). The following three classifications have become relatively well accepted:

Phonological Alexia

Phonological alexia is characterized by an inability to read pseudowords and some difficulty with low-frequency words (Beauvois and Derousne, 1979). High-frequency words are likely to be read correctly. Errors are usually visual errors; that is, the words identified are visually similar to the target words. Spelling may or may not be impaired, and aphasia may be absent. It is assumed that the patient with phonological alexia is impaired in the ability to use the letter-to-sound conversion rules of the language.

Deep Dyslexia

The patient with deep dyslexia makes predominantly semantic errors in oral reading; that is, the identified word is semantically related to the target word in some way. Visual and derivational errors (e.g., baker →''bakery'') also are made. Function words are misread much more often than contentives, and verbs are more difficult than adjectives, which are more difficult than nouns. The person with deep dyslexia also is unable to read pseudowords.

Surface Dyslexia

The syndrome of surface dyslexia is distinguished by poor ability to use grapheme-to-phoneme conversion rules, although there is a heavy reliance on these rules. Errors are phonologically similar to the target, and there is great sensitivity to spelling regularity. There is little sensitivity, however, to word meaning; the patient may match the meaning to the word he or she has identified, even though it may not fit in context.

Visual Agnosia

Visual agnosia is classically defined as a disorder of visual recognition secondary to acquired brain disease. Visual acuity is adequate, intelligence is normal, and aphasia is absent. It is assumed that the visual agnosias are produced by damage to the visual association cortex bilaterally in Brodmann's areas 18 and 19. Pure agnosia is rare; in fact, the aphasias, dyslexias, and apraxias are considered more common than the agnosias. However, the presence of a classic visual agnosia may contribute to acquired reading disorders.

In recent years, the category of visual agnosia has been broadened to include cortical blindness and the various imperceptions that are associated with brain injury. It is difficult to distinguish between pure visual agnosia and cortical blindness. It is assumed that cortical blindness is a loss of visual perception due to bilateral occipital or parietal-occipital lesions that destroy the primary visual cortex or optic radiation. Individuals diagnosed as having cortical blindness usually have blind areas (scotomae) in their visual fields.

In addition to pure agnosia and cortical blindness, many brain-damaged patients present with symptoms of hemispatial imperceptions, known as neglect, and hemiinattentions. The signs of neglect and inattention, usually seen on the left side of the body and associated with right brain damage, contribute to the broad category of visual imperception that affects the ability to read normally, as do the visual agnosias.

Types of Visual Agnosia

The cornerstone of the classic concept of visual agnosia is a failure to recognize objects through vision with a preserved ability to recognize them through touch and hearing. The implication is absence of a primary loss of vision as seen in cortical blindness. The classic concept of visual agnosia derives from Lissauer's (1890) description of a visual object agnosia. He divided the syndrome into two types, which are commonly but not universally accepted: apperceptive and associative visual agnosia.

Apperceptive agnosia is the more controversial of the two subtypes. It is assumed to occur in what is called the first stage of visual recognition in which perceived elements of the visual stimulus are synthesized into a whole. It is considered a mild but high level deficit in visual perception underlying the failure to recognize objects. Patients presenting with this disorder appear blind, although visual acuity is usually normal or near normal. Kirshner (1986) believes that in actuality apperceptive agnosia may be a recovery stage in true cortical blindness. Patients cannot match letters or words, nor can they copy them. The deficit produces a severe reading disorder.

Associative visual agnosia is a disorder of the second stage of visual recognition in that the meaning of a stimulus is appreciated by recall of previous visual experiences. This syndrome is more clearly defined than apperceptive agnosia. These patients also fail to recognize faces and colors, but they can describe the elements of drawings and make copies of these drawings. They cannot, however, recognize the picture or objects. Most individuals cannot recognize letters and words and have an alexia. Right homonymous hemianopsia and a short-term memory disturbance are often present. Bilateral occipital lesions are often present with an associative disorder.

THE NORMAL READER

To formulate treatment plans for acquired reading disorders, it is helpful to have some understanding of what is thought to occur during the normal reading process (i.e., to have a model). Marshall (1985) provides a flow diagram and explanation of an information-processing model of reading, as shown in Figure 24.1. In this model, the normal reader uses early visual analysis (EVA) to extract visual features from the stimuli. These are then fed through three distinct reading routes: the direct route, the lexical route, and the phonic route.

The Direct Route

Readers depending solely on the direct route have access only to their ''sight vocabulary.'' Use of the direct route is thought to occur by the EVA feeding a global mechanism called whole-word representations, or WWR. Visual stimulus information such as word length and overall configuration is processed in parallel and helps to locate representations of the

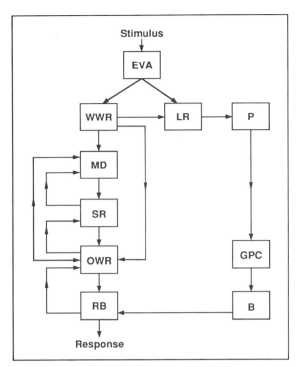

Figure 24.1. Mechanisms implicated in Marshall's model of normal reading. EVA = early visual analysis; WWR = whole word representations; LR = letter representation; P = graphemic parser; MD = morphological decomposition; SR = semantic representations; OWR = output word representations; GPC = grapheme-phoneme conversion; B = blender; RB = response buffer.

words. An arbitrary code is then generated that finds phonological representation of the word in the OWR (oral word representations). A feedback loop from the OWR to semantic representations accesses meaning. Readers depending only on the direct route may read regular and irregular words equally well. They may have difficulty interpreting homophones and classifying semantic information because of limited access to the lexical route. Nonsense words often cannot be read accurately because of poor use of the phonological route.

The Lexical Route

When this pathway is used WWR are fed to morphological decomposition (MD) where the whole words are segmented into potential base forms and affixes. This mechanism seems to operate primarily by rule generalization; words, therefore, may be segmented incorrectly at times. The segmented word form is then sent to semantic representation (SR) for a syntactic-semantic interpretation. A correctly segmented form will be matched and sent to OWR for phonological assignment. Incorrect morphological parsing prevents a match in SR, and the form is returned to MD for alternative parsing. When a match is made in SR, the segment is sent to OWR and then to the response buffer (RB). A reader using only the lexical route would not be able to read nonsense words aloud, would probably misread words with inflectional or derivational structure, and would have difficulty reading functor words and make frank semantic substitutions. Patients with *phonological alexia* and *deep dyslexia*, as described above, are thought to be depending primarily on the lexical route.

The Phonological Route

On activation of this route, letter recognition features are fed from the EVA to letter representations (LR), and abstract letter identities are assigned. Words are entered into the grapheme parser (P) after having been segmented into their component letters. During this stage the string of letters is segmented into graphemic chunks that will be identified as a single phoneme in real words or regularly spelled nonwords. This output is then sent to the grapheme-phoneme correspondence (GPC) rules, and each single or multicharacter phoneme is associated with the phoneme that is its most frequent realization. Words that contain irregular spellings will be misparsed during P and will be associated with an incorrect phonological code. The output of GPC is sent to the blender (B), where it is assigned an articulatory code. It then is sent to the RB to await final triggering for verbal output. Readers depending on the phonological route will misread irregularly spelled words and nonwords, often "regularizing" them. Semantic interpretation then depends on what the reader thought the word was. Readers with *surface dyslexia* are probably depending on the phonological route.

Automatic Versus Controlled Processing

Schneider and Shiffrin (1977) have theorized that most normal readers learn to use both automatic and controlled processing in reading. Good readers use primarily automatic processing, which implies a learned association in long-term memory that occurs with consistent training. It operates in parallel with other processes and does not require "cognitive attention." Controlled processing becomes necessary for new words or for comprehension of difficult text.

ASSESSMENT OF ACQUIRED READING DISORDERS

Patient History

With these clients, it is vital that a thorough "literacy history" be obtained. This should include educational levels, study habits in school, occupation and work habits, types of reading usually done daily, and, if the client can remember, what approach was used when he or she was taught to read. Listing what types of reading tasks the client must do to get along in his or her current routine and occupation, as well as listing what other kind of reading is desirable, is time well spent during the assessment.

Perceptual Testing

When confronted with a patient who might have visual agnosia or related visual imperceptual disorders, a systematic examination must be planned and executed by the speech-language pathologist. Other professionals should be called on to perform sections of the examination. The neurologist or neuroophthamologist may assist in completing the following assessments: (*a*) near and far point acuity of each; (*b*) visual fields; (*c*) binocular capacities, including accommodation suppression and diplopia; and (*d*) oculomotor functions. Once this initial examination is completed, investigation of possible visual agnosia or imperception problems may be assessed.

No standardized tests of visual agnosia are available, but Strub and Black (1985) have suggested the following procedure for identifying an apperceptive disorder: (*a*) Ask the patient to identify verbally a series of common objects presented visually; (*b*) if the patient fails to identify the object, allow him or her to manipulate the object; (*c*) it is assumed that if the patient readily identifies the object after manipulation with the use of kinesthetic cues, the visual disorder is an apperceptive agnosia; and (*d*) test the ability to match printed letters and words as well as copy them and say them. Failure points to an apperceptive disorder. The validity of the tasks is confounded by a coexisting aphasia or dementia in the patient.

An associative visual agnosia can be assessed by asking the patient to verbally identify an object and demonstrate its use. If the patient recognizes the object and can verify this by matching it to a like object as well as demonstrate its use, but cannot verbally identify it, the speech-language pathologist should suspect an associative agnosia. Again, aphasia or dementia may confound correct diagnosis.

Visual hemineglect usually can be established by having a patient copy a series of simple pictures like a clock or a plant (see Strub and Black, 1985, p. 24). The neglected portion of the drawing will be omitted or grossly distorted. Asking the patient to copy a series of letters on a piece of paper from left to right may also be used as a simple test of neglect. Omission or distortion of letters on one side of a page will suggest visual hemineglect.

Aphasia Batteries

Prior to planning a treatment program for the retraining of reading, assessment of the characteristics and severity of the deficit is necessary. Initial evaluation of the extent of impairment may be done as part of the total aphasia assessment by using any of several standardized aphasia batteries. Specifically, the Aphasia Language Performance Scales (ALPS) (Keenan and Brassell, 1975), the Minnesota Test for Differential Diagnosis of Aphasia (MTDDA) (Schuell, 1965), the Boston Diagnostic Aphasia Examination (BDAE) Goodglass and Kaplan, 1972), and the Western Aphasia Battery (WAB) Kertesz, 1982) each contain a section that enables the clinician to survey comprehension of single words, sentences, and short paragraphs. The Porch Index of Communicative Ability (PICA) (Porch, 1981) also tests comprehension at the sentence level, emphasizing nouns, verbs, and locatives. In addition, the MTDDA allows testing of visual matching skills and knowledge of the alphabet.

It should be noted, as a word of caution, that the research of Nicholas et al. (1986) using multiple sentence reading test items from widely used aphasia batteries as well as the RCBA (see below) demonstrated that the questions were often answered correctly by both normal and aphasic subjects who had not read the passages questioned. More comprehensive assessment is usually needed.

Comprehensive Assessment

Even if the client appears to be reading only at the single-word level, further assessment is usually necessary to define more clearly the deficits and locate the strengths or facilitators of successful reading. There are a limited number of assessments designed to explore reading skill in acquired brain injury. One such tool is the Reading Comprehension Battery for Aphasia (RCBA) (LaPointe and Horner, 1979). The RCBA enables the clinician to analyze patterns of errors such as visual, auditory, and semantic confusion. In addition, sentence and paragraph comprehension can be evaluated, although, as indicated above, results can be misleading.

Achievement Batteries

Although the standardized reading achievement batteries employed in school systems are not widely used in the practice of aphasia management, they can provide valuable information. Batteries such as the Gates-McGinite (Gates and MacGinite, 1978), The Stanford Diagnostic Reading Tests (Karlsen and Gardner, 1985), The California Achievement Reading Tests (1977), and The Woodcock Reading Mastery Test (1973) are helpful in planning interventions. These are useful especially with mildly impaired clients who aspire to reacquire skills at or near the premorbid level.

Oral Reading

Comprehension through silent reading is the most important skill to be evaluated in these clients, since this is the functional method of reading used by most people. Reading aloud, however, can be an important key in assessment and is the only way to categorize a disorder into one of the psycholinguistic classifications.

It has been suggested that word lists should be constructed to include high-frequency nouns; consonant-vowel-consonant (CVC) words organized according to vowel patterns; semantic groupings (e.g., fruits, clothing, sports), words with regular grapheme-phoneme conversion and words with potential for letter reversals and transpositions (Johnson, 1986). An experimental reading battery designed by Rothi and Moss (1985), called the Battery of Adult Reading Function, used word lists divided into regular words, rule-governed words, irregular words, functor words, and nonsense words. With testing designed in this manner, Rothi and Moss were able to delineate on which reading routes the reader was dependent and which routes were weak or unused. Treatment was then designed to strengthen the use of those routes.

Reading Rate

It is important to take a measure of speed of reading for text and to do a comprehension check after the measurement, especially with the client with the milder impairment. In this way it can be stated that the client reads at _____ words per minute with _____% comprehension.

Comprehension of Text

Clients who can read at a simple paragraph level should be evaluated as to comprehension and oral reading of text (Johnson, 1986; Weaver, 1988). Clinicians should have on hand several different reading passages at different grade levels. These should be about 500 words each, as research has shown that the quality of reading errors changes after the first 200 words, when the reader begins to develop meaning. The material should have a strong plot and identifiable theme. It should be something that the client can understand and relate to but that is new to him or her. A measure of comprehension should be done having the client, if possible, retell the story. This gives the clinician an idea of how well the reader remembers and interprets what is read. Reading rate can also be done with this material.

Error Analysis

The client should be asked to read the passages aloud after silent comprehension is measured. This can be recorded, and an error or miscue analysis can be performed later. According to Weaver (1988), the miscue analysis procedure may be used to determine the reader's strategies and the use of context. Questions should be asked concerning whether the miscue went with the preceding context or the following context, whether it preserved the essential meaning, and whether it was corrected. It is important to know that because it was corrected or because the miscue still preserved the essential meaning, no significant loss in comprehension occurred.

Cognitive-Linguistic Assessment

If the client can participate, testing of higher level cognitive functions is recommended. Questions need to be answered regarding such things as attention, reasoning, memory, and ability to access information not directly given in the text.

DECISIONS REGARDING INTERVENTION

Once the assessments and history are completed, the first decision must be whether treatment can significantly change the client's ability to read. This decision must be made on the basis of severity of the disorder, the client's motivation, and the presence of other complicating conditions such as memory deficit, visual disturbance, or severe deficit in other language modalities. If there is uncertainty, it should be presented honestly to the client and the family, and they must decide whether to participate. If only limited progress is predicted, the client must decide if the effort and expense involved are worth the predicted outcome. Aids and strategies to help the client who cannot read well should be presented at this time.

STIMULUS PARAMETERS

Most of us are deluged daily with printed matter. Thus, reading stimuli are readily available. Much of it may be inappropriate for a certain client, and great care must be taken in choosing suitable material. Compatible stimuli may include simple but common items from the environment such as menus, signs, maps, tickets, tourist brochures, telephone books, and directions printed for consumer information. A number of language workbooks that contain useful activities for aphasia therapy are available. There are also a few reading skills series that were designed for remedial classes and adult literacy classes that are most helpful. Appendix 24.1 lists published sources of selected stimuli.

Although materials are much more plentiful than they once were for adult reading training, the clinician must still individually design many of the activities presented in order to take into account the factors that will influence patient performance. These factors are listed below.

Frequency. Words that occur less frequently in the English language are often more difficult to read and understand than more frequently

occurring words (Halpern, 1965). The exception to this rule may be the connectors ("and") and functors ("but," "if") that occur frequently in our language but have been found to be difficult, especially for clients with agrammatism. Frequency is highly correlated with word length, abstractness, and familiarity in reading.

Length. In many cases, the longer words are more difficult. This variable is, however, greatly affected by frequency of occurrence and abstractness.

Imagery Value. Paivio et al. (1968) have compiled a long list of words ranked as to their rated "imagery value" or to what extent the word "evoked a mental image." Research by Marshall and Newcombe (1966), Richardson (1975), and Webb and Love (1983) has shown imagery level to be strongly correlated with success on reading tasks given to aphasic patients.

Other considerations, especially for the client with alexia without agraphia have been listed by Godwin (1983). These are size of print, density, typeface (use lowercase letters), spacing, and similarities of shape.

USE OF COMPUTERS AND OTHER EQUIPMENT

Access to computer technology and software programs does not guarantee success in retraining reading. It can, however, add variety to the necessary drills and sometimes save the clinician time in designing materials and tracking performance on certain tasks. Aaron and Baker (1991) caution that software be carefully selected with the following criteria in mind: (*a*) appropriateness for the ability level of the client; (*b*) interest level; (*c*) ease of use; and (*d*) cost. Appendix 24.1 includes listing of selected software programs for retraining reading.

Card readers such as the Language Master and the Voxcom may be valuable at the word or sentence level of reading training. Vocabulary may be tailored to the individual needs. The pictures and/or the written words may be put on the card and then the words recorded. The client then may be allowed independent time for drill work on this vocabulary or these sentences.

PERCEPTUAL TRAINING

Symptoms of cortical blindness, visual neglect, and inattention, as well as the rare cases of visual agnosia, are responsive both to spontaneous recovery and to training regimens (Gouvier and Warner, 1987). The spontaneous recovery of visuoperceptual disorders has been well documented in the neurological literature (Colombo et al., 1982; Hier et al., 1983; Meerwaldt, 1983). This literature suggests that most of the severe symptoms of hemiimperception of the right-brain-damaged patient resolve themselves within a year. Many patients recover faster than that, with major recovery occurring within the first 6 months followed by lesser increments of improvement. It may be that training programs can facilitate spontaneous recovery of visuoperceptual skills but offer little improvement in patients with profound and lasting imperceptual problems. If these perceptual problems underlie the acquired dyslexia in a significant way, training of higher reading-processing skills may be difficult and almost impossible.

Treatment regimens have been effective with a variety of reading problems. Zihl (1980) has indicated that cerebrovascular accident (CVA) patients with cortical blindness improved their ability to localize visual stimuli when they practiced looking in the direction of stimuli presented within the scotomae.

Zihl and VonCramon (1979) had 12 brain-injured individuals of various types practice identification of lights at the margins of their scotomae and found the scotomae were reduced in size. These studies suggest the possibility that visuoperceptual training regimens may be helpful in improving the occasional case of verified pure agnosia. Weinberg et al. (1982) employed training procedures involving the use of spatial coordinates for stimulus location and organization of stimuli into patterns, as well as the procedure for visual exploration, and found gains in visual analysis and organization in right-brain-damaged CVA patients free of neglect problems. In an early study, Lawson (1962) studied two right-brain-damaged CVA patients who were trained with reminders to "look left" and to use finger tracing to keep their place in reading activities. These simple procedures yielded improvement in the domain of reading but did not seem to improve the left spatial hemiimperception further.

The neuropsychological literature that has been reviewed suggests that a variety of training procedures are effective in remediating reading problems and visual imperception in the brain-damaged patient. It should be noted that the training research is directed primarily at left-side imperception associated with right brain damage. These patients have been particularly appropriate targets for intervention because such patients are free of aphasia for the most part, and the sparing of their verbal abilities can often be drawn on for compensation training. Information on left-brain-damaged individuals with acquired dyslexia is sorely needed to determine if visuoperceptual training procedures are as effective in improving reading and visual imperception impairment in these patients. Whatever the outcome, it appears that the reported training techniques have some validity in brain injury.

A question remains: What is the role of speech-language pathologists in the area of visuoperceptual training in the patient with a reading disorder? Research by Weinberg et al. (1977) has suggested that visual scanning procedures and cancellation training as outlined in the neuropsychological literature have a greater impact on visual spatial hemineglect than does routine occupational therapy alone. It may be that if the speech-language pathologist is faced with a patient with a reading disorder coexisting with visual spatial hemineglect, it would be appropriate to incorporate into the reading therapy one of the neuropsychological training paradigms that involve scanning and cancellation techniques. With improvement in visual imperception, the speech-language pathologist may then proceed to more traditional methods of dyslexia treatment.

SPECIFIC READING TASKS

The clinician must review the data from testing to determine the client's level of functioning. Is he or she at the visual matching level, single-word level, phrase level, sentence level, or paragraph level? Within this level, what length, frequency, abstraction level, contextual cues, and so on facilitate the comprehension? Is there a particular print size or a way of looking at the page (e.g., through a word window) that is facilitory? Answers to these questions will influence the choice of intervention targets.

It should be remembered in reading training that accurate comprehension of what is read is the principal goal, not accurate oral reading. Reading comprehension should be a generative process and should be facilitated by designing treatment tasks and selecting stimuli that allow cognitive interaction with the material (Wittrock, 1981).

Single-Word Level

For the client with a severe reading problem, it will be necessary to begin at the single-word level with recognition tasks. These will lead to more advanced tasks targeting comprehension. A true comprehension task requires the client to demonstrate in some way that the meaning of the word or words is understood, not merely the configuration recognized as a certain word in a closed-choice task. It is customary with aphasic patients to begin at a recognition level, aiming for true reading comprehension as therapy proceeds.

Recognition training is begun with matching tasks that require the client to match a written word to another written word, to an auditory stimulus, and finally to a picture. These are good starting tasks for the client learning single-word comprehension. If the client needs prior work on visual discrimination, then matching letter-to-letter and word-to-word tasks are very important. It is suggested that the client be required to meet a 100% criterion before moving from these discrimination tasks.

Though many clinicians (Darley, 1982; LaPointe, 1978; Schuell et al., 1964) recommend the tasks of pointing to letters named by the clinician or learning the alphabet by rote, we have not found these useful in retraining reading except in certain cases. For the client who has visual discrimination problems, time spent on this is necessary so that he or she may learn to scan and discriminate accurately and rapidly. The clients who benefit from spelling a word aloud to process it must also be adept with the alphabet letters, and these tasks are useful for them. Other clients do not, in our experience, benefit tremendously from the time spent on learning the names of the letters, and we recommend going to single words as soon as possible.

The matching tasks with words should use words that are relevant as possible. "Environmental notice" reading (e.g., restroom signs, exit, stop, push-pull) is very important to train early, and matching tasks with these signal words may be used initially. From there one may go to having the patient point to the word described that would fit with a certain picture. With all multiple-choice tasks, the choices should be limited to 2 or 3 initially and then increased to 8 or 10.

Comprehension at the single-word level can be begun using pictures in which there are many choices for targets. The clients must choose the object or concept in the picture referred to by the word shown. Verbs are a good choice, as gestures may be used to demonstrate comprehension. Early in word comprehension training, such words as "put," "give," "touch," "turn," and so on should be targeted because of their application in following written directions.

Single-word vocabulary training is aided by labeling also. The family of the client is asked to label objects around the house with their written names. In this way, the client is exposed to the words many times a day and associations are strengthened.

Opportunities should be designed for cognitive and functional interaction with the vocabulary. The number of words in the vocabulary should continue to be increased, as 90% comprehension is reached with a wide variety of choices. If the client has the verbal ability, the words should be accurately read aloud by this point. If possible, he or she should explain the meaning or give an example of situations in which one would find it or use it. If writing is possible, the client should be copying the words and then independently writing them to dictation and for labels.

Godwin (1983) has outlined a comprehensive program for the treatment of pure alexia (or alexia without agraphia). This four-stage program begins with letter- and word-recognition tasks. It takes the reader through phoneme-grapheme correspondence training to sentences with reduced print size and finally to the development of subskills to stabilize functional reading. For more severely impaired clients, this program appears well organized and quite useful. It has been empirically validated in the author's clinical practice with a small number of patients with pure alexia.

Oral Reading of Single Words

A treatment program to improve recognition and oral reading of single words has been designed by Rothi and Moss (1985). The Battery of Adult Reading Function is used to identify which reading routes need to be strengthened. The authors then suggest designs for activities that target each route. These are briefly summarized here.

Phonic Route. Nonwords or words that have direct grapheme-phoneme correspondence are used in the oral reading tasks. Accurate phonological decisions are the task objective.

Lexical Route. Exposure time for the words is limited to 500 to 600 milliseconds with a tachistoscope or as long as it takes to say it if exposing by hand. Stimuli should be real words that require a lexically based phonological analysis, not a semantic analysis.

Direct Route. A brief 350-millisecond exposure or a flash by hand exposure is used. Words should require a semantic analysis rather than a phonological analysis.

Phrase and Sentence Level

The client who has a single-word vocabulary of 50 to 100 nouns and verbs that can be easily comprehended is ready to combine those words for phrases and sentences. This may be begun by selecting pictures that depict images of noun-verb combinations that the client should know as separate words. He or she then may be shown the phrase or sentence and picture combination and hear them read aloud to him or he or she may read them aloud. The client then begins to match the sentences with the picture stimuli, and the number of foils are increased.

The client may now begin attempting to follow written directions. These may be at a very simple level dealing with movement of body parts or manipulation of objects on the desk in front of him or her. Complexity of the directions may be increased systematically using vocabulary, length, and syntax parameters to increase the difficulty level. Darley (1982) lists a suggested lexicon that may be taught as single words and then combined easily for following printed commands. Thorough understanding of the prepositions involved in movement commands is essential to their successful completion. If the client is misunderstanding the spatial relationships implied by various prepositions, these tasks will bring these misunderstandings to light.

As Shewan and Bandur (1986) point out, it is important to recognize that several research studies of sentence comprehension in the reading of aphasic patients have shown that certain kinds of sentences are more difficult to understand than others. If the client has the verbal ability, the words should be accurately read aloud by this point. If possible, he or she should explain the meaning or give an example of situations in which one would find it or use it. If writing is possible, the client should be copying the words and then independently writing them to dictation and labels.

A very useful therapy task comes from the research of Gardner et al. (1975) on aphasics' understanding of semantic and syntactic errors in reading. In their research, they had the subjects find the semantic and syntactic errors in sentences. They found the semantic errors were more easily identified by aphasic subjects. This finding was corroborated by our research on residual deficits in aphasics' reading (Webb and Love, 1983). This research task, we also discovered, becomes a valuable treatment task because it makes the client carefully read the sentences and analyze them while searching for the errors. The client who can find the more subtle syntactic errors of subject-verb agreement or pluralization is one who is reading closely and is becoming able to comprehend meaning at a deeper level than surface semantics.

Comprehension of questions seems to be one of the more difficult reading tasks for aphasic readers. It is advisable to check the client's comprehension very early through the use of written questions. In this way he or she may begin to become more familiar with some of the more difficult linguistic aspects of questions, such as the subject-verb inversion. At the early stages of therapy, the speech-language pathologist may be reading the questions aloud, but exposure should be visual also.

Yes/no questions about personal information (''Are you married?'' ''Is your home in Kentucky?'') are often the easiest to comprehend. *Wh*-questions are often difficult, and the meaning of each *wh*-word may have to be drilled separately. If the client cannot say or write the answers to *wh*-questions, he or she can often point to some aspect of a picture to show comprehension.

For the client to be able to read above a third- to fourth-grade level, he or she will need to be able to comprehend sentences that are semantically and syntactically complex. He or she may need some practice in breaking down complex sentences into component parts. The client may need to actually underline the key words. He or she may need extra help with special structures such as conditional clauses. The embedding of clauses beginning with such words as ''unless,'' ''except,'' ''after,'' and ''instead of'' may present comprehension challenges that he or she cannot meet without help. Length can be an important variable to control in the sentences. Research by Albert et al. (1981) and Schuell et al. (1964) has shown that reading comprehension is reduced in Broca's aphasia by increasing length, whereas Wernicke's patients may actually do better, especially if there is redundancy as a result.

Gardner and Zurif (1976) found that prepositional constructs were difficult for aphasic subjects. Shewan and Bandur (1986) reported that several studies have collectively shown that both anterior- and posterior-lesioned patients find nonreversible, simple, active, affirmative sentences relatively easy. Anterior-lesioned patients find semantic true/false easier than syntactic true/false. They found true/false easier than fill-in-the-blank with a similar hierarchy between semantic and syntactic tasks. Reversible simple, active, affirmative declaratives were most difficult for these patients. Posterior-lesioned clients performed equally well on both true/false sentence types, and fill-in-the-blank tasks were not more difficult for them. Information such as this should be considered important in treatment task design.

If the client has the verbal ability, the words should be accurately read aloud by this point. If possible, he or she should explain the meaning or give an example of situations in which one would find it or use it. If writing is possible, the client should be copying the words and then independently writing them to dictation and labels.

PARAGRAPH AND TEXT LEVEL

Clients who can read increasingly well at the sentence level should be moved into reading of text as soon as possible. One of the ways to begin working on paragraphs is to combine sentences on which the client has demonstrated good understanding into a short, one-paragraph story. If there is a breakdown, then the paragraph can be analyzed into its familiar component sentences. At this point, comprehension is best tested by simple multiple-choice or verbal questioning.

Pierce (1983) has shown that aphasics use a reading strategy based on subject-verb-object present-tense construction. He found that comprehension improves when additional surface structure markers are available to point out when exceptions to that strategy should be used ("For example, the man *has* walked to the store" or "The girl is *being* kissed by the boy"). Therefore, paragraphs including structures such as these might be used initially to help the client with lengthier material.

The clinician should try to increase gradually the length and the informational complexity of paragraphs. Informational complexity is a function of two things: number of details in the contextual material and the semantic and syntactic level of the material. It may be best to experiment with varying both—one at a time—when the client is ready for increased complexity. If the success is greater with a variation in one than with the other, this form of increased complexity should be used in the written material. If both are equal, the clinician may then try using paragraph-length material that has both a greater number of details and expanded semantic and syntactic complexity.

When the client is reading short paragraphs with about 75% comprehension, longer text may be attempted. The passages should be more than 200 words and should be at or below the grade level at which the patient reads on an instructional level, that is, comprehension at 45% to 55%. The Bormuth Close Readability Procedure could be used to determine the grade level of any text not already so designated (Weaver, 1988). With this procedure, the client can participate in choosing text to read and then help determine if it is too difficult. Because the procedure requires that the person fill in blanks put in the reading material by omitting words, a language deficit may prevent the client's active participation. In this case, the clinician can use readability formulas for teachers, such those as listed in Vacca and Vacca (1986).

Wittrock (1981) has written an excellent chapter on reading comprehension in which he discusses manipulations of written material that have been shown to facilitate comprehension in normal readers. Some of these may be applicable to the disabled aphasic reader when working at the paragraph or text level. He reports that giving goals and objectives to the reader prior to the reading of the text enhances comprehension and memory of the information relevant to the goal. Goals and objectives given immediately after the reading focus attention less narrowly and therefore tend to facilitate comprehension and memory more broadly. The findings are the same for questions inserted in the text.

The client should read both silently and, if possible, aloud. Various strategies to assess comprehension may be used, depending on the degree of language disorder. He or she may be asked to retell what has been read. Verbal or written questions concerning the material may be given with the client answering verbally, in writing, or using a multiple-choice format. The questions should go beyond mere details of facts presented in the text. They should help the person relate the material to personal experiences. Cognitive-linguistic processes such as association, deductive reasoning, sequencing, and analysis should be called into play when reading the material to answer the questions.

The client may need to learn various strategies to increase success on measures of comprehension. Underlining or highlighting important details may help memory and concentration. Those with serious memory limitations, as sometimes occurs with traumatic brain injury, may need to take notes while reading and be allowed to refer to the notes during questioning or retelling. Much help is often needed initially to help the client discriminate the important details or facts from the less critical.

If the client can read aloud, the clinician will be able to check the use of contextual cues for confirming and predicting. Good use of contextual cues will minimize errors that change essential meaning. If there seems to be poor use of context, the reader should be stopped at errors that change meaning and asked to analyze whether the error fits with the context read thus far. An explanation of why it is a misfit can be given if the reader does not know and then he or she can read it correctly.

If there is a pattern of decreased comprehension after a certain amount of text is read, the client can be taught to stop after reading a certain number of words or paragraphs. He or she then should take time to analyze what has been read to this point. This can be done semiindependently or with questions from the clinician or someone else reading with the client. The goal is the client's ability to use previous context to understand context that follows.

There are a few clients who comprehend lengthy material better if they are allowed to read it all at once rather than stopping to analyze it paragraph by paragraph. If the client cannot analyze the paragraphs, let him or her try this method. This reading of the story as a "gestalt" is the end goal, after all, for the clients who reach a reading skill level of contextual material. Use of the generative process of summarizing the material in their own language should be required, however, following this reading.

The client may have particular difficulty in monitoring and comprehension of context that did not seem evident in previous work at the sentence level. One exercise that may target this is to work on following written directions. There are workbooks that have tasks designed to provide material for this, and there are some that target the language of directions (see Laubach Literacy and the *Specific Skills Series* by Boning in Appendix 24.1). This works particularly well when there are multistep directions toward a particular outcome. If the client is aware of what the outcome should be, the activity has built-in reinforcement, since following the directions correctly leads to the desired outcome.

It should be stressed here and in the following section particularly that the client must commit a significant amount of time to reading and the reading assignments in order to progress. If the client does little beyond what is done in the treatment session or only works on reading 1 or 2 more hours each week, success is highly unlikely. It is therefore critical that the client has an understanding at the beginning of therapy that it requires a great individual effort. Only the well-motivated, determined person will have a good chance of improving reading after brain injury.

DEVELOPING THE SKILLS OF THE MILDLY IMPAIRED READER

Often the speech-language pathologist will be asked to work with a client who fits into the classification of "mildly impaired." This may be a client who has been in treatment and has gradually regained reading skill, or it may be a client who spontaneously recovered rapidly to a point of this residual deficit. This client is the one who can read at or near the premorbid grade level and comprehend shorter material well if allowed to read very slowly. This laborious approach, however, makes reading for pleasure or for one's work almost impossible. These clients, we have found, often demonstrate accompanying short memory deficits, difficulty with higher-level graphic tasks, and distractibility.

As reported previously (Webb, 1982), we have had success with a limited number of these clients using techniques taken from speech-reading training. Since that report, other techniques as taken from adult literacy education and study skills training have also been found by the first author to be successful with these clients.

Much of the training includes the client's learning to scan material to search out main ideas and skim unimportant details. Exercises are used to promote scanning and decrease recognition time in reading. Ann Arbor publishers (see Appendix 24.1) has several programs available, such as *Letter Tracking* and *Thought Tracking*, that improve purposeful scanning. Other scanning activities can be easily created by the clinician, such as scanning phone directories for certain names or scanning magazine or newspaper articles for certain details. The client should work until scanning is as accurate and fast as the clinician's scanning ability.

It is essential that the client emphasize strategies that allow cognitive interaction with the material. He or she should be taught to scan the material for a sense of what it concerns, find the main idea, and continually analyze what is being read to confirm what he or she thought it was about and try to predict what is coming next. This client may also have to stop at various points in the material and take notes or consciously summarize it mentally. Over time, however, this should be the method the reader uses automatically. Aaron and Baker (1991) point out that comprehension monitoring is a metacognitive process and, thus, difficult but very useful in improving reading comprehension. If a great deal of reading is used in the work setting or school work, therefore, the client may always need to take notes on reading material, especially if memory is a factor. Outlining may also be another good method, especially for the student.

Organizational strategies may be particularly relevant to the needs of these clients. They seem to lack the ability to organize and summarize the information gleaned from reading and the notes they took. Raphael (1984) offers an organizational strategy called the QAR, or Question-Answer-Relationship strategy. In training this method, the reader is provided experiences using three different sources of information. They are described to the client as (*a*) *Right There*: the answer can be found stated in the text; (*b*) *Think and Search*: the answer is in the text but not directly stated; and (*c*) *On My Own*: requires search of personal knowledge for the answer. When reading for a specific purpose or questions to answer, QAR would help the reader organize his or her approach.

Increasing Rate

Once the client is adept at the scanning, at searching for the main idea and confirmational details, and at summarizing with note taking, comprehension should improve with some decrease in reading time and effort. The laborious word-by-word reading of some clients still may greatly reduce speed of processing. Speed-reading training uses rapid fixation or perception exercises to force the reader to take in more information at one visual fixation. Flash cards, a tachistoscope, or a similar program on a computer can be used to present the words and phrases. Speed-reading texts such as *How to Read Better and Faster* (Lewis, 1978) contain exercises that can be used in this training. Some speed-reading trainers advocate the use of full pages of text that are scrolled at various rates rather than flashing words or phrases. If available, both kinds of exercises can be tried. Intensive practice must be done if progress is to be made.

It should also be understood by the clinician as well as the client that in *all* readers there is usually a trade-off between comprehension and speed. Thus, once a person increases speed, he or she must choose when to use the fastest reading and when to read more slowly so that comprehension will be maximized.

Teaching Phonics

Experience with the mildly impaired clients has demonstrated that some of them will improve enough to need some word-attack skills training so that an attempt may be made to "sound out" an unrecognized word. It should be emphasized to the clients that the time should not be taken for this activity if failure to pronounce the word does not reduce overall comprehension of the material. This is frequently true with character's names, cities, and so on. Rather than struggle, the reader should just call it "blank" or something else and proceed reading. If, however, the difficult words carry greater linguistic weight than this, it is useful to be able to try to pronounce it.

The clinician should first make sure the client knows the consonant sounds, because consonants facilitate pronunciation more than do vowels. The client can often figure out the word sounding out the consonants and guessing at the vowels.

There are only a few phonic rules that are consistent enough or that cover enough words to warrant spending a great deal of time on teaching, according to May and Elliott (1973). The consistent rules are listed below:

1. The VCE pattern. In one-syllable words containing two vowels, one of which is a final *e*, the first vowel usually represents a long vowel and the final *e* is silent.

2. The CV pattern. When there is only one vowel letter in a word or syllable and it comes at the end, it usually represents a long vowel.
3. The VC pattern. In either a word or syllable, a single vowel letter followed by a letter, digraph, or blend usually represents a short vowel sound.
4. The "g rule." When g comes at the end of words or just before a, o, or u, it sounds like /g/. Otherwise it has the /dz/ sound. *Get, give, begin,* and *girl* are important exceptions.
5. The "c rule." When c comes just before a, o, or u, it usually has the /k/ sound. Otherwise it usually has an /s/ sound.
6. The "r rule." The letter r usually modifies the short or long sound of the preceding vowel.
7. The VV pattern. In a word or syllable containing a vowel digraph, the first letter of the digraph usually represents a long vowel sound and the second is usually silent. This is fairly reliable for *ee, oa, ay, ea* and *ai* but not as reliable as others.

These rules regarding grapheme-phoneme conversion can be taught one by one to the client, and exercises can be given and incorporated into reading material. Work would continue on other aspects of reading simultaneously. Obviously, only the aphasic patient with retained ability for new learning would be a candidate for this training.

COMPENSATORY STRATEGIES

Many of the clients that we see for treatment will not be able to recover to their premorbid level of reading skill. Because it is true that a great many people in our population do not read in their work nor read much for pleasure, this impairment frequently does not interrupt routine. For those clients who did enjoy reading as an important part of their life, there are a few strategies that may assist.

Talking Books

The public library in most cities can help the client obtain "talking books." These were originally developed for the visually impaired but are available to anyone who can document an inability to read. The client is loaned a tape player and can check out or receive by mail a variety of tape-recorded reading material. This program has given much pleasure to reading-impaired adult clients. Books on tape are also readily available in bookstores now, frequently even for recently published works.

Reading Partners

The client may also recruit a friend or find a volunteer who will spend some time each day or each week reading to him or her. The newspapers, mail, magazines, novels, and so on may be chosen as desired material. At work, the mildly impaired reader may need to find a partner who will help read through material that must be digested rapidly.

FUTURE TRENDS

The reading disorders resulting from acquired brain damage remain a challenge to the clinician. As research in normal reading expands, it is likely that further elaboration of the mechanisms involved in reading will come forth and there will be acceptance of the model among reading specialists, researchers, and clinicians. When it is understood how normal reading occurs and when we know all the performance variables

that should be considered, we will be better able to define an aphasic individual's reading problem. There are many now who purport to do this, but there is little agreement among professionals about what is actually occurring.

It is also very likely that computers will play a greater role in the reading treatment of the future. As they become less expensive and more accessible to the clinicians and to the clients, many of the drill programs necessary in reading training will be presented via the computer. It will become easier for the clinician to design programs and to control variables such as vocabulary and length of exposure.

Technology will also advance the use of assistive devices for the impaired reader. There are now devices available for the blind that enable them to read text not translated into Braille. These scanners are passed over the text, and the print is converted into synthesized or digitized speech output. It is hoped that one day such devices would be more available as the technology improves and cost decreases. The aphasic person who cannot recover normal reading ability would then have opportunities for independence in reading that are now not possible.

References

Aaron, P. G., and Baker, C. (1991). *Reading disabilities in college and high school: Diagnosis and management.* Parkton, MD: New York Press, Inc.

Albert, M. L., Goodglass, H., Helm, N. A., Rubens, A. B. and Alexander, M. P. (1981). *Clinical aspects of dysphasia.* In G. E. Arnold, F. Winckel and B. D. Wyke (Eds.), *Disorders of human communication 2.* New York: Springer-Verlag.

Beauvois, M. F., and Derousne, J. (1979). Phonological alexia: Three dissociations. *Journal of Neurology, Neurosurgery, and Psychiatry, 42,* 1115–1124.

Benson, D. F. (1977). The third alexia. *Archives of Neurology, 34,* 327–331.

Benson, D. F. (1979). *Aphasia, alexia and agraphia.* New York: Churchill Livingston.

Benson, D. F., and Geschwind N. (1969). *The alexias.* In P. Vinken and G. Bruyn (Eds.), *Handbook of clinical neurology* (Vol. 4). Amsterdam: North-Holland.

California Achievement Tests: Reading. (1977). Monteray, VA: CTB/McGraw Hill.

Colombo, A., DeRenzi, E., and Genntilini, M. (1982). The time course of visual hemi-inattention. *Archives of Psychiatry and Neurological Sciences, 231,* 529–546.

Coltheart, M. (1978). Lexical access in simple reading tasks. In G. Underwood (Ed.), *Strategies of information processing.* London: Academic Press.

Coltheart, M. (1980). *Deep dyslexia,* London: Routledge & Kegan.

Darley, F. L. (1982). *Aphasia.* Philadelphia, PA: W. B. Saunders.

Davis, A. (1983). *A survey of adult aphasia.* Englewood Cliffs, NJ: Prentice-Hall.

Delis, D., Wapner, W., Gardner, H., and Moses, J. (1983). Right hemisphere and the organization of paragraphs. *Cortex, 19,* 43–50.

Deloche, G., Andrewsky, E., and Desi, M. (1982). Surface dyslexia: A case report and some theoretical implications to reading models. *Brain and Language, 15,* 12–31.

Friedman, R. B., and Albert, M. C. (1985). Alexia. In K. Heilman and E. Valenstein (Eds.), *Clinical neuropsychology.* New York: Oxford University Press.

Gardner, H., Denes, G., and Zurif, E. (1975). Critical reading at the sentence level in aphasia. *Cortex, 11,* 60–72.

Gardner, H., and Zurif, E. (1975). Bee but not be: Oral reading of single words in aphasia and alexia. *Neuropsychologica, 13,* 181–190.

Gardner, H., and Zurif, E. (1976). Critical reading of words and phrases in aphasia. *Brain and Language, 3,* 173–190.

Gates, A., and MacGinite, W. (1978). *Gates-MacGinite Reading Tests.* New York: Columbia University Press.

Godwin, R. (1983). The treatment of pure alexia. In C. Code and D. J. Muller (Eds.), *Aphasia therapy.* London: Edward Arnold (Publishers) Ltd.

Goodglass, H., and Kaplan, E. (1972). The Boston Diagnostic Aphasia *Examination*. In H. Goodglass and E. Kaplan (Eds.), *The assessment of aphasia and related disorders*. Philadelphia, PA: Lea & Febiger.

Gouvier, W. D. and Warner, M. S. (1987). Treatment of visual imperception and related disorders. In J. M. Williams and C. J. Long (Eds.), *The rehabilitation of cognitive disabilities* (pp. 109–122). New York: Plenum Press.

Halpern, H. (1975). Effects of stimulus variables on dysphasic verbal errors. *Perceptual Motor Skills*, 21, 291–295.

Hecaen, H., and Kremin, H. (1976). Neurolinguistic research on reading disorders resulting from left hemisphere lesions: Aphasic and "pure" alexias. In H. Whitaker and H. Whitaker (Eds.), *Studies in neurolinguistics* (Vol. 2). New York: Academic Press.

Hier, D. B., and Mohr, J. P. (1977). Incongruous oral and written naming; Evidence for a subdivision of Wernicke's aphasia. *Brain and Language*, 4, 115–126.

Hier, D. B., Mondlock, J., and Caplan, L. R. (1983). Recovery of brain abnormalities after right hemisphere stroke. *Neurology*, 33, 345–350.

Johnson, D. (1986). Remediation for dyslexic adults. In G. T. Pavlidus and D. F. Fisher (Eds.), *Dyslexia: Its neuropsychology and treatment*. New York: John Wiley.

Karlsen, B., and Gardner, F. (1985). *Stanford Diagnostic Reading Test* (3rd ed.). San Antonio, TX: The Psychological Corporation.

Keenan, J., and Brassell, E. (1975). *Aphasia Language Performance Scales*. Murfreesboro, TN: Pinnacle Press.

Kertesz, A. (1982). *The Western Aphasia Battery*. New York: Grune & Stratton.

Kirshner, H. S. (1986). *Behavioral neurology: A practical approach*. New York: Churchill Livingstone.

Kirshner, H. S., and Webb, W. G. (1982). Alexia and agraphia in Wernicke's aphasia. *Journal of Neurology, Neurosurgery and Psychiatry*, 45, 719–724.

LaPointe, L. (1978). Aphasia therapy: Some principles and strategies for treatment. In D. Johns (Ed.), *Clinical management of neurogenic communicative disorders*, Boston, MA: Little, Brown.

LaPointe, L., and Horner, J. (1979). *Reading Comprehension Battery for Aphasia*. Tigard, OR: CC Publications.

LaPointe, L., and Kraemer, I. (1983). Treatment of alexia without agraphia. In W. Perkins (Ed.), *Current therapy of communication: Language handicaps in adults*, New York: Thieme-Stratton.

Lawson, I. R. (1962). Visual-spatial neglect in lesions of the right cerebral hemisphere. *Neurology*, 12, 23–33.

Lewis, N. (1978). *How to read better and faster*. New York: T. Y. Crowell.

Lissauer, H. (1890). Ein fall von seelenblindheit nebst einen beitrag zur theorie derselben. *Archives of Psychiatry*, 20, 222–270.

Marshall, J. C. (1985). On some relationships between acquired and developmental dyslexias. In F. H. Duffy and N. Geschwind (Eds.), *Dyslexia: A neuroscientific approach to clinical evaluation*. Boston, MA: Little, Brown.

Marshall, J., and Newcombe, F. (1966). Syntactic and semantic errors in paralexia. *Neuropsychologia*, 4, 169–176.

Marshall, J. C., and Newcombe, F. (1973). Patterns of paralexia: A psycholinguistic approach. *Journal of Psycholinguistic Research*, 2, 175–186.

May, F. B. and Elliott, S. (1973). *To help children read: Mastery performance modules for teachers in training*. Columbus, OH: Charles C. Merrill.

Meerwaldt, J. D. (1983). Spatial disorientation in right handed infarction: A study of recovery. *Journal of Neurology, Neurosurgery and Psychiatry*, 46, 426–429.

Moyers, S. (1979). Rehabilitation of alexia: A case study. *Cortex*, 15, 139–144.

Newcombe, F., Hiorns, R., Marshall, J., and Adams, C. (1975). Acquired dyslexia: Patterns of deficit and recovery. *Outcome of severe damage to the central nervous system: A CIBA Foundation symposium*. New York: American Elsevier.

Nicholas, L. E., MacLennon, D. L. and Brookshire, R. H. (1986). Validity of multiple-sentence reading comprehension. *Journal of Speech and Hearing Disorders*, 51, 82–87.

Paivio, A., Yuille, J., and Madigan, S. (1968). Concreteness, imagery and meaningfulness values for 925 nouns. *Journal of Experimental Psychology*, Monograph Supplement, 76, 1, part 2.

Patterson, K., and Marcel, A. (1977). Aphasia, dyslexia, and the phonological coding of written words. *Quarterly Journal of Experimental Psychology*, 29, 307–318.

Pierce, R. (1983). Decoding syntax during reading in aphasia. *Journal of Communication Disorders*, 16, 181–188.

Porch, B. (1981). *The Porch Index of Communicative Ability*. Palo Alto, CA: Consulting Psychologists Press.

Raphael, T. E. (1984). Teaching learners about sources of information for answering comprehension questions. *Journal of Reading*, 27, 303–311.

Richardson, J. (1975). The effect of word imageability in acquired dyslexia. *Neuropsychologica*, 13, 218–288.

Rothi, L. G. and Moss, S. E. (1985). *Alexia/agraphia in brain damaged adults*. Paper presented at the Convention of the American Speech-Language-Hearing Association, Washington, DC.

Saffran, E. M., and Marin, O. S. M. (1977). Reading without phonology: Evidence from aphasia. *Quarterly Journal of Experimental Psychology*, 29, 515–525.

Saffran, E., Schwartz, M., and Marin, O. (1976). Semantic mechanisms in paralexia. *Brain and Language*, 3, 255–265.

Schneider, W., and Shiffrin, R. M. (1977). Automatic and controlled processing in vision. In D. LaBerge and S. J. Samuels (Eds.), *Basic process in reading: Perception and comprehension*. Hillsdale, NJ: Lawrence Erlbaum.

Schuell, H. (1973). *The Minnesota Test for Differential Diagnosis of Aphasia*. Minneapolis, MN: University of Minnesota Press.

Schuell, H., Jenkins, J. J., and Jimenez-Pabon, E. (1964). *Aphasia in adults: Diagnosis, prognosis and treatment*. New York: Harper & Row.

Shallice, R., and Warrington, E. K. (1975). Patterns of paralexia: A psycholinguistic approach. *Journal of Psycholinguistic Research*, 2, 195–199.

Shewan, C. M., and Bandur, D. L. (1986). *Treatment of aphasia: A language-oriented approach*. San Diego, CA: College Hill Press.

Strub, R., and Black, F. W. (1985). *Mental status examination in neurology* (2nd ed.). Philadelphia, PA: F. A. Davis.

Vacca, R. T., and Vacca, J. L. (1986). *Content area reading*. Boston, MA: Little, Brown.

Weaver, C. (1988). *Reading process and practice: From sociopsycholinguistic to whole language*. Portsmouth, NH: Heinemann Educational Books.

Webb, W. (1982). *Intervention strategies in mild reading disorders associated with aphasia*. Paper presented at the Annual Convention of the American Speech-Language-Hearing Association, Toronto, Canada.

Webb, W., and Love, R. (1983). The reading deficit in chronic aphasia. *Journal of Speech and Hearing Disorders*, 48, 164–171.

Weinberg, J., Diller, L., Gordon, W. A., Gerstman, L. A., Lieverman, A., Larkin, P., Hodges, G., and Ezarchi, O. (1977). Visual scanning training effect on reading related tasks in acquired right brain damage. *Archives of Physical Medicine and Rehabilitation*, 60, 491–496.

Weinberg, J., Piasetsky, E., Diller, L., and Gordon, W. (1982). Treating perceptual organization deficits in non-neglecting RBD stroke patients. *Journal of Clinical Neuropsychology*, 4, 59–75.

Wittrock, M. (1981). Reading comprehension. In F. Pirozzolo and M. Wittrock (Eds.), *Neuropsychological and cognitive processes in reading*. New York: Academic Press.

Woodcock Reading Mastery Tests. (1973). Circle Pines, MN: American Guidance Service.

Zihl, J. (1980). "Blindsight": Improvement of visual guided eye movements by systematic practice in patients with cerebral blindness. *Neuropsychologia*, 18, 71–77.

Zihl, J., and VonCramon, D. (1979). Restitution of visual functions in patients with cerebral blindness. *Journal of Neurology, Neurosurgery and Psychiatry*, 42, 312–322.

APPENDIX 24.1

Selected Tests, Treatment Programs, and Stimulus Material Resources

Adams, A., Flowers, A., and Woods, E. (1978). *Reading for survival in today's society* Vol. I. Santa Monica, CA: Goodyear Publishing.

Adult basic education and continuing education series. (1973). Naples, FL: Ann Arbor Publishers.

Bisset, J. D., and Fino, M. S. (1988). *Read all about it: Topics of interest to aphasic adults.* Tuscon, AZ: Communication Skill Builders. Boning, R. (1978). *Specific skill series.* Baldwin, NY: Barnell Loft.

Brain-Link Software. (no date). *Reading recognition: Serial 1.113.* Ann Arbor, MI.

Brown, V., Hammill, D., and Wiederhold, J. (1982). *Test of Reading Comprehension.* Los Angeles, CA: Western Psychological Services. Brubaker, S. (1982). *Sourcebook for aphasia.* Detroit, MI: Wayne State University Press.

Brubaker, S. (1983). *Workbook for reasoning skills.* Detroit, MI: Wayne State University Press.

Brubaker, S. H. (1984). *Workbook for language skills.* Detroit, MI: Wayne State University Press.

Davidson and Associates, Inc. (1988). *Speed reader* (for MS DOS/Apple). Torrance, CA.

Gates, A., and MacGinite, W. (1978). *Gates-MacGinite reading tests.* New York: Columbia University Press.

Gray standardized oral reading paragraphs. (1967). Indianapolis, IN: Bobbs-Merrill.

Halper, A., and Burns, M. (1989). *Treatment materials for auditory comprehension and reading comprehension.* Rockville, MD: Aspen Publishers.

Herman, E., and Everette, K. E. (1985). *Usage.* Moline, IL: Linguisystems.

Keenan, J. (1975). *A procedure manual in speech pathology with brain-injured adults.* Danville, IL: Interstate Printers and Publishers.

Keith, R. (1980). *Speech and language rehabilitation,* (Vol. I). Danville, IL: Interstate Printers and Publishers.

Keith, R. (1984). *Speech and language rehabilitation,* (Vol. II). Danville, IL: Interstate Printers and Publishers.

Kilpatrick, K. (1979). *Therapy guide for the adult with language and speech disorders* (Vol. II). Akron, OH: Visiting Nurse Service.

Kilpatrick, K. (1987). *Therapy guide for language and speech disorders: Vol. 5, reading comprehension materials.* Akron, OH: Visiting Nurse Service.

Kilpatrick, K., and Jones, C. (1977). *Therapy guide for the adult with language and speech disorders* (Vol. I). Akron, OH: Visiting Nurse Service.

Kuchinskas, G. A. (1984). *Reading through the fourth dimension* (software). Baldwin, NY: Barnell Loft.

Laugbach Literacy. (no date). *News for you.* Syracuse, NY: New Readers Press.

Martinoff, J., Martinoff, R., and Stokke, V. (1981). *Language rehabilitation: Reading.* Tigard, OR: CC Publications.

Morganstein, S., and Smith, M. C. (1982). *Thematic language stimulation.* Tucson, AZ: Communication Skill Builders.

Pavlak, S. A. (1985). *Informal tests for diagnosing specific reading problems.* West Nyack, NY: Parker Publishing Co.

Priven, J. (1986). *Reading and writing connection.* (software). Dimondale, MI: Hartley Courseware.

Sakiey, E., and Fry, E. (1984). *3000 instant words.* Providence, RI: Jamestown Publishers.

Stryker, S. (1975). *Speech after stroke.* Springfield, IL: Charles C. Thomas.

Traendly, C. (1980). *Aphasia rehabilitation reading.* Tigard, OR: CC Publications.

CHAPTER 25
Treatment of Writing Disorders in Aphasia

WALTER W. AMSTER AND JUDITH B. AMSTER

WRITING: A PROCESS DEFINITION

Historically, the ability to write has differentiated the rulers from the ruled and the privileged from the underprivileged. Under the best of circumstances, writing is a complex, demanding task. It assumes the presence of a knowledge base, the ability to organize and retrieve information, a language system in order to express one's thoughts about this information, a way to encode the information into appropriate graphophonological symbols, a willingness to adhere to the conventions of the written language system, and the motor ability to produce some sort of graphic or visual representation.

Stages of Writing

Current theory views writing as a process occurring in three major stages (Graves, 1975). The first, or "prewriting," stage has been relatively ignored in the literature concerning writing disorders in aphasia. It may be, however, the most significant in terms of treatment. Prewriting experiences focus on establishing motivation, calling on available schemas or scripts, and generating related vocabulary and ideas. Clear writing demands clear thinking. The implications for organizing thoughts and the potential benefit to overall cognition in the aphasia patient are provocative.

The second stage, that of "writing," is concerned with the reformulating of selected ideas and expressing them in appropriate and meaningful syntax and graphophonological form. The majority of traditional treatment approaches and related materials have focused on this stage, generally at the lower levels of letter formulation, spelling, and syntactical correctness.

The final stage in the writing process is that of "postwriting," or editing. Here, the writer is concerned with aspects of revision, elaboration, and transitions as well as with proofreading and editing the written product.

For the clinician, awareness of these stages in conjunction with an overall conceptual model can simplify the process of developing a treatment focus. In this regard, specific skills associated with each stage of the writing process have been adapted as shown below for aphasia treatment following the format of Wallace et al. (1987) and are presented below.

Prewriting Stage

Motivation to write
Preserved language
Retained reading ability
Ideation
Organization

Writing Stage

Producing words
Producing phrases
Producing sentences
Monitoring meaning
Monitoring intent
Written syntax
Written grammar
Written spelling
Punctuation
Copying
Handwriting
Spacing

Postwriting Stage

Editing and revising for meaning
Editing and revising for content
Editing and revising for organization
Proofing and correcting syntax
Proofing and correcting grammar
Proofing and correcting spelling
Proofing and correcting punctuation

As McNeil and Tseng (1990) indicate, models of normal writing can serve as legitimate heuristics for many neurogenic dysgraphias. The writing-process model offers the clinician a clinically sound, structured, but not limiting sequence for developing a treatment program in dysgraphia.

In the presence of aphasia, there is opportunity for one or all of the requisites for writing to be degraded. Writing, because of its complexity, is particularly vulnerable to even the most subtle neurological dysfunction. As a focus of research, the writing disorders associated with aphasia (dysgraphia, agraphia) have received minimal attention, other than the identification of their presence through the limited testing included in aphasia batteries.

Historically, writing disorders have not been useful in validating the localization of a lesion, as clear-cut symptomatology for aphasia classification, or as a primary communication mode. The treatment of writing disorders in aphasia and its efficacy have received even less formal attention, although writing has certainly been used in the clinical setting as an alternative means of expression for individuals with spoken language difficulty.

The unitary nature of aphasia suggests that improvement in one modality may work to the benefit of other damaged modalities. From this perspective, writing and its receptive corollary, reading, should be viewed not as extraneous or tangential activities but as part of the total language rehabilitation process.

Premises and Assumptions

This chapter is grounded on the following research and empirically based premises and assumptions:

1. That individuals with aphasia can improve in writing if provided with direct instruction
2. That people with aphasia retain the ability to understand and recall familiar schema or ''scripts''
3. That most current approaches to the treatment of writing disorders in aphasia focus at a microprocessing or ''bottom-up'' level of instruction
4. That the most effective procedures for retraining writing may be those that initiate instruction through a ''top-down'' or macroprocessing approach that exploits retained cognitive strengths
5. That the treatment of writing disorders should be viewed within a whole-language model of communication, and not taught as isolated, discrete skills

The present chapter is a departure from approaches to retraining writing skills presented in current treatment hierarchies. Rather, it incorporates constructs drawn from a discourse model of language and applied to writing improvement in aphasia.

RATIONALE FOR A MACROPROCESSING-MICROPROCESSING APPROACH TO WRITING DISORDERS

Basic factors that contribute to learning, such as the use of meaningful stimuli and relevant context, are valid in the presence or absence of aphasia. Some mention is made in current chapters on writing in aphasia (McNeil and Tseng, 1990; Rosenbek et al., 1989) as to the power of context and meaningfulness. However, the writing approaches presented as treatment models do not support this emphasis. Most focus at the level of isolated letter recognition and construction and move gradually toward spelling, writing of single words, and later writing of short phrases, activities that can be termed microprocessing tasks.

These ''bottom-up'' approaches to writing instruction for patients with aphasia, although they reflect necessary skills, do not take advantage of the potential benefits of meaning, context, and prior knowledge in maximizing the relearning process. The ability of individuals with aphasia to retain script knowledge (schema) was shown by Armus et al. (1989). These findings have significant implications for the structure of writing treatment. Writing treatment programs that incorporate microprocessing tasks such as improvement of spelling, syntax, and following written conventions as subordinate to the primary purpose of writing, that of communicating one's thought, are most consistent with current theories of writing instruction.

The present chapter views the writing process as having three components (Fig. 25.1): microprocessing, macroprocessing, and metacognitive processes. (Irwin [1991] views the reading process in a similar manner.)

An approach that addresses writing at the macroprocessing rather than the microprocessing level exploits the retained schema, prior knowledge, and motivation of the individual and offers the most logical point of entry for treatment.

CURRENT CONSIDERATIONS IN TREATING WRITING DISORDERS

Classification Approaches

Although it may be strikingly aberrant or mildly disturbed, the writing of aphasic patients should be viewed against a continuum of normal writing. Writing for most nonaphasic individuals is generally less fluent, more restricted, and less complex than spoken language. Further, it is a reflection of variables such as education, language ability, practice, and motivation. These variables also affect aphasic writing ability. They further preclude specificity concerning the nature of the writing disability associated with aphasia. However, there does appear to be a general agreement in the literature that fluency, severity, and syntactical involvement are the dimensions that most differentiate writing disorders. Differences between normal and aphasic populations have been found also in the proportion of errors made and their types (Sgaramella et al., 1991). These authors compared normals and individuals classified as Broca's aphasics, Wernicke's aphasics, and conduction aphasics. Higher proportions of word-level selection errors (substitutions, blends, neologisms, and omissions) were found for all three aphasic groups when compared with the normal writers.

The delineation of writing disorders by aphasia syndrome suggested by Goodglass (1981) may offer initial direction in setting expectations for written performance in given types of aphasia. When used to initiate a treatment hierarchy rather than to substantiate clinical classification of an aphasia, these syndrome clusters can serve a more useful purpose. In a similar approach, those classification systems that categorize the writing disorder based on neurological pathway models are also useful from a treatment perspective. In using such models to initiate treatment, the clinician should be attuned to the predominant features of the writing disorder, since these will direct the treatment design. Within this framework, writing disorders as well as reading disorders are classified as to the presumed language-processing function that has been disturbed. From a treatment orientation, phonological dysgraphia, lexical dysgraphia, and deep dysgraphia are the most relevant.

Information-processing models postulated in the study of dyslexia (Marshall and Newcombe, 1980) and in dysgraphia (Roeltgen and Heilman, 1985; Shallice, 1981) differentiate two primary pathways, those of phonological mediation and direct lexical access, for decoding and encoding written material. Under this assumption, a disruption in the ability to access stored phonemic information in writing (phonological dysgraphia) or in the alternate pathway of accessing the stored visual engram (lexical dysgraphia) may produce differentiating symptomatology. More important, these classifications, if valid, allow the retraining process to use the pathway assumed to be most functional. When access to both pathways appears to be compromised, a third classification, that of deep dysgraphia, is

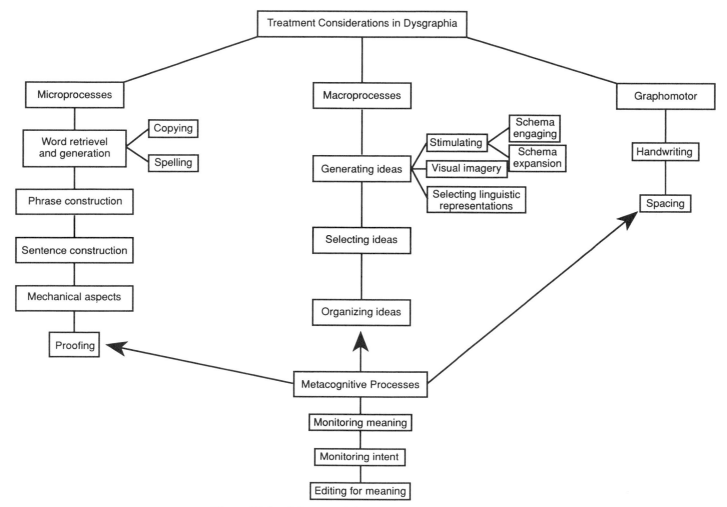

Figure 25.1.   A framework for writing treatment in aphasia.

suggested. In this instance, efforts to improve writing through conventional treatment may be nonproductive.

A fourth classification, apraxic dysgraphia may exist in association with the modality-processing dysgraphias. It may be the result of a graphomotor deficit in which selective impairment of letter formation is present. Current research suggests that there also may be a "letter imagery" impairment within apraxic dysgraphia (Crary and Heilman, 1988; Friedman and Alexander, 1989; Katz and Deser, 1991). The existence of a fifth classification, pure dysgraphia, not associated with any other neurological signs, remains a questionable, or at least an infrequently reported, finding (Chedru and Geschwind, 1972).

Efficacy of Treatment

Formal reports of improvement following treatment in writing are limited. However, available research suggests that changes in writing ability are correlated with general improvement in receptive and expressive language and reading. Positive differences were found following treatment in studies conducted by Basso et al. (1979), Butfield and Zangwill (1946), Haskins (1976), Katz and Nagy (1984), Vaughn (1986), and Wertz et al. (1981).

ASSESSMENT OF WRITING DISORDERS

Issues such as need and desire to write, possible vocational goals, premorbid writing status, and general educational level are factors that should be explored prior to initiating writing treatment goals. Further evaluation should include use of existing formal standardized evaluation procedures, adaptations of standardized writing tests available for the general population, and use of informal measures.

Formal Assessment

Few well-conceived, psychometrically sound measures of written ability are available for the nonaphasic individual. This condition is even more apparent with respect to writing tests for aphasic populations. To date, no comprehensive writing battery has been published for the aphasic population. Writing subtests contained within existing comprehensive aphasia batteries can provide initial data concerning severity of the writing disorder, the presence of syntactical deficits, and the level of fluency and nonfluency in writing. These are areas suggested by Rosenbek et al. (1989) as primary delineators of qualitative differences in the writing of individuals with aphasia. Writing subtests are included in the Minnesota Test of Differential Diagnosis of Aphasia (MTDDA) (Schuell, 1965); the Boston Diagnostic Aphasia Examination (BDAE) (Goodglass and Kaplan, 1983); the Western Aphasia Battery (WAB) (Kertesz, 1982); and the Porch Index of Communicative Ability (PICA) (Porch, 1981). Another measure, an "Experimental Neurogenic Dysgraphia Battery," was developed by McNeil and Tseng (1990). The information obtained from subtests such as these establishes general baseline data and therefore helps to develop initial guidelines for treatment.

Adaptation of Writing Tests Designed for Nonaphasic Populations

For the mild to moderately impaired individual, the clinician can obtain more specific writing assessment by using standardized instruments designed for nonaphasic adolescents. These tests can provide information at the macroprocessing level concerning (a) the individual's quality and quantity of ideas, (b) available vocabulary, and (c) organizational skills. Performance indicators at the microprocessing level assessing elements such as punctuation, capitalization, spelling, and syntax can also be obtained. One such measure, the Test of Written Language-2 (TOWL) developed by Hammill and Larsen (1988), can be used to document the presence or absence of appreciable writing problems, determine conditions that facilitate or retard an individual's writing ability, and identify gross areas of difficulty such as vocabulary, spelling, word usage, and thematic maturity (Hammill, 1990). An additional measure, the Picture Story Language Test (Myklebust, 1965), includes scales measuring the amount of writing produced, the correctness and complexity of syntax, and the abstract-concrete dimensions present in the writing. Another measure, the Test of Adolescent Language-2 (TOAL-2) (Hammill et al., 1987), offers measures of written vocabulary and written grammar. However, appropriate procedures and norms need to be developed if these measures are to be used with aphasic populations.

Informal Assessment

For the higher-functioning individual, a writing sample should be obtained. This sample can subsequently permit contextual evaluation at all levels of the writing process. The use of a writing sample allows for more in-depth appraisal of writing pragmatics and analysis of discourse and linguistic level performance (McNeil and Tseng, 1990).

The initial diagnostic results obtained from standardized and/or nonstandardized writing measures do not necessarily provide a definite path for developing a patient-specific treatment protocol. Rather, a more useful approach would be to employ the framework shown in Figure 25.1 and the skills listed earlier for each writing stage as areas that may require evaluation. Subsequently, results of all of these components can be used to formulate a comprehensive treatment plan.

Microprocessing-Level Assessment

At the microprocessing level, the clinician needs to establish the patient's performance with respect to (a) recognition and formulation of letters and words; (b) range of lexicon; (c) understanding of written syntactic elements; and (d) ability to string these units together into meaningful constructions. In

addition, rules of punctuation and capitalization need to be assessed.

Quantitative approaches are available for informal measurement of vocabulary and include use of the "type-token ratio" (Johnson, 1946). This procedure provides a comparison of the types of words used with the total number of words in a given passage. The ratio is derived mathematically from the formula of "type" (variety of words)/"token" (total number of words from which the ratio [TTR] is derived). Figure 25.2 shows the writing sample produced by a 57-year-old male classified as anomic aphasic on the WAB. This sample, which was obtained 2 weeks postonset, contains 22 types and 41 words, producing a TTR of .54.

The measurement of average sentence length (ASL) in a writing sample as described by Wallace et al. (1987) focuses on the increasing complexity of sentences generated by the individual. It allows for establishing a baseline and for ongoing evaluation of each new sample. The ASL in Figure 25.2 is obtained by counting the number of sentences (4) and dividing this by the total number of words used, producing an average sentence length of 10.3.

Quantitative and qualitative error analysis is a commonly used procedure that compares errors found in written productions with a list of grammatical, syntactic, spelling, and proofreading skills. The results of direct instruction in these deficits can be measured by a decrease in the percentage of errors produced as treatment progresses.

Macroprocessing-Level Assessment

Measurement of functioning at the macroprocessing level should include evaluation of written content including (a) accuracy, (b) ideas, and (c) organization (Cartwright, 1969). In Cartwright's Evaluation Scale, "accuracy" may range from little or no understanding of the topic to written productions in which all objectives of the communication are met. Likewise, "evaluation of ideas" provides a continuum from inadequate and unclear to pertinent and original. Aspects of "organization" vary from very poor relationship of ideas to ideas developed in logical and structured sequence. With some modifications for more severely impaired patients, Cartwright's scaling can offer a structured procedure for evaluating and monitoring writing improvement in the dysgraphic individual.

CURRENT APPROACHES TO TREATMENT

Most treatment approaches for writing disorders are based on the multimodality stimulation model provided by Schuell et al. (1964). That is, they include development of a task hierarchy, intervention at the level where a deficit occurs in the hierarchy, drill until acceptable criteria are reached, and movement to the next level of task difficulty. Within this treatment paradigm, an individual might be presented with the task of writing short phrases to dictation, having demonstrated ability to function at lower task levels such as writing single words to dictation.

In a similar vein, LaPointe (1977) outlined task hierarchies and provided a system for quantifying task performance in the "Base-10 Programmed Stimulation Treatment for Aphasic Writing." In this approach, the task is defined (e.g., writing two-word phrases from dictation), and the modality input and output are specified (e.g., auditory input, graphic output). Haskins (1976) has proposed a similar use of a multimodality

Two parties Are Having a picnic under a tree by a house a tree

a Boy is Flying a Kite by the Ocean

two people in a boat are sailing away.

a dog is near the boy who is flying the pole

Figure 25.2. Written language sample of the WAB "Picnic" scene.

sequence of tasks that begins at lower levels of functioning in writing (e.g., tracing, copying, writing letters) and progresses to formulating short sentences.

Additionally, approaches based on language-processing models (Wepman et al., 1960) have also formed the framework for treatment. Such models assume a linear pathway for language input, integration, and output, with levels of perceptual, associational, and conceptual functioning operating at each stage on which treatment hierarchies are derived (Rosenbek et al., 1989). For example, at the perceptual level, a task hierarchy might involve a progression of copying tasks from simple visual forms to written phrases.

These traditional approaches appear to be straightforward and valid treatment methods. McNeil and Tseng (1990) caution, however, that these treatment tasks, although helpful in structuring a treatment regimen, are without sufficient data on their effectiveness to allow their use "without careful vigilance." They do, however, offer guidelines and related instructional materials that can be incorporated into a more holistic approach for regaining writing skills.

WHOLE-LANGUAGE INTERVENTION

A rationale for treating the writing disorders associated with aphasia through a whole-language approach has been presented earlier in this chapter. Such an approach operationalizes the generally agreed-on value of context and meaning to the overall aphasia treatment program. In conjunction with the use of existing traditional treatment hierarchies, a whole-language model offers a comprehensive framework within which specific objectives and techniques can be developed for each patient. These procedures are discussed in the following sections as they occur in the stages of the writing process.

Treatment at the Prewriting Stage

Writing does not occur in isolation. For all writers, it requires motivation and stimulation in order to generate ideas. This is no less important for the individual with aphasia.

Stimulation activities involve recall and elaboration of existing schemata and selection of those that are of greatest interest, relevance, and familiarity to the patient. Use of oral receptive and expressive language in initiating discussions provides an opportunity for expanding or correcting limited or confused schemata. Ideas that are most relevant to the topic to be written about are expanded. Those that are unrelated are excluded. Once identified, ideas should be classified, ordered,

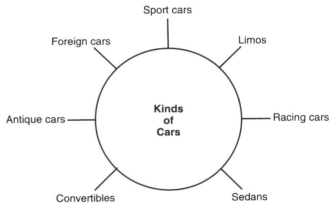

Figure 25.3. Visual map for brainstorming about types of cars.

and organized through techniques such as "brainstorming," in which thoughts about a topic are elicited. These ideas are then written down by the clinician or the patient and evaluated by both as to their relevance. Activities occurring in the prewriting stage provide significant opportunity to encourage divergent thinking. Further, valuable diagnostic indicators of cognitive functioning can be obtained during this stage based on patient output. For example, patients may demonstrate incorrect or incomplete schema as they attempt to generate ideas suggesting needed correction or expansion of existing schemata. Visual mapping or diagramming of important relationships can facilitate patient functioning. Such visual representations may enhance verbal understanding and clarify relationships among ideas. For example, Figure 25.3 shows a possible example of a visual map used during a discussion of cars. Conversely, linear visual diagramming activities are appropriate for talking and writing about events that occur in some chronological order (see Fig. 25.4). Diagrams that show superordinate and subordinate relationships (Fig. 25.5) are useful for classification activities (e.g., types of cars, kinds of jobs, organization of the family) at concrete and/or at more abstract levels. Direct instruction should be provided in recognizing high-frequency, simple organizational patterns of written materials. This can be accomplished through analysis of short paragraphs and development of graphic organizers as shown in Figure 25.6.

Throughout the process of oral and visual stimulation and brainstorming, the words, phrases, and sentences produced are recorded in some permanent form such as note cards, sentence strips, chart paper, or computer printout.

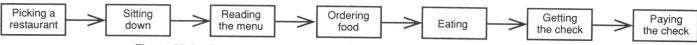

Figure 25.4. Diagram of linear relationships in a discussion of restaurant activities.

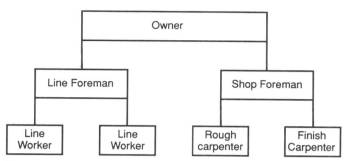

Figure 25.5. Diagram of superordinate-subordinate relationships in a work setting.

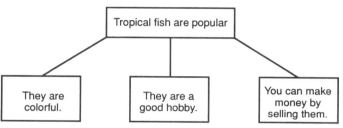

Figure 25.6. Graphic organizer for a short paragraph on tropical fish.

The patient's performance during this prewriting stage should be carefully observed. Direct instruction should be provided at any level at which the individual experiences difficulty (e.g., classifying, organizing, generating appropriate words, phrases, and sentences, visually recognizing appropriate written stimuli, maintaining a topic, and recognizing relevant or irrelevant ideas).

The prewriting stage is extremely valuable because of its inherent opportunities for language development through discussion and stimulation and the obvious cognitive and metacognitive activities that can occur. The careful attention to individual response and performance provides immediate information on which to base treatment. Opportunities should also be provided in reading and rereading words and phrases that have been produced and selected for writing about a given topic. Reading activities can be accompanied by copying the written stimuli, further reinforcing visual recognition and letter formulation. For individuals experiencing difficulty in copying because of graphomotor or letter imagery difficulty, the use of computers with adapted keyboards or of anagrams can be substituted. Tracing activities, as described by Haskins (1976), as a precursor to writing may also be of value for this population. The essential purposes of the prewriting stage—that is, generating and organizing ideas and developing language—remains primary. The motor aspects of writing, although important, serve only to support the prewriting activities.

The time spent at the prewriting stage will vary, depending on the individual's readiness, the level of functioning at which instruction can begin, and the need for intervention in deficient

macroprocessing skills. As treatment progresses and a pattern of response is accomplished, along with improvement of deficit areas that have been identified and treated, the length of time required to complete the prewriting stage can be reduced on the basis of clinical judgment.

Treatment at the Writing Stage

Graves (1975), in discussing the writing process approach, places the primary emphasis of this stage on the expression of meaning rather than on isolated "meaningless components." Deficits, of course, need to be treated, but this should be done within the context of meaning. The patient's writing productions, simple or complex as they may be, provide the guidelines for treatment.

The microprocessing components involved in functioning at this stage of the process are shown in Figure 25.1. Copying for the purpose of handwriting improvement and correctness of spelling receive little attention at the initial stage of intervention. When the need arises, individuals can refer to the previously recorded words elicited during the prewriting stage. Wallace et al. (1987) suggest that availability of these correct models reduces interruptions of the conceptualizing process necessary for coherent composing.

For individuals with difficulty in visual recognition or recall of words, procedures that incorporate visual-auditory-kinesthetic and tactile (VAKT) reinforcement, as developed by Fernald (1988), may be helpful. VAKT begins with tracing coupled with pronouncing the sounds of the word as the tracing occurs. In some cases, tactile reinforcement is provided through use of raised letters or roughened surfaces. The clinician will need to experiment with all or part of this approach and determine its possible value with each client.

Copying of clinician/patient-produced writing or materials that the patient is able to read can be an initial step for less able individuals. As progress is noted, elements of the passage can be omitted, beginning with single words and moving to phrases and simple sentences, leaving only the topic sentence intact. Because copying appears to be a well-preserved ability for many individuals with aphasia, it can serve a useful purpose when used within the context of a meaningful written production. When paired with oral rereading of the material following copying, considerable reinforcement can be provided.

The ability to formulate phrases and sentences is a critical element in the writing process. Initially, much of the stimuli will need to be presented by the clinician. The discussion should evolve from themes that are of interest to the group or individual. Group discussion concerning current events, personal experiences, or vocational or hobby interests can be generated by viewing stimulus pictures, reading newspaper articles orally, watching TV programs, listening to tapes, and role playing familiar experiential scripts. Brainstorming activities discussed in the preceding section will provide some clinician/patient-generated vocabulary, phrases, and possibly even short sentences that will have been written down. Expansion of these activities continues to take place during the writing stage.

During this stage, adaptations of the Fitzgerald Key Program (1966) may offer some methods for improving fluency and practice in the formulation and ordering of sentences. The Fitzgerald Key Program focuses on word classes as they are used in language. Phelps-Gunn and Phelps-Terasaki (1982), in reviewing the Fitzgerald approach, discuss its primary goals of (a) development of the semantic vocabulary and conceptual aspects of language and (b) stabilization of correct language form in the syntactic, morphological, and phonemic elements. Simple sentences can be created, copied, practiced, and read with more complex sentences evolving as new word classes are added. The "Key," as a visual system of illustrating the structure of written language, should be explored for use with dysgraphic patients. A similar approach, the Phelps Sentence Guide Program (Phelps-Terasaki and Phelps, 1980), offers treatment guidelines for sentence generation, elaboration, and ordering. It consists of hierarchical stages, beginning with simple sentences and progressing to paragraphs and stories. Columns are labeled to represent the parts of speech so that sentence structure is illustrated and can be referred to at all times. The clinician guides the development of syntactic relationships, reinforcing auditory and visual associations.

Modifications of the "Sentences and Other Systems" approach (Blackwell et al., 1978) can be used to provide instruction in (a) five basic sentence patterns; (b) expansion of these patterns into more complex sentences; and (c) analysis of written intent, style, and narrative voice. Based on transformational grammar, the program builds on developing and revising basic sentences such as "The girl ran" to creating more complex structures such as "The girl ate cookies."

Another method with treatment potential in dysgraphia bears the acronym "CATS" (Giordano, 1982). It provides instruction through (a) copying; (b) altering; (c) transforming; and (d) supplying a written response to a clinician-produced question. The writer initially copies simple sentences such as "I drink milk," or "I drink juice." At the altering stage, one word is substituted in a previously copied sentence ("I drink juice"/ "You drink juice"). The transforming stage requires making grammatical modifications in tense, number or gender and negative or interrogative forms. At the final stage, a question is generated and written by the clinician. It is then copied by the patient, who produces a written answer by the patient. Similar activities and exercises are available in most aphasia workbooks and computer programs. However, stimulus material generated by the patient, which focuses on topics of personal interest, would tend to be more motivating. The clinician is encouraged to review these available procedures and redefine them as necessary for the particular needs of the dysgraphic patient.

At higher performance levels, the development of short paragraphs can be accomplished through initial modeling by the clinician with input from the patient. Visual diagramming of ideas done previously during brainstorming activities in the prewriting stage can form a structure for (a) generating a topic sentence and (b) adding a few sentences to support or expand on the topic sentence. Copying of model paragraphs following this simple structure may be useful, and production of similar paragraphs can be attempted. Time will need to be spent on identifying and developing a topical statement and selecting and constructing supportive sentences. It may be necessary to provide sample sentences, having patients choose and order the most appropriate sentences. Opportunities abound in these activities for enhancing metacognitive processes through monitoring meaning, appropriateness, relevance, and organization of written ideas. At the initial stages, the use of short sentence patterns may be useful. Here the patient is asked to copy sentences, changing or filling in one word in the pattern and gradually progressing to more complex sentences with longer units to be changed. Exercises of this type are readily available in workbook and computer formats.

For some individuals, oral dictation of sentence patterns that are written down by the patient can follow the same sequence. Rereading and copying should be encouraged, as should reliance on visual stimuli to reduce dependence on oral stimuli. Computer programs with voice synthesizers can be very useful in addressing the needs of the patient with possible lexical access difficulties. The Language Master (Bell and Howell) and its accompanying phrase and sentence programs could be of use in providing auditory reinforcement of the written stimuli if computers are not available or not appropriate.

Such dictation activities, in the absence of visual stimuli, may place demands on the patient in terms of auditory processing, short-term auditory memory, and rapidity of graphomotor skills. Clinical judgment to determine their benefit will be required.

The clinician should be willing, during the actual writing stage, to accept mechanical and spelling errors and less important syntactic and grammatical errors, reserving attention to these for the final stage of postwriting.

Treatment at the Postwriting Stage

The focus of this stage is the process of revising to enhance and clarify the written product. As such, postwriting offers an excellent clinical opportunity to discuss aspects of clarity, ideation, relevance, and organization. Through semantic mapping procedures, expansion of the lexicon used can be encouraged. Correction of syntactic and grammatical errors to the degree possible and appropriate for the patient should also be included. Issues of spelling and proofreading for errors in punctuation and capitalization should be the final steps included in this stage.

THE LANGUAGE EXPERIENCE APPROACH IN THE WHOLE-LANGUAGE MODEL

Long recognized for its effectiveness with reading and writing disabled developmental learners, the Language Experience Approach (LEA) (Allen and Allen, 1966; Stauffer, 1970) provides an excellent structure for incorporating and operationalizing the writing process approach in the treatment of dysgraphia.

Unlike traditional workbook and drill approaches in aphasia treatment, Language Experience offers a high degree of interest for the individual. It draws on retained schema, is personalized, and allows immediate feedback and significant opportunity to incorporate all discourse modes, particularly reading. Further, it is adaptable to the patient's unique needs and is applicable in individual or group therapy. Often, the interaction of the group can enhance treatment activities.

Steps in the Language Experience Approach

An overview of procedures in the Language Experience Approach adapted for treatment in dysgraphia is presented below:

Step 1. Topics for writing are generated by the patient with stimulation from the clinician.

Step 2. Schema development and expansion activities are provided through listening, discussion, and visual stimulation.

Step 3. Ideas relevant to the topic are selected, classified, and organized through brainstorming activities, cuing through graphic organizers, visual mapping of relationships, and so on.

Step 4. Words, phrases, and possibly sentences related to the topic are elicited, written down by the clinician, and copied by the patient.

Step 5. Using the selected words, phrases, and sentences, the patient is encouraged to dictate ideas that are then written down by the clinician.

Step 6. Clinician and patient revise and edit to the degree necessary and possible, focusing on primary error targets that impede meaning.

Step 7. Clinician and patient read the corrected material aloud repeatedly with gradual ''fading'' by clinician.

Step 8. Patient copies material using writing, adapted computer keyboard, typewriter, or anagrams.

Step 9. Computer-generated printouts are made available for review and rereading outside the clinical setting.

Step 10. Further reinforcement can be provided through (*a*) tape recording the passage to assist in rereading activities; (*b*) creating flash cards, Language Master cards, or computer drills for reinforcing word and phrase recognition and spelling.

The amount of time spent in creating a written product will depend on the intervention needed to accomplish each step. The clinician should be willing to accept even minimal attempts, ''filling in the gaps'' as needed, until the patient can provide more input. Certainly, measures of patient improvement should be obtained at each step in the process. Areas in which progress should be monitored include (*a*) reduction in prompts needed; (*b*) decrease in targeted errors; (*c*) fluency of oral dictations, copying, writing, and reading; and (*d*) time needed to produce a final product.

Graphomotor Considerations

The intensive use of the Language Experience Approach provides extensive opportunity for improvement of graphomotor skills to the degree necessary and possible for the patient. Target areas for treatment of graphomotor difficulties should be those that most disturb overall legibility. Issues of spacing, letter size, and gross orthographical errors in letter formulation do require treatment. Direct instruction in these elements can be provided during the copying stages in the Language Experience activities. Additional isolated practice, if needed, can be provided through the use of workbooks and training materials. The patient should play a role in self-monitoring written productions for significant orthographical errors during the copy editing stages of the postwriting process.

The efficacy of computers and word processors should be explored for those patients for whom handwriting with the preferred or nonpreferred hand is extremely incapacitated. Further, the availability of adaptive keyboards, touch window screens, and other augmentative computer devices may allow patients with very restricted orthographical ability to benefit from the overall potential of the writing process.

COMPUTERS IN THE WRITING TREATMENT PROGRAM

With the proliferation of computers in the clinical and home setting and the development of instructional software developed specifically for use in the writing process, opportunities for enhancing patient performance are available. However, as Rosenbek et al. (1989) caution, ''The use of the microcomputer to treat aphasic writing to date has produced promise not proof.'' A further caveat is in order. Much of the available programming is at the drill and practice level. Although these materials may be useful, care must be taken in reviewing them for appropriateness with individuals who are aphasic.

The use of the computer at each stage of the writing process offers opportunities for drill and reinforcement of previously learned skills in clinical and extended settings. At the prewriting stage, the screen can be connected to an LCD (liquid crystal display) projection system to assist in brainstorming in a group setting. Ideas generated are printed out by the computer or filed on screen for expansion and organization. Programs that stimulate thinking, brainstorming, and organization of ideas have been developed (e.g., Milliken Writing Workshops: Prewriting, Postwriting); however, the complexity of these commercial programs may make them and similar materials unusable for all except the most mildly involved patient.

Word-processing programs can be very useful in the total writing process if their design and operation are carefully reviewed and found appropriate. The Language Experience Recorder (Teacher Support Software) provides a word-processing program that is especially valuable in the writing stage of the Language Experience Approach. It has small and large print capability and can be used in conjunction with a voice synthesizer for immediate feedback of what has been written. Of further use is its capacity to generate a type-token ratio (TTR) for written samples and to provide a large print hard-copy document.

Because of the variability found in aphasic writing, the clinician may find that developing programs through the use of authoring systems may be a necessity. The major advantages of these systems are that no programming skills are required and the system ''debugs'' itself following the author's instructions. The time spent in preparing these programs, although it may be considerable, will provide specific treatment tasks designed for the individual patient. Further, the use of voice synthesizers in conjunction with such programs allows for feedback and reinforcement, even in the absence of the clinician.

FUTURE TRENDS

With the increasing, if not as yet overwhelming, interest in the treatment of writing in aphasia, validation of existing approaches will need to be addressed. Concurrently, alternative approaches that view writing as part of the total communication process and that may offer positive treatment results will require inquiry. Comparative studies within and between treatments are critical to this process. Additionally, questions will need to be answered concerning if, and when, to initiate writing treatment and with whom.

The potential for improving oral language through the use of written language has yet to be measured under well-designed research paradigms. Similarly, we do not yet know how far the individual can travel in regaining some level of writing proficiency. Availability of this information will permit more accurate decisions as to which writing approaches to use for which writer. Investigation is needed concerning the role of the right hemisphere in the writing process. Results of such studies may provide treatment approaches that draw on right-hemisphere capabilities to facilitate writing. Continued advance can be expected in the use of iconic and other nonverbal symbols as a means for the severely impaired individual to graphically express his or her thoughts.

A call will certainly be heard for psychometrically sound and comprehensive measurement of writing in aphasic populations. The existence of such tests will undoubtedly drive research efforts and provide more defensible guidelines for intervention. Informal assessment techniques will need to be refined and given more structure, allowing for ongoing monitoring and changes in the therapeutic regimen specific to the identified needs of the patient. Programs for computer analysis of aphasic writing, such as those available for speech-sample analysis, should be developed. A large-scale database of this valuable, currently scattered information could be accumulated through networked systems and retrieved easily by researchers and clinicians.

At this juncture, clinicians need to explore various avenues of treatment in writing, and patients need to be given the opportunity to improve in what may be of significant value to them in the course of their treatment.

References

Allen, R. V., and Allen, C. (1966). *Language experiences in reading.* Chicago: Encyclopedia Brittanica Press.

Armus, S. R., Brookshire, R. H., and Nicholas, L. E. (1989). Aphasic and non-brain-damaged adults' knowledge of scripts for common situations. *Brain and Language, 36,* 518–528.

Basso, A., Capitani, E., and Vignolo, L. A. (1979). Influence of rehabilitation of language skills in aphasic patients: A controlled study. *Archives of Neurology, 36,* 190–196.

Benson, D. F. (1979). *Aphasia, alexia, and agraphia.* New York: Churchill Livingstone.

Blackwell, P. M., Engen, E., Fischgrund, J. E., and Zarcadoolas, C. (1978). *Sentences and other systems: A language and learning curriculum for hearing impaired children.* Washington, DC: The Alexander Graham Bell Association for the Deaf.

Butfield, E., and Zangwill, O. (1946). Re-education in aphasia: A review of 70 cases. *Journal of Neurology, Neurosurgery and Psychiatry, 9,* 75–79.

Cartwright, G. P. (1969). Written expression and spelling. In R. M. Smith (Ed.), *Teacher diagnosis of education difficulties* (pp. 95–117). Columbus, OH: Charles E. Merrill.

Chedru, F., and Geschwind, N. (1972). Writing disturbances in acute confusional states. *Neuropsychologia, 10,* 343–353.

Crary, M. A., and Heilman, K. M. (1988). Letter imagery deficits in a case of pure apraxic agraphia. *Brain and Language, 34,* 147–156.

Fernald, G. (1988). *Remedial techniques in basic school subjects.* Austin, TX: Pro-Ed.

Fitzgerald, E. (1966). *Straight language for the deaf.* Washington, DC: The Volta Bureau.

Friedman, R. B., and Alexander, M. P. (1989). Written spelling agraphia. *Brain and Language, 36,* 503–517.

Giordano, G. (1982). CATS exercises: Teaching disabled writers to communicate. *Academic Therapy, 18,* 236.

Goodglass, H. (1981). The syndromes of aphasia: Similarities and differences in neurolinguistic features. *Topics in Language Disorders, 1,* 1–14.

Goodglass, H., and Kaplan, E. (1983). *Boston Diagnostic Examination for Aphasia.* Philadelphia, PA: Lea & Febiger.

Graves, D. H. (1975). An examination of the writing process of seven year old children. *Language Arts, 56,* 312–319.

Hammill, D. D. (1990). Problems in written composition. In D. D. Hammill and N. R. Bartel (Eds.), *Teaching students with learning and behavior problems* (5th ed.). Boston, MA: Allyn & Bacon.

Hammill, D. D., Brown, V., Larsen, S., and Wiederholt, J. L. (1987). *The Test of Adolescent Language-2.* Austin, TX: Pro-Ed.

Hammill, D. D., and Larsen, S. (1988). *The Test of Written Language-2.* Austin, TX: Pro-Ed.

Haskins, S. (1976). A treatment procedure for writing disorders. In R. H. Brookshire (Ed.), *Proceedings of the Conference on Clinical Aphasiology* (pp. 192–199). Minneapolis, MN: BRK.

Irwin, J. W. (1991). *Teaching reading comprehension processes* (2nd ed.). Englewood Cliffs, NJ: Prentice-Hall.

Johnson, W. (1946). *People in quandaries: The semantics of personal adjustment.* New York: Harper & Row.

Katz, R. C., and Deser, T. (1991). Distinguishing representation deficits and processing deficits in a case of acquired dysgraphia. *Quarterly Journal of Experimental Psychology–Human-Experimental Psychology, 43A,* 249–266.

Katz, R. C., and Nagy, V. T. (1984). An intelligent computer-based spelling task for chronic aphasic patients. In R. H. Brookshire (Ed.), *Proceedings of the Conference on Clinical Aphasiology* (pp. 65–72). Minneapolis, MN: BRK.

Kertesz, A. (1982). *Western Aphasia Battery.* New York: Grune & Stratton.

Language Experience Recorder. Gainesville, FL: Teacher Support Software.

Language Master. Bell & Howell, Co., Chicago, IL.

LaPointe, L. L. (1977). Base-10 programmed stimulation: Task specification, scoring and plotting performance in aphasia therapy. *Journal of Speech and Hearing Disorders, 42,* 90–105.

Marshall, J. C., and Newcombe, F. (1980). The conceptual status of deep dyslexia: An historical perspective. M. Coltheart, K. Patterson, and J. C. Marshall (Eds.), *Deep dyslexia* (pp. 1–21). London: Routledge & Kegan Paul.

McNeil, M. R., and Tseng, C-H. (1990). Acquired neurogenic disorders. In L. L. LaPointe (Ed.), *Aphasia and related neurogenic language disorders* (pp. 147–176). New York: Thieme.

Milliken Writing Workshops: Prewriting and Postwriting. St. Louis, MO: Milliken Publishing Company.

Myklebust, H. R. (1965). *Picture Story Language Test.* New York: Grune & Stratton.

Phelps-Gunn, T., and Phelps-Teraskaki, D. (1982). *Written language instruction: Theory and remediation.* Rockville, MD: Aspen Systems Corporation.

Phelps-Terasaki, D., and Phelps, T. (1980). *Teaching written expression: The Phelps sentence guide program.* Novato, CA: Academic Therapy Publications.

Porch, B. E. (1981). *Porch Index of Communicative Ability* (3rd ed.). Palo Alto, CA: Consulting Psychologists Press.

Roeltgen, D. P., and Heilman, K. M. (1985). Review of agraphia and a proposal for an anatomically-based neuropsychological model of writing. *Applied Psycholinguistics, 6,* 205–230.

Rosenbek, J. C., LaPointe, L. L., and Wertz, R. T. (1989). *Aphasia: A clinical approach.* Austin, TX: Pro-Ed.

Schuell, H. (1965). *The Minnesota Test for Differential Diagnosis of Aphasia.* Minneapolis: University of Minnesota Press.

Schuell, H. (1974). The treatment of aphasia. In L. F. Sies (Ed.), *Aphasia theory and therapy: Selected lectures and papers of Hildred Schuell.* Baltimore, MD: University Park Press.

Schuell, H., Jenkins, J. J., and Jimenez-Pabon, E. (1964). *Aphasia in adults.* New York: Harper & Row.

Sgaramella, T. M., Ellis, A. W., and Semenza, C. (1991). Analysis of the spontaneous writing errors of normal and aphasic writers. *Cortex, 27,* 29–39.

Shallice, T. (1981). Phonological agraphia and the lexical route in writing. *Brain, 104,* 413–429.

Stauffer, R. G. (1970). *The language experience approach to the teaching of reading.* New York: Harper & Row.

Vaughn, G. (1986). *REMATE: Communication Outreach—Annual Report.* Birmingham, AL: Veterans Administration Medical Center.

Wallace, G., Cohen, S. B., and Polloway, E. A. (1987). *Language arts: Teaching exceptional students.* Austin, TX: Pro-Ed.

Wepman, J. M., Jones, L. V., Bock, R. D., and Van Pelt, D. (1960). Studies in aphasia: Background and theoretical formulations. *Journal of Speech and Hearing Disorders, 25,* 323–332.

Wertz, R. T., Weiss, D. G., Aten, J. L., Brookshire, R. H., Garcia-Bunuel, L., Holland, A. L., Kurtzke, J. F., LaPointe, L. L., Milianti, F. J., Brannegan, R., Greenbaum, H., Marshall, R. C., Vogel, D., Carter, J., Barners, N. S., and Goodman, R. (1981). Comparison of clinic, home, and deferred language treatment for aphasia: A Veterans Administration Cooperative Study. *Archives of Neurology, 43,* 653–658.

CHAPTER 26
The Nature and Treatment of Neuromotor Speech Disorders in Aphasia

PAULA A. SQUARE AND RUTH E. MARTIN

As early as 1825, the aphasiology literature cited the occurrence of a motor speech disorder resulting from insult or disease like that which caused aphasia. However, it had very different symptoms (Bouillaud, 1825). In aphasia, verbal comprehension, reading and writing, inner language, and possibly even intellect and memory were impaired (e.g., Jackson, 1868, as cited by Head, 1915; Marie, 1906; Wernicke, 1874). In individuals with the speech disorder, all of these abilities appeared to be *relatively* spared. The disorder was one of "articulated speech" (e.g., Broca, 1861; Kussmaul, 1877; Liepmann, 1913; Marie, 1906).

Table 26.1 provides a summary of selected clinical reports that have addressed this acquired disorder of "articulated speech" over the last 168 years. The nomenclature used to describe the acquired speech impairment was as diverse as were the descriptions of symptoms and pathophysiological, linguistic, and psychological constructs put forth to explain the disorder. Further, disagreements regarding the site of structural lesion underlying the "speech impairment" were, and continue to be, numerous. Among this controversy and terminological confusion, however, several major trends regarding the acquired impairment of articulated speech have consistently appeared. Many of these concepts are summarized in Table 26.1. First and foremost, the existence of a significant acquired motor speech disorder of sudden onset resulting from brain damage, the characteristics of which differed significantly from "impairment of internal language and intelligence" (aphasia) has been, and continues to be, widely acknowledged (e.g., Alajouanine et al., 1939; Bouillaud, 1825; Critchley, 1952; Darley, 1968; Dejerine, 1892; Schiff et al., 1983; Square et al., 1981, 1982, 1988; Square-Storer and Apeldoorn, 1991). Second, the articulatory impairment is thought to coexist in most cases with the impairment of aphasia (Ballarger, 1865; Jenkins et al., 1975; Marie et al., 1917; Schuell et al., 1964; Weisenberg and McBride, 1935; Wernicke, 1885), although the disorder can also appear in a pure form (Alajouanine et al., 1939; Dejerine, 1901; Goodglass and Kaplan, 1972; Marie et al., 1917; Schiff et al., 1983; Square and Mlcoch, 1983; Square et al., 1982, Square-Storer et al., 1988; Square-Storer and Apeldoorn, 1991). Third, there is a subgroup of patients with both disorders for whom treatment of the motor speech impairment should take precedence over the treatment of aphasia, although rehabilitation for both disorders is usually undertaken simultaneously (Darley et al., 1975; Square et al., 1985; Square et al., 1986; Square-Storer, 1989; Tonkovich and Peach, 1989; Wertz, LaPointe, and Rosenbek, 1984). Fourth, while aphasia generally was thought to arise from cortical lesions to the left hemisphere, the "articulatory disorder" was, in the 1800s and early 1900s, thought to be associated most often with subcortical damage, particularly to the white matter underlying Broca's area in the left hemisphere (e.g., Bouillaud, 1825; Dejerine, 1891, 1901; Lichteim, 1884–1885; Marie, 1906; Wernicke, 1885). Rarely, but sometimes, it was reported to occur with damage to the analogous area in the right hemisphere (e.g., Marie, 1906). But also in the 1800s, there were those of the opinion that the disorder could result from cortical damage. It was thought that aphasia was most likely to co-occur with cortical damage, especially to the left frontal lobe involving the third and sometimes the second convolution. (Lichteim, 1884–1885; Wernicke, 1874, 1885). The notion that cortical damage to the third left frontal convolution was responsible for the motor speech disorder was the prevailing one in North America in the 1900s (Bay, 1962; Denny-Brown, 1965; Goldstein, 1948; Shankweiler and Harris, 1966; Whitty, 1964;). Fifth, the character of this disorder was thought by many *not* to be paralytic/paretic (Bouillaud, 1825; Broca, 1861; Darley, 1968; Darley et al., 1975; Dejerine, 1901; Marie 1906; Shankweiler and Harris, 1966; Wertz et al., 1984) but, instead, somewhat akin to other movement disorders such as those associated with (*a*) cerebellar ataxia (Broca, 1861; Kussmaul, 1877; McNeil et al., 1989; McNeil et al., 1990); (*b*) lesions to or dysfunction of the extrapyramidal system (Marie et al., 1917; Naesser, 1982; Schiff et al, 1983; Square, 1981), with dystonic speech symptoms resulting (Alajouanine et al., 1939; Square, 1981; Square and Mlcoch, 1983); and/or (*c*) an apraxia affecting speech production (Bay, 1962; Darley, 1968; Whitty, 1964). Some aphasiologists specifically implicated left parietal cortical damage (Marie et al., 1917; Square, 1981; Square et al., 1982; Square-Storer and Apeldoorn, 1991), but most speculated that the apraxia was due to left frontal cortical damage, particularly to the third and sometimes second frontal convolutions (e.g., Alajouanine et al., 1939; Darley, 1977; Denny-Brown, 1965). Finally, a

Table 26.1.
Terminology Used to Denote the Acquired Speech Disorder of Sudden Onset Resulting for Brain Insult Like That Which Causes Aphasia

			Inner Language Preserved	Speech and/or Oral Motor Behavior	Site of Lesion
Bouillaud	1825	N/A	+	• No paralysis • Learned movements disrupted • Vegetative movements preserved	• White matter underlying frontal lobe
Broca	1861	Aphemia	+	• Verbal stereotypy • A kind of "locomotive ataxia" • No paralysis • Learned movements disrupted • Vegetative movements preserved	—
Laborde	1863	—		• Range of severity - Incapable of articulating a single word - Limited to stammering unintelligible sounds - Can write, but not perfectly	—
Trousseau	1864	Aphasia—a rare form	+	• Inability to speak • May ameliorate in 5 to 6 weeks	—
Ballarger	1865	Simple aphasia		• A more or less complete loss of speech • In some, the disorder impairs both speech and writing; in others, speech is impaired but writing is preserved • Involuntary speech is better than voluntary	—
Wernicke	1874	Motor aphasia		• Severe reduction in the capacity for oral expression and distortion of residual productions • Lesion causes more or less a total loss of motor word images	• Lesion of the verbomotor center
Wernicke	1874	Motor aphasia		• Power of expression totally affected in both its graphic and oral form	—
Kussmaul	1877	Ataxic aphasia	+	• Inability to speak • Cannot repeat	—
Lichtheim	1884–85	Cortical motor Subcortical motor	+	• Can no longer speak spontaneously, read aloud, repeat	• Three forms - Lesion of the center of "articulation imagery" (cortical motor) - Lesion to path linking center of articulation imagery and center of ideation - Lesion linking path of center of articulation imagery and inferior motor center (subcortical motor)

Author	Year	Term		Characteristics	Localization
Wernicke	1885	Subcortical motor aphasia	+	• Loss of images for articulated speech	• Subcortical
		Cortical motor aphasia	−	• Equivalent to "aphemia" of Broca • Can utter at most a few words	• Cortical—3rd frontal convolution
Pick	1892	Aphasic stuttering	—		—
Dejerine	1901	Pure subcortical motor aphasia	—	• Cannot produce a single word, spontaneously, reading, repeating, singing • Metalinguistic ability preserved—can take number of breaths for number of syllables or letters in a word	• Lenticular nucleus and anterior portion of internal capsule • Lucunary foci in putamen bilaterally • ∴ lesion to fibers coming from the 3rd frontal convolution
Dejerine	1901	True motor aphasia	−	• See Dejerine above	• Subcortical, see above
		Pure motor aphasia—an extrinsic form of aphasia	+		• Striated lenticular nucleus cutting fibers issuing from the 3rd frontal convolution
Marie	1906	Anarthria	+	• Speech is nil or incomprehensible • Metalinguistic skills for syllables, graphemes preserved • No paralysis • Disturbance of the movements peculiar to speech	—
Liepmann	1913	Apraxia		• A particular form of apraxia of the glossolabio-pharyngeal apparatus • Kinetic memory for speech is impaired	—
Marie, Foix, and Bertrand	1917	Complete anarthria	+	• Spontaneous and repeated speech are equally affected • Patient utters only inarticulate sounds • Speech may be regained through re-education but is jerky, spasmodic	• Putamen, caudate, capsulary segment, and white matter of posterior part of the frontal lobe
		Incomplete anarthria	+	• Speech is possible but difficult, deformed, incorrectly articulated • Repeated speech is not much better than spontaneous • In time, patient can imitate intonation and lip movement, but then dysarthria is revealed with the apraxia phenomenon	• Parietal cortical and subcortical = apraxia
Foix	1928	Broca's aphasia tending toward anarthria	−	• Ideomotor apraxia phenomenon	• Above plus head and foot of F$_3$

Table 26.1.
Terminology Used to Denote the Acquired Speech Disorder of Sudden Onset Resulting for Brain Insult Like That Which Causes Aphasia (*Contd.*)

		Inner Language Preserved	Speech and/or Oral Motor Behavior	Site of Lesion
Alajouanine, Ombredane, and Durrand	1939	+	• A disorder of articulatory realization • Three aspects whose respective importance seems variable—paralytic, dystonic, apraxic • Extrapyramidal signs • Pyramidal and extrapyramidal signs • Apraxia due to parietal involvement • Lower part of precentral gyrus or region deep to this area—cortical; apraxia; subcortical = dysarthria	—
Nathan	1947	—		
Goldstein	1948	— (Some agrammatism)	• Spontaneous speech severely diminished, motorically defective • Trial and error • Repetition may be somewhat better than spontaneous • Voluntary effort improves speech	• Cortical lesions
Critchley	1952	+ or –	• Disorder of articulate speech that is varied across patients and variable within patients • A defect of articulation rate and melody • Dysarthria and aphasia often co-occur	—
Russell and Espir	1961	+ or –	• Lesions involving lower part of Rolandic area	• Lesions involving lower part of Rolandic area
Bay	1962	+ or –	• Defect of movement of articulatory muscles and impaired tongue movement • Apraxia and spasticity	• Damage to the lower part of the central region
Luria	1964	+	• Breakdown of kinetic melodies of speech, i.e., skilled, sequential movements • Can position articulators but cannot move them smoothly from one articulatory position to another	• Posterior one-third of inferior portion of left frontal (secondary area)
		+	• Inability to position the articulators correctly because of impaired kinesthetic feedback • A form of oral apraxia • The harder the patient tries, the more difficulty he or she has articulating single sounds	• Inferior portion of the left precentral gyrus (secondary zone)

Apraxic dysarthria

Peripheral motor aphasia

Articulatory dyspraxia

Motor aphasia

Cortical dysarthria

Efferent motor aphasia

Afferent motor aphasia

Phonetic disintegration of speech

Author(s)	Year	Term		Characteristics	Lesion
		Dynamic aphasia		• Link between initial conception of verbal scheme and external speech is the primary problem • Paucity of spontaneous output • Comprehension, articulation, naming, and repetition are good	• Lesion of the left frontal lobe anterior to premotor area
Weisenberg and McBride	1964	Predominantly expressive aphasia	—	• Incoordination of cerebral and bulbary centers without paralysis • Speculated regarding relationship to dystonia, stuttering	—
Whitty	1964	Cortical dysarthria		• Transient cortical dysarthria basically apraxic in nature • Dysprosody	• Strictly frontal lesions at the base of Rolando undermining part of the 3rd and probably 2nd frontal convolution
Schuell et al. Jenkins et al.	1964	Aphasia with sensorimotor (somatosensory) involvement	—	• Severe reduction of vocabulary and reduced verbal retention span • Impaired perception and production of phonemic patterns • Normal articulation may be achieved for common words, phrases, and possibly short sentences • Speech breaks down in longer segments • Language breaks down in longer sentences and all but simple sentences	—
	1975	Aphasia with persisting dysfluency	—	• Mild language impairment • Articulation difficulties and persistent dysfluency • Patients can learn to control articulation and can even produce excellent articulation with conscience control	—
Denny-Brown	1965	Apraxia of vocal expression		• Variable speech production • Difficulty beginning a word • Special difficulty in making some types of syllables	• Cortical disturbance of the 3rd and 2nd frontal convolutions without involvement of the underlying white matter
Darley	1968	Apraxia of speech	±	• Inability to sequence the positioning of speech musculature • Prosodic deviances perhaps in compensation • Volitional difficulties make it an apraxia	—
Shankweiler and Harris	1968	Phonetic disintegration	+	• Speech is extremely effortful and slow • The "machinery" for producing sounds no longer • Not a dysarthria	• Cortical lesion due to stroke in the left hemisphere • Dysarthria is a different phenomenon restricted to lower levels of the motor system

Table 26.1.
Terminology Used to Denote the Acquired Speech Disorder of Sudden Onset Resulting for Brain Insult Like That Which Causes Aphasia (*Contd.*)

		Inner Language Preserved	Speech and/or Oral Motor Behavior	Site of Lesion
Goodglass and Kaplan	1972	+	• An isolated disorder of articulation • Initially cannot produce any speech sounds • Recovery yields slow and awkward articulation • Grammar and word finding are not impaired	• Subcortical lesion site interrupting final outflow of information from Broca's area to the speech effector system
Naeser et al.	1982	—	• Slow, dysarthric speech • Lasting right hemiplegia • Good comprehension and grammatical output	• Capsular-putamenal lesion sites with anterior-superior white-matter lesion extension
Schiff et al.	1983	+	• Severe dysarthria without aphasia • Initial muteness in many • Slow, effortful speech with articulation impairment • Prosody is slow, fragmented with reduced melodic transitions • Recitation, repetition, singing impaired • Transient buccofacial apraxia • Lower facial paralysis • Recovery to persistent dysarthria and/or dysprosody	• Left pars opercularis • Inferior pre-Rolandic gyrus • White matter deep to these areas

few French aphasiologists hypothesized that the motor speech disorder might in fact be a combination of **dystonic, paretic,** and **apraxic** components and that each patient's speech handicap was composed of differential proportions of each (Alajouanine et al., 1939).

The first purpose of this chapter is to demonstrate that neuromotor speech impairments are probable in many patients with acquired brain damage that also has resulted in aphasia, most probably because of the intimacy of the neural systems mediating linguistic and motoric behavior. This is especially true for those patients with subcortical frontal, cortical frontal, and/or midparietal cortical lesions. This view will be substantiated by literature on the neural control of motor behavior in both nonhuman primates and humans. Second, frameworks for establishing treatment goals for these neuromotor speech disorders will be presented. Third, facilitative techniques and treatment methods that have appeared in the literature will be described, and an attempt will be made to rationalize the neurophysiological basis for the effectiveness of each. Throughout, the literature regarding efficacy of treatment of motor speech disorders in aphasia will be reviewed, and questions that require investigation will be put forth. Finally, management of special motor speech conditions in aphasia will be considered. Our objectives are to provide for speech-language pathologists the background information necessary to understand and recognize the existence of significant motor speech handicaps in aphasia and to select appropriate management approaches based on the state of our science.

SPEECH MOTOR DISORDERS ACCOMPANYING APHASIA: NEUROANATOMICAL AND NEUROPHYSIOLOGICAL CONSIDERATIONS

Relatively little is known about the neural underpinnings of speech production. While local reflex circuits (for review, see Smith, 1992), brainstem centers (Grillner, 1982), subcortical nuclei of the basal ganglia and cerebellum (Darley et al., 1975; Kent et al., 1979), the thalamus (McLean et al., 1990), and a number of distinct cortical regions (Gracco and Abbs, 1987) have been implicated in speech, the roles of these structures in speech motor control remain unclear.

Our current lack of understanding of the neural correlates of speech production stems, in part, from the fact that speech is a uniquely human behavior. Whereas animal models and standard neurophysiological techniques have been employed extensively to study the neural control of behaviors that are shared by human and nonhuman species, such as vision, audition, and limb movement, it is more difficult to draw parallels between the neural control of vocalization and nonspeech orofacial behaviors in nonhuman species and the control of speech in humans. Nevertheless, since data from human lesion studies are limited in that lesion location and size cannot be precisely controlled, data from nonhuman studies may provide an important supplementary source of information pertaining to orofacial neural control.

One approach to elucidating the neural substrates of speech production is to view speech as the product of "multiple functional processes" (Gracco, 1991). These processes may include specification of a linguistic representation in terms of phonological or vocal tract parameters (Gracco, 1991; Perkell, 1980); programming (Gracco and Abbs, 1987) and initiation of movement sequences (Alexander et al., 1989); moment-to-moment monitoring and modulation of motor output through feedback and feedforward processes (Gracco and Abbs, 1985); and the coordinated activation of numerous muscles innervated by cranial and spinal motor nuclei. An understanding of the neural control of these component processes, based on data derived from studies of both humans and nonhuman primates, should provide a framework for making predictions about the neural organization of speech motor control. Such a perspective also should inform our considerations of the neural correlates of the motor speech deficits associated with aphasia (for discussion, see Kent, 1990).

Neural Control of Motor Behavior

Over the past two decades, a number of important insights into the neural control of motor behavior have emerged due, in large part, to technological advances in the field of neuroscience. For example, anatomical fiber-tracing techniques have revealed the intricate connections between the cerebral cortex and the subcortical nuclei in the primate (for example, see Schell and Strick, 1984; Wiesendanger and Wiesendanger, 1985a, 1985b). Application of single-neuron recording techniques and intracortical microstimulation (ICMS) has elucidated the functional organization of a number of cortical motor areas (for reviews, see Asanuma, 1989; Wiesendanger and Wise, 1992). And, data from regional cerebral blood flow (rCBF) (Roland, 1981) and positron emission topography (PET) studies (Metter et al., 1988a, 1988b) have contributed to our understanding of the dynamics of neural processing and neuropathophysiology.

One of the major concepts to emerge from recent neuroanatomical and neurophysiological studies is that *the motor cortex is made up of a number of spatially separate, functionally distinct cortical motor fields* (Dum and Strick, 1991; Muakkassa and Strick, 1979; Wiesendanger and Wise, 1992; Wise and Strick, 1984). These cortical motor fields are illustrated in Figure 26.1.

The primary motor cortex, or MI (Brodmann's area 4), located immediately rostral to the central sulcus, can be distinguished from the more rostral nonprimary motor cortex (Brodmann's area 6). Indeed, it has been suggested that the primary and nonprimary cortical regions play different roles in the regulation of movement. The nonprimary motor cortex has been implicated in the "programming" of complex, volitional movements, particularly in movement preparation and sensory guidance. In contrast, the primary motor cortex appears to control movement execution at a lower level of specification (for discussions, see Goldberg, 1985; Gracco and Abbs, 1987; Wise and Strick, 1984).

Based on anatomical and physiological studies in primates, the nonprimary motor cortex (Brodmann's area 6) has been further differentiated into a number of spatially separate, somatotopically organized regions, each of which projects to MI (Muakkassa and Strick, 1979). The two most prominent of these are a medial region, of which the supplementary motor area (SMA) is the major component, and a lateral region, known as the premotor area (PM) in human beings and the arcuate premotor area (APA) in the primate (for review, see Goldberg, 1985). Recent evidence suggests that SMA and PM are further differentiated into several fields (Wiesendanger and Wise,

Figure 26.1. Brodmann's areas of the human cerebral cortex. *A*, Lateral view. *B*, Medial view. Cortical motor fields are also indicated. MI = primary motor cortex; SMA = supplementary motor area; PM = premotor cortex; Area 44 = Broca's area.

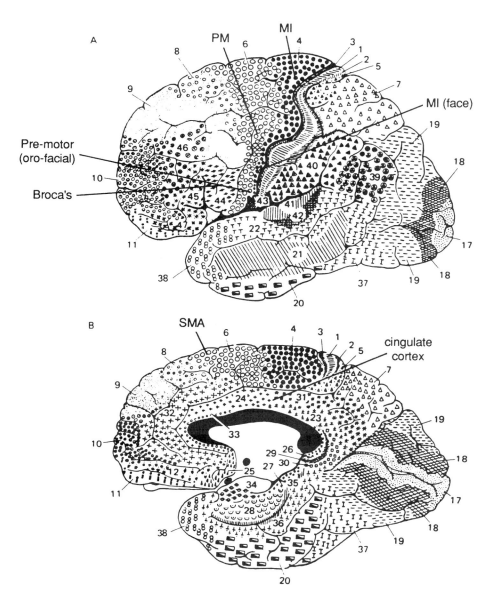

1992). In addition, two distinct cortical motor fields corresponding to Brodmann's areas 23 and 24, on the banks of the cingulate sulcus, have been proposed (Dum and Strick, 1991). This structural and functional differentiation of the motor cortex is consistent with the clinical observation that lesions involving grossly similar regions of the motor cortex often result in strikingly diverse constellations of motor deficits.

A second and related concept that has emerged in recent years is that *regions of the primary and nonprimary motor cortex are functionally linked to specific subcortical nuclei of the basal ganglia and cerebellum through a number of parallel circuits* (Asanuma et al., 1983; Schell and Strick, 1984; Wise and Strick, 1984). A common feature of these parallel circuits is that each receives inputs from a large region of cortex and projects back to a restricted cortical region.

Several such circuits involving basal ganglia and cerebellar inputs to motor cortex appear to be particularly important in motor control. The basal ganglia access the cortex through a number of segregated basal ganglia-thalamocortical circuits (for reviews, see Alexander and Crutcher, 1990; Alexander et al., 1986; DeLong, 1990; Evarts et al., 1984; Graybiel, 1990), one of which has been referred to as the ''motor circuit'' (Alexander et al., 1986). This is illustrated in Figure 26.2.

Within the motor circuit, MI, SMA, APA, and the somatosensory cortex each send topographical, largely nonoverlapping projections to the putamen, a region of the striatum (Alexander and Crutcher, 1990). (The striatum is believed to be the ''input stage'' of the basal ganglia.) This topographical arrangement is maintained as the putamen projects, in turn, to portions of the globus pallidus (GP) and substantia nigra (SN). Motor portions of the GP and SN send topographical projections to specific thalamic nuclei, particularly the VLo (nucleus ventralis posterior lateralis, pars oralis), and VLm (nucleus ventralis lateralis, pars medialis). As seen in Figure 26.3, the circuit is completed through projections from VLo and VLm to the SMA (Schell and Strick, 1984). Thus, a major output of the putamen is directed to the SMA. Furthermore, the prefrontal, parietal, and temporal association cortices project via the caudate to parts of the GP and SN, which project, in turn, to the anterior thalamic nuclei and then to the lateral precentral cortex (area 6) (for review, see Rolls and Johnstone, 1992). Thus, a major output of the caudate is directed to the PM (area 6).

There are two major circuits through which cerebellar output accesses the motor cortex (see Fig. 26.3). One circuit originates in the caudal portions of the deep cerebellar nuclei (e.g., the dentate, interpositus, and fastigial nuclei) and projects largely to area X of the thalamus in a somatotopic fashion (Asanuma et al., 1983; Schell and Strick, 1984). This is the area of thalamus that projects, in turn, to PM. Thus, a major output of the cerebellum is directed to the PM. A second, separate cerebello-thalamo-cortical system also has been described (Asanuma et al., 1983). This originates in the rostral parts of the deep cerebellar nuclei and projects largely to the VPLo (nucleus ventralis lateralis, pars oralis) of the thalamus. Outputs from this area of thalamus output directly to Ml. **Thus, there is a prominent cerebellar output to MI**. Regarding these parallel circuits, Schell and Strick (1984) have suggested that, "although the SMA and APA are interconnected with the motor cortex, it may be important to view the three cortical areas as components of functionally distinct efferent systems which are driven by largely separate subcortical nuclei" (p. 558).

Primary Motor Cortex (Ml)

Functional Organization.   Studies involving electrical stimulation of the cortical surface (Penfield and Rasmussen, 1950) were among the first to implicate MI in the control of movement (for review, see Evarts, 1986; Wiesendanger, 1986). These studies indicated that stimulation of different regions of MI evoked simple movements of discrete body regions, thus giving rise to the concept of the "excitable" cortex. They also showed that the lower limb, upper limb, and orofacial regions were represented in the medial, middle, and lateral regions of MI, respectively. Disproportionately large areas are devoted to representation of the face and hand.

Since those early studies, more refined stimulation techniques have revealed the detailed functional organization of MI (for discussion, see Wiesendanger, 1986). In particular, the use of intracortical microstimulation (ICMS) (Asanuma and Sakata, 1967) in nonhuman primates, in which very small currents are delivered to localized regions within the depths of the cortex, has provided a number of important insights regarding MI. For example, it has been shown that small currents delivered to MI activate single muscles or simple muscle synergies. This finding has led to the suggestion that MI is organized in terms of

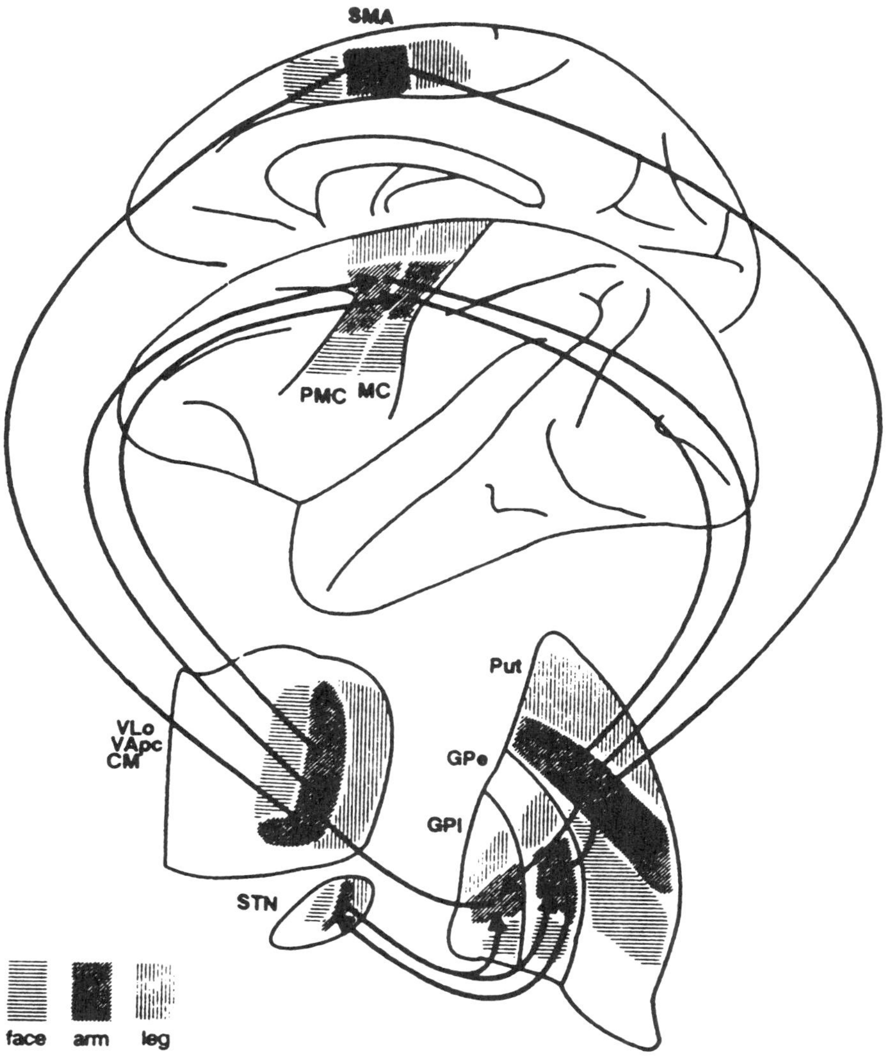

Figure 26.2.   Somatotopic organization of the "motor" circuit. Somatotopic subdivisions of each structure are indicated by differential shading. The arrows indicate the topographically organized pathways that link the respective "arm" representations at different stages of the circuit. Abbreviations: CM, centromedian nucleus; CPe, external segment of globus pallidus; GPi, internal segment of globus pallidus; MC, primary motor cortex; PMC, premotor cortex exclusive of the arcuate premotor area; Put, putamen; SMA, supplementary motor area; VApc, nucleus ventralis anterior pars parvocellularis; VLo, nucleus ventralis lateralis pars oralis.

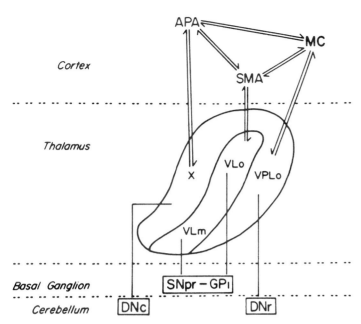

Figure 26.3. Summary of anatomical relationships between cerebellar and basal ganglia efferents and motor and premotor cortical areas. This diagram illustrates (*a*) the pathway from caudal portions of the deep cerebellar nuclei (DNc) to area X and the arcuate premotor area (APA); (*b*) the pathways from the pars reticulata of the substantia nigra (SNpr) and the internal segment of the globus pallidus (Gpi) to the thalamic nuclei and on to the supplementary motor area (SMA) and premotor cortex (PM); (*c*) the pathway from rostral portions of the deep cerebellar nuclei (DNr) to VPLo and the motor cortex (MC); and (*d*) the reciprocal connections between the MC, APA, and SMA.

"efferent microzones" (Wiesendanger, 1986). Each microzone represents a given muscle or elemental movement. Second, a given muscle or simple muscle synergy can be evoked from multiple, noncontiguous regions of MI. Finally, microzones representing different muscles overlap, giving rise to the concept that microzones are "nested" within MI (Kwan et al., 1978). In summary, these findings indicated that multiple, discrete efferent microzones represent a fundamental organizational principle of MI.

The functional implications of this organization have been discussed by a number of authors (Abbs and Welt, 1985; Barlow and Farley, 1989). It has been suggested, for example, that the organization of MI in terms of individual muscles or elemental movements may underly the fractionation of distal movements, most highly evolved in nonhuman and human primates. Further, the multiple, nested representations of muscles may provide a basis for the functional coupling of subsets of muscles and/or structures characteristic of complex, coordinated movements (e.g., the "coordinative structure" proposed by Fowler et al., 1980). The organization of MI also may underly the ability to generate a given elemental movement within the context of a variety of motor behaviors.

MI Inputs and Outputs. Because MI receives diverse inputs from both cortical and subcortical regions, it is believed to represent a "nodal point" within the motor system. It can be "addressed" through a variety of parallel and/or hierarchical circuits (for discussions, see Abbs and Welt, 1985; Gracco and

Abbs, 1987; Jones, 1987; Muakkassa and Strick, 1979; Smith, 1992; Wiesendanger, 1986). For example, MI receives prominent cortical inputs from a number of premotor fields, including SMA, PM, Brodmann's area 44, and the cingulate cortex (Muakkassa and Strick, 1979). As discussed previously, the basal ganglia and the cerebellum gain access to MI by way of these premotor inputs (Schell and Strick, 1984). MI also receives projections from Brodmann's areas 1 and 2 of the primary somatosensory cortex (SI) and from the posterior parietal areas. (Asanuma, 1989; Jones, 1987). The presence of such inputs suggests that MI has access to sensory information that has already undergone processing at the cortical level. In addition to these indirect sensory inputs to MI from somatosensory cortex, MI receives direct peripheral sensory inputs via thalamocortical fibers. Direct sensory inputs from the orofacial region are believed to project from the ventral posteromedial nucleus (VPM) of the thalamus to MI (Dubner et al., 1978). MI also receives a prominent cerebellar input via the VPLo of the thalamus (Schell and Strick, 1984).

The outputs from MI are equally diverse (for reviews, see Evarts, 1986; Wiesendanger, 1986). Both anatomical and physiological data from nonhuman and human primates (Kuypers, 1958a, 1958b; Sirisko and Sessle, 1983) have indicated that MI neurons project directly to motoneurons. This important finding has led to the suggestion that MI cells represent "upper motoneurons" that exert direct effects on motoneurons. In addition, MI projects to a number of cortical and subcortical regions in a distributed fashion, including the premotor cortex, thalamic nuclei, striatum, red nucleus, pontine nuclei, brain stem, and spinal cord dorsal and ventral horns (Wiesendanger, 1986). Wiesendanger (1986) has discussed the importance of these MI inputs to subcortical nuclei. He suggests that the activation of subcortical structures by motor cortex output may provide a means by which the accuracy of an evolving movement is checked in relation to stored "algorithms" resident in subcortical nuclei.

Role of Sensory Input to MI. As described above, MI receives prominent sensory inputs via the thalamus and the somatic sensory cortex. The extent of these sensory inputs to MI is reflected in the finding that many MI neurons are characterized by "receptive fields"; that is, they are activated when a particular region of the body is stimulated mechanically (Asanuma and Rosen, 1972). Moreover, for many MI neurons, there is a close spatial match between the receptive field and the body region in which movement is evoked when the neuron is stimulated electrically (Huang et al., 1989b; Murray and Sessle, 1992a).

A number of hypotheses have been advanced regarding the role of these relatively direct sensory inputs to MI in motor control. It has been suggested that they may provide a means by which movement synergies that are preprogrammed at subcortical levels are "fine-tuned" during motor execution in relation to incoming afferent information (for discussion, see Murray, 1989). Gracco and Abbs (1987) have suggested that the direct sensory inputs to MI via the thalamus and SI would be well suited for the "time-critical" processes of orofacial motor execution. They contrast these relatively direct sensory inputs with the contributions of the basal ganglia and cerebellum, which, they suggest, are involved preferentially in motor programming.

The effects of deafferentation on movement also suggest the importance of sensory input in motor control. Asanuma and Arissian (1984) found that unilateral lesions of SI and the dorsal column resulted in severe motor deficits that resembled the effects of MI lesions in some respects. Asanuma (1989) has suggested that afferent inputs to MI set the excitability levels of groups of MI neurons required for an upcoming movement and thereby provide for the fine control of distal movements. This concept is referred to as the "preferential bias theory."

Effects of Lesions to MI. Effects of lesions restricted to MI generally are consistent with the data from intracortical microstimulation studies and the multiple efferent microzone model of MI organization. As reviewed by Freund (1987), lesions of MI typically result in a contralateral **paresis,** most pronounced distally, which recedes rapidly, leaving a lasting deficit in the ability to perform fractionated movements involving the distal musculature. Evarts (1986) notes that even small MI lesions lead to impairment in the use of sets of muscles, not single muscles, for some, but not all, movements.

The question of whether lesions of MI result in spasticity remains controversial (for review, see Freund, 1987). While some have suggested that spasticity can result from lesions confined to MI, others contend that spasticity is related to damage to the premotor cortex (e.g., Brodmann's area 6). They attribute the more severe spasticity seen following capsular lesions to damage of fibers originating from the premotor areas, and not from MI.

Primary Motor Cortex Controlling Orofacial Function. Although current understanding of MI is based largely on studies of limb motor control, a small number of studies have provided insights into the functional organization of regions of MI involved in the control of orofacial motor behavior. Studies employing intracortical microstimulation (ICMS) in nonhuman primates have shown that the muscles of the face, jaw (particularly the jaw-opening muscles), tongue, and larynx (Hoffman and Luschei, 1980; Huang et al., 1988, Huang et al., 1989b; Murray and Sessle, 1992a; Zealear et al., 1983) are represented in the lateral regions of MI in a discontinuous, overlapping fashion. For example, Huang et al. (1988) found that the face representation (e.g., face MI) partly enclosed and overlapped the more lateral cortical regions controlling jaw and tongue muscles, and that a particular facial muscle was represented at multiple cortical sites. Whereas microstimulation evoked contralateral facial movements at most stimulation sites, ipsilateral responses also were found. Based on these findings, Huang et al. (1988) suggested that the close interrelationship of face, jaw, and tongue muscle representations, as well as the presence of both contralateral and ipsilateral responses, may allow for the necessary unilateral and bilateral integration of facial, jaw, and tongue movements that characterize most oral behaviors. Their results also indicated that the face motor cortex is organized in terms of multiple efferent microzones.

The functional significance of this region of MI in oral motor behavior has been suggested by a number of findings. First, the activity of neurons in the lateral precentral gyrus has been shown to be associated with performance of a number of oral behaviors in the primate, including a trained, steady bite-force task (Hoffman and Luschei, 1980) and trained tongue protrusion and biting (Murray and Sessle, 1992b, 1992c). Lesion studies also have demonstrated the significance of this cortical region. Luschei and Goodwin (1975) showed that bilateral ablation of

the face area of MI in the monkey disrupted the ability to maintain a low steady bite force. Murray et al. (1991) showed that inactivation of the tongue area of MI by reversible cooling resulted in a marked impairment in the ability to perform a trained tongue protrusion task but had only minor effects on performance of a trained biting task.

Studies in nonhuman primates also have indicated that regions of MI representing the orofacial musculature receive prominent sensory inputs. Hoffman and Luschei (1980) reported that the activity of neurons in the lateral precentral gyrus was modulated when a sinusoidal movement was imposed on the monkey's jaw. This finding suggests that MI neurons controlling jaw movements receive inputs from peripheral receptors. Further, different regions of the lateral precentral cortex appear to receive different sensory inputs. Neurons in the face (Huang et al., 1988, 1989b) and tongue (Murray and Sessle, 1992a) regions of primate MI are activated by light tactile stimulation of a small, discrete orofacial region. Unlike the limb motor cortex, few neurons in face and tongue MI are activated by deep mechanical stimulation, such as muscle stretch or pressure. In contrast, neurons in the jaw region of MI appear to receive deep sensory inputs and inputs from periodontal tissues (Murray and Sessle, 1992a). These findings are consistent with the view that superficial orofacial mechanoreceptors and tactile stimuli may be particularly important for the sensory guidance of orofacial movements, whereas stimulation of deep receptors may be preferentially important for the guidance of jaw movements. The prominent sensory inputs to face MI are of interest in relation to the proposal by Benke and Kertesz (1989) that damage to the postcentral cortex (i.e., sensory cortex) may be associated with a significant dysarthria.

Lateral PM and Area 44

The PM occupies the region of area 6 lateral to the SMA (for review, see Wise, 1985). It is bordered rostrally by prefrontal cortex, laterally by the Sylvian fissure, and caudally by MI. In the primate, PM is referred to as the arcuate premotor area (APA) (Schell and Strick, 1984). It has been suggested that, phylogenetically, PM is derived from insular cortex and that it represents a "protomotor" area, that is, a region of motor cortex where movements are specified at a relatively abstract level (Goldberg, 1985). Recent evidence suggests that PM is composed of a number of functionally distinct regions (Dum and Strick, 1991; Muakkassa and Strick, 1979; Mushiake et al., 1991; Wiesendanger and Wise, 1992).

Inputs and Outputs. PM receives cortical inputs from numerous sensory and association areas. In the primate, the posterior parietal association cortex, particularly area 7b (Godschalk et al., 1984), and the secondary somatosensory cortex (SII) (Godschalk et al., 1984) project to PM. PM also receives sensory inputs from visual and auditory areas (Wise, 1985). Thus, visual, somatic, and auditory sensory inputs have access to PM. PM also receives reciprocal inputs from MI (Godschalk et al., 1984; Pandya and Seltzer, 1982). As noted earlier, the major subcortical input to PM is from area X of thalamus, the region receiving cerebellar efferents. Thus, it has been suggested that the cerebellar nuclei "drive" PM (Schell and Strick, 1984).

PM projects topographically to MI, with the region lateral to the inferior end of the precentral sulcus projecting to the face region of MI in the monkey (Matelli et al., 1986; Muakkassa and Strick, 1979). Because PM receives input from sensory association areas and projects to MI, it has been suggested that PM uses sensory input to influence the activity of MI (Pandya and Seltzer, 1982). In particular, Muakkassa and Strick (1979) have suggested that APA (i.e., premotor area) may be part of a circuit through which area 7 of the parietal lobe gains access to MI during visually guided movements in the primate.

PM also projects reciprocally to SMA, to regions surrounding the lateral fissure, the cingulate cortex (Matelli et al., 1986), prefrontal cortex, and basal ganglia (Pandya and Barnes, 1987). In terms of descending projections to motor nuclei, it has been suggested that lateral PM does not have direct projections to motoneurons and that connections are generally indirect to reticular formation adjacent to motor nuclei (for discussion, see Abbs and Welt, 1985). However, Dum and Strick (1991) recently showed that neurons from a number of nonprimary motor areas in the primate, including APA, project directly to cervical segments of the spinal cord. The presence of these corticospinal neurons in PM suggests that, like MI and SMA, PM may represent a parallel pathway that influences motoneurons directly.

In contrast to PM, there has been relatively little study of the inputs and outputs of area 44. Area 44 receives projections from the posterior parietal and temporal cortical regions (for review, see Abbs and Welt, 1985). Muakkassa and Strick (1979) reported that there is a face representation in area 44 of the monkey. Abbs and Welt (1985) note that the efferent projections from area 44 to regions adjacent to the cranial motor nuclei are less dense and more diffuse than those originating from MI and PM and area 6. Thus, area 44 would be expected to exert less direct effects on motor execution than PM and MI.

Role of Sensory Input to PM.   It has been suggested that the role of PM in motor control is to use sensory inputs to organize or guide motor behavior (Wise, 1985). For example, the prominent input from area 7 of the posterior parietal cortex to PM suggests that PM is involved in visually guided movements. Indeed, PM neurons have been found to be preferentially active during visually guided, sequential limb movements in monkeys, whereas SMA neurons are preferentially active in relation to internally determined movements that are performed from memory (Mushiake et al., 1991).

Consistent with its prominent sensory inputs, PM neurons can be activated by tactile, visual, and/or auditory stimuli (for review, see Wise, 1985). For example, neurons in the lateral region of PM in the primate respond to tactile stimulation of the mouth (Rizzolatti et al., 1981). Moreover, regions of PM receive overlapping auditory-visual, auditory-somatic, or visual-somatic sensory inputs (Pandya and Seltzer, 1982). Thus, it has been suggested that PM may be involved in motor behaviors requiring integration of sensory inputs from different modalities.

Whereas PM has been implicated in motor behavior, recent evidence suggests that PM also may have a cognitive function. Watanabe (1992) examined single-neuron activity from the prefrontal and premotor cortex during a task in which a motor behavior and subsequent reward were associated with either auditory or visual cues. Consistent with previous studies, he found that PM neurons were characterized by cross-modal (auditory-visual) coding. Moreover, PM did not code the physical properties of the stimulus but rather its associative significance. Thus, Watanabe (1992) suggested that PM may code the behavioral significance of polymodal sensory inputs.

Lesions of PM.   Lesions of PM result in a number of sensorimotor deficits that are generally distinct from the symptoms of SMA and MI lesions. In primates, PM lesions result in a failure to respond to contralateral sensory stimuli (for review, see Pandya and Seltzer, 1982). Rizzolatti (1985) found that unilateral lesions of area 6 in the monkey resulted in failure to grasp food with the mouth when it was presented contralaterally, and hemiinattention. Lesions of PM in humans have been associated with deficits of complex movements. Freund (1987) notes that the patients reported by Foerster showed loss of kinetic melody, dissolution of context for composite movements, and disintegration of complex, skilled movements. Freund and Hummelsheim (1985) reported that lesions of PM were associated with limb-kinetic apraxia and a disturbance of movements requiring the temporal coordination of proximal muscles on both sides of the body.

PM and Orofacial Function.   Fulton (1949) suggested that the portion of PM inferior to the arcuate sulcus represents a premotor area for orofacial movements. This view has been supported by a number of lines of evidence. First, lesion studies in primates have implicated the lateral PM in complex oral motor behaviors, particularly those associated with food ingestion. Lesions of lateral PM and area 44 disrupt the coordinated movements of the lips, tongue, and jaw necessary for intraoral manipulation of food, mastication, and swallowing (Larson et al., 1980).

Stimulation studies also have suggested a role for this area in orofacial function. The area immediately lateral to face MI and adjacent to the Sylvian fissure has been designated the "cortical masticatory area" (CMA), based on the finding that electrical stimulation of this region evokes rhythmic jaw movements in the monkey (Huang et al., 1989a; Lund and Lamarre, 1974). Evidence from Huang et al. (1989a) indicated that rhythmical jaw movements are evoked by ICMS applied to four areas, including face MI, face SI, the principal cortical masticatory area (CMAp) located on the precentral gyrus lateral to face MI, and the deep CMA (CMAd) located on the inferior face of the frontal operculum. Further, these four regions where rhythmic jaw movements were evoked were characterized by different afferent inputs and different motor responses to ICMS. This suggests that these four areas may be differentially involved in the production and organization of mastication. Finally, stimulation of a region overlapping and immediately posterior to CMA has been reported to evoke swallowing in the monkey (Miller and Bowman, 1977).

Single-neuron recording studies also have implicated lateral PM in complex oral movements. Luschei et al., (1971) found that the activity of neurons in the precentral face area, including Brodmann's areas 6 and 4, was related to a visually cued, phasic bite task. The activity of other neurons was related to the oral movements associated with ingestion, but not to the bite task.

Role of the Lateral Precentral Cortex in Motor Speech Disorders

Human lesion studies have implicated the lateral precentral cortex (including Ml, PM, and Brodmann's area 44) and underlying white matter in the motor speech disorders associated with aphasia. Nevertheless, because lesions typically involve many cortical and subcortical structures, the differential contributions of MI, PM, area 44, and subcortical structures to motor speech impairments remain poorly understood (for discussion, see Tonkonogy and Goodglass, 1981).

Unilateral damage restricted to MI is traditionally thought to result in a mild, transient weakness of the contralateral tongue, lips, and lower face, with transient imprecise speech articulation (Abbs and Welt, 1985; Darley et al., 1975). However, Duffy and Folger (1986) and Hartman and Abbs (1989) have reported several cases of unilateral upper motor neuron (UUMN) dysarthria. A similar dysarthria has been reported following a subcortical lesion of the posterior limb of the internal capsule (Kennedy and Murdoch, 1989).

More extensive unilateral damage to the inferior region of the left MI (area 4) and subjacent white matter, particularly if it extends to the Rolandic operculum and insula (area 6), but sparing the rostral part of Broca's area and underlying white matter, can produce a speech deficit without major language impairment (Alexander et al., 1989; Baum et al., 1990; Damasio, 1991; Lecours and Lhermitte, 1976; Levine and Mohr, 1979; Pellat et al., 1991; Schiff et al., 1983; Tonkonogy and Goodglass, 1981). This speech deficit also has been reported following a largely subcortical lesion of the anterior limb of the internal capsule, between the head of the caudate and the putamen (Schiff et al., 1983). It is characterized by slow rate, effortful articulatory struggle, articulatory distortions, and disrupted prosody and, as indicated in Table 26.1, has been referred to by a number of terms, including aphemia (Schiff et al., 1983), apraxia of speech (Darley, 1968), and phonetic disintegration (Lecours and Lhermitte, 1976).

In attempting to interpret the symptomatology of "apraxia of speech," certain neuroanatomical and neurophysiological data merit consideration. First, it is noteworthy that apraxia of speech has been reported to result from lesions of the lateral PM and insula, regions that also have been implicated in the control of complex orofacial movements associated with ingestion, mastication, and swallowing in the primate. Moreover, the deficits seen following such lesions in humans, including slow, effortful, strugglelike movements and disintegration of complex movement sequences, bear certain similarities to the deficits of ingestive behavior seen following lesions of similar cortical regions in primates (for discussion, see Abbs and Welt, 1985). Second, it is important to consider that the lateral PM, implicated in apraxic deficits, receives prominent cerebellar and parietal afferent inputs. The cerebellar inputs to PM may be consistent with reports that apraxia of speech can be characterized by ataxic features (McNeil et al., 1989, 1990).

Bilateral perisylvian lesions involving the frontal and parietal opercula can produce a loss of voluntary control of the facial, masticatory, lingual, and pharyngeal musculature known as anterior operculum syndrome, or Foix-Chavany-Marie syndrome (Cappa et al., 1987; Mao et al., 1989). This is characterized by an automatic-voluntary dissociation, with preserved orofacial function for automatic behaviors and reflexes, except the gag reflex, which is absent. Speech is generally absent, and there is a pronounced dysphagia. Unilateral lesions involving the left frontal operculum, including Broca's area, the underlying white matter, and the lateral region of MI, result in a more complex disorder of both speech and language termed "Broca's area aphasia" or "small Broca's aphasia" (Alexander et al., 1989; Damasio, 1991; Mohr et al., 1975; Mohr et al., 1978). In contrast, true Broca's aphasia has been associated with more extensive damage to Broca's area, the surrounding premotor and prefrontal fields, underlying white matter, and the basal ganglia (Damasio, 1991; Mohr et al., 1975; Mohr et al., 1978; Tonkonogy and Goodglass, 1981).

Supplementary Motor Cortex

The SMA occupies the medial region of Brodmann's area 6, on the mesial surface of the hemispheres. It has been suggested that the SMA is derived from cingulate (limbic) cortex and, like PM, represents a "protomotor area" (Goldberg, 1985). It receives both cortical and subcortical inputs and is considered to be an area of cortical convergence, in that it receives projections from the primary and nonprimary motor cortex, cingulate cortex, and parietal and temporal cortical regions (for review, see Goldberg, 1985). As discussed earlier, the major subcortical input to SMA is from the VLo of the thalamus (Schell and Strick, 1984; Wiesendanger and Wiesendanger, 1985a). Because this is the region of thalamus receiving prominent globus pallidus and substantia nigra projections, the basal ganglia constitute the major subcortical input to SMA.

The efferent projections from SMA represent a cascading system (Jurgens, 1985). That is, SMA projects to a number of different levels, including MI bilaterally (Jurgens, 1985), PM, and the prefrontal, parietal, and cingulate cortex. The fact that SMA receives projections from the cingulate cortex and projects to MI has been taken to support the view that SMA is part of the system that "focuses limbic outflow onto motor executive regions, thus linking intention formation to programming and execution of specific acts" (Goldberg, 1985, p. 576). Subcortically, SMA makes connections with a number of nuclei of the thalamus, basal ganglia, and cerebellum. It has recently been demonstrated that SMA also makes direct corticospinal projections in the primate (Dum and Strick, 1991). Based on this finding, it has been suggested that the SMA has the potential to influence movement directly, independent of MI. Thus, outputs from SMA, PM, and MI may constitute distinct, parallel pathways through which movements are generated and controlled.

Functional Organization of SMA. Electrical stimulation of the SMA evokes complex multijoint movements and has been associated with transient arrest of ongoing motor activity (Fried et al., 1991; Penfield and Welch, 1951). SMA stimulation in epileptic patients has been reported to evoke an "urge" to perform a movement, or a feeling of anticipation that a movement is about to occur (Fried et al., 1991). These findings are consistent with the suggestion that the SMA is involved in establishing a "preparatory state" or "motor set" that precedes the execution of complex motor sequences (for discussions, see Kurata, 1992; Wise and Strick, 1984).

Another finding to emerge from stimulation studies is that the SMA is somatotopically organized, with the face, upper limb, and lower limb represented in a rostral to caudal direction within SMA (Brinkman and Porter, 1979; Kurata, 1992; see, however, Hummelsheim et al., 1986). Interestingly, neurons have been found in the most rostral areas of SMA that fire in relation to chewing and licking in the primate (Chen et al., 1991).

Single-neuron recording studies in awake monkeys have provided clues as to the role of the SMA in motor behavior. These investigations have shown that SMA neurons respond preferentially in relation to sequential motor behaviors, particularly if the movements are internally generated or self-initiated (Mushiake et al., 1991). Further, it appears that there are functionally distinct populations of neurons within SMA. Some neurons are similar to MI neurons, in that they are active in relation to movement execution. These have been termed "short lead neurons" (Chen et al., 1991; Wise and Strick, 1984). Other SMA neurons, called "long lead neurons" are active prior to movement onset and exhibit complex relations to movement execution (Chen et al., 1991). The activity of these neurons may be related to sensory stimuli, particularly if these sensory signals are cuing movement (Wise and Strick, 1984). Thus, the SMA has been implicated in the sensory guidance of movement.

Role of SMA in Speech Motor Control.   Cortical stimulation studies and human lesion data have implicated the SMA-basal ganglia system in the motor control of speech. Electrical stimulation of the cortical surface has been reported to evoke involuntary sustained or interrupted vocalization, speech arrest, slowing of speech, hesitations, word and syllable repetitions, and speech slurring and distortions (Chauvel et al., 1985; Fried et al., 1991; Penfield and Roberts, 1959; Penfield and Welch, 1951). Fried et al. (1991) indicated that vocalization, speech arrest, and slowing were evoked from the region immediately anterior to the face representation within SMA, and that vocalization was evoked only when stimulation was applied to the left hemisphere. This latter finding is consistent with the observation by Chauvel et al. (1985) that the probability of evoking vocalization was greater in the dominant hemisphere.

Lesions of the left SMA and/or cingulate cortex have been shown to result initially in a transient period of mutism and akinesia (Alexander et al., 1989; Damasio and Geschwind, 1984; Damasio and Van Hoesen, 1980; Jonas, 1981), which is more pronounced with bilateral lesions (Freund, 1987). As the mutism lifts, there is a paucity of speech (and motor behavior in general), and speech is delayed because of initiation difficulty. However, speech articulation is relatively intact and there are no overt signs of aphasia (Alexander et al., 1989; Damasio and Geschwind, 1984; Damasio and Van Hoesen, 1980). Damasio and Geschwind (1984) suggest that these symptoms reflect a reduced "drive" to communicate verbally and that the underlying deficit is motoric/affective and not primarily linguistic. Alexander et al. (1989) and Damasio and Geschwind (1984) reject the view that patients with lesions of the SMA have transcortical motor aphasia (Freedman et al., 1984) and suggest that damage to the medial aspect of the frontal lobes (i.e., SMA) results in a pattern of motor deficits and language recovery that is distinct from that associated with midfrontal lobe damage, giving rise to transcortical motor aphasia.

SMA lesions also have been reported to result in paroxysmal speech or palalalia, characterized by sudden involuntary vocalizations such as rhythmic repetitions of syllables, words and phrases (Alajounine et al., 1959; Jonas, 1981; Nagafuchi et al., 1991; Wallesch, 1990). Associated speech symptoms, including echolalia (Alexander et al., 1989; Jonas, 1981), "stuttering"

(Jonas, 1981), hesitations, perseverations, and word-finding difficulty, have been reported. SMA lesions also have been associated with reduced phonatory volume and aphonia (Jonas, 1981).

It is noteworthy that a number of the deficits resulting from SMA lesions also are associated with basal ganglia dysfunction. For example, akinesia is a primary deficit in both basal ganglia and SMA dysfunction. In relation to speech disorders, many of the speech symptoms associated with SMA lesions, such as dysfluency, akinesia, mutism, and aphonia, are present in Parkinson's disease (PD). This is consistent with the evidence that a major output of the basal ganglia is to the SMA (Schell and Strick, 1984).

Conversely, it has been suggested that certain motor deficits associated with basal ganglia dysfunction are related to a "functional deafferentation of the SMA (Rascol et al., 1992; Schell and Strick, 1984). This is supported by a recent study of regional cerebral blood flow (rCBF) in SMA and MI in akinetic PD patients (Rascol et al., 1992). These authors showed that PD patients whose akinesia was controlled by dopaminergic treatment had significant increases in blood flow in both MI and SMA associated with movement, whereas patients who were akinetic during "off" medication periods showed increases in MI only. Thus, it was suggested that akinesia in PD may be mediated by reduced subcortical drive of the SMA by the basal ganglia.

Parietal Lobe

The parietal lobe is characterized by a number of polysensory association areas that are believed to be critical for sensory integration of complex cognitive functions (for review, see Freund, 1987). Further, the links between the parietal and frontal lobes have been suggested to mediate the integration of sensory inputs in preparation of motor acts.

Lesions of the parietal lobe result in a number of sensorimotor deficits (Freund, 1987). For example, ideational, ideokinetic, tactile, and visuomotor apraxias have been reported following lesions of the posterior parietal lobe, or at its junction with the temporal and occipital lobes (for review, see Freund, 1987).

The role of the parietal lobe in speech motor control has been examined by Kimura and colleagues (Kimura, 1979, 1982; Mateer and Kimura, 1977). In a recent study, Kimura and Watson (1989) examined abilities of aphasic patients with anterior and posterior lesions to produce single and multiple speech and nonspeech oral movements. Patients with anterior lesions were impaired in their ability to reproduce single, nonverbal oral movements, and single isolated speech sounds, whereas patients with posterior lesions had difficulty only when they were required to produce multiple oral movements. Based on these findings, Kimura and Watson suggested that the region of the left hemisphere anterior to the Rolandic sulcus is critical for control at the "unit" level of movement, whereas the posterior region is involved in accurate selection of movements in multiple movement sequences. Further, they proposed a parietal system mediating praxic function and contrasted this with a temporal system mediating auditory control. Square-Storer and Apeldoorn (1991) reported one patient who had numerous symptoms of "apraxia of speech" but no aphasia as indicated by performance on standardized aphasia batteries. Computed tomography (CT) scan revealed that this patient had bilateral parietal lobe lesions. Although this patient was diagnosed as having apraxia of speech, his speech output differed from that of two other subjects who also had apraxia of speech but no clinically demonstrable aphasia. While the other two patients' speech was characterized by dysprosody, particularly slow rate and abnormal stress patterns, the parietal lobe-lesioned patient's speech pattern was characterized by relatively normal prosodic contours but frequent reattempts and false starts. Could it be that the other two patients had apraxia and dysarthria while the parietal-lesioned patient had true apraxia of speech?

Functional Effects of Structural Lesions

In the 1970s, dynamic methods for the study of regions of brain function were developed. With the advent of rCBF, it was possible to determine areas within the two hemispheres that were most active metabolically during certain behaviors (e.g., Soh et al., 1978). Dynamic recordings of brain metabolic activity were even further refined with the development of PET (c.f., Phelps et al., 1983).

Metter and colleagues used PET extensively to study glucose metabolism in resting aphasic patients with structural lesions confirmed by CT scan (Metter et al., 1981; Metter et al., 1982; Metter et al., 1983; Metter et al., 1985; Metter et al., 1986; Metter et al., 1987a; Metter et al., 1987b; Metter et al., 1988a; Metter et al., 1988b; Metter et al., 1989).

In this series of resting-state studies, several major findings regarding effects of structural lesions were replicated repeatedly. First, a lesion could cause hypometabolism in its environs only. Second, a structural lesion could cause diffuse hypometabolism throughout the left hemisphere. And, last, a structural lesion could cause remote hypometabolic effects. For the purposes of our discussion, the most salient of the remote effects were the following: (a) A subcortical lesion to the basal ganglia (Metter et al., 1988; Metter et al., 1988b) or the neostriatum (Illes et al., 1989) commonly resulted in hypometabolism within the speech motor control regions of the frontal lobe; and (b) ipsilateral cerebellar hemisphere hypometabolism is commonly associated with frontal lobe lesions (Metter et al., 1987b). These findings indicate that in many patients with aphasia and motor speech involvement, a static lesion to one motor center is capable of causing reduced function in other motor control centers.

Another important finding deriving from the PET studies undertaken by Metter and his group is that in all classifications of aphasia, there is significant temporoparietal hypometabolism. This finding has led to the resurgence of the hypothesis that aphasia may be a single entity; that is, in conduction, Broca's, and Wernicke's aphasia, despite the location of the static lesion, all classifications demonstrate similar patterns of hypometabolism in the temporoparietal regions. What differentiated the groups (classifications) was the presence and degree of coexisting prefrontal hypometabolism. In Broca's aphasia, there was significant prefrontal hypometabolism; in Wernicke's aphasia, there was prefrontal hypometabolism, though not to the extent found in Broca's aphasia; in conduction aphasia, two subgroups were identified, half with hypometabolism to Broca's area and half without, with none demonstrating prefrontal hypometabolism (Kempler et al., 1986). Metter and colleagues have speculated that the prefrontal hypometabolism factor differing syndromes of aphasia. Further, it was hypothesized that prefrontal hypometabolism may impose a motor deficit extrinsic to language functioning (Metter et al., 1987a). If, in fact, this motor deficit is the

distinguishing factor, it behooves us to develop motorically based treatments for "nonfluent" aphasia.

Summary and Implications for a Model of Motor Speech Disorders Accompanying Aphasia

The neuroanatomical and neurophysiological data presented here lead to a number of conclusions that are relevant to a discussion of motor speech deficits that accompany aphasia. First, a number of motor subsystems are found within the frontal and parietal lobes. Many of these same regions also have been implicated in language functions (Ojemann, 1988), and lesions to these areas frequently are associated with aphasia. Based on the intimacy of the neural structures that mediate linguistic and motoric functions, then, it is reasonable that motor speech deficits often accompany aphasia. Moreover, because these motor subsystems are functionally heterogeneous (distinct) and organized in parallel, various lesions may result in qualitatively different and/or functionally heterogeneous speech deficits, depending on the lesion site, extent, and remote effects. It is possible that what we have recently called "apraxia of speech" may not always be a unidimensional disorder but, instead, heterogeneous in constellations and predominance of symptoms (Rosenbek and McNeil, 1991; Square-Storer and Apeldoorn, 1991). For example, the neurophysiological data suggest that MI lesions impair motor execution and activation of distal musculature for fractionated movements. PM lesions, however, may result in impairments in the preparation of movement, programming of complex multiple movement sequences, kinetic melody, and use of sensory information to guide movements. As such, lesions involving both MI and PM may result in deficits of both motor programming and execution. Similarly, given the inputs of basal ganglia and cerebellum to MI via the premotor areas, deficits traditionally associated with pathology of these subcortical regions may be seen following lesions of the precentral cortex. This view is further substantiated by the results of the PET studies, which have demonstrated the functional linkages between spatially remote brain regions such as cerebellar and frontal regions. The controversy that has existed regarding the neuromotor speech disorder that frequently coexists with aphasia may, thus, be more clearly understood.

Apraxia of speech has been described as an articulatory-prosodic disorder due to brain damage in which the programming of speech movements with regard to their spatiotemporal aspects is impaired (Kent and Rosenbek, 1983) but in which there are not significant muscle strength, tone, or coordination impairments as observed in the dysarthrias (Darley et al., 1975). Recent studies have characterized apraxia of speech in terms of certain kinematic features. For example, apraxia of speech has been described as a movement disorder in which phase-plane relationships are disrupted (Forrest et al., 1991). This may be the underlying basis for the decoupling of normal spatiotemporal relations of speech movements (Itoh et al., 1979; Itoh et al., 1980; Kent and Rosenbek, 1983). McNeil and Adams (1990) and Robin et al. (1989) have speculated that the essence of the movement disorder is abnormal amplitude-velocity relations.[a]

---

[a] Adams (1990) suggested that abnormal velocity-amplitude relationships may be observed in apraxia of speech because of the slow rate of speech that is characteristic of the disorder. That is, normal speakers also demonstrate similar abnormal velocity-amplitude relationships when speaking at a slow rate.

All experienced aphasia clinicians, however, recognize that there is often an overriding coexisting dysarthriclike quality to the speech of patients whom we diagnose as having apraxia of speech. Indeed, over the years, apraxia of speech often has been referred to as a dysarthric condition. Many patients demonstrate an effortfulness of speech production and/or overriding voice and resonance qualities that are unlikely to be wholly apraxic in nature. Further, classical notions of apraxia indicate that automatic motor function is preserved whereas propositional movement is not, even when the same muscle collectives are called into play. In what we have traditionally labeled as apraxic-aphasic speakers, the automatic-volitional dichotomy of motor performance is only rarely observed (e.g., Wertz et al., 1984). Might it be that the automatic-volitional dichotomy is the essence of apraxia but the "apraxia of speech" we most commonly encounter is frequently complicated by dysarthric symptoms?

Although apraxia of speech is likely to occur with frontal subcortical and cortical lesions as well as midparietal lesions, it may coexist with other neuromotor speech disruptions that are dystonic, paretic, ataxic, and/or dysfluent (i.e., stutteringlike, in nature). Furthermore, the proportions and various combinations of these disorders will vary across individuals. An attempt to summarize our review of the literature regarding the neurophysiological control of motor speech within a clinically relevant framework is shown in Table 26.2. Suspected primary functional effects and expected speech symptoms arising from primary lesion sites are summarized. Table 26.2 represents a preliminary attempt to explain our understanding of the possible components that contribute to the impairment of articulated speech that may coexist with aphasia.

MANAGEMENT OF MOTOR SPEECH DISORDERS ACCOMPANYING APHASIA

The terminological confusion that has reigned regarding neuromotor speech deficits in aphasia has most probably biased both our assessment and treatment approaches. Because we have grouped the majority of patients into the diagnostic category of "apraxia of speech," we have tended to view patient differences as possibly being due to severity rather than combinations of primary and secondary pathophysiologies. Thus, treatment interventions have been advocated for severe, moderate, and mild apraxia of speech as shown in Table 26.3 (Wertz et al., 1984).

In the second column of Table 26.3, a critical analysis of the traditional approaches used for the enhancement of speech in patients with "acquired apraxia of speech" and aphasia indicates three assumed levels of intervention: (a) postural shaping, (b) postural shaping plus kinesthetic awareness for movement units, and (c) melodic or rhythmic flow and pacing approaches. We query whether, in fact, severity is the deciding factor in the appropriate selection of treatment approaches or whether, instead, it is the primary pathophysiology that is the determining factor. That is, are the postural shaping methods, especially those that use light tactile sensation, more appropriate for patients who cannot execute isolated phonemes and monosyllables? And, are melodic and rate control approaches more appropriate when any of the movement disorders/disruptions (apraxia, ataxia, dystonia), or combinations thereof, contribute significantly to speech breakdown? Most certainly, rate and rhythm approaches have been used widely in the treatment of movement disorders, particularly hypokinetic and ataxic dysar-

thria (Berry and Goshorn, 1983; Beukelman and Yorkston, 1978; Hanson and Metter, 1980, 1983; Helm, 1979; Yorkston and Beukelman, 1981), as well as apraxia of speech (Rubow et al., 1982; Simmons, 1978; Square-Storer, 1989; Wertz et al., 1984). The issue being raised here is whether these patients vary on a continuum of severity or whether they have different primary and secondary pathophysiologies for which different treatment methods may be preferentially effective.

Presented in Table 26.4 is a summary of the traditional approaches used for enhancement of speech among dysarthric speakers as derived principally from Yorkston et al. (1988). The similarities and differences between treatment approaches for what we have termed "apraxia of speech" and dysarthria are easily discerned from a comparison of Tables 26.3 and 26.4. There are two major differences. First, there is rarely a need to establish physiological support for speech in treatment approaches for the disorder we have termed apraxia of speech, whereas for dysarthric patients, rehabilitation directed at control and coordination of the respiratory, phonatory, and velopharyngeal systems is typical and often a necessary precursor prior to shifting to methods used for promoting oral tract spatial manipulations (articulation) and speech flow (rate and prosody). Second, for what we have termed severe and sometimes moderate apraxia of speech, it frequently has been inferred that there may be a need to focus on correct spatial parameters for individual phonemes or individual syllable production through tactile techniques such as phonetic placement or kinesthetic techniques such as phonetic derivation. For some dysarthric speakers, similar techniques are also needed, but generally, once adequate physiological support for speech has been obtained through work on the respiratory, phonatory, and velopharyngeal systems, contrastive articulation drills and intelligibility drills, examples of which are shown in Table 26.4, are the focus of treatment (Yorkston et al., 1988). It thus appears that severe apraxic speakers may be "more lost" in the oral cavity or are more likely to have an impaired guidance system for the spatial aspects of correct phoneme production than most dysarthric speakers.[b] Although the underlying cause is unknown, we do know, based on the clinical techniques used and reported to be successful, that the adult "apraxic" speaker may require more tactile and kinesthetic input to reestablish accurate articulation of "functional units" of speech (i.e., units of speech in which jaw, tongue, and lip movements are coordinated). Could it be that the postural shaping and kinesthetic enhancement techniques for short units of speech typically used with severe "apraxic" speakers help to reestablish the spatial coordinate system of the vocal tract and/or enhance the execution of functional units of speech? The questions posed in this section are those that need extensive investigation. Nonetheless, the differences in treatment approaches for what we have termed "apraxia of speech" and dysarthria are clear.

The similarities in treatment of apraxic and dysarthric speakers are also dramatic as demonstrated by a comparison of the information presented in Tables 26.3 and 26.4. That is, all other traditional therapeutic techniques for the two disorders are of one of two natures: postural shaping/kinesthetic awareness articula-

---

[b] MacNeilage (1970) suggested that speakers have an internalized spatial coordinate system of the vocal tract, and this spatial map is used to guide speech production. Could it be possible that a major deficit in patients with acquired apraxia of speech is a reduced ability to access or use their internalized spatial coordinate system of the vocal tract?

Table 26.2.
Functional Effects on Motor Speech Resulting from Damage to Various Sites in the Dominant Hemisphere

Lesion Site	Suggested Function	Analogous Existing Speech Classification	Speech Symptoms	Perceived Quality
FRONTAL CORTICAL LESION Primary motor cortex (area 4)	• Movement execution • Activation of distal musculature for fractional movements	• Pseudobulbar palsy • Upper motoneuron dysarthria	• Slow, effortful speech • Impaired spatial targeting within vocal tract	• Dysarthric • Spastic (?) • Paretic
Nonprimary Motor Cortex (Premotor area (areas 6, 44)	• Organization of motor output in relation to sensory information • Programming of complex, multiple movement sequences • "Kinetic melody" • Preparation for movement	• Apraxia of speech, aphemia • "Small" Broca's aphasia • Anterior operculum syndrome (with bilateral damage)	• Slow, effortful speech • Articulatory struggle and groping • Articulatory distortions • Dysprosody	• Apractic • Apraxic dysarthric
Supplementary motor area (area 6)	• Movement initiation • Scaling of motor output • Motor sequencing • Organization and preparation for internally generated motor behaviors	• Akinetic mutism • Proxysmal speech	• Initiation difficulty • Dysprosody • Akinesia • Dysphonia • Dysfluency • Palilalia • Mutism • Echolalia	• Dysfluent • Dysarthric • Dysphonic • Initially mute
FRONTAL SUBCORTICAL LESION Basal ganglia	• Facilitation or inhibition of cortically initiated movements • Modulation of frontal lobe functions • Role in preparation for movement	• Dysarthria, hyperkinetic	• Articulatory inaccuracy • Prosodic excess • Prosodic insufficiency • Reduced volume	• Dysarthric sometimes "Dystonic"
White matter underlying Broca's area	• Region of afferent and efferent projections with Broca's area.	• Dysarthria • Aphemia	• Slow, effortful speech • Impaired articulation	• Dysarthric • Apraxic
Cingulate cortex	• Role in engaging neocortex for ideational or propositional speech • Role in learned responses to emotional states	• Possible mutism	????	????
Insula	• Premotor association areas for orofacial behaviors	????	????	????
Internal capsule	• Carries ascending and descending projections from motor cortex	• Dysarthria	• Slow speech • Impaired articulation	• Dysarthric
PARIETAL CORTICAL LESION Midparietal lobe	• Complex motor sequencing	• "Apraxia of speech"	• Repetitions, reattempts • Articulation errors • No slowness; word, syllables, and vocalic nuclei of normal duration	• "Apraxic"

Table 26.3.
A Summary of the Traditional Speech Treatment Approaches for Patients with Apraxia of Speech of Different Degrees of Severity (Wertz et al., 1984) with Correlative Speculated Level of Intervention

Severity Level	Recommended Approach	Level of Intervention
SEVERE	Segmental/Syllabic Level Imitation with • Imitation • Phonetic placement • Phonetic derivation • Derivation + placement • Key word technique	Postural shaping (spatial targeting)
	Imitation of contrasts	Postural shaping/kinesthetic awareness (spatial targeting/movement units)
	Contrastive stress drills	Kinesthetic awareness; rate and melodic flow
MODERATE	Intersystemic facilitators • Tapping foot • Tapping leg • Finger counting • Finger tapping Intrasystemic facilitators • Pacing board	Rate and melodic flow Rate and melodic flow
MILD	Expanded contrastive stress drills	Rate and melodic flow

Table 26.4.
A Summary of the Traditional Speech Treatment Approaches for Patients with Acquired Dysarthrias (Yorkston et al., 1988) with Correlative Speculated Level of Intervention

Establishing Physiological Support for Speech
• Tone, strength
• Coordination of respiratory, phonatory, velopharyngeal

Articulatory Drills
• Vocal tract shaping/kinesthetic awareness of speech units
  Contrastive drills
    pin–bin
    day–may
  Intelligibility drills
    my, hi, buy, dye, sigh
    mail, Mel, mall, meal, mill, mole
    pan, ban, tan, can, ran, man
    lab, lack, lag, lap, lab, laugh

Rate and Stress Drills
• Melodic flow
• Rate control
  Rigid
    Pacing boards (Helm, 1979)
    Alphabet supplementation (Beukelman and Yorkston, 1978)
  Rhythmic cuing
    Computerized (Beukelman, 1983)
    Clinician-controlled reading rule (Yorkston and Beukelman, 1981)
  Other
    Delayed auditory feedback (Hanson and Metter, 1980)
    Oscilloscopic (Barry and Goshorn, 1983)
• Stress
    Natural stress patterning (Yorkston et al., 1988)

tory drills and techniques for enhancing the melodic flow, rhythm, and rate of speech. The latter category of techniques improve segmental production as well as rate and prosody. Although the treatment approaches may be summarized in this way, we by no means are indicating that what we have traditionally termed "apraxia of speech" is dysarthria or vice versa. What we are indicating is that the neuromotor speech disorder typically observed in aphasic patients is qualitatively different at some levels from those of our traditional dysarthria classifications (Darley et al., 1975), but also has elements that are strikingly similar to some of the characteristics observed in some of the dysarthrias.

We also are not attempting to diminish the fact that different treatment approaches are required for patients who are principally dysarthric or principally apraxic. However, it is our view that similarities exist when apraxic and dysarthric speakers have impairments to similar basic mechanisms guiding motor control. The similarities are due in large part to the intimacy of the interconnections of systems and the fact that the systems operate in parallel, as pointed out in the review of neurophysiological control of movement.[c]

Finally, the neuromotor speech disorder syndrome that usually accompanies aphasia is extremely heterogeneous and variable across patients with regard to pathophysiology and symptomatology. Hence, it may be necessary for treatment approaches to be guided more by the nature of the symptomatology and the correlative underlying pathophysiologies and their interactions rather than the name of the disorder. We have traditionally targeted treatment toward the underlying pathophysiology for dysarthric speakers (Rosenbek and LaPointe,

---

[c] Other discussions of the regulation of motor control include the following: (a) motor neurons, MI (c.f. Asanuma, 1989); (b) basal ganglia (DeLong and Georgopoulos, 1981; Marsden, 1982); (c) supplementary motor area (c.f. Goldberg, 1985); and (d) cerebellum (Thach et al., 1992).

1978, 1985; Yorkston et al., 1988). That is, rather than specifying treatments based on classification or type of dysarthria, such as hypokinetic, hyperkinetic, or spastic dysarthria, we have determined instead (a) what aspects of physiological support require modifications with regard to tone, strength, and so on; (b) how maximal physiological support for speech may be attained through coordination of speech subsystems, respiration, phonation, resonance, and articulation; (c) whether and when "articulation drills" need to be included; and (d) whether and when prosody and rate should be worked on. For patients with significant neuromotor speech disorder and aphasia, a similar approach may be advantageous rather than one that specifies treatment based on the labels of "apraxia of speech" and "dysarthria." This concept awaits empirical validation.

A Framework for Establishing Treatment Goals for the Neuromotor Speech Disorder

A possible alternative method to use of severity level for establishing treatment goals may be one that is based on the predominant observable deviant speech and orofacial control behaviors of the patient elicited under a variety of conditions. The assessment batteries proposed by Darley et al. (1975), Wertz (1978, 1985), Wertz et al. (1984), Yorkston et al. (1988) may form the basis for observing the predominant deficits of speech and orofacial motor control, or it may be that symptoms observed in spontaneous samples of propositional verbal output, when obtainable, provide the most useful information. We would recommend that analyses of propositional speech always be supplemented by the results of assessment batteries. That is, no one sample or battery should be used in isolation when developing a patient's treatment program.

Typical qualities of speech output of aphasic patients with motor speech dysfunction are shown in the first column of Table 26.5. The remaining two columns contain hypothetical information, all of which requires further empirical validation; nonetheless, based on the current state of knowledge, the information is inferentially logical. Table 26.5 represents a preliminary attempt to provide for clinicians a framework for deciding what approach(es) will most likely be most facilitative of improved speech motor control. In column two of Table 26.5, the specu-

lated underlying pathophysiologies associated with these symptoms are presented. It becomes immediately clear that a variety of deviant processes may underlie deviant speech behaviors, including spatial targeting deficits; abnormal tone and strength; reduced ability to sequence complex volitional movements; reduced ability to coordinate speech subsystems (i.e., to produce functional units of speech behavior); and reduced ability to scale movements with regard to range, rate, timing, and so on. The final column of Table 26.5 summarizes the treatment approaches that most logically would influence each symptom. The key concept here is that treatment aimed at one or several of three levels may be appropriate for the aphasic patient with neuromotor speech impairment. Again, those levels are postural shaping of the vocal tract, enhancement of kinesthesia for functional units of speech, and rhythmic flow and rate.

There are few formalized guidelines for selection of the most efficacious approach to treatment correlative to the constellation of symptoms observed and abilities preserved and lost. As shown in Table 26.3, an attempt was made by Wertz et al. (1984) to provide guidelines based on severity level and, as shown in Table 26.5, on predominance of speech symptoms. Nonetheless, there exist no empirical data to substantiate the validity of either approach for establishing treatment goals. We, like Wertz et al. (1984), advocate that a sufficient period of diagnostic treatment be administered to each patient to determine the most facilitative treatment approaches. The importance of diagnostic treatment is further highlighted by a case study published by Simmons (1978); her observations are summarized in detail in a subsequent section on formalized treatment approaches.

Current Issues in Speech Motor Control: Implications for Treatment

The current literature concerning speech motor control has provided us with several constructs. These include the role of sensory input, establishment of parameters of vocal tract involvement from existing multiple degrees of freedom; development of functional units of action; development of the ability for on-line shaping; and use of an internal oscillatory mechanism as a macrostructure controller of speech. Excellent discus-

Table 26.5.
Most Frequent Speech Symptoms Associated with the Neuromotor Speech Disorders in Aphasia Typically Called "Apraxia of Speech"

Symptoms	Possible Pathophysiological Processes	Probable Primary Facilitators
Perceived substitutions, distortions	Spatial targeting deficit	
Perceived omissions and additions	Reduced ability to regulate range, rate, and timing of movements	
Effortful speech	Increased tone	
Trial and error groping	A form of dysfluency and/or compensation	Postural shaping/kinesthesia
Slow speech		
Excess and equal stress	Reduced ability to sequence complex volitional movements	Rate and melodic flow
Repetitions		
More errors on polysyllabic stimuli		Rate and melodic flow
Inconsistent errors	Sustained postures especially vocalic nuclei	
Islands of error-free speech	Reduced ability to coordinate speech subsystems	

sions of these concepts are presented by Abbs (1989) and Gracco (1990). These constructs may explain the usefulness of many of the facilitative techniques employed in aiding the aphasic individual to regain control over his or her speech output. A brief discussion of sensory input and sensorimotor integration for motor speech control, followed by discussions of motor speech control constructs as they may relate to treatment approaches, are presented in this section.

Neurophysiological Control of Motor Speech Sensory Input and Sensorimotor Integration

Most treatments for motor speech disorders are aimed at providing or enhancing those sensory cues believed to be critical for the facilitation of speech production. As such, several questions regarding sensory inputs are of central importance to the present discussion: (*a*) What is the role of sensory information in normal and disordered speech motor systems? and (*b*) When certain sensory modalities and sensorimotor processes are disrupted following neurological damage, to what extent do alternate sensory processes take on "functional significance for speech"?

Both auditory and oral somatosensory signals have been implicated in the guidance and regulation of speech production. Both systems are endowed with receptors that appear to be sensitive to speech processes. For example, in the auditory system, certain acoustically and phonetically salient aspects of speechlike stimuli are coded in the discharge patterns of the auditory nerve (for review, see Sachs et al., 1982). In the case of oral sensation, the vocal tract is richly supplied with a variety of receptors, including epithelial mechanoreceptors, muscle spindles, temporomandibular joint afferents, baroceptors, and periodontal afferents (for reviews, see Kent et al., 1990; Smith, 1992). The potential importance of these receptors for motor speech regulation is suggested by a study by Johasson et al. (1988). They reported that mechanoreceptive afferents in the infraorbital nerve discharged in relation to facial movements associated with production of certain speech sounds.

One approach to elucidating the functional significance of sensory inputs in speech motor control has involved studying the effects of sensory deprivation. Long-term deprivation of auditory information, as occurs in the adventitiously deaf (i.e., persons who have lost their hearing following the development of speech and language), results in a gradual and dramatic reduction in speech intelligibility and naturalness (for review, see Kent and Adams, 1989). Data on the consequences of oral somatosensory deprivation are less compelling, although for patients with trigeminal sensory neuropathy, speech difficulties have been reported (Lecky et al., 1987).

Short-term sensory deprivation has been attempted experimentally through such manipulations as auditory masking and oral anesthesia (for reviews, see Kent et al., 1990; Smith, 1992). The major finding to emerge from this work is that, although these conditions are associated with alterations in the finer aspects of speech, normal speakers are able to produce highly intelligible speech in the face of sensory deprivation. Kent et al. (1990) interpret this finding as reflecting the fact that the internal standard for speech is intact and, hence, movements can be executed without full sensory feedback.

Another approach to studying the contribution of sensory inputs to speech production has involved disrupting or modifying the afferent signal, for example, using delayed auditory feedback or oral prostheses such as the bite block. It has been shown that subjects are able to produce acoustically satisfactory speech with the bite block, even on the first glottal pulse of phonation, that is, before auditory feedback is available to the speaker (Lindblom et al., 1979). However, under conditions of combined bite block and oral anesthesia, compensatory adjustments to the bite block are less immediate (for review, see Kent et al., 1990). This finding suggests that, when the physical environment within which speech movements are produced is altered, sensory feedback is necessary for accurate speech production.

Finally, the role of sensory feedback has been examined in studies in which unanticipated perturbations (e.g., loads) are applied to certain articulators during the production of speech sounds. For example, Abbs and Gracco (1984) applied perturbations to the lower lip during bilabial closing movements and reported compensatory movements of the upper lip. Further, they have shown that perturbations applied immediately preceding a movement onset give rise to compensatory adjustment of the primary articulators involved in the movement, whereas perturbations applied during the movement are associated with compensatory gestures of secondary articulators in order to achieve an acoustically equivalent output (Abbs, 1989). These studies have shown that normal speakers make adjustments for unanticipated perturbations; such perturbations have the potential to disrupt speech output, especially in the disordered system.

Enhancing Postural Shaping and Kinesthesia for the Reestablishment of Functional Units of Speech

For the patient who requires the reacquisition of functional units of speech (i.e., segments and syllables), a variety of facilitative approaches that help to reestablish accurate spatial targeting have been reported (Square-Storer, 1989a; Wertz et al., 1984). These have been written about extensively in the speech literature since the 1930s (Van Riper, 1939) and include **phonetic placement** and **phonetic derivation.** Explanations of these facilitative techniques as used with aphasic-apraxic patients are presented in detail by Square-Storer (1989b); Wertz et al. (1984). Phonetic placement techniques involve the use of descriptions of where (place) and how (manner, voice) sounds are made, the use of figures and models, imagery such as hissing for /s/, and/or manipulation of the orofacial musculature by the clinician. **Phonetic derivation** techniques are those that build on an orofacial skill already in the patient's repertoire. For instance, if the patient can pop his or her lips, this action may serve as the basis for providing both spatial and manner parameters for the production of /p/ and /b/. Or, using speech, a patient may be able to produce /s/ but not //. The // may be derived from /s/ by having the patient slowly draw his or her tongue posteriorly along the palate. Such methods bring to a conscience level of awareness both the spatial and kinesthetic cues of correct production of the segment being worked on. The key word technique may also be used. In this approach, a word that the patient can produce acceptably and that contains the target sound being worked on is produced by the patient while the clinician calls to his or her attention the feel (spatial and kinesthetic) of the sound. For instance, if the goal is volitional control over the production of /s/, and the patient can produce her husband's name, "Sam," the name would be used to enhance the feel of /s/.

We speculate that the use of phonetic placement and derivation techniques aid aphasic patients with neuromotor speech disorders to reestablish a corpus of **functional units** of (speech) action. As explained by Gracco (1990), even the production of an isolated vowel requires a functional unit of behavior in that adjustment of respiratory muscles, tension in the vocal folds, adjustments in the compliance of the oropharyngeal walls, shaping of the tongue, positioning of the jaw, elevation of the velum, and some lip shaping contribute in a coordinated fashion to the functional unit of behavior, the vowel. In normal adult speakers, these sets of functional action are firmly established. One way to view neuromotor speech pathologies is in terms of the number of degrees of freedom available to the impaired system. For example, in some cases of hyperkinesia characterized by extraneous movements, such movements may increase the degrees of freedom with which the system must contend to produce a given trajectory. However, in some cases of hypokinesia, the system may have far fewer degrees of freedom. As Gracco (1990) points out, the degrees of freedom available to the normal speaker are naturally limited by the fact that functional units of behavior have been firmly established. A possible positive symptom of neurological damage cortically and/or subcortically to the dominant frontal lobe is the alteration of functional units. Thus, reestablishment of functional units may be a goal of the treatments. It may be that work at the segmental and syllable level (vowel-consonant or consonant-vowel) using techniques such as phonetic placement and phonetic derivation helps the aphasic patient with neuromotor speech disorders to achieve this goal.

Imitation of contrasts is a therapeutic technique that seems to be useful once some functional units of speech have been established. This method is described comprehensively by Wertz et al. (1984). Advocated by Rosenbek and LaPointe (1978, 1985), the technique relies on integral stimulation ("Watch me. Listen to me.") for input, thus bringing to a conscious level of awareness the "look" and "sound" of the movement pattern. Wertz et al. (1984) stress that work should usually begin on a single target such as /s/ embedded in a variable CV or VC environment or minimally different "functional" units (e.g., say, sigh, so, see). The clinician stresses to the patient slowing the production of the syllables while *feeling the movement patterns*.

Imitation of contrast, such as see-tea, toe-sew, is also advised by Wertz et al. (1984) for aphasic patients with neuromotor speech deficits as well as by Yorkston et al. (1988) for dysarthric individuals. Both indicate the usefulness of producing numerous consonantal targets in a list in which the vowel nucleus remains stable (e.g., pie-die-I-sigh-rye-tie-lie-my). Such drills, when used with aphasic individuals with neuromotor speech deficits, may highlight for the patient a kinesthetic (conscious) awareness for movement units. As such, these exercises promote the reestablishment of sensorimotor contingencies of functional units. For example, in the CV sequence /s/ + vowel, production of /s/ varies in relation to vowel context (i.e., high-low-front-back). The sensorimotor specifications for /s/ in these various environments are different. Imitation of these contrasts may provide the opportunity for the system to experience the various sensorimotor specifications related to these functional units. Gracco (1990) describes motor programs as the assembly of functional units of action organized into larger systems. He stresses that, based on results of previous studies (Abbs et al.,

1984; Gracco, 1987), "a motor program is not a process but a set of *sensorimotor specifications* identifying the relative contribution of the vocal tract structures to the overall vocal tract configuration" (Gracco, 1990, p. 10).

The use of **contrastive stress drills** is advocated by many as a potent type of treatment (e.g., Rosenbek, 1983). Such drills can be thought of more as an approach to treatment rather than a facilitative technique but are discussed here because of their hypothesized underlying speech control mechanism, that being enhancement of an underlying **oscillatory mechanism**. Contrastive stress drills were first proposed by Fairbanks (1960) and popularized by Rosenbek (1976, 1985) for the treatment of acquired apraxia of speech. Question and answer dialogues that consist of short phrases centered on one or two phonemes are used. Thus, previously practiced functional units are embedded in connected interactive speech. Primary and secondary stress are the factors that are thought to promote improved speech movement. A typical dialogue may be as follows:

Clinician: What did you do?
Patient: I *ate* one.
Clinician: You ate three?
Patient: No, I ate *one*.
Clinician: Tom ate one.
Patient: No, *I* ate one.
Clinician: You drank one?
Patient: No, I *ate* one.
Clinician: You ate one!
Patient: Yes, *I* ate one.

A hierarchy for helping to ensure success for the patient is described fully by Wertz et al. (1984), and the reader is urged to consult that text.

The possible speech control mechanisms that may be reintegrated using this method are enhancement of an underlying oscillatory mechanism and, possibly, on-line shaping through reduced rate. With regard to the rhythm and stress aspects of such drills, Gracco (1990) notes that numerous aspects of motor behavior seem to be guided by an underlying internal oscillatory mechanism and that speech may be no exception. Over numerous kinematically recorded repetitions of phrases of normal speaking adults, there is an undeniable consistency in repetition suggesting "an underlying periodicity indicative of a rhythmic process" (p. 18). Further, it has been found that in normal speakers, the timing of the articulators reflects a system-level organization. That is, actions of individual articulators do not occur in isolation but, instead, react as a (functional) unit (e.g., Lofqvist and Yoshioka, 1981, 1984). We propose that contrastive stress drills may enhance the production of functional units in the context of enhanced rhythm and reduced rate. Further, it is speculated that the changing patterns of sentential stress in these drills may enhance flexibility in the motor programs. Wertz et al. (1984) state that "the contrastive stress drill may be one of the most potent techniques for stabilizing apraxic articulation and improving prosodic profiles" (p. 260). We speculate that this is so because a guiding rhythm is brought to consciousness and the system is required to make minimal prosodic changes within a constant phonetic environment.

Table 26.6.
Pacing and Rhythmic Approaches for the Treatment of Neuromotor Speech Deficits in Aphasia

- Metronomic pacing (Dworkin et al., 1988; Shane and Darley, 1978)
- Prolonged speech (Southwood, 1987)
- Finger counting (Simmons, 1978)
- Vibrotactile stimulation (Rubow et al., 1982)
- Singing (Keith and Aronson, 1975)
- Melodic intonation therapy (Sparks and Holland, 1976; Sparks et al., 1974)
- PROMPT (Square et al., 1985; Square et al., 1986)

Enhancing the Rhythmic Substrate and Slowing Motor Speech Production

Other therapeutic techniques that highlight the rhythmical aspects of speech and that may reestablish an internal oscillator have been used successfully with aphasic patients with neuromotor speech disorders. These are summarized in Table 26.6. Five will be discussed in this section as facilitation techniques: singing (Keith and Aronson, 1975); vibrotactile stimulation (Rubow et al., 1982); metronomic pacing (Dworkin et al., 1988; Shane and Darley, 1978); prolonged speech (Southwood, 1987); and use of the pacing board (Helm, 1979). In the next section, those rhythmic and pacing methods that constitute more formalized treatment programs, including finger counting (Simmons, 1978), melodic intonation therapy (Sparks and Deck, 1986), and PROMPT (Chumpelik [Hayden], 1984), will be discussed.

That singing may provide a facilitative substrate for motor speech production in nonfluent aphasic individuals has long been recognized (Head, 1926 [1963]). It is the opinion of Lebrun (1989), however, that this is only so for Broca's aphasic patients and not for patients designated as having apraxia of speech and minimal or no clinically discernible aphasia. Indeed, the one contemporary published case study documenting the facilitative effect of singing was of a patient with moderate to severe aphasia as measured by the Porch Index of Communicative Ability (PICA) (Porch, 1967) with a significant coexisting neuromotor speech disorder (Keith and Aronson, 1975). Singing therapy began after 3 weeks of traditional therapy in which limited gains were made. A cloze procedure was used whereby the patient completed a phrase by singing the final word. That is, the clinician would sing, "This is my _____," while pointing to his hand, and the patient would name the object, thus completing the sentence by singing, "hand." The patient was also encouraged to sing functional phrases such as "I want coffee," and "How are you?" The patient transferred the facilitative technique to her environment with rhythm and pitch patterns that had a definite musical quality. In less than a month, her PICA overall score improved by three points (from 7.93 to 10.99), and her verbal subtest score improved by seven points (from 3.55 to 10.55). A month later, the patient was doing well in speaking situations at home, although word-finding and grammatical errors were noticeable. She had completely given up singing as a facilitative approach but was using an enhanced melodic structure and slower rate in the natural context. Her verbal subtests on the PICA were almost two points higher (from 10.55 to 12.50) and her overall score almost one point higher (from 10.99 to 11.93). Keith and Aronson (1975) acknowledged that the "patient might have improved

to a similar extent had conventional therapy been continued or no therapy instituted at all" (p. 488), but, given their clinical acumen, they thought the case to be sufficiently noteworthy to report in the literature.

Another preliminary yet promising study of the effectiveness of rhythm, stress and pacing to promote articulatory accuracy in aphasic subjects with "apraxia of speech" was one that employed vibrotactile stimulation (Rubow et al., 1982). A 50 Hz vibration was applied to the volar surface of the index finger, and vibratory tactile stimulation was delivered for every syllable in three-syllable words. Because the clinician could control the timing, duration, and intensity (high or low) of the signal, the stimulation could indicate primary, secondary, and tertiary stress in three-syllable words such as "sensation." One subject was exposed to two alternating treatments: imitation treatment for a list of plosive-laden polysyllabic words (e.g., tobacco) and vibrotactile stimulation for a list of fricative-laden words (e.g., sensation). A 16-point multidimensional scoring system for the evaluation of apraxia of speech errors (Collins et al., 1980) was used to determine mean performance on both word lists pre- and posttherapy. At the beginning of treatment the mean score for both word lists was 5. After 14 sessions of treatment over 7 days, posttherapy scores indicated that the words trained using imitation improved only 1.9 points, whereas the wordlist trained using vibrotactile stimulation improved 5.8 points.

Other attempts have been made to use rhythm and pacing as facilitators of motor speech. Shane and Darley (1978) used a metronome paired with the reading of passages and set for three rates: normal speaking rate, a slower rate, and a faster rate. The external source of rhythm actually had a deleterious effect on accuracy of speech production compared with a control condition in which the metronome was not used. Further, there were no significant differences in articulation accuracy over the three rates. Despite these findings, Dworkin et al. (1988) used a metronome set at various speeds when treating a patient on the following tasks: a nonverbal neuromotor control task; alternate motion rates; word production; and sentence production in which sentences consisted of five words. Although no conjecture can be made about the facilitative effects of the metronome, it is interesting that these clinicians with exceptional backgrounds in the treatment of "apraxia of speech" used the approach. The patient improved on all tasks, but she may have also demonstrated such improvement without the metronome.

A study by Southwood (1987) of two patients who were considered to be principally apraxic, one mild and one moderate, provided quantifiable evidence of the facilitative effects of pacing. Southwood used the technique of **prolonged speech** in which speech rates were systematically reduced through conscious prolongation of vocalic nuclei. Systematic decreases in speech rate accompanied by visual guidance from a computer screen display resulted in substantially reduced speech errors. In a reversal phase, systematic increases in speaking rate resulted in an increase in errors. The prolonged speech technique, however, did not generalize, possibly because of its "bizarre" quality. Southwood recommended that, as in the prolonged speech program formulated for stutterers by Ingham (1983), generalization might be achieved if therapy directed at "naturalness" training is used as a supplement to the prolonged speech technique. It may be that the metronome and prolonged speech, like speech supplemented by gestures, "do nothing as grand as reorganizing neuromotor control, (but) they do slow the patient down, heighten rhythm and stress profiles, and they serve to remind the patient that he must attend to each syllable of an utterance" (Rosenbek, 1983, p. 53).

A similar facilitative effect may be derived with use of the pacing board (Helm, 1979). Such a board is approximately 13 inches long and is divided horizontally every 2 inches by a divider. Patients are trained to touch each consecutive square on the board for each unit of speech. Although we have no experimental data regarding the use of the pacing board with aphasic individuals with neuromotor speech disorders, the method is commonly considered for use by experienced clinicians (e.g., Wertz et al., 1984).

Although rhythmic and pacing facilitators are common in the treatment speech disorders in patients with aphasia accompanied by neuromotor speech deficits, it appears that the various methods may be tapping different processes. That is, some of these techniques are rigid pacing techniques, whereas others exaggerate the natural rhythm and stress patterns of the language. The rigid pacing techniques include the metronome, prolonged speech, and the pacing board. Those facilitators that enhance natural rhythm and stress include contrastive stress drills, vibrotactile stimulation, and singing. These later methods also slow rate, however. There do not exist in the literature any indications of the most effective of these techniques or indications of patient types for whom each is appropriate. Further, it is not known what aspect is facilitative—the pacing, the rhythm, or both. Clinical research addressing these issues is greatly needed.

Formalized Treatment Programs

Several formalized treatment approaches for neuromotor speech disorders in aphasia have appeared in the literature. These approaches have been of two types: **microstructural bottom-up approaches** and **macrostructural top-down approaches**. An issue of primary importance, then, is whether a patient requires a micro- or macro-structural approach to treatment in order to improve his or her motor speech control. That is, must functional units (i.e., speech segments and syllables) be reestablished and built on in order to improve functional verbal communication? Or, does the patient find the use of macrostructional approaches such as melodic intonation therapy (Berlin, 1976; Naeser and Helm-Estabrooks, 1985; Sparks et al., 1974; Sparks and Holland, 1976), PROMPT (Prompts for Restructuring Oral Muscular Phonetic Targets) (Chumpelik [Hayden], 1984; Square et al., 1985; Square et al., 1986; Square-Storer and Hayden, 1989), and integral stimulation for sentences administered in the eight-step continuum (Rosenbek et al., 1973) most facilitative? The unresolved issues are whether and/or for whom bottom-up microstructure versus top-down macrostructure methods of treatment should be employed. The bottom-up microstructure approaches include those methods that begin at either the nonverbal oromotor movement level or the segment-syllable level, with the most notable having been advocated by Dabul and Bollier (1976); Dworkin et al. (1988); Rosenbek (1983); and Wertz et al. (1984). As suggested above, we speculate that these bottom-up approaches aid the impaired system to (a) select the specific parameters to manipulate from the multiple degrees of freedom available to the pathological

speech system and/or increase the number of degrees of freedom; (b) establish and refine functional units of action; and (c) superimpose these functional units on a melodic line. The three best-known top-down or macrostructure approaches for the treatment of neuromotor speech disorders in aphasia are melodic intonation therapy (Naeser and Helm-Estabrooks, 1985); PROMPT (Square et al., 1985, 1986; Square-Storer and Hayden, 1989); and the eight-step task continuum as applied to functional sentences and phrases (Rosenbek et al., 1973). We speculate that these approaches help reestablish an underlying oscillatory rhythm, melody, and rate for speech production. The macro-approach of finger counting is less wellknown. It provides for the patient a rigid pacing for slowing of speech production. Each approach will be discussed in the next section.

Microstructural Approaches

Dabul and Bollier (1976) based their approach on the premise that the "apraxic" patient must first reestablish the ability to accurately attain articulatory postures at the phone level. Once the posturing for a particular "phone" is stabilized, reduplication of the consonant in the rapid reproduction of the "consonant + /a/" is prescribed. Once criterion level of rapid accurate reduplication at the level of 60 syllables per 15 seconds is achieved, production of the phone in monosyllable CVC or CVCV nonword combinations is advocated to establish volitional control of nonmeaningful syllable combinations. Finally, word attack skills are recommended in that it is assumed that the patient has acquired, through the previous exercises, a solid basic "vocabulary" of articulatory skills. Each sound in a word is attacked in isolation, and then the patient is encouraged to blend phonemes together.

Rosenbek (1983) and Wertz et al. (1984) do not present such a rigid approach to bottom-up treatment but do advocate an approach in which sounds are turned into syllables, and syllables are turned into words. The strength of their belief in this sort of building block approach is highlighted in the following quote from Rosenbek (1983): "Once the apraxic talker has begun to recall how sounds are made, to contrast those sounds with others, and to combine them into words and short phrases, traditional methods like imitation, placement and derivation can be replaced by methods that slow connected speech and heighten rhythm and stress profiles" (p. 52).

Dworkin et al. (1988) reported on a case in which a multiple probe design was applied to a therapeutic regimen that consisted of four levels of oromotor complexity, including nonverbal tongue tip raising and lowering with a bite block; performance of alternate motion rates on the syllables /ptk/ and /kpt/; isolated word training; and sentence training under two conditions, a stressed one and an unstressed one. The patient's performances improved on all tasks, but "these findings produced no evidence to suggest that successful performance at an earlier step in the treatment regimen generalized to later, ostensibly more complex, speech control activities" (p. 287). Although we can not infer that similar results would be found across subjects, this finding indicates that further research is warranted regarding the validity of and criteria for beginning treatment at the microlevel of speech for aphasic individuals with neuromotor speech disorders.

Macrostructural Approaches

There is evidence in the literature as well that certain top-down approaches may be effective for establishing functional speech in aphasic individuals with neuromotor speech disorders. That is, results of these approaches have demonstrated that a "building-block" approach to treatment is not always necessary. The most notable of these macrostructure techniques is melodic intonation therapy (MIT). The method of MIT is fully described by Sparks and Deck in Chapter 19 of this volume. Elements of inter- and intrasystemic organization (Luria, 1970; Rosenbek and LaPointe, 1978, 1985; Rosenbek et al., 1976) are incorporated into the intoning technique for phrase and sentence production. The intersystemic component consists of the hand gestures coupled with word production, while the intrasystemic aspect is reflected in the production of "intoned" rather than spoken speech. Meaningful phrases such as "I want coffee" and "Go to bed" are often produced fluently once a patient has worked through the various steps of the program. In our experience, performance is usually quite good throughout the program, but little empirical data exist regarding generalization. The startling aspect of this method is that even patients who appear to be totally "lost" in their vocal tracts and who have extreme difficulty initiating speech are greatly facilitated by this top-down approach. That is, there would appear to be no advantage to working on functional units of speech and building on those units for phrase production if, in fact, it could be empirically shown that MIT promotes generalization to novel productions. It appears that the macrostructure of the prosody enhanced by the intersystemic hand movement aids the patient in producing intelligible functional phrases. We must also consider whether the linguistic structure of the target phrases constitutes a facilitatory macrostructure for these aphasic patients. It has been our observation, as well as that of many others, that even severe Broca's patients who demonstrate some agrammatism and anomia produce fully syntactic utterances when facilitated by MIT if the syntactic structure of those utterances is simplistic. The question, then, is what aspect of this top-down approach accounts for the facilitative effect—the intersystemic hand tapping, the intrasystemic melodic speech, the linguistic template onto which the speech movements are fitted, or, most probably, all of the above in varying proportions?

The therapeutic benefits of MIT for nonfluent aphasic patients with good comprehension but minimal speech output were first reported by Albert et al. (1973). Three cases past the period of spontaneous recovery and for whom previous aphasia therapy had not improved speech output were reported. In each case, MIT treatment resulted in increased spontaneous output in the natural environment. One patient required only 2 weeks of treatment to progress from the use of six repetitive phonemes to full responses that were grammatically correct in his natural environment. The other two patients required approximately 11/2 months of treatment to progress from meaningless grunts and stereotyped phonemes to carrying on short but meaningful conversations. Each patient's posttreatment speech, however, was characterized as dysarthric or impaired with regard to articulation and prosody.

Several other reports, however, found that MIT was not effective as measured by improved language test scores for some nonfluent aphasic patients (Helm, 1979; Sparks et al., 1974). In an attempt to provide clearer guidelines for whom MIT was most appropriate, Naeser and Helm-Estabrooks (1985) undertook a study that examined site of lesion correlated with improved language test scores as derived from the Boston Diagnostic Aphasia Examination (BDAE) (Goodglass and Kaplan, 1972) following MIT treatment of eight patients who had also received CT scans.

Those patients who responded well to MIT, as measured by four subtests of the BDAE, had damage to left frontal motor and premotor areas and adjacent subcortical white matter, in combination with basal ganglia and capsular involvement in one patient. In other words, each of the patients had damage to the left cortical and some damage to subcortical motor speech control centers *without* involvement of Wernicke's area and/or the temporal isthmus. Of the four poor responders, three had the above sites of damage *plus* damage to Wernicke's area or the temporal isthmus. The fourth had a patchy frontal Broca's and premotor area lesion, which spared the periventricular white matter, and a small lesion deep to the motor cortex face region. Although the latter patient was termed a poor responder, it should be noted that this patient, *prior* to treatment, had an articulatory agility score of seven on the BDAE and, as such, was very different from the other seven subjects in that he was at ceiling on this measure. These results are impressive, and from them it may be inferred that MIT is an appropriate motor speech treatment for nonfluent aphasic subjects with severely restricted verbal output but *without* involvement to the dominant temporal lobe.

A macrostructural approach that used intersystemic reorganization in the form of fingercounting to mark the rhythmic flow of speech and a linguistic template of simple declarative sentences was reported by Simmons (1978). Although this was a single-case study and no known attempt to replicate the findings has been undertaken, this report is of great clinical significance because of the remarkable improvement and description of generalization of verbal expressive output demonstrated by the aphasic-apraxic subject. The subject had undergone 9 months of intensive language and speech therapy, showing steady improvement throughout. However, a plateau in performance was subsequently met for 5 months with no discernible improvement as measured by the PICA and subjective evaluation. During the 5-month period, various approaches to treatment were undertaken, including MIT, imitation, articulatory posturing, contrastive stress drills (Rosenbek, 1976), Ame-Rind (Skelly et al., 1974), and language master programming for production of utterances. Subsequent treatment was directed at the production of utterances of the linguistic form, "Pronoun + Verb + Preposition + Article + Noun." The patient was trained to hold up one finger for each word (finger counting) thus, producing one syllable for each finger raised. The training consisted of the five-task continuum shown in Appendix 26.1. Therapy was administered for 4 months with marked improvement in production of treated utterances. Generalization was demonstrated by the patient's outstanding improvement on the PICA verbal subtests of 21 percentile points. The patient was observed to transfer the finger-counting approach to her natural environment, and significant others commented on her increased sentence length and fluency.

Finger counting, like MIT, is an approach that couples intersystemic reorganization with a linguistic template. The two, coupled together, could have an interactive facilitative effect on the accuracy of verbal output in aphasic individuals with neuromotor speech disorders. Another additional possible explanation for the dramatic improvement demonstrated by this patient is that the rhythmic finger counting provides for the patient an internal tempo and possibly a rhythmic oscillation on which the speech stream may be superimposed. Might it also be that the limb movement helps to reestablish a paced oscillatory rhythm onto which the functional units of speech may be mapped? Further research is needed.

The application of PROMPT (Chumpelik [Hayden], 1984) produces similar successful results for the acquisition of a limited set of functional phrases and sentences (Square et al., 1985; Square et al., 1986; Square-Storer and Hayden, 1989). PROMPT is a tactile-kinesthetic method of treatment in which spatial targets are cued using orofacial prompts. Temporal flow and articulatory rate are regulated by the timing of delivery of spatial cues and by the pressure and duration of the cues. As temporal flow is regulated, the patient becomes consciously aware of the feel of dynamic speech movements (articulatory kinesthesia) as the clinician augments both the spatial and temporal parameters. The dynamic cues are delivered to the orofacial structures by the clinician while the patient produces a target utterance. The cues are gradually withdrawn until the patient can produce the utterance with no support.

Using single-case study designs and replication over four chronic severe Broca's patients with limited propositional output and severe neuromotor speech involvement, it was demonstrated that phrases can be "programmed in" for functional communication using this top-down macrostructure approach (Square et al., 1985; Square et al., 1986; Square-Storer and Hayden, 1989). According to reports from spouses, two patients generalized programmed (treated) phrases (e.g., "Stop it"; "I want more") to daily life. One patient was reevaluated 2 months after termination of treatment and was found to have retained the trained functional phrases with the same level of perceived efficiency as during treatment (Square-Storer and Hayden, 1989).

However, an important observation was that there was no generalization of speech skills to nontrained phrases among the four subjects who participated in the 4-week, 12-treatment session research protocols. One patient did continue in treatment after the experimental phase; he acquired approximately 20 additional functional phrases over the subsequent 3-month, twice-weekly period of treatment (Hayden, personal communication, 1986). Hayden (personal communication, 1992) reported that for a fifth nonexperimental patient, one who received two treatment sessions per week for 3 months followed by approximately one treatment session per week for an additional 9 months, generalization of speech control to untreated phrases elicited in treatment as well as to many novel phrases emitted by the patient in daily life occurred.

We speculate that PROMPT, like MIT and finger tapping strategies, provides for patients a linguistic template coupled with a paced rhythmic template and/or an oscillatory structure. In addition, for PROMPT only, spacial targets are superimposed upon the macrostructure provided by the oscillatory/linguistic maps. If, like Gracco (1990), we accept the definition of motor programs as, "a set of sensorimotor specifications which identify the relative contribution of vocal tract structures to overall vocal tract configuration" (p. 10), it logically follows that PROMPT probably provides for the patient the most salient

sensory information to correct the deviant programs that his or her system is internally generating.

In the application of PROMPT, not all possible prompts are delivered to the patient for every macrostructure. Instead, the master clinician constantly monitors performance and delivers only those prompts necessary to improve speech accuracy. What PROMPT appears to achieve in a very short time is the hardwiring of programs of several functional phrases in Broca's aphasic patients. The rapidity with which the phrases become hardwired is demonstrated in the learning curves of the subjects included in the previous experimental studies (Square et al., 1985; Square et al., 1986; Square-Storer and Hayden, 1989). That generalization to novel phrases may occur needs empirical validation. Another question that needs to be addressed is if, in fact, generalization occurs with PROMPT, is it of a sufficient quantity and quality to justify the costliness of one-on-one treatment for Broca's aphasic patients? A recent study has demonstrated that significant functional gains in information transfer can be made by chronic Broca's aphasic patients using generic aphasia and speech treatments concentrated over short periods of several months (Brindley et al., 1989). These gains were measured using the Functional Communication Profile of Sarno (1965) and, thus, reflect both verbal and nonverbal communication. Questions that arise are those related to cost-efficiency as well as consumer satisfaction. That is, is the cost of one-on-one neuromotor speech treatment justified based on increased consumer satisfaction? Further clinical research is needed.

The final macrostructure approach to treatment to be discussed is one of the first approaches reported in the contemporary literature for apraxia of speech. Rosenbek et al. (1973), when first reporting on the efficacy of their integral stimulation approach (i.e., "Watch me. Listen to me") within the context of their eight-step continuum of treatment for apraxia of speech, trained functional phrases in two of three aphasic patients with moderate to severe language and speech disturbance of not longer than 1-year duration. (The eight-step continuum prescribed by Rosenbek et al. is presented in Appendix 26.2.) Five phrases for training were individually selected for each patient based on their personal circumstances. No attempt was made to control for linguistic or phonetic complexity or for length. Both subjects acquired all five sentences within treatment. Carryover was informally assessed for one subject at 3 months posttreatment. At that time, carryover was evident for three of the five phrases. For both subjects, the most time-consuming step in therapy was Step 1, "Watch me. Listen to me," with simultaneous production with the clinician.

Deal and Florance (1978) essentially replicated the findings of Rosenbek et al. (1973) in their application of the eight-step continuum to four cases, three of whom were more than 1-year postonset. Two of the patients had essentially no functional speech at the beginning of treatment. One of these patients completed only 13 sessions but learned to produce three of the five trained sentences appropriately in her daily activities. The other patient completed 30 half-hour sessions over a 5-month period and had acquired 44 functional phrases. Another patient who used functional speech at times but relied most on gestural communication had replaced a large portion of the latter with functional verbal utterances after just 3 months of therapy. Finally, an acute patient who commenced therapy at 1 week postonset progressed so far that she was generating novel utterances from words acquired in trained utterances. Although a different learning criterion was used in the study by Deal and Florence (1978), they too found Step 1 to be the most laborious. Nonetheless, once criterion was achieved on the initial step, patients progressed rapidly. Further, Steps 1 through 4 seemed to constitute a unit, but not every patient needed all four of the steps. Step 8 was found useful for home programming.

The conclusion of Rosenbek and colleagues (1973) as well as of Deal and Florance (1978) was that the eight-step continuum could help restore some communicative ability to *some* severely apraxic patients. Selection criteria for the most appropriate patients were not specified with the exception of the description, *aphasic individuals who were severely limited in speech output.*

Choosing a Macro- Versus a Microstructural Approach

No empirical reports nor scholarly discussions exist in the literature regarding the selection of micro- versus macrostructural methods of treatment for neuromotor speech disorders in aphasia. In fact, to our knowledge, this is the first time in which these methods have been presented within this framework. It would seem logical, however, to start with a macrostructural approach when initiating treatment with the aphasic patient with significant speech involvement. First, we agree with Wertz et al. (1984) that it is extremely important to begin treatment on a positive note, and several of the macrostructural approaches such as PROMPT and MIT appear to have the power to rapidly facilitate the production of functional phrases in aphasic patients with neuromotor speech deficits. Second, there are indications in the literature that not all patients require a bottom-up approach. Several clinical reports have indicated that some aphasic patients with neuromotor speech deficits can transfer strategies from macrostructural approaches to control their speech in their natural environments (Albert et al., 1973; Deal and Florence, 1978; Hayden, personal communication, 1992; Rosenbek et al., 1973). Finally, bottom-up approaches require a time-consuming hierarchical process in which there is a time delay before functionality or patient selfcontrol of speech is reestablished. It appears prudent to provide the patient with control over several functional phrases of personal value as early as possible.

For some patients, it may be that progress is significant with macrostructural approaches. In these cases, there are no logical reasons to incorporate a microstructural regiment, although facilitative techniques may be applied liberally within the frameworks of macrostructural approaches. For other patients, especially those who appear to have the potential to achieve motor control over self-formulated discourse, it is our belief that microstructural approaches may be of great value. These approaches may be especially useful for patients with minimal aphasia coupled with keen insight about speech production and good self-evaluative skills.

A final issue that requires consideration is treating the left-hemisphere-lesioned patient whose language remains intact versus treating the aphasic individual with neuromotor speech deficits. Square-Storer et al. (1988) demonstrated empirically that apraxia of speech and aphasia were *distinct* disorders. It would, thus, seem logical that left-hemisphere-lesioned subjects with significant speech impairment and *no* or *relatively little* aphasia would require treatment approaches different from those subjects with aphasia complicated by a significant motor speech disorder. One conclusion that resonates in the clinical

treatment literature is that macrostructural treatment approaches that provide for the subject not only the rhythmic and rate structure but also a linguistic substrate are successful with *nonfluent aphasic* individuals. The efficacy studies of PROMPT were undertaken with patients classified as Broca's (Square et al., 1985, 1986) on the Western Aphasia Battery (Kertesz, 1982). The MIT reports of effectiveness were based on the performances of patients with aphasia and limited verbal output (Albert et al., 1973). The eight-step continuum was shown by Rosenbek et al. (1973) to be effective for patients with moderate aphasia and apraxia of speech, some of whom also demonstrated mild dysarthria. Simmons's finger-counting program with linguistic template was successful with an aphasic patient with apraxia of speech. To date, none has been reported to be successful with relatively pure neuromotor speech disorder following left-hemisphere lesion.

Again, common to each of the above successful techniques for aphasic-apraxic patients are three elements: rhythm, pacing, and linguistic templates. Extensive research is very much needed regarding the basis of success of the macrostructural approaches as well as for what type of patient each approach is most effective.

For patients with little or no aphasia but a significant motor speech impairment following left-hemisphere damage, it would appear that microstructural approaches that emphasize the establishment of functional units, parameter estimation, on-line shaping, and reestablishment of an underlying oscillatory mechanism may be most appropriate. Careful study of the writings of the eminent clinicians in this area, Wertz et al. (1984), indicates that this building-block approach is prescribed for the patient with minimal aphasia and a significant neuromotor speech disorder— what they call the mild and moderate apraxic patient.

Thus, guideposts have been established for the clinician with regard to selecting the most appropriate approaches to treatment for left-hemisphere-lesioned patients with neuromotor speech involvement both with and without aphasia. However, no empirically validated principles for selection have been reported. This is a fertile area for further research in our discipline.

A final word relates to treatment efficacy for chronic Broca's aphasic patients. Many of the above studies have demonstrated that such individuals progress in treatment even after many years postonset. A recent study further confirms this point (Brindley et al., 1989). More important, however, was the finding that of the five parameters measured using the Functional Communication Profile (Sarno, 1965)—movement, speech, understanding, reading, and other—the speech ratings followed by movement and reading improved most significantly following 3 months of intensive therapy of various generic types. Mean improvement on the speech subsection was 14%, with the other four sections improving from 1% to 6.5%. Such data are most convincing regarding the efficacy of treatment for aphasic patients who most likely also have significant neuromotor speech involvement.

Management of Special Motor Conditions

Brief mention must be made of two other conditions with probable motor underpinnings—mutism and recurrent utterances. For both conditions, there exist in the literature suggestions for management.

As cited previously, lesions to SMA and/or the cingulate cortex may result in mutism. Historically, there have appeared in the literature many reports of mutism evolving into aphasia marked by significant neuromotor speech dysfunction. Although the mutism is transitory and in most cases clears after several days (Albert et al., 1981; Crary et al., 1985; Mohr et al., 1978; Schiff et al., 1983), some patients are plagued by a more persistent disorder (Simpson and Clark, 1989). For patients with mutism that persists for more than several days and who also appear to have severe orofacial buccal apraxia, sometimes affecting respiration (Mitchell and Berger, 1975) and phonation (Marshall et al., 1988), it has been recommended that therapy focus initially on reestablishing volitional control of phonation (Simpson and Clark, 1989). Many of the techniques advocated for psychogenic mutism may be appropriate, such as shaping the voice from vegetative sounds (e.g., coughing or grunting) or stimulating the voice from humming. The cases reported by Simpson and Clark (1989) of protracted mutism were patients whose disorder evolved into aphasia with significant neuromotor speech involvement.

Another group of aphasic patients with coexisting neuromotor speech impairments are those with extremely limited speech output consisting almost exclusively of automatisms or recurrent utterances. It has recently been reported that such patients have lesion sites similar to those of patients with reduced, hesitant, poorly articulated, agrammatical speech except that the lesion sites of the group with stereotypies and/or no speech also included portions of the subcortical fasciculus and periventricular white matter near the body of the lateral ventricle (Naeser et al., 1989). From the time of Broca, one school of thought has been that speech automatisms result from selective damage to the mechanism responsible for the coordination of articulatory movement either by direct damage to the mechanism itself or by lack of activation of the mechanism by higher-level language processes (Blanken, 1991). On examination, many of these patients demonstrate a severe degree of trial-and-error groping and struggle when attempting to repeat words and sometimes even isolated phonemes. These are the patients designated by Wertz et al. (1984) as having severe apraxia of speech. We believe, similar to Blanken (1991), that patients with this deficit have stored, in a hypothetical ''articulatory buffer,'' a set motor program and, for one of two reasons, motor or linguistic, the stored program for the automatism can no longer be replaced or varied at will. Also, similar to Blanken, we believe that some patients whose speech is characterized by automatisms in the acute stage may evolve into apraxic speakers whereas others do not.

There have appeared in the literature two forms of treatment for such patients. Helm and Barresi (1980) put forth an approach that appears principally cognitive in nature: voluntary control of involuntary utterances (VCIU). The method capitalizes on patients reading words and phrases other than the stereotypy that they have been heard to utter at other times. Helm-Estabrook (1983) suggested that VCIU is a successful technique for patients with subcortical damage.

Stevens (1989), on the other hand, has demonstrated through clinical reports the effectiveness of her method, multiple input phoneme therapy (MIPT). The premise of MIPT is that verbal stereotypies are motoric in nature. If the motor program governing the stereotypy can be manipulated, the patient can gradually learn to produce some one-word functional responses and possibly even expand on these. From the phonemic structure of the stereotypy, monosyllabic words are constructed and, using a 22-step hierarchical program, are stabilized and brought under

control so that they can be used meaningfully. Reports of clinical success with severe Broca's and global patients using this motor speech treatment approach have been reported by Stevens (1989) and Stevens and Glaser (1983). The remarkable aspect of this treatment is that chronic patients have improved on both the Aphasia Quotient and the Cortical Quotient of the Western Aphasia Battery significantly, some up to 70 points, following treatment with this motor speech approach.

FUTURE DIRECTIONS

This chapter has raised more questions than answers. One central issue that has been clarified, however, is that left-hemisphere frontal lesions, both cortical and subcortical, most likely result in neuromotor deficits for speech production. This information also illuminates our understanding of the essence of the speech disorder that accompanies aphasia. Nonetheless, further and extensive research is needed in a number of areas.

Answers to the following questions are crucial to our clinical management of aphasic patients. Is there but one aphasia caused by damage to the temporal lobe? Are nonfluent aphasias simply aphasia complicated by motor speech impairment? What are the specific natures of the motor speech impairments accompanying frontal cortical and subcortical lesions to the dominant hemisphere—apraxic, dystonic, ataxic, paretic? When and for whom should microstructural versus macrostructural approaches to treatment be used? Is it true that the macrostructural approaches are successful for nonfluent aphasic patients for two reasons: *motoric* in that an oscillatory and rate mechanism is established and *linguistic* in that a template of semantic and syntactic structure is provided? How efficacious is each approach when studied empirically and with regard to increased verbal communication in the natural environment? When measures of social validation and consumer satisfaction are used in conjunction with measures of improvement on targets and standardized tests, are the treatments we administer efficacious and economically sound?

From the standpoint of issues regarding neuroanatomy and neurophysiology, we as a behavioral neuroscience must use more extensively the body of knowledge from the basic neurosciences to better understand the natures of neurological communication disorders. We must be much less influenced by static lesion correlated with symptomatology and endeavour to gain an appreciation of the dynamic aspects of brain functioning. Unfortunately like our predecessors, we have matched symptoms to lesion sites, sometimes clouding our understanding of aphasia and related disorders more than clarifying it (see Table 26.1). Finally, partnerships must be formed that undertake to integrate basic neurophysiology and the clinical science of communication disorders of neurogenic origin for the sake of advancement of both sciences. This chapter has been one attempt to interrelate these areas with the objective of enhancing our level of understanding regarding neuromotor speech disorders in aphasia.

Acknowledgments

We are grateful to Dr. Susan Shaiman, Ms. Joanne Winkel, and Ms. Debra Allison for their constructive comments on earlier versions of this manuscript; to the members of the Department of Communicative Disorders, Baycrest Geriatric Centre, Toronto, and particularly Ms. Regina Jokel, for their helpful assistance; to Ms. Janna Seto for preparation of the manuscript;

and to the Faculties of Medicine and Dentistry, University of Toronto, for their support for this project.

References

Abbs, J. H. (1989). Neurophysiologic processes of speech movement control. In N. Lass (Ed.), *Handbook of speech-language pathology and audiology* pp. 154–170. Toronto: B. Decker.

Abbs, J. H., and Gracco, V. L. (1984). Control of complex motor gestures: Orofacial muscle responses to load perturbation of the lip during speech. *Journal of Neurophysiology, 51,* 705.

Abbs, J. H., Gracco, V. L., and Cole, K. J. (1984). Control of multi-movement coordination: Sensorimotor mechanisms in speech motor programming. *Journal of Motor Behaviour, 16,* 195–232.

Abbs, J. H., and Welt, C. (1985). Lateral precentral cortex in speech motor control. In R. G. Daniloff (Ed.), *Recent advances in speech science.* San Diego, CA: College Hill Press.

Adams, S. G. (1990). *Rate and clarity of speech: An x-ray microbeam study.* Unpublished doctoral dissertation, University of Wisconsin—Madison.

Alajouanine, T., Castaigne, P., Sabouraud, O., and Contamin, F. (1959). Palilalie paroxystique et vocalizations itératives au cours de crises épileptiques par lésion intéressant l'aire motrice supplémentaire. *Revue Neuologique, 101,* 186–202.

Alajouanine, T., Ombredane, A., and Durand, M. (1939). *Le syndrome de désintegration phonétique dans l'aphasie.* Paris: Masson.

Albert, M. L., Goodglass, H., Helm, N. A., Rubens, A. B., and Alexander, M. P. (1981). Clinical aspects of dysphasia. In B. Arnold, F. Winckel, and B. Wyke (Eds.), *Disorders of human communication,* 2. New York: Springer-Verlag.

Albert, M. L., Spades, R. W., and Helm, N. A. (1973). Melodic intonation therapy for aphasia. *Archives of Neurology, 29,* 130–131.

Alexander, G. E., and Crutcher, M. D. (1990). Functional architecture of basal ganglia circuits: Neural substrates of parallel processing. *Trends in Neuroscience, 13,* 266–271.

Alexander, G. E., Delong, M. R., and Strick, P. L. (1986). Parallel organization of functionally segregated circuits linking basal ganglia and cortex. *Annual Review of Neuroscience, 9,* 357–381.

Alexander, M. P., Benson, D. F., and Stuss, D. T. (1989). Frontal lobes and language. *Brain and Language, 37,* 656–691.

Asanuma, H. (1989). *The motor cortex.* New York: Raven Press.

Asanuma, H., and Arissian, K. (1984). Experiments on functional role of peripheral input to motor cortex during voluntary movements in the monkey. *Journal of Neurophysiology, 52,* 212–227.

Asanuma, H., and Rosen, I. (1972). Topographical organization of cortical efferent zones projecting to distal forelimb muscles in the monkey. *Experimental Brain Research, 14,* 243–256.

Asanuma, H., and Sakata, H. (1967). Functional organization of a cortical efferent system examined with focal depth stimulation in cats. *Journal of Neurophysiology, 30,* 35–54.

Asanuma, H., Thach, W. T., and Jones, E. G. (1983). Distribution of cerebellar terminations in the ventral lateral thalamic region in the monkey. *Brain Research Review, 5,* 219–235.

Ballarger, J. (1865). De l'aphasie au point de vue psychologique. Aphasie avec terversion de la faculté du langage. In J. Ballarger (Ed.), *Recherches sur les maladies mentales.* Paris: Masson.

Barlow, S. M., and Farley, G. R. (1989). Neurophysiology of speech. In D. P. Kuehn, M. L. Lemme, and J. M. Baumgartner (Eds.), *Neural bases of speech, hearing and language* (pp. 146–200). Boston, MA: College Hill Press.

Baum, S. R., Blumstein, S. E., Naeser, M. A., and Palumbo, C. L. (1990). Temporal dimensions of consonant and vowel production: an acoustic and CT scan analysis of aphasic speech. *Brain and Language, 39,* 33–56.

Bay, E. (1962). Aphasia and non-verbal disorders of language. *Brain, 85,* 412–426.

Benke, T., and Kertesz, A. (1989). Hemispheric mechanisms of motor speech. *Aphasiology, 3,* 627–641.

Berlin, C. I. (1976). On melodic intonation therapy for aphasia. By R. W. Sparks and A. L. Holland. *Journal of Speech and Hearing Disorders, 41,* 298–300.

Berry, W. R., and Goshorn, E. L. (1983). Immediate visual feedback in the treatment of ataxic dysarthria: A case study. In W. R. Berry (Ed.), *Clinical dysarthria.* San Diego, CA: College Hill Press.

Beukelman, D. R., and Yorkston, K. M. (1978). Communication options for patient with brain stem lesions. *Archives of Physical Medicine and Rehabilitation, 59,* 337–340.

Blanken, G. (1991). The functional basis of speech automatisms (recurring utterances). *Aphasiology, 5,* 103–127.

Bouillaud, J. (1825). Recherches cliniques propres à demontrer que la perte de la parole correspond à la lésion des lobules antérieurs du cerveau, à confirmer l'opinion de M. GALL sur le siège de l'organe du langage articulé'. *Archives Générales de Mèdecine, 8,* 25–45.

Brindley, P., Copeland, M., DeMain, C., and & Martyn, P. (1989). A comparison of the speech of 10 chronic Broca's aphasics. *Aphasiology, 3,* 695–707.

Brinkman, C., and Porter, R. (1979). Supplementary motor area in the monkey. Activity of neurons during performance of a learned motor task. *Journal of Neurophysiology, 42,* 681–709.

Broca, P. (1861). Remarques sur le siège de la faculté de language suivies d'une observation d'aphémie. *Bulletin de la Société d'Anatomie, 6* (2e série), 330–357.

Cappa, S. F., Giudotti, M., Papagno, G., and Vignolo, L. A. (1987). Speechlessness with occasional vocalizations after bilateral opercular lesions: A case study. *Aphasiology, 1,* 35–39.

Chauvel, P., Bancaud, J., and Buser, P. (1985). Participation of the supplementary motor area in speech. *Experimental Brain Research, 58,* A14–A15.

Chen, D.-F., Hyland, B., Maier, V., Palmeri, A., and Wiesendanger, M. (1991). Comparison of neural activity in the supplementary motor area and in the primary motor cortex in monkeys. *Somatosensory and Motor Research, 8,* 27–44.

Chumpelik (Hayden), D. (1984). The PROMPT system of therapy. In D. Aram (Ed.), *Seminars in Speech and Language, 5,* 139–156.

Collins, M., Cariski, D., Longstreath, D., and Rosenbek, J. (1980). Patterns of articulatory behavior in selected motor speech programming disorders. In R. Brookshire (Ed.), *Clinical aphasiology: Conference proceedings* (pp. 196–208). Minneapolis, MN: BRK.

Crary, M., Hardy, T., and Williams, W. N. (1985). Aphemia with dysarthria or apraxia of speech. In R. Brookshire (Ed.), *Clinical aphasiology: conference proceedings* (pp. 113–125). Minneapolis, MN: BRK.

Critchley, M. (1952). Articulatory defects in aphasia. *Journal of Laryngology and Otology, 66,* 1–17.

Dabul, B., and Bollier, B. (1976). Therapeutic approaches to apraxia. *Journal of Speech and Hearing Disorders, 41,* 268–276.

Damasio, A. R. (1991). Aphasia. *New England Journal of Medicine, 326,* 531–539.

Damasio, A. R., and Geschwind, N. (1984). The neural basis of language. *Annual Review of Neuroscience, 7,* 127–147.

Damasio, A. R., and Van Hoesen, G. W. (1980). Structure and function of the supplementary motor area. *Neurology, 30,* 359.

Darley, F. L. (1968). *Apraxia of speech: 107 years of terminological confusion.* Paper presented to the American Speech and Hearing Association, Denver, CO.

Darley, F. L. (1975). Treatment of acquired aphasia. In W. Friedlander (Ed.). *Advances in Neurology, 7,* 112–145.

Darley, F. L. (1977). A retrospective review of aphasia. *Journal of Speech and Hearing Disorders, 42,* 161–169.

Darley, F. L. (1982). *Aphasia.* Philadelphia, PA: W. B. Saunders.

Darley, F. L., Aronson, A. E., and Brown, J. R. (1975). *Motor speech disorders.* Philadelphia, PA: W. B. Saunders.

Deal, J., and Florance C. (1978). Modification of the eight-step continuum for treatment of apraxia of speech in adults. *Journal of Speech and Hearing Disorders, 43,* 89–95.

Dejerine, J. (1892). Contribution à l'étude anatomo-pathologique et cliniques des différentes variétés de cécité verbale. *Mémoires de al Société de Biologie, 4,* 61.

Dejerine, J. (1901). Anatomie des centres nerveux. Parisi Rueff.

Dejerine, J. (1914). *Sémiologie des affections du système nerveux.* Paris: Masson.

Delong, M. R. (1990). Primate models of movement disorders of basal ganglia origin. *Trends in Neuroscience, 13,* 281–285.

Delong, M. R., and Georgopoulos, A. P. (1981). Motor functions of the basal ganglia. In V.B. Brooks (Ed.), *Handbook of physiology* (Sect. 1, Vol. 2, pp. 1010–1061). Bethesda, MD: American Physiological Society.

Denny-Brown, D. (1965). Physiological aspects of disturbances of speech. *Australian Journal of Experimental Biology and Medical Science, 43,* 455–474.

Dubner, R., Sessle, B. J., and Storey, A. T. (1978). *The neural basis of oral and facial function.* New York: Plenum Press.

Duffy, J. R., and Folger, W. N. (1986). *Dysarthria in unilateral central nervous system lesion: A retrospective study.* Paper presented at the Annual Convention of the American-Speech-Language and Hearing Association, Detroit, MI.

Dum, R. P., and Strick, P. L. (1991). The origin of corticospinal projections from the premotor areas in the frontal lobe. *Journal of Neuroscience, 11,* 667–689.

Dworkin, J. P., Abkarian, C. G., and Johns, D. F. (1988). Apraxia of speech: The effectiveness of a treatment regimen. *Journal of Speech and Hearing Disorders, 53,* 280–294.

Evarts, E. V. (1986). Motor cortex outputs in primates. In *Cerebral cortex, Vol. 5, Sensory motor areas and aspects of cortical connectivity* (pp. 217–241), New York: Plenum.

Evarts, E. V., Kimura, M., Wurtz, R. H., and Hikosake, O. (1984). Behavioral correlates of activity in basal ganglia neurons. *Trends in Neuroscience, 7,* 447–453.

Fairbanks, G. (1960). *Voice and articulation drillbook.* New York: Harper & Row.

Foix, C. (1928). Aphasias. In G. Roger, F. Widel, and P. Teissier (Eds.), *Nouveau traite de medecine.* Paris: Masson.

Forrest, K., Adams, S., McNeil, M., and Southwood, H. (1991). Kinematic, electromyographic, and perceptual evaluation of speech apraxia, conduction aphasia, ataxic dysarthria, and normal speech production. In C. Moore, K. Yorkston, and D. Beukelman (Eds.), *Dysarthria and apraxia of speech: Perspectives on management* (pp. 145–171). Baltimore, MD: Paul H. Brookes.

Fowler, C. A., Rubin, P., Remez, R. E., and Turvey, M. T. (1980). Implications for speech production of a general theory of action. In B. Butterworth (Ed.), *Language production* (pp. 373–420). New York: Academic Press.

Freedman, M., Alexander, M. P., and Naeser, M. A. (1984). Anatomic basis of transcortical motor aphasia. *Neurology, 40,* 409–417.

Freund, H.-J. (1987). Abnormalities of motor behavior after cortical lesions in humans. In S. Geiger, F. Plum, and V. Mountcastle (Eds.), *Handbook of Physiology, Vol. 5 , The Nervous System* (pp. 763–810). Bethesda, MD: American Physiological Society.

Freund, H.-J., and Hummelsheim, H. (1985). Lesions of premotor cortex in man. *Brain, 108,* 697–733.

Fried, I., Katz, A., McCarthy, G., Sass, K., Williamson, R., Spencer, S. S., and Spencer, D. D. (1991). Functional organization of human supplementary motor cortex studied by electrical stimulation. *Journal of Neuroscience, 11,* 3656–3666.

Fulton, J. F. (1949). *Physiology of the nervous system.* New York: Oxford University Press.

Godschalk, M., Lemon, R. N., Kuypers, H. G. J. M., and Ronday, H. K. (1984). Cortical afferents and efferents of monkey postarcuate area: An anatomical and electrophysiological study. *Experimental Brain Research, 56,* 410–424.

Goldberg, G. (1985). Supplementary motor area structure and function: Review and hypotheses. *Behavioral and Brain Sciences, 8,* 567–616.

Goldstein, K. (1948). *Language and language disturbances.* New York: Grune & Stratton.

Goodglass, H., and Kaplan, E. (1972). *The assessment of aphasia and related disorders.* Philadelphia, PA: Lea & Febiger.

Gracco, V. L. (1987). A multi-level control model for speech motor activity. In H. Peters and W. Hulstij (Eds.), *Speech motor dynamics in stuttering* (pp. 51–76). Wien, Austria: Springer-Verlag.

Gracco, V. L. (1990). Characteristics of speech as a motor control system. In G. Hammond (Ed.), *Cerebral control of speech and limb movements: advances in psychology* (Vol. 70, pp. 3–28). Amsterdam: North Holland.

Gracco, V. L. (1991). Sensorimotor mechanisms in speech motor control. In H. Peters, W. Hulstijn, and W. Starkweather (Eds.), *Speech motor control and stuttering* (pp. 53–76). New York: Elsevier Science Publishers.

Gracco, V. L., and Abbs, J. H. (1985). Dynamic control of the perioral system during speech: Kinematic analyses of autogenic and nonautogenic sensorimotor processes. *Journal of Neurophysiology, 54,* 418–432.

Gracco, V. L., and Abbs, J. H. (1987). Programming and execution processes of speech movement control: Potential neural correlates. In L. E. Keller and M. Gopnik (Eds.), *Symposium on motor and sensory language processes* (pp. 165–218). New Jersey: Lawrence Erlbaum.

Graybiel, A. M. (1990). Neurotransmitters and neuromodulators in the basal ganglia. *Trends in Neuroscience, 13,* 244–253.

Grillner, S. (1982). Possible analogies in the control of innate motor acts and the production of sound in speech. In S. Griller, B. Lindblom, J. Labker, and A. Persson (Eds.), *Speech motor control* (pp. 217–230). New York: Pergamon Press.

Hanson, W., and Metter, E. (1980). DAF as instrumental treatment for dysarthria in progressive supranuclear palsy: A case report. *Journal of Speech and Hearing Disorders, 45,* 268–276.

Hanson, W., and Metter, E. (1983). DAF speech rate modification in Parkinson's disease: A case report of two cases. In W. Berry (Ed.), *Clinical dysarthria.* San Diego, CA: College Hill Press.

Hartman, D. E., and Abbs, J. H. (1989). *Perceptual and physiological characteristics of unilateral upper motor neuron (UUMN) dysarthria.* Paper presented at the Annual Convention of the American Speech-Language-Hearing Association, St. Louis, MO.

Hayden (Chumpelik), D. (1986). Toronto Children's Centre, Speech Foundation of Ontario, Toronto, Ontario.

Hayden (Chumpelik), D. (1992). Toronto Children's Centre, Speech Foundation of Ontario, Toronto, Ontario.

Head, H. (1915). Hughlings Jackson on aphasia and kindred affections of speech. *Brain, 38,* 190.

Head, H. (1926 [1963]). *Aphasia and kindred disorders of speech* (Vol. 1). New York: Hafner.

Helm, N. (1979). Management of palilalia with a pacing board. *Journal of Speech and Hearing Disorders, 44,* 350–353.

Helm, N. A., and Barresi, B. (1980). Voluntary control of involuntary utterances: A treatment approach for severe aphasia. In R. Brookshire (Ed.), *Clinical aphasiology: Conference proceedings* (pp. 308–315). Minneapolis, MN: BRK.

Helm-Estabrooks, N. (1983). Treatment of subcortical aphasias. In W. Perkins (Ed.), *Language handicaps in adults* (pp. 97–103). New York: Thieme Stratton.

Hoffman, D. S., and Luschei, E. S. (1980). Responses of monkey precentral cortical cells during a controlled bite task. *Journal of Neurophysiology, 44,* 333–348.

Huang, C., Hiraba, H., Murray, G. M., and Sessle, B. J. (1989a). Topographical distribution and functional properties of cortically induced rhythmical jaw movements in the monkey (*Macaca fascicularis*). *Journal of Neurophysiology, 61,* 635–650.

Huang, C. S., Hiraba, H., and Sessle, B. J. (1989b). Input-output relationships of the pumary face motor cortex in the monkey (*Macaca fascicularis*). *Journal of Neurophysiology, 61,* 350–362.

Huang, C. S., Sirisko, M. A., Hiraba, H., Murray, G. M., and Sessle, B.J. (1988). Organization of the pumate face motor cortex as revealed by intracortical microstimulation and electrophysiological identification of afferent inputs and corticobulbar projections. *Journal of Neurophysiology, 59,* 796–818.

Hummelsheim, H., Wiesendanger, M., Bianchetti, M., Wiesendanger, R., and Macpherson, J. (1986). Further investigation of the efferent linkage of the supplementary motor area (SMA) with the spinal cord in the monkey. *Experimental Brain Research, 65,* 75–82.

Illes, J., Metter, E. J., Dennings, R., Jackson, C., Kemper, D., Hanson, W. (1989). Spontaneous language production in mild aphasia: Relationship to left prefrontal glucose hypometabolism. *Aphasiology, 3,* 527–537.

Ingham, R. J. (1983). *Stuttering and behaviour therapy: Current status and experimental foundations.* San Diego, CA: College Hill Press.

Itoh, M., Sasanuma, S., Hirose, H., Yosioka, H., and Yushigima, T. (1980). Abnormal articulatory dynamics in a patient with apraxia of speech. *Brain and Language, 11,* 66–75.

Itoh, M., Sasanuma, S., and Yushigima, T. (1979). Velar movements during speech in a patient with apraxia of speech. *Brain and Language, 7,* 227–239.

Jenkins, J., Jiminez-Pabon, E., Shaw, R., and Seefer, J. (1975). *Schuell's aphasia in adults,* (2nd ed.). New York: Harper & Row.

Johansson, R. S., Trulsson, M., Olsson, K. A., and Abbs, J. H. (1988). Mechanoreceptive afferent activity in the infraorbital nerve in man during speech and chewing movements. *Experimental Brain Research, 72,* 209–214.

Jonas, S. (1981). The supplementary motor region and speech emission. *Journal of Communicative Disorders, 14,* 349–373.

Jones, E. G. (1987). Ascending inputs to, and internal organization of, cortical motor areas. In G. Bock, M. O'Connor, and J. Marsh (Eds.), *Motor areas of the cerebral cortex.* CIBA Foundation Symposium, 132 (pp. 21–39). Chichester, Wiley.

Jurgens, U. (1985). Efferent connections of the supplementary motor area. *Experimental Brain Research, 58,* A1–A2.

Kann, J. (1950). A translation of Broca's original article on the location of the speech centre. *Journal of Speech and Hearing Disorders, 15,* 16–20.

Keith, R. L., and Aronson, A. E. (1975). Singing as therapy for apraxia of speech and aphasia: Report of a case. *Brain and Language, 2,* 483–488.

Kelly, J. P. (1985). Anatomical basis of sensory perception and motor coordination. In E. R. Kandel and J. H. Schwartz (Eds.), *Principles of Neural Science* (2nd ed., pp. 222-243). New York: Elsevier Science Publishing.

Kelso, J. A. S., and Tuller, B. (1984). Converging evidence in support of common dynamic principles for speech and movement coordination. *American Journal of Physiology*, 15, 928–935.

Kempler, D., Metter, E., Jackson, C., Hanson, W., Riege, W., Mazziota, J. C., and Phelps, M. A. (1986). Conduction aphasia: Subgroups based on behaviour, anatomy and physiology. In R. Brookshire (Ed.), *Clinical aphasiology: Conference proceedings* (Vol. 16, pp. 105–115). Minneapolis, MN: BRK.

Kennedy, M., Murdoch, B. E. (1989). Speech and language disorders subsequent to subcortical vascular lesions. *Aphasiology*, 3, 221–247.

Kent, R. D. (1990). The acoustic and physiologic characteristics of neurologically impaired speech movements. In W. Hardcastle and A. Marchal (Eds.), *Speech production and modelling* (pp. 365–401). Dordrecht: Kluwer Academic Publishers.

Kent, R. D., and Adams, S. G. (1989). The concept and measurement of coordination in speech disorders. In S. A. Wallace (Ed.), *Advances in Psychology: Perspectives on the Coordination of Movement* (Vol. 15, pp. 415–450). New York: Elsevier Science Publishing.

Kent, R. D., Martin, R. E., and Sufit, R. L. (1990). Oral sensation: A review and clinical prospective. In H. Winitz (Ed.), *Human communication and its disorders: A review.* (pp. 135–192). Norwood, N.J.: Ablex Publishing Corporation.

Kent, R. D., Netsell, R., and Abbs, J. H. (1979). Acoustic characteristics of dysarthria associated with cerebellar disease. *Journal of Speech and Hearing Research*, 22, 627–648.

Kent, R. D., and Rosenbek, J. C. (1983). Acoustic patterns of apraxia of speech. *Journal of Speech and Hearing Research*, 25, 231–249.

Kertesz, A. (1982). *Western Aphasia Battery*. New York: Grune & Stratton.

Kimura, D. (1979). Neuromotor mechanisms in the evolution of human communication. In H. D. Steklis and M. J. Raleigh (Eds.), *Neurobiology of social communication in primates* (pp. 197–219). New York: Academic Press.

Kimura, D. (1982). Left-hemisphere control of oral and brachial movements and their relation to communication. *Philosophical Transactions of the Royal Society of London*, B298, 135–149.

Kimura, D., and Watson, N. (1989). The relationship between oral movement control and speech. *Brain and Language*, 37, 565–590.

Kurata, K. (1992). Somatotopy in the human supplementary motor area. *Trends in Neuroscience*, 15, 159–160.

Kussmaul, A. (1877). Die St§rungen der Sprache. In *Ziemssen's Handbuch der speziellen Pathologie und Therapie*, 11, 1–300. Reprinted separately as *Die Störungen der Sprache. Versuch einer pathologie der Sprache*. Leipzig: Vogel (1881).

Kuypers, H. G. J. M. (1958a). Corticobulbar connexions to the pons and lower brain-stem in man. *Brain*, 81, 364–388.

Kuypers, H. G. J. M. (1958b). Some projections from the peri-central cortex to the pons and lower brain stem in monkey and chimpanzee. *Journal of Comparative Neurology*, 110, 221–255.

Kwan, H. C., Mackay, W. A., Murphy, J. T., and Wong, Y. C. (1978). Spatial organization of precentral cortex in awake primates II. Motor outputs. *Journal of Neurophysiology*, 41, 1120–1131.

Laborde. (1863). Discussion. *Bulletin Société Anatomique*, 376.

Larson, C. R., Byrd, K. E., Garthwaite, C. R., and Luschei, E. S. (1980). Alterations in the pattern of mastication after ablations of the lateral precentral cortex in rhesus monkeys. *Experimental Neurology*, 70, 638–651.

Lebrun, Y. (1989). Apraxia of speech: The history of a concept. In P. Square-Storer (Ed.), *Acquired apraxia of speech in aphasic adults* (pp. 3–19). London: Taylor & Francis.

Lecky, B. R. F., Hughes, R. A. C., and Murray, N. M. F. (1987). Trigeminal sensory neuropathy: A study of 22 cases. *Brain*, 110, 1463–1485.

Lecours, A. R., and Lhermitte, F. (1976). The "pure form" of the phonetic disintegration syndrome (pure anarthria); anatomo-clinical report of a historical case. *Brain and Language*, 3, 88–113.

Levine, D. N., and Mohr, J. P. (1979). Language after bilateral cerebral infarctions: Role of the minor hemisphere in speech. *Neurology*, 29, 927–938.

Lichtheim, L. (1884-1885). On aphasia. *Brain*, 7, 433–484.

Liepmann, H. (1913). Motorische, aphasie, und apraxie. *Transactions of the 17th International Congress of Medicine*, XI, 97–106.

Lindblom, B. E. F., Lubker, J. F., and Gay, T. (1979). Format frequencies of some fixed-mandible vowels and a model of speech motor programming by predictive stimulation. *Journal of Phonetics*, 7, 147–161.

Löfquist, A., and Yoshioka, H. (1981). Interarticulator programming in obstruent production. *Phonetica*, 38, 21–34.

Löfquist, A., and Yoshioka, H. (1984). Intersegmental timing: Laryngeal-oral coordination in voiceless consonant production. *Speech Communication*, 3, 279–289.

Lund, J. P., and Lamarre, Y. (1974). Activity of neurons in the lower precentral cortex during voluntary and rhythmical jaw movements in the monkey. *Experimental Brain Research*, 19, 282–299.

Luria, A. A. (1964). Factors and forms of aphasia. In A. V. S. De Reuck and M. O'Connor (Eds.), *Disorders of language*. London: Churchill.

Luria, A. A. (1970). *Traumatic aphasia: Its syndromes, psychology and treatment*. The Hague: Mouton.

Luschei, E. S., Garthwaite, C. R., and Armstrong, M. E. (1971). Relationship of firing patterns of units in face area of monkey precentral cortex to conditioned jaw movements. *Journal of Neurophysiology*, 34, 552–561.

Luschei, E. S., and Goodwin, G. M. (1975). Role of monkey precentral cortex in control of voluntary jaw movements. *Journal of Neurophysiology*, 38, 146–157.

MacNeilage, P. F. (1970). Motor control of serial ordering of speech. *Psychological Review*, 77, 182–196.

Mao, C. C., Coull, B. M., Golper, L. A. C., Rau, M. T. (1989). Anterior operculum syndrome. *Neurology*, 39, 1169–1172.

Marie, P. (1906). Révision de la question de l'aphasie: que fait-il penser des aphasies sous-corticales (aphasies pures)? *Semaine médicale*, 26, 493.

Marie, P., Foix, C., and Bertrand, I. (1917). Topographie cranio-cérébrale. *Annales de Médecine*, 55.

Marsden, C. D. (1982). The mysterious function of the basal ganglia: The Robert Wartenberg lecture. *Neurology*, 32, 514–539.

Marshall, R. C., Gandour, J., and Windsor, J. (1988). Selective impairment of phonation: a case study. *Brain and Language*, 35, 313–339.

Mateer, C., and Kimura, D. (1977). Impairment of nonverbal oral movements in aphasia. *Brain and Language*, 4, 262–276.

Matelli, M., Camarda, R., Glickstein, M., and Rizzolatti, G. (1986). Afferent and efferent projections of the inferior area 6 in the Macaque monkey. *Journal of Comparative Neurology*, 251, 281–298.

McLean, M. D., Dostrovsky, J. O., LEE, L., and Tasker, R. R. (1990). Somatosensory neurons in human thalamus respond to speech-induced orofacial movements. *Brain Research*, 513, 343–347.

McNeil, M. R., Adams, S. (1990). A comparison of speech kinematics among apraxic, conduction aphasic, ataxic dysarthric and normal geriatric speakers. In T. E. Prescott (Ed.), *Clinical Aphasiology*, (pp. 279–294). Austin, TX: Pro-Ed.

McNeil, M. R., Caligiuri, M., and Rosenbek, J. C. (1989). A comparison of labio-mandibular kinematic durations, displacements, velocities and dysmetrias in apraxic and normal adults. In T. E. Prescott (Ed.), *Clinical aphasiology* (pp. 173–179). Boston, MA: College Hill Press.

McNeil, M. R., Weismer, G., Adams, S., and Mulligan, M. (1990). Oral structure nonspeech motor control in normal dysarthric aphasic and apraxic speakers: Isometric force and static fine position control. *Journal of Speech and Hearing Research*, 33, 255–268.

Metter, E. J., Hanson, W. R., Kempler, D., Jackson, C., Mazziota, J., and Phelps, M. (1987a). Left prefrontal glucose hypometabolism in aphasia. In R. Brookshire (Ed.), *Clinical aphasiology* (Vol. 17, pp. 300–312). Minneapolis, MN: BRK.

Metter, E. J., Hanson, W. R., Riege, W. H., Jackson, C., Mazziotta, J., Phelps, M. E., Kuhl, D. E. (1985). Remote metabolic effects in aphasia stroke patients. In R. H. Brookshire (Ed.), *Clinical aphasiology* (Vol. 15, pp. 126–135). Minneapolis, MN: BRK.

Metter, E. J., Jackson, C. A., and Kempler, D. (1986). Left-hemisphere intracerebral haemorrhages studied by (F-18)-fluorodeoxyglucose PET. *Neurology*, 36, 1155–1162.

Metter, E. J., Kempler, D., Jackson, C., Hanson, W., Mazziota, J., and Phelps, M. (1989). Cerebellar glucose metabolism in Wernicke's and Broca's and conduction aphasias. *Archives of Neurology*, 46, 27–34.

Metter, E. J., Kempler, D., Jackson, C., Hanson, W., Riege, W., Camras, L., Mazziota, J., and Phelps, M. E. (1987b). Cerebellar glucose metabolism in chronic aphasia. *Neurology*, 37, 1599–1606.

Metter, E. J., Riege, W. R., Hanson, W. R., Jackson, C., Kempler, D., Van Lancker, D. (1988). Subcortical structures in aphasia: Analysis based on FBG, PET and CT. *Archives of Neurology*, 45, 1229–1234.

Metter, E. J., Riege, W. R., Hanson, W. R., Kuhl, D. E., Phelps, M. E., Squire, L. R. Wasterlain, C. G., and Benson, D. F. (1983). Comparison of metabolic rates, language and memory in subcortical aphasia. *Brain and Language*, 19, 33–47.

Metter, E. J., Riege, W. H., Hanson, W. R., Phelps, M. E., and Kuhl, D. E. (1982). Role of the caudate nucleus in aphasic language: Evidence from FDG-PET. *Neurology, 32,* A94.

Metter, E. J., Riege, W. H., Hanson, W. R., Phelps, M. E. and Kuhl, D. E. (1988b). Evidence for a caudate role in aphasia from FBG positron computed tomography. *Aphasiology, 2,* 33–43.

Metter, E. J., Wasterlain, C. G., Kuhl, D. E., Hanson, W. R., Phelps, M. E. (1981). FDG[18] positron emission computed tomography: A study of aphasia. *Annals of Neurology, 10,* 173–183.

Miller, A. J., and Bowman, J. P. (1977). Precentral cortical modulation of mastication and swallowing. *Journal of Dental Research, 56,* 1154.

Mitchell, R. A., and Berger, A. J. (1975). Neural regulation of respiration. *American Review of Respiratory Disease, III,* 206–224.

Mohr, J. P., Funkenstein, H. H., Finkelstein, S., Ressin, M. S., Duncan, G. W., and Davis, K. R. (1975). Broca's area infarction versus Broca's aphasia. *Neurology, 25,* 349.

Mohr, J. P., Pessin, M. S., Finkelstein, S., Funkenstein, H. H., Duncan, G. W., and Davis, K. R. (1978). Broca's aphasia: Pathologic and clinical. *Neurology, 28,* 311–324.

Muakkassa, K. F., and Strick, P. L. (1979). Frontal lobe inputs to primate motor cortex: Evidence for four somatotopically organized "premotor" areas. *Brain Research, 177,* 176–182.

Murray, G. M. (1989). *An analysis of motor cortex neural activities during trained orofacial motor behaviour in the awake primate (Macaca fascicularis).* Unpublished doctoral dissertation, University of Toronto.

Murray, G. M., Lin, L.-D., Moustafa, E., and Sessle, B. J. (1991). Effects of reversible inactivation by cooling of the primate face primary motor cortex on the performance of a trained tongue-protrusion task and a training biting task. *Journal of Neurophysiology, 65,* 511–530.

Murray, G. M., and Sessle, B. J. (1992a). Functional properties of single neurons in the face primary motor cortex of the primate I. Input and output features of tongue motor cortex. *Journal of Neurophysiology, 67,* 747–758.

Murray, G. M., and Sessle, B. J. (1992b). Functional properties of single neurons in the face primary motor cortex of the primate II. Relations with trained orofacial motor behavior. *Journal of Neurophysiology, 67,* 110, 221–255.

Murray, G. M., and Sessle, B. J. (1992c). Functional properties of single neurons in the face primary motor cortex of the primate III. Relations with different directions of trained tongue protrusion. *Journal of Neurophysiology, 67,* 775–785.

Mushiake, H., Inase, M., and Tanji, J. (1991). Neuronal activity in the primate premotor, supplementary, and precentral motor cortex during visually guided and internally determined sequential movements. *Journal of Neurophysiology, 66,* 705–718.

Naeser, M. A., Alexander, M. P., Helm-Estabrooks, N., Levine, H. L., Laughlin, S. A., and Geschwind, N. (1982). Aphasia with predominantly subcortical lesion sites. *Archives of Neurology, 39,* 2–14.

Naeser, M. A., and Helm-Estabrooks, N. (1985). CT scan lesion localization and response to melodic intonation therapy with nonfluent aphasia cases. *Cortex, 21,* 203-223.

Naeser, M. A., Palumbo, C. L., Helm-Estabrooks, N., Stiassny-Eder, D., and Albert, M. (1989). Severe nonfluency in aphasia. *Brain, 112,* 1–38.

Nagafuchi, M., Aoki, Y., Niizuma, H., and Okita, N. (1991). Paroxysmal speech disorder following left-frontal brain damage. *Brain and Language, 40,* 266–273.

Nathan, P. W. (1947). Facial apraxia and apraxic dysarthria. *Brain, 70,* 449–478.

Ojemann, G. (1988). Effects of cortical and subcortical stimulation on human language and verbal memory. In F. Plum (Ed.), *Language, communication and the brain* (pp. 101–115). New York: Raven Press.

Pandya, D. N., and Barnes, C. L. (1987). Architecture and connections of the frontal lobe. *Frontal lobes revisited* (pp. 41–72). New York: IRBV Press.

Pandya, D. N., and Seltzer, B. (1982). Association areas of the cerebral cortex. *Trends in Neuroscience, 5,* 386–390.

Pellat, J., Gentil, M., Lyard, G., Vila, A., Tarel, V., Moreau, O., and Benabio, A. L. (1991). Aphemia after a penetrating brain wound: A case study. *Brain and Language, 40,* 459–470.

Penfield, W., and Rasmussen, T. (1950). *The cerebral cortex of man* (1st ed.). New York: MacMillan.

Penfield, W., and Roberts, L. (1959). *Speech and brain-mechanisms.* Princeton, NJ: Princeton University Press.

Penfield, W., and Welch, K. (1951). The supplementary motor area of the cerebral cortex: A clinical and experimental study. *American Medical Association Archives of Neurology and Psychiatry, 66,* 289–317.

Perkell, J. S. (1980). Phonetic features and the physiology of speech production. In B. Butterworth (Ed.), *Language production* (pp. 337–372). London: Academic Press.

Phelps, M. E., Schelbert, H. R., and Mazziota, J. C. (1983). Positron computed tomography for studies of myocardial and cerebral function. *Annals of Internal Medicine, 98,* 339–359.

Pick, A. (1892). Beitrage zur Lehre von den Storungen der Sprache. *Archiv für Psychiatrie ünd Nervenkrankheiten, 23,* 896.

Porch, B. E. (1967). *The Porch Index of Communicative Ability.* Palo Alto, CA: Consulting Psychologists Press.

Rascol, O., Sabatini, U., Celsis, P., Montastruc, J. L., and Chollet, F. (1992). Activation of the supplementary motor area in akinetic patients with Parkinson's disease: Regional cerebral blood flow changes in the "ON" and "OFF" conditions. *Movement Disorders, 7,* (Suppl. 1), 147.

Rizzolatti, G. (1985). Neurological deficits following the removal of postarcuate cortex in macaque monkeys. *Experimental Brain Research, 58,* a9.

Rizzolatti, G., Scandolara, C., Gentilucci, M., and Camarda, R. (1981). Response properties and behavioural modulation of "mouth" neurons in the postarcuate cortex (area 6) in macaque monkeys. *Brain Research, 225,* 421–424.

Robin, D. A., Bean, C., and Folkins, J. W. (1989). Lip movement in apraxia of speech. *Journal of Speech and Hearing Research, 42,* 512–523.

Roland, P. E. (1981). Somatotopic tuning of postcentral gyrus during focal attention in man. *Journal of Neurophysiology, 46,* 744–754.

Rolls, E., and Johnstone, S. (1992). Neurophysiological analysis of striatal function. In G. Vallar, S. Cappa, C. Wallesch (Eds.), *Neurophysiological disorders associated with subcortical disorders* (pp. 61–97). Oxford: Oxford Press.

Rosenbek, J. C. (1976). *Treatment of apraxia of speech: Prevention, facilitation and reorganization.* Paper presented at the Annual Meeting of the American Speech and Hearing Association, Houston, TX.

Rosenbek, J. C. (1983). Treatment for apraxia of speech in adults. In W. H. Perkins (Ed.), *Dysarthria and apraxia* (pp. 49–57). New York: Thieme-Stratton.

Rosenbek, J. C. (1985). *Treating apraxia of speech.* In D. F. Johns (Ed.), *Clinical management of neurogenic communicative disorders* (pp. 267–312). Boston: Little Brown.

Rosenbek, J. C. and McNeil, M. R. (1991). A discussion of the classification in motor speech disorders: Dysarthria and apraxia of speech. In C. Moore, K. Yorkston, and D. Beukelman (Eds.), *Dysarthria and apraxia of speech* (pp. 289–295), Baltimore, MD: Paul H. Brookes.

Rosenbek, J. C., Collins, M., and Wertz, R. (1976). Intersystemic reorganization for apraxia of speech. In R. Brookshire (Ed.), *Clinical aphasiology: Conference proceedings* (pp. 255–260). Minneapolis, MN: BRK.

Rosenbek, J. C., and LaPointe, L. L. (1978, 1985). The dysarthrias: Description, diagnosis and treatment. In D. F. Johns (Ed.), *Clinical management of neurogenic communicative disorders.* Boston, MA: Little, Brown.

Rosenbek, J. C., Lemme, M. L., Ahern, M. B., Harris, E. H., and Wertz, R. T. (1973). A treatment for apraxia of speech in adults. *Journal of Speech and Hearing Disorders, 38,* 462–472.

Rubow, R. T., Rosenbek, J. C., and Collins, M. J. (1982). Vibrotactile stimulation for intersystemic reorganization in the treatment of apraxia of speech. *Archives of Physical Medicine and Rehabilitation, 63,* 150–153.

Russell, W., and Espir, M. (1961). *Traumatic aphasia.* London: Oxford Press.

Sachs, M. B., Young, E. D., and Miller, M. I. (1982). Encoding of speech features in the auditory nerve. In R. Carlson and B. Granstrom (Eds.), *The representation of speech in the peripheral auditory system* (pp. 115–130). New York: Elsevier.

Sarno, M. T. (1965). Functional communication profile. *Archives of Physical Medicine and Rehabilitation, 46,* 101–107.

Schell, G. R., and Strick, P. L. (1984). The origin of thalamic inputs to the arcuate premotor and supplementary motor areas. *Journal of Neuroscience, 4,* 539–560.

Schiff, H. B., Alexander, M. P., Naeser, M. A., and Galaburda, A. M. (1983). Aphemia: Clinical–anatomic correlates. *Archives of Neurology, 40,* 720–727.

Schuell, H., Jenkins, J., and Jimenez-Pabon, E. (1964). *Aphasia in adults.* New York: Harper & Row.

Shane, H. C., and Darley, F. L. (1978). The effect of auditory rhythmic stimulation on articulatory accuracy in apraxia of speech. *Cortex, 14,* 444–450.

Shankweiler, D., and Harris, K. S. (1966). An experimental approach to the problem of articulation in aphasia. *Cortex, 2,* 287–292.

Simmons, N. N. (1978). Finger counting as an intersystemic reorganizer in apraxia of speech. In R. H. Brookshire (Ed.), *Clinical aphasiology: Conference proceedings* (pp. 174–179). Minneapolis, MN: BRK.

Simpson, M. B., and Clark, A. R. (1989). Clinical management of apractic mutism. In P. Square-Storer (Ed.), *Acquired apraxia in aphasic adults* (pp. 241–266). London: Taylor & Francis.

Sirisko, M. A., and Sessle, B. J. (1983). Corticobulbar projections and orofacial and muscle afferent inputs to neurons in primate sensorimotor cerebral cortex. *Experimental Neurology, 82,* 716–720.

Skelly, M., Schensky, L., Smith, R., and Foust, R. (1974). American Indian Sign (Amerind) as a facilitation of verbalization for the oral verbal apraxia. *Journal of Speech and Hearing Disorders, 39,* 445–456.

Smith, A. (1992). The control of orofacial movements in speech. *Critical Reviews in Oral Biology and Medicine, 3,* 233–267.

Soh, K., Larsen, B., Skinhoj, E., and Lassen, N. A. (1978). Regional cerebral blood flow in aphasia. *Archives of Neurology, 35,* 625–632.

Southwood, H. (1987). The use of prolonged speech in the treatment of apraxia of speech. In R. Brookshire (Ed.), *Clinical aphasiology* (pp. 277–287). Minneapolis, MN: BRK.

Sparks, R., and Deck, J. (1986). Melodic intonation therapy. In R. Chapey (Ed.), *Language intervention strategies in adult aphasia* (pp. 320–332). Baltimore, MD: Williams & Wilkins.

Sparks, R., Helm, N., and Albert, M. (1974). Aphasia rehabilitation resulting from melodic intonation therapy. *Cortex, 10,* 303–316.

Sparks, R., and Holland, A. (1976). Method: Melodic intonation therapy. *Journal of Speech and Hearing Disorders, 41,* 287–297.

Square, P. A. (1981). *Apraxia of speech in adults: Speech perception and production.* Unpublished doctoral dissertation, Kent State University, OH.

Square, P., Chumpelik (Hayden), D., and Adams, S. (1985). Efficacy of the PROMPT system of therapy for the treatment of acquired apraxia of speech. In R. Brookshire (Ed.), *Clinical aphasiology: Conference proceedings* (pp. 319–320). Minneapolis, MN: BRK.

Square, P., Chumpelik (Hayden), D., Morningstar, D., and Adams, S. (1986). Efficacy of the PROMPT system of therapy for the treatment for the apraxia of speech. A follow-up investigation. In R. Brookshire (Ed.), *Clinical aphasiology: Conference proceedings* (pp. 221–226). Minneapolis, MN: BRK.

Square, P. A., Darley, F. L. and Sommers, R. K. (1981). Speech perception among patients demonstrating apraxia of speech, aphasia and both disorders. In R. Brookshire (Ed.), *Clinical aphasiology: Conference proceedings* (pp. 83–88). Minneapolis, MN: BRK.

Square, P. A., Darley, F. L., and Sommers, R. K. (1982). An analysis of the productive errors made by pure apractic speakers with differing loci of lesions. In R. Brookshire (Ed.), *Clinical aphasiology: Conference proceedings* (pp. 245–250). Minneapolis, MN: BRK.

Square, P. A., and Mlcoch, A. G. (1983). The syndrome of subcortical apraxia of speech: Acoustic analysis. In R. Brookshire (Ed.), *Clinical aphasiology: Conference proceedings* (pp. 239–243). Minneapolis, MN: BRK.

Square-Storer, P. A. (1987). Acquired apraxia of speech. In H. Winitz (Ed.), *Human communication and its disorders: A review—1987* (pp. 88–166). Norwood, NJ: Ablex Publishing Corp.

Square-Storer, P. A. (1989a). Traditional therapies for apraxia of speech—reviewed and rationalized. In P. Square-Storer (Ed.), *Acquired apraxia of speech in aphasic adults* (pp. 145–161). London: Lawrence Erlbaum.

Square-Storer, P. A. (1989b). *Acquired apraxia of speech in aphasic adults: Theoretical and clinical issues.* London: Taylor & Francis.

Square-Storer, P. A., and Apeldoorn, S. (1991). An acoustic study of apraxia of speech in patients with different lesion loci. In C. Moore, K. Yorkston, and D. Beukelman (Eds.), *Dysarthria and apraxia of speech: Perspectives on management* (pp. 271–288). Baltimore, MD: Paul H. Brookes.

Square-Storer, P. A., Darley, F. L., and Sommers, R. K. (1988). Speech processing abilities in patients with aphasia and apraxia of speech. *Brain and Language, 33,* 65–85.

Square-Storer, P., and Hayden (Chumpelik), D. (1989). PROMPT treatment. In P. Square-Storer (Ed.), *Acquired apraxia of speech in aphasic adults* (pp. 190–219). London: Lawrence Erlbaum.

Stevens, E. R. (1989). Multiple inputs phoneme therapy. In P. Square-Storer (Ed.), *Acquired apraxia of speech in aphasic adults* (pp. 220–238). London: Lawrence Erlbaum.

Stevens, E., and Glasser, L. (1983). Multiple input phoneme therapy: An approach to severe apraxia and expressive aphasia. In R. Brookshire (Ed.), *Clinical aphasiology,* (pp. 148–155). Minneapolis, MN: BRK.

Thach, W. T., Goodkin, H. P., and Keating, J. G. (1992). The cerebellum and the adaptive co-ordination of movement. *Annual Review of Neuroscience, 15,* 403–442.

Tonkonogy, J., and Goodglass, H. (1981). Language function, foot of the third frontal gyrus, and rolandic operculum. *Archives of Neurology, 38,* 486–490.

Tonkovich, J. D., and Peach, R. K. (1989). What to treat: Apraxia of speech, aphasia or both. In P. Square-Storer (Ed.). *Acquired apraxia of speech in aphasic adults: theoretical and clinical issues,* (pp. 115–144). London: Lawrence Erlbaum.

Trousseau, A. (1861-1864). *Clinique Médicale de l'Hôtel–Dieu de Paris.* Paris: Masson.

Van Riper, C. (1939). *Speech correction: Principles and methods.* Englewood Cliffs, NJ: Prentice-Hall.

Wallesch, C.-W. (1990). Repetitive verbal behaviour: Functional and neurological considerations. *Aphasiology, 4,* 133–153.

Watanabe, M. (1992). Frontal units of the monkey coding the associative significance of visual and auditory stimuli. *Experimental Brain Research, 89,* 233–247.

Weisenberg, T., and McBride, K. E. (1935). *Aphasia: A clinical and psychological study.* New York: Commonwealth Fund.

Weisenberg, T., and McBride, K. E. (1964). *Aphasia.* New York: Commonwealth Fund. Reprinted by Hafner Publishing Company, New York, 1964.

Wernicke, C. (1874). *Der aphasische symptomenkomplex.* Breslau: Cohn & Weigert.

Wernicke, C. (1885). Die neueren Arbeiten Über Aphasie. *Fortschritte der Medizin, 3,* 824–830.

Wertz, R. T. (1978, 1985). Neuropathologies of speech and language: An introduction to patient management. In D. F. Johns (Ed.), *Clinical management of neurogenic communicative disorders.* Boston, MA: Little, Brown.

Wertz, R. T., LaPointe, L. L. and Rosenbek, J. C. (1984). *Apraxia of speech in adults: The disorder and its management.* New York: Grune & Stratton.

Whitty, C. W. M. (1964). Cortical dysarthria and dysprosody of speech. *Journal of Neurology, Neurosurgery, and Psychiatry, 27,* 507–510.

Wiesendanger, M. (1986). Redistributive function of the motor cortex. *Trends in Neuroscience, 93,* 120–125.

Wiesendanger, M., and Wise, S. P. (1992). Current issues concerning the functional organization of motor cortical areas in non-human primates. In P. Chauvel, A. V. Delgado-Escueta, et al. (Eds.), *Advances in Neurology, 57,* 117–134.

Wiesendanger, R., and Wiesendanger, M. (1985a). The thalamic connection with medial area 6 (supplementary motor cortex) in the monkey. *Experimental Brain Research, 59,* 91–104.

Wiesendanger, R., and Wiesendanger, M. (1985b). Cerebello-cortical linkage in the monkey as revealed by transcellular labeling with the lectin wheat germ agglutinin conjugated to the marker horseradish peroxidase. *Experimental Brain Research, 59,* 105–117.

Wise, S. P. (1985). The primate premotor cortex: Past, present, and preparatory. *Annual Review of Neuroscience, 8,* 1–19.

Wise, S. P., and Strick, P. L. (1984). Anatomical and physiological organization of the non-primary motor cortex. *Trends in Neuroscience, 7,* 442–446.

Yorkston, K. M., and Beukelman, D. R. (1981). Ataxic dysarthria: Treatment sequences based on intelligibility and prosodic considerations. *Journal of Speech and Hearing Disorders, 46,* 398–404.

Yorkston, K. M., Beukelman, D. R., and Bell, K. R. (1988). *Clinical management of dysarthric speakers.* Boston, MA: College Hill Press.

Zealear, D. L., Hast, M. H., and Kurago, Z. (1983). Functional organization of the primary motor cortex controlling the face, tongue, jaw, and larynx in the monkey. In I. R. Titze and R. C. Scherer (Eds.), *Vocal fold physiology: Biomechanics, acoustics and phonatory control* (pp. 57–73). Denver, CO: Denver Center for the Performing Arts.

APPENDIX 26.1

Hierarchy for Finger Tapping Therapy[a]

1. Patient watches and listens as clinician says each word of sentence, holding one finger up for every word.
2. Unison production.
3. Client production with mimed verbal production by clinician or unison finger counting by clinician.
4. Patient counts off words while choosing written words in proper sequence.

5. Clinician presents a question to which the patient must respond with the practiced sentence using finger counting.

[a] As specified by Simmons, N. N. (1978). Finger counting as an intersystemic reorganizer apraxia of speech. In R. H. Brookshire (Ed.), *Clinical aphasiology: Conference proceedings.* Minneapolis, MN: BRK.

APPENDIX 26.2

Eight-Step Task Continuum with Integral Stimulation[a]

1. Integral stimulation ("Watch me," "Listen to me") followed by unison production.
2. Integral stimulation. Clinician supports patient's delayed response with mime.
3. Integral stimulation. Patient produces response without support.
4. Integral stimulation followed by successive unsupported productions by patient.

5. Written stimulus with unison production.
6. Written stimulus is provided but is removed before patient responds.
7. Utterance is elicited by a question.
8. Utterance is elicited in role playing.

[a] As specified by Rosenbek, J.C., Lemme, M. L., Ahern, M. B., Harris, E. H., and Wertz, R. T. (1973). A treatment for apraxia of speech in adults. *Journal of Speech and Hearing Disorders, 38,* 462–472.

SECTION FOUR
REMEDIATION OF RELATED DISORDERS

CHAPTER 27
Management of Dysphagia Poststroke

JERI A. LOGEMANN

This chapter is designed to provide a perspective on research in dysphagia poststroke in the context of our understanding of normal swallow physiology and neurophysiology, and to describe appropriate techniques for assessment and treatment of oropharyngeal swallow disorders after stroke.

HISTORICAL PERSPECTIVE ON DYSPHAGIA RESEARCH IN STROKE PATIENTS

Over the past 30 years, research on swallowing disorders poststroke has evolved from studies of a few stroke patients (Donner, 1974; Silbiger et al., 1967) included in a heterogeneous population of neurogenically impaired dysphagic patients to studies of carefully defined patients with specified lesions in the central nervous system (Barer, 1989; Logemann et al., 1989; Robbins and Levine, 1988). In parallel with this progression from heterogeneous to more homogeneous populations of stroke patients examined at uncontrolled times poststroke, investigators have begun to examine dysphagic stroke patients at selected times postictus (Bisch et al., 1991; Gordon et al., 1987; Lazarus et al., 1991; Robbins and Levine, 1988). Studies have also progressed from limited descriptions of swallow disorders derived from observations of radiographic studies (Donner, 1974; Silbiger et al., 1967; Veis and Logemann, 1985) to measurements of specific bolus movements, such as oral transit times, or of oral-pharyngeal movement parameters, such as durations of airway closure and cricopharyngeal opening (Lazarus et al., 1991; Robbins and Levine, 1988). To some extent, research in poststroke dysphagia has paralleled the development of research in normal swallow physiology, which has also developed from observations of oropharyngeal function and bolus transit in heterogeneous groups of normal subjects (Ardran and Kemp, 1951; Blonsky et al., 1975; Bosma, 1957) to more precise measurements of swallow physiology, using specified bolus types and carefully selected age-controlled normal subjects (Bisch et al., 1991; Cook et al., Dodds et al., 1989; Dodds et al., 1990; Jacob et al., 1989; Kahrilas et al., 1992, 1993; Logemann et al., 1992). These research developments in normal swallow physiology and dysphagia poststroke have significant potential for (a) expanding our knowledge of normal neurophysiology of deglutition; (b) measuring efficacy of existing treatment techniques with dysphagic stroke patients; and (c) defining new evaluation and treatment strategies for swallowing disorders resulting from stroke.

SWALLOW DISORDERS BY SITE OF LESION

The body of knowledge on swallow abnormalities resulting from stroke at specific sites in the central nervous system is just evolving (Barer, 1989; Celifarco et al., 1990; Delgado, 1988; Logemann and Kahrilas, 1990; Meadows, 1973; Smith and Dodd, 1990; Wade and Hewer, 1987). There is, however, adequate information to begin to understand the types of swallow disorders exhibited by patients with isolated lesions in the brain stem, subcortical regions, and left and right hemispheres of the cerebral cortex. The discussion below is based on data from our studies of patients at 3 weeks poststroke who have suffered a single infarct with no prior history of stroke or other neurological disorders or damage to the head and neck, and who have been otherwise apparently healthy until their stroke. Medical complications, preexisting medical problems, and medications can affect the severity of swallowing problems poststroke, as discussed in the section entitled, "Effects of Other Factors on Swallowing Function and Recovery in the Stroke Patient."

Effects of Lesions in the Brain Stem

Lesions in the lower brain stem (medullary region) generally result in significant oropharyngeal swallow impairment because of the location of the major swallow centers (nucleus tractus solitarius and nucleus ambiguous) within the medulla (Jean and Car, 1979; Miller, 1982). Patients with unilateral medullary lesions typically exhibit functional or near-normal oral control with significantly impaired triggering and neuromotor control of the pharyngeal swallow. Specifically, these patients often exhibit what appears to be an absent pharyngeal swallow in the first week postictus. As the pharyngeal swallow begins to appear (usually in the second week poststroke), there is a significant delay in triggering the pharyngeal swallow (often 10 to 15 seconds or more). When the pharyngeal swallow triggers, these patients exhibit (a) reduced laryngeal elevation and anterior motion, which contributes to reduced opening of the cricopharyngeal region, with the symptom of residual food collecting in the pyriform sinuses, particularly on one side; and (b) unilateral pharyngeal weakness, which further contributes to the residual food remaining in the pyriform sinus on one side. Some patients also exhibit unilateral adductor vocal fold paresis. While these patients often exhibit significant dysphagia requiring nonoral intake at 1 to 2 weeks poststroke, by 3 weeks poststroke their swallow has often recovered sufficiently to be functional and allow full oral intake. In general, the more severe the swallow abnormalities at 2 to 3 weeks postictus, and the more medical complications present, the longer the swallow recovery period. After medullary stroke, some patients will not recover functional swallowing for 4 to 6 months poststroke.

Examination of pharyngeal swallow measures at 12 and 24 weeks poststroke in medullary stroke patients whose swallow was functional at 3 weeks postictus reveals that, although their swallow is functional (i.e., they are eating a full, normal diet orally with no aspiration and only small amounts of residue in the pyriform sinuses), their measures of pharyngeal movement during swallow are just outside the normal range.

Effects of Subcortical Stroke

Subcortical lesions may affect motor as well as sensory pathways to and from the cortex. Subcortical stroke usually results in mild delays in oral transit times (3 to 5 seconds), mild delays (3 to 5 seconds) in triggering the pharyngeal swallow, and mild to moderate impairments in timing of the neuromuscular components of the pharyngeal swallow. A small number of these patients exhibit aspiration as a result of the pharyngeal swallow delay. Their recovery of full oral intake may take 3 to 6 weeks poststroke, if no medical complications are present, and longer if medical problems, such as diabetes or pneumonia, are present.

Effects of Stroke in the Cerebral Cortex

Patients with lesions in the left or right hemisphere of the cerebral cortex display differences in swallow function, as described below. To date, swallow disorders characteristic of various areas within each hemisphere have not been examined.

Stroke within the left hemisphere of the cerebral cortex can result in apraxia for swallow, which can range from mild to severe, and usually accompanies some degree of oral apraxia. Apraxia of swallow is characterized by delay in initiating the oral swallow with no tongue motion in response to presentation of a bolus in the mouth or by mild to severe searching motions of the tongue prior to initiating the swallow. Generally, patients with swallow apraxia exhibit better swallow function when eating automatically without any verbal commands to swallow. Left cortical stroke patients also usually exhibit mild oral transit delays (3 to 5 seconds) and mild delays in triggering the pharyngeal swallow (2 to 3 seconds). Usually, the pharyngeal swallow itself is motorically normal in these patients.

In contrast with the left cortical stroke patient, the patient who has suffered a stroke in the right hemisphere exhibits mild oral transit delays (2 to 3 seconds) and slightly longer pharyngeal delays (3 to 5 seconds). When the pharyngeal swallow triggers in these patients, laryngeal elevation may be slightly delayed, contributing to aspiration before or as the pharyngeal swallow is triggering. Despite both verbal and physical prompting, right-hemisphere patients often have difficulty integrating therapy or compensatory strategies into their oral feeding, including postural compensations such as the chin-down head position, because of their cognitive disorders and relative inattention. For this reason, patients suffering a right cortical stroke may be later in returning to oral intake.

Effects of Multiple Strokes

Patients who have suffered multiple strokes often exhibit more significant swallowing abnormalities. Their oral function may be slower with many repetitive tongue movements and oral transit times of over 5 seconds. Delay in triggering the pharyngeal swallow is also usually more severe (+ 5 seconds). When the pharyngeal swallow triggers, these patients may exhibit reduced laryngeal elevation and reduced closure of the laryngeal vestibule/entryway, resulting in penetration of food into the laryngeal entrance, as well as unilateral weakness of the pharyngeal wall, resulting in residual food remaining on the pharyngeal wall and in the pyriform sinus on the affected side. Often their attention is affected, and their ability to use therapy strategies and to focus on the task of eating and swallowing is also impaired.

Recovery of Swallow Poststroke

Little data exist on recovery of swallow after stroke in specific locations in the brain stem or cortex (Barer, 1989; Wade and Hewer, 1987). An ongoing study of recovery in first-time stroke patients (infarct only), underway at Northwestern University and the Rehabilitation Institute of Chicago, indicates that in these noncomplicated stroke patients, recovery is steady, vigorous, and rapid, with all subjects to date (85 patients) returning to full oral intake by 6 weeks postictus, regardless of site of lesion. However, even when these patients return to full oral intake, their temporal measures of swallow physiology, such as duration of airway closure and cricopharyngeal opening, and the temporal relationship between these actions do not return to entirely normal values as compared with age-matched controls. This would indicate that the swallow mechanism is never quite the same poststroke, and may help to explain why swallow dysfunction is more severely affected when or if the patient later suffers a second or third stroke.

Recovery is most rapid in the first 3 weeks poststroke, indicating the need to evaluate the stroke patient's swallow function in the first week and reevaluate it at 3 to 4 weeks poststroke. This is particularly important if a nonoral feeding is inserted in the first few days poststroke. The patient may no longer need this nonoral nutritional support at 3 to 4 weeks postonset.

Because the criteria for entry to this investigation are very narrow, excluding patients with a history of any factors that might affect swallow function, as outlined in the next section, the population of stroke patients studied represents only approximately 10% of the total stroke admissions to the two institutions in any one year. However, the resulting data represent (as much as possible) only the effect of the infarct on the patient's swallow function. The preliminary data from this study indicate that the patient's prior medical history and any complications that arise in the patient's poststroke care are more important contributors to the patient's poststroke swallow function and recovery than previously acknowledged.

Effects of Other Factors on Swallowing Function and Recovery in the Stroke Patient

A number of other factors in the patient's medical history or medical management can affect his or her swallow ability poststroke (Wright, 1985). Tracheostomy during the acute stroke phase may worsen the patient's swallowing problem, particularly if the tracheostomy cuff is kept inflated. Inflating the tracheostomy cuff for long periods of time can create tracheal irritation but also produces a greater friction on the tracheal wall as the larynx tries to elevate, potentially reducing laryngeal elevation more than a tracheostomy tube with the cuff deflated (Buckwalter and Sasaki, 1984; Nash, 1988). Particularly in older patients (over age 80) whose laryngeal elevation is already reduced, tracheostomy may contribute to further reduction in laryngeal elevation and closure during the swallow. Long-term tracheostomy (more than 6 months) can contribute to reduced closure of the airway during the swallow, since the sensory receptors under the vocal folds are not stimulated by airflow. In addition, an open tracheostomy tube does not permit the buildup of subglottic pressure during swallow, which is thought to facilitate airway closure. When the patient who is tracheotomized is swallowing, he or she should be taught to lightly cover the external end of the tracheostomy during the swallow to facilitate more normal vocal fold closure and airway protection.

Some medications given to the stroke patient may worsen any poststroke swallowing disorders. Antidepressant medications in particular may slow swallow coordination and increase the severity of swallow disorders. The interaction of medications may cause xerostomia (dry mouth), which makes swallowing more difficult (Hughes et al., 1987).

Other concurrent medical problems, such as long-standing diabetes, can increase the severity or prolong recovery of swallowing function because of the potential for myopathies and neuropathies that may affect pharyngeal muscle coordination and range of motion. Any prior history of transient ischemic attacks (TIAs), prior strokes, or other neurological damage may increase the stroke patient's chances for significant swallow problems or worsen their severity. It is important that the speech-language pathologist investigate the patient's medical history carefully from chart review and from family/patient interview to identify factors that may pertain to the patient's dysphagia and recovery. In this way, patient/family counseling regarding recovery can be more realistic.

To date, no age effects on swallow function poststroke have been identified. The age of the stroke patient does not appear to affect recovery potential. Minor differences in oropharyngeal swallow function have been identified in older normal subjects (ages 60 to 80) (Tracy et al., 1989). These older subjects exhibited a significantly longer pharyngeal delay time than younger subjects, though the difference was only a fraction of a second. No differences in amount of residue were observed between the older and younger subjects. Studies of oropharyngeal swallow physiology in normal male subjects over age 80 indicate a significant reduction in range of hyoid and laryngeal movement as compared with young men ages 21 to 30 (Logemann, 1993a).

EVALUATION OF SWALLOW POSTSTROKE

Optimally, oropharyngeal swallow poststroke should be evaluated first at the bedside with a clinical assessment and then radiographically (Chen et al., 1990; Dodds et al., 1990a, b; Gresham, 1990; Logemann, 1983a, 1986a, 1993b; Simmons, 1986; Soren et al., 1988).

Bedside/Clinical Examination

The initial bedside examination can be conducted as soon as 24 hours poststroke, as long as the patient is alert and awake.

The bedside clinical examination is designed to define the patient's medical history, oromotor function, and need for further in-depth physiological testing, such as radiographic studies and cognitive and behavioral characteristics, because they may affect safe and efficient swallowing and successful eating. The patient's behavioral characteristics are assessed at the bedside to determine the patient's ability to maintain adequate oral intake, as well as to cooperate with the radiographic study and use various compensatory and therapy strategies. A patient whose attention wanders and cannot focus on the task of eating may have difficulty getting adequate oral intake, despite normal or near-normal swallow physiology.

Oromotor assessment completed during the bedside assessment is designed to look at the status of oral anatomy including symmetry of structures, level and nature of oral secretions, and locations of any pooled secretions, in addition to the range, rate, strength, and coordination of movements of the lips, tongue, jaw, palate, and larynx. The patient is asked to do a variety of voluntary tasks with each of the target structures (e.g., spread and round the lips, protrude and retract the tongue, wipe the lips with the tongue) so that the movement characteristics of each structure can be examined. Assessment of chewing is usually best done using a 4 × 4 inch gauze pad rolled into a cigarette shape with one end dipped into a pleasant-tasting liquid. The excess liquid can be squeezed from the gauze and the damp end of the gauze placed in the patient's mouth, the dry end protruding from the patient's lips. The patient can be asked to move the gauze over to his or her teeth, to chew on the gauze, and to move it to the other side of his or her mouth and chew on it. In this way, the oral coordination for mastication can be examined without risk of the patient's accidentally losing food into the pharynx and aspirating it.

The oromotor assessment also includes evaluation of laryngeal function through definition of vocal quality, phonation time, loudness control, and strength of the volitional cough and throat clearing. A gurgly voice quality has been associated with aspiration in some patients and should be carefully observed (Horner et al., 1988; Linden and Siebens, 1983). Hoarseness may indicate a unilateral vocal fold paralysis or other laryngeal dysfunction leading to aspiration during the swallow, which requires further otolaryngological assessment. The oromotor assessment should also include an oral sensory evaluation that begins with evaluation of the palatal and gag reflexes. The palatal reflex is triggered when a cold stimulus is rubbed on the anterior surface of the soft palate. The reflexive response is elevation and retraction of the soft palate to contact the posterior pharyngeal wall, and this response can be used to assess rate and range of motion of the soft palate. The gag reflex can be used to assess pharyngeal wall contraction. When the gag is triggered by contact of a foreign body (e.g., finger, tongue blade, or laryngeal mirror), with the posterior tongue or posterior pharyngeal wall, the larynx and pharynx elevate and the pharyngeal walls contract strongly to eject the noxious stimulus from the pharynx back into the mouth. Pharyngeal wall contraction should be symmetrical. Asymmetrical contraction indicates a unilateral weakness in the pharyngeal wall. Designed as the protective mechanism for vomit and reflux (both foreign bodies when brought up to the pharynx from the stomach), the gag reflex cannot be used to predict the presence of normalcy of a swallow. No neurophysiological relationship has been established between presence of a gag reflex and presence of a normal oropharyngeal swallow. In fact, many normal individuals have no gag reflex, or they have a variable gag reflex.

Orosensory examination should also include evaluation of the patient's awareness of the light touch of a cotton swab in the mouth. This testing can define areas of poor oral sensation. Food or liquid should normally be placed in areas of best sensation.

At the end of the bedside/clinical examination, the clinician should have a good understanding of the patient's ability to focus on the task and follow directions, as well as the patient's level of alertness, cooperation, and orosensory and oromotor characteristics as applied to eating and swallowing. What is missing from this assessment is information on the patient's pharyngeal swallow physiology. The radiographic study is designed to define pharyngeal anatomy and swallow physiology, thereby determining efficiency of the swallow, the etiology for any aspiration that may occur, and the efficacy of treatment strategies. If the clinician thinks the stroke patient's swallowing disorder is solely oral, with no pharyngeal involvement, then a radiographic study is not necessary. However, if any pharyngeal dysfunction is suspected, a radiographic study should be completed.

Radiographic Evaluation

The radiographic evaluation of the dysphagic stroke patient has two purposes: (a) to define the nature of the anatomy and physiology of the oropharyngeal swallow and (b) to examine the effects of treatment strategies on the safety and efficiency of the swallow and recommend strategies for optimal management of the dysphagia (Logemann, 1993b). The radiographic study is not done to determine *if* the patient aspirates but *why* (i.e., the anatomy or physiology that causes food or liquid to enter the airway below the vocal folds).

Optimally, during the radiographic study, the patient should be seated upright in a normal eating position and viewed radiographically in the lateral plane. The patient's posture should be a comfortable one, enabling a view of the oral cavity and pharynx from the soft palate superiorly to the bottom of the cervical esophagus inferiorly, and from the lips anteriorly to the posterior pharyngeal wall. If the oral cavity and pharynx cannot be viewed simultaneously, the pharynx should be examined first, since the oral cavity and its function can be examined at the bedside. The foods to be given to the dysphagic stroke patient should be standardized in terms of volume and viscosity. Our typical protocol includes two swallows each of 1 mL, 3 mL, 5 mL, and 10 mL of thin liquids, cup drinking of thin liquids, 1 mL of chocolate pudding mixed with barium in a formula of two-thirds pudding to one-third barium (Esophatrast®), and one-fourth of a Lorna Doone cookie coated with the barium pudding for contrast. During the liquid swallows of measured volumes, the patient is told to hold the liquid in the mouth until instructed to swallow. Volumes of 1 mL and 3 mL are presented on a spoon; 5- and 10-mL amounts are placed (not squirted) in the mouth with a syringe. If the patient has reduced lip closure, larger measured volumes (5 and 10 mL) cannot be given because of spillage from the mouth. With cup drinking, the patient is asked to take three to four sequential swallows from the cup. When the cookie is presented, the patient is instructed to chew the cookie and swallow whenever he or she is ready. The patient is given liquids initially because

there is no risk that liquid will block the airway, if aspirated, and it is more easily expectorated.

If the patient aspirates at any time during the radiographic study, or if the patient exhibits a highly inefficient swallow without aspiration, treatment strategies are introduced to improve swallow efficiency or eliminate the aspiration. Such strategies include (a) postural techniques that redirect food flow or change pharyngeal dimension; (b) increased sensory input; (c) swallow maneuvers that apply voluntary control to selected aspects of swallow physiology; or (d) changes in bolus viscosity (i.e., thick liquids, purees, etc.). Generally, postural techniques and swallow maneuvers are both attempted before a particular food consistency (such as thin liquid) is eliminated, since the goal of the radiographic study is to identify conditions under which the patient can retain oral intake on all food consistencies, rather than eliminating a particular food, such as thin liquids, from the diet.

Table 27.1 presents one example of a typical protocol for presentation of treatment strategies in the radiographic study of a stroke patient, with the goal of eliminating aspiration. The example given is of a right cortical stroke patient with a delayed pharyngeal swallow that causes aspiration before the pharyngeal swallow is triggered. In this example, the patient aspirates on swallows of 3 mL of thin liquid during the pharyngeal swallow delay. The first strategy attempted is the chin-down posture, which was chosen because it narrows the entrance to the airway and puts the epiglottis in a more overhanging position to protect the airway. The chin-down posture also widens the vallecular space in some individuals, thus increasing the chance of retaining the bolus in the valleculae during the pharyngeal delay, rather than allowing it to fall into the airway. In this example, the chin-down posture is effective in eliminating aspiration on swallows of 3 mL and 5 mL of thin liquids. But aspiration returns at 10 mL because the volume overwhelms the postural effect. Rather than simply eliminating larger volumes of thin liquids, the patient is taught the breath-hold maneuver (the supraglottic swallow) to close the airway before and during the swallow. In this way, the patient will not aspirate even if liquid drips into the airway entrance during the pharyngeal delay. Because this patient has had a right cortical cerebrovascular accident (CVA), the breath hold is combined with the chin-down posture to reduce confusion. Some patients may need a combination of chin down and breath hold to prevent aspiration during drinking of thin liquids.

Some patients who have had right cortical strokes cannot learn to integrate the supraglottic swallow into their swallow regimen. In that case, the patient would be limited to 5-mL (teaspoon) amounts of liquid orally and would be restricted from cup drinking. By introducing treatment strategies directed at improving specific swallowing disorders into the radiographic study, the clinician can document the effects of these strategies and recommend that the patient continue to receive oral intake while using the various successful treatment techniques. In this way, the patient maintains oral intake rather than eliminating some or all food consistencies from the diet. Generally, selected postural techniques and increased sensory input are introduced first because they do not require significant learning or cognitive ability and are easy to do without creating fatigue. Swallow maneuvers are used only when the patient cannot successfully swallow with postures alone. These tech-

Table 27.1.

Example of a Radiographic Protocol for a Right Cortical Stroke Patient with Delayed Triggering of the Pharyngeal Swallow[a]

Number of Swallows	Amount/ Consistency	Posture, Maneuver	Swallowing Problem
2	1 mL thin liquid	None	Delayed pharyngeal swallow
1	3 mL thin liquid	None	Delayed pharyngeal swallow—aspiration
2	3 mL thin liquid	Chin down	Delayed pharyngeal swallow—no aspiration
2	5 mL thin liquid	Chin down	Delayed pharyngeal swallow—no aspiration
1	10 mL thin liquid	Chin down	Delayed pharyngeal swallow—aspiration
2	10 mL thin liquid	Chin down, supraglottic swallow	Delayed pharyngeal swallow—no aspiration
2	1 mL pudding[b]	Chin down, supraglottic swallow	Delayed pharyngeal swallow—no aspiration
2	¼ cookie[b] (Lorna Doone)	Chin down, supraglottic swallow	Delayed pharyngeal swallow—no aspiration

[a] Two swallows of each volume are given unless the patient aspirated. Two swallows with each therapy strategy are given.
[b] These strategies may not be needed with thicker foods. However, the right CVA patient may become too confused by using strategies during liquid swallows, but not during swallows of other foods, and may need to use these strategies at all times on all swallows in order to remain safe.

Table 27.2.

Postural Techniques Appropriate for Each Swallow Disorder and the Effect of the Posture on Pharyngeal Dimensions or Bolus Flow

Disorder Observed on Fluoroscopy	Posture Applied	Effect of Posture
Inefficient oral transit (Reduced posterior propulsion of bolus by tongue)	Head back	Uses gravity to clear oral cavity
Delay in triggering the pharyngeal swallow (Bolus past ramus of mandible but pharyngeal swallow is not triggered)	Head down	Widens valleculae to prevent bolus entering airway; narrows airway entrance
Reduced tongue base retraction (Residue in valleculae)	Head down	Pushes tongue base backward toward pharyngeal wall
Unilateral laryngeal dysfunction (Aspiration during swallow)	Head down	Places epiglottis in more posterior, protective position
Reduced laryngeal closure (Aspiration during the swallow)	Head rotated to damaged side	Increases vocal-fold closure by applying extrinsic pressure; narrows laryngeal entrance
Reduced pharyngeal contraction (Residue spread throughout pharynx)	Lying down on one side	Eliminates gravitational effect on pharyngeal residue
Unilateral pharyngeal paresis (Residue on one side of pharynx)	Head rotated to damaged side	Eliminates damaged side from bolus path
Cricopharyngeal dysfunction (Residue in pyriform sinuses)	Head rotated	Pulls cricoid cartilage away from posterior pharyngeal wall, reducing resting pressure in cricopharyngeal sphincter

niques are described in more detail in the section on "Treatment Procedures" in this chapter.

Table 27.2 presents the various available postural strategies and their effects on swallow disorders. In general, postural techniques change the direction of food flow and/or change the dimensions of the pharynx.

Additional bolus types may be introduced in the radiographic study to define the patient's ability to swallow varying bolus consistencies (see Table 27.3). If thick liquids will be given to the patient, it is suggested that liquids be evaluated radiographically to be sure that the patient can successfully manage thickened liquids. Any number of foods and liquids can be given during the radiographic study by mixing them with barium. However, the clinician must also be aware that only a limited number of swallows can be examined, and those that will pro-

vide the greatest information about the patient's swallow physiology and treatment efficacy should be presented. Usually, the patient's radiographic exposure time should be limited to approximately 5 minutes. Ordinarily, 25 to 30 swallows can be examined during a 5-minute assessment.

The clinician participating in the videofluoroscopic study of oropharyngeal swallow should receive minimal radiation exposure as long as radiation precautions are used. These include wearing a lead apron, a lead collar to cover the thyroid, a badge to register the amount of radiation exposure, and, if desired, lead goggles. If available, a mobile lead shield can be positioned between the clinician and the patient to provide additional protection. Such shields are used regularly by radiologists when doing radiographic studies involving injections given to the patient.

Table 27.3.
Bolus Consistencies and the Swallow Problems for Which They Are Most Appropriate

Food Consistencies	Disorders for Which These Foods Are Most Appropriate
Thin liquids	Reduced tongue base retraction Reduced pharyngeal wall contraction Reduced laryngeal elevation Reduced cricopharyngeal opening
Thickened liquids Purees and thick foods, including thickened liquids	Oral tongue dysfunction Delayed pharyngeal swallow Reduced laryngeal closure at the entrance Reduced laryngeal closure throughout

Other Assessment Techniques

A number of other instrumental assessment techniques are available to evaluate various aspects of oral or pharyngeal swallow physiology in the stroke patient. Some of these techniques offer the opportunity for biofeedback during therapy. Each procedure answers specific clinical questions regarding the patient's swallowing function. In selecting a particular evaluation strategy, the clinician should determine the clinical questions to be answered with each patient, and thereby identify the appropriate assessment procedure.

Ultrasound is a noninvasive imaging procedure (using high-frequency sound waves) that enables visualization of the oral cavity, particularly the tongue, during swallow (Shawker et al., 1984; Stone and Shawker, 1986). Ultrasound enables the clinician to visualize tongue movements over time and to provide the patient with biofeedback during therapy. Because ultrasound is noninvasive, it can be used over a long period of time and repeatedly. Ultrasound is limited, currently, to visualization of the oral cavity during swallow. Thus, ultrasound cannot answer clinical questions regarding pharyngeal swallow physiology.

Fiberoptic endoscopic examination of swallow (FEES) involves placement of a 3.5-mm fiberoptic bundle transnasally so that the pharynx is viewed from above (Langmore et al., 1988). This superior view of the pharynx enables the clinician to visualize the bolus coming over the back of the tongue and entering the pharynx prior to the triggering of the pharyngeal swallow. Prior to the swallow, as the bolus comes into view over the base of the tongue, the clinician can determine the presence of a pharyngeal delay and the duration of that delay. Oral function cannot be seen. During the pharyngeal swallow, the image disappears, so that the actual pharyngeal swallow cannot be assessed. After the swallow, as the pharynx and larynx lower and relax, the larynx and pharynx return to view, and the clinician can identify residual food remaining in the valleculae or pyriform sinuses, as well as any aspiration of this residue after the swallow. Aspiration of saliva before or after the swallow can also be visualized. The fiberoptic bundle can be lowered to contact the laryngeal vestibule so that laryngeal sensation can be tested directly.

FEES can also be used to provide biofeedback to the patient learning airway closure techniques, as the vocal folds can be visualized from above during breath-hold maneuvers, prior to the swallow. The patient will be able to visualize vocal-fold position. FEES has the disadvantage of requiring nasal placement of a tube, which is not possible in all stroke patients because of behavioral factors or nasal obstruction.

Pharyngeal manometry also involves placement of a tube transnasally. In the case of manometry, this tube contains several pressure sensors (usually 1 cm long) at spaced intervals (Dodds et al., 1987; McConnel et al., 1988). When the tube is in place, the sensors will register pressure changes as the bolus passes each of them, or as any pharyngeal structure contacts them. Unfortunately, without simultaneous videofluoroscopy, manometry in the pharynx is difficult, if not impossible, to interpret, since without x-ray, the position of the manometric sensors cannot be identified in relation to pharyngeal structures. In addition, manometry alone does not define movement patterns of the pharynx to enable identification of pharyngeal movement abnormalities, nor does it define the presence or timing of aspiration. Manometry does provide information about the pressure generated within the pharynx and transmitted to the bolus itself during the pharyngeal swallow.

Surface electromyography can be used to identify the presence of a swallow but cannot be used to identify specific swallowing abnormalities in the oral or pharyngeal stage of deglutition.

TREATMENT PROCEDURES

The treatment plan for the dysphagic stroke patient should be developed after the patient's swallow physiology has been carefully studied and abnormalities identified. The key to effective swallowing rehabilitation is directing therapy management at the abnormal components of the oropharyngeal swallow (Logemann, 1983a, 1986b, 1993).

Swallowing therapy can be direct or indirect. Direct therapy uses the presentation of food during attempts to swallow; various treatment strategies are used. Indirect therapy involves muscle exercises to improve the range of motion, coordination, and strength of movements involved in swallowing, or uses swallow practice on specific techniques without giving food (i.e., using saliva). In general, indirect therapy is used when it is unsafe for the patient to swallow any food consistency.

Swallowing therapy can also be divided into compensatory management versus therapy strategies. In general compensatory management is under the control of the clinician and requires minimal cognition or direction following on the part of the patient. In contrast, therapy strategies are designed to change swallow physiology and involve sensory stimulation, exercise programs, and swallow maneuvers.

Compensatory Management

Compensatory management uses techniques that affect the symptoms of the swallow disorders without, necessarily, changing the actual swallow physiology. Compensatory strategies include changes in posture, changes in bolus volume or viscosity, and changes in feeding procedures.

Five postural changes have been described that affect the bolus flow through the oral cavity and pharynx or pharyngeal dimensions (Logemann, 1983a; Logemann et al., 1989; Shanahan, 1991; Welch et al., 1993). Each of these postures is successful in improving swallow efficiency or safety in particular swallow disorders. These postures and their effects on pharyngeal dimensions or bolus flow are presented in Table 27.2. Postural techniques can be highly effective strategies in eliminating aspiration or improving the efficiency of the swallow (Rasley et al., 1993). Horner et al. (1988) report elimination of aspiration 80% of the time with the use of postural techniques in stroke patients.

Changing bolus volume can improve swallow physiology in some stroke patients. Many stroke patients exhibit significant difficulty swallowing small bolus volumes, such as saliva (1 to 3 mL), or swallowing large bolus volumes (10 to 20 mL), as in cup drinking. Providing a variety of bolus volumes during the radiographic study will enable the clinician to identify the bolus volume most effective for each patient.

Changes in bolus viscosity will also change the speed of bolus flow (normal transit times are slower on thicker foods), and thus some viscosities are more easily swallowed in the presence of particular swallow abnormalities. For example, the patient with a delay in triggering the pharyngeal swallow typically exhibits greater difficulty, as evidenced by coughing, on thin liquids than on thick liquids and purees. This difference occurs because thin liquids move more rapidly and splash into the pharynx and potentially into the open airway during the pharyngeal delay, whereas thicker foods slide more slowly and often remain in the valleculae during the pharyngeal delay, not entering the airway. Patients with other swallow disorders may find purees more difficult. For example, the patient with a cricopharyngeal dysfunction has greater difficulty with thick foods, such as purees, and is more easily able to handle thin liquids. In this case, thin liquids drain through even a small cricopharyngeal opening, while thicker foods will tend to get caught in the opening, clogging and preventing flow. Table 27.3 presents a list of food consistencies and the swallow disorders for which they are most appropriate.

The manner in which stroke patients are fed can increase efficiency or safety of oral intake, or decrease intake and increase the danger of aspiration, particularly in the multistroke patient, or the stroke patient with dementia. In general, if the patient is distractible, he or she should be positioned in a quiet room with no auditory or visual distractions during meals. The feeder should position himself or herself on the patient's most functional side and position food within the patient's visual field. Giving the patient several seconds to become acclimated to the food smells can increase appetite and the desire to eat and swallow. When positioning food in the patient's mouth, the feeder should be sure to place food in the area of greatest oral sensation and monitor the volume per swallow to assure that the patient is not given larger amounts than he or she can handle. The feeder should observe the patient's neck for laryngeal elevation to assure that the patient has completed a swallow before presenting a new bolus. In some cases, several dry swallows should be encouraged to clear the pharynx. Feeding staff should be trained to stop feeding the patient if the

patient exhibits any abnormal behaviors or difficulty swallowing, including coughing or breathing difficulties, and to immediately contact the swallowing therapist. The swallowing therapist's role is to train and supervise the feeding staff.

Therapy Strategies

Therapy strategies fall into one of three categories: sensory stimulation, exercise programs, and swallow maneuvers (Heimlich, 1983; Kahrilas et al., 1992; Kahrilas et al., 1991; Lazzara et al., 1986; Logemann and Kahrilas, 1990; Selley, 1985).

Sensory stimulation is generally appropriate for the patient with swallow apraxia or with generally reduced oral sensation. Increasing sensory stimulation may be accomplished by presentation of a cold or warm bolus, by increasing the downward pressure of the spoon on the patient's tongue as the food is being presented, or by presenting foods with strong flavors or textures. These techniques usually improve the oral onset of the swallow and may improve the speed of triggering of the pharyngeal swallow. For some patients, presentation of a bolus requiring chewing will also facilitate faster oral onset and increased oral motion. For other patients, self-feeding is the key to initiation of the oral activity for swallowing.

Two techniques for increasing oral sensation have been used specifically to improve the speed of triggering of the pharyngeal swallow: **thermal/tactile stimulation** and the **suck-swallow.** Both techniques provide increased oral sensation prior to the patient's attempt to initiate the swallow. In the case of thermal/tactile stimulation, a size 00 laryngeal mirror is placed in ice and then rubbed five times up and down against the anterior facial arch on one side, with good contact of the entire back surface of the laryngeal mirror to the oral tissue. This stimulation is repeated on the other side, and then the patient is presented with a small amount of liquid and asked to swallow. Or the patient is encouraged to swallow without the presentation of liquid. In either case, the purpose of the stimulation is to provide an alerting stimulus to the nervous system so that when the patient attempts to initiate a swallow, the triggering of the pharyngeal swallow will be faster. There is some carryover of this stimulation from one swallow to the next over a sequence of three to four swallows. The clinician can time the effect of the stimulation by placing the index finger lightly under the chin and the two middle fingers lightly on the front of the neck and defining the time elapsed between the onset of the oral swallow (as indicated by contraction of submandibular muscles) and laryngeal and hyoid elevation (indicating the onset of the pharyngeal swallow). The time between these two events should be no more than 1 second. In therapy, thermal/tactile stimulation is generally done every third or fourth swallow for a sequence of 20 to 40 swallows. Usually, the pharyngeal delay diminishes so that at the end of the session, the delay is shorter than it was at the beginning. Patients can learn to do this stimulation themselves, or family members can be taught to provide it.

The suck-swallow technique involves producing an exaggerated suck with lips closed and exaggerated vertical back-tongue motion prior to a swallow attempt. The sucking action pulls saliva to the back of the mouth and seems to improve triggering of the pharyngeal swallow, again by providing increased oral sensation before a swallow attempt. The exaggerated suck-swallow can be done using a popsicle or by keeping the patient's lips closed and asking him or her to produce significant suction of saliva back into the mouth.

For some stroke patients, **chewing** provides the additional oral sensation required to reduce the pharyngeal delay. These patients exhibit less pharyngeal delay on boluses requiring chewing. When asked to chew liquids, these patients also present less delay than when swallowing liquids without the chewing behavior.

Exercise programs may be provided to improve the range of lip, tongue, and jaw motion after stroke; to improve the coordination of lip and tongue motion; to improve vocal-fold adduction; and to improve laryngeal elevation and tongue base retraction. Range-of-motion exercises for the lips, tongue, and/or jaw can be presented for unilateral or bilateral weakness. All range-of-motion exercises involve moving the target structure as far as possible in the desired direction, holding the structure extended in that direction for several seconds, and then relaxing. Resistance exercises, using a tongue blade between the lips or against the tongue, can also be used to improve range of motion. Adduction exercises can be used to improve movement of the normal vocal fold in the presence of a unilateral vocal-fold paresis, and the falsetto exercise (sliding up scale to the highest squeaky voice producible) can be used to improve laryngeal elevation. Tongue base retraction can be improved by asking the patient to do range-of-motion exercises that involve pulling the tongue straight back in the mouth as far as possible. The effortful swallow (described below) can also serve as a range-of-motion exercise for the tongue base. Chewing exercises can be done with gauze by rolling a 4-inch gauze pad into a cigarette shape and dipping one end into liquid to provide a pleasurable flavor. With the damp end of the gauze roll in the patient's mouth, the patient can lateralize the gauze to the teeth, bite on it, rotate it back onto the teeth with the tongue, move the gauze to the opposite side of the mouth, and repeat the action. In this way, the patient can work on coordination of tongue and jaw motion for mastication without risk of losing food into the pharynx prematurely and aspirating.

Swallow maneuvers, another category of swallow therapy, involve the application of voluntary control to specific components of the pharyngeal swallow. The **supraglottic swallow** involves voluntary closure of the vocal folds before and during the swallow. The patient is directed to inhale, hold the breath, swallow while holding the breath, and cough when the swallow is finished (before inhaling again). Some patients find it easier to inhale, exhale slightly, hold the breath, swallow while breath holding, and then cough. The breath hold closes the vocal folds before and during the swallow. The **super supraglottic swallow** creates closure of the entrance to the airway (between the arytenoids and the base of the epiglottis) before and during the swallow. This maneuver uses the same sequence of directions as the supraglottic swallow, except the patient is also asked to bear down hard when holding the breath. The effort of bearing down tilts the arytenoids forward to contact the base of the epiglottis, closing the entrance to the airway. The **Mendelsohn Maneuver** uses information on the role of hyolaryngeal anterior-superior motion in the normal opening of the upper esophageal sphincter to gain volitional control over the duration of cricopharyngeal opening by teaching the patient to prolong maximal elevation of the larynx during the swallow. The patient is asked to feel his or her Adam's apple or voice box move up and down during swallow. When patients are aware of this, they are asked to swallow normally again and as they feel their larynx reach the top of their neck during the swallow, to grab the larynx with their neck muscles (not their hand), and to keep the larynx elevated for several seconds. The effort of maintaining laryngeal elevation results in greater laryngeal movement and wider and longer upper esophageal sphincter opening. The **effortful swallow** is designed to increase posterior tongue base motion and tongue pressure during the pharyngeal swallow and to improve clearance of the bolus from the valleculae. To elicit the Effortful Swallow, the patient is instructed to squeeze hard with all of the "mouth and throat muscles" during the swallow. All of these swallow maneuvers require cognitive ability and direction following. For the most part, patients requiring these maneuvers are most often those who have had brain stem strokes and who have the cognitive ability to learn and implement the maneuvers. Swallow maneuvers in general require more effort and will fatigue the patient faster than techniques such as changes in head or body posture.

Factors Affecting Treatment Selection

A number of patient characteristics affect the selection of treatment techniques to be used in management of a dysphagic stroke patient (Logemann, 1990). Many stroke patients fatigue quickly, especially in the first few weeks poststroke, and are unable to sustain the muscle effort required for use of a swallow maneuver, such as a supraglottic swallow, during a meal. Sometimes this problem can be managed by more frequent, smaller meals. Another option is to use these procedures in therapy but not implement them on a regular basis during eating.

If a patient's swallowing problem can be compensated for with postures or diet changes, no direct therapy may be needed. However, some stroke patients have linguistic or cognitive problems that make their use of even head postures difficult on a consistent basis. Occasionally, stroke patients exhibit behavioral problems that make their use of *any* treatment paradigms difficult, even postures. The clinician should look at all of these characteristics of the patient in defining the patient's dysphagia management plan.

MULTIDISCIPLINARY TEAM

Management of dysphagia in the stroke patient requires multidisciplinary input from assessment through treatment.

Assessment

A variety of assessment techniques may be used in the stroke patient, as discussed earlier. These techniques require the joint involvement of the speech-language pathologist, the otolaryngologist (endoscopy), the gastroenterologist (manometry), or the radiologist (videofluoroscopy).

Dietary/Nutritional Management

In the management of the patient's nutritional needs, the dietitian is essential. When recommendations are needed regarding nonoral feeding during the initial recovery stages in dysphagia after stroke, the dietitian and the patient's attending physician will discuss the various alternatives for nutritional intake, taking into account the patient's medical status, gastrointestinal function, finances, and behavior. Throughout the patient's recovery, the various members of the dysphagia rehabilitation team will interact in decision making regarding swallowing treatment and return to oral intake.

Nonoral feeding plays an important role in dysphagia rehabilitation. It provides patients with adequate calories and hydration to support their recovery and rehabilitation. Nutrition should never be compromised in the process of management of a swallowing disorder. Rather, nutritional support should be provided to facilitate the patient's recovery and rehabilitation back to full oral intake. When presenting the need for nonoral feeding or supplements to the patient and family, it is important to stress the value of both nutrition and hydration, as well as the temporary nature of these methods. Any nonoral feeding can be discontinued as soon as the patient is ready to resume oral intake.

Physical and Occupational Therapy

Physical and occupational therapy input is important in providing seating devices and positioning appropriate for the patient's swallowing disorders and assistive devices to facilitate hand-to-mouth coordination in those patients able to provide self-feeding.

Medical and Surgical Management

Medical and surgical intervention for dysphagia is generally not needed in the stroke patient unless the swallowing problems fail to recover with therapy (Blitzer et al., 1988; Butcher, 1982). If a patient is chronically aspirating his or her own secretions, despite significant and aggressive therapy over a prolonged period, surgical management may be needed. There are techniques available for airway diversion, vocal-fold suturing, or epiglottic pull-down, which can, in some cases, eliminate chronic aspiration by preventing material from entering the airway. The ultimate solution for chronic aspiration leading to repeated pneumonia is total laryngectomy. These procedures are used only infrequently in cases of stroke-induced dysphagia after prolonged therapy has been found to be unsuccessful and the patient's general health is severely compromised by the chronic aspiration.

PATIENT/FAMILY COUNSELING AND FOLLOW-UP

Teaching the patient and family about normal swallow physiology and the nature of the stroke patient's dysphagia is critical to their support of and participation in a therapy program. Involvement of the family in management of the patient can be helpful in many cases. At the very least, enlisting the family's support for the patient as he or she progresses through therapy is often critical to continued high motivation. Families can participate in therapy by providing encouragement for repeating exercises or by actually participating in direct therapy such as providing thermal/tactile stimulation. If the dysphagic patient has a slower recovery, reevaluation by radiography or other instrumental techniques is usually needed to document recovery and move the patient to a more normal diet. Usually, this follow-up occurs approximately 3 to 4 weeks after the initial assessment but may be as much as 2 to 3 months later. If a patient's progress is extremely slow or the patient's function plateaus, exhibiting no improvement for at least 1 month, the clinician may decide to dismiss the patient from direct therapy and to reassess his or her function in 3 to 6 months. Because there are significant gaps in our knowledge base regarding recovery rates for specific neural damage, it is impossible to say that a patient will never recover swallow ability. Rather, the clinician should schedule the patient for a reevaluation after a period of time without therapy to determine any improvement in status. Many stroke patients will recover swallow function 3 to 12 months after their stroke.

FUTURE TRENDS IN DYSPHAGIA MANAGEMENT POSTSTROKE

In the next 10 years, I believe we can look forward to expansion of our knowledge base regarding the effects of specific stroke loci in the central nervous system on swallow physiology and the impact of therapy procedures on these swallow disorders. It is likely that additional diagnostic procedures will be applied to the study of dysphagia poststroke and that we will develop a much larger database on the effects of age on normal oropharyngeal swallow physiology in contrast to the effects of stroke and other types of neural damage. Part of this database will include normal measures against which stroke patients' oropharyngeal range of motion and coordination can be compared.

With an increased number of stroke patients placed on neurological treatment protocols to reduce the neural damage in the immediate poststroke period and eliminate the long-term effects of stroke, it is possible that the severity of dysphagia will decrease in stroke patients and that the rate of swallow recovery will increase in the acute care period. All of these projections will depend on an increased number of investigators focusing on normal swallow and swallow physiology after stroke.

Acknowledgment

This research was funded by NIH grants ROI NS 28525 and NIH ROI DC 00550.

References

Ardran, G. M., and Kemp, F. (1951). The mechanism of swallowing. *Proceedings of the Royal Society of Medicine, 44,* 1038–1040.

Barer, D. H. (1989). The natural history and functional consequences of dysphagia after hemispheric stroke. *Journal of Neurology, Neurosurgery and Psychiatry, 52,* 236–241.

Bisch, E. M., Logemann, J. A., Rademaker, A. W., Lazarus, C., and Kahrilas, P. J. (1991, November). *Pharyngeal effects of bolus temperature.* Paper presented at American Speech-Language-Hearing Association (ASHA) Annual Convention.

Blitzer, A., Krespi, Y., Oppenheimer, R., and Levine, T. (1988). Surgical management of aspiration. *Otolaryngologic Clinics of North America, 21,* 743–750.

Blonsky, E., Logemann, J., Boshes, B., and Fisher, H. (1975). Comparison of speech and swallowing function in patients with tremor disorders and in normal geriatric patients: A cinefluorographic study. *Journal of Gerontology, 30,* 299–303.

Bosma, J. (1957). Deglutition: Pharyngeal stage. *Physiological Reviews, 37,* 275–300.

Buckwalter, J. A., and Sasaki, C. T. (1984). Effect of tracheostomy on laryngeal function. *Otolaryngologic Clinics of North America, 17,* 41–48.

Butcher, R. (1982). Treatment of chronic aspiration as a complication of cerebrovascular accident. *Laryngoscope, 92,* 681–685.

Celifarco, A., Gerard, G., Faegenburg, D., and Burakoff, R. (1990). Dysphagia as the sole manifestation of bilateral strokes. *American Journal of Gastroenterology, 85*(5), 610–613.

Chen, M., Ott, D., Peele, V., and Gelfand, D. (1990). Oropharynx in patients with cerebrovascular disease: Evaluation and videofluoroscopy. *Radiology, 176*(3), 641–643.

Cook, I. J., Dodds, W. J., Dantas, R. O., Kern, M. K., Massey, B. T., Shaker, R., and Hogan, W. J. (1989). Timing of videofluoroscopic, manometric events and bolus transit during the oral and pharyngeal phases of swallowing. *Dysphagia, 4,* 8–15.

Delgado, J. J. (1988). Paralysis, dysphagia and balance problems associated with stroke. *Journal of Neuroscience Nursing, 20*(4), 260.

Dodds, W. J., Kahrilas, P. J., Dent, J., and Hogan, W. J. (1987). Considerations about pharyngeal manometry. *Dysphagia, 1,* 209–214.

Dodds, W. J., Logemann, J. A., and Stewart, E. T. (1990a). Radiological assessment of abnormal oral and pharyngeal phases of swallowing. *American Journal of Roentgenology, 154,* 965–974.

Dodds, W. J., Stewart, E. T., and Logemann, J. A. (1990b). Physiology and radiology of the normal oral and pharyngeal phases of swallowing. *American Journal of Roentgenology, 154,* 953–965.

Dodds, W. J., Taylor, A. J., Stewart, E. T., Kern, M. K., Logemann, J. A., and Cook, I. J. (1989). Tipper and dipper types of oral swallows. *American Journal of Roentgenology, 153,* 1197–1199.

Donner, M. (1974). Swallowing mechanism and neuromuscular disorders. *Seminars in Roentgenology, 9,* 273–282.

Gordon, C., Hewer, R. L., and Wade, D. T. (1987). Dysphagia in acute stroke. *British Medical Journal,* 15 August, 411–414.

Gresham, S. L. (1990). Clinical assessment and management of swallowing difficulties after stroke. *Medical Journal of Australia, 153,* 397–399.

Heimlich, H. (1983). Rehabilitation of swallowing after stroke. *Annals of Otology, Rhinology and Laryngology, 92,* 357–359.

Horner, J., Massey, E., Riski, J., Lathrop, D., and Chase, K. (1988). Aspiration following stroke: Clinical correlates and outcomes. *Neurology, 38,* 1359–1362.

Hughes, C. V., Baum, B. J., Fox, P. C., Marmary, Y., Yeh, C. K., and Sonies, B. C. (1987). Oral-pharyngeal dysphagia: A common sequelae of salivary gland dysfunction. *Dysphagia, 1,* 173–177.

Jacob, P., Kahrilas, P., Logemann, J., Shah, V., and Ha, T. (1989). Upper esophageal sphincter opening and modulation during swallowing. *Gastroenterology, 97,* 1469–1478.

Jean, A., and Car, A. (1979). Inputs to the swallowing medullary neurons from the peripheral afferent fibers and the swallowing cortical area. *Brain Research, 178,* 567–572.

Kahrilas, P. J., Lin, S., Logemann, J. A., Ergun, G. A., and Facchini, F. (1993). Deglutitive tongue action: Volume accommodation and bolus propulsion. *Gastroenterology, 104,* 152–162.

Kahrilas, P. J., Logemann, J. A., and Gibbons, P. (1992). Food intake by maneuver: An extreme compensation for impaired swallowing. *Dysphagia, 7,* 155–159.

Kahrilas, P. J., Logemann, J. A., Krugler, C., and Flanagan, E. (1991). Volitional augmentation of upper esophageal sphincter opening during swallowing. *American Journal of Physiology, 260 (Gastrointestinal and Liver Physiology, 23),* G450–456.

Kahrilas, P. J., Logemann, J. A., Lin, S., Ergun, G. A. (1992). Pharyngeal clearance during swallowing: A combined manometric and videofluoroscopic study. *Gastroenterology, 103,* 128–136.

Langmore, S. E., Schatz, K., and Olsen, N. (1988). Fiberoptic endoscopic examination of swallowing safety: A new procedure. *Dysphagia, 2,* 216–219.

Lazarus, C., Logemann, J. A., Kahrilas, P. J., Rademaker, A., and Pajak, T. (1991, November). *Effects of bolus volume, viscosity and repeated swallows in normals and stroke patients.* Paper presented at ASHA Annual Convention.

Lazzara, G., Lazarus, C., and Logemann, J. A. (1986). Impact of thermal stimulation on the triggering of the swallowing reflex. *Dysphagia, 1,* 73–77.

Linden, P., and Siebens, A. (1983). Dysphagia: Predicting laryngeal penetration. *Physical Medicine and Rehabilitation, 64,* 281–284.

Logemann, J. (1983a). *Evaluation and treatment of swallowing disorders.* San Diego, CA: College Hill Press.

Logemann, J. A. (1983b). Treatment of swallowing disorders. In W. H. Perkins (Ed.), *Phonologic and articulatory disorders.* New York: Thieme-Stratton.

Logemann, J. A. (1986a). *Manual for videofluoroscopic evaluation of swallowing.* San Diego, CA: College Hill Press.

Logemann, J. A. (1986b). Treatment of aspiration related to dysphagia: An overview. *Dysphagia, 1,* 34–38.

Logemann, J. A. (1990). Factors affecting ability to resume oral nutrition in the oropharyngeal dysphagic individual. *Dysphagia, 4,* 202–208.

Logemann, J. A. (1993a). *Effects of aging on the swallowing mechanism.* Paper presented at the International Geriatrics Society, Budapest.

Logemann, J. A. (1993b). Manual for videofluoroscopic evaluation of swallowing. Austin, Tx: Pro-Ed.

Logemann, J. A., and Kahrilas, P. J. (1990). Relearning to swallow post CVA: Application of maneuvers and indirect biofeedback: A case study. *Neurology, 40,* 1136–1138.

Logemann, J. A., Kahrilas, P. J., Cheng, J., Pauloski, B. R., Gibbons, P. J., Rademaker, F. W., and Lin, S. (1992). Closure mechanisms of the laryngeal vestibule during swallowing. *American Journal of Physiology, 262 (Gastrointestinal and Liver Physiology, 25),* G338–344.

Logemann, J., Kahrilas, P., Kobara, M., and Vakil, N. (1989). The benefit of head rotation on pharyngoesophageal dysphagia. *Archives of Physical Medicine and Rehabilitation, 70,* 767–771.

McConnel, F. M. S., Cerenko, D., and Mendelsohn, M. (1988). Manofluorographic analyses of swallowing. *Otolaryngologic Clinics of North America, 21*(4), 625–635.

Meadows, J. (1973). Dysphagia in unilateral cerebral lesions. *Journal of Neurology, Neurosurgery and Psychiatry, 36,* 853–860.

Miller, A. J. (1982). Deglutition. *Physiologic Review, 62,* 129–184.

Nash, M. (1988). Swallowing problems in the tracheotomized patient. *Otolaryngologic Clinics of North America, 21,* 701–709.

Pommerenke, W. (1928). A study of the sensory areas eliciting the swallowing reflex. *American Journal of Physiology, 84,* 36–41.

Rasley, A., Logemann, J. A., Kahrilas, P. J., Rademaker, A. N., Pauloski, B., and Dodds, N. J. (1993). Prevention of barium aspiration during videofluoroscopic swallowing studies: Value of change in posture. *American Journal of Roentgenology, 160,* 1005–1009.

Robbins. J., and Levine, R. (1988). Swallowing after unilateral stroke of the cerebral cortex: Preliminary experience. *Dysphagia, 3,* 11–17.

Selley, W. G. (1985, November). Swallowing difficulties in stroke patients: A new treatment. *Age and Ageing,* pp. 361–365.

Shanahan, T. (1991, November). *Effects of chin down posture on aspiration in dysphagic patients.* Paper presented at ASHA Annual Convention.

Shawker, T. H., Sonies, P. C., and Stone, M. (1984). Sonography of speech and swallowing. In R. Sanders and M. Hill (Eds.), *Ultrasound annual* (pp. 237–260). New York: Raven.

Silbiger, M., Pikielney, R., and Donner, M. (1967). Neuromuscular disorders affecting the pharynx: Cineradiographic analysis. *Investigative Radiology, 2,* 442–448.

Simmons, K. (1986). Dysphagia management means diagnosis, exercise, reeducation. *Journal of the American Medical Association, 255,* 3209–3212.

Smith, D. S., and Dodd, B. A. (1990). Swallowing disorders in stroke. *Medical Journal of Australia, 153,* 372–373.

Soren, R., Somers, S., Austin, W., and Bester, S. (1988). The influence of videofluoroscopy on the management of the dysphagic patient. *Dysphagia, 2,* 127–135.

Stone, M., and Shawker, T. H. (1986). An ultrasound examination of tongue movement during swallowing. *Dysphagia, 1,* 78–83.

Tracy, J., Logemann, J., Kahrilas, P., Jacob, P., Kobara, M., and Krugler, C. (1989). Preliminary observations on the effects of age on oropharyngeal deglutition. *Dysphagia, 4,* 90–94.

Veis, S., and Logemann, J. (1985). The nature of swallowing disorders in CVA patients. *Archives of Physical Medicine and Rehabilitation, 66,* 372–375.

Wade, D., and Hewer, R. (1987). Motor loss and swallowing difficulty after stroke: Frequency, recovery, and prognosis. *Acta Neurology Scandinavia, 76,* 50–54.

Welch, M. V., Logemann, J. A., Rademaker, A. W., and Kahrilas, P. J. (1993). Changes in pharyngeal dimensions effected by chin tuck. *Archives of Physical Medicine and Rehabilitation, 74,* 178–181.

Wright. A. (1985). An unusual but easily treatable cause of dysphagia and dysarthria complicating stroke. *British Medical Journal, 291,* 1412–1413.

CHAPTER 28
Communication Disorders Associated with Right-Hemisphere Brain Damage

PENELOPE S. MYERS

Patients with damage confined to the right hemisphere may have a variety of cognitive and perceptual problems including deficits in attention, visual perception, and communication. Not all patients with right-hemisphere damage (RHD) have communication impairments, but it is generally accepted that those who do are not aphasic. Their command over basic linguistic structures is usually adequate, and they may do well in superficial or straightforward conversation. Their communication problems typically become apparent in more complex communicative events in which verbal and nonverbal contextual cues must be used to assess and convey communicative intent. Before discussing their problems in detail, it might be useful to draw a very general portrait of a typical RHD patient, Mr. Smith.

An initial and fairly casual encounter with Mr. Smith may leave the visitor with an overly optimistic picture of his cognitive and communicative capacity. Questions about the weather, treatment by the hospital staff, the quality of the food, and so on will elicit responses that seem not only linguistically accurate but appropriate as well. He may seem a bit less responsive and may speak in a monotone, but these characteristics might easily be attributed to fatigue and to the general effects of his recent trauma. The visitor may even be cheered by Mr. Smith's occasional jocularity and blithe assurances about resuming all aspects of his former life.

During subsequent visits, however, the very factors that led to a firm belief in his full recovery seem suspect. He may deny a need for rehabilitative services, refusing to take his physical limitations seriously. His assessment of his capabilities may be at odds with his progress in simple self-care. He may be unable to groom himself properly or to figure out how to put on his shirt. He may talk about returning to work next week yet be unable to transfer himself from bed to wheelchair. Once in his wheelchair, he may demonstrate difficulty finding his way to the nearby nurses' station or back to his room.

He may have trouble recognizing friends and may deny that they have visited him before. In extended conversation, he may seem excessively bound up in himself. He may not respect conversational rules. He may interrupt, fail to assess, and appear not to care about his listener's reaction. He may not maintain eye contact, and he may seem wholly unresponsive to the

emotional tone of verbal and nonverbal messages. His tendency to personalize abstract topics, his seeming difficulty in grasping the point of a conversation, and his tendency to digress furthers the impression either that he is confused or that he operates in isolation during conversation.

His jocularity will now strike a discordant note, and he may trivialize topics by focusing on tangential and unnecessary detail. Although quick to provide a response, he may take an excessive amount of time to actually answer substantive questions. He may seem verbose and disorganized. The patient's responses, then, may seem inefficient and lacking an organizational base. His ready answers may seem impulsive, produced without internal reflection.

In short, despite an apparently adequate linguistic system, many RHD patients neither respond to nor participate in communicative events as they once did. The near-universal refrain of friends and families associated with communicatively impaired RHD adults is, ''He does talk, but it isn't the same.''

As this portrait suggests, some RHD patients not only have communication impairments but may also suffer from a variety of other cognitive and perceptual impairments. Regardless of whether these deficits affect communication directly or indirectly, the clinician must recognize their potential impact on the patient.

NONLINGUISTIC DEFICITS

Nonlinguistic deficits associated with RHD include left-sided neglect, attentional deficits, and visuoperceptual problems. These disorders can co-occur and can affect communication. They are discussed in the following sections.

Neglect and Attention

Unilateral or hemispatial neglect is a complex disorder in which patients fail to report, respond, or orient to stimuli on the side opposite their brain lesion (the contralesional side), despite the motor and sensory capacity to do so (Heilman et al., 1983). Although it may occur with left-hemisphere damage (LHD), neglect is usually longer lasting, more severe, and more common in individuals with RHD lesions (Mesulam, 1985; Ogden, 1985). Once thought to occur subsequent to parietal lesions, neglect has been found to occur with frontal, temporal, parietal, and subcortical lesions (Horner et al., 1989; Mesulam, 1981, 1985; Vallar and Perani, 1986). Neglect may occur in the visual, tactile, auditory, or olfactory senses, or in combinations thereof, but it is most common in the visual modality.

RHD patients with neglect fail to attend to left-sided input— that is, to input in contralesional space. They may not notice the phone ringing on the left side of the room, nor eat food on the left side of their trays, nor notice people on the left side of their beds. More severe manifestations of neglect may include failure to recognize their paralyzed or weakened limbs as their own (''I'd be all right if I had my own arm'').

Patients with neglect have problems attending to stimuli not only in contralesional space but also in ipsilesional space (i.e., the same side as their brain lesion). In addition, they may fail to attend and respond to the left side of stimuli presented in the middle of their visual space (Gainotti et al., 1986).

Neglect has a motor as well as a sensory component. For example, RHD patients with neglect may not include left-sided detail in their drawings. They may not be able to dress or groom themselves properly because they fail to reach over to the contralesional side of their bodies.

Most theories of neglect hold that it is a deficit in attention (see Bisiach et al., 1981, and Bisiach et al., 1979, for an alternative hypothesis). The types of attention implicated in neglect include (*a*) *arousal* (Coslett et al., 1987; Heilman et al., 1978; Heilman et al., 1984b); (*b*) *sustained attention* (Bub et al., 1990); (*c*) the capacity to *disengage attention* from ipsilesional space (Heilman et al., 1985; Posner et al., 1984); and (*d*) *selective and directed attention* (Mesulam, 1981; Rapcsak et al., 1989). RHD patients without demonstrable neglect may also experience attention deficits. Each type of attention disorder is discussed briefly below.

Attention Deficits

Arousal.   RHD patients with neglect have been called hypoaroused, and studies comparing them with LHD patients suggest they are generally less attentive to external stimuli and less aroused or alert (Coslett et al., 1987; Heilman et al., 1978; Howes and Boller, 1975). Studies of the physiological correlates of arousal such as galvanic skin response (GSR) indicate that RHD subjects have significantly lower GSRs to pain and to emotional material than do nonlesioned controls and aphasic subjects (Heilman et al., 1978; Morrow et al., 1981). RHD subjects have slower reaction times (RTs) in response to simple visual and auditory stimuli, such as a point of light or a simple tone, compared with LHD and non-brain-damaged (NBD) subjects (Benson and Barton, 1970; Dee and Van Allen, 1973; Howes and Boller, 1975), suggesting a reduction in arousal or general attention. In functional terms, RHD patients may need more intense stimulation or more time to get ready to attend than other populations of brain-damaged patients with focal lesions.

Sustained Attention.   Reaction time (RT) tasks have been conceptualized as measures of general attention and/or of vigilance. Subjects must be ready to respond to stimuli that occur at unpredictable or random intervals. To measure attention adequately, RT tasks elicit many responses that require sustained attention over long periods of time. A recent study by Bub et al. (1990) found that both LHD and RHD subjects had slower

RTs to an auditory stimulus than NBD controls, suggesting some problems in vigilance. In addition, they found that the RHD subjects' performance became slower and more variable as the task progressed, while the performance of LHD subjects improved. The authors concluded that vigilance is not selectively impaired by RHD but that sustained attention may be. This result supports the clinical impression that some RHD patients have difficulty sustaining attention during therapy, a factor that may affect their progress.

Disengagement.   Deficits in the capacity to disengage attention from ipsilesional space is another way of saying that RHD patients with neglect have difficulty attending to left-sided stimuli when their attention is captured by right-sided stimuli. For example, Mark et al. (1988) tested RHD subjects with neglect on two versions of a cancellation task. Subjects were asked to cancel (i.e., draw a line through) short lines randomly distributed on a sheet of paper. In a second task they were asked to cancel the lines by erasing them. It was found that they canceled more lines in the second task as the stimuli were progressively removed (erased) than in the first task.

According to Posner (1980) and Posner et al. (1980), attention to visual stimuli can shift without actual eye movement. This is called covert attention. RHD patients may have difficulty shifting their attention from stimuli that have attracted their attention (disengaging) and may have problems in *preparing* to shift their attention (shifting covert attention). These problems have also been found in RHD patients with neglect in response to auditory stimuli (Farah et al., 1989), although they may be more prominent in the visual modality. In a cross-modal study of attention in RHD subjects, Robin and Rizzo (1989) found that impairments in orienting and disengaging attention were particularly evident in response to visual (versus auditory) stimuli.

These findings suggest that RHD patients with neglect may have problems shifting attention from stimuli on the right in addition to problems in directing attention to the left. Thus, clinicians should take into account the level of right-sided stimulation present in tasks designed to measure or alleviate left-sided neglect.

Directed and Selective Attention.   Problems in directed attention manifest themselves as difficulty in orienting to left-sided stimuli with the intention of acting on it. According to Mesulam (1981), neglect may impair exploration of space by disrupting the motor sequences (including eye movements) necessary for exploring and manipulating stimuli in contralesional space. Thus, patients with neglect may fail to perform tasks that require them to visually explore left-sided space or tasks that involve movements on both sides of the body (e.g., cooking, combing hair, brushing teeth, dressing).

Impaired selective attention may affect the capacity to recognize stimulus significance (Mesulam, 1981). Patients with neglect may have difficulty selecting relevant stimuli or filtering out distractors. The signs of neglect may increase (and performance deteriorate) as the selective attention demands of tasks increases (Rapcsak et al., 1989).

Effect of Attention Deficits on Communication

Attentional impairments have cognitive consequences that may affect all levels of experience, including communication. That is, attention deficits may impair the appreciation of the verbal and visual cues that specify the context within which communication takes place. Patients may be less able to shift attention, actively or covertly, when listening to conversation or observing situations. They may be less able to sustain attention and to attend selectively to stimuli anywhere in the stimulus array. Thus, they may not be able to attend selectively to important information and may be overwhelmed by complex narratives. Finally, attention deficits may place demands on the patient's internal resources such that as tasks become more difficult, cognitive resources are strained. These potential effects will be addressed more thoroughly in the section on ''Extralinguistic Disorders.''

Evaluation of Neglect

Evaluation of neglect involves establishing its presence and severity. Most tests of neglect can be considered tests of attention. Professionals participating in the evaluation of neglect include physicians, occupational therapists, neuropsychologists, and speech pathologists. The presence of neglect can be established in a variety of informal sensory and motor tasks described below.

Sensory neglect can be tested by *bilateral simultaneous stimulation* in which patients are presented with stimuli on both sides of their bodies. The stimulation may be tactile (e.g., tapping the shoulders) or visual (e.g., a point of light presented in the left and right peripheral vision). If, after initially noting the two sets of stimuli, the patient ''extinguishes'' or fails to report the presence of the stimulation on the left, left-sided neglect is said to be present.

Typical motor tests of neglect include cancellation,. scanning, line bisection, and drawing tasks. *Cancellation tasks* require patients to look at an array of stimuli (e.g., lines, letters, or numbers) that are randomly distributed on a sheet of paper (Albert, 1973). The patient is asked to cross out all occurrences of the stimuli by marking through or canceling them with a pen. Neglect is measured by the number of left-sided stimuli missed by the patient. Generalized attention deficits may be measured by the number missed, regardless of their spatial location. Because the target stimuli do not differ from each other, this type of cancellation task is considered simple.

Complex cancellation tasks involve selective attention. The stimuli may be two or three different shapes (e.g., letters or numbers) in different colors. The patient is asked to cancel occurrences of only one of the shapes in a particular color—that is, to select and cancel only instances of a particular target that conjoins the feature of shape and color. For example, patients may be asked to cancel only red triangles in an array of red and blue triangles and squares. Selective attention deficits may exacerbate neglect in complex cancellation or visual search tasks and may further impair attention in nonneglect patients. Thus, patients may omit only left-sided stimuli in a simple cancellation task but may miss targets on the right and may miss more targets on the left in a complex cancellation task. By using simple and complex tasks, the influence of selective attention on the patient's neglect can be assessed.

Scanning tasks require patients to scan an array of letters, numbers, or objects in which instances of a target stimulus are embedded (e.g., finding all the instances of the letter ''A'' in a line of random letters). Typically, the stimuli are arranged in a horizontal line or set of lines rather than randomly distributed

on a page. Neglect is measured by the number of target stimuli missed by the subject to the left of the midline. Scanning tasks are often given to assess the influence of neglect on reading.

Line bisection tasks require patients to bisect a straight horizontal line by drawing a vertical line through the center of the line. Neglect may be measured by how far to the right of center the patient's vertical line is. Line bisection helps establish the degree to which the patient's sense of space is skewed to the right. Several recent studies of line bisection have found that there is tremendous variability in the normal population in accuracy of line bisection, and that in patients with neglect, the shorter the line, the more accurate they are in judging its center (Halligan et al., 1990; Halligan and Marshall, 1988; Marshall and Halligan, 1989; Tegner et al., 1990).

The effects of neglect on reading can be measured by asking patients to *read compound words or sentences* presented at their visual midline. The effects of neglect on writing can be assessed by asking patients to *write or copy a short paragraph.* Patients may omit the left half of sentences and words read aloud (e.g., ''house'' for ''greenhouse''), and their writing samples may contain excessive left-sided margins, iterations, and/or omissions of letters and words.

Finally, patients may be asked to *draw from memory or copy symmetrical objects* such as a clock face, a flower, a man, or collections of objects in a simple scene. Neglect is measured by the number of left-sided details and/or objects omitted from the patient's drawings. Drawings may also be inspected for overall structure and integration of object parts.

Based on results of testing neglect by line bisection, drawing from memory, copying, reading, and writing in 106 RHD stroke patients, Horner et al. (1989) reported that no single task in isolation identified neglect in all subjects. This suggests that combinations of tasks should be administered to establish the presence of neglect. Severity can be estimated by combinations of scores on the informal tests mentioned above. In scoring neglect, clinicians should note inattention to right- as well as left-sided detail as a measure of attention.

Establishing the presence and severity of neglect is important in the management of RHD communication disorders for several reasons. It helps clarify whether or not reading and writing deficits are linguistically or perceptually based. It helps establish the patient's capacity to attend to visual stimuli in other diagnostic and therapy materials. Finally, as a reflection of a general attention deficit, neglect may interfere in the patient's general level of arousal, readiness to respond, and ability to produce and sustain effortful, directed attention, regardless of whether external stimulation is visual. As such, neglect may interfere in the cognitive operations involved in communication.

It should be emphasized that some RHD patients will have impaired attention of one type or another without demonstrating signs of neglect. Thus, all RHD patients should be tested for attentional deficits, and the results should be included in family counseling and taken into account in evaluating and treating RHD communication impairments. Additional tests of attention can be found in published materials designed for traumatic brain-injury patients and in the literature on cognitive rehabilitation (see Sohlberg and Mateer, 1989, for a review of attentional deficits subsequent to brain injury).

Treatment of Neglect

Management of neglect revolves around the issue of treating the symptom or the cause. That is, should one attempt to alleviate the symptoms by trying to force the patient to attend to left-sided input, or should one address attention itself? Treatment of symptoms is rarely successful. Verbally cuing the patient to look to the left or highlighting stimuli on the left (e.g., drawing a red line down the left margin of a printed page) rarely translates into an internal or self-cue by the patient.

If one accepts that various types of attention are a significant factor in neglect and in RHD deficits in general, then it makes sense to work on attention directly in tasks designed to increase the level of arousal, vigilance, and selective attention capacity. Any task that requires patients to attend to the occurrence of simple, but unpredictable, stimuli may increase their capacity for vigilance (e.g., listening for a target word in a word list). Selective attention may be addressed by the modifying tasks designed for evaluating neglect. Additional tasks for treating attentional deficits subsequent to brain injury can be found in published materials (see Baines and Robinson, 1991; Sohlberg and Mateer, 1986, 1987).

Increasing attention to the left side of space may be most effectively addressed by designing tasks in which patients internalize the need to look to the left. For example, rather than cuing them to the left in visual search tasks, one could tell them the number of targets they must find without telling them where to look. Without telling them where to look, clinicians can encourage patients to continue the search until the total number is found. This technique may be best used with real objects such as colored cubes that patients themselves can count to chart their progress. Cubes can be placed on a flat board divided into quadrants. One may begin such a search-and-find task with as few as two cubes of a single color. Task difficulty can be increased by changing cube placement (i.e., placing cubes to the left as well as the right of midline, then in the lower left as well as the upper left quadrant); by increasing the number of cubes; and by having target cubes differ in color from foils. This type of task has been described in detail by Myers and Mackisack (1990). The advantage of such a task is that it instills the need to search to the left without external cuing, thus increasing the potential for generalization. A second advantage noted clinically is that it appears to increase patients' general level of attention and as such may be a good introduction to therapy for cognitive and communication impairments.

In addition to addressing attention directly, one needs to counsel patients about their neglect and attentional disorders; discuss the effects of neglect on activities of daily living, including communication; and, if necessary, demonstrate the problems in a way that enables patients to overcome possible denial. Families should be included in understanding the effects of these impairments on communication.

Visuoperceptual Deficits

RHD is associated with various visuoperceptual deficits including problems in object recognition, constructional tasks, and spatial orientation. Not all RHD patients have visuoperceptual impairments. Those who do often have neglect as well.

Object Recognition

RHD is not typically associated with problems in identifying or using real objects (Damasio, 1985; Kertesz, 1983). That is, RHD patients do not have visual agnosia. They are usually unimpaired in recognizing pictures of isolated objects presented in natural or prototypic views (DeRenzi and Spinnler, 1966; Layman and Green, 1988; Warrington and James, 1967). RHD patients' object recognition deficits surface under conditions in which stimuli have been degraded. For example, they may have problems with figure-ground tasks such as identifying overlapping figures (DeRenzi et al., 1969; DeRenzi and Spinnler, 1966; Hier and Kaplan, 1980; Warrington and Taylor, 1973). They may have trouble identifying objects depicted in unusual orientations or of unusual size (Humphries and Riddoch, 1984; Layman and Green, 1988; Warrington and Taylor, 1973, 1978). They may not be able to identify incomplete or fragmented figures (DeRenzi and Spinnler, 1966; Mackisack et al., 1987; Myers, 1979; Myers et al., 1985; Warrington and James, 1967; Warrington and Taylor, 1973).

What all this means is that RHD patients may have no trouble identifying objects in their everyday activities. They may, however, have difficulty when the visual system is taxed by confusing input, such as closely spaced or overlapping pictured objects and people.

Constructional Apraxia

The term "constructional apraxia" refers to deficits in specific visuomotor tasks such as drawing or block design. The presence of this disorder is established by asking patients to draw simple objects and complex figures and to copy block designs. Both LHD and RHD patients may be impaired in copying and drawing, but there are important differences between their performances. In studies of constructional apraxia, subjects are almost always right-handed, so LHD subjects draw with their nondominant hand, whereas RHD subjects use their preferred hand. The drawings of LHD patients tend to be more primitive but similar in form and spatial organization to those of NBD subjects. The drawings of RHD patients, on the other hand, tend to be fragmented, scattered, and spatially disorganized. They may contain excessive detail and iteration of lines on the right and omissions of detail on the left. Object parts may be mislocated (e.g., a chimney coming out of the side of a house). Unlike the drawings of LHD patients, those of RHD patients may not benefit from a model or from cuing, nor may the drawings improve over time (Swindell et al., 1988).

The failure of RHD subjects to benefit from cuing, and the finding that drawing deficits may be correlated with perceptual deficits in RHD subjects but not in LHD subjects, has suggested to some investigators that RHD drawing deficits may be based on perceptual impairments (Griffiths and Cook, 1986; Hecaen and Assal, 1970; Kim et al., 1984; Mack and Levine, 1981; Villa et al., 1986; Warrington and Rabin, 1970). That is, constructional apraxia in RHD patients may reflect impairments in spatial organization and integration, as opposed to a motor or motor programming deficit. This possibility suggests that compared with LHD and NBD adults, RHD patients may not perceive visual detail, may not have the same internal representation of the spatial organization of object parts, and/or may have specific deficits in integrating object parts.

Spatial Orientation Deficits

RHD patients may have difficulty following familiar routes, orienting to maps, learning mazes, pointing to body parts, and performing spatial memory tasks (DeRenzi et al., 1977; Newcombe et al., 1987; Newcombe and Russell, 1969; Ratcliff and Newcombe, 1973). These deficits are not necessarily related to impaired mental imagery nor to disorientation. For example, finding cities on a map may depend on prior experience and education of subjects. Many adults have a rather fuzzy picture of geography, and this fact should be taken into account in testing RHD patients on map orientation.

Patients who cannot follow familiar routes or learn new ones are said to have "topological disorientation." Often they compensate by verbal cues ("Go left after the fourth door past the nurses' station"). The ability to compensate argues against the kind of general disorientation associated with confusion and memory loss. Unlike patients with Alzheimer's disease who find themselves confused about why they are in a specific room, uncertain how they got there, or how they will get back, RHD patients will set off with a specific destination in mind but be uncertain of the route. The source of route-finding problems is not clear. It may be related to deficits in the internal representation of space. More likely, patients have trouble recognizing familiar landmarks and learning new ones because they do not attend to visual cues.

Route-finding problems are not unique to RHD. LHD patients with parietal lesions may have similar difficulties during the acute phase of their illness (Teuber, 1963). On the other hand, specific problems in abilities such as discriminating the direction of lines or matching the location of targets are more strongly associated with right-hemisphere damage than with left-hemisphere damage (Benton et al., 1978; Kim et al., 1984; Magnussen et al., 1987), suggesting that RHD patients, particularly those with neglect, may be impaired in some aspects of spatial judgment.

Effects of Visuoperceptual Deficits on Communication

Difficulty in drawing, in finding one's way around familiar routes, and in making sense of ambiguous pictured objects may appear to have little to do with communication. Indeed, aside from possible interference in recognizing pictured therapy materials, visuoperceptual problems may not have any immediate impact on communication.

However, visuoperceptual impairments may be related to cognitive deficits that do affect communication. That is, visuoperceptual problems may reflect more general cognitive problems. The connections between attentional, perceptual, and cognitive deficits subsequent to RHD may be very important to our understanding of RHD patients' communicative disorders. For example, in a typical visual discrimination task, patients are asked to match a geometric or nonsense figure to one of several figures that differ in as few as one or two attributes or features from the target. Problems in recognizing which features matter may be related to selective attention deficits. Impaired selective attention can also affect appreciating which details matter in narrative discourse. That is, visuoperceptual deficits may not just be visual and may be part of a larger cognitive deficit that is independent of modality.

Problems in spatial organization, noted in constructional apraxia, may also reflect a more general problem in organizing

and integrating many other types of information. A relationship between visuoperceptual deficits and cognitive impairments is supported by two studies (Benowitz et al., 1990; Moya et al., 1986). Both studies found RHD subjects significantly impaired relative to NBD controls in recalling details, in abstracting the relationships among events or characters, and in drawing appropriate inferences about narrative stories. Subjects were also asked to copy a series of figures such as a cube and a complicated geometric form. Drawings were scored for details, for overall organization and form, and for left neglect. Even when the effects of lesion size, age, education, and atrophy were held constant, there were significant correlations between impairments in abstracting information from narratives and constructional apraxia in subjects' drawings. The fact that deficits in narrative discourse correlated positively with visuospatial deficits suggested to the authors the possibility that the "appreciation of spatial configurations and the comprehension of interrelationships among elements in narrative material may to some extent require a common mechanism" (p. 240). They went on to suggest that the identification of constructional apraxia in RHD patients may be indicative of a more "pervasive cognitive deficit." Thus, problems in organizing visuospatial information may be related to problems organizing narrative information.

Evaluation and Treatment

Evaluation and treatment of visuoperceptual deficits are typically in the province of occupational therapists. It is a good idea for speech pathologists to keep current with patients' visuoperceptual deficits and to be aware of the potential effects of such deficits on their performance in speech-language therapy for two reasons: (*a*) The deficits may interfere with visual recognition of stimulus materials; and (*b*) they may reflect more general problems in some of the cognitive operations involved in narrative communication, such as integration and organization.

LINGUISTIC DEFICITS

Description

Some RHD patients may make errors on straightforward expressive and receptive language tasks such as naming, word discrimination, following simple commands, word definitions, verbal fluency, and reading and writing. There is general agreement that their errors on aphasia batteries do not mirror those of aphasic patients (Archibald and Wepman, 1968; Deal et al., 1979; Eisenson, 1962). Linguistic deficits are not considered a major source of RHD communication impairments for several reasons. First, when found, they tend to be mild. Second, they do not appear to have an impact on the constellation of extralinguistic communication impairments in this population (see the following section).

Studies of linguistic impairments have reported conflicting results. Several studies of auditory comprehension have found that RHD subjects are impaired in sentence comprehension as measured by tasks similar to the Token Test (Adamovich and Brooks, 1981; DeRenzi and Vignolo, 1962; McNeil and Prescott, 1978; Swisher and Sarno, 1969). Several other studies have found no differences between NBD controls and RHD patients on these tasks (Cappa et al., 1990; Cavalli et al., 1981).

Several studies of naming have found that RHD subjects are impaired in single-word naming relative to NBD controls (Diggs and Basili, 1987; Gainotti et al., 1981; Joanette et al., 1983), whereas others have not (Cappa et al., 1990; Rivers and Love, 1980). Hier and Kaplan (1980) and Rivers and Love (1980) found that RHD and NBD controls performed comparably on a word-definition task, but Joanette et al. (1983) did not find this result.

Some investigations of verbal fluency (e.g., naming as many members as possible from a given category such as "animals") have found RHD subjects significantly impaired relative to NBD subjects (Diggs and Basili, 1987; Schechter et al., 1985; Schneiderman and Saddy, 1988), whereas others have not (Cappa et al., 1990; Cavalli et al., 1981).

Factors other than linguistic deficits can affect performance on some linguistic tasks. Neglect has been noted as a factor in some studies of naming. For example, Myers (1992) found that RHD subjects with little or no neglect did not differ significantly from NBD controls in naming single objects, whereas those with greater degrees of neglect did. Similarly, Gainotti et al. (1979) found that significant differences between the performance of RHD and NBD controls on a naming task disappeared when the effects of neglect were controlled.

Spatial and/or visuoperceptual deficits could also be a factor in responses to tests like the Token Test (DeRenzi and Vignolo, 1962) in which patients must scan an array of shapes and use color and shape in responding to verbal commands. Verbal discrimination tasks that require scanning an array of closely positioned objects may also pose visuoperceptual problems for RHD patients. In addition, writing impairments at the sentence and paragraph level—which may include spelling errors, omission and/or iteration of graphemes and words, and impaired use of margins (Metzler and Jelinek, 1977)—may be confounded by neglect, attentional problems, and visuoperceptual deficits.

Summary

The available data suggest that word discrimination, naming, and other straightforward language tasks may present problems for RHD patients, but the problems are relatively mild, are not indicative of aphasia, and may not affect communication ability significantly. In addition, visuospatial deficits, neglect, and attentional impairments have been cited as possible contaminating factors in some studies investigating linguistic disorders in RHD subjects (Adamovich and Brooks, 1981; Archibald and Wepman, 1968; Swisher and Sarno, 1969).

In general, RHD patients are able to structure sentences and paragraphs according to the rules of their language. They do not have particular problems in retrieving words, and they make few paraphasic errors. However, their control over linguistic structure may belie a more general problem with language use at the narrative level of communication. These deficits will be explored in the section on "Extralinguistic Deficits."

Evaluation and Treatment

Control over the structure of language should be tested to rule out aphasia subsequent to RHD. When doing so, care should be taken to distinguish between problems that are linguistic versus extralinguistic in nature. Subtests from aphasia batteries designed to test language in constructions that are essentially context-free are useful in assessing straightforward

language functions (e.g., ask patients to follow verbal commands rather than to interpret paragraphs). Complex and closely spaced visual stimuli in the response field should be avoided. Naming should be assessed by verbal definition as well as by picture naming. Errors should be examined in light of visuoperceptual and attentional deficits identified in nonlinguistic tasks. If the clinician feels certain that the patient has a language problem rather than, or in addition to, attentional or perceptual deficits, treatment should follow the traditional approaches used in management of aphasia. Treatment of reading and writing impairments subsequent to neglect should include the suggestions set forth in the section on neglect.

EXTRALINGUISTIC DEFICITS

Although RHD patients typically do not have aphasia, many of them do have communication disorders. Extralinguistic deficits represent the heart of their communication problems. The term "extralinguistic" refers to factors that affect communication but are not linguistic in nature. The extralinguistic aspects of communication essentially specify the context within which communication takes place and allow one to understand and convey intentions, emotional tone, and implied meaning. These aspects of communication extend communicated meaning beyond the literal or surface structure of words and sentences. Context is conveyed through an array of sensory cues such as gesture, body language, facial expression, and prosodic contour, as well as through the choice and grouping of words themselves. Extralinguistic cues allow us to interpret what is meant from what is said and to understand such things as the relative formality of an exchange, the emotional tone of narratives, the roles played by participants in a conversation (e.g., peer versus subordinate), and whether someone is being funny or sarcastic or serious. These same cues allow us to express our own intended meanings.

Some RHD patients appear to have difficulty using these cues to understand the implied meaning of complex narratives. Thus, they may miss the theme or point of a story. They may not recognize relationships among characters or the motives behind their actions. They may not respond to the emotions expressed by characters or conveyed by other artistic conventions used in dramas, films, narratives, and other art forms.

In conversation, RHD patients may not understand humor or the subtleties of irony. They may miss the main points a speaker is making because they focus on unimportant details and have difficulty integrating information into an overall theme. They may not attend to a speaker's facial expression, tone of voice, the prosodic cues that convey emotion, or the physical setting in which the communicative act takes place.

They may also have difficulty expressing their own intended meaning. Their speech may be inefficient and uninformative and lack specificity. They may have problems getting to the point they are trying to make. Finally, they may have difficulty using the extralinguistic cues that convey emotion through gesture and prosody.

Most studies of RHD communication disorders have provided descriptions of deficits and specified the conditions under which deficits may be observed, but few have addressed the general mechanisms that may underlie those deficits. Indeed, the term "right-hemisphere communication disorders" refers to anatomy rather than to impaired cognitive processes. Without hypotheses about the origin of these problems, management remains at the level of treating the symptoms rather than the cause. One such hypothesis is presented below.

Inference Deficit

As pointed out by Myers (1992), early attempts to specify underlying mechanisms tended to postulate specific relationships between isolated deficits and right-hemisphere functions. For example, based on documented RHD deficits, it was suggested that the right hemisphere might (a) play a special role in detecting absurd or humorous content (Gardner, 1975); (b) be specialized for mediating emotion (Bear, 1983; Burns et al., 1985; Gainotti, 1972; Silberman and Weingartner, 1986); (c) be uniquely organized for the appreciation of figurative language (Gardner and Denes, 1973; Van Lancker and Kempler, 1987); and (d) be organized for storing and processing personally familiar proper nouns (Van Lancker et al., 1991).

Some more parsimonious explanations for RHD patients' communicative impairments have been developed. These explanations range from impairments in "holistic pattern recognition" (Van Lancker et al., 1991) to diminished ability to evaluate the "gestalt or form of linguistic entities" (Wapner et al., 1981). Recently, Myers (1991) suggested that most RHD communication deficits may be explained by an underlying "inference deficit." An advantage of the term "inference deficit" is that it removes anatomy from the picture by referring to a cognitive impairment. Another advantage is that it encompasses the total symptomatology of RHD by integrating attentional and perceptual deficits with impairments in communication. In this way, communication impairments can be conceived of as the cognitive outcome of attentional and perceptual deficits subsequent to RHD.

According to Myers (1992), "An inference is a hypothesis about sensory data such that input is not only sensed, but interpreted." Initial inferences are beliefs or hypotheses about sensations. Later stage inferences are hypotheses based on those initial beliefs. Thus, a viewer might interpret a picture of a man wearing a purple robe and a crown and holding a scepter as a king. The inference that he is a king is a hypothesis about the intended meaning of the visual image.

There are many levels of inference. In the above example, organizing the visual image into the form of a human is an inference, and determining that the image is that of a man is another inference. In general, the type of communication impairments experienced by RHD patients suggests that inference breaks down at a later stage of processing rather than at the level of translating light rays into shapes or sound waves into phonemes.

Inferences depend on at least four operations:

1. *Attention* to individual cues
2. *Selection* of relevant cues
3. *Integration* of relevant cues with one another
4. *Association* of cues with prior experience

In the above example, the color of the man's hair would be considered an irrelevant cue. Relevant cues include the crown, the robe, the scepter, and perhaps the color purple. These combined cues create the context from which the inference of royalty is made. That is, the elements not only must be recognized but must be sorted for relevance, and those considered

relevant must be combined or integrated to create a context, pattern, or meaning beyond the superficial recognition of color, form, light, and shadow. The combined cues can be associated with prior experience. These operations are not necessarily sequentially ordered but are more likely to occur in parallel.

In similar fashion, recognizing the intended meaning of verbal communication requires that one go beyond the superficial, literal, or referential meaning of individual words to their implied or inferred meaning. In addition to the four components listed above, inference generation also involves operations such as the ability to integrate verbal information into an overall structure or theme, to generate alternative meanings, and to revise original hypotheses or inferences based on new contextual information.

The possibility that RHD communication disorders are caused by an underlying "inference deficit" is a useful hypothesis or framework through which to explore the apparently disparate RHD communication symptoms and to address their management. The literature documenting RHD extralinguistic communication deficits includes certain recurring themes that include impairments in:

1. Producing informative content
2. Integrating narrative information
3. Generating alternative meanings
4. Comprehending and expressing emotion
5. Comprehending and producing prosody

These deficit areas are related to one another and are possibly all related to deficits in generating inferences. They are addressed separately in the following sections.

Producing Informative Content

When families state that RHD patients "talk, but it isn't the same," they are often referring to the reduced level of information contained in the patients' conversational speech. That is, RHD patients may produce as many or more words than NBD adults, but what they say conveys less information. Studies investigating informative content of narratives typically ask subjects to paraphrase stories or to produce narratives in response to pictured scenes and stories. They have found that RHD subjects' narratives contain fewer concepts, less relevant concepts, and less specific information than those of NBD subjects (Bloom et al., 1992; Cimino et al., 1991; Diggs and Basili, 1987; Joanette et al., 1986; Myers and Brookshire, 1994; Urayse et al., 1991).

Conversational output of RHD patients may also suffer from reduced informative content but not from lack of words. As one patient said, "I know the point I want to reach, but as I get there my mind, like a vacuum cleaner, sucks up every thought along the way and spews it out." RHD patients' conversational expression has been described as hyperfluent and digressive (Roman et al., 1987; Sherratt and Penn, 1990; Trupe and Hillis, 1985). In reviewing their RHD subjects' picture descriptions, Tompkins and Flowers (1985), for example, noted that low concept scores were overwhelmingly associated with excessive verbal output, reflecting "repetitiveness" and "irrelevant comments" (p. 529). The tangential comments made by RHD patients may not be off the topic altogether, but their presence signals difficulty in getting to the point the patient wants to express. For example, asked what had happened to her and why she was in the hospital, one patient responded:

''My husband saw I wasn't in bed, and he found me in the clothes that I came to the hospital in, same robe and gown and everything. And we have a very thick rug, what they call a sculptured pattern with swirls and all that. It goes down to the base—fiber base, about two, more than two inches down deep. . . .''

Her comments about the carpet continued. They are tangential but related—related to the fact that although she had fallen on the floor, the cause of her hospitalization was a stroke, not the blow to her head, since the carpet softened the fall. She was unable to make her point explicitly, and thus her listener was burdened with having to fill in the missing information.

Digressive and inefficient output may be related to impaired appreciation of listener needs. It is interesting to note that Rehak et al. (1992a) found RHD subjects particularly impaired relative to NBD controls in judging the effects of tangentiality on conversational partners. Their lack of sensitivity to the interference of tangential remarks may be a reflection of insensitivity to their own tendencies in this direction.

Occasionally, tangential or irrelevant output appears to be a reflection of uncertainty about the intended meaning of events. Failing to infer the examiner's intended meaning when asked to describe a pictured scene, one RHD patient discussed the size and weight of the paper, its plastic coating, and the type of pen used to create the drawing, but he did not describe the action depicted in the picture. Prompted by a further explanation of the request, the patient was able to generate a more informative narrative.

Occasionally, uncertainty will cause RHD patients to confabulate. In retelling stories with surprise or nonsensical endings, RHD subjects have been known to make up details that would make the events more plausible (Wapner et al., 1981). Confabulation is not a typical response but is one that may arise when patients are confronted by events they find confusing. Their confusion may be related to difficulty in extracting the implicit meaning of situations and conversations.

Many studies investigating narrative-level deficits have used pictured scenes and story sequences to elicit original narratives. It is possible that narratives based on visual stimuli result in lower informative content because RHD subjects have problems perceiving what is in the pictures. However, several studies of scene description have demonstrated that RHD patients do not have problems recognizing objects and people in scenes as visually complex as Norman Rockwell illustrations. For example, Mackisack et al. (1987), Myers (1992), and Myers and Brookshire (1994) found that RHD subjects were as accurate as NBD controls in labeling items contained in such pictured scenes. Furthermore, the latter two studies manipulated the visual and inferential characteristics of the pictured stimuli to determine the relative effects of visual and inferential complexity on subjects' responses. They found that the level of inference required to interpret a scene significantly impaired performance. Visual complexity, as measured by the number of objects and people in the scenes, had no effect on performance of either the NBD group or the RHD group. In addition, reduced informative content has also been found in response to verbal narrative passages (Cimino et al., 1991; Wapner et al., 1981), suggesting that this impairment is not restricted to visual input but crosses the visual and verbal modalities.

Summary

Digressive output and reduced informative content appear to be related to impaired capacity to infer the meaning of *external* events, and to deficits in recognizing, selecting, integrating, and organizing *internal* thoughts and information. As a result, RHD patients may produce as many or more words than NBD adults, but they may say less. They may delete episodes in a story or cloud relevant information with trivial comments. They may be confused by situations or requests and may attempt to cover their confusion by confabulation. They may not recognize or may be unable to accommodate their listeners' needs in conversation. Finally, they may fixate on irrelevant details and have problems marshaling important facts into a coherent structure. Without a structure to guide them, they may digress and even wander off the topic.

Integrating Narrative Information

Problems in generating an organizing principle or macrostructure for narrative discourse relate to deficits in integrating contextual information (Hough, 1990; Kaczmarek, 1984; Wapner et al., 1981). As explained by Brownell (1988) and Hough (1990), understanding the theme or overall gist of narratives involves the extraction of meaning from individual sentences and the *integration* of their meaning into the context supplied by the other sentences. Similarly, interpreting pictured scenes or real situations involves the extraction of individual objects and their integration with one another. Integration of discrete items with one another is one of the operations involved in inference generation.

Impaired ability to extract and integrate bits of information can be demonstrated by patient descriptions of the familiar ''Cookie Theft'' picture from the Boston Diagnostic Aphasia Examination (Goodglass and Kaplan, 1983). The ''Cookie Theft'' scene depicts a series of disasters taking place in a kitchen. A mother stands distractedly washing dishes at an overflowing sink, her back to two children who are attempting to steal cookies from a high cupboard as their stool tips over. Adequate interpretation of the scene (i.e., the overall implication of disaster) involves inference, which as stated earlier, involves the selection and integration of cues and their association with prior experience. Selecting and integrating relevant cues results in inferences about *individual* elements depicted in the scene from which is built the overall theme or macrostructure. For example, calling the woman a ''mother'' (versus a ''woman'') is an inference based on recognizing and integrating individual cues such as the appliances that suggest a kitchen, her apron, and the children behind her. Determining that the children are not just ''reaching for cookies,'' but stealing them, requires the integration of the action of the boy reaching in the cookie jar with the action of the girl who has her finger to her mouth in the gesture of ''shhh.'' RHD patients may say the boy has his hand in the jar, and the girl has her finger to her mouth, without combining the two actions into the inference of ''stealing.''

RHD patients often begin their descriptions of this picture by discussing irrelevant details such as the garden outside the window or the cups on the counter. This tendency demonstrates a problem in selecting relevant information, which further inhibits interpretation or inference. Selecting relevant cues is the first step in generating inferences. Myers (1979) and Myers and Linebaugh (1980) found that RHD subjects produced significantly fewer "interpretive" or inferential concepts in describing the "Cookie Theft" picture compared with NBD controls. They noted that RHD subjects tended to list individual elements without explicitly connecting them to each other or to the central focus of the action. Much of what they listed was irrelevant to the central theme or action.

This latter observation has been documented in several other studies. For example, Mackisack et al. (1987) found that RHD subjects labeled more than twice as many items as NBD controls when describing Norman Rockwell illustrations. Similarly, when Hough (1990) asked subjects to interpret the theme of short verbal narratives, she found that RHD subjects tended to list information and "retained isolated pieces of paragraph data rather than integrating this information to deduce the meaning of the narratives" (p. 271). In a discussion of narrative discourse deficits, Brownell et al. (1986) state, "Where normal listeners are concerned to weave a coherent interpretation of an entire discourse so that each component jibes with the broader reality, RHD patients are often stuck with, or are satisfied with, a limited and piecemeal understanding" (p. 319).

These impairments may occur even at the level of organizing individually printed sentences into paragraphs (Delis et al., 1983). RHD deficits in such tasks support the notion that RHD patients may have difficulty integrating isolated pieces of information (Brownell, 1988; Joanette et al., 1986). Piecemeal processing (i.e., listing objects in pictures or pieces of narratives verbatim) may be related to or caused by failure to integrate information.

Integration deficits also occur in perceptual impairments associated with RHD. As noted earlier, impaired integration of visuospatial information may be a factor in constructional apraxia. That is, a patient may know the components of an object such as a clock but fail to integrate them into an overall structure. Thus, the hands and numbers may appear to be trailing off outside the clock face, suggesting that the patient has the pieces but cannot put them together.

At the level of narrative comprehension and production, one not only must integrate individual elements (e.g., sentences) but also must infer the semantic links between sentences or the links between actions presented in pictured stories. That is, not all the links are explicitly stated or depicted (Brownell, 1988; Joanette et al., 1986). Narrative discourse, then, requires the extraction and integration of individual units of meaning (explicit and implicit) into a larger whole. Impairments in this process affect the comprehension and production of narrative discourse subsequent to RHD.

Summary

Extraction and integration of relevant contextual features with one another are two of the components of inference generation. Deficits in these operations affect communicative ability by making it difficult for patients to comprehend the gist of conversation and narratives and to express their own main points and intentions. As a result, they may not follow conversational paths or the themes of narratives. They may produce discourse that is inefficient and lacking in structure while burdening the listener with trying to ascertain the point they are trying to make. These deficits may be related to impairments in attention and perception. Attentional deficits may inhibit the ability to filter irrelevant information and recognize important contextual cues. Deficits in organizing and integrating component features into coherently structured drawings at the perceptual level may be related to impaired integration of units of narrative content and to impairments in generating a narrative macrostructure. As a result, some RHD patients may have difficulty not only in comprehending externally presented extralinguistic information but also in filtering, integrating, and organizing internal information in such a way as to generate efficient narrative expression.

Generating Alternative Meanings

As stated earlier, inferencing involves the selection and integration of elements and their association with prior experience. Out of this process, we create new or alternate meanings for our initial sensory impressions. Thus, in the example of the picture of the king (referred to in the section on "Inference Deficit") one impression of the picture is that of a man in a purple robe. An alternate impression is that the man is a king. Alternate meanings are forms of inference. An inference deficit can affect communication in context—that is, at the level of connected discourse. However, there is also evidence that RHD patients have difficulty generating alternative meanings for isolated, noncontextual information. This suggests that deficits in generating alternative meanings may be an independent problem, not restricted to situations calling for inferences.

For example, studies have demonstrated impairments in generating alternative meanings for single words that are not embedded in context (Brownell et al., 1984; Brownell et al., 1990; Gardner and Denes, 1973). Individual words may evoke a denotative or connotative meaning. Denotative meanings are similar to dictionary definitions and are appropriate for words taken out of context where further interpretation is not called for. Connotative meanings refer to alternative, nonliteral, or interpretive meanings. Thus, for example, the denotative meaning of the word "lion" is "animal that lives in Africa." Its connotative meanings may include "regal," "king of the jungle," "ferocious," or even "MGM." These nonliteral meanings can be considered *alternates* to those that everyone would agree on.

Brownell et al. (1984) asked RHD, LHD, and NBD subjects to group the two of three words in a given set that were closest in meaning. The words could be grouped according to either connotative or denotative meanings. Results demonstrated that the RHD group relied on denotative meanings, and the aphasic group relied largely on connotative meanings. NBD controls were more flexible and made judgments based on both types of meaning. Similarly, Brownell et al. (1990) found that RHD patients were impaired in appreciating both metaphoric and *nonmetaphoric* alternative meanings of single words. As Brownell et al. (1990) suggest, these impairments "may not be restricted to metaphor; rather they may be but one reflection of a more pervasive impairment affecting appreciation of different types of alternative meanings" (p. 376).

RHD patients tend to respond to the literal, rather than to the intended (alternate), meanings of idioms and metaphor (Myers and Linebaugh, 1981; Van Lancker and Kempler, 1987; Winner and Gardner, 1977). For example, asked to match a picture to an idiomatic phrase such as, "He has a heavy heart," Winner and Gardner (1977) found that RHD subjects tended to point to a literal depiction of the idiom (a man carrying a very large and heavy heart) rather than to the alternate or metaphoric depiction (a many crying).

Indirect requests also may be misinterpreted by RHD patients. In these cases, generating an alternative meaning for the words one hears depends on appreciating the context in which the request is made. For example, taken literally, the question "Can you open the window?" represents an inquiry about a person's physical capacity. The intended or alternate meaning is a request for someone to open the window. The context (e.g., the temperature of the room) specifies the meaning of the words. Several investigations have found that RHD subjects are impaired in interpreting indirect requests represented in pictures (Foldi, 1987; Hirst et al., 1984) and in paragraphs (Weylman et al., 1989).

Metaphoric language, idiomatic expressions, the connotative meaning of individual words, and indirect requests share a common feature. They must be associated with one's prior experience to be understood. It may be that RHD patients may have difficulty relating these speech acts to prior personal knowledge of such acts. Support for deficits in associating current information with prior experience comes from studies of verbal fluency in which the ability to generate members of a given category is tested.

These studies have investigated the capacity to generate members of *uncommon* categories that rely on less automatic retrieval than does a common category such as "animals." For example, Diggs and Basili (1987) found that RHD subjects produced significantly fewer uses for given objects (e.g., bricks) compared with NBD controls. Hough et al. (1994) found that RHD subjects performed comparably to NBD controls in generating members of common categories but were significantly impaired in generating members of uncommon categories such as "things to take on a camping trip." As Hough et al. (1994) point out, subjects must appeal to their store of previous experience to generate members of such categories. That is, to list what to take on a camping trip, one must be able to retrieve a memory of some prior experience with camping—from what one has read or experienced personally. Similarly, previous experience is crucial to produce additional meanings for the word "lion" or an alternate meaning for the phrase "He hit the roof."

Impairments in the ability to generate alternatives and to relate words, phrases, and situations to prior experience may make conversation difficult. Some RHD patients respond only to the most literal and superficial meanings of the words they hear, and, as a result, they may miss the point or misinterpret certain communicative events.

Deficits in the capacity to revise original interpretations are another source of problems in the accurate interpretation of conversations and narratives. Sometimes, one must change one's original interpretation of sentences or events to accommodate new information. Revisions are closely tied to generating alternative meanings, since they represent new or different interpretations.

One way that this possibility has been investigated is in the study of humor. Clinically, RHD patients may appear to have problems appreciating humor, and these problems have been documented in several studies (Dagge and Hartje, 1985; Gardner et al., 1975). Problems in revising original interpretations have been invoked to explain these deficits. Brownell et al.

(1983) investigated the cognitive aspects of humor and suggested that appreciation of humor involves sensitivity to two elements: surprise and coherence. Surprise occurs in the punchline of a joke, and coherence occurs when the punchline is integrated back into the body of the joke. Integrating the punchline into the foregoing context entails the *revision* of original expectations. Brownell et al (1983) found that when asked to select the punchline for a joke from a set of foils, RHD patients were selectively impaired in appreciating coherence but not surprise. That is, they tended to choose a funny ending for a joke but not one that jibed with the previous context. Bihrle et al. (1986) found the same results in a cartoon completion task. In reviewing their results relative to accounts of RHD deficits in narrative tasks, Bihrle et al. (1986) state, "In these tasks RHD patients seem to appreciate isolated meanings, but they cannot consider the importance of relevant information for revising their initial interpretation" (p. 409). Thus, deficits in humor may have a cognitive, rather than an affective, basis—one that may impair humor but that is based on deficits in integrating information and revising interpretations.

Impaired ability to revise expectations also may be a factor in RHD patients' problems in following conversations. For example, Kaplan et al. (1990) found that RHD subjects were impaired in interpreting whether conversational remarks between two speakers were to be taken literally. Nonliteral remarks occurred when one speaker was making fun, being sarcastic, or telling a white lie. Understanding the intended meaning of these nonliteral remarks required reinterpreting them in light of previous information.

Similarly, Brownell et al. (1986) found that RHD subjects were impaired at interpreting the meaning of sentence pairs when misleading information was presented in the first as opposed to the second sentence, as in the example, "Barbara became too bored to finish the history book. She had already spent five years writing it." Taken in isolation, the first sentence implies that Barbara is reading a book rather than writing one. The position of the misleading sentence affected RHD subjects' performance more than it did the controls' performance. When misleading information was presented first, RHD subjects had more difficulty than NBD subjects in revising their original interpretations to accommodate the information contained in the second sentence. The authors concluded that RHD patients may have particular difficulty in the effortful task of revising expectations generated by initially acquired information.

Impairments in revision have even been found in a lexical task that required revising the lexical function of a single word. Schneiderman and Saddy (1988) found that RHD subjects had difficulty inserting a word into a well-formed sentence when the word altered the lexical status of one of the words in the sentence. Sentence construction was such that word insertions were of two types. The first type left the original interpretation of the sentence intact (e.g., inserting the word "red" in the sentence "I see a rose"). The second type altered the lexical function of a word and thus required that the original interpretation of the sentence be revised (e.g., inserting the word "daughter" into the sentence, "Cindy saw her take his drink"). RHD subjects had particular difficulty and were more impaired than LHD subjects when they had to revise the original meaning of sentences to perform the task. The authors suggest that the apparent rigidity of RHD subjects on the sentence revision condition of their task might have "repercussions in all cases of semantic reinterpretation, whether at the sentential (sentence) or at the discourse level'' (p. 51).

Deficits in revising expectations may have a significant impact on the patient's capacity to follow the flow of events. We are continually confronted with new information that alters our original interpretations. For example, we hear an introduction to a news story that is meant to capture our attention such as, ''And next we'll hear about some boys who've really learned to fly,'' and then find that the story is about a track and field event, not about boys who have sprouted wings or are flying airplanes. We must revise as we participate in the twists and turns in everyday events and conversations. For the RHD patient, such seemingly automatic revisions may take extra effort and may not be made at all, so that new information is processed inadequately and entire meanings are missed.

Summary

Some RHD patients have demonstrated impairments in appreciating figurative language (metaphor, idioms, proverbs) and other nonliteral forms of language such as indirect requests. Their deficits may relate to impaired appreciation of information that specifies the context within which figurative language is communicated. In addition, these deficits may be related to a more fundamental deficit in generating alternative meanings that may be independent of contextual processing. Problems in generating alternatives have been found in context-free language tasks and in tasks for which subjects had to apply previous experience to novel situations (i.e., generating members for uncommon categories). Deficits in generating alternative meanings may be independent of generating inferences, but it affects the process.

The ability to revise original interpretations in light of new information is crucial to accurate comprehension of intended meaning. Deficits in this ability make participation in conversation difficult. RHD patients may be unsure if someone is being sarcastic, telling the truth, or making a joke. They may not be able to infer a character's motives in a movie or book as new information unfolds. They may not appreciate humor or even irony that requires the reinterpretation of previously gleaned information. Like generating alternative meanings, revisions require effort, attention, and a certain mental flexibility.

Comprehension and Expression of Emotion

Given their impairments in appreciating and producing extralinguistic cues, it is not surprising that RHD patients may have difficulty interpreting and expressing emotional content. In addition, they may speak in a monotone, may seem unresponsive, and may appear to have little reaction to their illness. These symptoms have been referred to as the ''indifference'' reaction (Denny-Brown et al., 1952). Reduced response to emotional material coupled with reduced emotional expression (''flattened affect'') has led researchers to investigate possible emotional or affective disorders subsequent to RHD. Several investigators have suggested that the right hemisphere plays a special role in processing emotional content and that RHD alters patients' internal emotional states (Bear, 1983; Silberman and Weingartner, 1986; Tucker, 1981).

It is possible, however, that deficits in the appreciation of emotional material are due to a cognitive, rather than to an affective, disorder. The operations involved in interpreting emo-

tional content are much the same as those involved in generating inference. Emotional tone or ''affect'' is conveyed through extralinguistic cues such as facial expression, body language, gesture, narrative cues, and the prosodic features of speech. These cues must be recognized, combined, and associated with prior experience. The following sections review the literature on emotional processing deficits and explore the issue of their basis.

Alterations of Emotional State

Evidence for an underlying emotional disorder in RHD patients stems from several sources. Gainotti (1972) explored emotional reactions of 160 RHD and LHD patients by investigating their response to failure. LHD patients generally had strong, even catastrophic, reactions, whereas RHD patients appeared to be relatively unaffected by the stress of failure. Inspired by such findings, a number of studies have investigated mood disorders in stroke patients, but the results have been conflicting.

Some studies have suggested that RHD patients with anterior lesions are ''unduly cheerful'' (''hypermania''), whereas anterior LHD patients are depressed (Robinson et al., 1984a; Robinson et al., 1984b). Other studies have found depression following stroke regardless of side of lesion (Sinyor et al., 1986). House et al. (1990) found no evidence that RHD was associated with hypermania in their sample of 73 stroke patients. Folstein et al. (1977) found that RHD patients had a syndrome of apathy and difficulty in concentration.

At this point, evidence of an association between altered internal emotional states and site of lesion following stroke is inconclusive. Indifference and ''flattened affect'' may be associated with decreased arousal (Heilman et al., 1978). That is, RHD patients may be indifferent because they are less aware of and less responsive to external stimuli, regardless of whether or not the stimuli are emotional.

Facial Expression Deficits

Comprehension of Facial Expression. Decreased arousal and attention may affect patients' responses to the nonverbal cues that signify emotional expression. Numerous studies have reported that RHD patients have difficulty interpreting facial expressions depicting emotions (Benowitz et al., 1983; Blonder et al., 1991; Borod et al., 1986; Bowers et al., 1985; Cancelliere and Kertesz, 1990; Cicone et al., 1980; DeKosky et al., 1980). It is uncertain whether these deficits represent an emotional disorder or a perceptual one. Most studies investigating the interpretation of facial expression present faces in isolation without other contextual cues to specify the emotion. The expression must thus be determined by inspection and analysis of the spatial characteristics of facial features such as how close the eyebrows are, how wide the eyes are, and the degree to which the corners of the mouth are upturned. This type of perceptual feature analysis depends on spatial or ''metric'' judgments, which may be in the province of the intact right hemisphere (Kosslyn, 1987, 1988). Furthermore, individual features must be combined with one another to arrive at an accurate judgment. Deficits in identifying emotional expression may thus arise from deficits in spatial judgment and feature integration, rather than from an emotional deficit, although the ultimate result may be an interference in emotional comprehension.

Production of Facial Expression. Studies investigating the production of nonverbal emotional expression have produced conflicting results. Borod et al. (1986) and Buck and Duffy (1981), for example, found that RHD patients were impaired relative to LHD and NBD controls in spontaneously producing emotional facial expression in response to slides depicting emotional situations. In a similar task, Mammucari et al. (1988) found no differences in emotional expression between LHD and RHD subject groups, both of which had less facial expression than NBD controls.

The effects of facial paresis were not controlled for in the above studies. In addition, it is important to recognize that reduced *comprehension* of emotional stimuli may be a factor in reduced spontaneous facial expression. For example, in the above studies, subjects' facial expressions were monitored as they observed slides and films. Presumably, their responses depended on comprehension of the stimuli as well as on the ability to translate comprehension into expression, although this variable was not analyzed.

Comprehension of Emotional Content

Comprehension of emotion has been assessed by asking patients to (*a*) match emotions depicted in stories with those depicted in scenes (Cicone et al., 1980); (*b*) answer questions in response to pictured stories that are neutral or emotional (Bloom et al., 1992); (*c*) identify the emotions depicted in pictured scenes (Cancelliere and Kertesz, 1990); and (*d*) identify the emotions depicted in sentences that describe emotions (Blonder et al., 1991). RHD patients are impaired relative to NBD controls in many of these tasks.

Evidence that a cognitive as opposed to an emotional deficit is responsible for these findings comes from a closer inspection of the tasks by which "emotional" deficits are elicited. Determining the emotional valance of situations, expressions, and narratives involves the four operations involved in inference—that is, recognition, selection, and integration of cues, and their association with prior experience. Often, determining the emotional tone of a story or scene requires a greater number of inferences than does interpreting emotionally neutral stimuli. One not only must infer the actions and overall theme but also infer the emotional response of the characters. For example, "He went into the house" is inferentially less complex than "He stole into the house."

Most studies documenting problems in inferring emotions from stimuli have not included comparable tasks designed to test subjects' capacity to infer nonemotional or neutral content (e.g., DeKosky et al., 1980; Benowitz et al., 1983; Blonder et al., 1991; Cancelliere and Kertesz, 1990; Cicone et al., 1980). Studies that have done so have produced mixed results. Ostrove et al. (1990), for example, found no significant differences in accuracy between RHD and NBD controls in a task in which subjects had to answer questions about the emotional state of the main character and what he might do next in a simple story. In fact, RHD subjects were impaired relative to controls only in response to stories with neutral (versus emotional) content.

Bloom et al. (1992) compared the number of content units produced by RHD, LHD, and NBD subjects in response to pictured story sequences, the contents of which were either neutral, spatial, or emotional. The authors found that RHD subjects had a selective deficit in producing emotional contents.

However, a look at the story sequences in each condition suggests that the stimuli were not comparable in cognitive complexity. The neutral condition depicted a familiar procedure (frying eggs). The spatial condition depicted a boy getting on a stool to take books from a shelf. There were no surprises or revisions required in analyzing the action. The emotional story depicted a girl playing with her dog, the dog getting run over, and her reaction to this event. The sequence contains surprise and requires subjects to infer emotional response as well as action. Thus, it is difficult to know if the findings relate to emotional content independent of inferential complexity.

Functionally, RHD subjects may have trouble interpreting emotional content, whether it be the expression on the face of their conversational partner or the emotional impact of what he or she is trying to express. These deficits could be the result of failure to attend to and analyze cues and problems in producing the inferences that flow from them.

Verbal Expression of Emotional Content

Most studies of the expression of emotional content involve a comprehension task, making it hard to know if subjects' impairments are based on failure to comprehend or to express emotions or both. Cimino et al. (1991) circumvented this problem by investigating the spontaneous verbal expression of emotional content. They asked RHD and NBD subjects to recall episodes from their own lives in response to a cue word. Cue words were emotional or neutral. Responses were rated by independent judges for level of emotionality and specificity. Not surprisingly, RHD responses were rated as less specific than those of NBD subjects regardless of type of cue word. Although the emotional cue words produced higher emotionality ratings than neutral cues for both groups, the RHD patients' reports were rated as significantly less emotional than those of the NBD subjects. Interjudge reliability for rating specificity of content ranged from 0.89 to 0.95. However, reliability for rating emotionality ranged from 0.61 to 0.76, which is lower than the usual standard for acceptable reliability. These differences suggest that judging the degree to which a response is emotional is not an easy task.

Impaired prosodic production in some RHD patients has also led to the impression that they have difficulty expressing emotions. This topic will be addressed in the section on prosody.

Summary

RHD patients may have problems both in interpreting and in expressing emotional content. However, it is not clear that they have an affective disorder per se. Studies investigating emotional status following stroke have produced conflicting results. Emotional "indifference" may be a component of a more general attention deficit that reduces responsiveness to the external environment. Reduced responsiveness may impair the appreciation of the extralinguistic cues from which one can infer the emotional valance of situations and narratives. In addition, perceptual impairments in spatial judgment and feature integration may contribute to impaired ability to identify emotional facial expression. These attentional, perceptual, and cognitive factors may result in an alteration of the patient's internal emotional state and, hence, create an affective disorder, but that issue remains unexplored.

Comprehension and Production of Prosody

The prosodic features of speech convey both emotional and linguistic information. Alterations in pitch, volume, duration of utterances, and duration of pause time between words create intonational patterns that add extralinguistic information to linguistic content. The moods conveyed include not only emotional states but also intents such as sarcasm and irony. RHD patients may be impaired in their appreciation and expression of these prosodic features of speech.

Initial investigations of prosodic disturbances suggested that the deficits were the outcome of an emotional disorder, and terms such as "auditory *affective* agnosia" were used to describe the problem (Heilman et al., 1975). Recent research investigating the complicated array of phenomena that may contribute to impaired prosodic processing suggests that prosodic deficits are not the result of an emotional disturbance.

Prosodic Comprehension

Most studies investigating comprehension of prosody have used a paradigm in which subjects listen to neutral sentences expressed with an emotional overlay and identify the mood conveyed by the speaker. In such studies, Heilman et al. (1975) and Tucker et al. (1977) found that RHD subjects were more impaired than LHD subjects in identifying and discriminating emotional prosody. RHD subjects have also been found to be impaired in discriminating emotions in tasks in which speech was filtered so that prosodic features remained while words did not (Denes et al., 1984; Heilman et al., 1984a; Lalande et al., 1992; Tompkins and Flowers, 1985). These results appear to point to an affective disturbance.

However, RHD subjects may also have impaired comprehension of linguistic or *nonaffective* prosody—that is, the prosodic features used to convey (*a*) different types of sentences (e.g., declarative, interrogative, or exclamatory); (*b*) different word meanings through use of emphatic stress (e.g., distinguishing "greenhouse" from "green house"); and (*c*) linguistic stress markers that can alter sentence meanings ("John wants the *red* bike" versus "*John* wants the red bike") (Bryan, 1989a; Heilman et al., 1984a; Weintraub et al., 1981). These findings suggest that RHD prosodic comprehension impairments extend to the nonaffective or propositional aspects of speech. Interestingly, even in a study on discriminating emotional prosody, Tompkins and Flowers (1985) found that most of the RHD subjects' errors occurred on discriminating nonemotional stimuli.

The cause of impaired prosodic comprehension is uncertain, but because it extends to nonemotional material, it is unlikely the result of an affective disorder. It may be due to a deficit in detecting changes in tonal patterns. Tompkins and Flowers (1985), for example, found that RHD subjects with impairments in prosodic comprehension were also impaired relative to LHD and NBD subjects on a tonal memory task. And Tompkins (1991) found that RHD subjects with poor tonal memory scores had slower reaction times in judging prosodically conveyed moods than other RHD subjects. In a series of psychoacoustic tasks, Robin et al. (1987) found that RHD was more closely associated with impaired pitch discrimination and matching than with impaired temporal processing (i.e., discriminating auditory gaps between stimuli).

Impaired attention may be another factor in prosodic comprehension deficits. The tasks used to assess prosodic comprehension make particular demands on attention. In many studies, subjects must listen to sentences but dissociate meaning from tone, forcing them to divide their attention in the performance of a rather unnatural task. Considering that neglect is associated with attention deficits, it is interesting to note that RHD subjects with neglect have difficulty with such tasks (Heilman et al., 1975; Tompkins and Flowers, 1985; Tucker et al., 1977), yet those without neglect may not (Schlanger et al., 1976).

Prosodic judgments by RHD subjects may improve when the task becomes less difficult. Tompkins (1991) found that increased semantic redundancy in the form of a word suggesting a given emotion improved accuracy of LHD, RHD, and NBD subjects in judging the mood conveyed in a short paragraph. The redundancy also improved RHD subjects' prosodic judgments of neutral sentences that followed the paragraphs. Improvements in response to easier tasks support a cognitive rather than an emotional basis for impaired prosodic comprehension.

The extent to which patients suffer from difficulty in prosodic comprehension in everyday life is not clear. In ongoing conversation, it is impossible to separate the factors that may cause problems in interpreting conversational remarks. It may be that impaired prosodic processing is a contributing factor in that prosody represents just one more aspect of the overall context within which the message is contained. Laboratory efforts to investigate prosodic deficits by their nature attempt to control for the variables that operate in natural conversation. RHD subjects are impaired in tasks designed to assess comprehension of prosody when it is devoid of linguistic content, and in tasks in which prosody is incongruent with linguistic content. These tasks force patients to select and detect relevant features, to attend to two things at once, and to ignore one thing while attending to another. Thus, it is uncertain whether prosodic impairments in the laboratory reflect true deficits in processing prosodic aspects of conversations. It is likely, however, that some RHD patients do fail to attend to these important extralinguistic cues. The severity of the deficit may vary with the level of redundancy of contextual information specifying the intended meaning of the speaker.

Prosodic Production

The clinical impression of flattened affect accompanied by monotone conversational speech in some RHD patients led to studies investigating the possibility of impaired prosodic production. Production of prosody, both emotional and linguistic, has been tested by asking subjects to repeat or read neutral sentences with a specified emotional tone, to imitate the prosodic production of a speaker, and to spontaneously produce emphatic stress. Prosodic productions have been analyzed perceptually and acoustically. The findings from these studies, particularly those using acoustic analysis, have been mixed, and the issue of whether RHD patients as a group have impaired prosodic production remains unresolved.

Studies using perceptual ratings of judges have found RHD impairments in producing emotional prosody (Ross and Mesulam, 1979; Tucker et al., 1977) and linguistic stress (Behrens, 1988; Weintraub et al., 1981). The problem with perceptual judgments is that there may be great variability among ratings. For example, in preparing stimuli for a study of prosodic perception, Tompkins (1991) noted that five judges agreed on the emotional tone of only 64 of 192 sentences produced by three NBD speakers.

Acoustic measures may be more reliable, but there is disagreement in the literature about which measures to use and about the existence of RHD impairments. Productions are judged by analysis of the speech wave relative to rate, amplitude, and fundamental frequency. An early acoustic study (Kent and Rosenbek, 1982) found that RHD patients had a fast rate, reduced acoustic contrast, and reduced energy in frequencies above 500 Hz. Behrens (1988) found that at the word level, RHD and NBD subjects did not differ significantly in their ability to convey linguistic stress, although RHD subjects used fewer of the cues used by NBD subjects to do so (e.g., amplitude, duration, and fundamental frequency changes).

At the sentence level, Shapiro and Danly (1985) found that RHD subjects with anterior and central damage had less pitch variation and a reduced intonational range in expressing both linguistic and emotional prosody. They found that RHD patients with right posterior damage had exaggerated pitch variation and intonational range (hyperprosody). The finding of hyperprosody in the RHD posterior group was challenged by Colsher et al. (1987), who suggested that the abnormal pitch variance (both excessive and reduced) might be related to differences in the mean pitch levels of the two groups. They suggested that mean pitch should be divided into the measure of variability to normalize or "relativize" it. Reevaluation of the Shapiro and Danly (1985) data in such a way resulted in a reversal of the original findings. That is, anterior patients had near-normal variability of pitch, while posterior patients had slightly reduced variability (Colsher et al., 1987). Thus, even within a study, methods of measurement can affect outcome.

Behrens (1989) also looked at sentence-level prosodic productions that signaled different sentences types and found that RHD subjects differed from NBD controls in several, but not all, measures of overall pitch contour and pattern. Finally, in a sentence repetition task, Ryalls et al. (1987) found no significant differences between their RHD and NBD subjects in mean fundamental frequency, frequency range, overall sentence duration, and several other complicated frequency measures.

Interestingly, despite their failure to find differences, Ryalls et al. (1987) noted that when listening to the tapes of their RHD subjects, they thought they heard deviations from a normal speech pattern—deviations that their acoustic measures did not demonstrate. The changes they thought they heard were changes about which some of their subjects complained (i.e., reduction in pitch range and in volume). Subjects even said that their voices sometimes felt "hoarse" and "strangled." Kent and Rosenbek (1982) found that their RHD patients had a tendency toward indistinct articulation and mild to moderate hypernasality—measures not addressed in most acoustic studies. These impressions suggest that impaired prosody may be part of a motor execution disorder (e.g., dysarthria) rather than a deficit at the level of motor planning.

Summary

Prosodic comprehension and production deficits may occur subsequent to RHD. Prosodic comprehension impairments are not restricted to emotional prosody and may include linguistic or propositional prosodic deficits. Whether prosodic compre-

hension deficits found in the laboratory translate into prosodic deficits in natural conversations is not clear. Prosodic comprehension deficits may be related (a) to impaired tonal perception and (b) to attentional deficits in response to tasks designed to isolate prosodic from linguistic information.

Prosodic production impairments may also exist in some RHD patients. Clinical impressions of impaired prosody have been difficult to quantify. It is possible that dysarthria plays a role in prosodic production of some RHD patients, although this possibility has not been formally addressed in studies of prosodic disturbance.

Effect of Extralinguistic Deficits on Communication

Deficits in the use and appreciation of extralinguistic cues may interfere with accurate interpretation of narrative content, emotional valance, conversational exchange, and discourse production. These extralinguistic deficits are likely the cognitive outcome of the attentional and perceptual deficits specified earlier in this chapter. Decreased arousal and impaired selective attention may impair the appreciation of key contextual cues— verbal, visual, and prosodic. Reduced attention may make the effort required for generating alternative meanings and revising original interpretations difficult. Impaired organizational abilities at the perceptual level may be associated with impairments in organizing narratives, such that patients respond to piecemeal aspects of communicative events rather than integrating them with one another. Deficits in integration may affect revision abilities. When they occur, these deficits are usually pervasive, crossing the visual and verbal modalities. Together, such deficits may decrease patients' capacity to generate inferences about the intended meaning of communicative events and may interfere in their ability to express their own intended meaning efficiently.

Interference Versus Loss

Aphasia is generally conceptualized not as a loss of language but as an interference in its efficient operation. Similarly, an inference deficit may be considered an interference or impairment in the ability to generate inferences, rather than a loss of the ability. That is, inference deficits may surface only in tasks that tax attentional and cognitive capacities, and they may be present to different degrees among patients or not present at all.

Indeed, in a task designed to investigate the ability to generate inferences from simple premises such as "The bird is in the cage" (Premise 1) and "The cage is under the table" (Premise 2), RHD and NBD subjects did not differ in their ability to arrive at the inference the "bird is under the table" (McDonald and Wales, 1986). Like NBD subjects, RHD patients were able not only to store the first two premises verbatim but also to generate simple inferences based on the meaning of the stored information.

RHD patients may not experience difficulty with the structure of simple stories and procedural discourse (e.g., explaining activities such as how to fry an egg) (Ostrove et al., 1990; Rehak et al., 1992b; Roman et al., 1987). They also may not experience difficulty when the text is very explicit and very redundant (Brookshire and Nicholas, 1984; Stachowiak et al., 1977; Tompkins, 1991).

Effortful interpretations have been measured in several ways, and RHD subjects have been found to be more impaired when implied meaning is more difficult to ascertain. Myers and Brookshire (1994), for example, found that RHD subjects were less impaired in producing accurate concepts in response to pictures that contained simple inferences compared with those that were inferentially complex. Hough (1990) found that RHD subjects were less accurate and identified fewer story themes when the central theme was presented in an unexpected format (i.e., at the end of a narrative rather than at the beginning). Tompkins (1991) suggested that the better-than-expected performance of RHD subjects on judging the mood of an orally presented story may have been due to methodological factors that decreased the cognitive burden of the task (i.e., extensive pretask instruction and practice).

As these studies suggest, RHD communication disorders may occur only in situations where patients' attentional perceptual, and cognitive resources are taxed. Hence, the observation that in simple interactions where meaning is explicit, RHD patients may appear to have normal conversational skills. In more complex exchanges, however, they may have problems inferring intended meaning from contextual cues and in producing efficient narrative expression.

Finally, the issue of severity is important. RHD patients differ from each other in severity of deficit, which may affect the degree to which they demonstrate communicative deficits. As yet, there are no tests that measure severity of deficit for all of the extralinguistic deficits that may affect RHD patients.

Evaluation of Extralinguistic Deficits

Extralinguistic deficits represent the heart of communication deficits associated with RHD. Not every RHD patient will have communication impairments, so the primary goal in evaluation is establishing the presence or absence of deficits. If the patient has communication impairments, their severity and nature should be documented. Commercially available assessment tools (Bryan, 1989b; Burns et al., 1985) can be used in conjunction with some of the informal approaches described below.

Patient Interview

The purpose of the interview is to establish rapport and to obtain a sample of patients' conversational speech that can be assessed for content and structure. Establishing rapport with RHD patients is particularly crucial for several reasons. First, they may not recognize or may deny their problems. They may wonder why they are seeing a speech-language clinician when their speech sounds fine to them. Second, families often support patients' denial unwittingly by exhibiting their relief that the patient "can talk." If patients have communication problems, families may not be immediately aware of them. One way of addressing denial is to explain in the initial interview that all stroke patients are tested for communication deficits, to agree with patients that they may not have any problems, and to explain that communication consists of more than speech and language.

Another reason patients may be resistant is that they *are aware* of some of their deficits (perhaps they have trouble following TV shows or have noticed problems in reading or in following complex conversations). They may be afraid to admit to these problems in the face of family relief that they can talk (and hence "do not have communication problems"). They may fear they are mentally unbalanced or generally confused. Their fears can be allayed by clinician assurances that the communication difficulties may be due to specific causes that have nothing to do with their mental stability. The clinician can help patients overcome denial by demonstrating some specific problems they may have and by explaining that help is available. In the author's experience, fear is as powerful a factor as denial in inhibiting rehabilitative progress. Explaining and demonstrating problems to the patient can decrease fear, make problems seem more manageable, and increase insight and cooperation.

The second goal of the interview is to obtain a sample of conversational speech on audio- or videotape that can be reviewed for structure and content. Questions should address patients' orientation, their assessment of their problems, their daily activities, something about their work history or personal lives, and their plans for the future. The interview thus addresses memory, orientation, and insight. Responses can be assessed for the degree to which they observe pragmatic rules of conversation (i.e., turn taking, listener burden, etc.) and the degree to which content is informative, organized, and efficient.

Picture Description

A pictured scene that tells a story or depicts a situation can be used to elicit narrative discourse for the evaluation of extralinguistic deficits. Commercially available pictures such as the "Cookie Theft" picture from the Boston Diagnostic Aphasia Examination (Goodglass and Kaplan, 1983) can be used. A list of concepts for that picture generated by NBD subjects was collected by Yorkston and Beukelman (1980) and broken down into "interpretive" and "literal" concepts by Myers (1979). An interpretive score is arrived at by dividing the total number of concepts by the number of interpretive concepts. As a guideline, Myers and Linebaugh (1980) found the mean percent of interpretive concepts was 26.5 for a sample of RHD patients and 48.9 for NBD subjects. The concepts are listed in Appendix 28.1, and sample responses and scores are provided in Appendix 28.2. This scoring system represents only one method of scoring narrative verbal output. It captures only some of the potential deficits, and because the concepts are those mentioned by a small number of NBD subjects in a single study, it does not represent all the concepts a patient might mention. Its advantages are that the concepts are data based and that the scoring system has been found to establish differences between NBD and RHD patients in several studies. It can be adapted as clinicians see fit and used during treatment as a probe task to measure progress in therapy.

A picture description task enables the clinician to quickly assess patients' abilities to attend to and interpret contextual or extralinguistic information. It has several advantages over asking patients to retell stories: (*a*) It elicits a more spontaneous production; (*b*) it does not involve memory; and (*c*) concepts missed by the patient can be pointed out by directing the patient's attention to the visually present contextual cues. Transcribed picture descriptions can also be evaluated by techniques of discourse analysis (see Sherratt and Penn, 1990; Urayse et al., 1991) or other types of concept analysis (see Nicholas and Brookshire, 1993).

Treatment of Extralinguistic Deficits

As discussed in the section on "Nonlinguistic Deficits," stimulating recovery of function may be addressed by working directly on attention and neglect, since it is presumed these are some of the underlying causes of extralinguistic impairments. In general, treatment for extralinguistic deficits should address deficits in the four stages of generating inferences mentioned earlier. The goal of most of the tasks described below is compensation for deficits as opposed to stimulating recovery of function. Most of the tasks involve teaching patients new strategies for responding to extralinguistic information and generating inferences. That is, a clinician may train patients to consciously analyze what was once apprehended more automatically by teaching them to *attend to cues,* to *select relevant cues,* to *integrate relevant cues with one another,* and to *associate cues with prior experience.* By so doing, one might improve patients' ability to understand what is meant from what is said and to improve the degree to which verbal expression is informative.

There are no published studies on the efficacy of a given treatment technique for RHD communication deficits. There is hardly agreement about the nature of the deficits themselves. Thus, clinicians must be creative in designing tasks and evaluating their impact on communication. A good source of tasks is the research literature from which we have gleaned descriptions of RHD deficits. What follows are some suggestions based on that literature and on the author's clinical experience with patients who have extralinguistic deficits. This is not intended to be an exhaustive list of tasks but rather some examples of directions to follow in designing therapy techniques and materials. It is assumed that clinicians will use the techniques mentioned elsewhere in this book to establish cuing hierarchies and to probe patient progress. Tasks designed to increase patient abilities to generate alternative meanings and integrate information are considered useful in increasing the amount of informative content in patients' verbal expression. Treatment of emotional deficits can be addressed in these same tasks if one adopts the position that emotional deficits stem from the same source as narrative-level deficits. Evaluation and treatment of prosodic deficits are discussed separately.

Generating Alternative Meanings

Any task that requires patients to demonstrate their knowledge of nonliteral meanings can be used to improve ability to generate alternate meanings. Patients can be asked to interpret metaphoric or idiomatic expressions by matching them to pictures depicting literal or metaphoric interpretations (see Winner and Gardner, 1977). Or they may be asked to explain the events in simple two-sentence narratives in which the events turn on an idiomatic expression or an indirect request (see Myers and Linebaugh, 1981). It is not necessarily a good idea to ask patients to explain or define idioms, since this can be a difficult task for NBD adults (Myers and Mackisack, 1986).

Patients can also be asked to generate members of uncommon categories (see Diggs and Basili, 1987; Hough et al., 1994). They may be asked to specify the ways in which objects are similar or dissimilar, to group words according to their connotative and denotative meanings, or simply to express alternate meanings for single words.

Table 28.1.
Noun Phrase Categories

Pictured accurate	A noun phrase that accurately refers to a person or object depicted in the picture
Pictured wrong	A noun phrase that inaccurately or imprecisely refers to a person or object in the picture
Inferred accurate	A noun phrase that refers to a person, object, or abstract concept whose function or meaning is accurately inferred from the context of the picture
Inferred wrong	A noun phrase that refers to a person, object, or abstract concept whose function or meaning is inaccurately inferred from the context of the picture

From Myers, P. S. (1992). The effect of visual and inferential complexity on the verbal expression of non-brain-damaged and right-hemisphere-damaged adults. Doctoral dissertation, University of Minnesota. *Dissertation Abstracts International, 53,* 03B.

Impairments in revising assumptions may be treated in tasks that require patients to integrate new narrative information such as choosing the correct punchline for a joke or the correct ending to a story. Stimuli similar to those created by Brownell et al. (1986) and by Kaplan et al. (1990) can be used to assess patients' ability to use contextual information to reinterpret simple stories.

Integrating Narrative Content

The capacity to structure narrative content can be addressed by asking patients to organize printed sentences into a story or pictures into a logical sequence. Stimuli can vary in number of details and in how explicit or implicit the content is.

Pictured scenes can be used as stimuli in treating problems in interpreting and integrating narrative discourse. The stimuli can vary in level of inference required from simple action pictures to more inferential pictures that contain less explicit, and even emotional, material. Patients can be asked to "tell what is happening" in the picture, and responses can be scored for comprehension of content (theme) and amount of informative content. Suggestions for quantifying the level of informative content include counting the number of "content units" as described in the literature (see Nicholas and Brookshire, 1993); using other methods of discourse analysis; or counting the number and type of noun phrases according to the operational definitions in Table 28.1.

Problems in scene interpretation can be addressed by helping the patient to analyze the picture—that is, by overt instruction for what was once a more automatic task. Patients can be asked to do the following:

1. Label the items in the picture.
2. Specify the relevant or significant items.
3. Point to items that are related.
4. Explain the relationships among items.

Stimuli for this type of task may be pictured or in the form of a narrative or story. Stories should be printed to avoid taxing memory and to avoid arguments about story contents.

Another way to help patients structure and integrate narrative expression is by asking them to answer divergent questions on current topics of interest (e.g., ''Do you think there should be tighter gun control laws?''). Answers can be tape recorded, transcribed, and rated according to how integrated, complete, efficient, related, and coherent the answer is. Problems in each of these areas can then be worked on separately.

Prosodic Deficits

Evaluation. Prosodic comprehension can be assessed by asking patients to interpret the emotional content of neutral sentences or by asking them to distinguish between words with varying emphatic stress. In the former task, a tape of sentences such as ''The boy came home'' can be read with varying types of emotional prosody such as surprise, sadness, or happiness, and patients can be asked to identify the emotion contained in the phrase. For linguistic stress, the clinician can ask the patient to point to a picture that represents a given word such as ''white house'' versus ''Whitehouse.''

Prosodic production is difficult to assess. For perceptual judgments, clinicians must rely on subjective judgments of others, which can be cumbersome and potentially unreliable. If the clinician is convinced that such testing is necessary, he or she can ask patients to read neutral sentences of the type described above with a specified emotional overlay. The recorded sentences can be played for judges who identify the emotion the patient was attempting to express. Acoustic measures are more objective but may not be available to clinicians. And, as noted, the literature is not clear on the best acoustic measures to use.

Treatment. Treatment for prosodic deficits is not considered by the author to be a priority in patient management, since these deficits are probably the least of the patient's communication problems. Training comprehension of other contextual cues is likely to be a more effective way of treating deficits in prosody. In addition, since the source of prosodic production deficits is uncertain (motor planning versus motor execution), treatment may be a waste of client effort.

FUTURE DIRECTIONS

It is hoped that the description of deficits and the framework in which they have been placed in this chapter will encourage clinicians to design innovative therapy techniques. Future directions for research include (*a*) furthering our understanding of the connections between nonlinguistic and extralinguistic deficits; (*b*) development of better assessment measures; (*c*) studies on prognosis and recovery patterns subsequent to RHD; and (*d*) studies on the efficacy of treatment techniques that include increasing our knowledge of the cues that facilitate performance.

Acknowledgment

The author would like to acknowledge the helpful comments made by Shelley Brundage and Joe Duffy on earlier versions of this chapter.

References

Adamovich, B. L., and Brooks, R. L. (1981). A diagnostic protocol to assess the communication deficits of patients with right hemisphere damage. In R. H. Brookshire (Ed.), *Clinical aphasiology: Conference proceedings* (pp. 244–253). Minneapolis, MN: BRK.

Albert, M. L. (1973). A simple test of visual neglect. *Neurology, 23,* 658–664.

Archibald, T. M., and Wepman, J. M. (1968). Language disturbances and nonverbal cognitive performance in eight patients following injury to the right hemisphere. *Brain, 91,* 117–130.

Baines, K. A., and Robinson, R. L. (1991). *Exercises for right hemisphere rehabilitation: Attentional processing and visual reorganization.* Austin, TX: Pro-Ed.

Bear, D. M. (1983). Hemispheric specialization and the neurology of emotion. *Archives of Neurology, 40,* 195–202.

Behrens, S. J. (1988). The role of the right hemisphere in the production of linguistic stress. *Brain and Language, 33,* 104–127.

Behrens, S. J. (1989). Characterizing sentence intonation in a right hemisphere-damaged population. *Brain and Language, 37,* 181–200.

Benowitz, L. I., Bear, D. M., Rosenthal, R., Mesulam, M. M., Zaidel, E., and Sperry, R. W. (1983). Hemispheric specialization in nonverbal communication. *Cortex, 19,* 5–11.

Benowitz, L. I., Moya, K. L., and Levine, D. N. (1990). Impaired verbal reasoning and constructional apraxia in subjects with right hemisphere damage. *Neuropsychologia, 28,* 231–241.

Benson D. F., and Barton, M. I. (1970). Disturbances in constructional ability. *Cortex, 6,* 19–46.

Benton, A. L., Varney, N. R., and Hamsher, K. (1978). Visuospatial judgment: A clinical test. *Archives of Neurology, 35,* 364–367.

Bihrle, A. M., Brownell, H. H., and Powelson, J. (1986). Comprehension of humorous and nonhumorous materials by left and right brain-damaged patients. *Brain and Cognition, 5,* 399–411.

Bisiach, E., Capitani, E., Luzzatti, C., and Perani, D. (1981). Brain and the conscious representation of outside reality. *Neuropsychologia, 19,* 543–551.

Bisiach, E. Luzzatti, C., and Perani, D. (1979). Unilateral neglect, representational schema and consciousness. *Brain, 102,* 609–618.

Blonder, L. X., Bowers, D., and Heilman, K. M. (1991). The role of the right hemisphere in emotional communication. *Brain, 114,* 1115–1127.

Bloom, R. L., Borod, J. C., Obler, L. K., and Gerstman, L. J. (1992). Impact of emotional content on discourse production in patients with unilateral brain damage. *Brain and Language, 42,* 153–164.

Borod, J. C., Koff, E., Lorch, M. P., and Nicholas, M. (1986). The expression and perception of facial emotion in brain-damaged patients. *Neuropsychologia, 24,* 169–180.

Bowers, D., Bauer, R. M., Coslett, H. B., and Heilman, K. M. (1985). Processing of faces by patients with unilateral hemisphere lesions. *Brain and Cognition, 4,* 258–272.

Brookshire, R. H., and Nicholas, L. E. (1984). Comprehension of directly and indirectly stated main ideas and details in discourse by brain-damaged and non-brain-damaged listeners. *Brain and Language, 21,* 21–36.

Brownell, H. H. (1988). The neuropsychology of narrative comprehension. *Aphasiology, 2,* 247–250.

Brownell, H. H., Michel, D., Powelson, J., and Gardner, H. (1983). Surprise but not coherence: Sensitivity to verbal humor in right-hemisphere patients. *Brain and Language, 18,* 20–27.

Brownell, H. H., Potter, H. H., Bihrle, A. M., and Gardner, H. (1986). Inference deficits in right brain-damaged patients. *Brain and Language, 27,* 310–321.

Brownell, H. H., Potter, H. H., Michelow, D., and Gardner, H. (1984). Sensitivity to lexical denotation and connotation in brain damaged patients: A double dissociation? *Brain and Language, 22,* 253–265.

Brownell, H. H., Simpson, T. L., Bihrle, A. M., Potter, H. H., and Gardner, H. (1990). Appreciation of metaphoric alternative word meanings by left and right brain-damaged patients. *Neuropsychologia, 28,* 375–383.

Bryan, K. L. (1989a). Language prosody and the right hemisphere. *Aphasiology, 3,* 285–299.

Bryan, K. L. (1989b). *The Right Hemisphere Language Battery.* Leicester, England: Far Communications.

Bub, D., Audet, T., and LeCours, A. R. (1990). Re-evaluating the effect of unilateral brain damage on simple reaction time to auditory stimulation. *Cortex, 26,* 227–237.

Buck, R., and Duffy, R. J. (1981). Nonverbal communication of affect in brain-damaged patients. *Cortex, 6,* 351–362.

Burns, M. S., Halper, A. S., Mogil, S. I. (1985). *Clinical management of right hemisphere dysfunction.* Rockville, MD: Aspen Publications.

Cancelliere, A. E. B., and Kertesz, A. (1990). Lesion localization in acquired deficits of emotional expression and comprehension. *Brain and Cognition, 13,* 133–147.

Cappa, S. F., Papagno, C., and Vallar, G. (1990). Language and verbal memory after right hemispheric stroke: A clinical-CT scan study. *Neuropsychologia, 28,* 503–509.

Cavalli, M., De Renzi, E., Faglioni, P., and Vitale, A. (1981). Impairment of right brain-damaged patients on a linguistic cognitive task. *Cortex, 17,* 545–556.

Cicone, M., Wapner, W., and Gardner, H. (1980). Sensitivity to emotional expressions and situations in organic patients. *Cortex, 16,* 145–158.

Cimino, C. R., Verfaellie, M., Bowers, D., and Heilman, K. M. (1991). Autobiographical memory: Influence of right hemisphere damage on emotionality and specificity. *Brain and Cognition, 15,* 106–118.

Colsher, P. L., Cooper, W. E., and Graff-Radford, N. (1987). Intonational variability in the speech of right-hemisphere damaged patients. *Brain and Language, 32,* 379–383.

Coslett, H. B., Bowers, D., and Heilman, K. M. (1987). Reduction in cerebral activation after right hemisphere stroke. *Neurology, 37,* 957–962.

Dagge, M., and Hartje, W. (1985). Influence of contextual complexity on the processing of cartoons by patients with unilateral lesions. *Cortex, 21,* 607–616.

Damasio, A. R. (1985). Disorders of complex visual processing: Agnosias, achromatopsia, Balint's syndrome, and related difficulties of orientation and construction. In M. Mesulam (Ed.), *Principles of behavioral neurology* (pp. 259–288). Philadelphia, PA: F. A. Davis.

Deal, J., Deal, L., Wertz, R. W., Kitselman, K., and Dwyer, C. (1979). Right hemisphere PICA percentiles: Some speculations about aphasia. In R. H. Brookshire (Ed.), *Clinical aphasiology: Conference proceedings* (pp. 30–37). Minneapolis, MN: BRK.

Dee, H. L., and Van Allen, M. W. (1973). Speed of decision-making processes in patients with unilateral cerebral disease. *Archives of Neurology, 28,* 163–166.

DeKosky, S. T., Heilman, K. M., Bowers, D., and Valenstein, E. (1980). Recognition and discrimination of emotional faces and pictures. *Brain and Language, 9,* 206–214.

Delis, D., Wapner, W., Gardner, H., and Moses, J. (1983). The contribution of the right hemisphere to the organization of paragraphs. *Cortex, 19,* 43–50.

Denes, G., Caldognetto, E. M., Semenza, C., Vagges, K., and Zettin, M. (1984). Discrimination and identification of emotions in human voice by brain-damaged subjects. *Acta Neurologica Scandinavia, 69,* 154–162.

Denny-Brown, D., Meyer, J. S., and Horenstein, S. (1952). The significance of perceptual rivalry resulting from parietal lesion. *Brain, 75,* 433–471.

DeRenzi, E., Faglione, P., and Previdi, P. (1977). Spatial memory and hemispheric locus of lesion. *Cortex, 13,* 43–50.

DeRenzi, E., Scotti, G., and Spinnler, H. (1969). Perceptual and associative disorders of visual recognition. *Neurology, 19,* 634–642.

DeRenzi, E., and Spinnler, H. (1966). Visual recognition in patients with unilateral cerebral disease. *Journal of Nervous and Mental Disease, 142,* 515–525.

DeRenzi, E., and Vignolo, L. A. (1962). The Token Test: A sensitive test to detect receptive disturbances in aphasics. *Brain, 85,* 665–678.

Diggs, C., and Basili, A. G. (1987). Verbal expression of right cerebrovascular accident patients: Convergent and divergent language. *Brain and Language, 30,* 130–146.

Eisenson, J. (1962). Language and intellectual modifications associated with right cerebral damage. *Language and Speech, 5,* 49–53.

Farah, M. J., Wong, A. B., Monheit, M. A., and Morrow, L. A. (1989). Parietal lobe mechanisms of spatial attention: Modality-specific or supramodal? *Neuropsychologia, 27,* 461–470.

Foldi, N. S. (1987). Appreciation of pragmatic interpretation of indirect commands: Comparison of right and left hemisphere brain-damaged patients. *Brain and Language, 31,* 88–108.

Folstein, M. R., Maiberger, R., and McHugh, P. R. (1977). Mood disorder as a specific complication of stroke. *Journal of Neurology, Neurosurgery and Psychiatry, 40,* 1018–1020.

Gainotti, G. (1972). Emotional behavior and hemispheric side of lesion. *Cortex, 8,* 41–55.

Gainotti, G., Caltagirone, C., and Miceli (1979). Semantic disorders of auditory language comprehension in right brain-damaged patients. *Journal of Psycholinguistic Research, 8,* 13–20.

Gainotti, G., Caltagirone, C., Miceli, G., and Masullo, C. (1981). Selective semantic-lexical impairment of language comprehension in right brain-damaged patients. *Brain and Language, 13,* 201–211.

Gainotti, G., D'Erme, P., and DeBonis, C. (1989). Components of visual attention disrupted in unilateral neglect. In J. W. Brown (Ed.), *Neuropsychology of visual perception* (pp. 123–144). Hillsdale, NJ: Lawrence Erlbaum.

Gainotti, G., D'Erme, P., Monteleone, D., and Silveri, M. C. (1986). Mechanisms of unilateral spatial neglect in relation to laterality of cerebral lesions. *Brain, 109,* 599–612.

Gardner, H. (1975). *The shattered mind.* New York: Knoph.

Gardner, H., and Denes, G. (1973). Connotative judgements by aphasic patients on a pictorial adaptation of the semantic differential. *Cortex, 9,* 183–196.

Gardner, H., Ling, P. K., Flamm, L., and Silverman, J. (1975). Comprehension and appreciation of humorous material following brain damage. *Brain, 98,* 399–412.

Goodglass, H., and Kaplan, E. (1983). *The Boston Diagnostic Aphasia Examination.* Philadelphia, PA: Lea & Febiger.

Griffiths, K., and Cook, M. (1986). Attribute processing in patients with graphical copying disability. *Neuropsychologia, 24,* 371–383.

Halligan, P. W., Manning, L., and Marshall, J. C. (1990). Individual variation in line bisection: A study of four patients with right hemisphere damage and normal controls. *Neuropsychologia, 28,* 1043–1051.

Halligan, P. W., and Marshall, J. C. (1988). How long is a piece of string? A study of line bisection in a case of visual neglect. *Cortex, 24,* 321–328.

Hecaen, H., and Assal, G. (1970). A comparison of constructive deficits following right and left hemisphere lesions. *Neuropsychologia, 8,* 289–303.

Heilman, K. M., Bowers, D., Coslett, H. B., Whelan, H., and Watson, R. T. (1985). Directional hypokinesia: Prolonged reaction times for leftward movements in patients with right hemisphere lesions and neglect. *Neurology, 35,* 855–859.

Heilman, K. M., Bowers, D., Speedie, L., and Coslett, H. B. (1984a). Comprehension of affective and nonaffective prosody. *Neurology, 34,* 917–921.

Heilman, K. M., Scholes, R., and Watson, R. T. (1975). Auditory affective agnosia. *Journal of Neurology, Neurosurgery and Psychiatry, 38,* 69–72.

Heilman, K. M., Schwartz, H. D., and Watson, R. T. (1978). Hypo-arousal in patients with the neglect syndrome and emotional indifference. *Neurology, 28,* 229–232.

Heilman, K. M., Valenstein, E., and Watson, R. T. (1984b). Neglect and related disorders. *Seminars in Neurology, 4,* 209–219.

Heilman, K. M., Watson, R. T., Valenstein, E., and Damasio, A. (1983). Localization of lesions in neglect. In A. Kertesz (Ed.), *Localization in neuropsychology* (pp. 471–492). New York: Academic Press.

Hier, H., and Kaplan, J., (1980). Verbal comprehension deficits after right hemisphere damage. *Applied Psycholinguistics, 1,* 279–294.

Hirst, W., LeDoux, J., and Stein, S. (1984). Constraints on the processing of indirect speech acts: Evidence from aphasiology. *Brain and Language, 23,* 26–33.

Horner, J., Massey, E. W., Woodruff, W. W., Chase, K. N., and Dawson, D. V. (1989). Task-dependent neglect: Computed tomography size and locus correlations. *Journal of Neurological Rehabilitation, 3,* 7–13.

Hough, M. (1990). Narrative comprehension in adults with right and left hemisphere brain-damage: Theme organization. *Brain and Language, 38,* 253–277.

Hough, M. S., May, M. J., and DeMarco, S. (1994). Categorization skills in right hemisphere brain-damage for common and goal-derived categories. In M. Lemme (Ed.), *Clinical aphasiology* (Vol. 22). Austin, TX: Pro-Ed.

House, A., Dennis, M., Warlow, C., Hawton, K., and Molyneux, A. (1990). Mood disorders after stroke and their relation to lesion location. *Brain, 113,* 1113–1129.

Howes, D., and Boller, F. (1975). Simple reaction time: Evidence for focal impairment from lesions in the right hemisphere. *Brain, 98,* 317–332.

Huber, W., and Gleber, J. (1982). Linguistic and nonlinguistic processing of narrative in aphasia. *Brain and Language, 16,* 1–18.

Humphries, G. W., and Riddoch, M. J. (1984). Routes to object constancy: Implications from neurological impairments of object constancy. *Quarterly Journal of Experimental Psychology, 36A,* 385–415.

Joanette, Y., Goulet P., Ska, B., and Nespoulous, J-L. (1986). Informative content of narrative discourse in right-brain-damaged right-handers. *Brain and Language, 29,* 81–105.

Joanette, Y., Lecours, A. R., Lepage, Y., and Lamoureux, M. (1983). Language in right-handers with right-hemisphere lesions: A preliminary study including anatomical, genetic, and social factors. *Brain and Language, 20,* 217–248.

Kaczmarek, B. L. J. (1984). Neurolinguistic analysis of verbal utterances in patients with focal lesions of the frontal lobes. *Brain and Language, 21,* 52–58.

Kaplan, J., Brownell, H., Jacobs, J. R., and Gardner, H. (1990). The effects of right hemisphere damage on the pragmatic interpretation of conversational remarks. *Brain and Language, 38,* 315–333.

Kent, R. D., and Rosenbek, J. C. (1982). Prosodic disturbance and neurologic lesion. *Brain and Language, 15,* 259–291.

Kertesz, A. (1983). Right-hemisphere lesions in constructional apraxia and visuospatial deficit. In A. Kertesz (Ed.), *Localization in neuropsychology* (pp. 445–470). New York: Academic Press.

Kim, Y., Morrow, L., Passafieume, D., and Boller, F. (1984). Visuoperceptual and visuomotor abilities and locus of lesion. *Neuropsychologia, 22,* 177–185.

Kosslyn, S. M. (1987). Seeing and imagining in the cerebral hemispheres: A computational approach. *Psychological Review, 94,* 148–175.

Kosslyn, S. M. (1988). Aspects of a cognitive neuroscience of mental imagery. *Science, 240,* 1621–1626.

Lalande, S., Braun, C. M. J., Carlebois, N., and Whitaker, H. A. (1992). Effects of right and left hemisphere cerebrovascular lesions on discrimination of prosodic and semantic aspects of affect in sentences. *Brain and Language, 42,* 165–186.

Layman, S., and Green, E. (1988). The effect of stroke on object recognition. *Brain and Cognition, 7,* 87–114.

Mack, J. L., and Levine, R. N. (1981). The basis of visual constructive disability in patients with unilateral cerebral lesions. *Cortex, 17,* 512–532.

Mackisack, E. L., Myers, P. S., and Duffy, J. R. (1987). Verbosity and labeling behavior: The performance of right hemisphere and non-brain-damaged adults on an inferential picture description task. In R. H. Brookshire (Ed.), *Clinical aphasiology* (Vol. 17, pp. 143–151). Minneapolis, MN: BRK.

Magnussen, S., Johnsen, T., and Reinvang, I. (1987). Interaction between local and global visual orientation signals in subjects with unilateral brain lesions. *Neuropsychologia, 25,* 989–993.

Mammucari, A., Caltagrione, C., Ekman, P., Friesen, W., Gainotti, G., Pizza-miglio, L., and Zoccolotti, P. (1988). Spontaneous facial expression of emotions in brain-damaged patients. *Cortex, 24,* 521–533.

Mark, V. W., Kooistra, C. A., and Heilman, K. M. (1988). Hemispatial neglect affected by non-neglected stimuli. *Neurology, 38,* 1207–1211.

Marshall, J. C., and Halligan, P. W. (1989). When right goes left: An investigation of line bisection in a case of visual neglect. *Cortex, 25,* 503–515.

McDonald, S., and Wales, R. (1986). An investigation of the ability to process inferences in language following right hemisphere brain damage. *Brain and Language, 29,* 68–80.

McNeil, M. R., and Prescott, T. E. (1978). *The Revised Token Test.* Baltimore, MD: University Park Press.

Mesulam, M. (1981). A cortical network for directed attention and unilateral neglect. *Annals of Neurology, 10,* 307–325.

Mesulam, M. (1985). Attention, confusional states, and neglect. In M. Mesulam (Ed.), *Principles of behavioral neurology* (pp. 125–168). Philadelphia, PA: F. A. Davis.

Metzler, N., and Jelinek, J. (1977). Writing disturbances in patients with right cerebral hemisphere lesions. In R. H. Brookshire (Ed.), *Clinical aphasiology: Conference proceedings* (pp. 214–225). Minneapolis, MN: BRK.

Morrow, L., Vrtunsk, P. B., Kim, Y., and Boller, E. (1981). Arousal responses to emotional stimuli and laterality of lesion. *Neuropsychologia, 19,* 65–71.

Moya, K. L., Benowitz, L. I., Levine, D. N., and Finklestein, S. (1986). Covariant deficits in visuospatial abilities and recall of verbal narratives after right hemisphere stroke. *Cortex, 22,* 381–397.

Myers, P. S. (1979). Profiles of communication deficits in patients with right cerebral hemisphere damage. In R. H. Brookshire (Ed.), *Clinical aphasiology: Conference proceedings* (pp. 38–46). Minneapolis, MN: BRK.

Myers, P. S. (1991). Inference failure: The underlying impairment in right hemisphere communication disorders. In T. Prescott (Ed.), *Clinical aphasiology* (Vol. 20, pp. 167–180). Austin, TX: Pro-Ed.

Myers, P. S. (1992). The effect of visual and inferential complexity on the verbal expression of non-brain-damaged and right-hemisphere-damaged adults. Doctoral dissertation, University of Minnesota, *Dissertation Abstracts International, 53,* 03B.

Myers, P. S., and Brookshire, R. H. (1994). The effects of visual and inferential complexity on the picture descriptions of non-brain-damaged and right-hemisphere-damaged adults. In M. Lemme (Ed.), *Clinical aphasiology* (Vol. 22). Austin, TX: Pro-Ed.

Myers, P. S., and Linebaugh, C. W. (1980, November). *The perception of contextually conveyed relationships by right brain-damaged patients.* Paper presented to the American Speech-Language-Hearing Association Convention, Detroit, MI.

Myers, P. S., and Linebaugh, C. W. (1981). Comprehension of idiomatic expressions by right-hemisphere-damaged adults. In R. H. Brookshire (Ed.), *Clinical aphasiology: Conference proceedings* (pp. 254–261). Minneapolis, MN: BRK.

Myers, P. S., Linebaugh, C. W., and Mackisack, E. L. (1985). Extracting implicit meaning: Right versus left hemisphere damage. In R. H. Brookshire (Ed.), *Clinical aphasiology* (Vol. 15, pp. 72–82). Minneapolis, MN: BRK.

Myers, P. S., and Mackisack, E. L. (1986). Defining single versus dual definition idioms: The performance of right hemisphere and non-brain-damaged adults. In R. H. Brookshire (Ed.), *Clinical aphasiology* (Vol. 16, pp. 267–274). Minneapolis, MN: BRK.

Myers, P. S., and Mackisack, E. L. (1990). Right hemisphere syndrome. In L. L. LaPointe (Ed.), *Aphasia and related neurogenic language disorders* (pp. 177–195). New York: Thieme Medical Publishers.

Newcombe, F., Ratcliff, G., and Damasio, H. (1987). Dissociable visual and spatial impairments following right posterior cerebral lesions: Clinical, neuropsychological, and anatomical evidence. *Neuropsychologia, 25,* 149–161.

Newcombe, F., and Russell, W. R. (1969). Dissociated visual perceptual and spatial deficits in focal lesions of the right hemisphere. *Journal of Neurology, Neurosurgery and Psychiatry, 32,* 73–81.

Nicholas, L., and Brookshire, R. L. (1993). A system for scoring main concepts in the discourse of non-brain-damaged and aphasic speakers. In M. Lemme (Ed.), *Clinical aphasiology* (Vol. 21). Austin, TX: Pro-Ed.

Ogden, J. A. (1985). Anterior-posterior interhemispheric differences in the loci of lesions producing visual hemineglect. *Brain and Cognition, 4,* 59–75.

Ostrove, J. M., Simpson, T., and Gardner, H. (1990). Beyond scripts: A note on the capacity of right hemisphere-damaged patients to process social and emotional content. *Brain and Cognition, 12,* 144–154.

Posner, M. I. (1980). Orienting of attention. *Quarterly Journal of Experimental Psychology, 32,* 3–25.

Posner, M. I., Snyder, C. R., and Davidson, B. J. (1980). Attention and the detection of signals. *Journal of Experimental Psychology: General, 109,* 160–174.

Posner, M. I., Walker, J. A., Friedrich, F. J., and Raphal, R. D. (1984). Effects of parietal lobe injury on covert orienting of visual attention. *Journal of Neuroscience, 4,* 1863–1864.

Rapcsak, S. Z., Verfaellie, M., Fleet, W. S., and Heilman, K. M. (1989). Selective attention in hemispatial neglect. *Archives of Neurology, 46,* 178–182.

Ratcliff, G., and Newcombe, F. (1973). Spatial orientation in man: Effects of left, right, and bilateral posterior cerebral lesions. *Journal of Neurology, Neurosurgery and Psychiatry, 36,* 448–454.

Rehak, A., Kaplan, J. A., and Gardner, H. (1992a). Sensitivity to conversational deviance in right-hemisphere-damaged patients. *Brain and Language, 42,* 203–217.

Rehak, A., Kaplan, J. A., Weylman, S. T., Kelly, B., Brownell, H. H. (1992b). Story processing in right-hemisphere-brain damaged patients. *Brain and Language, 42,* 320–336.

Rivers, D. L., and Love, R. J. (1980). Language performance on visual processing tasks in right hemisphere lesion cases. *Brain and Language, 10,* 348–366.

Robin, D. A., and Rizzo, M. (1989). The effect of focal cerebral lesions on intramodal and cross modal orienting of attention. In T. Prescott (Ed.), *Clinical aphasiology* (Vol. 18, pp. 61–74). Austin, TX: Pro-Ed.

Robin, D. A., Tranel, D., and Damasio, H. (1987, October). *Deficits in temporal and spectral perception following focal cerebral damage.* Presented at the Academy of Aphasia, Phoenix, AZ.

Robinson, R. G., Kubos, K. L., Starr, L. B., Rao, K., and Price, T. R. (1984a). Mood disorders in stroke patients: Importance of location of lesion. *Brain, 107,* 81–93.

Robinson, R. G., Starr, L. B., Lipsey, J. R., Rao, K., and Price, T. R. (1984b). A two-year longitudinal study of poststroke mood disorders: Dynamic changes in associated variables over the first six months of follow-up. *Stroke, 15,* 510–517.

Roman, M., Brownell, H. H., Potter, H. H., Seibold, M. S., and Gardner, H. (1987). Script knowledge in right hemisphere-damaged and normal elderly adults. *Brain and Language, 31,* 151–170.

Ross, E. D., and Mesulam, M. M. (1979). Dominant language functions of the right hemisphere? Prosody and emotional gesturing. *Archives of Neurology, 36,* 561–569.

Ryalls, R., Joanette, Y., and Feldman, L. (1987). An acoustic comparison of normal and right-hemisphere-damaged speech prosody. *Cortex, 23,* 685–694.

Schechter, I., Korn, C., Yungreis, A., Koren, R., Sternfeld, R., Motlis, H., and Bergman, M. (1985). The word retrieval fluency test: What does it assess? *Scandinavian Journal of Rehabilitation Medicine* (Suppl 12), 76–79.

Schlanger, B. B., Schlanger, P., and Gerstman, L. J. (1976). The perception of emotionally toned sentences by right hemisphere-damaged and aphasic subjects. *Brain and Language, 3,* 396–403.

Schneiderman, E. I., and Saddy, J. D. (1988). A linguistic deficit resulting from right-hemisphere damage. *Brain and Language, 34,* 38–53.

Shapiro, B. E., and Danly, M. (1985). The role of the right hemisphere in the control of speech prosody in propositional and affective contexts. *Brain and Language, 25,* 19–36.

Sherratt, S. M., and Penn, C. (1990). Discourse in a right-hemisphere brain-damaged subject. *Aphasiology, 4,* 539–560.

Silberman, E. K., and Weingartner, H. (1986). Hemispheric lateralization of functions related to emotion. *Brain and Cognition, 5,* 322-353.

Sinyor, D., Jacques, P., Kaloupek, D. G., Becker, R., Goldenberg, M., and Coopersmith, H. (1986). Poststroke depression and lesion location: An attempted replication. *Brain, 109,* 537–546.

Sohlberg, M. M., and Mateer, C. A. (1986). *Attention process training (APT).* Pyallup, WA: Association for Neuropsychological Research and Development.

Sohlberg, M. M., and Mateer, C. A. (1987). Effectiveness of an attention training program. *Journal of Clinical and Experimental Neuropsychology, 9,* 117–130.

Sohlberg, M. M., and Mateer, C. A. (1989). *Introduction to cognitive rehabilitation.* New York: Gilford Press.

Stachowiak, F-J., Huber, W., Poeck, K., and Kerschensteiner, M. (1977). Text comprehension in aphasia. *Brain and Language, 4,* 177–195.

Swindell, C. S., Holland, A. L., Fromm, D., and Greenhouse, J. B. (1988). Characteristics of recovery of drawing ability in left and right brain-damaged patients. *Brain and Cognition, 7,* 16–30.

Swisher, L. P., and Sarno, M. T. (1969). Token Test scores of three matched patient groups: Left brain-damaged, right brain-damaged without aphasia, and non-brain-damaged. *Cortex, 5,* 264–273.

Tegner, R., Levander, M., and Caneman, G. (1990). Apparent right neglect in patients with left visual neglect. *Cortex, 26,* 455–458.

Teuber, H-L. (1963). Space perception and its disturbances after brain injury in man. *Neuropsychologia, 1,* 47–57.

Tompkins, C. A. (1991). Redundancy enhances emotional inferencing by right- and left-hemisphere-damaged adults. *Journal of Speech and Hearing Research, 34,* 1142–1149.

Tompkins, C. A., and Flowers, C. R. (1985). Perception of emotional intonation by brain-damaged adults: The influence of task processing levels. *Journal of Speech and Hearing Research, 28,* 527–538.

Trupe, E. H., and Hillis, A. (1985). Paucity vs. verbosity. Another analysis of right hemisphere communication deficits. In R. H. Brookshire (Ed.), *Clinical aphasiology* (Vol. 15, pp. 83–96). Minneapolis, MN: BRK.

Tucker, D. M. (1981). Lateral brain function, emotion, and conceptualization. *Psychological Bulletin, 89,* 19–46.

Tucker, D. M., Watson, R. T., and Heilman, K. M. (1977). Discrimination and evocation of affectively intoned speech in patients with right parietal disease. *Neurology, 27,* 947–950.

Urayse, D., Duffy, R. J., and Liles, B. Z. (1991). Analysis and description of narrative discourse in right-hemisphere-damaged adults: A comparison with neurologically normal and left-hemisphere-damaged aphasic adults. In T. Prescott (Ed.), *Clinical aphasiology* (Vol. 19, pp. 125–138). Austin, TX: Pro-Ed.

Vallar, G., and Perani, D. (1986). The anatomy of unilateral neglect after right-hemisphere stroke lesions. A clinical/CT-scan correlation study in man. *Neuropsychologia, 24,* 609–622.

Van Lancker, D. R., and Kempler, D. (1987). Comprehension of familiar phrases by left but not by right hemisphere damaged patients. *Brain and Language, 32,* 265–277.

Van Lancker, D. R., Klein, K., Hanson, W., Lanto, A., and Metter, E. J. (1991). Preferential representation of personal names in the right hemisphere. In T. Prescott (Ed.), *Clinical aphasiology* (Vol. 20, pp. 181–190). Austin, TX: Pro-Ed.

Villa, G., Gainotti, G., and DeBonis, C. (1986). Constructive disabilities in focal brain-damaged patients. Influence of hemispheric side, locus of lesion, and coexistent mental deterioration. *Neuropsychologia, 24,* 497–510.

Wapner, W., Hamby, S., and Gardner, H. (1981). The role of the right hemisphere in the appreciation of complex linguistic materials. *Brain and Language, 14,* 15–33.

Warrington, E. K., and James, M. (1967). Disorders of visual perception in patients with localized cerebral lesions. *Neuropsychologia, 8,* 457–487.

Warrington, E. K., James, M., and Kinsbourne, M. (1966). Drawing disability in relation to laterality of cerebral lesion. *Brain, 89,* 53–82.

Warrington, E. K., and Rabin, P. (1970). Perceptual matching in patients with localized cerebral lesions. *Neuropsychologia, 8,* 457–487.

Warrington, E. K., and Taylor, A. M. (1973). The contribution of the right parietal lobe to object recognition. *Cortex, 9,* 152–164.

Warrington, E. K., and Taylor, A. M. (1978). Two categorical stages of object recognition. *Perception, 7,* 695–705.

Weintraub, S., Mesulam, M. M., and Kramer, L. (1981). Disturbances in prosody: A right-hemisphere contribution to language. *Archives of Neurology, 38,* 742–744.

Weylman, S. T., Brownell, H. H., Roman, M., and Gardner, H. (1989). Appreciation of indirect requests by left- and right-brain-damaged patients: The effects of verbal context and conventionality of wording. *Brain and Language, 36,* 580–591.

Winner, E., and Gardner, H. (1977). The comprehension of metaphor in brain damaged patients. *Brain, 100,* 719–727.

Yorkston, K. M., and Beukelman, D. R. (1980). An analysis of connected speech samples of aphasic and normal speakers. *Journal of Speech and Hearing Disorders, 45,* 27–36.

APPENDIX 28.1

Literal and Interpretive Concepts for the "Cookie Theft" Picture[a]

Literal Concepts

two	has finger on mouth
children (kids)	children behind her
little	sink
boy (kid)	dishes
girl (kid)	faucet
standing	water
stool (footstool)	overflowing (going over)
three-legged	onto the floor
on the floor	dirty dishes left
reaching up	puddle
cookies	lawn
shelf	sidewalk
cupboard	house next door
with the open door	by the boy
window	reaching up

Interpretive Concepts

brother	wobbling
sister	hurt himself
taking (stealing)	for himself
for his sister	cookie jar
handing to sister	asking for cookie
laughing	saying "shhhh"
mother	trying (not trying) to help
washing (doing)	drying (wiping)
feet getting wet	ignoring
	general statement about
in the kitchen	disaster

Scoring:
1. Count each concept only once
2. Add number of literal concepts
3. Add number of interpretive concepts
4. Divide number of interpretive by total concepts

[a](Concepts adapted from Yorkston and Beukelman (1980). Divided into literal and interpretive concepts by Myers (1979).

APPENDIX 28.2

Sample "Cookie Theft" Descriptions

RHD Patient

"Looks like a lady *washing dishes* and gettin' ready for dishes. And the *sink* is *going over*. And that looks like a drive and that's a *window*, and that's a curtain. And the *faucet*, and it looks like it's going over anyway. And a *kid* on a *footstool*, putting dishes away, I guess. Kitchen *cupboard*, *cookie jar*. And a *girl*, and a *boy* on a stool. And there's—look like a bunch of trees here and long grass, and that's it."

Score: No. Interpretive Concepts: 2

No. Literal Concepts: 9

Total Concepts: 11

% Interpretive: 2/11 = 18%

NBD Adult

"This is a *woman washing* or wiping *dishes*. And the *sink* is *overflowing* while the *children* are trying to get into the *cookie jar*. And the *stool* on which the *boy* is standing is about to turn over. There's a *little girl* watching him. The *mother's* not paying any attention to the water. It's spilling on the *kitchen floor*."

Score: No. Interpretive Concepts: 4

No. Literal Concepts: 9

Total Concepts: 13

% Interpretive: 4/13 = 30%

CHAPTER 29

Management of Neurogenic Communication Disorders Associated with Dementia

KATHRYN A. BAYLES

Dementia is a syndrome associated with numerous diseases, infections, toxins, and trauma. Because many of the causes of dementia are reversible, irreversibility of the syndrome must never be presumed without careful review of the case history and diagnostic procedures. Whereas speech-language pathologists may be instrumental in identifying individuals with reversible dementia, their role is primarily with patients having irreversible dementia associated with primary degenerative brain diseases. Irreversible dementia is characterized by chronic progressive deterioration of intellect, memory, personality, and communicative function. The most common disease associated with irreversible dementia is Alzheimer's disease (AD), accounting for approximately half of all dementia cases. Vascular dementia, caused by many small infarctions, accounts for approximately 20% of the cases, and AD and vascular dementia are thought to co-occur in another 15% (Tomlinson, 1977). Another commonly occurring dementing disease is Parkinson's disease (PD), although not all patients with idiopathic PD develop dementia. In the early literature, reports of the prevalence of dementia in PD patients ranged from 2% (Patrick and Levy, 1922) to 77% (Lewy, 1923). More recently, when researchers have used the *Diagnostic and Statistical Manual-III* (DSM-III) criteria for dementia to diagnose its presence in PD patients, the reported rates have been lower (Lees and Smith, 1983).

PROFILES OF DEMENTIA PATIENTS

To introduce the clinician to the behavioral changes associated with dementia in AD, PD, and vascular disease patients, three case histories have been included: first, the history of an AD patient; second, a patient with PD; and third, a patient with vascular dementia (Table 29.1).

Profile of an AD Patient

Bill was 69 years old when he first visited the neurology clinic. He came at the urging of his wife, Jean, who was convinced something was seriously wrong. As a way of introducing the clinical staff to Bill's problems, Jean described the events of the previous weekend, emphasizing them as typical of Bill's behavior for the past 4 months. Jean explained she and Bill had been invited by old friends to a small dinner party, an

Table 29.1.
Conditions Associated with Irreversible Dementia

Parkinson's disease
Creutzfeldt-Jacob disease
Progressive supranuclear palsy
Progressive subcortical gliosis
Pick's disease

Huntington o Disease

anniversary celebration. Although Bill had been sociable and gregarious all his life, he was apathetic about the party and had to be coaxed to go. Jean had planned to purchase a floral arrangement en route to the party and asked Bill, who was driving, to stop at the flower shop. Even though Bill had been to the florist shop on many occasions, he had to ask Jean for directions. During the purchase of the flowers, Bill gave the clerk the wrong amount of money and argued about who had made the error. When they returned to their car, Bill was irritable and asked to go home. Jean encouraged him to go to the party, and reluctantly he complied. At the party, Bill had difficulty remembering the names of several old friends and the names of his friend's children. Throughout dinner, he made irrelevant comments and failed to acknowledge the party as an anniversary celebration. Several people asked Jean if Bill was ill, expressing concern about his confusion. On the way home, Bill asked where the flowers were, having forgotten they had been given as an anniversary gift.

The apathy, irritability, difficulty with recent and remote memory, and disorientation experienced by Bill typify AD patients and are the symptoms frequently noticed in casual encounters. If the affected individual is tested by a neuropsychologist, intellectual deficits are apparent. AD symptomatology is formally specified in the *Diagnostic and Statistical Manual III - Revised* (American Psychiatric Association, 1987) and is as follows: dementia, insidious onset and progressively degenerative course, and exclusion of all other specific causes of dementia by history, physical examination, and laboratory tests.

The changes in Bill's behavior resulted from neuropathological and neurochemical aberrations in the brain. Neuritic plaques, neurofibrillary tangles, and areas of granulovacuolar degeneration are widely, although not uniformly, distributed (Tomlinson,

1977), predominantly in the temporal and frontal lobes, the hippocampus, and adjacent areas. The denser the distribution of morphological changes, the more severe the dementia. In parieto-occipital areas changes are less apparent and are least common in inferior frontal and inferior occipital gyri (Tomlinson, 1982).

Neuritic plaques are aggregations of neurons with an amyloid core surrounded by a ring of granular material. Neurofibrillary tangles, the most characteristic morphological change, occur when fibers within the cell become twisted in a helical fashion. The nucleus of cells with neurofibrillary tangles is normal except for twisted tubules in the cytoplasm of the cell body. "Granulovacuolar degeneration" is a term describing the accumulation within the cell of both granular debris and fluid-filled empty spaces. Such morphological changes interfere with nerve transmission at the cellular level. To date, scientists are uncertain of their cause, but in recent years they have been considered a possible by-product of a malfunction in the cholinergic system (Gottfries et al., 1983; Whitehouse et al., 1981).

The cholinergic system is a neuronal network that transmits nerve impulses through acetylcholine. Enzymes necessary for the manufacture of acetylcholine, choline acetyltransferase, and acetylcholinesterase have been found to be reduced by 80% in AD patients (Bowen et al., 1981; Davies, 1983; Reisine et al., 1978). Curiously, reduction is marked in those brain areas with the greatest concentration of neuritic plaques, neurofibrillary tangles, and granulovacuolar degeneration. Of interest to scientists is the connection between cortical changes and subcortical nuclei containing cholinergic neurons, particularly the nucleus basalis of Meynert (Coyle et al., 1983). This nucleus is a major component of the substantia innominata located beneath the globus pallidus. About 70% of the cholinergic activity in the cortex appears to reside in terminals with cell bodies located in this nucleus. In AD patients, extensive reduction of cholinergic neurons has occurred within the nucleus basalis, a finding that has led researchers to theorize a relation between lack of cortical cholinergic input and the development of neuritic plaques, neurofibrillary tangles, and granulovacuolar degeneration. Other evidence supporting the cholinergic deficit theory of AD is that drugs interfering with the action of acetylcholine in normal subjects cause memory impairment (Drachman and Leavitt, 1974; Innes and Nickerson, 1970). In addition to the loss of acetylcholine, reductions are apparent in other neurochemicals, among them dopamine, and serotonin.

Profile of a PD Patient with Dementia

Ruth, an administrative assistant to a medical school dean, was 65 at the time of the neurological examination. She described herself as having been depressed for several months, but she had failed to seek medical advice until a tremor developed in her left hand. While taking her medical history, the doctor discovered Ruth had been sleeping poorly, had stopped going to church and bridge club, and was frequently absent from work. The neurologist recommended Ruth be examined by a neuropsychologist who found her to have episodic memory deficits, psychomotor retardation or slowness in the ability to think, visuospatial deficits, and difficulty processing complex new information. The findings of the neurologist and neuropsychologist led to a diagnosis of idiopathic PD with mild dementia.

Idiopathic parkinsonism accounts for 85% of the cases, and postencephalitic, a form occurring after encephalitis, accounts for the remaining 15% (Pollock and Hornabrook, 1966). The classic symptoms of rigidity, rest tremor, and bradykinesia (slowness of movement) are consequent to degeneration of the dopaminergic neurons in the basal ganglia, subcortical structures involved in the control of movement. Dopamine is a neurotransmitter involved in the initiation of movement. PD patients have difficulty initiating movement and commonly have a slow shuffling gait, flexed posture, and an inexpressive masklike face.

AD-like degenerative changes have been found in the brains of PD patients with dementia (Hakim and Mathieson, 1979; Hirano and Zimmerman, 1962), but it is unclear whether all PD patients have such changes. Results of recent positron emission tomography (PET) studies indicate that in addition to the known loss of dopamine in the nigrostriatal system, abnormal metabolic processes exist throughout the parkinsonian brain (Kuhl et al., 1984). This reduction in cerebral glucose metabolism in PD patients (18% average decrease) is similar to the general reduction in cerebral glucose metabolism in AD patients. Finally, choline acetyltransferase activity in the cortex of PD patients is reduced in apparent proportion to dementia severity (Ruberg et al., 1982). Several investigators suggest there may be two forms of PD (Boller et al., 1979; Garron et al., 1972; Lieberman et al., 1979): a motor disorder without dementia in which changes are limited to subcortical structures and a second form in which dementia is associated with motor dysfunction and both cortical and subcortical changes.

Profile of a Vascular Dementia Patient

Donna was 63 when first evaluated in the neurology clinic. On the previous day she had experienced faintness followed by confusion and difficulty walking. She was brought to the clinic by her son, who reported her to be "quite good on some days but bad on others." Donna reported having had several episodes of faintness during the previous 8 months. In this same period, dependence on her son and his family had gradually increased. Going to church was Donna's main out-of-the-home activity. Unlike in the past, however, she no longer discussed the sermons or people she met while at church.

Patients with dementia, subsequent to multiple infarctions, form a much less homogeneous population than AD or PD patients. The behavioral profile of each of these patients depends on the distribution of brain lesions, which varies markedly among individuals. Vascular dementia patients typically have a history of hypertension, previous strokes, abrupt onset of mental change with stepwise deterioration, and focal neurological signs. Brain damage results from a variety of thrombotic and embolic cerebrovascular diseases.

One method of classifying vascular dementia patients is to separate them according to the location of major infarctions and the size of blood vessels affected (Cummings and Benson, 1983). When the major infarctions are cortical, patients may exhibit amnesia, visuospatial deficits, and aphasia. Major subcortical infarctions frequently are associated with memory impairment and psychomotor retardation. When the small arteries of the basal ganglia, thalamus, and internal capsule are obstructed, the patients may be described as having lacunar state

(Cummings and Benson, 1983); 70-80% of patients with lacunar state have an associated dementia (Brown et al., 1972; Celesia and Wanamaker, 1972). Vascular dementia patients are sometimes confused with PD patients because both have extrapyramidal symptomatology.

Differentiating Demented from Aphasic Stroke Patients

In the last decade, speech-language pathologists and other professionals responsible for the care of dementia patients have recognized the existence of communication deficits in dementia patients regardless of the stage of the syndrome (Bayles, 1984; Bayles et al., in press; Cummings, 1990). In early dementia, when personality changes are subtle and intellectual deficits are mild, communicative impairment is mild, but as the neuropathological and neurochemical changes become more pronounced, deficits in linguistic communication become more pronounced. This is not to say that all aspects of linguistic communication or intellectual functioning are affected to the same degree, that a one-to-one relation exists between communicative and intellectual deficits. Relations between mental functions and the nervous system are not so easily characterized. For example, the nervous system is so constructed that certain intellectual and linguistic processes are applied in an automatic unconscious fashion, perhaps because they are better learned, more predictable or simpler. Other intellectual and linguistic processes (generally those representing the sum of many mental operations such as memory, attention, and perception) require conscious attention. Those processes requiring many mental operations are the most likely to be impaired early in the dementia syndrome.

A simple way to predict whether a particular communicative function will be impaired early in the dementia syndrome is to consider the degree to which the function is routine and dependent on environmental sensitivity and memory. Communicative functions such as object naming, reciting the alphabet, and sentence completion are not likely to be affected, whereas functions involving semantic analysis, the ability to relate meaning to situation, and generation of names of items within a category are affected.

When the criteria for predicting communicative functions likely to be affected early in dementia are considered in relation to types of linguistic knowledge, semantic and pragmatic communicative functions emerge as having greater early vulnerability. Phonological and syntactic rules generally are applied automatically, unlike most semantic and pragmatic rules. Indeed, dementia patients are well known for their ability to correctly apply phonological and syntactic rules until quite late in the syndrome (Bayles and Boone, 1982; Bayles and Kaszniak, 1987; Schwartz et al., 1979; Whitaker, 1976).

Are Dementia Patients Aphasic?

To answer this question, specification must be made of what is meant by the term "aphasia." Aphasia comes from Greek and means "without speaking." According to Webster, it is the partial or total loss of the ability to articulate ideas in any form resulting from brain damage. The inability to articulate ideas in any form sounds more like the communicative behaviors of dementia patients. Benson (1979a) paraphrased the similar definitions of Nielsen (1936), Geschwind (Benson and

Geschwind, 1971), Darley (1975), and Adams and Victor (1977), defining aphasia as "the loss of, or impairment of, language caused by brain damage" (p. 5). In his definition, Benson has specified the denotative meaning of the term, but the connotative, or that which is implied, is extensive and generally considered by speech-language pathologists as part of the denotative meaning. People familiar with only the denotative meaning, and there are many in other professions, and people partial to the medical tradition of using terms according to their translations from Greek, use the term "aphasia" to describe changes in communicative functions experienced by dementia patients as well as stroke patients. Dementia patients have language impairment caused by brain damage. Of course, the brain damage is different from that typically associated with aphasia because it is caused by chronic progressive degenerative brain disease that eventuates in generalized intellectual deterioration.

The term "aphasia" also connotes abrupt onset of linguistic impairment, an inappropriate description of the course of linguistic dissolution seen in dementia patients. Most patients with aphasia experience abrupt onset of linguistic impairment as a consequence of stroke or traumatic brain injury, but patients with nonvascular dementia experience insidious loss of communicative function. Vascular dementia patients are exceptional because they may exhibit sudden dramatic change in communicative function when an infarction occurs in brain areas specialized for language.

Finally, the diagnosis of aphasia connotes linguistic impairment disproportionate to intellectual impairment. Unlike dementia patients, aphasia patients frequently express nonlinguistically what they cannot express linguistically. The disparity between intellectual and linguistic abilities was the characteristic Halpern et al. (1973) chose to emphasize when they described the linguistic impairment of dementia as "the language of generalized intellectual impairment."

In summary, most speech-language pathologists do not believe the linguistic impairment associated with dementia should be called aphasia. For them, aphasia is associated with a group of syndromes differing markedly from the pattern of communicative impairment observed in dementia patients. Thus, for purposes of clarity, the term "aphasia" will be used in this chapter to refer to sudden loss of communicative function due to focal brain damage.

Types of Patients Who Are Likely to Be Confused with Each Other

The AD patient is unlikely to be confused with patients who have nonfluent aphasia because AD spares the motor strip throughout most of the disease and affected individuals are verbally fluent. More likely to be confused are AD and fluent aphasia patients. Also contributing to the confusion is the fact that aphasic stroke patients may have memory deficits, which are the primary characteristics of AD patients.

The following series of discourse samples are from an AD patient who was followed for several years; these samples reveal the disease effects on linguistic communication. The devastation of semantic content and verbal output is apparent. Note, however, the relative preservation of grammar.

Sample 1—Year 1

E: Now I'd like you to look at that picture there.

S: Too many children.

E: Yes, I'd like you to tell me everything you can about that. Describe what's happening in the picture.

S: Well, here's a man reading something. It's happening, but he's not looking at the reading. See he's looking someplace else, and he's he's talking to these beautiful ladies here, and also reading his own paper beside. And here's his little boy. Isn't he cute?

E: Describe what's happening there.

S: Well the father's gotten a little tired of reading all this, see, so he's just getting rid of that, one at a time as they march past him going to their own reading or whatever else they do. (laugh) That's real good. And he has his own great big, great great big newspaper. And then he has a few down here like this. Two feet for all that. That's a cute thing right there. (laughing)

E: Okay, do you want to say anything else about that?

S: No, I don't think anything needs to be seen on it.

E: Okay, great.

S: There's a man that thinks maybe something else might be, but he's left everything alone except his newspaper. So everything is all right with him. Don't you think?

E: Yeah.

S: He's he's keeping some of the papers with his teeth. (laughs)

E: All right, thanks.

Sample 2—Year 3

E: Describe what's going on in this picture, and say what you would like to about that.

S: Well, they look like the pictures that uh don't want to be pick-picketed or or made made up into an odd creature in in the meantime.

E: Is there anything else that you want to say about that?

S: Yes, they do. They they they they they actually look so actable that it makes you want to run away for some reason or other. But um they have their their special aqualelge over. The way people take uh take uh an (actoba) that they don't even know anything about. But they just don't try to bother with these other people who have their.

E: Okay, great, thank you.

Sample 3—Year 5

E: Tell me about this picture. What can you tell me about that picture?

S: Yes. Mmhm. It must be a ah, ah, somebody that really thought themselves really gone and close way.

E: What's happening in this picture?

S: No.

E: What's happening in this picture?

S: Well, there's that's something that we'd be supplied with it, but usually goes away with a.

E: Okay. Good

Phenomena Common in Aphasia and Dementia

Memory Deficits of AD and Aphasia Patients

The AD patient suffers particular impairment in working memory and the episodic and semantic subsystems of declarative memory (Bayles and Kaszniak, 1987). The span of working memory gradually shrinks; the episodes of daily life are not recorded, and conceptual knowledge becomes less accessible. The impairments of memory are apparent regardless of whether the clinician uses linguistic or nonlinguistic memory tasks.

Because brain areas critical for language also have a role in memory function (Squire, 1987), a stroke will cause deficits in language and memory. Unlike AD patients, however, the memory deficits of aphasic patients are more likely apparent when the clinician uses linguistically oriented memory tasks (Butters et al., 1970; Goodglass, 1970).

Recent research suggests that individuals with aphasia and lesions primarily anterior to the Rolandic fissure have particular impairment of long-term verbal memory, whereas individuals with aphasia and lesions primarily posterior to the Rolandic fissure have particular impairment of short-term verbal memory (Beeson, 1990; Risse et al., 1984).

Beeson (1990) characterized the differences in memory of aphasic stroke patients with anterior and posterior lesions as "differential impairments of working memory" (p. 73). In patients with anterior lesions, the central executive component of working memory likely is impaired. The central executive initiates the processes of information retrieval from long-term memory. Thus, these individuals have difficulty bringing information into working memory. In patients with posterior lesions, damage may occur to the articulatory loop system, thereby making it difficult to rehearse information so that it can be maintained in working memory.

Aphasic stroke and dementia patients are best differentiated in terms of memory by tasks that evaluate encoding, free recall, cued recall, and recognition using stimuli that are linguistic and nonlinguistic. Aphasic patients typically perform better on cued recall and recognition segments than do dementia patients because their greater intellectual capacity has enabled them to better process and remember test stimuli (Grober and Buschke, 1987), particularly nonlinguistic stimuli.

If dementia patients do not have aphasia, they do, nonetheless, have some of the same communication problems seen in aphasia patients: anomia, verbal perseveration, dysfluency, jargon, and circumlocution.

Anomia

In the early stages, dementia patients are most likely to be anomic in spontaneous discourse (Critchley, 1964; Stengel, 1964) and have difficulty generating names of items within a category on verbal fluency tasks (Appell et al., 1982; Bayles and Tomoeda, 1983; Martin and Fedio, 1983; Rosen, 1980a).

Some dispute exists about the effects of AD on confrontation naming ability. Whereas impairment in confrontation naming is common in AD patients and often proportionate to severity of dementia, some mildly demented individuals may have severe naming deficits, and some severely demented individuals may have mild naming deficits (Bayles and Trosset, 1992).

AD patients are more likely to name a real object correctly than a picture or line drawing (Kirshner et al., 1984). Bayles et al. (1990) observed that presentation of the real object facilitated naming in AD patients; however, the facilitation effect of 27% was modest.

Perseveration

Perseveration is the involuntary repetition of a previous response occurring in the absence of the original stimulus. It is associated with all types of brain damage, as well as damage in many anatomical areas (Buckingham et al., 1979; Hudson, 1968; Luria, 1965). In a study of verbal perseveration of dementia patients, repetition of ideas was found to be the most common form, more common than sound, word, and phrase repetition or use of interjections and filler words (Bayles et al., 1985). Further, as the dementia worsened, the frequency of verbal perseverations increased.

Dysfluency

Dysfluency may characterize the speech of individuals with subcortical pathology and dementia (Cummings, 1990). For example, patients with PD may be very slow in their production of words and have difficulty initiating speech. The involuntary movements and muscle spasms typical of Huntington's patients make coordination of the processes necessary for fluent speech production difficult.

Jargon

In the advanced stages of the dementia syndrome, some patients produce jargon. Others are mute or use meaningful words in a nonmeaningful way (Obler, 1983). The different late-stage manifestations likely result from unique patterns of morphological and neurochemical change. As yet, however, the relation of linguistic performance to distribution and degree of morphological change and neurochemical alterations is not well understood.

Circumlocution

Talking around an idea or failing to express it explicitly is circumlocution. Circuitous output is associated most commonly with anomic aphasia; that is, when the desired word is not available, the individual will attempt to substitute a description. Clinical experience suggests the circumlocution of dementia patients is slightly different from that seen in aphasia patients. Whereas aphasia patients know what they want to say but have difficulty producing the desired word, dementia patients are likely to have forgotten their linguistic intention or are unable to think of meaningful discourse. An analysis of the discourse of AD patients followed longitudinally revealed that circumlocutions were rare.

In summary, when the language behaviors thought to be present in both aphasia and dementia are scrutinized, subtle differences become apparent, differences due in many cases to the effects of progressive intellectual deterioration in dementia patients. It is the presence of intellectual deterioration and its linguistic consequences that necessitates a different testing approach for dementia patients than those traditionally employed with aphasia patients.

ASSESSMENT OF DEMENTIA

Whereas patients with focal brain lesions will show marked impairment primarily in the psychological function or functions subserved by the affected brain tissue, dementia patients experience deficits in all higher order mental processes. To detect dementia early, the clinician will need an extensive case history containing information about any neuropsychological changes. The patient cannot be considered a reliable informant because episodic memory deficit is an inherent feature of AD and other dementing diseases. Interviewing the primary caregiver, usually the spouse, is advantageous. As part of a longitudinal study of

the effects of AD on language, the primary caregivers of 99 AD patients were interviewed about early linguistic and nonlinguistic symptomatology (Bayles, 1991). Caregivers commonly reported memory deficits, word-finding problems, difficulty with finances, and trouble writing letters as antedating the medial diagnosis of the disease.

Identifying the individual at risk for developing dementia demands that the clinician consider whether current behavior is congruent with the individual's premorbid intellectual ability. For example, an individual whose clinical performance on intellectual tasks was average, but who was a Phi Beta Kappa in college, would be suspect. Such an individual would be expected to perform above average. Premorbid intelligence can be estimated using demographic information (Barona et al., 1984; Wilson et al., 1979).

A condition that may cause the performance of the individual to look like dementia is depression, often referred to as pseudodementia. Therefore, it is important to consider screening the patient at risk for dementia for depression and enlisting the assistance of colleagues knowledgeable of geriatric depression. Typically depressed patients will complain about their deficits and perform inconsistently on tasks of similar difficulty (Wells, 1980). Two scales useful for screening individuals for depression are the Hamilton Rating Scale (Hamilton, 1960) and the Beck Depression Inventory (Beck et al., 1961). The Hamilton Rating Scale (Hamilton, 1960, 1967) is an interview-based rating scale composed of a 17-item inventory of symptoms, both physical and psychological, which are rated for severity by one or two clinicians. The Beck Depression Inventory (Beck et al., 1961) is a self-report instrument composed of 21 items. The psychometric value of the measure has been studied by several investigators who report it as having sufficient internal consistency for use in research and screening applications with elderly adults (Gallagher et al., 1983; Miller and Seligman, 1973).

AD and vascular disease co-occur in about 15% of the population of dementia patients, making it important to consider the possibility of vascular disease in the patient suspected of having dementia. The Hachinski Ischemic Scale (Hachinski et al., 1975) is widely used to identify individuals with symptoms typically associated with vascular disease and stroke. The scale comprises 13 features associated with vascular disease and stroke, such as history of hypertension, focal neurological signs, and abrupt onset. Each feature is evaluated and points are accumulated for those present. Individuals who have seven or more points are considered at risk for vascular disease. A shortened version of the scale has evolved (Rosen et al., 1980) and has been demonstrated to be valid for distinguishing vascular disease.

Another factor the clinician should consider in assessing dementia is whether drugs could be causing the observed mental changes. The average elderly individual fills 13 prescriptions annually (Besdine, 1982) and takes six drugs at any point in time. Many frequently prescribed drugs cause changes in mental status. Ask about drug regimen during examination of the patient.

Neuropsychological Tests Sensitive to Dementia

Neuropsychological investigation of dementia patients has a longer and richer history than investigation of communicative

Table 29.2.
List of Neuropsychological Measures Efficacious for Use with Dementia Patients

Memory
Wechsler Memory Scale (WAIS) (Wechsler, 1945)
Revised Wechsler Memory Scale (Russell, 1975)
Benton Revised Visual Retention Test (Benton, 1974)
The Guild Memory Test (Crook et al., 1980)
Fuld Object Memory Evaluation (Fuld, 1980, 1981)
New York University Memory Test (Osborne et al., 1982)

Perception
Benton Facial Recognition Test (Benton and Van Allen, 1968)
Benton Line Orientation Test (Benton et al., 1978)

Intelligence
Wechsler Adult Intelligence Scale (WAIS) (Wechsler, 1958)
Wechsler Adult Intelligence Scale–Revised (Wechsler, 1981)

Attention
Auditory Digit Span (as contained in WAIS)
Visual Letter (Talland and Schwab, 1964)
Digit Cancellation Task (Lewis and Kupke, 1977)

Abstraction and Cognitive Flexibility
WAIS Similarities Subtest
WAIS Comprehension Subtest
Wisconsin Card Sorting Test (Berg, 1948)
Picture Absurdities of Stanford-Binet (Terman and Merrill, 1973)

Construction Ability
WAIS Block Design Subtest

functions, and several neuropsychological tests have been identified as sensitive to dementia. Memory deficits occur early and become increasingly prominent as the syndrome develops (Fuld, 1978; Hagberg, 1978; Logue and Wyrick, 1979; Miller and Lewis, 1977; Rosen, 1983). Certain perceptual processes also are affected early, most notably visuospatial processsses (Mayeux et al., 1981; Rosen, 1983). Generally, neuropsychologists recommend testing a variety of cognitive functions, among them memory, visuospatial perception, and general intelligence. It is beyond the scope of this chapter to review all the neuropsychological tests used with dementia patients, but many measures having a reputation for sensitivity to early dementia are listed in Table 29.2. Readers interested in a more in-depth discussion are referred to Kaszniak's (1985) review in the book

Neuropsychological Assessment of Neuropsychiatric Disorders

A logical question clinicians might ask about neuropsychological tests is how useful they are for identifying the etiology of dementia. Unfortunately, although many are sensitive to the presence of dementia, their usefulness for differentiating etiology is limited. Generally, the prominent tests used to identify dementia—the Wechsler Adult Intelligence Scale (Wechsler,1955, 1958, 1981) tests of intelligence, the Luria (Christensen, 1975; Golden, 1981) and the Halstead-Reitan (Halstead, 1940; Reitan, 1955, 1964)—were developed for other purposes. Although experienced clinicians may come to associate subtle differences in performance patterns with particular etiologies, standard profiles for patients with different dementing illnesses

do not exist. Many clinicians have created their own dementia battery by combining subtests from the prominent neuropsychological batteries with ones they have developed.

Another appropriate clinical question is whether the detection of dementia always requires the administration of a long test battery. The answer is no. Many clinicians include in their armamentarium a short, simply administered measure of mental status. Several measures have been demonstrated to be sensitive to dementia and provide clinicians with an index of dementia severity: Mini-Mental State Examination (Folstein et al., 1975); Global Deterioration Scale (Reisberg et al., 1982); orientation and memory examination (Blessed et al., 1968), which has been modified for American patients by Fuld (1978); Short Portable Mental Status Questionnaire (Pfeiffer, 1975); Mental Status Questionnaire (Kahn et al., 1960); and Mattis Dementia Rating Scale (Coblentz et al., 1973; Mattis, 1976).

Language Tests Sensitive to Dementia

A battery for testing the communicative functions of dementia patients must assess the effects of intellectual deterioration, particularly memory deficits, on communication. The task of deciding which measures to include would be simpler if the constitutive rules of one linguistic domain, but not the others, could be said to depend on consciously applied intellectual and memorial functions. However, within each linguistic domain, variability exists in the degree to which the rules composing the domain can be applied without the communicator's awareness. Nonetheless, it is true that certain of the domains, notably the pragmatic and semantic, appear to have greater dependence on conscious thought and intellectual integrity than the phonological and syntactic and are therefore more vulnerable to effects of dementing illness. The face validity of this observation is more convincing when the realization is made that phonological and syntactic decisions are not made consciously by adults, except in unusual situations.

Conversely, to form an appropriate communicative intention, which is an integral part of the pragmatic use of language, the speaker must take into account the context, topic, amount of shared information existing between conversants, interspeaker relationships and time available. Assessment of so many variables requires complex information processing, healthy memory and the ability to relate perceptions to past experience. Thus, certain aspects of pragmatic functioning are dependent on perceptual and mnestic integrity. For these reasons, measures of semantic and pragmatic reasoning also should be included in a test battery for patients suspected of having dementia.

Tasks most sensitive to the dementia syndrome are those that are active, nonautomatic, or generative or that depend on logical reasoning. Active nonautomatic tasks require the patient's mental and linguistic involvement in a creative way, such as in object description, story retelling, defining concepts, and explanation of sentence meaning.

Automatic tasks are those asking for responses that are overlearned (i.e., recitating days of the week, counting, saying the alphabet).

When individuals have to conceive of and produce, either in writing or orally, a series of related ideas or examples of objects in a category, they are performing a generative task. An example of such a task in the FAS Verbal Fluency Test (Borkowski et al., 1967) is one in which an individual must think of as many words as possible beginning with the letters F, A, and S in 1 minute. Dementia patients are impoverished in their ability to call forth answers or develop strategies to think of examples (Bayles et al., 1989). As a consequence, they perform more poorly on a generative naming task, particularly in the early stages, than on a task of confrontation naming (Bayles and Tomoeda, 1983; Bayles and Trosset, 1992).

The Similarities subtest of the Wechsler Adult Intelligence Scale (Wechsler, 1955, 1958, 1981) is an example of a measure of reasoning in which the individual has to form a conclusion based on perceiving similarities or differences between two or more items. Another example of a reasoning task is explaining proverbs.

In 1991, Bayles and Tomoeda published a test battery that was designed for the purpose of quantifying the communication disorder associated with AD. The battery is called the Arizona Battery for Communication Disorders of Dementia (ABCD) and provides information about linguistic comprehension, linguistic expression, verbal episodic memory, mental status, and visuospatial construction. The battery contains 14 subtests that can be given individually or together to obtain an overall score.

The ABCD was standardized on 100 individuals: 50 AD subjects and 50 normal control subjects. All standardization study participants were residents of southern Arizona, were Caucasian, and met the following criteria: had no history of previous neurologic or psychiatric disorder, were not clinically depressed, had sufficient visual acuity to read newsprint, had sufficient hearing acuity to pass a speech discrimination test with 80% or better accuracy, had no history of alcohol or drug abuse, were literate, and spoke English as a first language. No significant differences existed between the AD and normal control subjects in age, education, handedness, or estimated intelligence. The AD patients were diagnosed according to the NINCDS-ADRDA research task force criteria (McKhann et al., 1984).

The ABCD subtests were found to correlate highly with three widely accepted measures of dementia severity: the Global Deterioration Scale (Reisberg et al., 1982), the Mini-mental State Examination (Folstein et al., 1975), and the Block Design subtest of the Wechsler Adult Intelligence Scale (Wechsler, 1981).

The ABCD provides a cutoff score for each of the subtests below which an individual could be considered to have performed subnormally. The cutoff value approximates the fifth percentile of normal performances. Best among the subtests for screening for AD were the verbal episodic memory tasks: free recall, total recall, and recognition components of the Word Learning Subtest and the Story Retelling Subtest.

In the Story Retelling subtest (Bayles and Tomoeda, 1991) subjects are asked to tell the following story immediately after hearing it and later after having taken several other tests.

> While a lady was shopping, her wallet fell out of her purse, but she did not see it fall. When she got to the check-out counter, she had no way to pay for her groceries. So she put the groceries away and went home. Just as she opened the door to her house, the phone rang and a little girl told her that she had found her wallet. The lady was very relieved.

Whereas normal elders retold 13.4 units of information from the story (SD = 3.2), mild AD patients retold 7.1 (SD = 3.8), and moderate AD patients retold 3.4 (SD = 3.2). In the delayed

condition, normal elders remembered 11.1 units of information (SD = 5.4), but mild AD patients recalled an average of only 0.9 information units (SD = 3.2), and moderate AD patients could not recall anything about the story (SD = 0).

MANAGEMENT OF DEMENTIA PATIENTS

The speech-language pathologist has a critical role in the management of dementia patients in relation to diagnosis, monitoring development of the syndrome, identifying most effective means of communicating with the dementia patient, assessing efficacy of pharmacological and other therapies, and counseling the family. Measures of communicative function have been demonstrated to be effective for identifying the presence of early dementia and as such should be used in screening the elderly. Early identification is extremely valuable for patients with reversible dementia, as well as for those with irreversible dementia. Patients with reversible dementia need treatment, and patients with irreversible dementia and their families need information about how to maximize communicative performance.

In both AD and PD patients, the dementia syndrome can develop slowly, with patients remaining in the mild stage for many years. Consider the benefit to the caregiver of information about how to maximize the communicative capability of the mildly affected patient. Clinical experience has demonstrated improvement in interpersonal relations between the caregiver and the patient when the caregiver understands the nature of the linguistic and intellectual problems experienced by the patient. In the early stages of dementia, families are generally ignorant of neuropathology and its consequences and frequently misinterpret the behaviors of the affected individual. When the apathy, depression, confusion, forgetfulness, and other features of early dementia are explainable, caregivers become more objective and less likely to feel angry toward the affected individual.

In addition to educating the family about communication deficits of their loved one, clinicians should explore the efficacy of various techniques for improving the communicative functioning of the patient. One aspect of exploration should be evaluation of the communicative skills of the caregiver. Many caregivers have sensory deficits and communication habits detrimental to effective communication. To improve communication with the dementia patient, the caregiver generally needs instruction about the process of communication. For example, most individuals lack an understanding of the difference between speech and language or the varied knowledge needed for appropriate communication. They are unaware of variables under their control when communicating with the dementia patient, variables such as the topic, amount of new information, amount of redundancy, speaking rate, number of conversants, complexity of syntax, and word choice. Although reports of empirical studies demonstrating the beneficial effects on dementia patients of manipulation of these communication variables are as yet unavailable, results of studies on other populations, as well as clinical experience, suggests they may have a significant effect.

Many reasons can be given for knowing the extent of the development of the dementia syndrome in an individual, among them making decisions about living arrangements, as well as economic, financial, and social matters. Periodic evaluation of

Table 29.3.
Effects of Dementing Illnesses on Communication

	EARLY STAGES
Sounds:	Used correctly
Words:	May omit a meaningful word, usually a noun, when talking in sentences. May report trouble thinking of the right word. Vocabulary is shrinking
Grammar:	Generally correct
Content:	May drift from the topic. Reduced ability to generate series of meaningful sentences. Difficulty comprehending new information. Vague
Use:	Knows when to talk, although may talk too long on a subject. May be apathetic, failing to initiate a conversation when it would be appropriate to do so. May have difficulty understanding humor, verbal analogies, sarcasm, and indirect and nonliteral statements
	MIDDLE STAGES
Sounds:	Used correctly
Words:	Difficulty thinking of words in a category. Anomia in conversation. Difficulty naming objects. Reliance on automatisms. Vocabulary noticeably diminished
Grammar:	Sentence fragments and deviations common. May have difficulty understanding grammatically complex sentences
Content:	Frequently repeats ideas. Forgets topic. Talks about events of past or trivia. Fewer ideas
Use:	Knows when to talk. Recognizes questions. May fail to greet. Loss of sensitivity to conversational partners. Rarely corrects mistakes
	LATE STAGES
Sounds:	Generally used correctly, but errors are not uncommon
Words:	Marked anomia. Poor vocabulary. Lack of word comprehension. May make up words and produce jargon
Grammar:	Some grammar is preserved but sentence fragments and deviations common. Lack of comprehension of many grammatical forms
Content:	Generally unable to produce a sequence of related ideas. Content may be meaningless and bizarre. Subject of most meaningful utterances is the retelling of a past event. Marked repetition of words and phrases
Use:	Generally unaware of surroundings and context. Insensitive to others. Little meaningful use of language. Some patients are mute; some are echolalic

communicative function is an excellent way to monitor behavioral change. Performance on language tests has been shown to correlate strongly with severity of dementia, and assessment of communicative functions is noninvasive and easily accomplished. In addition to providing the family with important information about the patient's status, measures of communicative function can provide researchers with critical information about the effectiveness of various therapies, particularly pharmacologic. Finally, speech-language pathologists, as communication experts, have a responsibility to advise families of the effects on communication of irreversible dementing illnesses.

Effects of Dementing Illnesses on Communication

When families know what to expect, coping is easier, even though deterioration of function will be inexorable. As the wife of a dementia patient said, "The hardest part was not knowing what to expect and being embarrassed and angry." An outline of changes in communicative function, according to stage of dementia and used by the author with families of patients, is given in Table 29.3.

Forms of Language Difficult for Dementia Patients

Close inspection of the nature of linguistic dissolution in dementia may suggest to the reader language forms likely to be difficult for dementia patients, for example, verbal analogies. Comprehension of analogies requires attention, verbal memory, and associative reasoning, processes particularly affected in dementing illnesses. Other problematic forms are the use of sarcasm and open-ended questions. Comprehension of sarcasm

requires sensitivity to context and past experience. Open-ended questions are difficult because dementia patients lack the ability to think of possible answers. Rather than ask an individual, "What would you like to do this afternoon?" it is preferable to provide simple options, as in "Would you like to watch television or go for a walk?" The memory limitations of dementia patients make processing of long complex discourse and accurate interpretation of indefinite reference hard. Thus, rather than saying, "They will come to dinner," specify who. Finally, the concrete and familiar are easier to comprehend than the abstract. Advise caregivers to use familiar words, talk slowly, and whenever possible, limit to two the number of individuals in a conversation.

FUTURE TRENDS

Reports of communication disorders associated with dementia have existed in the literature since the turn of the century, but only in the last decade have researchers demonstrated communicative impairment to be an integral feature of the dementia syndrome. Still needing definition, however, are differences in patient communication profiles according to etiology of the dementia. That is, understanding is lacking of how AD, Huntington's, and PD patients of equivalent dementia severity differ in communicative competency. Then, too, research is lacking about intragroup differences. For example, a question remains as to why AD begins in some individuals with a progressive aphasia (Green et al., 1990; Kirshner et al., 1984; Poeck and Luzzatti, 1988; Pogacar and Williams, 1984). It is widely recognized that the distribution of pathology within the two cerebral hemispheres can be asymmetrical, however, the cause of this asymmetry is not understood.

To date, no investigator has reported on the relation between patient differences in communicative abilities in the end stages of AD, nor have deficits in linguistic communication in life been related to the distribution of pathology at post mortem examination. Understanding is lacking about why some individuals become mute, and others become palilalic and echolalic.

In addition to extending our understanding of differences in communicative functioning in dementia patients, researchers of the future will likely study efficacy of various treatment strategies. To date, no results of treatment studies have been published. Perhaps treatment by speech-language pathologists has not received much attention because researchers have had a pessimistic view of diseases like AD and Huntington's, and only recently has dementia been widely recognized as associated with PD. However, dementia develops very slowly in many individuals, and often years elapse before the individual is noticeably impaired in casual encounters. As recognition grows of the slow dementing course of many patients, more research energy is likely to be directed to learning how to maximize the communicative performance of individuals with dementia. Therapy may markedly improve the existence of patients who remain in the mild stages for several years. As professionals, we must be committed to improving the existence of these individuals and their families insofar as is possible.

References

Adams, R. D., and Victor M. (1977). *Principles of neurology*. New York: McGraw-Hill.

American Psychiatric Association. (1987). *Diagnostic and statistical manual of mental disorders* (3rd ed.). Washington, DC: American Psychiatric Association.

Appell, J., Kertesz, A., and Fisman, M. (1982). A study of language functioning in Alzheimer's patients. *Brain and Language, 17,* 73–91.

Barona, A., Reynolds, C., and Chastain, R. (1984). A demographically based index of premorbid intelligence for the WAIS-R. *Journal of Clinical Consulting Psychology, 52,* 885–887.

Bayles, K. A. (1984). Language and dementia. In A. Holland (Ed.), *Language disorders in adults*. San Diego, CA: College Hill Press.

Bayles, K. A. (1991). Alzheimer's disease symptoms: Prevalence and order of appearance. *Journal of Applied Gerontology, 10,* 419–430.

Bayles, K. A., and Boone, D. R. (1982). The potential of language tasks for identifying senile dementia. *Journal Speech and Hearing Disorders, 47,* 210–217.

Bayles, K. A., Caffrey, J. T., Tomoeda, C. K., and Trosset, M. W. (1990). Confrontation naming and auditory comprehension in Alzheimer's patients. *Journal of Speech Language Pathology and Audiology, 14,* 15–20.

Bayles, K. A., and Kaszniak, A. W. (1987). *Communication and cognition in normal aging and dementia*. Austin, TX: Pro-Ed.

Bayles, K. A., Salmon, D. P., Tomoeda, C. K., Jacobs, D., Caffrey, J. T., Kaszniak, A. W., and Troster, A. I. (1989). Semantic and letter category naming in Alzheimer's patients: A predictable difference. *Developmental Neuropsychology, 5,* 335–347.

Bayles, K. A., and Tomoeda, C. K. (1983). Confrontation and generative naming abilities of dementia patients. In R. H. Brookshire (Ed.), *Clinical Aphasiology Conference Proceedings*. Minneapolis, MN: BRK.

Bayles, K. A., and Tomoeda, C. K. (1991). *Arizona Battery for Communication Disorders of Dementia*. Tucson, AZ: Canyonlands Publishing.

Bayles, K. A., Tomoeda, C. K., Kaszniak, A. W., Stern, L. Z., and Eagans, K. K. (1985). Verbal perseveration of dementia patients. *Brain and Language, 25,* 102–116.

Bayles, K. A., Tomoeda, C. K., and Trosset, M. W. (1992). Relation of linguistic communication abilities of Alzheimer's patients to stage of disease. *Brain and Language, 42,* 454–472.

Bayles, K. A., and Trosset, M. W. (1992). Confrontation naming in Alzheimer's patients: Relation to disease severity. *Psychology of Aging, 7,* 197–203.

Beck, A. T., Ward, C. H., Mendelson, M., Mock, J., and Erbaugh, J. (1961). An inventory for measuring depression. *Archives of General Psychiatry, 4,* 53.

Beeson, P. M. (1990). *Memory impairment associated with stroke and aphasia*. Unpublished doctoral dissertation. University of Arizona, Tucson, AZ.

Benson, D. F. (1979a). *Aphasia, alexia, and agraphia*. London: Churchill Livingstone.

Benson, D. F., and Geschwind, N. (1971). Aphasia and related cortical disturbances. In A. B. Baker and L. H. Baker (Eds.), *Clinical neurology*, New York: Harper and Row.

Benton, A. L., and Van Allen, M. W. (1968). Impairment in facial recognition in patients with cerebral disease. *Cortex, 4,* 344–358.

Benton, A. L. (1974). *Revised Visual Retention Test: Clinical and experimental application*, (4th ed.). New York: Psychological Corporation.

Benton, A. L. Varney, N. R., and Hamsher, K. (1978). Visuospatial judgment: A clinical test. *Archives of Neurology, 35,* 364–367.

Berg, E. A. (1948). A simple objective test for measuring flexibility in thinking. *Journal of General Psychology, 39,* 15–22.

Besdine, R. W. (1982). The data base of geriatric medicine. In J. W. Ross and R. W. Besdine (Eds.), *Health and diseases in old age*. Boston, MA: Little, Brown.

Blessed, G., Tomlinson, B. E., and Roth, M. (1968). The association between quantitative measures of dementia and of senile changes in the cerebral grey matter of elderly subject. *British Journal of Psychiatry, 114,* 797–811.

Boller, F., Mizutani, T., Roessmann, V., and Gambetti, P. (1979). Parkinson's disease, dementia, and Alzheimer's disease: Clinical pathological correlations. *Annals of Neurology, 7,* 329–335.

Borkowski, J. G., Benton, A. L., and Spreen, O. (1967). Word fluency and brain damage. *Neuropsychologia, 5,* 135–140.

Bowen, D. M., Davison, A. N., and Sims, N. (1981). Biochemical and pathological correlates of cerebral aging and dementia. *Gerontology, 27,* 100–101.

Brown, G., La, V., and Wilson, W. P. (1972). Parkinsonism and depression. *Southern Medical Journal, 65,* 540–545.

Buckingham, H. W., Whitaker, H., and Whitaker, H. A. (1979). On linguistic perseveration. In H. Whitaker and H. A. Whitaker (Eds.), *Studies in Neurolinguistics* (Vol 4). New York: Academic Press.

Butters, N., Samuels, I., Goodglass, H., and Brody, B. (1970). Short-term visual and auditory memory disorders after parietal and frontal lobe damage. *Cortex, 6,* 440–459.

Celesia, G. G., and Wanamaker, W. M. (1972). Psychiatric disturbances in Parkinson's disease. *Diseases of the Nervous System, 33,* 577–583.

Christensen, A. (1975). *Luria's neuropsychological investigation*. New York: Spectrum.

Coblentz, J. M., Mattis, S., Zingesser, L. H., Kasoff, S. S., Wisniewski, H. M., and Katzman, R. (1973). Presenile dementia: clinical evaluation of cerebrospinal fluid dynamics. *Archives of Neurology, 29,* 299–308.

Coyle, J. T., Price, D. L., and DeLong, M. R. (1983). Alzheimer's disease: a disorder of cortical cholinergic innervation. *Science, 219,* 1194–1219.

Critchley, M. (1964). The neurology of psychotic speech. *British Journal of Psychiatry, 110,* 353–364.

Crook, T., Gilbert, J. G., and Ferris, S. (1980). Operationalizing memory impairment for elderly persons: The Guild Memory Test. *Psychology Research, 47,*1315–1318.

Cummings, J. L. (Ed.). (1990). *Subcortical dementia*. New York: Oxford University Press.

Cummings, J. L., and Benson, D. F. (1983). *Dementia: A clinical approach*. Boston, MA: Butterworths.

Darley, F. L. (1975). Treatment of acquired aphasia. In W. J. Friedlander (Ed.). *Advances in neurology* (Vol. 7). New York: Raven Press.

Davies, P. (1983). An update on the neurochemistry of Alzheimer disease. In R. Mayeux and W. G. Rosen (Eds.), *The dementias*. New York: Raven Press.

Drachman, D. A., and Leavitt, J. (1974). Human memory and the cholinergic system: a relationship to aging. *Archives of Neurology, 30,* 113–121.

Folstein, M. F., Folstein, S. E., and McHugh, P. R. (1975). "Mini-mental state": a practical method for grading the mental state of patients for the clinician. *Journal of Psychiatric Research, 12,* 189–198.

Fuld, P. A. (1978). Psychological testing in the differential diagnosis of the dementias. In R. Katzman, R. D. Terry, and K. L. Bick (Eds.), *Alzheimer's disease: Senile dementia and related disorders*. New York: Raven Press.

Fuld, P. A. (1980). Guaranteed stimulus-processing in the evaluation of memory and learning. *Cortex, 16*, 225–271.

Gallagher, D., Breckenridge, J., Steinmetz, J., and Thompson, L. (1983). The Beck Depression Inventory and research diagnostic criteria: congruence in an older population. *Journal of Consulting and Clinical Psychology, 51,* 945.

Garron, D. C., Klawans, H. L., and Narin, F. (1972). Intellectual functioning of persons with idiopathic parkinsonism. *Journal of Nervous and Mental Disease, 154,* 445–452.

Golden, C. J. (1981). A standardized version of Luria's neuropsychological tests: a quantitative and qualitative approach to neuropsychological evaluation. In S. B. Filskov and T. J. Boll (Eds.), *Handbook of clinical neuropsychology.* New York: John Wiley and Sons.

Goodglass, H., Gleason, J. B., and Hyde, B. (1970). Some dimensions of auditory language comprehension in aphasia. *Journal of Speech and Hearing Research, 13,* 595–606.

Gottfries, C., Adolfsson, R., Aquilonius, S., Carlsson, A., Eckernas, S., Nordberg, A., Oreland, L., Svennerholm, L., Wiberg, A., and Winblad, A. (1983). Biochemical changes in dementia disorders of Alzheimer type. *Neurobiology of Aging, 4,* 261–271.

Green, J., Morris, J. C., Sandson, J., McKeel, D. W., and Miller, J. W. (1990). Progressive aphasia: a precursor of global dementia? *Neurology, 40,* 423-429.

Grober, E. and Buschke, H. (1987). Genuine memory deficits in dementia. *Developmental Neuropsychology, 3,* 13–36.

Hachinski, V. C., Iliff, L. D., DuBoulay, G. H., McAllister, A. L., Marshall, J., Russell, R. W., and Symon, L. (1975). Cerebral blood flow in dementia. *Archives of Neurology, 32,* 632.

Hagberg, B. (1978). Defects of immediate memory related to the cerebral blood flow distribution. *Brain and Language, 5,* 366–377.

Hakim, A. M., and Mathieson, G. (1979). Dementia in Parkinson's disease: a neuropathologic study. *Neurology, 29,* 1209–1214.

Halpern, H., Darley, F. L., and Brown, J. R. (1973) Differential language and neurologic characteristics in cerebral involvement. *Journal of Speech and Hearing Disorders, 38,*162–173.

Halstead, W. C. (1940). Preliminary analysis of grouping behavior in patients with cerebral insults by the method of equivalent and non-equivalent stimuli. *American Journal of Psychiatry, 96,* 1263–1294.

Hamilton, M. (1960). A rating scale for depression. *Journal of Neurological Neurosurgery and Psychiatry, 23,* 56.

Hamilton, M. (1967). Development of a rating scale for primary depressive illness. *British Journal of Social Psychology, 6,* 278.

Hirano, A., and Zimmerman, H. M. (1962). Alzheimer's neurofibrillary changes. *Archives of Neurology, 7,* 227–242.

Hudson, A. J. (1968). Perseveration, *Brain, 91,* 571–582.

Innes, I. R., and Nickerson, N. (1970). Drugs inhibiting the action of acetylcholine on structures innervated by postganglionic parasympathetic nerves (antimuscarinic or atropinic drugs). In A. G. Gilman, L. S. Goodman, and A. Gilman (Eds.), *The pharmacologic basis of therapeutics,* (4th ed.). New York: Macmillan.

Kahn, P., Goldfard, A., Pollak, M., and Peck, A. (1960). Brief objective measures for the determination of mental status in the aged. *American Journal of Psychiatry, 117,* 326–328.

Kaszniak, A. W. (1985). Neuropsychology of dementia. In I. Grant and K. Adams (Eds.), *Neuropsychological assessment of neuropsychiatric disorders.* New York: Oxford.

Kirshner, H. S., Webb, W. G., and Kelly, M. P. (1984). The naming disorder of dementia. *Neuropsychologia, 22,* 23–30.

Kirshner, H. S., Webb, W. G., Kelly, M. P., and Wells, C. E. (1984). Disturbance: An initial symptom of cortical degeneration and dementia. *Archives of Neurology, 41,* 491–496.

Kuhl, D. E., Matter, E. J., and Riege, W. H. (1984). Patterns of local cerebral glucose utilization determined in Parkinson's disease by the fluorodeoxyglucose method. *Annals of Neurology, 15,* 419–424.

Lees, A. J. and Smith, E. (1983). Cognitive deficits in the early stages of Parkinson's disease. *Brain, 106,* 257–270.

Lewis, R., and Kupke, T. (1977). The Lafayette Clinic repeatable neuropsychological test battery: Its development and research applications. Paper presented at annual meeting of Southeastern Psychological Association. Hollywood, FL.

Lewy, F. H. (1923). *Monographs of Neurological Psychiatry, 34,* 32.

Lieberman, A., Dziatolowski, M., Kupersmith, M., Serby, M., Goodgold, A., Korein, J., and Goldstein, M. (1979). Dementia in Parkinson disease. *Annals of Neurology, 6,* 355–359.

Logue, P., and Wyrick, L. (1979). Initial validation of Russell's revised Wechsler Memory Scale: A comparison of normal aging versus dementia. *Journal of Consulting and Clinical Psychology, 47,* 176–178.

Luria, A. R. (1965). Two kinds of motor perseveration in massive injury of the frontal lobes. *Brain, 88,* 1–10.

Martin, A., and Fedio, P. (1983). Word production and comprehension in Alzheimer's disease: The breakdown of semantic knowledge. *Brain and Language, 19,* 124–141.

Mattis, S. (1976). Mental status examination for organic mental syndrome in the elderly patient. In R. Bellack and B. Karasu (Eds.), *Geriatric psychiatry.* New York: Grune and Stratton.

Mayeux, R., Stern, Y., Rosen, J., and Levanthal, J. (1981). Depression, intellectual impairment and Parkinson's disease. *Neurology, 31,* 645–650.

McKhann, G., Drachman, D., Folstein, M., Katzman, R., Price, D., and Stadlan, E. M. (1984). Clinical diagnosis of Alzheimer's disease: Report of the NINCDS-ADRDA work group under the auspices of the Department of Health and Human Services task force on Alzheimer's disease. *Neurology, 34,* 939-944.

Miller, E., and Lewis, P. (1977). Recognition memory in elderly patients with depression and dementia: a signal detection analysis. *Journal of Abnormal Psychology, 86,* 84–86.

Miller, W. R., and Seligman, M. E. P. (1973). Depression and the perceptions of reinforcement. *Journal of Abnormal Psychology, 82,* 62.

Nielsen, J. M. (1936). *Agnosia, apraxia and aphasia: Their value in cerebral localization.* Los Angeles, CA: Los Angeles Neurological Society.

Obler, L. K. (1983). Language and brain dysfunction in dementia. In S. Segalowitz (Ed.), *Language functions and brain organization.* New York: Academic Press.

Osborne, D. P., Brown, E. R., and Randt, C. T. (1982). Qualitative changes in memory function: Aging and dementia. In S. Corkin, K. L. Davis, J. H. Growdon, E. Usdin, and R. L. Wurtnam (Eds.), *Alzheimer's disease: A report of progress (Aging,* Vol. 19). New York: Raven Press.

Patrick, H. T., and Levy, D. M. (1922). Parkinson's disease: A clinical study of one hundred and forty-six cases. *Archives of Neurology and Psychiatry, 7,* 711–720.

Pfeiffer, E. (1975). A short portable mental status questionnaire for the assessment of organic brain deficit in elderly patients. *Journal of the American Geriatric Society, 23,* 433–441.

Poeck, K., and Luzzatti, C. (1988). Slowly progressive aphasia in three patients, *Brain, 111,* 151–168.

Pogacar, S., and Williams, R. S. (1984). Alzheimer's disease presenting as slowly progressive aphasia. *Rhode Island Medical Journal, 67,* 181–185.

Pollock M., and Hornabrook, R. W. (1966). The prevalence, natural history and dementia of Parkinson's disease. *Brain, 89,* 429–488.

Reisberg, B., Ferris, S. H., DeLeon, M. J., and Crook, T. (1982). The global deterioration scale (GDS): An instrument for the assessment of primary degenerative dementia (PDD). *American Journal of Psychiatry, 139,* 1136-1139.

Reisine, T. D., Yamamura, H. I., Bird, E. D., Spokes, E., and Enna, S. J. (1978). Pre- and postsynaptic neurochemical alterations in Alzheimer's disease. *Brain Research, 159,* 477–481.

Reitan, R. M. (1955). Investigation of the validity of Halstead's measures of biological intelligence. *Archives of Neurological Psychiatry, 78,* 28–35.

Reitan, R. M. (1964). Psychological deficits resulting from cerebral lesions in man. In J. M. Warren and K. Akert (Eds.), *The frontal granular cortex and behavior,* New York: McGraw-Hill.

Risse, G. L., Rubens, A. B., and Jordan, L. S. (1984). Disturbances of long-term memory in aphasic patients. *Brain, 107,* 605–617.

Rosen, W. G. (1980). Verbal fluency in aging and dementia. *Journal of Clinical Neuropsychology, 2,* 135–146.

Rosen, W. G. (1983). Neuropsychological investigation of memory, visuoconstructional, visuoperceptual, and language abilities in senile dementia of the Alzheimer's type. In R. Mayeux and W. G. Rosen (Eds.), *The dementias,* New York: Raven Press.

Rosen, W. G., Terry, R. D., Fuld, P. A., Katzman, R., and Peck, A. (1980). Pathological verification of ischemic score in differentiation of dementia. *Annals of Neurology, 7,* 486–488.

Ruberg, M., Ploska, A., and Javoy-Agid, F. (1982). Muscarinic binding and choline acetyltransferase activity in parkinsonian subjects with reference to dementia. *Brain Research, 232,* 129–139.

Russel, E. N. (1975). A multiple scoring method for the assessment of complex memory functions. *Journal of Consulting and Clinical Psychology, 43,* 800–809.

Schwartz, M., Marin, O., and Saffran, E. (1979). Dissociations of language functions in dementia: A case study. *Brain and Language*, 7, 277–306.

Squire, L. R. (1987). *Memory and brain*. New York: Oxford University Press.

Stengel, E. (1964). Speech disorders and mental disorders. In A. V. S. DeReuck and M. O'Connor (Eds.), *Disorders of Language* (Ciba Foundation Symposium). Boston, MA: Little, Brown.

Talland, G. A., and Schwab, R. S. (1964). Performance with multiple sets in Parkinson's disease. *Neuropsychologia*, 2, 45–53.

Terman, L. M., and Merrill, M. A. (1973). *Stanford-Binet Intelligence Scale. Manual for the Third Revision, Form L-M*. Boston: Houghton Mifflin.

Tomlinson, B. E. (1977). The pathology of dementia. In C. E. Wells (Ed.), *Dementia*. Philadelphia: F. A. Davis.

Tomlinson, B. E. (1982). Plaques, tangles, and Alzheimer's disease. *Psychological Medicine*, 12, 449–459.

Wechsler, D. (1945). A standardized memory scale for clinical use. *Journal of Psychology*, 19, 87–95.

Wechsler, D. (1955). *Manual for the Wechsler Adult Intelligence Scale*. New York: Psychological Corporation.

Wechsler, D. (1958). *The measurement and appraisal of adult intelligence*, (4th ed.). Baltimore, MD: Williams & Wilkins.

Wechsler, D. (1981). *Wechsler Adult Intelligence Scale-Revised Manual*. New York: Psychological Corporation.

Wells, C. E. (1980). The differential diagnosis of psychiatric disorders in the elderly. In J. Cole and J. Barrett (Eds.), *Psychopathology in the aged*. New York: Raven Press.

Whitaker, H. (1976). A case of the isolation of the language function. In H. Whitaker and H. A. Whitaker (Eds.), *Studies in neurolinguistics* (Vol. 2). New York: Academic Press.

Whitehouse, P. J., Price, D. L., Clark, A. W., Coyle, J. T., and DeLong, M. R. (1981). Alzheimer disease: evidence for selective loss of cholinergic neurons in the nucleus basalis. *Annals of Neurology*, 10, 122–126.

Wilson, R. S., Rosenbaum, G., and Brown, G. (1979). The problem of premorbid intelligence in neuropsychological assessment. *Journal of Clinical Neuropsychology*, 1, 49–53.

CHAPTER 30
Communication Disorders Associated with Closed Head Injury

MARK YLVISAKER AND SHIRLEY F. SZEKERES

CLOSED HEAD INJURY AS A DISABILITY CATEGORY

Since we wrote our chapter for the second edition of this book in 1985, closed head injury (CHI) has become well established as a disability category in rehabilitation for adults and, more recently, under the more general heading "traumatic brain injury" (TBI), in special education for children. The number of designated head injury rehabilitation programs in the United States increased from fewer than 50 in 1980 to more than 900 in 1990. Today, large numbers of speech-language pathologists work exclusively or primarily with individuals with CHI in a variety of clinical environments, whereas in 1980 this was a relatively esoteric subspecialty.

The rapid expansion of CHI outcome research, intervention literature, and clinical services over the past 15 years can only partially be explained by the growth in numbers of individuals who survive severe injuries. Indeed, many professionals consider CHI and TBI to be at best misleading as disability categories because they are actually *etiology* categories, identifying potential causes of varied disability, not the disability itself. In this respect, these categories are comparable to stroke or perinatal asphyxia, events that may or may not produce disability. Furthermore, as with stroke and perinatal asphyxia, constellations of communicative strengths and weaknesses potentially associated with CHI are extremely varied, depending on the nature, location, and severity of the injury, as well as characteristics of the individual who is injured. Therefore, clinicians should expect not only great diversity within this group but also substantial overlap between CHI and other categories of adult neurogenic communication disorder, such as aphasia, dementia, and right-hemisphere syndrome. Despite many commonalities among survivors of severe CHI (described below), these important considerations should prevent thoughtful clinicians from approaching intervention in this area with a rigidly "curricular" orientation.

In this discussion, CHI will be considered a brain injury in which the primary mechanism of damage is a blunt blow to the head, associated with acceleration/deceleration forces (Levin et al., 1982). Contact of a moving skull with a surface or of a moving object with the skull may cause skull distortion and

fracture and is traditionally thought to be responsible for *coup* (site of contact) and *contrecoup* (opposite side) brain contusion. Neurobehavioral deficits associated with these lesions vary with the site of impact and therefore cannot explain central tendencies within the population as a whole. Rather, damage associated with differential movements within the skull, both brain-skull and brain-brain movements created by inertial forces (especially rotational inertia), often plays the greatest role in determining outcome and best explains population commonalities. This type of injury is possible even in the absence of a blow to the head if the skull is accelerated and/or decelerated rapidly (e.g., shaken baby syndrome) (Gennarelli et al., 1982). TBI is a more inclusive category than CHI, including penetrating missile injuries in which focal damage is related to the site of penetration and which are more strongly associated with aphasia than is CHI (Newcombe, 1969). As defined by the new federal education law, PL 101-476 (Individuals with Disabilities Education Act, 1990), TBI includes injury to the brain acquired after birth and associated with an external cause. However, some state departments of education have made TBI an even broader category when applied to special education, including stroke, tumor, anoxia, toxic encephalopathy, meningitis, encephalitis, and other causes of noncongenital brain injury.

In severe CHI, brain-skull differential movement in the area of bony prominences within the skull can cause surface contusion and laceration as well as deeper shearing of axons (diffuse axonal injury) and blood vessels (subdural and intracerebral hematoma). Regardless of site of impact in high-speed CHI, focal contusion as well as axon shearing are often concentrated within anterior and inferior frontal and temporal lobe structures bilaterally because of their adjacency to sharp, irregular surfaces inside the skull (Alexander, 1987; Courville, 1937; Katz, 1992). Damage to these areas explains many of the commonly observed neurobehavioral symptoms that negatively affect communication after CHI, including depressed executive control over cognitive and communicative functions (prefrontal damage), impaired social perception (prefrontal damage, particularly right hemisphere), and generally reduced behavioral self-regulation (prefrontal, frontolimbic, and anterior temporal damage). The relative infrequency of specific aphasic syndromes in CHI is in part a consequence of the smooth interior surface of the skull adjacent to the traditional language centers in the brain. Neuronal shearing is also often concentrated in the brain stem and corpus callosum, contributing to initial coma and subsequent attentional deficits and slowed mental processing (Adams et al., 1982).

Secondary damage in CHI includes slowly developing hemorrhages and localized or widespread swelling and edema, both of which contribute to increased intracranial pressure which can be acutely life threatening and contributes to morbidity in those who survive. In addition, hypoxic-ischemic injury and abnormal neurotransmitter surges, both common secondary consequences of severe CHI, often pick out specific vulnerable structures, notably the hippocampus bilaterally, thereby contributing to memory and new learning problems after the injury (Katz, 1992). This is an especially ominous consequence for young people who face substantial new learning challenges in school and on the job. Tragically, the vast majority of individuals with CHI are children, adolescents, and young adults.

Given the variety of pathophysiologic mechanisms in CHI, many of which are related to site of impact, it is understandable that there are no consistent outcome profiles with respect to communication or any other domain of behavior: Any function can be spared or impaired—and to any degree—in CHI. Heterogeneity is increased by diversity in pretraumatic intelligence, educational and vocational levels, age, personality, and coping styles as well as by variation in posttraumatic environments, support systems, and emotional and behavioral reactions of the individual. These observations underscore the extreme importance of customizing assessment procedures and intervention goals and methods for this group. However, clinical observations supported by a growing outcome literature seem to converge on a number of unifying themes with respect to communication outcome following CHI. These themes are discussed below.

Infrequency of Aphasia

Although symptoms of aphasia are often present early in recovery and, in some cases, specific aphasias do persist, aphasia defined in terms of the classical syndromes is relatively uncommon in CHI (Heilman et al., 1971), including severe CHI (Sarno, 1980, 1984; Sarno et al., 1986). Anomia, which can be associated with a wide variety of brain lesions, is often reported to be the primary residual aphasic symptom in the absence of general cognitive disruption (Heilman et al., 1971; Levin et al., 1981; Sarno, 1980, 1984; Thomsen, 1975). Generalized and persistent expressive and receptive language impairment is generally associated with widespread diffuse injury that also produces global cognitive deficits (Levin et al., 1981).

Nonaphasic Communication Disorders

Communication challenges following CHI are most often "nonaphasic" in nature; that is, they coexist with intact speech, reasonably fluent and grammatical expressive language, and comprehension adequate to support everyday interaction. Depending on the severity of injury, stage of recovery, and particular focus of research, the characteristic communication profiles following CHI have been variously referred to as "the language of confusion" (Halpern et al., 1973), "nonaphasic language disturbances" (Prigatano, 1986), "cognitive-language disturbances" (Hagen, 1981), and "subclinical aphasia" (Sarno,

1980, 1984). Sarno (1984) found that although a distinct minority of a consecutive series of 69 severely injured individuals admitted to an inpatient rehabilitation facility could be diagnosed with aphasia, *all* of the patients were found to have some combination of subclinical language deficits, including impaired confrontation naming, word fluency, and comprehension of complex oral commands. She did not evaluate their interactive competence with increasing cognitive and social demands, factors that clinicians, teachers, and family members often identify as major contributors to communication breakdowns after CHI.

The overlapping collections of communication deficits highlighted by these investigators have been grouped by the American Speech-Language-Hearing Association under the heading "cognitive-communicative impairment" (ASHA, 1988). Long-term disturbances within this category include:

- Disorganized, tangential, wandering discourse, including conversational and monologic discourse (e.g., spoken or written narratives)
- Imprecise language and word-retrieval difficulties
- Disinhibited, socially inappropriate language; hyperverbosity; ineffective use of social and contextual cues

or

- Restricted output, lack of initiation
- Difficulty comprehending extended language (spoken or written), especially under time pressure; difficulty detecting main ideas
- Difficulty following rapidly spoken language
- Difficulty communicating in distracting or stressful environments
- Difficulty reading social cues and flexibly adjusting interactive styles to meet situational demands
- Difficulty understanding abstract language, including indirect or implied meaning
- Inefficient verbal learning and verbal reasoning

Any combination of these changes in the comprehension and expression of language, particularly in demanding social contexts, can substantially affect life after CHI. The success of an individual's social, vocational, familial, and academic reintegration rests on the recovery of effective communication. For example, families routinely report that it is easier to adjust to physical disability in a loved one with CHI than to personality changes manifested in stressful and unsatisfying communication (Livingston and Brooks, 1988). Vocational success similarly relies on the individual's ability to interact effectively with peers, supervisors, and possibly customers (Brooks et al., 1987). Finally, social relationships and academic performance are frequent victims of the language and communication challenges associated with CHI (Ylvisaker, 1992).

Effects of Prefrontal Damage

Many, but not all, of the symptoms listed above are associated with prefrontal damage (Alexander et al., 1989; Stuss and Benson, 1986). For example, both right- and left-hemisphere prefrontal structures are associated with regulation (initiation, inhibition, direction) of behavior, including communication behavior; with organization of language into coherent discourse; and with control over attentional and memory processes to make them useful in daily life. Both left- and right-hemisphere orbital frontal damage has been associated with personality changes, including disinhibition, volatility, and verbal "dysdecorum" (Alexander et al., 1989). Right frontal lobe damage has been associated with more specific pragmatic deficits, such as (*a*) decreased ability to produce appropriate paralinguistic accompaniments to speech, including gesture and facial expression as well as prosody in speech; (*b*) decreased ability to comprehend prosodic features in the speech of others and to interpret indirect pragmatic intents, including humor, sarcasm, metaphor, and other indirect meanings; and (*c*) inattention to context, including social context, resulting in socially inappropriate behavior (Alexander et al., 1989). Although it is certainly possible to escape prefrontal injury in CHI, its frequency and its profound impact on communicative effectiveness combine to give it and its general neurobehavioral correlate, executive system dysfunction, an important heuristic role in organizing intervention planning in CHI (Ylvisaker, 1992).

Age of Onset

In contrast to stroke, the highest risk group for CHI consists of active, risk-taking adolescents and young adults. Because many severely injured survivors were still in school or had just begun vocational exploration at the time of the injury, rehabilitation goals and the overall flavor of rehabilitation differ in important ways from stroke rehabilitation.

In this chapter, we will address selected issues in assessment and intervention associated with communication impairments that have their basis in more general cognitive, psychosocial, and executive system disruption. It is useful for speech-language pathologists to broaden their traditional professional horizons and see these clinical issues as falling under two broad interdisciplinary umbrellas: cognitive rehabilitation and social skills intervention. The issues that we have selected for discussion do not come close to covering the entire territory. Furthermore, we have given an admittedly biased perspective on intervention, based on our combined 30 years in the field, on a considerable body of efficacy research in related fields, and on an extremely small body of efficacy literature in head injury rehabilitation. In a number of other publications, we have developed these themes in greater detail than is possible in this chapter (e.g., Szekeres et al., 1987; Ylvisaker et al., in press b; Ylvisaker et al., 1992; Ylvisaker et al., in press c; Ylvisaker et al., 1987; Ylvisaker and Urbanczyk, 1990).

COGNITION

A conceptual framework helps clinicians to avoid a haphazard and inefficient "workbook" approach to treatment, facilitates communication among professionals and between clinicians and clients, promotes systematic observation and program evaluation, and serves as a source of intervention principles and procedures. Because of the complexity of cognition and the relationships among its components, the development of a coherent and manageable framework for cognitive-communicative intervention becomes a major challenge. This challenge is increased by the competing theoretical descriptions of cognition and its development (Dodd and White, 1980; Flavell, 1985; Siegler, 1986).

We have borrowed most heavily from information-processing theories because of the comprehensiveness of that approach and the clinical usefulness of its categories. From one information-processing perspective, cognition is viewed broadly as the processing of information for particular purposes and within specific mental structures and environmental constraints (Dodd and White, 1980). In our clinical work, we have found it productive to describe cognitive functioning and recovery in terms of three general aspects of cognition: processes, systems, and functional-integrative performance. Each of the processes and systems relates in identifiable ways to language and communication. The value of this framework will be highlighted in treatment discussions later in this chapter.

Component Processes

Component processes include mental activities or operations involved in taking in, interpreting, encoding, storing, retrieving, and making use of knowledge or information, and generating a response. Inferences about what cognitive activities or operations have occurred are based on the nature of people's behavior in relation to the information that they receive, and from their explanations of what they have done. For example, if a person is given a list of words in random order and the recall output is in categories, it is assumed that a covert organizing process was used (either deliberately or automatically). Component processes (or categories of processes) can be grouped under the headings attending, perceiving, learning/memory, organizing, reasoning, and problem solving. There is, of course, a certain amount of arbitrariness in any system used to classify cognitive processes.

Interaction among processes presents a diagnostic challenge to clinicians working with individuals with cognitive impairment. For example, attention, organization, memory, and executive control are all dynamically interrelated in most acts of cognitive processing. A problem in any of these areas can easily masquerade as a problem in any of the other areas. Furthermore, improvement in any of the areas easily supports improvement in the others, both in normal human development and in adult processing. Because of the complexity within each of the processes and their dynamic interaction, it is misleading to suggest a hierarchy of processes, with, for example, attending at the bottom and reasoning at the top. In normal cognitive development, all processes undergo gradual maturation beginning in early infancy (Flavell, 1985). Related to this developmental principle is the everyday observation that some attentional tasks are extremely demanding and some reasoning tasks are extremely simple. For these and other reasons, it is a mistake to look for or create a hierarchical curriculum for cognitive rehabilitation, beginning with purportedly simple processes and progressing to purportedly more complex processes. Indeed, sometimes improvements in purportedly higher processes (e.g., organizing schemes) are needed to effect improvement in purportedly lower processes (e.g., attention).

Attending

Attending is holding objects, events, words, or thoughts in consciousness. It includes basic alertness as well as the active selection of information from the environment and from storage for further processing. Attentional control, including selecting the focus of attention and maintaining, shifting, and dividing attention, is influenced by the individual's perceptual and affective set, his or her immediate and long-term goals, and the nature of the stimuli (e.g., intensity, novelty). Executive control over attentional processes increases with cognitive development and is often a victim of prefrontal injury in CHI. Impaired attentional processes can negatively affect a variety of communication processes, including word retrieval, maintenance of coherent discourse, and comprehension of extended units of language (spoken or written).

Perceiving

Perception is the recognition of features of stimuli and relations among the features. It is affected by preexisting knowledge; by context; by the intensity, complexity, and duration of the stimuli; and by the significance and familiarity of the stimuli for the perceiver. Visual-perceptual deficits can have a predictably negative effect on reading and also reduce communicative effectiveness by interfering with the reception of social cues.

Memory/Learning

Memory/learning is a complex three-stage process. The *encoding* stage involves the construction of an internal representation of an event. One many encode specific selected information from the event itself, aspects of the context, co-occurring internal experiences, and the interpretation of the event (Hintzman, 1978). The encoding process may be involuntary, in which case the orientation is to an activity, such as playing a game, and memory or learning is a by-product (Smirnov, 1973). This is sometimes referred to as "incidental learning." Alternatively, encoding may be voluntary or deliberate, in which case the intention to remember something prompts one to select or create a strategy or operation to achieve that cognitive goal. Prefrontal injury easily impairs this executive control over memory processes and may therefore significantly reduce the effectiveness of voluntary or deliberate learning.

The *storage* stage involves holding information over time in what is thought to be a highly organized system (Smith, 1978). Efficient storage is more likely if the information is significant and is well attended to, understood, integrated into existing knowledge and experience, and well organized (Brown, 1975, 1979). Although brain injury can result in relatively rapid decay of information, this aspect of learning is the least likely to be impaired in CHI.

The *retrieval* stage involves the transfer of information from long-term storage to consciousness. Retrieval may be as effortless as producing familiar words during relaxed conversation and as unintentional as nearly continuous attention to sad or stressful information. On other occasions, retrieval may be the result of an intensive directed search of one's knowledge base. Recognition memory is typically the simplest type of retrieval and occurs when the stimulus is present and must only be identified (e.g., true/false or multiple-choice questions). Cued recall is the retrieval of information in response to cues (e.g., *wh*-questions, category cues, phoneme cues). In free recall, the information must be retrieved in the absence of cues. Differential performance on free recall, cued recall, and recognition memory tasks helps to sort out the encoding and retrieval contributions to a manifest memory problem.

An extremely common profile following CHI includes fairly good recovery of pretraumatically acquired knowledge and skill combined with substantial difficulty learning new information. The new learning problem can result from medial temporal lobe damage to those structures responsible for consolidation of new memories, from prefrontal injury that may interfere with executive control over memory processes (deliberate learning), or from impairment in any of the other cognitive processes

or systems that contribute to the processing of information (Levin et al., 1988). In extreme cases, the coherence of discourse can be affected by memory problems. Any degree of impairment can negatively affect the learning efficiency of a young person returning to school or vocational training after CHI.

Organizing

Organizing processes include analyzing information, identifying relevant features, comparing for similarities and differences, classifying/categorizing/associating, sequencing, and integrating information into larger units (e.g., main ideas, themes, scripts, or higher-level categories). Organizational problems, which are believed to be common after CHI, may result from lost organizing schemes or from inadequate executive control over available schemes (prefrontal injury). In either case, discourse may ramble, comprehension of extended text may be weak, and searches for words may be inefficient and ineffective.

Reasoning

Reasoning is the process of considering evidence and making inferences or drawing conclusions. In deductive reasoning, inferences are drawn on the basis of formal relations among propositions (e.g., syllogistic reasoning). Inductive reasoning involves direct inferences from experience (e.g., scientific generalizations). Analogical reasoning (one of the most common and powerful types of reasoning in everyday life) allows us to draw inferences indirectly from experience by using known relationships to explain or predict different but related phenomena. Evaluative reasoning involves considering the merits of ideas, courses of action, things, or people in relation to explicit or assumed criteria, and making judgments of value on the basis of these considerations.

From a somewhat different perspective, reasoning can be divided into *convergent* thinking (the search for main ideas, central themes, and single conclusions) and *divergent* thinking (creative exploration of alternative possibilities, relevant information, examples of concepts or rules, and the like).

Problem Solving

Problem solving, which occurs when a goal cannot be reached without special (cognitive) effort, is a complex activity involving a variety of types of reasoning, domain-specific knowledge, and a disposition to be independent and strategic. Organized, deliberate problem solving includes identifying and clarifying obstacles in relation to one's goal, gathering and considering information relevant to solving the problem, exploring possible solutions, weighing their merits, selecting the best solution, executing the plan, and evaluating the results of that choice. Each of the types of reasoning mentioned above is a component of mature problem solving. *Judgment* is a decision to act based on available information, which includes prediction of consequences.

In light of the large number of personal problems created by CHI, it is tragic and ironic that the part of the brain associated with organized problem solving is often injured, rendering that individual relatively weak in the function most needed to deal with daily challenges. Impairment of any type of reasoning, reduction in stored knowledge of rules, roles, and routines, and generally weakened self-regulatory functions can contribute to ineffective problem solving. Social judgment is often further compromised by specific right frontal lobe damage, which is associated with impaired social perception and associated social communication problems (Alexander et al., 1989).

Component Systems

Component cognitive systems are organized structures composed of basic and acquired processes and information.

Working Memory

Working memory is a storage or holding ''space'' where conscious coding and other operations occur. Information in working memory is that which is being attended to. This short-term memory is of limited structural capacity. However, the *functional* capacity of the system is increased by making operations automatic and also by deliberately organizing pieces of information into single ''chunks.'' Although reduction in structural capacity of working memory is not among the most common consequences of CHI, individuals in whom working memory is impaired profit from maximally effective organizing processes and from as much routine in their lives as possible.

Long-Term Memory (Knowledge Base)

Long-term or permanent memory is a highly organized system of stored knowledge and memories. Memory can be subclassified in a variety of ways. One of the most popular begins with a distinction between declarative and procedural memory. Declarative memory includes semantic memory (knowledge of objects, people, events, word meanings, rules, scripts, and other types of information that are not associated with specific times and places in one's life) and episodic memory (memory for autobiographical information—memories associated with specific times, places, and personal experiences) (Tulving, 1972). Procedural memory or knowledge includes learned motor and perceptual skills as well as behavioral routines, each of which may be accessible only through performing the skill or routine (e.g., riding a bike, playing a video game) (Mayes, 1988).

Stored knowledge plays a critical role in nearly every human activity, including comprehending and remembering new information. Although knowledge and skill acquired before a head injury are often recovered in the weeks and months after the injury despite substantial new learning problems, this recovery may be quite incomplete. Indeed, it is not uncommon for individuals with CHI to have unusual profiles of knowledge and skill, with gaps at relatively low levels and preserved islands at relatively high levels. This adds to the necessity of flexibility and creativity in assessment and intervention.

Executive System

With respect to cognitive functioning, the executive component is responsible for identifying one's strengths and weaknesses, setting goals, planning and organizing cognitive behavior designed to achieve the goals, initiating and inhibiting behavior, monitoring and evaluating the results, and solving problems that are encountered (strategic behavior). The executive system (or ''central processor'') can direct processing (e.g., attending, perceiving, organizing) and the selection of strategies in relation to immediate and long-term goals.

The frequency of prefrontal injury in CHI brings executive functions to center stage in rehabilitation that targets cognitive, communicative, and general behavioral dysfunction. Clinicians must carefully distinguish between impaired processes and impaired executive control over those processes. Process-specific exercises are predictably ineffective if the problem is largely self-regulation or executive control over the process.

Response System

The response system controls all output, such as speech, facial expression, and fine- and gross-motor activity, including motor planning.

Functional-Integrative Performance

Functional-integrative performance of ''real-life'' tasks and activities (e.g., dressing, conversing, reading a novel) involves a complex interaction of the entire cognitive mechanism, personality and motivational variables, and the environment. The importance of highlighting functional-integrative performance in cognitive rehabilitation is underscored by the common clinical observation that many individuals fail to spontaneously transfer improved functioning at the level of isolated component processes and systems to the complex real-life activities that give rehabilitation its meaning. Because people process information for particular purposes and within particular environmental constraints, it is critical to include functional-integrative performance in a rehabilitation-relevant definition of cognition.

The potential for variation in performance of complex environmental interactions is great, making it difficult to measure improvement in real-world functioning. Therefore, in addition to the cognitive categories described above, it is useful to track functional performance of real-world tasks along the following dimensions:

Efficiency: Rate and duration of performance (e.g., time needed to read a chapter or describe an event) and amount accomplished (e.g., number of pages read, length of lecture attended to, number of utterances in a monologic discourse)
Level: Complexity, abstractness, and developmental/academic level of the task
Scope: The variety of contexts in which performance can be maintained at a given level
Manner: Qualities of task performance, such as dependence (needing cues) versus independence; impulsiveness versus reflectiveness; rigidity versus flexibility

Use of the Framework in Planning Intervention

We have found that these distinctions among and within processes, systems, and functional performance facilitate more precise identification of individuals' strengths and weaknesses, which results in customized treatment plans and more effective treatment. For example, adults with CHI often present with apparent attentional problems that interfere with conversational flow. J. N. and M. M. were two such clients. To isolate the underlying disturbance, we varied the difficulty and interest level of discourse and the mode of presentation (e.g., purely verbal versus verbal supported by pictures). In the case of J. N., there was no difference in the quality of conversation as a function of this variation. Consequently, his treatment focused on strategies to maximize his ability to attend and to request assistance from his communication partner if necessary. M. M.'s conversational ability improved sharply when discourse was simplified and supported by situational and picture cues. Treatment in his case targeted growth of the semantic knowledge base and language comprehension, as well as counseling of communication partners.

FACILITATING CHANGE IN PERFORMANCE

Cognitive Development

The literature on cognitive development (briefly reviewed by Ylvisaker et al., 1992) and on transfer of cognitive skill (reviewed by Singley and Anderson, 1989) provides useful information concerning variables that are significant in promoting cognitive growth and, derivatively, in the selection of treatment goals that are productive in achieving higher levels of cognitive-communicative functioning. As noted earlier, cognitive development involves the simultaneous growth of major aspects of cognition, with gains in any area mutually supporting development in other areas. Therefore, therapy cannot be structured as a hierarchical or serial-order progression through developmentally ordered cognitive processes.

The developmental literature does, however, highlight some fundamental features of cognitive development that may be necessary for higher-level functioning. Major changes during development involve expansion of the knowledge base, increases in attention and memory capacity (either structural or functional), increases in the efficiency of information processing, and the development of metacognitive awareness, which is closely related to the increasing use of cognitive strategies. Additionally, a gradual decentration in perception and thinking occurs. This makes possible the consideration of an increasingly large number and variety of features of an object, event, or person, as well as the ability to think hypothetically and consider alternative possibilities and alternative perspectives (nonegocentrism) (Flavell, 1985). Therefore, there is reason to concentrate intervention on improved processing efficiency, growth of the knowledge base (including concepts, organizing schemas, and strategies), and improved executive functions (including metacognitive awareness, self-direction, and strategic thinking). By borrowing from the developmental literature, we do not wish to endorse the validity of the regression hypothesis following brain injury. We do know, however, that impaired cognitive processes and systems following severe CHI make it difficult to deal strategically with complex and abstract information and tasks. This is also a characteristic of earlier developmental periods. Knowing how children develop into abstract and strategic thinkers can guide our selection of treatment goals for adults. The clinical challenge is to design tasks that are respectful of an adult's maturity, self-concept, and pretraumatic levels of functioning while at the same time rebuilding cognitive skills necessary for resuming adult thinking and activity.

Transfer of Cognitive Skill

The experimental literature on transfer of cognitive skill in normally functioning adults is very pessimistic with respect to spontaneous transfer or generalization (e.g., Singley and Anderson, 1989). For example, rules and principles of mathematics or logic learned in the context of one type of problem are characteristically not transferred by college students to other

types of problem to which the rules apply. With this as background, it is no wonder that the primary lesson from careful efficacy research with a wide variety of clinical populations and areas of intervention is that performance can readily be improved under laboratory conditions but with little or no transfer to other tasks or settings. This is consistent with the common clinical observation in brain-injury rehabilitation that individuals whose performance improves from poor to excellent in *decontextualized* cognitive drill (e.g., workbook or computer exercises) often continue to perform badly in real-world tasks that appear to engage the same cognitive processes that improved in therapy.

Despite a broad-based movement in the direction of appropriately contextualized intervention for other disability groups—including family-based services for infants and preschoolers with disabilities, classroom-based services for school-age children, and supported employment and community-based supports for adults with developmental disabilities—rehabilitation professionals have been slow to provide meaningful contexts in their cognitive services for individuals with CHI. There are three distinct solutions to this critical problem: (*a*) Follow the traditional acquisition-stabilization-generalization model of intervention, with acquisition and stabilization occurring in nonfunctional tasks and settings but with heavy emphasis on generalization to functional tasks and settings. This may be appropriate for individuals who are capable of a sufficient degree of abstract thinking to effect the transfer. (*b*) Alternatively, skills can be targeted from the outset with functional, meaningful tasks and also progress quickly from therapy settings to natural settings. This approach is most critical for people who are very concrete and may therefore acquire associations in decontextualized training that actually *interfere* with generalization. (*c*) In either case, there is great value in focusing on the individual's "strategic attitude"—that is, on the disposition to be actively involved in problem solving and in transfer of skill from training tasks to other tasks and settings. This is discussed below.

Structures, Skill, and Knowledge

Approaching cognitive rehabilitation through decontextualized drill and practice (e.g., multitrial workbook or computer exercises) assumes in most cases that the process or function that is exercised is a skill than can be strengthened with practice and once improved will support improved performance of any task that engages that process or function. Unfortunately, this assumption is frequently invalid. For example, working memory is often drilled as a skill (e.g., having clients repeat series of numbers or unrelated words) but is more likely a fixed-capacity structure that cannot be strengthened with exercise as though it were a mental muscle (although functional capacity can be increased with organizing strategies). Similarly, organizing processes are often drilled with decontextualized exercises (e.g., workbook exercises with categories, sequences, and associations) but are best understood as including two types of domain-specific knowledge (information and organizing schemas). For example, a stock boy knows how to categorize items in a supermarket and a librarian knows how to categorize books, but no matter how knowledgeable and effective they may be in their own domain, neither can be assumed to be an effective organizer in the other's domain. Other cognitive targets (e.g., problem solving) are best understood as a complex combination of skill, strategic attitude, and domain-specific knowledge, all operating within fixed cognitive structures. To be effective, intervention must be sensitive to all of these components.

Failure to consider these issues easily leads inexperienced clinicians to address this clinical territory by identifying an impaired cognitive function and creating tasks (that lack personal relevance and are removed from natural settings) to exercise the function. This model of cognitive intervention is comparable to prevailing practices in language therapy and special education in the 1960s and 1970s—practices that were subsequently found to be relatively ineffective for most children with language and learning disability, in large part because of the failure of transfer. The clinical bottom line is that individuals who wish, for example, to be better organized must practice organizing in contexts (activities and settings) in which they need to be better organized; people who wish to be better problem solvers must practice solving real-world problems in contexts in which it is important for them to be good problem solvers. Decontextualized cognitive drill and practice, although potentially a useful activity in which to highlight cognitive strengths and deficits and identify components of functioning that require attention, must give way to functional, contextualized, personally relevant intervention as the cornerstone of brain-injury rehabilitation.

STAGES OF "RECOVERY"

The word "recovery" has been placed in quotation marks in this heading because of its potential to suggest misleadingly that a common outcome after CHI is return to pretrauma levels of function in every respect. This is certainly not true, and therefore "Stages of Improvement" may be a better heading (Kay and Lezak, 1990). Because intervention goals, priorities, and procedures vary dramatically with general levels of cognitive and behavioral functioning, and because the process of "recovery" can be very protracted after CHI (compared, for example, with recovery after stroke), there is value in outlining stages that differ qualitatively from an intervention perspective. Furthermore, an understanding of typical stages of improvement helps treatment staff, family members, and individuals with CHI to place in perspective behaviors that would otherwise be most distressing. However, any discussion of stages must be sensitive to the varied patterns and rates of improvement experienced by different individuals.

The Rancho Los Amigos (RLA) Hospital Levels of Cognitive Recovery (Hagen, 1981), an eight-stage recovery scale, is widely used for this purpose. From an even more general perspective, we have found it useful to base rehabilitation program development on three very broad stages: early, middle, and late.

Early Stage (RLA 2–3)

This stage begins with the first generalized responses to environmental stimuli and ends with stimulus-specific responses (e.g., visual tracking, localizing to sound), recognition of some common objects through appropriate use of the object (if motorically capable), and comprehension of some simple commands in context. From a cognitive perspective, this is often called the sensory or coma stimulation stage of rehabilitation, currently a controversial and hotly debated field of intervention.

Zasler and colleagues (1991) presented a useful review of these themes and a conservative approach to coma management.

Middle Stage (RLA 4–6)

This stage begins with heightened alertness and increased activity combined with some degree of confusion and disorientation, which may include agitated behavior unrelated to environmental provocation. It ends with a reduction in confusion, which is manifested by adequate orientation and behavior that is generally goal directed in a familiar environment. This is the stage of rehabilitation in which the environment as well as group and individual therapy sessions are simplified, structured, and focused so as to reduce confusion and promote adaptive behavior and progressively increasing ability to process information and communicate effectively.

Late Stage (RLA 7, 8, and Beyond)

This stage begins with an adequate, though perhaps superficial and fragile, orientation to important aspects of life and ends with the individual's ultimate level of neurologic improvement, which may or may not include cognitive and communicative deficits that are functionally impairing. This is the stage of rehabilitation in which environmental supports are gradually withdrawn for purposes of helping individuals to become maximally independent and to learn how to compensate for and adjust to the remaining deficits. It is also the stage of refinement of skills with a focus on effective information processing and social communication in real-world settings and with real-life demands. Neurologic improvement after severe CHI can continue (at a decelerating rate) for many months and even years in some cases. Beyond that, there is no specific upper limit to learning, compensation, and adjustment that can be facilitated by creative clinicians and can substantially affect successful living.

In this chapter, we will discuss assessment and treatment issues related to the middle and late stages of recovery.

GENERAL PRINCIPLES OF TREATMENT

From this broad framework, together with our experience working with several hundred individuals with CHI, we have isolated a small number of principles that are critical in designing treatment programs. The concrete application of the principle varies with the stage of recovery.

1. Success, resulting from planned compensation and appropriately adjusted expectations, facilitates progress while building a positive self-concept.
2. The systematic gradation of activities, demands, and support ("scaffolding"; Wood et al., 1976), carefully adjusted to meet individual needs with withdrawal of support as individuals demonstrate increased capacity, facilitates improvement.
3. Generalization to real-world settings and activities must be a central component of intervention. The model could be either (*a*) focusing intensively on generalization after a skill has been acquired in a clinical context or (*b*) focusing on generalization from the outset, using functional activities and a variety of settings and everyday people. Furthermore, individuals should be addressed as strategic problems solvers, actively involved in the process of generalization.
4. Sensitivity to executive system themes must be part of therapy sessions and the rehabilitative environment in general. This includes engaging individuals with CHI in self-appraisal, goal setting, deci-

sion making, planning and organizing, monitoring and evaluating, and practical problem solving in a variety of functional contexts.

5. Integration of treatment (including daily interaction and behavioral intervention) among all staff and family members facilitates the individual's orientation, learning, and generalization of learned skills. A key role for speech-language pathologists is to train everyday people (family, friends, and direct-care staff) in basic communicative competencies.

6. Whenever possible, personally meaningful activities and natural settings should be selected for cognitive and communicative intervention. Although individual sessions can be useful for diagnostic therapy, for training in personally sensitive areas, and for highly specific interventions, group therapy and community-based intervention are necessary components of social skills and social cognition therapy and for generalization training.

7. As much as possible, tasks should be designed that are consistent with the individual's pretraumatic personality, interests, and educational/vocational background as well as goals for the future.

ASSESSMENT

In certain respects, assessment of individuals with CHI is a particularly perilous and complex process and therefore merits a discussion that would take us beyond the scope of this chapter. Our few comments on the subject are intended to place in perspective the various approaches to assessment and to highlight the limitations of strictly formal assessment of individuals with CHI. (See Groher and Ochipa [1992] for a discussion of the importance and limitations of formal language testing after CHI.)

Aphasia batteries are certainly useful for those clients with specific language impairment. The primary limitation of aphasia tests in CHI, however, is that they are insensitive to communication impairment associated with prefrontal (executive system) injury. It is well established that prefrontal damage, including bilateral damage, is compatible with average or above average results of intelligence and language tests in adults (Stuss and Benson, 1986) and children (Mateer and Williams, 1991; Welsh and Pennington, 1988). Furthermore, there are reports in the neuropsychological literature of individuals with known prefrontal lesions performing within normal limits on neuropsychological tests *specifically designed to detect impaired performance related to prefrontal injury* (Bigler, 1988; Eslinger and Damasio, 1985; Stuss and Benson, 1986).

The fundamental paradox of executive system assessment is that by presenting prestructured tasks removed from real-world goals and in a simplified environment, the examiner eliminates the possibility of evaluating how effectively the individual can perceive and interpret real-world situations; creatively plan, initiate, monitor, and evaluate behavior designed to achieve personal goals; and adjust to real-world challenges (Lezak, 1982). That is, examiners and the examination situation function as ''prosthetic frontal lobes'' (Stuss and Benson, 1986). This is an explanation for the common report from clinicians and family members that individuals who score well on language tests after CHI nevertheless may communicate ineffectively in social contexts or fail to handle the language demands of school or other demanding environments. Alternatively, individuals with specific language skill deficiencies associated with more posterior damage may perform poorly on tests but surprisingly well in familiar vocational or social contexts.

There are several important ways in which the conditions of formal testing may prevent examiners from identifying functionally impairing deficits after CHI (Ylvisaker et al., in press a).

1. The neat and quiet environment of testing may compensate for problems with attention and concentration.
2. A series of short testing sessions may compensate for problems with endurance, perseverance, and fatigue.
3. Tests that do not measure learning from one session to the next may compensate for serious memory and learning problems.
4. Clear instructions and explanations of test items may compensate for difficulties with initiation, inhibition, task orientation, flexible reorientation to new tasks, and problem solving.
5. The supportive interactive manner of the examiner may compensate for motivational difficulties or inability to deal with interpersonal stress.
6. Test items that fail to present real-life amounts of information or rate of delivery may compensate for a generalized inefficiency in information processing.
7. Tests that assess pretraumatically acquired information or rules easily create unrealistic expectations for new learning.
8. Formal tests fail to measure the crucial ability to generalize newly acquired skills or strategies from one setting to another. This is not to suggest that a clear picture of optimal performance is undesirable. Rather, it is to caution clinicians that formal test results may lack ecological validity, necessitating the use of functional real-world observations to complete the assessment.

Even cleverly designed real-world tasks often place much of the executive burden of the task on the evaluator. For example, giving the client a certain amount of money and asking him to purchase a list of items in a shopping mall within a limited amount of time is a useful evaluation of certain aspects of planning, organizing, and communicating. However, *any* task that begins with the evaluator saying, in effect, ''This is what I would like you to do and here are the rules,'' removes from the client the need to identify the situation and the behavior appropriate in the situation—a critical aspect of executive functioning often weak after prefrontal injury.

For these reasons, formal cognitive and communicative assessment after CHI must be supplemented by careful observation of the individual in a variety of settings, by a thorough interview of significant everyday people in his or her life, and by ongoing diagnostic therapy. Informal observation in selected settings reveals the effects of varying environmental conditions and stressors on the appropriateness of communication and the efficiency of processing. A careful family interview that focuses on the individual's behavior in familiar environments often reveals behaviors at both the highest and lowest ends of functioning. A period of diagnostic therapy is often necessary to sort out which of the manifest problems are primary and which secondary, to determine which intervention procedures are most effective, and to assess the individual's rate of new learning and ability to generalize from one setting to another. Furthermore, self-awareness of deficits and their implications as well as general metacognitive and executive system recovery are often revealed only in the process of diagnostic intervention. Hartley (1990, 1992) provided an excellent framework and many useful procedures for functional communication assessment after CHI. Ylvisaker and Szekeres (1989) presented a variety of procedures designed to probe executive functions in an ecologically valid manner.

Assessment designed to facilitate treatment planning is best understood as an ongoing process of testing hypotheses—with the hypotheses relating to the client's profile of strengths and weaknesses, to situational variability, and to the usefulness of possible intervention strategies. Ylvisaker and colleagues (1990 and 1992) presented a number of procedures for testing hypotheses regarding cognitive-communicative functioning after CHI. Useful questions to guide an assessment of cognitive-communicative functioning include the following.

Language Comprehension

What is the individual's receptive vocabulary level? Are there gaps in the semantic knowledge base? How is language comprehension affected by systematically increasing processing demands: increased length and complexity of utterances, increased rate of presentation, increased amount of information to be processed, increased environmental interference, and increased interpersonal stress in conversational exchanges? Language comprehension includes reading as well as auditory comprehension. Real-world processing demands should be simulated, which, in the case of a college student, would include reading appropriate textbooks and listening to extended lectures.

Language Expression

What is the individual's unstressed expressive vocabulary level? How do varying forms of stress affect naming and word retrieval? Can the individual organize reasonably large amounts of information for organized, fluent, and complete expression (focusing on *coherence* more than cohesion in discourse)? Is conversation coherent, flexible, adequately creative, and socially appropriate? Are there difficulties either initiating or inhibiting social interaction? What cognitive and social variables influence conversational competence? Prutting and Kirchner (1987) presented a useful taxonomy for identifying conversational strengths and weaknesses. Mentis and Prutting (1991) described useful procedures for analyzing the coherence of monologic discourse. Language expression includes writing as well as speaking.

Integrative Language and Verbal Reasoning

How well organized is the semantic system (e.g., real-world scripts, associations, categories)? Can the individual detect subtleties of meaning? Efficiently form new verbal concepts? Use language to draw conclusions, solve problems, explore alternatives, generate interpretations? Are these integrative abilities used spontaneously in natural settings?

Verbal Memory and New Learning

Can the individual selectively attend, concentrate, and shift and divide attentional focus? What is the structural capacity of working memory (e.g., digit span)? Does the individual store and retrieve newly learned information or rules over extended periods of time? Make effective use of feedback in verbal learning? Spontaneously use strategies to facilitate learning? Profit from strategies suggested by others? Store and retrieve daily events (episodic memory)? What variables appear to be particularly related to memory efficiency: attention? interest

level? perceptual modality? familiarity? inherent organization of information to be learned? context? personal importance? mnemonic strategies?

MIDDLE-STAGE INTERVENTION

Although there is great variability among individuals with CHI at any stage of improvement, the dominant cognitive and behavioral characteristics at this stage are confusion, restricted ability to process information, and weak regulation of behavior (possibly culminating in unprovoked agitation). More specifically, many individuals have difficulty focusing and maintaining attention to the most salient aspects of a situation; perceiving events, including social events, accurately; encoding, storing, and retrieving new information; retrieving information already stored in the knowledge base; organizing information, language, and behavior; planning, organizing, initiating, and monitoring behavior in the pursuit of personal goals; controlling emotional responses; and solving problems as they arise in daily life.

The general goals of cognitive intervention at this stage are to decrease confusion, improve orientation, increase processing abilities (including organized thinking), increase goal-directed behavior, reestablish access to semantic and episodic memories, and gradually increase awareness of the new profile of strengths and limitations. This is accomplished by (*a*) creating a highly structured, orderly, predictable, and supportive environment that by itself promotes adaptive behavior; (*b*) withdrawing this structure and support as quickly as possible to prevent learned dependence and to promote independent problem solving and decision making; and (*c*) engaging the individual in structured tasks that are carefully arranged along several dimensions of difficulty and complexity so that success is guaranteed and processing abilities can be systematically regained (see below). Specific communication goals generally include decreasing tangential and rambling discourse, increasing the appropriateness of conversation, improving comprehension of increasingly long and complex segments of language, improving the organization of the semantic knowledge base, and improving word-retrieval abilities.

If these symptoms of language disorders are grounded in more general cognitive disruption at this stage, treatment may not be most effectively directed at the symptom but rather at more general dimensions of cognitive processing and organization. Later in this section, we provide illustrations of therapy tasks that are consistent with this orientation.

Environmental Intervention

An individual's environment at this stage of rehabilitation typically consists of (*a*) the nursing unit, the routines on the unit, and the staff and family members who are the everyday communication partners in that setting; (*b*) other hospital areas, such as the dining and recreational areas and the interactions that occur there; (*c*) therapy areas, the treating staff, and their interactions with the patient; and (*d*) possibly home and the interactions that occur there. The amount of time spent with therapists, especially just with the speech-language pathologist, is very small relative to the number of waking hours in the week. This fact, combined with the important premise that any experience or interaction has the potential to increase orientation, sense of success, adaptation, organization, and processing efficiency—or, alternatively, contribute to confusion, behavioral outbursts, anger, fear, and withdrawal—strongly suggests that speech-language pathologists should team with behavioral psychologists and others to ensure that activities throughout the day are well designed to meet the patient's cognitive and behavioral needs and that everyday people in the environment are well oriented and trained in communicative and behavioral competencies. Ylvisaker and colleagues (1993) described in detail a program designed to create well-trained communication partners for individuals with CHI.

The keys to successful environmental intervention include (*a*) sufficient consistency of routine and familiarity of settings and staff to prevent confusion; (*b*) selection of activities (including activities of daily living and recreational activities) that approach but do not exceed the individual's ability to process the information and organize a response; (*c*) interactive styles and approaches to behavioral outbursts that are effective and consistent among staff and family members; and (*d*) as much active decision making and problem solving as is possible for the individual at that time. In most head-injury rehabilitation centers, a log or memory book system is used at this stage to facilitate recovery of orientation and memory as well as to promote communication among staff members and between staff and family. For severely disoriented individuals, the book may include schedules, maps, photographs of significant people, and possibly also photographs of the patient engaged in daily routines.

During the confused stages of improvement, orientation activities occur throughout the day. They include (*a*) listening to and repeating (in as conversational a manner as possible) personally meaningful orienting information; (*b*) learning how to use calendars, log books, schedules, photographs, maps, and the like to gain orientation; (*c*) frequently reviewing events from the recent past and plans for the immediate future; and (*d*) creating time lines that include personally significant life events. In addition, nurses, other health care workers, and family members are trained to create a structured therapeutic experience out of any daily activity, including recreational and self-care activities.

Structured Activities

Speech-language pathologists (and others) can promote cognitive-communicative recovery through functional-integrative activities that focus the individual's attention, systematically increase the ability to process information, promote access to the knowledge base, and facilitate organized and appropriate behavior and decision making in increasingly varied and complex contexts. Clinicians need not, and in most case should not, restrict their intervention at this stage to specifically linguistic targets or auditory-verbal activities.

Functional activities can, then, be selected on the basis of the individual's interests and strongest receptive and expressive modalities (often visual input and motor output). It is useful to involve patients in selecting the activity (stopping short of causing stress and confusion by giving too many choices), in part to increase their engagement in rehabilitation but also to begin gradually to target decision making and other executive functions in therapy. The primary responsibility of treatment staff is to engage patients in highly structured activities in such a way as to guarantee successful performance and gradually and systematically to increase task demands as indicated by improvements in functioning.

Activities that are appropriate for this process of systematically organizing and gradually challenging the processing mechanism include concrete visual-perceptual-motor tasks (e.g., helping to sort clothing, collectibles, or other personally meaningful items), simplified but meaningful vocational tasks, simple video games, self-care tasks, craft projects, simple meal preparation, and high-interest board and card games. Verbal activities may include reading of (or selective listening to) cartoons, greeting cards, letters from family and friends, and high-interest newspaper or magazine stories (reading or listening for specific pieces of information); describing familiar scripts (e.g., pretrauma work or recreational routines) in an organized manner; and describing personally significant people, places, events, or things, possibly using an organizational guide to promote completeness and coherence of the description. These activities are embedded in the context of natural respectful conversation (e.g., "Could you tell me about your home, starting with things in your living room?" or "Could you tell Joe about the cartoon that we read this morning?" or "Let's read the letter from your brother and find out when he is coming"). The functionality and personal relevance of the task contribute to motivation as well as to transfer of training.

The therapeutic effect of these activities comes through the gradual and systematic increase in the demands that the activity places on the individual's processing and self-regulatory systems. Each of the following variables represents a continuum of difficulty that should be considered in designing tasks.

1. *Perceptual Variables:* Sensory-integrative requirements, environmental distractions, visual complexity, rate of presentation
2. *Cognitive Variables:* Attention span and endurance, familiarity of the activity, number and variety of elements to be arranged, sequential organization, planning, memory, time limits, cognitive flexibility, decision making, problem solving, safety judgment, self-monitoring, and self-evaluation
3. *Linguistic Variables:* Specific language comprehension and expression factors
4. *Psychosocial Variables:* Initiation, interpersonal relations, frustration tolerance

Staff (and family members) can promote improvement of cognitive processes and systems during these functional activities by prompting patients to maintain attention, scan stimuli for relevance to the task at hand, observe other people's performance, use external memory aids, create an organized work space, take time to think and act, explain why events occur, predict consequences of acts, and describe feelings and perceptions. Furthermore, staff should use these meaningful activities as occasions to model deliberate thinking, reasoning, problem solving, self-questioning, self-instructing (e.g., "I'll have trouble remembering that; I'd better write it down"), and self-evaluation (e.g., "Let's make sure that we have all of the ingredients in"). This modeling begins to set the stage for deliberate compensatory behavior later in recovery.

Cognitive-Communicative Activities

During the confused stages of a patient's recovery, clinicians may also focus specifically on one or more cognitive processes or systems with the ultimate goal of improving communication. Organization is often a primary intervention target in cognitive-communicative intervention because of the pervasiveness of organizational impairments at this stage, the strong connection between cognitive organization and effective language comprehension and expression, and the well-documented relation between effective organization and efficient learning (encoding, storage, and retrieval) of new information (Bjorkland, 1985; Brown, 1975; Lange, 1978; Levin et al., 1988; and many others). If a person recognizes a familiar organizational pattern of some sort in information to be processed and uses that pattern or scheme in encoding, storing, and retrieving the information, memory/new learning is enhanced (Brown, 1975, 1979). For example, presenting objects that are related within a category system (e.g., some fruits and some vegetables, both of which are foods) will facilitate memory only if the individual understands and recognizes that category system. All environmental interactions become more efficient and less confusing when one is able to perceive organization in events or impose it where it is lacking. Therefore, it is useful for clinicians to understand organization and clearly differentiate organizational schemes so that they can highlight them effectively.

Organization may be understood as a product, process, or conceptual structure. As a *product,* organization is an identifiable and stable relationship that exists among ideas, objects, people, or events in a set (Mandler, 1967). Prominent organizational schemes that can be identified in our daily living, school, and work activities include perceptual similarity (e.g., color, shape, size); semantic similarity (e.g., superordinate categories); functional use (e.g., items used to perform a specific task); specific real-event scripts (e.g., the typical sequence of events involved in eating at a restaurant); general lie scripts or commonalities across the life span (e.g., attending elementary and high school; beginning employment; getting married); hierarchical discourse structure (e.g., main idea and details); narrative schemes (e.g., story grammar); alphabetical order; and others. Schemes may also be combined—for example, including narrative illustrations in a book that is largely organized according to a main idea-detail outline form.

As a *conceptual structure,* organization is the way in which ideas are interrelated in semantic memory. When a person identifies and benefits from an organizational scheme inherent in stimuli or independently imposes a scheme on stimuli (e.g., tells a well-organized story), it can be inferred that the scheme (e.g., story grammar) is present in semantic memory and that it serves as a frame for processing information or manipulating the environment.

Organization as a *process* is a complex activity involving the entire processing mechanism. Organizing can be the active process one carries out while assimilating and encoding information (input organization); the directed process of retrieving information; or the process of organizing information for coherent expression, for goal-directed behavior, or for arranging objects in the environment (output organization). All organizing activity is directed by goals and constrained by the knowledge and organizing schemes stored in long-term memory as well as by the context of action. Imposing organization is dependent not only on knowledge of organizing schemes but also on a functional executive system.

Confused patients in the middle stages of recovery often need help in reestablishing access to their knowledge base; reestablishing, stabilizing, and using organizing schemes; controlling their attention; deliberately searching for and retrieving

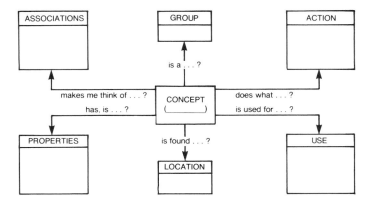

Figure 30.1. Feature analysis guide.

information and words; and evaluating the relevance and adequacy of information before a response is formulated. That is, these individuals need practice in organized thinking.

Feature Analysis

Feature analysis is an organized thinking procedure that we use to facilitate (*a*) deliberate control of attention, (*b*) organized information retrieval and word retrieval, (*c*) monitoring of the relevancy and adequacy of information about a topic, and (*d*) organized formulation of verbal output. Any of these goals may be primary for a specific client. For example, if the goal is attentional control, the individual may be challenged to retrieve information that is relevant to only one feature category. The procedure is based on leading theories regarding the organization of concepts in semantic memory (e.g., Smith, 1978).

In the initial phase of treatment, analysis of basic-level concepts (Rosch, 1977) is prompted using these feature categories: group (superordinate category), action, use, location, properties/ parts, and strong semantic and experiential associations. Figure 30.1 illustrates one possible visual representation that can be used to guide the analysis. The objectives at this phase are attentional control, increasingly deep reflection on a feature in focus, organized retrieval of information, and monitoring of responses for relevance and adequacy. Since the ultimate goal is to reestablish an organized semantic knowledge base and/or organized retrieval of information from that knowledge base, the analysis always proceeds in the same clockwise fashion.

When attentional control is adequate, the goal is to learn the procedure, including labels or descriptors for each of the boxes on the guide. Prompting and cuing are as frequent as needed and may range from yes/no questions (recognition memory) to *wh*-questions (cued recall) to general encouragement to think more deeply (free recall). The responsibility for structuring the analysis and evaluating responses is gradually shifted from clinician to client.

It is important that individuals not simply retrieve information because requested to or as an end in itself. Rather, the information retrieved should be put to use (consistent with the premise that cognitive behavior is goal directed). We practice the organized use of the information gathered in a feature analysis in a variety of ways, including (*a*) writing a descriptive paragraph, (*b*) writing a narrative, (*c*) comparing concepts (i.e., similarities and differences exercises), and (*d*) problem-solving exercises. Following a feature analysis with one of these tasks not only gives a point to the feature analysis exercise but also illustrates for clients the value of a solid knowledge base for producing good descriptions and for solving problems.

A useful goal for individuals at this stage of recovery is that they learn the procedure to the point of completing an analysis independently and with reasonable thoroughness and relevance. Throughout, we focus attention on missing information and how that information could be acquired (e.g., ask someone; use a reference book). During later stages of treatment, individuals may deliberately use this procedure as a strategy for searching their knowledge base for information or for words.

Developing Knowledge and Use of Organizing Schemes

Table 30.1 outlines a variety of organizing schemes and describes examples of meaningful activities designed to highlight the schemes and to develop awareness of their usefulness. The final column of Table 30.1 includes suggested questions designed to prompt reflection on the effectiveness of the organizing scheme in relation to the goal of the practical activity and to promote application to other real-life situations. This metacognitive aspect of the organizational activities should be gradually phased in over the middle stages of recovery. One goal of the metacognitive questioning is to prepare individuals for the possible need to use these organizing schemes deliberately as compensatory strategies later in recovery if organization continues to be an area of relative impairment.

Rebuilding specific event scripts (e.g., personally meaningful vocational or home routines; eating in a cafeteria; going to a bank, a movie, or a grocery store) is especially important for individuals who are confused. The individual may need to repeat a sequence of events (simulated or real) to reestablish a stable script, complete with socially conventional behavior. Watching a video with on-line or delayed narration, role playing, describing pictured events, and practicing the script in real-world contexts may all be used to facilitate this development. After a stable script is established, individuals need to practice dealing with variations in the sequence of events. There is an important sense in which this type of organization is more basic in guiding thinking, talking, and acting than more abstract types of organization, such as categories, perceptual similarities, and the like, which are the focus of many cognitive rehabilitation workbooks.

Individuals Who Do Not Progress Beyond Confused Stages of Recovery

Some people with severe injuries do not progress beyond the confused stages of recovery. Because of persistent confusion and very shallow processing, they continue to require a highly structured and simplified environment and well-trained family members and direct care staff in order to maintain orientation, initiate socially meaningful behavior, inhibit challenging behavior, and communicate effectively. The quality of life for these individuals can be enhanced through intensive training in a limited set of social behaviors (e.g., greetings, social requests), everyday routines, and avocational activities. To be successful, training that takes place in a rehabilitation center must be guided by the social and avocational realities of the proposed discharge destination. Rehabilitative programming often includes the following:

1. Developing and practicing routines that will serve to structure the day (e.g., time to get up, shower, dress, eat breakfast). Often, posted checklists continue to be needed indefinitely to complete routines in the proper sequence.
2. Selecting and practicing recreational activities. The following sequence is illustrative: Help the individual select a small number of games that are appropriate to his or her age, interests, and ability; practice playing the games, with adaptations of the rules if necessary; if rules are adapted, attach a typed description of adaptations to the game box so that other partners can play appropriately; attach a list of the games to the lap tray or some other likely place; prompt the individual to initiate the activity with varied partners—this may require rehearsing specific sentences, such as "Would you like to play . . . ?" Termination sentences may also be practiced, such as "Maybe we could play again sometime"; these sentences may themselves be attached to the lap tray to serve as cues. Finally, family members or staff should receive instruction and counseling so that they are accepting of limited avocational goals and are knowledgeable about the selected activities.
3. Using chained activities, or activities that cannot be completed in one day (e.g., craft projects) to help maintain orientation to the recent past and to provide day-to-day linking.
4. Encouraging the individual to make collections (e.g., audio tapes, baseball cards, figurines) to heighten a sense of permanence and provide enjoyment and topics for conversation (Gobble and Pfahl, 1985).

For individuals with a severe initiation impairment, prosthetics may be considered, for example, a tastefully printed note placed on a wheelchair lap tray inviting others to join the individual in a favored activity. Individuals with severe inhibition impairment may need to live in a "child-proofed" environment with staff or family members well trained in redirection procedures.

LATE-STAGE INTERVENTION

Individuals in the late (postconfusion) stages of cognitive and behavioral recovery are adequately oriented to their environment, act in a generally goal-directed manner, and process information in sufficient depth to learn new information and routines and to avoid the appearance of grossly inappropriate behavior. The combination of growing metacognitive awareness, improved self-regulation, and an emerging profile of residual strengths and weaknesses supports the consideration of training in the deliberate use of strategic procedures to compensate for ongoing deficits.

Residual cognitive, communicative, and behavioral impairments in adults with CHI vary with the nature and severity of the injury and preinjury status. Some combination of the following challenges is frequently observed: ineffective control over attentional and perceptual processes (e.g., difficulty maintaining, shifting, and dividing attentional focus; difficulty searching and scanning in an organized manner; difficulty attending to a variety of perceptual and social cues simultaneously); inefficient memory/learning (possibly affecting any memory process or type of memory, including deliberate use of memory strategies); relatively marked deterioration in language comprehension caused by increases in the amount, complexity, and abstractness of language and in the rate of presentation; word-retrieval problems; poorly organized behavior and language expression; shallow reasoning and problem solving; impulsive and socially awkward behavior; inflexible thinking and behavior; and relatively weak executive functions (including

Table 30.1.
Reestablishing Organized Semantic Memory[a]

Organizational Schema (means for attaining the goal)	Task and Goal	Activity	Reflections[b]
Perceptual Similarity (e.g., color, shape, size, texture, rhyme)	"The shop asked us to organize these leftover pieces of sandpaper so they can easily be found. Let's find a good way to do this."	1. Label small boxes for different grains (extra fine, fine, medium, etc.). 2. Sort the pieces according to their "texture" and put them into the labeled boxes. 3. Call out the textures and time how quickly they can be found.	How did you sort? Why this way? Was it "good"? In what other situations might one sort by texture? What would have happened if you had sorted by size? How could this help you remember where your tools or other possessions are kept or at least help you always locate them?
Semantic Similarity (e.g., superordinate category, opposites)	"We got a job to set up the layout of a new department store. We have to make it easy for customers to find what they want."	Make a floor plan specifying the location of departments. Place labeled items into the departments, grouping them by similarity (e.g., TVs, stereos, radios) in one area, but subgrouped within the area. Make display arrangement to entice people to buy (e.g., comfortable chair, flowers, glass of wine and stereo).	How did you arrange the store? Why did you use that arrangement? In what other situations would you group things this way? When would this arrangement be inconvenient? How could knowing this arrangement help your memory of a visit to a store? How did the display arrangement differ from the floor arrangement?
Function (use)	"We are moving furniture into a new house. We have to arrange the living room for TV watching and conversation."	Make a floor plan and arrange labeled blocks representing the furniture. Then rearrange them for special occasions, such as a cocktail party, Tupperware party, etc.	How were the items arranged for each activity? Why did you have to change them? How is this different from a department store arrangement?
Main Idea and Topic (discourse structure)	"We will present today's news to the orientation group." (Watch a videotaped news item or listen to an audiotaped news item.)	Listen to the tape. Fill in a form answering Who, What, When, Where, Why, and What happened questions and identifying the main idea. Relate the news item to another person using the diagram as notes.	How did the form help you remember? When wouldn't the form help? How did you stay so organized and coherent when you related the news item?

Table 30.1.
Reestablishing Organized Semantic Memory (*Continued*)

Organizational Schema (means for attaining the goal)	Task and Goal	Activity	Reflections[a]
Story Schema	"We will share a short story or TV show with ( ) who was unable to see or hear it."	Watch the videotape of a TV show or listen to an audiotape of a radio show. Fill out a schema diagram, including characters, setting, and episodes. Retell the story using the organizational diagram as a cue.	How did this form help you remember? How is the information arranged? Why is this arrangement good for a story? Would it be good for a math book? Why not?
General Life Scripts (abstracted common life events)	"We will write our autobiographies and present a 'this is your life' program"	Fill out a form with labeled boxes of common life events (birth, school, marriage, job) and uncommon significant events (e.g., head injury). Using the form as a guide, write the autobiography and then present it formally in a radio program format.	How did the form make writing more organized? How could the form help reconstruct the past? How is your autobiography organized (e.g., chronologically)? How did the written preparation help the oral presentation?
Specific Event Scripts (e.g., going to a restaurant, going to the dentist)	"We will explain to (*a small child*) what it will be like when he has to go to the dentist."	Fill in a form with relevant information about the situation to prepare what you are going to say to the child: ● Who will be there ● Sequence of expected events and actions ● Expected layout of the room and some variations Then using the guide, explain to a child or explain in a role-playing situation.	How did this form help you? Why wouldn't a general life script help you? How is your explanation to the child organized? Why would this help you remember what has happened to you?

[a] Possible probe questions to develop metacognition, understanding, and awareness.

self-awareness, goal setting, planning/organizing, self-initiating or inhibiting, self-monitoring and evaluating, and strategic thinking).

The general purpose of cognitive intervention at this stage is to help people to overcome cognitive barriers to the achievement of their goals in their natural environment. The goal is to rehabilitate people, not cognition. Rehabilitative options include (*a*) exercising impaired cognitive processes if there is reason to believe that such exercise will result in functionally meaningful improvement in real-world performance; (*b*) helping individuals to acquire procedures designed to compensate for deficits that are likely to persist; (*c*) identifying ideal teaching procedures so that educational and vocational professionals can efficiently teach domain-specific knowledge and skill; (*d*) helping everyday people design accommodations in their behavior and in the environment to compensate for the cognitive deficits of the individual with CHI; and (*e*) helping family members, employers, teachers, and the individual understand

and adjust to persistent changes in cognitive and related behavioral and communicative functioning.

During the 1980s, there was considerable enthusiasm for process-specific retraining exercises as a solution to chronic cognitive challenges caused by severe CHI. A large number of retraining programs were developed, many of which used the computer as a medium for presenting the retraining tasks (see, for example, Sohlberg and Mateer, 1989). More recently, professional enthusiasm for this approach has waned, in part because many investigations into the effectiveness of this approach have failed to show that the improvements in cognitive functioning generated by retraining exercises (a) are sufficient to make a difference in everyday tasks; (b) generalize to everyday settings; (c) are maintained over meaningful periods of time; (d) could not have been achieved in a more cost-effective manner with a functional approach; and (e) have a direct effect on communicative effectiveness (Berrol, 1990; Butler and Namerow, 1988; Schacter and Glisky, 1986). Ben-Yishay and Prigatano's (1990) cautions about "the computer approach" are particularly noteworthy, because both of these clinician/investigators were earlier associated with rehabilitation programs that highlighted computerized cognitive retraining exercises. Limited effectiveness of direct, decontextualized cognitive retraining exercises should not be surprising in light of the generally weak outcomes using this approach in general education and special education (reviewed by Mann, 1979) and the decades of accumulating evidence that transfer of cognitive skill is severely limited in people with no brain injury (reviewed by Singley and Anderson, 1989).

In discussion of late-stage cognitive intervention, we will emphasize compensatory strategies and applied, functional cognitive intervention. This selection should not be taken to imply abandonment of process-specific approaches. One reason for caution with respect to the restoration-versus-compensation debate is that one can never be certain that improvements following restoration exercises are not a result of the individual fashioning compensations for himself or herself or that improvements following compensation exercises are not a result of restoration of function occasioned by the compensation tasks. We simply urge clinicians to be appropriately skeptical of decontextualized cognitive exercises, knowing that this approach has a history of disappointing its proponents in the long run (Hresko and Reid, 1988; Kavale and Mattson, 1983; Mann, 1979).

Teaching Compensatory Strategies

Many cognitive and communicative consequences of severe CHI persist despite intensive remedial efforts. These consequences easily create obstacles to academic, vocational, and social success—obstacles that necessitate a greater degree of strategic proficiency than would be required in the absence of a brain injury. Unfortunately, the parts of the brain associated with strategic thinking and behavior are often themselves injured in CHI. Therefore, intervention designed to equip individuals with strategic procedures for overcoming obstacles is at the same time extremely important and extremely tricky.

Compensatory strategies are simply procedures—sometimes unconventional—that an individual deliberately uses to achieve goals that cannot be achieved without such special effort. Although the ultimate goal of intervention is habituation of the procedures so that their use need not consume limited attentional resources, we emphasize the word "deliberate" in order to distinguish this sense of "strategy" from the general notion of organized behavior (which is often referred to as a strategy even if not deliberate) and also from instructional or treatment strategies that are procedures used by therapists.

Strategies designed to compensate for cognitive deficits may involve the use of external aids (e.g., memory book, printed reminders, maps, alarm watch). Alternatively, a person might compensate using overt behavior (e.g., requesting clarification or repetition) or covert behavior (e.g., self-reminders, mental rehearsal or elaboration, structured thinking procedures, such as the Feature Analysis Guide [Fig. 30.1]). Appendix 30.1 includes a large number (by no means exhaustive) of strategic procedures that appropriately selected individuals can use to compensate for selected cognitive and communicative deficits.

It is tempting to conceive of teaching strategies as no different from other teaching; that is, the clinician identifies the client's needs, selects an appropriate strategy, selects appropriate teaching procedures, teaches the strategy, and monitors and evaluates the outcome. The client's role is, then, to follow the clinician's lead and acquire the strategic procedure. However, if strategies are what strategic people do, then this model of teaching must be thought of as *antistrategic strategy intervention,* because all of the truly strategic, problem-solving behavior is assumed by the clinician. In denying the client the right to participate in the strategic aspects of strategy learning, the clinician might inadvertently contribute to the client's learned helplessness—that is, passive reliance on others to solve critical problems posed by cognitive and communicative weakness. Furthermore, not only does this model of teaching fail to promote truly strategic behavior, it also have been found to fail the litmus tests of generalization and maintenance when applied to a variety of populations of impaired learners (Flavell, 1985; Pressley and associates, 1990).

There is clinical wisdom, therefore, in following Pressley's advice to structure strategy intervention around a model of a good strategy user (Pressley et al., 1989). Such a model not only serves to identify a variety of diverse goals that may be components of this intervention but also helps to separate reasonable from risky candidates for strategy intervention. Truly strategic people have the following characteristics:

- They have goals to which strategies are relevant.
- They know that their performance needs to be enhanced, that strategies enhance performance, and that they are capable of using strategies.
- They know when, where, and why to use specific strategic procedures.
- They monitor and evaluate the effectiveness of their performance so that being strategic is its own reward.
- They know a number of procedures, can select the procedure most relevant to a particular challenge, and can flexibly modify it as needed or create new procedures.
- They use strategic procedures frequently so that the procedures become relatively automatic and require little effort or planning.
- They have adequate "space" in working memory so that they can think about the task at hand and strategic procedures at the same time.
- They are not so impulsive that they act before considering a strategic maneuver.
- They are not so anxious that they neglect strategic behavior because of their focus on fear of failure.

- They have the support of teachers, employers, and family members to use strategies.
- They know enough about the subject at hand that they can meaningfully use strategies to learn more.

Ideal candidates for strategy intervention are individuals who have specific goals; are aware of their deficits and needs; have sufficient metacognitive maturity to think about thinking, communicating, and other cognitive issues; are disposed to strategic behavior (e.g., like to play games of strategy); have adequate attentional resources; are motivated; have reasonable self-control; and live in supportive environments. College students returning to school after a mild to moderate injury often fall into this category. Individuals who are extremely weak in many of these dimensions may not be candidates for strategy intervention, except perhaps in the limited sense of acquiring helpful routines that involve external aids (e.g., using printed schedules or maps). Most people with CHI fall between these two extremes, which means that strategy intervention must include attempts to improve a variety of areas of functioning related to strategic behavior. Because of the large number of complex factors involved in being strategic, it is unlikely that there ever will be a "test of candidacy for strategy intervention." Therefore, clinicians must simply be attentive to all of these dimensions in their diagnostic intervention with clients.

Selection of the areas for compensation and of specific strategic procedures must involve active engagement of the client, which frequently includes a tension between his or her natural strategic inclinations and the judgment of the clinician. Brainstorming and experimentation with alternative strategies (described in Table 30.2) help to resolve this tension. The ultimate test of the appropriateness of the strategy is spontaneous use and improved performance in natural settings. Intervention will inevitably fail if clients do not see the usefulness of the strategy relative to their goals or if the strategy does not fit the individual's overall style of learning, interacting, and coping. For example, it is quixotic at best to expect a shy and generally noninteractive person to enthusiastically adopt an input control strategy that requires him to request that speakers slow down or clarify and simplify their language. Variables to be reviewed in negotiating the selection of strategies include whether the procedure is used spontaneously; whether its degree of complexity and abstractness fits the client's cognitive level; how difficult the procedure is to use relative to its payoff; whether it fits the client's profile of neuropsychological strengths; whether it fits the client's personality; and whether it specifically addresses obstacles to the individual's concrete goals.

Table 30.2 outlines a set of intervention procedures that we have found useful in working with individuals with CHI. The three phases are very roughly sequential but should not be considered mutually exclusive. For example, attempts to promote improved awareness of strengths and weaknesses (part of Phase I) often continue throughout a client's entire rehabilitation program. In addition, work on generalization should begin before a procedure is habituated in a clinical setting.

In summary, our experience in helping individuals with CHI to become increasingly strategic underscores the importance of the following principles of strategy intervention: (*a*) Intervention should be embedded in natural, meaningful activities and settings, with strategic procedures specifically related to the client's goals; (*b*) intervention should be intensive and long term; (*c*) goals should be modest; (*d*) the environment as a whole should be supportive of and promote strategic thinking and strategic behavior. Although there are reports in the head-injury literature regarding the effectiveness of teaching strategies as individual procedures designed to improve one specific aspect of functioning, there is scant empirical evidence to support the effectiveness of strategy intervention, as we have described it, in head-injury rehabilitation. There is, however, a growing body of positive evidence in the educational psychology literature (reviewed by Pressley and associates, 1990), which Pressley (1993) has attempted to apply to the field of cognitive intervention after CHI. Ylvisaker and Szekeres (1989) outlined a number of procedures designed to promote improvements in executive functions, which are close relatives to strategic behavior. Meichenbaum (1993) discussed the application of another related set of intervention procedures, cognitive behavior modification, to head-injury rehabilitation.

Memory

Treatment of memory deficits requires careful analysis of the nature and extent of the memory disturbance. The conceptual terrain covered by the general term "memory" is vast and has been mapped in a variety of useful ways (e.g., Dodd and White, 1980; Hintzman, 1978). We will discuss treatment in relation to some of these mappings, but the distinctions should not be thought to represent diagnostic categories (i.e., discrete memory disorders).

Memory Processes: Encoding, Storage, and Retrieval

If an individual has difficulty encoding information, treatment is directed toward manipulating the encoding situation in such a way as to increase the probability that the information will be represented and retained. It has been well established that information is better retained if it is attended to and perceived, is thoroughly understood, has a coherent organization that fits the conceptual framework of the individual, can be integrated into stored knowledge, is personally significant, and has a defined context (Brown, 1975, 1979).

Controlling Input. The objective of training is to ensure that perception and comprehension occur. We encourage individuals to identify breakdowns in comprehension using techniques similar to those listed in Table 30.2. Clients must then learn to control the presentation of information using appropriate "input control" and comprehension strategies (see Appendix 30.1 for examples).

Identifying Organization in the Information. We encourage individuals to scan the information for inherent organization. Inherent organization includes scripts, temporal sequence, categories, main ideas or themes, and the structure identified by who, what, where, when, and why questions.

Imposing Organization. If there is no apparent organization in the information to be remembered or the organization is inadequate, we encourage individuals to impose their own organizing scheme. For example, if one observes an event that would be worth reporting later, it may be helpful to classify the event as a joke or tragedy. We use role playing and videotaped vignettes as stimulus materials for this activity.

Integrating New with Old Information (Elaboration). If the joke or tragedy mentioned above could be related to a previously experienced funny story or tragic experience, the new information will thereby be made more memorable. We

Table 30.2.
Teaching Compensatory Strategies[a]

Note: These phases of intervention are not necessarily hierarchical or mutually exclusive.

Phase I: General Strategic Thinking

A. Metacognitive-Awareness

Goals: Clients will discriminate effective from ineffective performance; become aware of their strengths and weaknesses; recognize implications of their deficits.

Rationale: Given the frequency of frontolimbic and right-hemisphere damage in CHI, self-awareness is frequently compromised. Individuals are unlikely to acquire and use procedures designed to compensate for problems that they do not recognize as problems.

Procedures

1. *Objective:* Improve the client's perception of successful versus unsuccessful task performance. Illustrate successful and unsuccessful performance of a functional task through role play or on videotape. With the client, analyze the performances in sufficient detail that the client can identify the features that account for successful versus unsuccessful performance.

2. *Objective:* Improve the client's ability to perceive functional impairments. Individually, request that the client make note of specific deficits of other clients in the program or of individuals observed on tape. Discuss these observations. Planned peer teaching is useful. Discuss the effects of CHI on cognitive and social functioning. If appropriate, read and discuss literature on the effects of CHI.

3. *Objective:* Improve the client's awareness of his or her own strengths and weaknesses. Videotape the client in activities designed to reveal strong and weak areas of functioning. (Alternatively, use role play.) Review the tapes (beginning with strong performance), first without commentary, subsequently inviting comments about what was done well and what needs improvement. Gradually turn over to the client the responsibility for stopping the tape when problems are noted. *Note:* Considerable desensitizing may be needed before video self-viewing is possible.

4. *Objective:* Improve the client's understanding of the relation between deficits and long-term goals. Discuss in concrete detail the individual's long-term goals and expectations. Jointly create a list of specific skills and resources needed to achieve these goals. Jointly identify the skills that are present and those that are weak relative to this goal.

Note: These metacognitive discoveries are facilitated if the activities are personally meaningful and intimately connected to the client's goals.

B. Value of Being Strategic

Goal: Clients will recognize the importance of being strategic and will identify the characteristics of strategic people.

Rationale: Because the ultimate goal of this intervention is to promote strategic thinking and strategic behavior in general—not simply to teach specific strategic behaviors as routines—it is important that the client understand what it is to be strategic and that these are valuable attributes.

Procedures

1. *Objective:* Improve the client's understanding of strategy. Using games, sports, or other relevant models, clarify the concept of strategy as something that one does to achieve goals when there are obstacles.

2. *Objective:* Heighten the client's appreciation of strategic behavior. Together with the client, identify several individuals who are known to be very strategic (e.g., sports heroes, military heroes). Discuss why they are considered heroic. Clinicians should also clearly model their own strategic behavior and discuss the value of their own strategies.

3. *Objective:* Improve the client's understanding of the behaviors that are part of being strategic. Using models relevant to the client (e.g., military, sports, or business analogies), brainstorm about the characteristics of people who are known to be very strategic. Include high level of motivation and initiative; ability to identify and clarify obstacles to goals; ability to plan procedures to overcome obstacles; ability to monitor and evaluate performance; willingness to engage in ongoing problem solving.

Phase II: Selecting Specific Strategic Procedures

Goal: Clients will identify specific procedures useful in overcoming important personal obstacles.

Rationale: It is important that clients participate in the selection of strategic procedures that they will use and that the procedures be truly useful in achieving their goals.

Procedures

1. Use group brainstorming procedures to identify possible strategies.

2. Use "product monitoring" tasks to test the value of strategies. Have the client perform a task with and without the strategy or with a variety of different strategies. Objectively compare the results. (Video analysis may be useful here.)

3. Have advanced clients demonstrate the value of certain procedures or offer testimonials.

4. Discuss the widespread use of compensatory procedures (lists, memos, tape recorders, and so forth) by people who do not have brain injury.

Phase III: Teaching Specific Strategies

Note: If the discovery procedures in Phase II (e.g., brainstorming and product monitoring) are effective, there may be little need for specific teaching procedures.

Procedures:

A. *Modeling:* The steps in the strategy can be modeled by the therapist or by a peer, or by means of videotape or other media. Modeling is initially accompanied by overt verbalization of the strategy by the model. The client then rehearses the strategy with gradually decreasing cues and self-talk.

B. *Direct Instruction:* The carefully programmed behavioral teaching procedures of direct instruction can be used to teach strategies. If this is the only approach used, however, it is likely that the best result will be the acquisition of a learned sequence of behaviors (which may be a desirable outcome), without positive movement in the direction of becoming a strategic person.

C. *Functional Practice:* However the strategy is acquired, it must be frequently rehearsed in natural settings using functional activities.

Table 30.2.
Teaching Compensatory Strategies *(Continued)*

Phase IV: Generalization and Maintenance

Generalization of strategic behavior beyond the context of training is a combined consequence of the perceived utility of the strategy for the individual, the inherent generalizability and utility of the strategy, widespread environmental support for strategic behavior and thinking, and specific teaching procedures designed to enhance generalization.

Note 1: Generalization includes generalized use of specific strategies as well as strategic behavior in general.

Note 2: Generalization may not be a separate phase if the acquisition stage takes place in the context of functional activities and natural settings. This is particularly important for very concrete people.

Note 3: Generalization may be a relatively unimportant phase of intervention if the individual has acquired a strategic attitude and actively seeks occasions for transfer.

Note 4: Some individuals may need environmental reminders indefinitely to use their strategic procedures.

1. *Objective:* Improve the client's discrimination of situations that require or do not require a given strategy.
   - Use videotaped scenes or role playing to illustrate the correct use of a strategy in an appropriate situation, inappropriate use of the strategy, and failure to use the strategy when appropriate. Discuss the conditions that require the strategy.
   - Use short videotaped scenes to train the client in efficient and accurate judgments as to whether a strategy is appropriate in a context.
2. *Objective:* Increase the client's spontaneous use of strategies in varied situations.
   - Include family members, work supervisors, and teachers in strategy intervention to (*a*) provide varied opportunities for the use of specific strategies and of strategic behavior in general, (*b*) reinforce the client's use of strategies, and (*c*) model strategic behavior themselves.
   - Ask clients to keep a log in which they record their successes and failures in strategy use. Make generalization an explicit goal.
3. *Objective:* Increase the client's acceptance of strategic behavior.
   - Ensure that the client is successful using strategies.
   - Promote emotional acceptance of strategic behavior by using whatever motivating procedures work (e.g., personal images or metaphors, testimonials, and the like).

have individuals practice associational strategies of this sort with the same role-playing episodes or videotaped vignettes.

Using Context. We encourage individuals to scan the environment for salient features (e.g., people, objects, locations) that can later be used as cues for retrieval of target information within that context.

Using External Aids. We encourage individuals to use memos, memory books, tape recorders, and the like as needed to compensate for severely impaired memory or to support independent functioning in a demanding environment. Effective use of note-taking strategies often requires additional training in summarizing thoughts into key words or phrases, or in using outlining or diagramming techniques.

Retrieval is enhanced when the cues present at encoding—including strategies as well as contextual cues—are also present in the retrieval situation (''encoding specificity,'' Tulving and Thomson [1973]). Clients should therefore practice reconstructing the context of encoding. Furthermore, if a particular approach to encoding/retrieval can become habituated, the likelihood increases that the same scheme will be used for both tasks. It is valuable to use consistent forms or visual representations of strategies to highlight the cognitive process that we wish to take place at encoding and retrieval. Finally, directed searches of memory are enhanced if individuals are aware of the encoding strategies they typically use and can systematically review those strategies in the search. The Feature Analysis procedure (Fig. 30.1) is one such search strategy. Others are listed in Appendix 30.1.

Episodic Versus Semantic Memory

Individuals with relatively depressed episodic memory may have an adequate knowledge base, yet are not able to maintain ongoing recall of personal experiences. There are the people who have what is popularly referred to as amnesia. Some of these individuals have difficulty retrieving significant biographical information from the distant past as well (retrograde amnesia). In the case of such severe episodic impairments, we help clients reconstruct their past with printed or pictured time lines of significant life events. Furthermore, at any time we may ask the client to bring to consciousness any feelings, opinions, or other reactions that stimulate the formation of episodic memories. Memory books and other mnemonic strategies enhance orientation and retrieval for less severely impaired individuals.

Other clients evidence severely depressed semantic knowledge despite relatively intact retrieval of daily events. Treatment for these individuals is radically different from treatment that is appropriate for those with episodic memory problems. The key to treatment is reeducation, which may include teaching vocabulary, general information, and other academic content. Appropriate materials may include academic textbooks. We frequently recommend remedial community college courses for those individuals who were college educated pretraumatically.

Input Modality

Visual and auditory memory can be differentially impaired following CHI. When this is the case, we encourage the individual to recode information into the stronger modality. For example, verbal information can be represented in diagrams or images.

Involuntary Versus Deliberate Memory

If executive control over memory processes is significantly impaired, it is unreasonable and counterproductive to approach memory intervention from a strategic perspective. Such clients—often those with prefrontal injury—may be confused by deliberate approaches to memory that require a degree of metacognitive awareness and planning that is simply unavailable. Learning is enhanced when the goal is not to remember but rather to complete a concrete, personally meaningful task. As with young children, learning is a by-product of interesting and personally meaningful activities. The *stated* goal for these clients should always be the end product of the activity (versus learning something). The clinician's job is to design the activity so that the information to be remembered is processed deeply and therefore more likely to be remembered in the absence of deliberate memory strategies.

If the individual's performance is not depressed by deliberate attempts to remember, then strategy intervention as discussed earlier is applicable.

Working Memory

Structural capacity of working memory (that which is measured by digit span) is not among the most commonly impaired aspects of memory in CHI. However, the ability to increase the *functional* capacity of working memory using organizational strategies often is affected. Attempts to expand the capacity of working memory by means of repetitive drill with digit sequences or similar stimuli are rarely successful (Moffat, 1984). Rather, we attempt to increase the functional capacity by means of semantic (grouping by meaningful units), syntactic, or melodic chunking, or by increasing knowledge in a specific domain.

Organization

Treatment procedures that target impaired organization during the middle stages of recovery were discussed earlier. Treatment at the late stages of recovery is directed primarily toward improving organization as a process. Late-stage therapeutic activities require clients to impose organization on their thinking, behavior, or verbal expression in contexts that progressively require more organizing activity and to use organized thinking procedures strategically. The organizing schemas described earlier may now be used as deliberate compensatory strategies.

Tasks include planning and executing increasingly complex functional-integrative activities that relate to the individual's social, educational, or vocational goals. Language organizational tasks may include telling or writing narratives; writing descriptions of people, objects, and events; writing themes on increasingly complex topics; teaching others to play games or perform specific tasks; writing speeches to persuade or convince; writing letters of application; writing resumes; and the like.

We have created a number of forms, flowcharts, checklists, diagrams, outlines, and other visual representations of task organization that may be helpful for individual clients. At this stage of intervention, clients are expected to use these organizational guides independently. These forms also help individuals to work cooperatively in groups and to give the therapy team a common vocabulary and set of procedures to promote generalization.

Problem Solving and Practical Reasoning

Investigations of problem-solving expertise have identified three salient characteristics of effective problem solvers: (*a*) They attempt to clarify the problem before attempting to solve it; (*b*) they attempt to relate the problem at hand to more general representations of problems stored in memory, thereby defining the set of relevant information and making available helpful analogies to other problem-solving situations; (*c*) they develop a plan to explore possible solutions (Dodd and White, 1980). This research suggests that attempts to help people become better problem solvers should focus considerable attention on the "front-end" aspects of the process—"What exactly is the problem? What kind of problem is this? Is it similar to other difficult situations that you or others have faced? What has worked in those cases?"—versus the "tail-end" aspects—"Tell me what you would do in this situation."

Other investigations of the cognitive processes involved in problem solving indicate that there is a fierce "domain specificity" to problem-solving effectiveness (Singley and Anderson, 1989). This is in part because effective problem solving presupposes specific knowledge of the content in question as well as of the considerations that are relevant in that domain. It is for these reasons that great problem solvers, like General Montgomery in military history, Yogi Berra in baseball, Stephen Hawking in astrophysics, and the champion videogame player at the local arcade, are unlikely to be useful consultants in the others' domains. That is, their problem-solving wizardry is not a context-independent skill that they could apply with equal effectiveness across domains. Rather, they have learned how to think clearly about problems in their domain of interest, and they know a great deal about that domain.

Unfortunately, most "cognitive retraining" programs that focus on problem solving are incompatible with these two important principles. First, these exercises tend to focus on the tail-end ("What would you do if . . . ?") of the reasoning process. Clinicians are familiar with individuals with CHI who might be able to answer questions of this sort adequately because of recovered knowledge of reasonable choices in common situations, but who nevertheless are very weak practical problem solvers because of some combination of (*a*) difficulty recognizing that they are in a real-world problematic situation; (*b*) difficulty clearly defining the problem; (*c*) difficulty marshaling relevant information and analogies to think clearly about the problem; and (*d*) difficulty considering a variety of solutions and their relative merits. Second, because cognitive retraining exercises tend not to be embedded in a personally meaningful context (content and setting), there is little reason to believe that improvements in problem solving will transfer from the domain of training to educational, vocational, and social real life. For this reason, one must be skeptical of the overreliance on videogames, workbooks, and related activities as the basis for improving problem solving.

Therapy settings and activities can be used to help individuals acquire an organized procedure for thinking about important problems. Ideally, these discussions and exercises take place in groups to capitalize on the social cues present in groups, the divergent thinking that is likely with several participants, and the peer coaching and feedback that is possible only in groups. In structured therapy sessions, we encourage organized thinking about problems, using the following format:

1. *Problem identification:* "Briefly, what is the problem?"
2. *Problem classification:* "What kind of problem is this? Is it similar to other tough situations you have faced?"
3. *Goal identification:* "What will you gain by solving this problem?"
4. *Identification of relevant information:* "What do you need to know to solve this problem? Do you have any experience with problems like this that will be helpful?"
5. *Identification of possible solutions:* "What could you possibly do to solve this problem?"
6. *Evaluation of solutions:* "What is good or bad about each of these possibilities?" *Consider:* Effective? Able to do it? Enough time? Like to do it? Break any rules? Worked in the past? Effects on others? Yourself? The environment?
7. *Decision:* "What is the smartest thing to do?"
8. *Formulation of a plan:* "Exactly how do you plan to accomplish this?"
9. *Monitoring and evaluating the outcome:* "Did it work? Are you satisfied? Any new problems?"

Organized, deliberate problem solving is thus a multistage process that involves several distinct types of thinking as well as considerable declarative knowledge: convergent isolation of main ideas (parts 1, 3); divergent (flexible, creative) thinking (parts 4, 5, 6); reflection on relevance (part 4); classification (part 2); analogical reasoning (parts 2, 4, 6); convergent, deductive reasoning (part 7); executive goal setting (part 3); executive planning and organizing (part 8); and executive monitoring and evaluating (part 9). One of the values of integrative problem-solving exercises of this sort is that it creates a functional context within which to practice a variety of types of thinking and reasoning that clinicians might otherwise be tempted to exercise with nonmeaningful workbook exercises.

Although clients might use this format as a worksheet to think through certain problems, it is unreasonable to expect anybody, brain injured or otherwise, to routinely be this organized and deliberate in everyday problem solving. Therefore, an important component of problem-solving intervention is real-world coaching, in which the clinician helps the client identify areas of greatest weakness in real-world problem solving (possibly failure to clarify the problem or consider past experience) and ways to overcome these critical weaknesses in practical problem solving. The clinician must be skilled at modeling the appropriate steps in the process and at catching real problems as they arise (in or out of therapy sessions) and using these occasions to strengthen this type of thinking. Furthermore, everyday people (family members, direct care staff, employers) should be sensitized to their role in promoting more effective problem solving.

FUTURE TRENDS

In this chapter, we have outlined a perspective on rehabilitation of individuals with cognitive-communicative impairment after CHI. Because this is a chapter and not a book, we have omitted many important areas of intervention. Most notably, we have said very little about social cognition and social skills, aspects of functioning that figure prominently in community reintegration after CHI. Elsewhere we have presented a framework and procedures for addressing social skills in individuals with TBI (Ylvisaker et al., 1992 b; Ylvisaker et al., in press b).

In our "Future Trends" discussion for the previous edition of this book, we optimistically anticipated that within the next

decade, assessment tools and intervention techniques would be validated for this population, pharmacologic intervention for disorders of cognition and behavior would substantially improve outcome, and resources would become available for long-term work and living arrangements specifically designed to meet the needs of young adults with significant challenges after severe CHI. Seven years later, our assessment of progress is not encouraging. Although there has been useful work in designing and validating formal assessment tools, controversies and theoretically questionable clinical practices continue to abound in the field of cognitive rehabilitation; the impact of pharmacology on cognitive and psychosocial outcome continues to be largely a promise; and resources to support individuals in their home, community, and work environments are sorely lacking.

On the positive side, a naive expectation that computer exercises could substantially improve the vocational and social life of individuals with serious cognitive and psychosocial challenges has given way to a more sober awareness that chronic cognitive and communicative problems must ultimately be addressed in the individual's real-world context. A shift in the focus of postacute rehabilitative services—including those provided by speech-language pathologists—from a medical, facility-based model to a community-based support model (discussed by Kneipp and Paul-Cohen, 1993, and Williams, 1993) will surely be a welcome development over the next decade. This, however, necessitates a fundamental change in the way rehabilitative services are understood and funded in this country.

References

Adams, J. H., Graham, D. I., Murray, L. S., and Scott, G. (1982). Diffuse axonal injury due to non-missile head injury in humans: An analysis of 45 cases. *Annals of Neurology, 12,* 557–563.
Alexander, M. P. (1987). Syndromes in the rehabilitation and outcome of closed head injury. In H. S. Levin, J. Grafman, and H. M. Eisenberg (Eds.), *Neurobehavioral recovery from head injury* (pp. 192–205). New York: Oxford.
Alexander, M. P., Benson, D. F., and Stuss, D. T. (1989). Frontal lobes and language. *Brain and Language, 37,* 656–691.
American Speech-Language-Hearing Association (ASHA) (1988, March). The role of speech-language pathologists in the identification, diagnosis, and treatment of individuals with cognitive-communicative impairments. *ASHA, 30,* 79.
Ben-Yishay, Y., and Prigatano, G. P. (1990). Cognitive remediation. In M. Rosenthal, E. Griffith, M. Bond, and J. D. Miller (Eds.), *Rehabilitation of the adult and child with traumatic brain injury* (pp. 393–409). Philadelphia, PA: F. A. Davis.
Berrol, S. (1990). Issues in cognitive rehabilitation. *Archives of Neurology, 47,* 219–220.
Bigler, E. D. (1988). Frontal lobe damage and neuropsychological assessment. *Archives of Clinical Neuropsychology, 3,* 279–297.
Bjorkland, D. (1985). The role of conceptual knowledge in the development of organization in children's memory. In M. Pressley and C. Brainerd (Eds.), *Basic processes in memory development* (pp. 103–134). New York: Springer-Verlag.
Brooks, N., McKinlay, W., Symington, C., Beattie, A., and Campsie, L. (1987). Return to work within the first seven years of severe head injury. *Brain Injury, 1,* 5–19.
Brown, A. L. (1975). The development of memory: Knowing, knowing about knowing, and knowing how to know. In H. W. Reese (Ed.), *Advances in child development and behavior* (Vol. 10, pp. 103–152). New York: Academic Press.
Brown, A. L. (1979). Theories of memory and problems of development, activity, growth, and knowledge. In F. I. M. Craik and L. Cermak (Eds.),

Levels of processing and memory (pp. 225–258). Hillsdale, NJ: Lawrence Erlbaum.

Butler, R. W., and Namerow, M. D. (1988). Cognitive retraining in brain injury rehabilitation: A critical review. *Journal of Neurologic Rehabilitation, 2,* 97–101.

Courville, C. B. (1937). *Pathology of the central nervous system.* Mountain View, CA: Pacific Press.

Dodd, D., and White, R. M., Jr. (1980). *Cognition: Mental structures and processes.* Boston, MA: Allyn & Bacon.

Eslinger, P. J., and Damasio, A. R. (1985). Severe disturbance of higher cognition following bilateral frontal lobe oblation: Patient EVR. *Neurology, 35,* 1731–1741.

Flavell, J. H. (1985). *Cognitive development* (2nd ed.). Englewood Cliffs, NJ: Prentice-Hall.

Gennarelli, T. A., Thibault, L. E., Adams, J. H., Graham, D. I., Thompson, C. J., and Macincin, R. P. (182). Diffuse axonal injury and traumatic coma in the primate. *Annals of Neurology, 12,* 564–574.

Gobble, E. M., and Pfahl, J. C. (1985). Career development. In M. Ylvisaker (Ed.), *Head injury rehabilitation: Children and adolescents* (pp. 411–426). Austin, TX: Pro-Ed.

Groher, M. E., and Ochipa, C. (1992). The standardized communication assessment of individuals with traumatic brain injury. *Seminars in Speech and Language, 13,* 252–262.

Hagen, C. (1981). Language disorders secondary to closed head injury. *Topics in Language Disorders, 1,* 73–87.

Halpern, H., Darley, F. L., and Brown, J. R. (1973). Differential language and neurologic characteristics in cerebral involvement. *Journal of Speech and Hearing Disorders, 38,* 162–173.

Hartley, L. L. (1990). Assessment of functional communication. In D. E. Tupper and K. D. Cicerone (Eds.), *The neuropsychology of everyday life: Assessment and basic competencies* (pp. 125–168). Boston, MA: Kluwer Academic Publishers.

Hartley, L. L. (1992). Assessment of functional communication. *Seminars in Speech and Language, 13,* 264–279.

Heilman, K. M., Safran, A., and Geschwind, N. (1971). Closed head trauma and aphasia. *Journal of Neurology, Neurosurgery and Psychiatry, 34,* 265–269.

Hintzman, D. L. (1978). *The psychology of learning and memory.* New York: W. H. Freeman Co.

Hresko, W. P., and Reid, D. K. (1988). Five faces of cognition. Theoretical influences on approaches to learning disabilities. *Learning Disability Quarterly, 4,* 211–216.

Katz, D. I. (1992). Neuropathology and neurobehavioral recovery from closed head injury. *Journal of Head Trauma Rehabilitation, 7,* 1–15.

Kavale, K., and Mattson, P. (1983). "One jumped off the balance beam": Meta-analysis of perceptual-motor training. *Journal of Learning Disabilities, 16,* 165–173.

Kay, T., and Lezak, M. (1990). The nature of head injury. In D. W. Corthell (Ed.), *Traumatic brain injury and vocational rehabilitation* (pp. 21–65). Menomonie, WI: University of Wisconsin, Stout.

Kneipp, S., and Paul-Cohen, M. S. (1993). Community-based services and supports for individuals with traumatic brain injury. *Seminars in Speech and Language, 14,* 32–42.

Lange, G. (1978). Organization-related processes in children's recall. In P. Ornstein (Ed.), *Memory development in children* (pp. 101–128). Hillsdale, NJ: Lawrence Erlbaum.

Levin, H. S., Benton, A. L., and Grossman, R. G. (1982). *Neurobehavioral consequences of closed head injury.* New York: Oxford University Press.

Levin, H. S., Goldstein, F. C., High, M. M., and Williams, D. (1988). Automatic and effortful processing after severe closed head injury. *Brain and Language, 7,* 283–297.

Levin, H. S., Grossman, R. G., Sarwar, M., and Meyers, C. A. (1981). Linguistic recovery after closed head injury. *Brain and Language, 12,* 360–374.

Lezak, M. D. (1982). The problem of assessing executive functions. *International Journal of Psychology, 17,* 281–297.

Livingston, M. G., and Brooks, D. N. (1988). The burden on families of the brain injured: A review. *Journal of Head Trauma Rehabilitation, 3*(4), 6–15.

Mandler, G. (1967). Organization and memory. In K. W. Spence and J. T. Spence (Eds.), *The psychology of learning and motivation* (Vol. 1). New York: Academic Press.

Mann, L. (1979). *On the trail of process: A historical perspective on cognitive processes and their training.* New York: Grune & Stratton.

Mateer, C. A., and Williams, D. (1991). Effects of frontal lobe injury in childhood. *Developmental Neuropsychology, 7,* 359–376.

Mayes, A. (1988). *Human organic memory disorders.* New York: Cambridge University Press.

Meichenbaum, D. (1993). The "potential" contribution of cognitive behavior modification to the rehabilitation of individuals with traumatic brain injury. *Seminars in Speech and Language, 14,* 18–30.

Mentis, M., and Prutting, C. A. (1991). Analysis of topic as illustrated in a head-injured and a normal adult. *Journal of Speech and Hearing Research, 34,* 583–595.

Moffat, N. (1984). Strategies of memory therapy. In B. Wilson and N. Moffat (Eds.), *Clinical management of memory problems* (pp. 63–88). Rockville, MD: Aspen Systems.

Newcombe, F. (1969). *Missile wounds of the brain.* London: Oxford University Press.

Pressley, M. (1993). Teaching cognitive strategies to brain-injured clients: The good information processing perspective. *Seminars in Speech and Language, 14,* 1–16.

Pressley, M. and Associates. (1990). *Cognitive strategy instruction that really improves children's academic performance.* Cambridge, MA: Brookline Books.

Pressley, M., Borkowski, J. G., and Schneider, W. (1989). Good information processing: What is it and what education can do to promote it. *International Journal of Educational Research, 13,* 857–867.

Prigatano, G. P. (1986). *Neuropsychological rehabilitation after brain injury.* Baltimore, MD: Johns Hopkins University Press.

Prutting, C. A., and Kirchner, D. M. (1987). A clinical appraisal of the pragmatic aspects of language. *Journal of Speech and Hearing Disorders, 52,* 105–119.

Rosch, E. (1977). Classification of real-world objects: Origins and representations in cognition. In P. N. Johnson-Laird and P. C. Watson (Eds.), *Thinking: Readings in cognitive science.* New York: Cambridge University Press.

Sarno, M. T. (1980). The nature of verbal impairment after closed head injury. *Journal of Nervous and Mental Disease, 169,* 685–692.

Sarno, M. T. (1984). Verbal impairment after closed head injury: Report of a replication study. *Journal of Nervous and Mental Disease, 172,* 475–479.

Sarno, M. T., Buonaguro, A., and Levita, E. (1986). Characteristics of verbal impairment in closed head injured patients. *Archives of Physical Medicine and Rehabilitation, 67,* 400–405.

Schacter, D. L., and Glisky, E. L. (1986). Memory remediation: Restoration, alleviation, and the acquisition of domain-specific knowledge. In B. Uzzell and Y. Gross (Eds.), *Clinical neuropsychology of intervention* (pp. 257–282). Boston, MA: Martinus Nijhoff Publishing.

Siegler, R. (1986). *Children's thinking.* Englewood Cliffs, NJ: Prentice-Hall.

Singley, M. K., and Anderson, J. R. (1989). *The transfer of cognitive skill.* Cambridge, MA: Harvard University Press.

Smirnov, A. (1973). *Problems in psychology and memory.* New York: Plenum Press.

Smith, E. (1978). Theories of semantic memory. In W. Estes (Ed.), *Linguistic functions in cognitive theory.* Hillsdale, NJ: Lawrence Erlbaum.

Sohlberg, M., and Mateer, C. (1989). *Introduction to cognitive rehabilitation: Theory and practice.* New York: Guilford Press.

Stuss, D. T., and Benson, D. F. (1986). *The frontal lobes.* New York: Raven Press.

Szekeres, S. F., Ylvisaker, M., and Cohen, S. (1987). A framework for cognitive rehabilitation therapy. In M. Ylvisaker and E. M. R. Gobble (Eds.), *Community reentry for head injured adults* (pp. 87–136). Austin, TX: Pro-Ed.

Thomsen, I. V. (1975). Evaluation and outcome of aphasia in patients with severe head trauma. *Journal of Neurology, Neurosurgery and Psychiatry, 38,* 713–718.

Tulving, E. (1972). Episodic and semantic memory. In E. Tulving and W. Donaldson (Eds.), *Organization of memory* (pp. 382–403). New York: Academic Press.

Tulving, E., and Thomson, D. (1973). Encoding specificity and retrieval processes in episodic memory. *Psychological Review, 80,* 352–373.

Welsh, M. C., and Pennington, B. F. (1988). Assessing frontal lobe functioning in children: Views from developmental psychology. *Developmental Neuropsychology, 4,* 199–230.

Williams, J. M. (1993). Supporting families after head injury: Implications for the speech-language pathologist. *Seminars in Speech and Language, 14,* 44–59.

Wood, D., Bruner, J., and Ross, G. (1976). The role of tutoring in problem solving. *Journal of Child Psychology and Psychiatry, 17,* 89–100.

Ylvisaker, M. (1992). Communication outcome following traumatic brain injury. *Seminars in Speech and Language, 13,* 239–250.

Ylvisaker, M., Chorazy, A., Cohen, S., Nelson, J., Mastrelli, J., Molitor, C., Szekeres, S., and Valko, A. (1990). Rehabilitative assessment following head injury in children. In M. Rosenthal, E. Griffith, M. Bond, and J. D. Miller (Eds.), *Rehabilitation of the adult and child with traumatic brain injury* (pp. 558–592). Philadelphia, PA: F. A. Davis.

Ylvisaker, M., Feeney, T. J., and Urbanczyk, B. (1993). Developing a positive communication culture for rehabilitation: Communication training for staff and family members. In C. J. Durgin, N. D. Schmidt, and L. J. Fryer (Eds.), *Staff development and clinical intervention in brain injury rehabilitation* (pp. 57–85). Gaithersburg, MD: Aspen Publishers.

Ylvisaker, M., Hartwick, P., Ross, B., and Nussbaum, N. (in press a). Cognitive assessment. In R. Savage and G. Wolcott (Eds.), *Educational programming for children and young adults with acquired brain injury.* Austin, TX: Pro-Ed.

Ylvisaker, M., and Szekeres, S. (1989). Metacognitive and executive impairments in head injured children and adults. *Topics in Language Disorders, 9,* 34–49.

Ylvisaker, M., Szekeres, S., Haarbauer-Krupa, J., Urbanczyk, B., and Feeney, T. (in press b). Speech and language intervention. In R. Savage and G.

Wolcott (Eds.), *Educational programming for children and young adults with acquired brain injury.* Austin, TX: Pro-Ed.

Ylvisaker, M. S., Szekeres, S. F., and Hartwick, P. (1992a). Cognitive rehabilitation following traumatic brain injury. In M. Tramontana and S. Hooper (Eds.), *Advances in child neuropsychology* (Vol. 1, pp. 168–218). New York: Springer-Verlag.

Ylvisaker, M., Szekeres, S. F., Hartwick, P., and Tworek, P. (in press c). Cognitive intervention. In R. Savage and G. Wolcott (Eds.), *Educational programming for children and young adults with acquired brain injury.* Austin, TX: Pro-Ed.

Ylvisaker, M., Szekeres, S., Henry, K., Sullivan, D., and Wheeler, P. (1987). Topics in cognitive rehabilitation. In M. Ylvisaker (Ed.), *Community re-entry for head injured adults* (pp. 137–215). Austin, TX: Pro-Ed.

Ylvisaker, M., and Urbanczyk, B. (1990). The efficacy of speech-language pathology intervention: Traumatic brain injury. *Seminars in Speech and Language, 11,* 215–225.

Ylvisaker, M., Urbanczyk, B., and Feeney, T. J. (1992b). Social skills following traumatic brain injury. *Seminars in Speech and Language, 13,* 308–321.

Zasler, N. D., Kreutzer, J. S., and Taylor, D. (1991). Coma stimulation and coma recovery: A critical review. *NeuroRehabilitation, 1,* 33–40.

APPENDIX 30.1

Examples of Compensatory Strategies for Patients with Cognitive Impairments

Attention and Concentration

A. External Aids
1. Use a timer or alarm watch to focus attention for a specified period
2. Organize the work environment and eliminate distractions
3. Use a written or pictorial task plan with built-in rest periods and reinforcement; move a marker along to show progress
4. Place a symbol or picture card in an obvious place in the work areas as a reminder to maintain attention

B. Internal Procedures
1. Set increasingly demanding goals for self, including sustained work time
2. Self-instruct (e.g., ''Am I wandering? What am I supposed to do? What should I be doing now?'') (Written cue cards may be needed for these during training period.)

Orientation (to Time, Place, Person, and Event)

A. External Aids
1. Use a log or journal book or tape recorder to record significant information and events of the day
2. Refer to pictures of persons who are not readily identified (carry pictures attached to logbook)
3. Use appointment book or daily schedule sheet
4. Use alarm watch set for regular intervals
5. Refer to maps or pictures for spatial orientation; make maps with landmarks

B. Internal Procedures
1. Select anchor points or events during the week and then attempt to reconstruct either previous or subsequent points in time (e.g., ''My birthday was on Wednesday and that was yesterday, so this must be Thursday'')
2. Request time, date, and similar information from others, when necessary
3. Scan environment for landmarks

Input Control (Amount, Duration, Complexity, Rate, and Interference)

A. Auditory
1. Give feedback to speaker (e.g., ''Please slow down; speed up; break information into smaller 'chunks''')
2. Request repetition in another form (e.g., ''Would you please write that down for me?'')

B. Visual
1. Request longer viewing time or repeated viewings; request extra time for reading
2. Cover parts of a page and look at exposed areas systematically, as in a ''clockwise direction'' or ''left to right''
3. Use finger or index card to assist scanning and to maintain place
4. Use symbol to mark right and left margins of written material or top and bottom segments as anchors in space
5. Use large-print books or talking books
6. Request a verbal description
7. Remove an object from its setting to examine it; then return it to the original setting and view it again
8. Place items in best visual field and eliminate visual distractors
9. Turn head to compensate for field cut

Comprehension and Memory Processes

A. Use self-questions (e.g., ''Do I understand? Do I need to ask a question? How is this meaningful to me? How does this fit with what I know?''). Periodically look for GMCs (gaps, misconceptions, or confusion) by summarizing or explaining and checking back with speaker, a written source, or reference material

B. Build ''frames'' or background for new information that is of particular significance or interest. Read summaries and general textbooks and ask knowledgeable persons about topic of special interest (a procedure in building frames)

C. Use a study guide for extended discourse material (e.g., SQ 3R procedure—survey, question, read, recite, review)

D. Make charts and graphs of important relationships in textual material

E. Use external memory aids (e.g., tape recorder, logbook, notes, memos, written or pictured time lines)

F. Rehearse: Covert or overt; auditory-vocal or motor (pantomime)

G. Organization: Scan for or impose some order on incoming information

H. Mnemonics: Method of loci, rhymes, imagery (meaningful and novel associations)

I. Use diagrams or forms that facilitate deeper encoding of information and its subsequent retrieval

J. Relate the information to personal life experiences and current knowledge. Use semantic knowledge of basic scripts (e.g., going to a restaurant, buying groceries) to help reconstruct previous events

K. Project and describe situation in which target information will be needed or used

L. At retrieval reconstruct environment in which information was received

M. Verbalize visual-spatial information (e.g., ''X is to the left of Y''). Visualize verbal information in graphs, pictures, cartoons, or action-based imagery

N. Keep items in designated places

Word Retrieval

A. Search lexical memory according to various categories and subcategories (e.g., person: family)

B. Describe the concept; circumlocute freely (talk about or around subject)

C. Use gestures or signs

D. Attempt to generate a sentence or use a carrier phrase

E. Search letters or sounds of the alphabet (more effective in retrieving members of a limited category, such as names)

F. Describe perceptual attributes and semantic features of the concept

G. Draw the item

H. Attempt to write the word

I. Create an image of the object in a scene; then attempt to describe the scene

J. Attempt to retrieve the overlearned opposite

K. Free associate with image in mind

L. Associate persons' names with physical characteristics or a known person of the same name

Thought Organization and Verbal Expression

A. Use a structured thinking procedure (e.g., ''feature analysis guide,'' Fig. 30.1)

B. Use knowledge of scripts to generate real or imagined descriptions of experiences (narratives)

C. Construct a time line to maintain appropriate sequence of events

D. Note topic in any conversation; self-question about the main point of expression; alert others before shifting a topic abruptly

E. Watch others for feedback as to whether your words are confusing: Watch facial expression, and so forth, or directly ask listeners, ''Am I being clear?''

F. Rehearse important comments or questions and listen to self

G. Set limits of time or allowable number of sentences in any one turn

Reasoning, Problem Solving, Judgment

A. Use a problem-solving guide

B. Use self-questioning for alternatives or consequences. (''What else could I do?'' ''What would happen if it did that?'')

C. Look at possible solutions from at least two different perspectives

D. Scan environment for cues as to appropriateness or inappropriateness of a behavior (e.g., facial expression of others; signs like ''No Smoking''; formality vs. informality of setting)

E. Set specific times or places for behaviors that are appropriate only in specified situations

F. Actively envision situations to which successful procedures can be generalized

Self-Monitoring

A. Use symbols or signs, placed in obvious places, or alarms that mean ''pause'' or ''stop'' or ''Am I doing what I should be doing?''

B. Use book or notebook with cards inserted at selected places with self-monitoring cues (e.g., ''Summarize what you read'')

C. Pair specific self-instruction with the associated emotion (e.g., ''Calm down'' when angry)

Task Organization

A. Use task organization checklist: materials, sequenced steps, time line, evaluation of results. Check each when completed

B. Prepare work space and assign space as task demands

PROFESSIONAL CONSIDERATIONS

CHAPTER 31
Applying Research Principles to Language Intervention

CONNIE A. TOMPKINS

Most clinicians value the intuitive, artistic nature of our endeavors. But many also recognize that effective clinical management cannot proceed by intuition alone. As Kearns (1993) suggests, ''. . . failure to apply scientific thinking and measurement during the clinical process is surely as misguided as leaving our empathy, clinical intuition, and caring attitudes behind as we enter the clinical arena'' (p. 71). This chapter advocates a scientific approach to clinical decision-making, emphasizing primarily the clinician's role as a consumer of research information. Other sections recount the advantages of a systematic approach to treatment planning and implementation and suggest ways in which clinicians can contribute to the professional database. Finally, some future trends in the application of research principles to clinical intervention are considered.

DEFINITIONS AND PERSPECTIVES

Nature of Research and Science

To set the stage for this discussion, let us review briefly some relevant terminology, and consider several focal aspects of research and scientific inquiry. Research can be viewed as a process of asking and answering questions, which is structured by a set of criteria and procedures for maximizing the probability of attaining reliability, validity, and generality of results. Each of these factors affects the confidence one can have in the findings and conclusions reported for a research effort.

Reliability refers to the stability, consistency, or repeatability of findings. The well-known types include observer reliability (inter- and intra-) and test-retest reliability. These or related indicators (e.g., parallel/alternate forms reliability) should be assessed whenever standardized instruments or nonstandardized probes are used to measure performance.

Another important concept in the interpretation of reliability is *standard error*. Standard error reflects the precision of specific statistics (means, medians, correlations, proportions, differences between means, etc.) by estimating the random fluctuations in those statistics that would be obtained if they were derived on repeated occasions. Relatedly, a statistic called the

standard error of measurement estimates the consistency with which particular tests would measure performance on repeated administrations. The larger the standard error relative to the magnitude of the obtained scores, the more difficult it is to tell whether an individual score is truly different from some other score (e.g., whether there is a change after treatment). It is beyond the scope of this chapter to discuss the calculation and interpretation of various standard error statistics. For more information see, for example, Kerlinger (1967).

Two other less familiar forms of reliability will also be considered briefly. The first, *internal consistency reliability*, reflects the homogeneity of test items. Acceptable levels should be demonstrated whenever items are summed to generate a ''total score'' measure of a single construct, such as ''syntactic comprehension'' or ''naming ability.'' If the items to be added together do not measure the same thing, combining them into a single score is like comparing the proverbial apples and oranges. *Procedural reliability* data indicate the consistency with which the experimental conditions or treatment procedures themselves are implemented in a research study. Also known as reliability of the independent variable, procedural reliability is often neglected in the language intervention literature. We will return to this concept in another section of the chapter.

Validity refers to ''truth'' of measurement. Perhaps the definition of validity can best be illustrated by the following question: Are we measuring what we think we are measuring? Many of us assume that, once documented, validity is an inherent and invariant property of specific tests and measurements. However, the term applies better to the inferences we derive from tests and measurements: The conclusions we wish to draw, the individuals we tested, and the procedures we followed all influence claims of validity. The familiar types of validity for tests and measurement instruments are content, criterion (predictive and concurrent), and construct validity.

Several forms of validity are important for designing and evaluating research as well. *Internal validity* reflects how confidently we can attribute any changes observed to the experimental treatments or conditions themselves, rather than to artifacts or confounding variables (Campbell and Stanley, 1966). *Exter-*

Table 31.1.
Some Key Scientific Principles and Values

Testability: propositions and questions are specific enough to be evaluated.
Replicability: reported detail is sufficient to allow findings to be reproduced.
Objectivity: dogmatism and bias are rejected; counterevidence and alternative interpretations are sought.
Systematicity: theories and experiments are evaluated and developed in a logical, orderly way.
Tentativeness: the possibility and sources of error are recognized; the elusiveness of answers is understood.
Concern for clinical significance: the importance and/or relevance of outcomes is evaluated.
Concern for protection of human subjects: the welfare of those participating in research projects is paramount.

---

nal validity involves the *generality*, or representativeness, of the conclusions (Campbell and Stanley, 1966) and concerns the extent to which findings can be expected to apply to particular populations, settings, or treatment and measurement variables.[a] It is important to remember that reliability is necessary for, but does not guarantee, validity. Ventry and Schiavetti (1980) give an example of a scale that is consistently off by one-half pound: It is a reliable instrument, but not a valid one.

Knowledge of methods to maximize reliability and validity is essential for conducting and evaluating research, and a later section of this chapter will examine some reliability and validity concerns specific to language intervention studies. But as Chial (1985) reminds us, a commitment to science is also a state of mind. Some principles at the heart of a scientific orientation are summarized in Table 31.1. The penultimate entry in the table, which focuses on clinical significance, deserves brief comment here. A concern for clinical significance calls for judgment of the relevance or meaningfulness of effects. Is a statistically significant performance change of 5% following intervention a *clinically important* difference? There is no easy answer, as the importance of a change depends on such factors as the specific behaviors being targeted, the client's level of functioning, and the nature of the treatment goals. But the question of clinical significance is one that both researchers and clinicians should keep in mind. We will also return to this issue later in the chapter.

Value of Science to Clinicians

Why should clinicians care about research and science? At least five reasons come immediately to mind. First, we need to think critically to be wise consumers of anything in life. For our purposes, the point applies to the published data and continuing education information that we consume professionally. There may be a tendency to accept at face value anything that is published or presented at a professional conference, especially by someone who is known as an authority. One needs to learn how to evaluate research in order to guard against this type of halo effect (Perkins, 1985). Second, the principles and skills of science guide efficacious clinical practice. Diagnosis and treatment have long been viewed as exercises in hypothesis-testing. In every session, the clinician should develop pertinent questions or hypotheses, postulate relationships, decide how to assess them (reliably and validly), and collect and interpret the data. Third, clinicians can make important contributions to the database that forms the foundation of our diagnostic and treatment activities. The effects, effectiveness, and efficiency of various assessment

and treatment approaches cannot be assumed, and clinical research is badly needed. Fourth, and relatedly, clinicians are ethically responsible for evaluating the impact of their services (ASHA, 1992). In this vein, Rosenbek et al. (1989, p. 12) assert "...untested treatments are immoral, therefore clinical practice must include clinical experimentation." Finally, a scientific approach kindles informed curiosity and keeps us growing and thinking professionally. A scientific attitude may help to stave off "burnout," as searching for another question or pursuing a different hypothesis helps to keep life interesting. The next sections of this chapter will highlight clinicians as both consumers and potential producers of research.

CLINICIAN AS RESEARCH CONSUMER

Our role as consumers of research information is one of the most important that we can adopt. Participating in continuing education efforts is laudable but worth little if we simply soak up or disseminate information without critical evaluation.

Questions to Ask in Evaluating Research

The literature is replete with contributions describing general principles for evaluating published material and presentations. I will recapitulate some here, in the form of 12 questions for the consumer, with examples and elaboration specific to neurologic or aging populations. Most of these questions can be asked of "basic" and "treatment efficacy" research; they have been culled primarily from Kent (1985a), Silverman (1985), and Ventry and Schiavetti (1980).[b]

1. *Are convincing rationales and hypotheses provided?* The weight given to rationales and hypotheses varies depending on their sources, which can include critical examination of prior literature, knowledge of normal processes, and of course, clinical observation and intuition. Most sound rationales and hypotheses originate from more than one of these roots. A rationale such as "I wonder what would happen if . . ." clearly needs support and development from other sources; but in most instances, each of us must decide whether a convincing case is presented for the questions asked or the hypotheses provided.

2. *Are research questions answerable?* From the perspective of research evaluation, an answerable question is one that is explicitly specified. A well-specified question is like an appropriately written behavioral objective. There is an obvious difference between clinical goals such as "improving auditory comprehension" and "achieving 85% comprehension of yes/no questions about implied main ideas in spoken eighth-grade level paragraphs." The latter is more measurable. To take an-

---

[a] The factors that compromise internal and external validity in research can also affect the validation of a test instrument; for examples consult Franzen (1989).

[b] Some of these issues have been elaborated further by Tompkins (1992).

other example, the old standard efficacy question, "Does aphasia treatment work?" lacks operational specificity and is probably impossible to answer in any one or several studies. A more answerable question would indicate the nature of the treatment, the types of patients to whom it is to be applied, and the criteria for determining if it has "worked."

3. *Do clients studied represent group(s) they are meant to represent?* Using an example from aphasia, Darley (1972) emphasized long ago that researchers must define and operationalize what they mean by "aphasia." Neither poor performance on an aphasia examination nor the occurrence of one or more "strokes" is sufficient evidence to render the diagnosis of aphasia. Several other varieties of nonaphasic language disturbance follow damage to the central nervous system, and this diagnostic distinction is more than a simple semantic distinction. We would not expect traditional aphasia treatments to benefit someone with an isolated dysarthria, or someone whose language impairments are embedded in an assortment of other cognitive problems such as confusion and severe memory disorder. To address this question, the criteria, rationales, and reliability for judgments about essential diagnoses and characteristics (e.g., fluent vs. nonfluent aphasia) should be reported. For qualitative or subjective judgments in particular, it would be desirable to have independent verification by someone who did not have a stake in the outcome of the study.

4. *Are subjects sufficiently described for assessing the believability, replicability, and generality of results?* Again drawing on aphasia to illustrate, a number of variables may influence results in treatment studies, such as duration of aphasia, severity of deficits, aphasia type, etiology, prior neurological and psychiatric history, sensory and motor status, and literacy (Rosenbek et al., 1989; Shewan, 1986). Similar sets of factors affect research with other neurologically impaired populations, and some are also relevant for characterizing communication behaviors of normally aging adults. Of course, any component skills or prerequisites for processing and responding to treatment or probe stimuli (e.g., visual and auditory perceptual abilities) should be specified and measured as well.

Brookshire (1983) suggests a minimum list of descriptors for aphasic patients in his treatise on the subject of subjects. Others (e.g., Rosenbek, 1987; Rosenbek et al., 1989; Tompkins et al., 1990) have offered additional possibilities and discussed novel ways to operationalize some of the tried-and-true descriptors (see Table 31.2). It is not practical, or even necessary, to expect all of these variables to be described in every study. However, given more specifically operationalized indicators, consumers can more easily determine how to apply the results, and investigators can better attempt replication and extension of the reported findings. As Brookshire (1983) notes, including characteristics such as those discussed here is also important for the internal validity of a study. If such factors are not reported, consumers cannot rule out the possibility that the results have been influenced in unintended ways. Detailed subject information is critical as well if we are to begin formulating hypotheses about why certain people do not respond as expected, or about which individuals might benefit most from particular interventions.

5. *Are (treatment) procedures, conditions, and variables adequately specified?* This question most obviously refers to replicability, but if specification is inadequate, it may also raise internal validity concerns that diminish confidence in the results. The essential aspects of procedures and conditions, and the opera-

tional definitions of dependent (outcome) and independent (predictor) variables, should be clearly presented. Some important characteristics of the independent variable (the treatment) for aphasia treatment trials include the type and training of the clinician, amount of treatment, type of treatment, intensity of treatment, and choice of the no-treatment comparison condition (Rosenbek et al., 1989; Shewan, 1986). Procedures, criteria or decision rules, and responses should also be described as precisely as possible. In addition, if several conditions are contrasted, clear operational distinctions should be provided.

6. *Are (treatment) procedures, conditions, and variables reliable and valid?* Let us focus first on *reliability* issues. As mentioned earlier, the reliability (and validity) question can be asked of standardized measures. Often, however, psychometrically sound measures are not appropriate or available, and investigators develop or modify measures of their own.

When these specialized measures are used, researchers should provide the best data they can to address reliability concerns. Test-retest reliability of the outcome measures and consideration of standard error statistics are crucial in studies of treatment effects, as we need to be able to determine whether observed changes can be attributed to the intervention rather than to unstable measurements. An estimate of test-retest characteristics can be made from multiple assessments taken in the baseline (preintervention) phase of single-subject experiments, and repeated measures can be taken for a similar purpose prior to implementing experimental procedures or treatments in a group study. The appropriate standard error statistic can be calculated and evaluated as well.

Interobserver and intraobserver reliability for dependent and independent variables, assessed in each phase of a study, are just as crucial. Dependent variable reliability data are needed to ensure that scoring of the dependent measures is objective and repeatable. Without evidence of acceptable agreement between independent judges, and of consistent scoring by the same judge, the research consumer has to question whether idiosyncratic decisions or unintentional bias could have affected the results. Independent variable reliability data are essential to demonstrate that all aspects of the independent variable (e.g., treatment) have been delivered consistently and as intended. Thus, evidence of procedural reliability for various aspects of the treatment, such as the timing and selection of cues or prompts, and the accuracy and delivery of feedback, should also be documented in a research report (see examples in Bourgeois, 1992; Massaro and Tompkins, 1993).

A variety of issues and procedures in observer reliability assessment have been discussed by Kearns and his colleagues (Kearns, 1990, 1992; Kearns and Simmons, 1988; McReynolds and Kearns, 1983). One caveat to note here is that correlation coefficients, which are often reported to document reliability, are unacceptable indices to demonstrate it. Correlation only indicates association, and two sets of scores may be highly associated (e.g., subjects who score high one time also score high the second time) but still significantly different (see, e.g., Wertz et al., 1985). Another point is that levels of chance agreement should be considered when evaluating the acceptability of reliability indices (see Kearns, 1990, 1992).

We turn now to *validity* issues to continue illustrating the question posed above. Silverman (1985) indicates that a validity assessment should ask whether the observations made are appropriate for answering the questions asked, and whether the

Table 31.2.
Some Useful Descriptive Information About Neurologically Impaired Persons

Brookshire (1983) re: aphasia	Age Education Gender Premorbid handedness Source of subjects	Etiology Time postonset Severity of aphasia Type of aphasia Lesion location

Rosenbek (1987)	*Risk Factors*
	  Smoking
	  Drinking
	  Obesity
	  Diabetes
	  Hypertension
		Other Medical
		  Factors
		  Medications
		  Seizures

Rosenbek et al. (1989)	Willingness to practice Ability to learn Ability to generalize Ability to retain	

Tompkins et al.
   (1990)
	Physiological indices of
	   aging
	Estimated premorbid
	   intelligence
	Auditory processing
	   abilities
	Personality/attitudinal
	   variables
	Social integration/social
	   support	

investigator observed and described what he wished to.[c] Thus, consumers should scrutinize the choice of outcome measures and treatments selected to achieve the stated goals. For example, if the goal of study is to assess a person's knowledge of particular syntactic constructions, would it be appropriate to rely on a test that requires spoken production of those constructions? It probably would not be appropriate unless it could be demonstrated that the person's knowledge is not masked by other problems of response formulation and execution. The validity of the connection between treatment and outcome measure is also paramount. As a hypothetical example, one would question whether reading comprehension, as an outcome goal, would be expected to improve with an oral reading treatment. Thus, examiners should justify the link between their independent and dependent variables. The validity of specially designed measures can be enhanced by providing evidence and logical arguments about the choice of items included, and by assessing their internal consistency reliability, to determine whether the items are measuring the same thing.

The last statement recalls an earlier maxim: Reliability is necessary (though not sufficient) for ensuring validity. The validity of a treatment also depends in part on demonstrating procedural reliability or compliance with the experimental protocol.[d] Wertz (1992) raises the issue of compliance in treatment studies, but his point applies to other kinds of research as well. Deviations from a protocol partway through a study, such as modifying selection criteria to include more patients, relaxing

the amount of treatment or practice provided, or changing the clinician, can vitiate the validity of a research effort.[e]

A special validity problem in studies of neurologically impaired persons is how to control for spontaneous recovery in evaluating treatment outcome. This will be discussed in question 9 below.

7. *Is the behavior sample adequate?* Three senses of adequacy are considered here. The first concerns repeated measurement with the same instrument or task, which was emphasized above. Typically, one-shot measurement is not sufficient. Repeated measurements may be needed to assess the stability of pretreatment baseline performance, to gather data to approximate test-retest reliability before initiating a treatment or experimental manipulation, and/or to observe the timing or pattern of change over the course of a study. The second sense of adequacy refers to the number of observations in each task. Generally, the more observations or items included in a measure, the more reliable that measurement will be. Brookshire and Nicholas (in press) demonstrated this point, showing that discourse measures based on single (short) speech samples were less stable than those based on a combination of samples. The third sense of adequacy refers to collecting multiple indicators at each measurement occasion, including measures indexing treated behaviors and conditions as well as untreated behaviors and conditions. Multiple measurements are needed in treatment studies to assess whether an effect has generalized beyond that specifically trained.

8. *Are precautions taken to reduce potential (even unknowing) examiner bias?* It is well documented that biases can be introduced by experimenters' expectations about the outcome

---

[c] Under these guidelines, it should be clear that point 3 above bears on the validity of subject selection.

[d] Assessing procedural reliability would also be important for studies comparing treatments; treatment delivery would need to be monitored to ensure that the treatments remained distinct.

---

[e] But a later section of this chapter will point out the flexibility of single-subject experimental designs, when modifications are analytically motivated and systematically applied.

of their research. Some possible controls for bias include keeping the experimenter blind to each individual subject's group, whenever possible, and having different people provide treatment and evaluate treatment data. Another check is achieved when interobserver reliability is high for selecting subjects, adhering to procedures, scoring outcomes, and judging the existence and magnitude of treatment effects.

9. *Are data interpreted appropriately?* Two facets of this question will be considered. One element concerns whether the results could be due to something other than the factors that the investigator is interested in. This is an issue of internal validity. Threats to internal validity probably can never be ruled out entirely, but their possible influence should be acknowledged and discussed, and interpretations should be appropriately cautious.

It is beyond the scope of this chapter to review all threats to internal validity (see discussions in Campbell and Stanley, 1966 and Ventry and Schiavetti, 1980; for a more general reference on alternative interpretations, see Huck and Sandler, 1979), but several major threats will be discussed here from the perspective of language intervention research. One that is important in group treatment trials is the composition of no-treatment control groups. A randomly assigned control group is essential for demonstrating efficacy in group studies (Wertz, 1992). But because it is generally believed that it is unethical to deny treatment, this crucial condition is rarely met.[f] Rather, control groups are typically self-selected, consisting of patients who live in remote areas, who elect not to participate, or who cannot pay for treatment. A self-selected control group may differ from the treatment group in critical ways, and the consequence is that differences in outcome between treatment and control groups may not be attributable to the treatment. A related difficulty centers around differential dropout from the study. There are a variety of reasons that patients drop out of treatment studies: They may be too ill or too severely impaired to participate; they may have improved sufficiently that they no longer want treatment; they may not be aware of a continued need for treatment; they may not like the treatment they are receiving. Any of these sorts of factors may make the groups unequal, thus biasing the results of the study.

Another difficult problem for the internal validity of neurological research is a possibility of concurrent other treatments and/or prior treatments interacting with the treatment of interest. Perhaps the other treatments paved the way, bringing the subject to the point at which he was ready to profit from the intervention being evaluated. This is one example of an order effect; more generally, the order and sequence with which conditions are applied may influence the reported results. Sequence and order effects may even affect results on a day-to-day basis. For example, if conditions are arranged in a fixed order or sequence, fatigue or warm-up effects may adversely affect some performances and not others. Conditions should be randomized or counterbalanced in group studies and in across-subject replications of single-subject designs.

The influence of spontaneous recovery is nature's version of an "interacting treatments" problem. Physiological improvement brings about behavior change that is difficult to separate from that which we would like to attribute to our treatments. Some researchers have tried to skirt the issue by conducting their treatment investigations in neurologically stable patients, years beyond the presumed effects of spontaneous recovery. One limitation of this approach is that we do not know how long spontaneous recovery persists, particularly for traumatically brain-injured persons. Another concern is that most of our treatment is delivered in the period shortly after the injury, so it is imperative to evaluate the effectiveness of treatment in patients who may still be undergoing neurological restitution.

For a large group treatment trial, random assignment to treatment and control groups is one solution. Then the effects of spontaneous recovery are assumed not to differ between groups (Wertz, 1992). However, random assignment does not ensure equality. It might also be important to measure several behaviors that are approximately equal in difficulty to the target behaviors, but that the treatment is not expected to influence. If the recovery curve is steeper for treated behaviors than for untreated functions, treatment may be responsible for the changes.[g] Multiple baseline designs (McReynolds and Kearns, 1983), which track untreated behaviors while others are treated, can provide evidence of this sort in individual subjects. Each time that treatment is applied to a previously untreated behavior, the slope of change for that behavior should accelerate if treatment is exceeding the influence of spontaneous recovery. Single-subject experimental designs that allow reversal and reinstitution of treatment effects for the same behavior in the same individuals (McReynolds and Kearns, 1983) can also provide convincing evidence of the influence of treatment over spontaneous recovery.

A related issue in interpreting the results of intervention studies concerns a general attention effect. It might be argued that apparent treatment effects have resulted from the time and attention given to the patient, rather than from the content or process of treatment. The simultaneous measurement of treated and untreated behaviors can help to address this issue. Taking repeated measurements in a pretreatment baseline phase, where patients are being given time and attention, can also help to dilute this threat.

Another set of potential problems in attributing results to the experimental conditions involves the influence of factors that have demonstrated relationships to language and cognitive performance in non-neurologically-impaired persons. Some of these include age, hearing ability, medical risk factors, education/premorbid intelligence, and literacy (see Tompkins, 1992, for elaboration). It is important to remember that not all "errors" are due to a patient's neurological condition. A good example of this point comes from Yorkston and colleagues (Yorkston et al., 1990; Yorkston et al., 1993), who demonstrated that certain measures of word usage and grammatical complexity differed for non-brain-damaged adults differing in socioeconomic status. Similarly, Tompkins et al. (1993) found that several connected speech attributes thought to characterize adults with right hemisphere brain damage did not distinguish their speech samples from those of normally aging persons. The lesson is that findings for neurologically impaired persons must be evaluated against the appropriate control data and expectations.

---

[f] Wertz, Weiss, Aten et al. (1986) solved this dilemma by including a deferred treatment group, whose progress during the no-treatment phase could be analyzed as control data.

[g] However, another dilemma is that we do not know whether the rate, timing, or extent of spontaneous recovery is comparable for different behaviors or functions. Lesser change in an untreated function may simply represent a difference in the "recovery schedule," or in the complexity of the treated and untreated behaviors.

The last statement exemplifies the second facet of the interpretive question: given what we already know, does the interpretation ring true? Evaluating interpretations at this level requires knowledge or access to current theory and data and a sense of their validity and replicability.

10. *Are maintenance and generalization programmed and probed in treatment efficacy studies?* This is related to the earlier point about adequate behavior sample and multiple measures. It is important to plan treatments to maximize the likelihood of their generalizing (see discussions in Kearns, 1989; Thompson, 1989) and to assess whether treatment effects do in fact generalize to untrained exemplars and to other ecologically valid measures, situations, and conversational partners. Kearns (1993) indicates that generalization planning involves "comprehensive, multifaceted evaluation; the establishment of generalization criteria; incorporation of treatment strategies that might facilitate generalization; continuous measurement and probing for functional, generalized improvements; and, when necessary, extending treatments to additional settings, people and conditions until targeted levels of generalization occur." If generalization beyond the treated tasks is not apparent, the treatment effects may not be very meaningful. Similarly, maintenance of treatment gains should be assessed. It is rare for long-term maintenance data, much more than a few weeks after the end of treatment, to be provided in language intervention studies; evaluating maintenance over extended time intervals should become a priority.

11. *Are individual subject characteristics related to the reported outcomes?* Individual performance should be analyzed in group data, and factors that appear to contribute to success or failure need to be evaluated. Most clinical manipulations, like pause insertion or speech rate reduction, affect some people and not others (e.g., Nicholas and Brookshire, 1986). To apply findings to other individuals, it is important to try to identify what characterizes those with good and poor response.

12. *Is there some attempt to evaluate the meaningfulness or importance of changes attributed to the experimental manipulations?* We return to the issue of clinical significance here and raise the related concept of "effect size." Metter (1985) has suggested that some neurologists' skepticism about aphasia treatment efficacy is due to concerns about the relevance of specific improvements in treated deficits to real-life, functional goals. Goldstein (1990) reviews several approaches for examining clinical significance, including normative comparisons of target performance and subjective evaluations of changes effected. Results of these types of assessments have begun to appear in some language intervention research. For example, normative comparison data in the aphasia literature have been gathered by assessing the frequency of requests for information by neurologically intact adults in conversations with unfamiliar partners (Doyle et al., 1989) and by examining non-brain-damaged adults' usage of social conventions (Thompson and Byrne, 1984). Studies by Doyle, Goldstein, and Bourgeois (1987) and Massaro and Tompkins (1993) exemplify two varieties of subjective evaluation, examining listeners' ratings of the adequacy of selected communication parameters following language intervention. Whitney and Goldstein (1989) used a hybrid approach, in which subjective evaluations were made of aphasic adults' speech samples intermixed with samples from non-brain-damaged control speakers.

Table 31.3.
Scientific Steps in the Diagnostic Process

1. Define and delimit the problem.
2. Develop hypotheses to be tested; know what evidence is needed to evaluate them.
3. Develop procedures to test hypotheses systematically.
4. Collect the data: minimize bias and maximize validity.
5. Analyze the data: score and organize objectively.
6. Interpret the data: evaluate meaningfulness; support or reject hypotheses.
7. Generalize from data: reason from the evidence to draw tentative conclusions.

When a clinical intervention is not expected to lead directly to an ultimate outcome, several other measures of "importance" can be reported. Analysis of effect size has a precise statistical meaning (e.g., Cohen, 1977), but the idea is to determine how "large" or meaningful some statistically significant difference really is. Wertz (1991) suggests evaluating the size of a difference between groups of scores by examining their distributions for overlap or separation. This could be done by calculating the 95% confidence intervals for each set of scores, using standard error estimates. Another way to assess the importance or strength of an experimental effect is to set a predetermined difference criterion, designating a change of at least one or two standard deviation units, or a doubling or tripling of baseline performance, as clinically meaningful. To convey some indication of the strength of an observed group effect, researchers can report the number or percentage of subjects in a group study whose performance conforms to the overall, average pattern and/or who achieve the designated criterion for meaningful change.

THE CLINICIAN AS RESEARCHER

Science and Clinical Decision Making

Although some clinicians may shudder at the thought of "doing research," effective diagnosis and treatment are modeled on the principles that guide scientific inquiry. Parallels between research and treatment have been noted by many (e.g., Kent, 1985b; Silverman, 1985; Warren, 1986). For example, Nation and Aram (1984, p. 54) suggest that careful diagnosis is like conducting a "mini research project." Table 31.3 illustrates the scientific nature of the diagnostic process (after Nation and Aram) by laying out the chain of diagnostic steps that parallel scientific problem solving. This theme is not at all new. Many years ago, Johnson et al. (1963) emphasized diagnosis as a hypothesis-testing process, guided by principles of critical thinking, special observation skills, and impartial, precise, and reliable observation.

Clinically accountable treatment, which can be documented as effective, is guided by these same procedures and principles. Each session, we can and should define a problem, develop and test hypotheses, collect good data, evaluate the results, and then determine the next questions to pursue. Using a hypothesis-testing model, we would gather initial information about our patients from a range of sources, form our best guesses regarding the nature of functional strengths and weaknesses and what can be done to ameliorate them, and then test and refine these hypotheses. We would systematically manipulate the demands of our tasks, such as the level and type of information processing required, against the background of our knowledge about a patient's compensatory abilities, premorbid skills, environmental supports, and so forth.

To conclude, Silverman (1985) suggests that a scientific approach to clinical management involves four principles: specifying clear objectives; posing answerable or testable hypotheses and questions; observing systematically; and remaining aware of the tentative nature of the findings. I would add a fifth: justifying the choice of measures and treatments as appropriate to our patients' needs and our clinical goals. If we strive to adopt these principles, our clinical efforts should be more precise, and our patients can only benefit.

Contributing to the Scientific Database

Clinicians can contribute meaningfully to their professional literature, although there may be obstacles along the way (cf. Schumacher and Nicholas, 1991; Warren et al., 1987). Two avenues are probably most feasible for interested clinicians, particularly if they seek collaborative relationships with established research consultants. The first is to evaluate the effectiveness of their own interventions. The second is to contribute more generally to information in the field, helping to provide much-needed data through original studies or replications and extensions of existing work.

Clinicians Evaluating Their Own Interventions

Single-subject or within-subject experimental designs (e.g., McReynolds and Kearns, 1983) are probably the most appropriate designs for clinicians wishing to evaluate their treatments. Single-subject experimental designs are not glorified case studies. Well-conceived single-subject designs are built around the important components of scientific inquiry, such as operational definitions, attention to reliability and validity, and control of extraneous variables. The designs should incorporate repeated measurements of observable, operationally defined target behaviors, with independent scoring of a portion of those behaviors by more than one examiner, to demonstrate objectivity and consistency. Stable preintervention baseline data, collected on the clearly specified dependent variables, are used as reference points for evaluating the efficacy of replicable interventions conducted with well-defined subjects. The effects of these interventions are evaluated continuously within and across design phases (e.g., baseline, treatment, return to baseline, or maintenance), behaviors, and/or patients. Although tightly controlled and well suited to maximize internal validity, the designs also allow flexibility in treatment when a need for modification becomes apparent (Connell and Thompson, 1986; Kearns, 1986a; McReynolds and Thompson, 1986).

Investigators unfamiliar with single-subject designs may equate them with pretest-posttest studies, but the two designs are quite dissimilar. In a pretest-posttest design, a target behavior (e.g., reading comprehension) is measured once before treatment, an intervention is applied, and then the target behavior is measured again. This is a weak form of evidence about a treatment's effects; in fact, some would not grant it the status of evidence because of the inherent threats to the internal validity of the design (for further discussion see Campbell and Stanley, 1966; Ventry and Schiavetti, 1980).

Single-subject experimental designs are discussed in detail in a number of sources (e.g., Connell and Thompson, 1986; Kearns, 1986a; McReynolds and Kearns, 1983; McReynolds and Thompson, 1986). Kent (1985a) provides a useful table illustrating a variety of research questions together with some of the single-subject designs that are appropriate for addressing those questions. Examples of studies using these designs with neurologically impaired persons are also available in the aphasiology literature (cf., Bellaire et al., 1991; Doyle et al., 1991; Kearns, 1986b; Kearns and Potechin Scher, 1989; Massaro and Tompkins, 1993; Thompson and Byrne, 1984; Whitney and Goldstein, 1989).

Despite the strength of these designs for examining treatment efficacy, the ultimate clinical concern, there remain relatively few published examples. Perhaps the difficulty of implementing controlled research in a clinical environment is partly responsible for this situation. In describing their efforts to evaluate a treatment approach for a fluent aphasic patient, clinicians Schumacher and Nicholas (1991) recount a variety of problems that they faced when conducting research in their clinical setting. They question the feasibility of single-subject research in the clinical arena, unless a clinician is provided with release time for research or with assistance for collecting and analyzing data. Warren et al. (1987) suggest that the major difference between typical clinical procedure and rigorous study is the time required to conduct behavior probes in the no-treatment phases. In addition, designing and implementing generalization probes outside the treatment setting takes time and planning. Despite these barriers, Schumacher and Nicholas (1991) and Warren et al. (1987) clearly believe that clinicians can generate worthwhile research in certain conditions. Those who have the drive to tackle a research problem, and who consult with knowledgeable researchers before starting, could probably evaluate a number of questions in their clinical settings, particularly if they enlist assistance in scoring, checking scoring reliability, and the like. If several clinicians in one shop are interested, they can share these tasks. Or graduate students from local university programs can be recruited and trained to assist. Some of the kinds of studies that clinicians can probably implement most readily are described in the next section.

If a full-blown research project is too daunting given day-to-day responsibilities and time constraints, clinicians can still make their own treatments more rigorous by incorporating the scientific principles discussed thus far into their own treatment. To recapitulate, these include operationally specifying the nature of the client's abilities and the treatment plans; maximizing reliability and validity of measurement and treatment implementation; collecting an adequate behavior sample, including repeated measurements; attempting to control for extraneous factors like spontaneous recovery; programming for and measuring generalization to untreated behaviors and settings; assessing the maintenance of behavior change after treatment ends; examining potential factors related to success or failure; and assessing social validity to determine whether any changes effected have "made a difference." The more clinicians attend to these elements, the more confident they can be in interpreting the results of their own interventions, leading to more accountable service delivery.[h]

---

[h] Of course, as Kent and Fair (1985) warn, equating science with effective clinical problem-solving may dilute or trivialize the meaning of the former, and misrepresent or overlook some of what occurs in the latter.

Clinicians Contributing More Generally to Professional Literature

There are several avenues that I consider most feasible for clinicians who wish to contribute to our clinical database: evaluating efficacy of established treatment programs; replicating or extending existing studies; analyzing factors that may be important in interpreting assessment data or in implementing treatments; and gathering comparative performance data from persons without neurological impairments. Each of these is considered briefly below.

Evaluating Efficacy of Established Programs. Numerous treatment programs exist, and are recommended to clinicians, with only cursory efficacy data. Clinicians are well situated to evaluate these sorts of programs. One model of this kind of work is provided by Conlon and McNeil (1991), who examined the efficacy of Visual Action Therapy (Helm-Estabrooks et al., 1982) for globally aphasic adults. When attempting to evaluate these programs, clinicians may note that procedural specification is inadequate to allow consistent treatment delivery. In this case, a good deal of planning and work must go into the project up front to specify stimulus choices, cuing/prompting criteria and hierarchies, scoring procedures, and the like. However, after that it becomes a much simpler matter to carry out the treatment program and to use it with other potential candidates. An example of this approach can be found in Massaro and Tompkins (1993), who operationalized a Feature Analysis treatment program (Szekeres et al., 1987) that has been recommended for traumatically brain-injured patients. Massaro and Tompkins also gathered some data about the program's efficacy with two patients.

Conducting Replication and Extension Studies. Replication and extension studies are particularly lacking in the speech-language pathology research base. This is important in part because so much of our research has been done on small samples of subjects, who exhibit a limited range of characteristics. Attempting to replicate the findings from an already published project with another sample of subjects, or to extend the study using different subjects, stimuli, or settings, is an excellent way for a clinical researcher to begin. Some recent examples of replication and extension studies can be found in Beard and Prescott (1991); Bloise and Tompkins (1993); and Kimelman and McNeil (1987). The study reported by Kearns and Potechin Scher (1989) presents an even less frequent phenomenon: replication and extension by the original investigators. Often, publications do not contain sufficient detail to allow replication, so an investigator wishing to replicate a study may need to contact the original authors for specific materials and procedures.

Analyzing Factors That Influence Delivery and Interpretation of Assessments of Treatments. Questions about the content, procedures, or interpretation of assessment tools have motivated a variety of clinical research. These kinds of questions typically stem from clinical observation; as such, they are good candidates for the interested clinical investigator. In one example, Nicholas et al. (1986) evaluated a number of reading comprehension batteries and documented the extent to which the comprehension questions could be answered without reading the associated passages. In other work, Nicholas et al. (1989) revised and standardized the administration and scoring procedures for the Boston Naming Test, which had been inadequately specified. They also reported extended normative data

for their revision. Another set of inquiries has focused on whether hypothetically important elements of treatment programs have an effect in practice. For example, several studies have examined whether the "new information" principle of PACE therapy (Promoting Aphasics' Communicative Effectiveness; Davis and Wilcox, 1985) has observable effects on narratives elicited from aphasic adults (Bottenberg and Lemme, 1991; Brenneise-Sarshad et al., 1991).

Gathering Normative Comparison Data. Judgments of our patients' abilities and performance should be made against a backdrop of knowledge about the nonneurological factors that may influence performance on language and cognitive tasks. Among the possible influences, noted earlier, are factors like age, education, socioeconomic status, physical health, or hearing impairment; however, few relevant data are available. Clinicians can design protocols to gather group data as a partial response to this need. Some examples are provided by Parr (1992), who examined everyday reading and writing practices of normal adults; Hansen and McNeil (1986), who studied writing with the nondominant hand; Elman et al. (1991), who documented the influence of education on judgments of nonneurologically impaired adults' writing and drawing samples; Tompkins et al. (1993), who assessed some characteristics of performance in normally aging adults' picture descriptions; and Yorkston et al. (1990, 1993), who reported on the discourse performance of non-brain-damaged subjects who were similar in terms of socioeconomic status to the "typical" traumatically brain-injured patient.

Of course, practical concerns affect the kinds of questions or problem areas that one can study. Time demands and the need for consultation and support personnel have already been emphasized; having equipment and facilities on hand is also important. For group data collection, the availability of subjects is a major issue. Funding may also be a concern, but some studies, particularly those evaluating established treatments, could probably be run as part of routine clinical practice (e.g., Kearns, 1986b; Massaro and Tompkins, in press). In the end, personal interests and the perceived value of the research may be the most important motivators for clinicians deciding to embark on the research enterprise.

Some Competencies for Clinician-Investigators

A clinician-investigator should be able to formulate answerable questions that have practical significance, and to make the necessary observations, with acceptable levels of validity and reliability, to offer tentative answers. This presumes current knowledge in the content area (e.g., the nature of neurological disorders and their treatment; the nature of normal language and cognition) as well as familiarity with guidelines for evaluating research. Persistence and tolerance for imperfection would be important personality characteristics, because, as Warren (1986) reminds us, there is no "perfect design" for any study. Compromises are usually necessary, in research as well as in clinical endeavors. Most clinicians will feel more confident about the effects of particular compromises in their research plans after consulting with an expert.

Initiating a Research Project

When clinicians decide that they have the appropriate interests, competencies, and supports, they can begin developing their research projects. The first step is to hone the idea that sparked interest in the investigation. This can be accomplished by reviewing the available literature, to see what aspects of the research problem have not been addressed adequately, or at all. Computerized databases such as PsycLIT, PsychINFO, and Medline and abstract journals such as *Psychological Abstracts* and *Index Medicus* will help clinicians to locate the relevant literature. The *Clinical Aphasiology* publications (e.g., Lemme, 1993; Prescott, 1989, 1991a, 1991b) are particularly valuable references for those studying adult neurologic communicative disorders.

While reviewing the relevant literature, the clinician should try to determine what factors point to the need for further investigation in an area of interest. For example, control for spontaneous recovery or examiner bias may be in doubt; the operationalization of the dependent measures may be debatable; or the findings may have limited generality given the size and characteristics of the subject sample. A project can be developed to rectify particular issues of concern or to replicate and extend findings in research that is essentially sound.

Planning can proceed by focusing on the questions that have been outlined for research consumers. Brainstorming with other clinicians about the best ways to operationalize and measure variables, or about how to minimize factors that might confound the results, is a useful activity. It is also helpful to run the initial ideas and plans by someone with research expertise, as suggested previously. Pilot-testing the methods on at least a few subjects is recommended as well; even experienced investigators generally identify wrinkles that remain to be ironed out during initial feasibility testing.

Finally, in the planning phase, investigators should contact their institution's Research and Human Rights Committee, Institutional Review Board, or similar committee, to ascertain what procedures they should follow to obtain approval for the project. Typically, these committees ask for a description of the intent, general procedures, and risks and benefits of the proposed research, along with specific precautions taken to protect the patients' rights. A detailed consent form, spelling out these elements for the patients, is also essential.

Opportunities for Funding and Consultation Assistance

Funding may be an important consideration, either for partial salary coverage in order to obtain release time to plan and conduct a project, or for paying research assistants or subjects. A variety of funding opportunities that may be available for clinician-investigators, depending on their level of expertise. Several are outlined below; interested readers should contact the organizations listed for further information.

(*a*) The American Speech-Language-Hearing Foundation (ASHF) has for a number of years sponsored New Investigator awards for those who have recently completed their latest degree program. (*b*) The American Speech-Language-Hearing Association (ASHA) periodically compiles a resource entitled *Profiles of Funding Sources*; the fourth edition was published in 1991. This publication provides a geographic guide to corporate and private foundations with a history of supporting research in communication disorders. (*c*) Graduate students in our program have received individual grant support from the Alzheimer's Disease and Related Disorders Association, the American Association of University Women, and the Sigma Xi Research Society. (*d*) The National Institutes of Health (NIH) Small Grants Program (R03) provides 2 years of funding to support pilot projects and feasibility research for investigators with limited research experience. Language researchers would most likely apply for NIH funding from the National Institute on Deafness and Other Communication Disorders (NIDCD), but some projects might be fundable by the National Institute on Aging (NIA) or the National Institute of Mental Health (NIMH). (*e*) Finally, internal institutional funding may be available. Some hospitals and rehabilitation centers sponsor competitions for funding, or release time, to encourage staff research efforts. The Department of Veteran's Affairs Research Advisory Group (RAG) program supports newly recruited junior investigators by providing funds for initiating research efforts. And many universities grant seed monies for pilot projects expected to lead to larger efforts. A clinician-investigator's project, sponsored by a faculty member, might be partially fundable in this way.

The value of consulting assistance has been emphasized repeatedly in this chapter. The way to get the most out of a consultative relationship is to consult before beginning a project rather than trying to salvage mistakes later. But best laid plans being what they are, a good consultant may be able to help rescue some elements of an errant project after the fact as well. A clinician-investigator should not be afraid to seek help with a project by contacting people with the appropriate expertise.

There are a variety of avenues for identifying potential consultants. ASHF has sponsored several workshops on treatment efficacy research. Attending such conferences is valuable for both continuing education and networking purposes, but even reading the conference proceedings can point clinicians toward experts who might be willing to serve as research consultants. University faculty or master clinicians who publish their work would be good contacts as well. Professional journals list their authors and reviewers, and a Grants Directory distributed by ASHA's Research Division designates speech and language researchers who have received grants; these would also be good sources of possible expert consultants.

Selling the Administration on Your Research Plans

It would be necessary for investigators in most clinical settings to garner administrative support for their research efforts. Silverman (1985, p. 269) provides the following arguments for convincing administrators that research is beneficial to them.

"1. Accountability is an important consideration. Research assessing the impact of your clinical program (therapy outcome research) on the communicatively handicapped could be used by your administrator or administrators to demonstrate its value to various groups, including: (a) administrators of the institution in which the program is located, (b) potential consumers of the services offered, i.e., the communicatively handicapped and their families, (c) third parties who are paying for the services, e.g., voluntary organizations, governmental agencies, and insurance companies, (d) governmental agencies and private foundations that award grants, and (e) the community.

"2. Evaluating your clinical programs systematically will provide you with information you need to maximize their effectiveness. If you do not systematically evaluate the impact of your clinical programs on your clients, how can you tell if they are achieving their objectives?

"3. The presence of an ongoing clinical research program is likely to bring local, state, national, and international recognition to the institution that should help in attracting grants and gifts from individuals, private foundations, and governmental sources."

Warren, a clinician and an administrator, also points out the value of efficacy data for demonstrating accountability to quality assurance evaluators and third-party payers (Warren et al., 1987). The costs involved can be justified by emphasizing the enhanced confidence with which outcomes can be linked to the treatments provided.

FUTURE TRENDS IN APPLICATION OF RESEARCH PRINCIPLES TO INTERVENTION

Level of Outcome and Clinical Significance

Clinical significance and meaningfulness of outcomes have been recurrent themes in this chapter. These concerns have also become important from a reimbursement perspective. It is anticipated that the future will see more attention to documenting the clinical importance of changes effected by interventions.

Most clinical aphasiologists would probably agree that our ultimate goal should be to enhance communicative effectiveness or adequacy in real-life interactions. However, we also know that there are typically a number of steps along the way to ultimate, clinically significant outcomes. In this regard, Campbell and Bain (1991) contrast ultimate outcomes with intermediate outcomes, which are believed to be prerequisite for progressing toward ultimate goals, and with instrumental outcomes, which may lead to other outcomes without additional intervention. An example of an intermediate goal for a fluent aphasic patient might be to control excessive verbal output as a prerequisite for maximizing eventual language comprehension and production. A potential instrumental goal might be to establish a compensatory strategy that is assumed to have broad applicability for functional communication, such as referring to an external memory aid.[i] Taking another tack, Schwartz and Whyte (1992) discuss interventions in the framework proposed by the World Health Organization (1980), which distinguishes among impairment, disability, and handicap. Impairment refers to specific deficits, such as agrammatic output. Disability refers to the impact of impairments on specific skills (e.g., agrammatism, apraxia of speech, and dysarthria will affect the ability to speak). Handicap reflects the effects of disabilities on social roles. If, for example, severely dysarthric speech affects a person's ability to function in everyday situations, a handicap is present. Thus, the concept of "handicap" in this perspective is related to functional communicative adequacy or ultimate outcomes.

Research and clinical intervention in aphasia has tended to focus at the level of impairment, or sometimes disability, rather than social communicative functioning (Schwartz and Whyte, 1992). As indicated earlier, this may contribute to the poor opinion of our profession held by some neurologists and other medical personnel. It is certainly important for us to implement and evaluate interventions that target more ecologically valid outcomes, such as conversational exchanges, whenever possible. One obvious dilemma is that intermediate or prerequisite goals, and impairments or disabilities, may be legitimate treat-

ment targets, especially in the early postonset stage. When treatments are not intended or expected to result immediately in clinically significant gains, it will be incumbent on investigators to specify the eventual pathway from their treatment focus to the desired end result, indicating why or how their treatment goal should be an important step along the way to some more relevant outcome. Another problem is that ultimate outcomes are difficult to define and operationalize, with the consequence that they are difficult to measure. Achieving generalization to everyday settings and tasks and documenting social validity are two possible ways to demonstrate the functionality of outcomes, especially if the effects have staying power. To examine the durability of clinically important effects, investigators should begin to assess clinical significance or social validity using data from several phases of treatment studies, including data collected during maintenance probes.

Social validity assessments are in their infancy, so standards and criteria for conducting them are not well defined. The future will see more attempts to develop a rigorous technology for determining social validity. The concerns of reliability, validity, and generality are paramount here as they are in any measurement effort. Questionnaires and rating scales should be constructed so that the resulting data are sound. Silverman (1985) discusses several other critical factors such as the design of the social validity tasks; numbers and characteristics of raters, including their knowledge of subject group or time of sample; and selection of the scaling method. One salient question (Campbell and Dollaghan, 1992; Goldstein, 1990; Tompkins, 1992) has to do with the choice of the "gold standard" for a normative comparison approach to determining clinical significance. When patients are severely impaired, a standard might be chosen to approximate communicative performance of a milder, but functional, aphasic communicator. For mildly involved patients, a normal criterion may be appropriate. Whatever the comparison group, though, we will be more careful to specify the subject matching factors that we consider relevant. The common practice of matching comparison and treatment subjects only for chronological age and gender will be recognized as insufficient. As procedural issues are being sorted out, much more work will also be needed to assess the correspondence between these sorts of social validity data and other measures of communication performance in the natural environment.

Documenting functional status has recently taken on more practical urgency (Warren et al., 1991). Rapidly escalating health care costs and concern about cost accountability have instigated a search for outcome measures that can be used to cut rehabilitation expenditures. A variety of generic rating scales have been proposed to quantify "functional outcome" (see Warren et al., 1991). These scales are being advocated not only for documenting quality of services and reimbursement rates but also for determining eligibility for services. Unfortunately, issues of reliability, validity, and sensitivity to change have, for the most part, been inadequately addressed in the development and application of these scales (AHSA, 1990; Kearns, 1993). ASHA is in the process of validating a more extensive functional communication measure for adults (Fratalli, 1991), an important step given the likelihood that the focus on "functional outcome" will continue to encompass both clinical and reimbursement issues.

---

[i] It is difficult to identify instrumental outcomes in language intervention because we have little information about which cognitive or linguistic abilities would allow other goals to be reached without further treatment (Campbell and Bain, 1991). Generalization data are necessary to test the assumption that an instrumental outcome has been achieved.

Intervention Efforts Focused on Communication Partners

Targeting communication partner behaviors, as well as those of the patients, is a relatively untapped but potentially important direction in treatment research. After all, communication is an interactive process, and its success hinges on the interplay between participants. Turning some attention to the neurologically intact member of a communicative dyad would have considerable ecological validity in the sense emphasized above. Some recent interest in targeting communication partners has been documented in the literature. For example, Simmons et al. (1987) evaluated an intervention to diminish inappropriate partner behaviors, such as interrupting before the aphasic participant had time to respond. Flowers and Peizer (1984) reported a system designed to quantify partner strategies and to identify those that were more or less successful in communicative exchanges, so that they could be addressed in treatment.

Relatedly, the future may also see more efforts to train communication partners as intervention agents (cf., Bourgeois, 1991). This approach may accomplish several goals simultaneously: It can put the treatment in the natural environment, free some of the clinician's time, and allow more treatment to be delivered than would otherwise be feasible or affordable. It may also empower communication partners by giving them some specific things to do in the event of communication breakdown.

Obviously, there may be a number of pitfalls to either of these approaches. The clinician would have to invest time to train the communication partners and to monitor delivery of treatment and/or evaluation of responses. Personalities and prior patterns of interaction between communication partners also may mitigate against these methods or diminish their effectiveness. In addition, it may be difficult to get reimbursement for services that target communication partners, unless creative outcome measures are employed. Of course, rigorous evaluation of efficacy will be necessary, as it is for any language intervention approach. Despite these possible drawbacks, the potential benefits of interventions targeting the neurologically intact communication partner are likely to spur further exploration in the future.

CONCLUSION

This chapter emphasizes parallels between research and clinical decision making and encourages clinicians to adopt a scientific orientation to clinical management. A scientific approach makes our clinical efforts more accountable, more rigorous, and more interesting and allows us to get the most from our continuing education experiences. For clinicians dedicated to providing the best possible services to their patients, it is difficult to imagine more worthwhile goals.

Acknowledgments

Preparation of this chapter was supported in part by National Institute on Deafness and Other Communication Disorders Grant DC00453. Kristie Spencer and Maura Mullane Timko also provided invaluable assistance.

References

American Speech-Language-Hearing Association. (1990). *Report of the advisory panel to ASHA's functional communication measures project*. Rockville, MD: American Speech-Language-Hearing Association.

American Speech-Language-Hearing Association. (1992). Code of Ethics. *ASHA, 34* (March, Suppl. 9), 1–2.

Beard, L. C., and Prescott, T. E. (1991). Replication of a treatment protocol for repetition deficit in conduction aphasia. In T. E. Prescott (Ed.), *Clinical aphasiology* (Vol. 19, pp. 197–208). Austin, TX: Pro-Ed.

Bellaire, K. J., Georges, J. B., and Thompson, C. K. (1991). Establishing functional communication board use for nonverbal aphasic subjects. In T. E. Prescott (Ed.), *Clinical aphasiology* (Vol. 19, pp. 219–227). Austin, TX: Pro-Ed.

Bloise, C. G. R., and Tompkins, C. A. (1993). Right brain damage and inference revision, revisited. In M. L. Lemme (Ed.), *Clinical aphasiology* (Vol. 21, pp. 145–155). Austin, TX: Pro-Ed.

Bottenberg, D., and Lemme, M. L. (1991). Effect of shared and unshared listener knowledge on narratives of normal and aphasic adults. In T. E. Prescott (Ed.), *Clinical aphasiology* (Vol. 19, pp. 109–116). Austin, TX: Pro-Ed.

Bourgeois, M. S. (1991). Communication treatment for adults with dementia. *Journal of Speech and Hearing Research, 34*, 831–844.

Bourgeois, M. S. (1992). Evaluating memory wallets in conversations with patients with dementia. *Journal of Speech and Hearing Research, 35*, 1344–1357.

Brenneise-Sarshad, R., Nicholas, L. E., and Brookshire, R. H. (1991). Effects of apparent listener knowledge and picture stimuli on aphasic and non-brain-damaged speakers' narrative discourse. *Journal of Speech and Hearing Research, 34*, 168–176.

Brookshire, R. H. (1983). Subject description and generality of results in experiments with aphasic adults. *Journal of Speech and Hearing Disorders, 48*, 342–346.

Brookshire, R. H., and Nicholas, L. E. (in press). Test-retest stability of measures of connected speech in aphasia. In M. L. Lemme (Ed.), *Clinical aphasiology* (Vol. 22). Austin, TX: Pro-Ed.

Campbell, D. T., and Stanley, J. C. (1966). *Experimental and quasi-experimental designs for research*. Chicago: Rand McNally.

Campbell, T. F., and Bain, B. (1991). How long to treat: A multiple outcome approach. *Language, Speech, and Hearing Services in Schools, 22*, 271–276.

Campbell, T. F., and Dollaghan, C. (1992). A method for obtaining listener judgments of spontaneously produced language: Social validation through direct magnitude estimation. *Topics in Language Disorders, 12*, 42–55.

Chial, M. R. (1985). Scholarship as process: A task analysis of thesis and dissertation research. In R. D. Kent (Ed.), *Seminars in speech and language: Vol. 6. Application of research to assessment and therapy* (pp. 35–54). New York: Thieme-Stratton.

Cohen, J. (1977). *Statistical power analysis for the behavioral sciences*. New York: Academic Press.

Conlon, C. P., and McNeil, M. R. (1991). The efficacy of treatment for two globally aphasic adults using visual action therapy. In T. E. Prescott (Ed.), *Clinical aphasiology* (Vol. 19, pp. 185–195). Austin, TX: Pro-Ed.

Connell, P. J., and Thompson, C. K. (1986). Flexibility of single-subject experimental designs. Part III: Using flexibility to design or modify experiments. *Journal of Speech and Hearing Disorders, 51*, 214–225.

Darley, F. L. (1972). The efficacy of language rehabilitation in aphasia. *Journal of Speech and Hearing Disorders, 37*, 3–21.

Davis, G. A., and Wilcox, M. J. (1985). *Adult aphasia rehabilitation: Applied pragmatics*. San Diego: College Hill Press.

Doyle, P. J., Goldstein, H., and Bourgeois, M. S. (1987). Experimental analysis of syntax training in Broca's aphasia: A generalization and social validation study. *Journal of Speech and Hearing Disorders, 52*, 143–155.

Doyle, P. J., Goldstein, H., Bourgeois, M. S., and Nakles, K. (1989). Facilitating generalized requesting behavior in Broca's aphasia: An experimental analysis of a generalization training procedure. *Journal of Applied Behavior Analysis, 22*, 157–170.

Doyle, P. J., Oleyar, K. S., and Goldstein, H. (1991). Facilitating functional conversational skills in aphasia: An experimental analysis of a generalization training procedure. In T. E. Prescott (Ed.), *Clinical aphasiology* (Vol. 19, pp. 101–241). Austin: Pro-Ed.

Elman, R. J., Roberts, J. A., and Wertz, R. T. (1991). The effect of education on diagnosis of aphasia from writing and drawing performance by mildly aphasic and non-brain-damaged adults. In T. E. Prescott (Ed.), *Clinical aphasiology* (Vol. 20, pp. 101–110). Austin, TX: Pro-Ed.

Flowers, C. R., and Peizer, E. R. (1984). Strategies for obtaining information from aphasic persons. In R. H. Brookshire (Ed.), *Clinical aphasiology: Conference proceedings 1984* (pp. 106–113). Minneapolis, MN: BRK.

Franzen, M. D. (1989). *Reliability and validity in neuropsychological assessment*. New York: Plenum.

Fratalli, C. (1991). *Functional communication scales for adults*. Rockville, MD: American Speech-Language-Hearing Association.

Goldstein, H. (1990). Assessing clinical significance. In L. B. Olswang, C. K. Thompson, S. F. Warren, and N. J. Minghetti (Eds.), *Treatment efficacy research in communication disorders* (pp. 91–98). Rockville, MD: American Speech-Language-Hearing Foundation.

Hansen, A. M., and McNeil, M. R. (1986). Differences between writing with the dominant and nondominant hand by normal geriatric subjects on a spontaneous writing task: Twenty perceptual and computerized measures. In R. H. Brookshire (Ed.), *Clinical aphasiology* (Vol. 16, pp. 116–122). Minneapolis, MN: BRK.

Helm-Estabrooks, N., Fitzpatrick, P. M., and Barresi, B. (1982). Visual action therapy for global aphasia. *Journal of Speech and Hearing Disorders, 47*, 385–389.

Huck, S. W., and Sandler, H. M. (1979). *Rival hypotheses: Alternative interpretations of data based conclusions*. New York: Harper & Row.

Johnson, W., Darley, F. L., and Spriestersbach, D. C. (1963). *Diagnostic methods in speech pathology*. New York: Harper & Row.

Kearns, K. P. (1986a). Flexibility of single-subject experimental designs. Part II: Design selection and arrangements of experimental phases. *Journal of Speech and Hearing Disorders, 51*, 204–214.

Kearns, K. P. (1986b). Systematic programming of verbal elaboration skills in chronic Broca's aphasia. In R. C. Marshall (Ed.), *Case studies in aphasia rehabilitation* (pp. 225–244). Austin, TX: Pro-Ed.

Kearns, K. P. (1989). Methodologies for studying generalization. In L. V. McReynolds and J. Spradlin (Eds.), *Generalization strategies in the treatment of communication disorders*, Toronto: B. C. Decker.

Kearns, K. P. (1990). Reliability of procedures and measures. In L. Olswang, C. Thompson, and S. Warren (Eds.), *Treatment efficacy research in communication disorders* (pp. 71–90). Rockville, MD: American Speech-Language-Hearing Foundation.

Kearns, K. P. (1993). Functional outcome: Methodological considerations. In M. L. Lemme (Ed.), *Clinical aphasiology* (Vol. 21, pp. 67–72). Austin, TX: Pro-Ed.

Kearns, K. P. (1992). Methodological issues in treatment research: A single-subject perspective. *Aphasia treatment: Current approaches and research opportunities* (pp. 1–16). Washington, D.C.: National Institute on Deafness and Other Communication Disorders.

Kearns, K. P., and Potechin Scher, G. (1989). The generalization of response elaboration training effects. In T. E. Prescott (Ed.), *Clinical aphasiology* (Vol. 18, pp. 223-245). Boston, MA: College Hill Press.

Kearns, K. P., and Simmons, N. N. (1988). Interobserver reliability and perceptual ratings: More than meets the ear. *Journal of Speech and Hearing Research, 31*, 131–136.

Kent, R. D. (1985a). Science and the clinician: The practice of science and the science of practice. In R. D. Kent (Ed.), *Seminars in speech and language: Vol. 6. Application of research to assessment and therapy* (pp. 1–12). New York: Thieme-Stratton.

Kent, R. D. (Ed.). (1985b). *Seminars in speech and language: Vol. 6. Application of research to assessment and therapy*. New York: Thieme-Stratton.

Kent, R. D., and Fair, J. (1985). Clinical research: Who, where, and how? In R. D. Kent (Ed.), *Seminars in Speech and Language: Vol. 6. Application of Research to Assessment and Therapy*(pp. 23–34). New York: Thieme-Stratton.

Kimelman, M. D. Z., and McNeil, M. R. (1987). An investigation of emphatic stress comprehension in adult aphasia: A replication. *Journal of Speech and Hearing Research, 30*, 295–300.

Lemme, M. L. (Ed.). (1993). *Clinical aphasiology* (Vol. 21). Austin, TX: Pro-Ed.

Massaro, M., and Tompkins, C. A. (in press). Feature analysis for treatment of communication disorders in traumatically brain-injured patients: An efficacy study. *Clinical aphasiology* (Vol. 22). Austin, TX: Pro-Ed.

McReynolds, L., and Kearns, K. P. (1983). *Single-subject experimental design in communicative disorders*. Baltimore, MD: University Park Press.

McReynolds, L. V., and Thompson, C. K. (1986). Flexibility of single-subject experimental designs. Part I: Review of the basics of single-subject designs. *Journal of Speech and Hearing Disorders, 51*, 194–203.

Metter, E. J. (1985). Issues and directions for the future: Speech pathology - A physician's perspective. In R. H. Brookshire (Ed.), *Clinical aphasiology* (Vol. 15, pp. 22–28). Minneapolis, MN: BRK.

Nation, J. E., and Aram, D. M. (1984). *Diagnosis of speech and language disorders* (2nd ed.). Boston, MA: College Hill.

Nicholas, L. E., and Brookshire, R. H. (1986). Consistency of the effects of rate of speech on brain-damaged adults' comprehension of narrative discourse. *Journal of Speech and Hearing Research, 29*, 462–470.

Nicholas, L. E., Brookshire, R. H., MacLennan, D. L., Schumacher, J. G., and Porazzo, S. A. (1989). Revised administration and scoring procedures for the Boston Naming Test and norms for non-brain-damaged adults. *Aphasiology, 3*(6), 569–580.

Nicholas, L. E., MacLennan, D. L., and Brookshire, R. H. (1986). Validity of multiple-sentence reading comprehension tests for aphasic adults. *Journal of Speech and Hearing Disorders, 51*, 82–87.

Parr, S. (1992). Everyday reading and writing practices of normal adults: Implications for aphasia assessment. *Aphasiology, 3*, 273–284.

Perkins, W. H. (1985). From clinical dispenser to clinical scientist. In R. D. Kent (Ed.), *Seminars in speech and language: Vol. 6. Application of research to assessment and therapy* (pp. 13–22). New York: Thieme-Stratton.

Prescott, T. E. (Ed.). (1989). *Clinical aphasiology* (Vol. 18). Boston, MA: College Hill.

Prescott, T. E. (Ed.). (1991a). *Clinical aphasiology* (Vol. 19). Austin, TX: Pro-Ed.

Prescott, T. E. (Ed.). (1991b). *Clinical aphasiology* (Vol. 20). Austin, TX: Pro-Ed.

Rosenbek, J. C. (1987). Unusual aphasias: Some criteria for evaluating case studies in aphasiology. In R. H. Brookshire (Ed.), *Clinical aphasiology* (Vol. 17, pp. 357–361). Minneapolis, MN: BRK.

Rosenbek, J. C., LaPointe, L. L., and Wertz, R. T. (1989). *Aphasia: A clinical approach*. Austin, TX: Pro-Ed.

Schumacher, J. G., and Nicholas, L. E. (1991). Conducting research in a clinical setting against all odds: Unusual treatment of fluent aphasia. In T. E. Prescott (Ed.), *Clinical aphasiology* (Vol. 19, pp. 267–277). Austin, TX: Pro-Ed.

Schwartz, M. F., and Whyte, J. (1992). Methodological issues in aphasia treatment research: The big picture. *Aphasia treatment: Current approaches and research opportunities* (pp. 17–23). Washington, D.C.: National Institute on Deafness and Other Communication Disorders.

Shewan, C. M. (1986). The history and efficacy of aphasia treatment. In R. Chapey (Ed.), *Language intervention strategies in adult aphasia* (2nd ed., pp. 28–43). Baltimore, MD: Williams & Wilkins.

Silverman, F. H. (1985). *Research design and evaluation in speech-language pathology and audiology* (2nd ed.). Englewood Cliffs, NJ: Prentice-Hall.

Simmons, N. N., Kearns, K. P., and Potechin, G. (1987). Treatment of aphasia through family member training. In R. H. Brookshire (Ed.), *Clinical aphasiology* (Vol. 17, pp. 106–116). Minneapolis, MN: BRK.

Szekeres, S. F., Ylvisaker, M., and Cohen, S. B. (1987). A framework for cognitive rehabilitation therapy. In M. Ylvisaker and E. R. Gobble (Eds.), *Community re-entry for head injured adults* (pp. 87–136). Boston, MA: College Hill Press.

Thompson, C. K. (1989). Generalization research in aphasia: A review of the literature. In T. E. Prescott (Ed.), *Clinical aphasiology* (Vol. 18, pp. 195–222). Boston: College Hill Press.

Thompson, C. K., and Byrne, M. E. (1984). Across setting generalization of social conventions in aphasia: An experimental analysis of "loose training." In R. H. Brookshire (Ed.), *Clinical aphasiology: Conference proceedings 1984* (pp. 132-144). Minneapolis, MN: BRK.

Tompkins, C. A. (1992). Improving aphasia treatment research: Some methodological considerations. *Aphasia treatment: Current approaches and research opportunities* (pp. 37–46). Washington, D.C.: National Institute on Deafness and Other Communication Disorders.

Tompkins, C. A., Boada, R., McGarry, K., Jones, J., Rahn, A. E., and Ranier, S. (1993). Connected speech characteristics of right hemisphere damaged adults: A re-examination. In M. L. Lemme (Ed.), *Clinical aphasiology* (Vol. 21, pp. 113–122). Austin, TX: Pro-Ed.

Tompkins, C. A., Jackson, S. T., and Schulz, R. (1990). On prognostic research in adult neurogenic disorders. *Journal of Speech and Hearing Research, 33*, 398–401.

Ventry, I. M., and Schiavetti, N. (1980). *Evaluating research in speech pathology and audiology: A guide for clinicians and students*. Reading, MA: Addison-Wesley.

Warren, R. L. (1986). Research design: Considerations for the clinician. In R. Chapey (Ed.), *Language intervention strategies in adult aphasia* (2nd ed., pp. 66–80). Baltimore, MD: Williams & Wilkins.

Warren, R. L., Gabriel, C., Johnston, A., and Gaddie, A. (1987). Efficacy during acute rehabilitation. In R. H. Brookshire (Ed.), *Clinical aphasiology* (Vol. 17, pp. 1–11). Minneapolis, MN: BRK.

Warren, R. L., Loverso, F. L., and DePiero, J. (1991). The relationships among level of measurement, generalization, and reimbursement. In T. E. Prescott (Ed.), *Clinical aphasiology* (Vol. 19, pp. 163–170). Austin, TX: Pro-Ed.

Wertz, R. T. (1991). Predictability: Greater than p < .05. In T. E. Prescott (Ed.), *Clinical aphasiology* (Vol. 19, pp. 21–30). Austin, TX: Pro-Ed.

Wertz, R. T. (1992). A single case for group treatment studies in aphasia. *Aphasia treatment: Current approaches and research opportunities* (pp. 25–36). Washington, D.C.: National Institute on Deafness and Other Communication Disorders.

Wertz, R. T., Shubitowski, Y., Dronkers, N. F., Lemme, M. L., and Deal, J. L. (1985). *Word fluency measure reliability in normal and brain damaged adults*. Paper presented at the American Speech-Language-Hearing Association convention, Washington, DC.

Wertz, R. T., Weiss, D. G., Aten, J. L., Brookshire, R. H., Garcia-Bunuel, L., Holland, A. L., Kurtzke, J. F., LaPointe, L. L., Milianti, F. J., Brannegan, R., Greenbaum, H., Marshall, R. C., Vogel, D., Carter, J., Barnes, N. S., and Goodman, R. (1986). Comparison of clinic, home, and deferred language treatment for aphasia: A Veterans Administration cooperative study. *Archives of Neurology, 43*, 653–658.

Whitney, J. L., and Goldstein, H. (1989). Using self-monitoring to reduce disfluencies in speakers with mild aphasia. *Journal of Speech and Hearing Disorders, 54*, 576–586.

World Health Organization. (1980). International classification of impairments, disabilities and handicaps. Geneva.

Yorkston, K. M., Farrier, L., Zeches, J., and Uomoto, J. M. (1990). *Discourse patterns in traumatically brain injured and control subjects*. Paper presented at the American Speech-Language-Hearing Association convention, Washington, DC.

Yorkston, K. M., Zeches, J., Farrier, L., and Uomoto, J. M. (1993). Lexical pitch as a measure of word choice in narratives of traumatically brain injured and control subjects. *Clinical aphasiology* (Vol. 21, pp. 165–172). Austin, TX: Pro-Ed.

CHAPTER 32
Interdisciplinary Team Intervention

MICHAEL L. KIMBAROW

The student reading this comprehensive textbook as part of a course in aphasia might well believe that the communication deficits exhibited by aphasic patients are of paramount importance to the individual and his or her family. The intensive academic and clinical preparation in communication disorders may also lead to the belief that the profession of speech-language pathology is the singlemost important discipline concerned with assessment and remediation of the aphasic person's deficits (Rothberg, 1981).

After graduating with their Master's degree, many new clinicians enter their first job convinced that speech-language pathology services take precedence over all other disciplines when treating aphasia. Clinical reality dictates a rapid reassessment of this position. New clinicians learn quickly that they are but one of many professionals charged with the care of the aphasic patient.

Treating an aphasic patient is a daunting task. Whether one works in an acute care hospital, a rehabilitation center, a nursing home or the patient's own home, the communicative, physical, and emotional deficits associated with aphasia demand a remarkable level of skill, knowledge, and training to treat the patient successfully. The new clinician might appropriately ask how it is possible to address all of the patient's problems and achieve the treatment goals in the limited amount of time he or she spends with the patient each day. Fortunately, in many practice settings there is a team of professionals charged with rehabilitation of the aphasic patient. The ''team'' approach to working with an aphasic person recognizes the interrelationships among the individual's communicative, cognitive, emotional, and physical disabilities. Teams treat the aphasic individual as a ''whole person'' and not as someone exhibiting a set of isolated deficits.

It is virtually impossible to establish a single definition of a treatment team. Each practice setting has a unique team identity and defines the responsibilities of team members according to the specific goals and structure of the clinical program. Consequently, this chapter will address general principles and issues of team management as a way of introducing readers to the professional situations they are likely to encounter in their work with aphasic patients.

PERSPECTIVES ON TEAM MANAGEMENT

The concept of team care for persons exhibiting chronic illness has been a cornerstone of rehabilitation theory and practice for many years (Halstead, 1976). Longevity, however, does not constitute a mandate for its continued application in treatment of the aphasic person. Support for the team approach is evident in current recommended practice patterns in speech-language pathology. Practice patterns are, in turn, driven by regulatory and financial considerations and, most important, by the needs of patients and their families.

Recommended Practice Patterns

In addition to their language impairments, aphasic patients may also demonstrate a host of related disorders such as (a) hemiplegia or hemiparesis, (b) impaired activities of daily living (ADLs), (c) visual-perceptual deficits, (d) psychosocial adjustment problems, (e) depression, (f) dysphagia, and (g) cognitive disorders (e.g., attention, memory, or problem-solving deficits). The presence of any one of these associated disorders may interact with the aphasic person's language deficit, thereby complicating the recovery process. For example, depression may interfere with a patient's motivation and participation in therapy, or difficulties with fine-motor control may interfere with the patient's ability to communicate in writing. It is incumbent on the speech-language pathologist to use the information offered by other professionals with expertise in assessment and management of these related disorders to develop an appropriate treatment plan for the patient (Brookshire, 1992; Wertz et al., 1984).

The American Speech-Language-Hearing Association (ASHA) supports the use of the team approach. The National Joint Committee for the Communicative Needs of Persons with Severe Disabilities (of which the ASHA is a member) observed that ''delivery of intervention services . . . requires the collaboration and competence of families and professionals and paraprofessionals from many disciplines'' (1992, p. 5). The ASHA guidelines for managing patients with language and/or cognitive-communicative disorders recommend that speech-language pathologists become competent in ''designing and implementing an intervention plan that is coordinated and integrated with other services'' (American Speech-Language-Hearing Association, 1991, p. 23).

Health Care Funding Issues

To maximize the return on investment of the health care dollar, payers expect and have the right to demand that rehabilitation services are provided in a fiscally responsible manner. Aphasia rehabilitation is both labor intensive and time intensive. Consequently, government or private insurers accept a significant financial burden when they agree to support therapy. The current emphasis on controlling escalating health care costs directly influences practice patterns in rehabilitation and effectively mandates a team approach to working with individuals with chronic illness. It is a widely held belief that using a team approach reduces the length of stay in treatment and is regarded as de facto evidence that a program is operating efficiently and effectively (Diller, 1990).

Until recently, there has been little agreement on how to measure rehabilitation program effectiveness. Efforts are now underway toward defining program effectiveness through measurement of functional outcomes for the patient. It appears that interdisciplinary evaluation of functional outcomes measures will be the barometer against which reimbursement rates will be established to support long-term rehabilitation (Fratelli, 1992; Wilkerson et al., 1992). It is believed that coordinated efforts in functional assessment and treatment of the aphasic patient will lead to shorter stays in therapy and result in better outcomes than if the patient is treated in an isolated manner by each of the team members (Griffin, 1990).

Patient/Family Perspectives

Patients and their families are the front-line consumers of speech-language pathology services. They have a right to expect the most effective and efficient treatment methods be used in the rehabilitation process. Patients need consistency and benefit most when the efforts of the team are coordinated. Behavior change is likely to occur when everyone working with the patient establishes identical response requirements (Olson and Henig, 1983).

It is a truism that the lives of patients and families are permanently altered following a stroke. Consequently, service providers are obligated to minimize the demands placed on the family and to ease the burden of adjusting to the disability as much as possible. The team approach, at the very least, eliminates the need for the family to meet with each separate discipline involved in the patient's program. Information is channeled through the physician or case manager, enabling the family to conserve time and energy for addressing the many issues they have to face poststroke.

MEMBERS OF THE TEAM

A rehabilitation team is composed of individuals brought together for the express purpose of improving the functional capacity of patients to enhance their quality of life. The actual composition of the team varies by individual program. However, the team draws from a roster including patient and family, primary professionals, and supporting disciplines.

Patient/Family

The one obligatory member of any rehabilitation team is the patient/family. The team's existence and purpose is defined by the problems and needs of the patient. Consequently, it is critical that patient and family participate in the team management process. The patient and family must be included in all decisions regarding the goals of the therapy program. This is considered so important that in order for rehabilitation programs to become accredited, they must demonstrate that the patient or his or her representative has reviewed and approved on the plan of care (Commission on Accreditation of Rehabilitation Facilities, 1991; Health Care Finance Administration, 1989; Joint Commission on Accreditation of Health Care Organizations, 1991).

Regulatory requirements aside, there is a more compelling rationale for including the patient in all aspects of treatment planning. Functional goals are more likely to be met if patient and family are engaged in the process and understand their responsibilities in implementing the program (Bach-y-Rita and Bach-y-Rita, 1990). Actively involving the patient and family in the team helps to restore their sense of control and often results in increased motivation in therapy (Tanner, 1980).

Primary Professionals

Rehabilitation programs bring a number of disciplines together for the common purpose of improving the patient's life. Primary professionals are almost always involved in one way or another with patient care. It is beyond the scope of this review to provide a detailed description of the responsibilities and functions of each team member. The intent is to introduce the speech-language pathologist to the other disciplines represented on the treatment team and to provide a sense of the traditional role each team plays in the rehabilitation process.

Physical Therapist

The physical therapist (PT) evaluates, prevents, and manages disorders of human motion with the goal of maximizing functional independence and healthful life-style. This traditionally includes working with patients to improve strength and range of motion of muscles of the trunk and upper and lower extremities. Physical therapists work with patients to restore mobility. This may involve instructing patients in the use of a wheelchair and how to transfer off the chair or teaching them how to walk with a cane.

Occupational Therapist

Occupational therapists (OTs) are traditionally concerned with improving the patient's sensory-motor, perceptual, and neuromuscular functioning. OTs promote functional independence in ADLs such as cooking, personal grooming, and feeding. They are skilled in creating and training patients to use assistive/adaptive devices to help with ADLs. Occupational therapists often go into patients' homes and identify and make necessary environmental physical modifications to assist the patient in achieving functional independence (e.g., lowering kitchen counters and installing seats and handrails in the shower for a wheelchair-dependent patient).

Neuropsychologist

The neuropsychologist is a specialist in test administration and interpretation of higher- and lower-level cognitive/mental functioning. The neuropsychologist provides information to the team on the patient's attentional abilities, memory functions, and learning potential in therapy. Test batteries often include assessment of attention, memory, visual perception, nonverbal and verbal intelligence, and verbal functions (Lezak, 1976). Neuropsychologists often will provide recommendations on how to work through a patient's cognitive deficits to achieve program goals.

Social Worker

The social worker traditionally works with the patient and family to assist them in their psychosocial adjustment to stroke. The social worker evaluates family support systems. This information assists the rehabilitation team in understanding the interaction between the patient's social situation and the disability and how it may influence his or her response in therapy. The social worker helps the patient and family cope with the process of recovery and assists with referrals to appropriate community agencies. The social worker may provide counseling to members of the rehabilitation team to assist in coping with difficult-to-treat patients or issues of staff burnout.

Physiatrist

Physiatrists are medical doctors specializing in rehabilitation medicine. They are responsible for medical management of rehabilitation patients and have ultimate responsibility for the patient's recovery. Physiatrists arrange for consultations to other medical specialists and serve as the liaison between the rehabilitation program and the patient's personal physician.

Rehabilitation Nurse

Rehabilitation nurses provide direct and indirect care to patients to prevent further disability and to restore lost ability. They establish a therapeutic environment to assist the patient with recovery. Rehabilitation nurses monitor and prevent medical complications that may interfere with recovery. They reinforce activities taught by other team members and establish their own goals to ameliorate the physical and emotional discomfort of the patient (Boucher, 1989; Ditmar, 1989).

Vocational Rehabilitation Counselor

Vocational rehabilitation counselors (VRCs) evaluate the patient's potential for employment. They match patients to jobs based on education aptitude skill and level of functioning. VRCs monitor the patient's progress in relation to job placement and work closely with the team and community to assist the patient with his or her reentry into the work place.

Supporting Team Members

Supporting members of the rehabilitation team are called on to address specific patient needs. This is not to suggest that their contributions carry less weight than primary team members; it simply recognizes that not all patients have deficits requiring their particular professional expertise.

Audiologist

The audiologist will be called on to evaluate a patient for a suspected hearing loss. The audiologist may recommend and prescribe hearing aids and instruct patients, families, and team members in use and care of the aid. They may also plan and conduct an aural rehabilitation program as necessary to improve the patient's auditory perceptual/comprehension skills.

Recreational Therapist

The recreational therapist (RT) will work with the patient to structure leisure activities with a decidedly therapeutic benefit. The RT will assist patients in developing new hobbies appropriate to their functional status to improve the quality of their leisure activities on discharge.

Educational/Reading Specialists

Educational/reading specialists may be called on when a patient prepares to return to school. They assist the patient in establishing learning readiness skills and may also develop a program to address specific reading disorders.

Rehabilitation Engineers

Rehabilitation engineers are specialists in the design and development of enabling technology for disabled individuals. They may create assistive devices, and they often work with the speech-language pathologist and occupational therapist in the design of augmentative/alternative communication systems.

INTERDISCIPLINARY TEAM MANAGEMENT

Interdisciplinary team management of aphasic patients presents both opportunities and challenges to the speech-language pathologist. However, in most cases, there is little formal preparation available to teach the clinician how to be a team member. The following is intended to briefly review the model of interdisciplinary team care, the role of the speech-language pathologist on the team, and the communication process within the team.

Philosophy of Interdisciplinary Intervention

Members of an interdisciplinary team collaborate on defining program goals for the patient and the methods for achieving those objectives. The goals of the team supersede the goals of each individual discipline. One is likely to encounter an interdisciplinary team approach in a rehabilitation center with a well-defined philosophy of patient care.

Interdisciplinary teams are rooted in the belief that once a patient's problems have been identified, all of the appropriate disciplines work in concert to achieve the goals of the program. This sometimes results in team members crossing professional boundaries and working on areas outside of their scope of practice. For example, a collective team goal might be to return an aphasic patient to functional independence in the home. The speech-language pathologist may determine that improving word retrieval will move the patient toward this desired outcome. The speech-language pathologist may then review word-retrieval cuing strategies for all members of the team to use when working with the patient. Similarly, the physical therapist may recommend that all team members position the patient in a manner that facilitates improvement in muscle strength and control necessary for the patient to relearn how to walk. There is continuity and consistency in how the patient is treated, no matter who the patient works with (Cohen and Titonis, 1985).

Serving on an interdisciplinary team requires that individual disciplines relinquish a certain amount of professional territory. For the first-time team member, this is probably the most discomforting aspect of team membership. There is comfort in a clearly defined professional scope of practice. However, discomfort is rapidly replaced with tolerance and acceptance of blurring of professional lines with the realization that the patient is the ultimate beneficiary of the approach. It makes wonderful sense to treat the aphasic individual as a "whole" person and not a collection of isolated deficits.

Role of the Speech-Language Pathologist

The speech-language pathologist usually works with the aphasic patient longer than most of the other members of the team. Consequently, clinicians often find themselves in the role of case manager. Case managers assume a leadership role in developing and coordinating treatment plans with other professionals (American Speech-Language-Hearing Association, 1991) Case managers often arbitrate areas of professional conflict within the team and ensure that the team is working synergistically on behalf of the patient. They also serve as liaisons between the patient/family and treatment team.

Speech-language pathologists usually communicate effectively with their aphasic patients so, it is logical for them to transmit information between the patient and the team. However, the speech-language pathologist may also assist the team in achieving its program goals by sharing strategies with team members for instructing and communicating with the patient. The value of this to the ultimate success of the program cannot be overstated.

Communication Among Team Members

Each facility has its own unique method of facilitating communication among team members. There are, however, two basic communication modes used in the team management approach.

Team Meetings

Team meetings are an effective means for gathering all rehabilitation services in one place to ensure timely and accurate information exchange. The frequency of team meetings is dictated by each facility's policies and procedures and may also be dictated by patient's needs.

Traditionally, a team meeting is held after all members of the evaluation team have completed their testing. The purpose of the initial meeting is to review the diagnosis and establish a prognosis for the patient. The team typically establishes the program goals for the patient at this time. A case manager may be identified based on the particular needs of the patient.

Patient and family members should be encouraged to participate in the initial team meeting. However, some facilities conduct a separate patient/family conference. This provides an opportunity for the rehabilitation team to engage in the problem-solving process beforehand and typically results in a more cogent presentation to the family.

Once the patient is actively engaged in the program, teams may meet as frequently as once a week or as infrequently as once a month. The goals of these interim meetings are to review the patient's progress and to adjust goals as needed. When the patient is ready to leave the program, a discharge meeting is conducted during which the team reviews recommendations for follow-up care with the patient/family.

Documentation

All team members working with the patient are required to document their treatment and meeting activities. Accrediting agencies look for evidence of coordination and communication among team members. Typically, this will take the form of a chart note in which the clinician indicates the day and time the communication occurred and a summary of what was discussed.

If it is impossible to communicate directly with other members of the team (e.g., if services are provided in the home), the next best alternative is to establish a written document that all team members are required to review and signoff on, indicating they are aware of the goals and objectives of the other team members. The drawback to relying on written treatment plans is there is no guarantee that all team members will actually read the goals and objectives established by the other members. It is the responsibility of the team leader to ensure this doesn't happen.

PROFESSIONAL CONSIDERATIONS

The ideal of interdisciplinary intervention would suggest that all members of the team work cohesively and to best serve the needs of the aphasic patient. Clinical practice requires acknowledgment of the exceptions to smooth implementation of the team model.

More than one clinician has found himself or herself reviewing an evaluation report written by the neuropsychologist only to find that the patient has been administered the Boston Diagnostic Aphasia Examination or the Western Aphasia Battery. The speech-language pathologist may well wonder if he or she should administer the same test, give another examination, or simply rely on the information provided in the neuropsychology report. To complicate matters further, the report may also indicate the nature of the patient's aphasic impairment as interpreted by the neuropsychologist. There may even be recommendations for what to work on in therapy.

Unfortunately, there is no easy resolution to this situation. It is within the scope of the practice of neuropsychology to administer a battery of tests to evaluate a patient's cognitive/linguistic deficit. It is also clearly within the scope of the practice of the speech-language pathologist to do so as well. The best and most effective resolution to this potential conflict is to communicate directly with the neuropsychologist to reach an accord on how to avoid duplication of services to the patient. It is also essential for the speech-language pathologist to clearly establish the scope of practice regarding the evaluation and treatment of the aphasic patient (American Speech-Language-Hearing Association, 1990). As independent service providers we are responsible for establishing the treatment plan (with physician approval but not prescription) and do not practice under the direction of neuropsychology.

There are additional scope-of-practice conflicts regarding the domain of cognitive retraining of neurologically impaired patients. The diagnosis and remediation of cognitive disorders are identified in the scope of practice of the professions of speech-language pathology, neuropsychology and occupational therapy. The resolution of these professional crossovers is beyond the scope of this chapter. However, Griffin (1990) offered a timely piece of advice when she stated, "The mindset of the profession [speech-language pathology] must turn to one of collaboration with other practitioners rather than competition about who will provide the service." (p. 34). Her observation is in the best tradition of the interdisciplinary model. As long as interprofessional conflicts are resolved with the best care for the aphasic patient in mind, everyone wins.

FUTURE TRENDS IN INTERDISCIPLINARY INTERVENTION

It is always interesting to look forward and prognosticate on where things will end up in one's profession. It appears there will always be a place for the interdisciplinary approach in aphasia treatment, and there will always be a place on the team for the speech-language pathologist. However, the next decade promises significant changes in the health care delivery system in the United States and, with these changes, significant shifts in how speech-language pathologists will deliver services. Clinicians will increasingly find they are working with aphasic patients in their own home (Batey and Horton, 1992; Kurent, 1989). The challenges of coordinating care through a team approach when team members have little face-to-face contact are obvious.

As the United States moves toward Universal health care, there will be increased reliance on managed systems of health care service delivery, such as health maintenance organizations (HMOs) and preferred provider organizations (PPOs), as a method to control costs (Cornett, 1988; Kenkel, 1988). It remains to be seen how these programs will approach long-term rehabilitation and how they will use rehabilitation services. One newly emerging trend in this regard is the advent of the transdisciplinary team approach to intervention.

According to Melvin (1989), in the transdisciplinary model one member of the team acts as the primary therapist with other members of the team serving in a consultant like capacity. The cost savings of using one professional to carry out a treatment program are obvious. However, there is no evidence demonstrating that this model of care results in improved functional status for the patient. This will clearly challenge professional scope-of-practice issues and ethical issues, and it remains to be seen if the transdisciplinary approach will take hold (King and Titus, 1993).

Finally, there is a great need for research in the efficacy of the interdisciplinary approach to rehabilitation (American Speech-Language-Hearing Association, 1992). I expect we will soon find the answers to some of the burning questions regarding what aspects of interdisciplinary intervention work and who benefits most from the team approach.

References

American Speech-Language-Hearing Association. (1990 April). Major issues affecting the delivery of services in hospital settings: Recommendations and strategies. *ASHA, 32*, 67–70.

American Speech-Language-Hearing Association. (1991). Guidelines for speech-language pathologists serving persons with language, socio-communicative, and/or cognitive communicative impairments. *ASHA, 33* (Suppl. 5), 21–28.

American Speech-Language-Hearing Association. (1992, March). *Report and Research Plan for the National Center for Medical Rehabilitation Research.* Rockville, MD: American Speech-Language-Hearing Association.

Bach-y-Rita, P, and Bach-y-Rita, E. (1990). Hope and active patient participation in the rehabilitation environment. *Archives of Physical Medicine and Rehabilitation, 71*, 1084–1085.

Batey, J. M., and Horton, A. M. (1992, April). Home care: The future is now. *ASHA, 34*, 45–47.

Boucher, J. (1989). Nursing process. In S. Ditmar (Ed.), *Rehabilitation nursing: Process and application.* St. Louis, MO: C. V. Mosby.

Brookshire, R. H. (1992) *An introduction to neurogenic communication disorders* (4th ed). St. Louis, MO: Mosby Year Book.

Cohen, S. B., and Titonis, J. (1985). Head injury rehabilitation: Management issues. In M. Ylvisaker (Ed.), *Head injury rehabilitation: Children and adolescents.* San Diego, CA: College Hill Press.

Commission on Accreditation of Rehabilitation Facilities. (1991). *Standards manual for organizations serving people with disabilities.* Tuscon, AZ: Commission on Accreditation of Rehabilitation Facilities.

Cornett, B. S. (1988, September). Speech-language pathologists and audiologists, and HMOs: Status and outlook. *ASHA, 30*, 64–67.

Diller, L. (1990) Fostering the interdisciplinary team, fostering research in a society in transition. *Archives of Physical Medicine and Rehabilitation, 71*, 275–278.

Ditmar, S. (1989) Rehabilitation team. In S. Ditmar (Ed.), *Rehabilitation nursing: Process and application.* St. Louis, MO: C. V. Mosby.

Fratelli, C. M. (1992). Functional assessment of communication: Merging public policy with clinical views. *Aphasiology, 6*, 63–83.

Griffin, K. M. (1990, Fall/Winter). Interdisciplinary collaboration means professional viability. *Texas Journal of Audiology and Speech Pathology, 16*, 33–35.

Halstead, L. S. (1976). Team care in chronic illness: A critical review. *Archives of Physical Medicine and Rehabilitation 61*, 507–511.

Health Care Finance Administration. (1989). *Medical outpatient physical therapy and comprehensive outpatient rehabilitation facility manual.* Section 502, Transmittal No. 87. Baltimore, MD: Health Care Finance Administration.

Joint Commission on Accreditation of Health Care Organizations. (1991). *Accreditation manual for hospitals.* Chicago, IL: Joint Commission on Accreditation of Health Care Organizations.

Kenkel, P. J. (1988, July 29). Managed care will dominate within a decade—experts. *Modern Healthcare,* p. 31.

King, J. C., and Titus, M. N. (1993). Prescriptions, referrals, and the rehabilitation team. In J. A. Delisa and B. M. Gans (Eds.), *Rehabilitation medicine: Principles and practice.* Philadelphia, PA: J. B. Lippincott.

Kurent, H. (1989, December). Future trends in healthcare. *ASHA, 31*, 40–42.

Lezak, M. (1976). *Neuropsychological assessment.* New York: Oxford University Press.

Melvin, J. L. (1989). Status report on interdisciplinary medical rehabilitation. *Archives of Physical Medicine and Rehabilitation, 70*, 273–277.

National Joint Committee for the Communicative Needs of Persons with Severe Disabilities. (1992, March). Guidelines for meeting the communication needs of persons with severe disabilities. *ASHA 34*(Suppl. 7), 1–8.

Olson, D. A., and Henig, E. (1983). *A manual of behavior management strategies for brain injured adults.* Chicago, IL: Rehabilitation Institute of Chicago.

Rothberg, J. S. (1981). The rehabilitation team: Future directions. *Archives of Physical Medicine and Rehabilitation, 62*, 407–410.

Tanner, D. C. (1980). Loss and grief: Implications for the speech-language pathologist and audiologist. *ASHA, 22*, 916–928.

Wertz, R. T., LaPointe, L. L., and Rosenbek, J. C. (1984). *Apraxia of speech in adults: The disorder and its management.* Orlando, FL: Grune & Stratton.

Wilkerson, D. L., Batavia, A. I., and DeJong, G. (1992). Use of functional status measures for payment of medical rehabilitation services. *Archives of Physical Medicine and Rehabilitation, 73*, 111–120.

CHAPTER 33
Epilogue: The Future—A Continued Commitment to Excellence

ROBERTA CHAPEY

According to Albert Schweitzer, good consists in maintaining, assisting, and enhancing life. We, as aphasiologists, continually seek to maintain, assist, and enhance life in the hope that we can make a greater difference in the lives of those whom we serve. Toward that end, we have amassed a surprisingly detailed fund of information about stroke symptomatology, assessment, intervention, and prevention. But what we have today will be obsolete tomorrow. The best practice for today may not be the best practice for tomorrow. Therefore, we must work with a multidisciplinary approach and expect, indeed strive, for *change*. "Progress" must continue to be "our most important product." Both providers and recipients of health care must join in a cooperative effort to spread the application of existing knowledge and to improve the quality of knowledge and the quality of all health care services. It is hoped this will include heightening of our clinical problem-solving and decision-making skills. We continue to need the following:

● To promote greater acceptance of a philosophy of the quality of life for the elderly and the disabled. The goal of medical care should be to improve the quality of life of each individual.
● To develop better health-related quality of life (QOL) measures that assess dimensions of physical function, mental or cognitive function, emotional or psychological function, social and role function, disease symptoms, life satisfaction, and perception of well-being in each individual in order to monitor change in those who need our care (Mac Keigan and Pathak, 1992). The objective of health care should be to reduce the individual's disability as well as his or her discomfort.
● To increase public awareness of aphasia therapy as an *essential* human service.
● To heighten the involvement of businesses, corporations, and communities in stroke rehabilitation.
● To initiate more research geared to the prevention of stroke.
● To develop better physical access for the handicapped.
● To develop a philosophy of custody for the elderly.
● To develop a greater number and higher quality of hospice care for stroke and aphasia victims.
● To develop more elderhostels for aphasic patients.
● To develop better assistive technology and rehabilitation technology.

● To develop more relevant and accurate measurements of change in communication.
● To develop more effective and efficient assessment protocols that will facilitate differential diagnoses and choice of intervention goals.
● To initiate more research on the structure and function of long-term memory and of working memory and the role of each in cognitive, pragmatic, and linguistic abilities.
● To increase research to foster a better understanding of semantic, syntactic, pragmatic, and cognitive processing.
● To develop new multidisciplinary innovative approaches to long-term care.
● To initiate more research geared to effective rehabilitation of stroke and aphasia.
● To develop more functionally relevant alternative treatment models.
● To develop a clearer understanding of motivation and its relationship to intervention outcomes.
● To develop more reliable and valid measures of the social network and support resources of clients (Tompkins et al., 1990).
● To initiate more research that will analyze the interaction between treatment methods and client characteristics and type of therapist most likely to succeed at various approaches.
● To increase research that will foster a better understanding of semantic, syntactic, pragmatic, and cognitive processing.
● To heighten ASHA's responsibility to the profession and to our customers. ASHA needs to help its members stay alive professionally "not only to adapt to change that has already occurred, but also to see change coming; to be creative; to stimulate thoughts and feelings about what is new and different; to be pioneers; to set the pace, not lag behind" (Melby, 1992, p. 2464). (Melby is addressing hospital pharmacists.) ASHA needs to set national standards, to teach us tools of continuous quality improvement, and to determine critical pathways of adaptation and survival (Melby, 1992). To be successful, ASHA needs to be full of excitement, energy, and change. It needs to develop a compelling view of the future, define a specific market, and pursue it aggressively (Melby, 1992). Our professional organization needs to be skilled at identifying the "big picture" while surpassing the competition in the basics of service delivery (Melby, 1992). According to Melby (1992):

The successful organization in the future will have as its mindset continuous quality improvement and a focus on customers—both its own (members) and those whom its members represent (patients). It will have a governance structure capable of reacting to a rapidly changing environment. It will be an organization that sorts out and coordinates the special interests of segments of its membership that may disagree on its direction and priorities. The organization will make its mark in the international marketplace (p. 2466).

As a profession, we continue our search for excellence through the 1990s and the 21st century. Health care will be *the* economic, political, and social issue of the future. "If we cannot demonstrate that we are adding value—to society, to health care, and to each and every consumer—we may have outlived our usefulness" (Melby, 1992, p. 2466). As a group, we, the membership, need to create and promote our vision of the future (Melby, 1992).

References

Mac Keigan, L., and Pathak, D. (1992). Overview of health related quality-of-life measures. *American Journal of Hospital Pharmacists, 49,* 2236–2245.

Melby, M. (1992). ASHP and its customers. *American Journal of Hospital Pharmacists, 49,* 2462–2466.

Tompkins, C., Jackson, S. and Schulz, R. (1990). On prognostic research in adult neurologic disorders. *Journal of Speech and Hearing Research, 33,* 398–401.

Figure and Table Credits

Figure 1.1. From Damasio, H. (1981). In M. T. Sarno (Ed.), *Acquired aphasia*. New York: Academic Press.

Figure 2.1. From Metter, E. J., and Hanson, W. R. (1985). Brain imaging as related to speech and language. In J. Darby (Ed.), *Speech evaluation in neurology*(pp. 123-160). New York: Grune & Stratton.

Figure 3.1. From Palumbo, C. L., Alexander, M. P., Naeser, M. A. (1992). CT scan lesion sites associated with conduction aphasia. In S. Kohn (Ed.), *Conduction aphasia*(pp. 51-76). New York: Lawrence Erlbaum Associates. Reprinted with permission.

Figure 3.4. From Naeser, M. A., Palumbo, C. L., Helm-Estabrooks, N., Stiassny-Eder, D., and Albert, M. L. (1989). Severe non-fluency in aphasia: Role of the medial subcallosal fasciculus plus other white matter pathways in recovery of spontaneous speech. *Brain, 112*, 1-38. Reprinted with permission.

Figure 3.5. From Naeser, M. A. (in press). Neuroimaging and recovery of auditory comprehension and spontaneous speech in aphasia. In A. Kertesz (Ed.), *Localization and neuroimaging in neuropsychology*(2nd ed.). Orlando, FL: Academic Press. Reprinted with permission.

Figure 3.6. From Naeser, M. A. (in press). Neuroimaging and recovery of auditory comprehension and spontaneous speech in aphasia. In A. Kertesz (Ed.), *Localization and neuroimaging in neuropsychology*(2nd ed.). Orlando, FL: Academic Press. Reprinted with permission.

Figure 3.7. From Naeser, M. A., Helm-Estabrooks, N., Haas, G., Auerbach, S., and Srinivasan, M. (1987). Relationship between lesion extent in "Wernicke's area" on CT scan and predicting recovery of comprehension in Wernicke's aphasia. *Archives of Neurology, 44*, 73-82. Reprinted with permission.

Figure 3.8. From Naeser, M. A., Helm-Estabrooks, N., Haas, G., Auerbach, S., and Srinivasan, M. (1987). Relationship between lesion extent in "Wernicke's area" on CT scan and predicting recovery of comprehension in Wernicke's aphasia. *Archives of Neurology, 44*, 73-82. Reprinted with permission.

Figure 3.9. From Naeser, M. A., Gaddie, A., Palumbo, C. L., and Stiassny-Eder, D. (1990). Late recovery of auditory comprehension in global aphasia: Improved recovery observed with subcortical temporal isthmus lesion versus Wernicke's cortical area lesion. *Archives of Neurology, 47*, 425-432. Reprinted with permission.

Figure 3.10. From Naeser, M. A., Gaddie, A., Palumbo, C. L., and Stiassny-Eder, D. (1990). Late recovery of auditory comprehension in global aphasia: Improved recovery observed with subcortical temporal isthmus lesion versus Wernicke's cortical area lesion. *Archives of Neurology, 47*, 425-432. Reprinted with permission.

Figure 3.11. From Naeser, M. A., Gaddie, A., Palumbo, C. L., and Stiassny-Eder, D. (1990). Late recovery of auditory comprehension in global aphasia: Improved recovery observed with subcortical temporal isthmus lesion versus Wernicke's cortical area lesion. *Archives of Neurology, 47*, 425-432. Reprinted with permission.

Figure 3.12. From Naeser, M. A., Gaddie, A., Palumbo, C. L., and Stiassny-Eder, D. (1990). Late recovery of auditory comprehension in global aphasia: Improved recovery observed with subcortical temporal isthmus lesion versus Wernicke's cortical area lesion. *Archives of Neurology, 47*, 425-432. Reprinted with permission.

Figure 3.13. From Naeser, M. A., Palumbo, C. L., Helm-Estabrooks, N., Stiassny-Eder, D., and Albert, M. L. (1989). Severe non-fluency in aphasia: Role of the medial subcallosal fasciculus plus other white matter pathways in recovery of spontaneous speech. *Brain, 112*, 1-38. Reprinted with permission.

Figure 3.14. From Naeser, M. A., Palumbo, C. L., Helm-Estabrooks, N., Stiassny-Eder,

D., and Albert, M. L. (1989). Severe non-fluency in aphasia: Role of the medial subcallosal fasciculus plus other white matter pathways in recovery of spontaneous speech. *Brain, 112*, 1-38. Reprinted with permission.

Figure 3.15. From Naeser, M. A., Palumbo, C. L., Helm-Estabrooks, N., Stiassny-Eder, D., and Albert, M. L. (1989). Severe non-fluency in aphasia: Role of the medial subcallosal fasciculus plus other white matter pathways in recovery of spontaneous speech. *Brain, 112*, 1-38. Reprinted with permission.

Figure 3.16. From Naeser, M. A., Palumbo, C. L., Helm-Estabrooks, N., Stiassny-Eder, D., and Albert, M. L. (1989). Severe non-fluency in aphasia: Role of the medial subcallosal fasciculus plus other white matter pathways in recovery of spontaneous speech. *Brain, 112*, 1-38. Reprinted with permission.

Figure 3.17. From Naeser, M. A., Palumbo, C. L., Helm-Estabrooks, N., Stiassny-Eder, D., and Albert, M. L. (1989). Severe non-fluency in aphasia: Role of the medial subcallosal fasciculus plus other white matter pathways in recovery of spontaneous speech. *Brain, 112*, 1-38. Reprinted with permission.

Figure 3.18. From Naeser, M. A., Frumkin, N. L., Fitzpatrick, P., and Palumbo, C. L. (submitted 1992). CT scan lesion sites and good response versus poor response with melodic intonation therapy -- A report of eight cases. Reprinted with permission.

Figure 3.19. From Naeser, M. A., Frumkin, N. L., Fitzpatrick, P., and Palumbo, C. L. (submitted 1992). CT scan lesion sites and good response versus poor response with melodic intonation therapy -- A report of eight cases. Reprinted with permission.

Figure 3.20. From Naeser, M. A., Frumkin, N. L., Baker, E. H., Nicholas, M., Palumbo, C. L., and Alexander, M. P. (submitted 1992). CT scan lesion sites in severe nonverbal aphasia patients appropriate for treatment with a computer-assisted visual communication program (C-ViC). Reprinted with permission.

Figure 3.21. From Naeser, M. A., Frumkin, N. L., Baker, E. H., Nicholas, M., Palumbo, C. L., and Alexander, M. P. (submitted 1992). CT scan lesion sites in severe non-verbal aphasia patients appropriate for treatment with a computer-assisted visual communication program (C-ViC). Reprinted with permission.

Figure 9.1. From Shewan, C. M., and Bandur, D. L. (1986). *Treatment of aphasia: A language-oriented approach*(p. 10). Austin, TX: Pro-Ed.

Figure 9.2. From Shewan, C. M., and Bandur, D. L. (1986). *Treatment of aphasia: A language-oriented approach*(p. 16). Austin, TX: Pro-Ed.

Figure 9.3. From Shewan, C. M., and Bandur, D. L. (1986). *Treatment of aphasia: A language-oriented approach*(p. 18). Austin, TX: Pro-Ed.

Figure 9.4. From Shewan, C. M., and Bandur, D. L. (1986). *Treatment of aphasia: A language-oriented approach*(p. 43). Austin, TX: Pro-Ed.

Figure 9.5. From Shewan, C. M., and Bandur, D. L. (1986). *Treatment of aphasia: A language-oriented approach*(p. 174). Austin, TX: Pro-Ed.

Figure 9.6. From Shewan, C. M., and Bandur, D. L. (1986). *Treatment of aphasia: A language-oriented approach*(p. 256). Austin, TX: Pro-Ed.

Figure 9.7. From Shewan, C. M., and Bandur, D. L. (1986). *Treatment of aphasia: A language-oriented approach*(p. 257). Austin, TX: Pro-Ed.

Appendix 9.1. From Shewan, C. M., and Bandur, D. L. (1986). *Treatment of aphasia: A language-oriented approach*(p. 26). Austin, TX: Pro-Ed.

Appendix 9.2. From Shewan, C. M., and Bandur, D. L. (1986). *Treatment of aphasia: A language-oriented approach*(p. 257). Austin, TX: Pro-Ed.

Figure 11.1. From Wepman, J. M., Jones, L. U., Bock, R. D., and Van Pelt, D. (1960). Studies in aphasia: Background and theoretical formulations. *Journal of Speech and Hearing Disorders, 25*323-332.

Figure 11.3. From Chapey, R. (1983). Language-based cognitive abilities in adult aphasia: Rationale for intervention. *Journal of Communication Disorders, 16*, 405-424.

Figure 17.1. From Yorkston, K. (Ed.). (1992). *Augmentative communication in the medical setting*(pp. 329-330). Tuscon, AZ:

Communication Skill Builders. Copyright 1992 by Communication Skill Builders. Reprinted by permission.

Figure 17.2. From Hux, K., Beukelman, D. R., and Garrett, K. Copyright 1992 by D. R. Beukelman. Reprinted by permission.

Figure 17.5. From Garrett, K., Beukelman, D. R., and Low-Morrow, D. (1989). A comprehensive augmentative communication system for an adult with Broca's aphasia. *Augmentative and Alternative Communication, 5*, 57. Copyright 1989 by Williams & Wilkins. Reprinted by permission.

Figure 17.6. From Garrett, K., Beukelman, D. R., and Low-Morrow, D. (1989). A comprehensive augmentative communication system for an adult with Broca's aphasia. *Augmentative and Alternative Communication, 5*, 57. Copyright 1989 by Williams & Wilkins. Reprinted by permission.

Figure 17.7. From Garrett, K., Beukelman, D. R., and Low-Morrow, D. (1989). A comprehensive augmentative communication system for an adult with Broca's aphasia. *Augmentative and Alternative Communication, 5*, 59. Copyright 1989 by Williams & Wilkins. Reprinted by permission.

Figure 17.8. From Garrett, K., Beukelman, D. R., and Low-Morrow, D. (1989). A comprehensive augmentative communication system for an adult with Broca's aphasia. *Augmentative and Alternative Communication, 5*, 58. Copyright 1989 by Williams & Wilkins. Reprinted by permission.

Figure 22.1. From Rapp, B., and Caramazza, A. (1991). Lexical deficits. In M. Sarno (Ed.), *Acquired aphasia*(2nd ed., p. 188). New York: Academic Press. Reprinted with permission.

Figure 22.2. From Thompson, C. K., McReynolds, L. V., and Vance, C. (1982). Generative use of locatives in multiword utterances in agrammatism: A matrix training approach. In R. H. Brookshire (Ed.), *Clinical Aphasiology Conference proceedings*(p. 292). Minneapolis, MN: BRK. Reprinted with permission.

Figure 22.4. From Garrett, M. F. (1984). The organization of processing structure for language production: Application to aphasic speech. In D. Caplan, A. R. Lecours, and A. Smith (Eds.), *Biological perspectives on language*(p. 174). Cambridge, MA: MIT Press. Reprinted with permission.

Figure 22.5. From Mitchum, C. C., and Berndt, R. S. (1992).

Figure 22.6. From Doyle, P. J., Oleyar, K. S., and Goldstein, H. (1991). Facilitating functional conversational skills in aphasia: An experimental analysis of a generalization training procedure. In T. Prescott (Ed.), *Clinical aphasiology*(Vol. 19, p. 234). Austin, TX: Pro-Ed. Reprinted with permission.

Figure 24.1. From Marshall, J. C. (1985). On some relationships between acquired and developmental dyslexias. In F. H. Duffy and N. Geschwind (Eds.), *Dyslexia: A neuroscientific approach to clinical evaluation*. Boston, MA: Little, Brown. Reprinted with permission.

Figure 26.1. Adapted from Kelly, J. P. (1985). Anatomical basis of sensory perception and motor coordination. In E. R. Kandel and J. H. Schwartz (Eds.), *Principles of Neural Science*(2nd ed.). New York: Elsevier Science Publishing. Used with permission.

Figure 26.2. From Alexander, G. E., and Crutcher, M. D. (1990). Functional architecture of basal ganglia circuits: Neural substrates of parallel processing. *Trends in Neuroscience, 13*, 266-271. Reproduced with permission.

Figure 26.3. From Schell, G. R., and Strick, P. L. (1984). The origin of thalamic inputs to the arcuate premotor and supplementary motor areas. *Journal of Neuroscience, 4*, 557. Reproduced with permission.

Table 30.1. From Ylvisaker, M., Szekeres, S., Henry, K. Sullivan, D., and Wheeler, P. (1987). Topics in cognitive rehabilitation. In M. Ylvisaker (Ed.), *Community re-entry for head injured adults* (pp. 137-215). Austin, TX: Pro-Ed.

Table 30.2. Modified from Haarbauer-Krupp, J., Henry, K., Szekeres, S., and Vlvisaker, M. (1985). Cognitive rehabilitation therapy: Late stages of recovery. In M. Ylvisaker (Ed.), *Head injury rehabilitation: Children and adolescents* (pp. 318-319). Austin, TX: Pro-Ed. Reprinted with permission.

Appendix 30.1. Modified from Haarbauer-Krupp, J., Henry, K., Szekeres, S., and Ylvisaker, M. (1985). Cognitive rehabilitation therapy: Late stages of recovery. In M. Ylvisaker (Ed.), *Head injury rehabilitation: Children and adolescents* (pp. 318-319). Austin, TX: Pro-Ed. Reprinted with permission.

Table 31.3. After Nation, J.E., and Aram, D.M. (1984). *Diagnosis of speech and language disorders* (2nd ed.). Boston, MA: College Hill Press.

Author Index

Subject Index

Page numbers followed by "f" denote figures; those followed by "t" denote tables.